10 Update in Intensive Care and Emergency Medicine

Edited by J. L. Vincent

W0043749

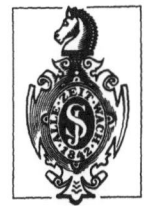

10   Update in Intensive Care
and Emergency Medicine

Edited by J.L. Vincent

Update 1990

Edited by
J. L. Vincent

With 192 Figures and 108 Tables

Springer-Verlag
Berlin Heidelberg New York London
Paris Tokyo Hong Kong

Prof. Jean Louis Vincent   Clinical Director
                           Department of Intensive Care
                           Erasme Hospital
                           Free University of Brussels
                           Route de Lennik 808
                           B-1070 Brussels, Belgium

ISBN-13: 978-3-540-52269-0   e-ISBN-13: 978-3-642-84125-5
DOI: 10.1007/978-3-642-84125-5

Library of Congress Cataloging-in-Publication Data

Update 1990 / edited by J. L. Vincent. (Update in intensive care and emergency medicine ;
ISBN-13: 978-3-540-52269-0 . : alk. paper) 1. Critical care medicine-Congresses.
2. Emergency   medicine-Congresses. I. Vincent,   J. L. II. Series. RC86.2.U63 1990
616′.028-dc20

2119/3140-5 4 3 2 1 0 – Printed on acid-free paper

Contents

Cardiopulmonary Resuscitation

Cerebral Crisis

Gastro-Intestinal Crisis

Sedation of the Critically Ill

Fluids and Electrolytes – Endocrine Function

Evaluation of Intensive Care

List of Contributors

Abramson, N. S.
Resuscitation Research Center, University
of Pittsburgh, 3434 Fifth Avenue,
Pittsburgh, PA 15260, USA

Allgöwer, M.
North Western Injury Hospital Centre,
University of Manchester, Oxford Road,
Manchester M13 9PT, United Kingdom

Barvais, L.
Department of Anesthesiology, Erasme
University Hospital, Route de Lennik 808,
1070 Brussels, Belgium

Baumgartner, J. D.
Infectious Diseases, C.H.U. Vaudois,
1011 Lausanne, Switzerland

Bausch, R.
Department of Cardiology,
Remscheid Hospital, Burgerstrasse 211,
5630 Remscheid, Germany

Beaufils, F.
Department of Pediatric Intensive Care,
Robert Debré Hospital, 75019 Paris,
France

Bennett, D.
Intensive Care Unit,
The Middlesex Hospital, Mortimer Street,
London W1N 8AA, United Kingdom

Bergbom-Engberg, I.
Department of Anesthesiology, Sahlgren's
Hospital, University of Gothenburg,
413 45 Gothenburg, Sweden

Bion, J.
Department of Anaesthetics, Queen
Elizabeth Hospital, Birmingham B15 2TH,
United Kingdom

Bone, R. C.
Department of Internal Medicine,
St Luke's Medical Center, 1753 West
Congress Parkway, Chicago, IL 60612,
USA

Bossaert, L. L.
Department of Intensive Care, U. Z.
Antwerpen, Wilrijkstraat 10, 2520 Edegem,
Belgium

Brandolese, R.
Institute of Occupational Medicine,
University of Padova, Italy

Braschi, A.
Department of Anesthesia, Policlinico
S. Matteo, Piazzale Golgi 2, 27100 Pavia,
Italy

Braughler, J. M.
Clinical Research Director, The Upjohn
Company, 526 Jasper Street, Kalamazoo,
MI 49007, USA

Brown, R. C.
Department of Internal Medicine,
St Luke's Medical Center, 1753 West
Congress Parkway, Chicago, IL 60612,
USA

Byrne, A. J.
Adult Intensive Care, Queen's Medical
Center, University Hospital, Nottingham
NG7 2UH, United Kingdom

Calame, A.
Department of Pediatrics, C.H.U. Vaudois,
1011 Lausanne, Switzerland

Calvin, J. E.
Heart Institute, Ottawa Civic Hospital,
1053 Carling Avenue, Ottawa, Ontario
K1Y 4E9, Canada

Carpentier, F.
Department of Intensive Care, C.H.U.
Grenoble, BP 217 X, 38043 Grenoble
Cédex, France

Cerra, F. B.
Department of Surgery, University of
Minnesota Medical School, 516 Delaware
Street SE, Minneapolis, MN 55455, USA

Chyatte, D.
Division of Neurosurgery, Yale University
School of Medicine, 333 Cedar Street,
New Haven, CT 06510, USA

Clark, C. J.
Department of Bacteriology, Royal
Infirmary, Glasgow G4 OSF,
United Kingdom

Clergue, F.
Department of Anesthesiology, G.H.
Pitié Salpêtrière, 43 Bld de l'Hôpital,
75651 Paris Cédex 13, France

Cloud, M.
Lilly Research Laboratories, Eli Lilly
Company, Lilly Corporate Center,
Indianapolis, IN 46285, USA

Conti, G.
Istituto di Anestesia e Rianimazione,
Universita "La Sapienza", 00161 Roma,
Italy

Coppel, D. L.
Intensive Care Unit,
Royal Victoria Hospital, Grosvenor Road,
Belfast BT12 6BA, United Kingdom

Costantino, D.
Department of Anesthesia, Ospedale
Maggiore, Via F. Sforza 35, 20122 Milano,
Italy

Cotev, S.
Department of Anesthesiology, Hadassah
University Hospital, P.O.Box 12000,
Jerusalem 91120, Israel

Dantzker, D. R.
Pulmonary and Critical Care Medicine,
Health Science Center, 6431 Fannin,
Suite 1274, Houston, TX 77030, USA

Daoud, P.
Department of Pediatric Intensive Care,
Robert Debré Hospital, 75019 Paris,
France

Dean, J. M.
Pediatric Intensive Care, Primary
Children's Medical Center, 4529 South
Parkview Drive, Salt Lake City, UT 84124,
USA

De Boeck, H.
Intensive Care Unit, A.Z. V.U.B.,
Laarbeeklaan 101, 1090 Brussels, Belgium

Deby-Dupont, G.
Department of Anesthesiology, C.H.U.
Liège, Sart Tilman B35, 4000 Liège 1,
Belgium

Dechamps, P.
Division of Intensive Care, St Pierre
University Hospital, rue Haute 322,
1000 Brussels, Belgium

Dhainaut, J. F.
Department of Intensive Care, C.H.U.
Cochin Port Royal, 27 Faubourg St
Jacques, 75674 Paris Cédex 14, France

Dick, W. F.
Department of Anesthesia, Johannes
Gutenberg-Universität, Langenbeckstrasse 1,
6500 Mainz, Germany

Downs, J. B.
Department of Anesthesiology, University
of South Florida, 12901 Bruce B. Downs
Boulevard, Tampa, FL 33612-4799, USA

Dragsted, L.
Department of Anesthesia, Herlev
Hospital, University of Copenhagen,
2730 Herlev, Denmark

Dugernier, T.
Intensive Care Unit, Clinique St Pierre,
1340 Ottignies, Belgium

Eyer, S.
Department of Surgery, University of
Minnesota Medical School, 516 Delaware
Street SE, Minneapolis, MN 55455, USA

Fahrenkrog, U.
Department of Cardiology,
Remscheid Hospital, Burgerstrasse 211,
5630 Remscheid, Germany

Farquhar, I. K.
University Department of Anaesthesia,
Queen's Medical Center, Nottingham NG7
2UH, United Kingdom

Fawer, C. L.
Department of Pediatrics, C.H.U. Vaudois,
1011 Lausanne, Switzerland

Faymonville, M. E.
Department of Anesthesiology, C.H.U.
Liège, Sart Tilman B35, 4000 Liège 1,
Belgium

Flameng, W.
Department of Cardiac Surgery,
AZ St Raphaël Provisorium 1,
Minderbroedersstraat 17, 3000 Leuven,
Belgium

Foëx, P.
Nuffield Department of Anaesthetics,
Radcliffe Infirmary, Woodstock Road,
Oxford OX2 6HE, United Kingdom

Gasparetto, A.
Istituto di Anestesia e Rianimazione,
Universita "La Sapienza", Roma, Italy

Gattinoni, L.
Institute of Anesthesia, University of
Milan, Via Donizetti 106, 20052 Monza
(Milano), Italy

Gauthier, M.
Pediatric Intensive Care Unit, Ste Justine
Hospital, 3175 Côte Sainte-Catherine,
Montreal H2T 1C5, Canada

Gemmell, C. G.
Department of Bacteriology,
Royal Infirmary, Glasgow G4 0SF,
United Kingdom

George, T. M.
Division of Neurosurgery, Yale University
School of Medicine, 333 Cedar Street,
New Haven, CT 06510, USA

Gervais, H. W.
Department of Anesthesia, Johannes
Gutenberg-Universität, Langenbeckstrasse 1,
6500 Mainz, Germany

Ghouri, A. F.
Department of Anesthesiology,
Washington University Medical Center,
660 South Euclid Avenue, St Louis,
MO 63110, USA

Gisvold, S. E.
Department of Anesthesia, University
Hospital, 7006 Trondheim, Norway

Glauser, M. P.
Infectious Diseases, C.H.U. Vaudois,
1011 Lausanne, Switzerland

Goenen, M.
Intensive Care Unit, St. Luc University
Hospital, Avenue Hippocrate 10,
1200 Brussels, Belgium

Goldfrank, L.
Emergency Medical Services, New York
University Medical Center, First Avenue
and 27th Street, New York, NY 10016,
USA

Gorman, D.
North Western Injury Hospital Centre,
University of Manchester, Oxford Road,
Manchester M13 9PT, United Kingdom

Greig, P. D.
Gastro-Intestinal Transplantation, Toronto
General Hospital, 200 Elizabeth Street,
Toronto, Ontario M5G 2C4, Canada

Guignier, M.
Department of Intensive Care, C.H.U.
Grenoble, BP 217 X, 38043 Grenoble
Cédex, France

Haefeli, W.
Department of Intensive Care, University
Hospital, 4031 Basel, Switzerland

Häggmark, S.
Department of Anesthesiology, University
of Umea, 90185 Umea, Sweden

Haljamäe, H.
Department of Anesthesiology, Sahlgren's
Hospital, University of Gothenburg,
413 45 Gothenburg, Sweden

Hall, E. D.
Clinical Research Director, The Upjohn
Company, 526 Jasper Street, Kalamazoo,
MI 49007, USA

Hallenberg, B.
Department of Anesthesiology, Sahlgren's
Hospital, University of Gothenburg,
413 45 Gothenburg, Sweden

Hamy, I.
Department of Intensive Care, C.H.U.
Cochin Port Royal, 27 Faubourg St
Jacques, 75674 Paris Cédex 14, France

Hartmann, J.-F.
Department of Pediatric Intensive Care,
Robert Debré Hospital, 75019 Paris,
France

Hedenstierna, G.
Department of Clinical Physiology,
University Hospital, 751 85 Uppsala,
Sweden

Hermans, P.
Division of Infectious Diseases, St Pierre
University Hospital, Rue Haute 322,
1000 Brussels, Belgium

Herrmann, M.
Infectious Disease Division, Hôpital
Cantonal, Rue Micheli-du-Crest,
1211 Genève 4, Switzerland

Heyndrickx, G.
Cardiovascular Center, O.L. Vrouw
Ziekenhuis, 9300 Aalst, Belgium

Hillman, K.
Department of Intensive Care,
The Liverpool Hospital, P.O. Box 103,
Liverpool 2170 NSW, Australia

Hinds, C. J.
Department of Anesthesia,
St Bartholomew's Hospital, West
Smithfield, London EC1A 7BE,
United Kingdom

Hoffman, W. D.
Department of Critical Care Medicine,
National Institute of Health, Building ID
Room 10D48, Bethesda, MD 20892, USA

Hohner, P.
Department of Anesthesiology, University
of Umea, 90185 Umea, Sweden

Iotti, G.
Department of Anesthesia, Policlinico
S. Matteo, Piazzale Golgi 2, 27100 Pavia,
Italy

Jacquet, L.
Intensive Care Unit, St. Luc University
Hospital, Avenue Hippocrate 10,
1200 Brussels, Belgium

Jansen, J. R. C.
Department of Pulmonary Disease,
Erasmus University, P. O. Box 1738,
3000 DR Rotterdam, The Netherlands

Jivegård, L.
Department of Anesthesiology, Sahlgren's
Hospital, University of Gothenburg,
413 45 Gothenburg, Sweden

Johnston, J. R.
Intensive Care Unit,
Royal Victoria Hospital, Grosvenor Road,
Belfast BT12 6BA, United Kingdom

Kinsella, J.
Department of Bacteriology,
Royal Infirmary, Glasgow G4 0SF,
United Kingdom

Koyama, K.
Department of Emergency Medicine,
University of Tsukuba School of Medicine,
2-1-1 Amakubo, Tsukuba City, Ibaraki 305,
Japan

Lacroix, J.
Pediatric Intensive Care Unit, Ste Justine
Hospital, 3175 Côte Sainte-Catherine,
Montreal H2T 1C5, Canada

Lamy, M.
Department of Anesthesiology, C.H.U.
Liège, Sart Tilman B35, 4000 Liège 1,
Belgium

Langer, M.
Department of Anesthesia,
Ospedale Maggiore, Via F. Sforza 35,
20122 Milano, Italy

Leeman, M.
Department of Intensive Care, Erasme
University Hospital, Route de Lennik 808,
1070 Brussels, Belgium

LeJemtel, T. H.
Cardiovascular Research Laboratory,
Albert Einstein College of Medicine,
1300 Morris Park Avenue,
Bronx, NY 10461, USA

Lenhart, F. P.
Department of Anesthesiology, Klinikum
Grosshadern, 8000 München 70, Germany

Levy, G. A.
Gastro-Intestinal Transplantation, Toronto
General Hospital, 200 Elizabeth Street,
Toronto, Ontario M5G 2C4, Canada

Lew, D. P.
Infectious Disease Division, Hôpital
Cantonal, Rue Micheli-du-Crest 24,
1211 Genève 4, Switzerland

Little, R.A.
North Western Injury Hospital Centre,
University of Manchester, Oxford Road,
Manchester M13 9PT, United Kingdom

Löllgen, H.
Department of Cardiology,
Remscheid Hospital, Burgerstrasse 211,
5630 Remscheid, Germany

Luce, J.M.
Chest Service, San Francisco General
Hospital, P.O. Box 0841, San Francisco,
CA 94143-0841, USA

Mancebo, J.
Department of Intensive Care, Hospital
de la Santa Creu I Sant Pau, Av St Antoni
Ma Claret 167, 08025 Barcelona, Spain

Marbet, G.A.
Department of Intensive Care, University
Hospital, 4031 Basel, Switzerland

Marini, J.J.
Department of Critical Care Medicine, St
Paul Ramsey Medical Center, 640 Jackson
Street, St Paul, MN 55101-2595, USA

Means, E.D.
Clinical Research Director, The Upjohn
Company, 526 Jasper Street, Kalamazoo,
MI 49007, USA

Mebazaa, A.
Department of Anesthesiology, Lariboisière
Hospital, 2 rue Ambroise Paré, 75475 Paris
Cédex 10, France

Milic-Emili, J.
Meakins-Christie Laboratories, McGill
University, Montreal, Canada

Mills, A.K.
Department of Anesthesiology,
Washington University Medical Center,
660 South Euclid Avenue, St Louis,
MO 63110, USA

Mingat, J.
Department of Intensive Care, C.H.U.
Grenoble, BP 217 X, 38043 Grenoble
Cédex, France

Natanson, C.
Department of Critical Care Medicine,
National Institute of Health, Building ID
Room 10D48, Bethesda, MD 20892, USA

Negro, F.
Department of Surgery, University of
Minnesota Medical School, 516 Delaware
Street SE, Minneapolis, MN 55455, USA

Nelson, L.D.
Surgical Intensive Care, Vanderbilt
University, 218 Medical Center South,
Nashville, TN 37232, USA

Nichols, A.J.
Department of Pharmacology, Smith Kline
Beecham Plc, P.O. Box 1539, King of
Prussia, PA 19406-0939, USA

Nisi, R.
Cardiovascular Research Laboratory,
Albert Einstein College of Medicine, 1300
Morris Park Avenue, Bronx, NY 10461,
USA

Oudemans-van Straaten, H.M.
Department of Intensive Care,
O.L.V. Ziekenhuis, le Oosterparkstraat 179,
1091 HA Amsterdam, The Netherlands

Pansard, J.L.
Department of Anesthesiology, G.H.
Pitié Salpêtrière, 43 Bld de l'Hôpital,
75651 Paris Cédex 13, France

Park, G.R.
Anesthesia and Intensive Care,
Addenbrooke's Hospital, Hills Road,
Cambridge CB2 2QQ, United Kingdom

Payen, D.
Department of Anesthesiology,
Lariboisière Hospital, 2 rue Ambroise Paré,
75475 Paris Cédex 10, France

Payen, M.C.
Division of Infectious Diseases, St Pierre
University Hospital, Rue Haute 322,
1000 Brussels, Belgium

Pelosi, P.
Institute of Anesthesia, University of
Milan, Via Donizetti 106, 20052 Monza
(Milano), Italy

Pepe, P.E.
Emergency Medical Services, Baylor
College of Medicine, 1 Baylor Plaza,
Houston, TX 77030, USA

Pesenti, A.
Institute of Anesthesia, University of
Milan, Via Donizetti 106, 20052 Monza
(Milano), Italy

Piantadosi, C. A.
Department of Medicine, Duke University
Medical Center, Durham, NC 27710, USA

Pollard, B. J.
Department of Anesthesia, Manchester
Royal Infirmary, Oxford Road,
Manchester M13 9WL, United Kingdom

Quinn, K.
Anesthesia and Intensive Care,
Addenbrooke's Hospital, Hills Road,
Cambridge CB2 2QQ, United Kingdom

Reiz, S.
Department of Anesthesiology,
University of Umea, 90185 Umea, Sweden

Reynaert, M. S.
Intensive Care Unit, Clinique St Pierre,
1340 Ottignies, Belgium

Ritz, R.
Department of Intensive Care, University
Hospital, 4031 Basel, Switzerland

Robotham, J. L.
Department of Anesthesiology, The Johns
Hopkins Hospital, Blalock 15, Baltimore,
MD 21205, USA

Rocco, M.
Istituto di Anestesia e Rianimazione,
Universita "La Sapienza", 00161 Roma,
Italy

Roine, R. O.
Department of Neurology,
Helsinki University Central Hospital,
00290 Helsinki, Finland

Rosen, D. A.
Department of Anesthesia, Mott Children's
Hospital, Room C4139, Box 0800,
Ann Arbor, MI 48109-0800, USA

Rosen, K. R.
Department of Anesthesia, Mott Children's
Hospital, Room C4139, Box 0800,
Ann Arbor, MI 48109-0800, USA

Rosenthal, M. H.
Intensive Care Units, Stanford University
Hospital, Stanford, CA 94305, USA

Rossi, A.
Department of Anesthesia and Intensive
Care, City Hospital, Padova, Italy

Rouby, J.-J.
Surgical Critical Care Unit, G.H.
Pitié Salpêtrière, 43 Bld de l'Hôpital,
75651 Paris Cédex 13, France

Ruckdeschel, G.
Department of Anesthesiology, Klinikum
Grosshadern, 8000 München 70, Germany

Ruffolo, R. R. Jr.
Department of Pharmacology, Smith Kline
Beecham Plc, P.O. Box 1539, King of
Prussia, PA 19406-0939, USA

Scheidegger, D.
Department of Anesthesia, Kantonsspital,
4031 Basel, Switzerland

Schmid-Schönbein, H.
Department of Physiology, RWTH
Klinikum, Pauwelsstrasse, 5100 Aachen,
Germany

Schremmer, B.
Department of Intensive Care, C.H.U.
Cochin Port Royal, 27 Faubourg St
Jacques, 75674 Paris Cédex 14, France

Schreuder, J. J.
Department of Anesthesiology,
University Hospital, P.O. Box 1918,
6201 BX Maastricht, The Netherlands

Settels, J. J.
Department of Pulmonary Disease,
Erasmus University, P.O. Box 1738,
3000 DR Rotterdam, The Netherlands

Shapira, Y.
Department of Anesthesiology, Hadassah
University Hospital, P.O. Box 12000,
Jerusalem 91120, Israel

Sheiner, P. A.
Gastro-Intestinal Transplantation, Toronto
General Hospital, 200 Elizabeth Street,
Toronto, Ontario M5G 2C4, Canada

Shohami, E.
Department of Anesthesiology, Hadassah
University Hospital, P.O. Box 12000,
Jerusalem 91120, Israel

Silverman, H. J.
Department of Critical Care Medicine,
University of Maryland at Baltimore,
10 South Pine Street, Baltimore,
MD 21201, USA

Simon, C.
Department of Anesthesia, Kantonsspital,
4031 Basel, Switzerland

Singer, M.
Intensive Care Unit,
The Middlesex Hospital, Mortimer Street,
London W1N 8AA, United Kingdom

Sonnenblick, E. H.
Cardiovascular Research Laboratory,
Albert Einstein College of Medicine,
1300 Morris Park Avenue, Bronx,
NY 10461, USA

Spoendlin, M.
Department of Intensive Care, University
Hospital, 4031 Basel, Switzerland

Sprung, C. L.
Department of Anesthesiology,
Kiryat Hadassah, P.O. Box 12000,
91120 Jerusalem, Israel

Stoutenbeek, C. P.
Department of Intensive Care, O.L.V.
Ziekenhuis, 1e Oosterparkstraat 179,
1091 HA Amsterdam, The Netherlands

Strack van Schijndel, R.J.M.
Department of Intensive Care, Academisch
Ziekenhuis, De Boelelaan 1117,
1007 MB Amsterdam, The Netherlands

Sturk, A.
Laboratory for Medical Biochemistry,
Rockefeller University, 1230 York Avenue,
New York, NY 10021, USA

Sylin, P.
Department of Anesthesiology, Erasme
University Hospital, Route de Lennik 808,
1070 Brussels, Belgium

Takata, M.
Department of Anesthesiology, The Johns
Hopkins Hospital, Blalock 15, Baltimore,
MD 21205, USA

Takeda, M.
Department of Pharmacy, Tsukuba
University Hospital, 2-1-1 Amakubo,
Tsukuba-shi, Ibaraki 305, Japan

Teboul, J.L.
Medical ICU, CHU Le Kremlin-Bicêtre,
Paris, France

Tenaillon, A.
Department of Intensive Care, C.H. Louise
Michel, Quartier du Canal Courcouronnes,
91014 Evry Cédex, France

ten Cate, J. W.
Laboratory for Medical Biochemistry,
Rockefeller University, 1230 York Avenue,
New York, NY 10021, USA

Thijs, L. G.
Department of Intensive Care, Academisch
Ziekenhuis, De Boelelaan 1117,
1007 MB Amsterdam, The Netherlands

Thompson, W. L.
Lilly Research Laboratories, Eli Lilly
Company, Lilly Corporate Center,
Indianapolis, IN 46285, USA

Tokics, L.
Department of Clinical Physiology,
University Hospital, 751 85 Uppsala,
Sweden

Unertl, K. E.
Department of Anesthesiology, Klinikum
Grosshadern, 8000 München 70, Germany

Van Deventer, S.J.H.
Laboratory for Medical Biochemistry,
Rockefeller University, 1230 York Avenue,
New York, NY 10021, USA

Van Dyck, M.
Intensive Care Unit, St. Luc University
Hospital, Avenue Hippocrate 10,
1200 Brussels, Belgium

Van Hoeyweghen, R.A.F.
Department of Intensive Care,
U.Z. Antwerpen, Wilrijkstraat 10,
2520 Edegem, Belgium

Versprille, A.
Pulmonary Diseases, Erasmus Universiteit,
Postbus 1738, 3000 Rotterdam,
The Netherlands

Vesconi, S.
Department of Anesthesia, Ospedale
Maggiore, Via F. Sforza 35, 20122 Milano,
Italy

Vincken, W.
Intensive Care Unit, A.Z. V.U.B.,
Laarbeeklaan 101, 1090 Brussels, Belgium

Voerman, H.J.
Department of Intensive Care, Academisch
Ziekenhuis, De Boelelaan 1117,
1007 MB Amsterdam, The Netherlands

von Planta, M.
Department of Internal Medicine,
Kantonsspital, Petersgraben 4, 4031 Basel,
Switzerland

Wachter, R.M.
Chest Service, San Francisco General
Hospital, P.O. Box 0841, San Francisco,
CA 94143-0841, USA

White, P.F.
Department of Anesthesiology,
Washington University Medical Center,
660 South Euclid Avenue, St Louis,
MO 63110, USA

Wilson, J.J.
Intensive Care Unit, Royal Victoria
Hospital, Grosvenor Road,
Belfast BT12 6BA, United Kingdom

Yamashita, M.
Department of Emergency Medicine,
University of Tsukuba School of Medicine,
2-1-1 Amakubo, Tsukuba City, Ibaraki 305,
Japan

Yates, D.W.
Emergency Medicine, Hope Hospital,
Eccles Old Road, Salford M6 8HD,
United Kingdom

Yau, E.H.S.
Department of Anesthesia,
St Bartholomew's Hospital, West
Smithfield, London EC1A 7BE,
United Kingdom

Multiple Organ Failure

Synergetic Order and Chaotic Malfunctions of the Circulatory Systems in Multiple Organ Failure*
Breakdown of Cooperativity of Hemodynamic Functions as Cause of Acute Microvascular Pathologies

H. Schmid-Schönbein

Introduction: Towards an Understanding of the Physiological and Pathological Forms of Synergetic Cooperativity of the Cardiovascular Subsystems

"Synergetics" and "chaos theory" [1-4] prove to be extremely helpful in comprehending the order and stability of biological processes, defining deterministic cooperativity ("synergetic order") as emaneting from the controlled flow of energy and matter in restricted compartments. "Chaos theory" is rapidly gaining interest among medical theoreticians and medical practitioners for three reasons: 1. there is increasing awareness that biological processes are subject to fundamental regularities – but also to the inherent unpredictabilities – of many dynamic "multiphase systems" (v.i.) studied in chemistry and physics, 2. functional cooperativity, previously thought to be the privilege of biological systems, also exists in chemical and physical systems, bears the trait for catastophic reactions which are deterministic yet unpredictable and 3. new, and generally applicable criteria for the establishment of stability of processes (and for their breakdown) are in progress of being developed. Already now, the comprehension of a broad spectrum of endogeneously stable and coherent processes, and the knowledge of destabilizing mechanisms in the cooperativity of intravascular, extravascular and intracellular process is of potential practical interest to intensive care and emergency medicine.

The present review starts from the assumption (detailed in [5]) that the intact circulatory system of the blood constituents (macrocirculation, microcirculation, extravascular percolation due to the process of filtration and reabsorption) can be interpreted as a large ensemble of simple dynamic systems that are "coherent" in behavior. Mechanical "coherence" (in the synergetic sense of the word) in a system of connected conduits follows from the simple laws of communicating tubes, but there is also "chemical coherence" of the processes in which the blood constituents take part (v.i.).

In close analogy to the synergetics of "amplified physical processes" (e.g. Lasers and superconductors, explained in [1] and [2]), a "rectification process" takes place in the erythrocytes subjected to shear forces while perfusing microscopic vessels with dimensions smaller than their resting diameter. As detailed in [5],

---

* Dedicated to Prof. Ilja Prigogine, Brussels, in admiration.

this process of entropy driven subordination of erythrocytes to the existing set of physical forces (each cell following a principle of minimum energy expenditure) induces large scale cooperativity and coherence of all moving erythrocytes and thereby "amplifies" and "stabilizes" their motion. Moreover, since more than 95% of the mechanical energy supplied by the heart is dissipated in the terminal vascular beds [5], erythrocyte orientation in shear is the most important, but by no means the only rectification process in the circulatory bed. It does, however, minimize the frictional energy dissipation unavoidably associated with the perfusion of a narrow blood conduits and thence helps to conserve a large portion of the "power" generated in the heart not only in the microvessels, but also in the venous bed. By this effect, it helps to "stabilize" the dynamic process of the perpetual motion of the blood. Since not only the intravascular, but also the interstitial convective transport processes are "powered" by the "rectified" flow of energy, stability of flow also exerts control over the stability of chemical reactions in these two compartments. Moreover, by keeping their "milieu exterieur" in stable order, stable perfusion of the interstitial space therefore helps to maintain the intracellular integrity.

The cooperativity and coherence of rectified flow in the entire systemic circulation therefore stabilizes:

1. the directionality of vascular perfusion and interstitial percolation;
2. the distribution of flows (ordered attendance of blood constituents to individual vells segments and to the interstitial spaces; and
3. the biochemical processes taking place in the different parts of the large interstitial compartment by strongly favoring stable "linear" and by effectively inhibiting unstable or "non-linear" catalyzed reactions.

"Synergetics" and "chaos theory" are so far concerned with relatively simple dynamic systems; we are just beginning to extrapolate the regularities found in them to the much more complex ensembles of dynamic systems found in the biological world. This is justified under the assumption that 1. we subdivide the organism into "limited compartments" as the site of a controlled flow of energy and matter and 2. that we regard "processes" and their power (flow of energy in unit time) rather than "reactions" and their kinetics. As will be discussed later, the concept of a "dissipative structure" (see section IV and appendix) is very helpful for this purpose: we will take the entire cardiovascular system as one such cooperative "dissipative structure", but also the interstitial space (including the lymphatic system) and the intracellular spaces. Their efficacy, their internal and external cooperativity and their stability is primarily based on the maintenance of a "boosted steady state" (see section IV) and on the tight control over the "economical" dissipation of energy for any given process.

"Synergetic order" is in jeopardy of breakdown (or of "destabilization") for two possible reasons, namely by inadequate energy content or by uncontrolled energy flow. For the former state, in which a previously existing order is "lost", and the components operate incoherently and thence in an indeterminate fashion ("infrasynergetic chaos"). Uncontrolled flow of energy through "dissipative structures", however, overtaxes the "ordering potentials" of the synergetic components, and there is a transgression into another type of chaotic behavior, which has been termed "deterministic chaos" [3, 4]. For this state, the term "suprasynergetic chaos" appears appropriate (see section II).

The physiological order of the entire organism (a synergetic cosmos) is based on strict cooperativity of biomechanical and biochemical processes. As will be seen, the phenotype of "multiorgan failure", of "circulatory shock" and of the host of abnormal biochemical abnormalities plagueing intensive care and emergency medicine can be reduced to a combination of "infrasynergetic chaos" in the mechanical domain, "suprasynergetic chaos" in the biochemical domain and to breakdown of the physiological cooperativity between these two domains due to local "divergence phenomena".

Synergetic Order in Dynamic Biological Systems

"Synergetic" and "chaos" theory help to transcend the reductionist phase of biological research. The last two hundred years of biomedical research were dominated by the analysis of isolated components of biological systems (organisms, organs, tissues, cells and molecules). As a rule, the biological functions and their pathological deviations were comprehended as *"reactions"* between individual partners, their mutual interdependency as in potentiating or inhibiting, accelerating or depressing each other were always considered; the time has now come to think in terms of dynamic *processes*.

As will be shown, in synergetic dynamic systems, the "boosted steady state" guarantees 1. a more or less stable "order" of processes associated with continuous flow of energy and matter, 2. the spontaneous subordination of subsystems to a stable arrangement of elements. The "stability" however, proves to be quite sensitive to disturbances, since it can either break down or "die down" (when the flow of energy and matter is insufficient), when it experiences "blow out" or when the transfer is becoming too large to be compatible with order. To cope with these potentials of well organized multiphase systems, the paradoxical yet vividly descriptive name "dissipative structure" was invented [3], since the macroscopic order in a synergetic system assumes often a characteristic pattern. Dissipative structures are labile; the apparently stationary configuration being always in danger to "implode" or to "explode".

The dynamics of highly non-linear mechanical and chemical reactions in simple dynamic systems are the topic of synergetics and chaos theory [4]; many contributions came from pure mathematicians who developed the formal treatment of apparently "catastrophical" reactions [7]. The choice of the word "chaos" in these theories in many respects violates one's linguistic intuition because the term was formerly associated with "states of utter confusion, completely wanting in order, sequence, organization or predictable operation" (Websters dictionary). Following Haken [2], who speaks about the transients "from chaos to order onto chaos", the present author therefore proposes to refer to the physiological processes of biological systems as being "synergetically ordered" ("synergetic cosmos"), delineating the normal functional state from two pathological domains, namely "infrasynergetic chaos" and "suprasynergetic chaos".

The first state is defined either as the unorganized state of primordial matter or as the defective states of previously existing order after the flow of energy and matter becomes insufficient to induce synergy; it could also be called "indeterminate chaos". The term "suprasynergetic chaos" is identical in meaning to "deterministic chaos" in the conventional connotation of "chaos theory".

"Attractor Processes" and "Dissipative Structures"

Simple *reactions* in the physical domain (e.g. mass transports by convection or diffusion) and in the chemical domain (formation of a product upon collision of two molecules or atoms) can be described by simple "laws". However, in order to understand the behavior of complex processes (and thence of the synergy of subsystems of an organism), it must be taken as fact that the symptoms one perceives from them are the reflection of "dynamic processes" rather than of simple reactions. "Synergetics" have paved the way for such a novel "dialogue" with nature (to use a term by Prigogine [3]) and it is essential to understand the often unusual semantics of this new paradigmatic system ("structures", "order parameters", "attractors", "divergence phenomena") dealing with "processes in" rather than with "properties of" dynamic systems. For example, the term "dissipative structure" reflects the emanation of a highly ordered stream of energy and matter (see Appendix). "Attractors" have to be viewed as "powered processes" rather than as "forces", their efficacy depends on the flow of energy in unit time (Nm/s) or the "work" performed in them (power multiplied by time, Nm). "Strong attractors" guarantee stable, or "one-dimensional" processes, in the cardiovascular system they dominate even the directionality of apparently unrelated processes. Systems which are well "boosted" (the dynamic steady state of which is *far* from thermodynamic equilibrium) allow processes to occur which are referred to as only having one "attractor". However, if systems are displaced *closer* to their thermodynamic equilibrium (or to their static steady state), the stability can be further endangered by the action of so called "strange attractors". Again, we have to perceive this in the realm of "competing processes": they were termed "strange" because their *power* (absolute, or relative that of the principle attractor process) is 1. highly sensitive to the boundary condition and therefore 2. highly non-linear in their kinetics. The rheological potentials of the blood, especially its tendency to undergo reversible and irreversible "phase transitions" (fluid-solid) predispose them for the leading role in "strange attractor processes" destabilizing the motion of blood. It is noted in parentheses already here that the beneficial role of "hemorheological therapies" (especially hemodilution) must probably be seen in this context: they strengthen the power of the „strong attractor" of the cardiovascular system (the cardiac work) and they attenuate the efficacy of rheological "strange attractors" in the microcirculation.

The Concept of a "Boosted Steady State"

A descriptive picture of the term "steady state" in a synergetic context is that of an elevated reservoir of energy and matter (for example water dammed to provide a stable reservoir for irrigational purposes and for transferring its potential energy into electric energy). The pressure built-up in the example of an energized wind sleeve (see Appendix) (as well as that in the arterial side of the systemic circulation) also represents a situation that the present author proposes to call "boosted steady states". In biological systems, both intracellularly and in the blood plasma, "chemical energy" is "stored" in synthetized macromolecules (lipids, glycogen, and most importantly, highly specialized proteins), mechanical energy is "stored" in the pressurized arterial system (in essence in the conformational energy of the compliant blood containers), electrical energy is "stored" in the membrane potentials. Transport processes (the heart as a pump, membranal pumps) replenish the amount of energy that is continuously being lost in dissipative processes. The present author suggests the term "boosted steady state" to paraphrase the (phasically shifting) equilibrium between *input* of energy (in unit time) and energy dissipated in unit time. By a host of control mechanism, the *flow rate* of energy and matter through compartments of finite size is closely matched to "biological requirements", it is perhaps trivial to state that such control is conditio sine qua non for both the adaptability and the stability of synergetic systems with a wide range of "process velocities".

Synergetics has uncovered an important regularity of many dynamic systems in the "boosted steady state", namely that they have the potential for highly coherent, cooperative and "self organized" performance, the ability to find spontaneously a high level of efficacy provided that the system is kept "boosted", i.e. removed far from its thermodynamic equilibrium. There is increasing evidence that "synergetic systems" in this sense are an automatic emanation (latin manare: to flow) of the unavoidable entropy generation in dissipative structures [3, 4]. "Chance" and "necessity" can be linked by the genetically determined directionality of energy transfer processes. This directionality is instituted by the macroscopic and microscopic "structure" of components and follows from the principle of minimum energy expenditure. By a process akin to "trial and error", this results in amplified "efficacy" of the energy flow to continuously voided "energy sinks".

There is a wide spectrum of "stabilities" on the energy flow in biological processes, and "periodically driven" processes such as that of the cardiovascular system are endogenously immune to be "destabilized" by weak attractors when there is a mechanism that links energy input to energy dissipation. This is achieved by the close mechanical coupling of venous return to cardiac output (v.i.). In understanding the problems associated with cardiovascular instability in critically ill patients, one must appreciate that – on the other hand – this system is always very close to, in fact "only one heartbeat away" from its thermodynamic equilibrium: cardiac standstill bringing the arterial pressure (and thence the only energy content) down to that of the veins. Periodically energized synergetic systems can be "robust" only provided they are dominated by exclusively one "strong attractor process". Stability is bound to be lost 1. when its influence vanishes and 2. when several, often weakly acting attractors compete for the effectuation of the flow of energy and matter.

Non-nutritional Functions of the Blood and Flow Destabilization

The synergetics of nutritional and non-nutritional functions of the blood differ in principle: while the former thrive on flow stability, the latter require flow destabilization to allow chemical synergy. For a comprehensive discussion of the "synergetics" of all blood flow in a fully comprehensive fashion, the multiplicity of functions has to be considered. It is perhaps trivial to state that all hemostatic and host defense reactions are associated with phase transitions from "quasi-fluid" to "quasi-solid" and with localized losses of blood fluidity and/or blood motion [9]. In large parts, the specific and unspecific humoral defense reactions result from the "immobilization" of potentially hostile microorganisms that have penetrated the body (or more specifically the extracellular compartment). Once they reside in the extravascular spaces, they find ideal conditions for parasitic life, for survival and reproduction. Unless immobilized by reactions that impede their motion in the blood stream, the extracellular interstitial flow and the lymph-flow, these microorganisms would be readily transported within the cardiovascular system.

From a rheological point of view, the dissemination of microbiological organisms is impeded by reactions and processes that bear dynamic similarity to explosive chemical reactions. They can only be understood in their biological dynamics if understood as "processes" in flow reactors: the reactive plasma must be delivered to, but should not escape from the site of reaction. For this purpose the blood is endowed with properties that allow just that, namely to undergo "fluid-solid-phase transitions" [11]. While trivial from a biochemical point of view it is of utmost rheological interest to note that the precursor *reaction* in the plasmatic coagulation system (enzyme cascade) is triggered by F XIIa, is capable of initiating the multienzyme network of the fibrinolytic system, the alternate pathway of the complement system and the kinin-system [12]. Which of the *processes* is then started depends on the mechanical conditions: flow rate assuming a pivotal role "regulating" the site, the directionality and the rate of the autocatalytically amplification determining blood components *in vivo*. More specifically, the stability or instability of the flow exclusively governs whether or not enzymatically amplified reactions and thence chemically highly *unstable* processes actually do taken place in the large extravascular components of the body.

It is often overlooked that the cellular defense mechanism, taken over by granulocytes is not only based on phagocytosis, but in part on hemodynamic effects exerted by plugging and marginating granulocytes [11]. There are intricate relationships between all biochemical processes (proteolytic, oxidative) and the biomechanical events controlling microvascular blood flow: in the vessels, strictly laminar flow guarantees the course of linear reactions ("scavenging reactions" between proteases and their inhibitors) (Fig. 1). Conversely, all forms of "separated flow" (vortex formation, microvascular stasis, to and from movements equivalent to "infrasynergetic" or indeterminate mechanical chaos) invariably induce shift from the synergetically ordered chemical scavenging reactions to "explosive" biochemical reactions. "Separated flow" (stasis in small, vortex flow in large compartments) proves to be the absolute prerequisite for the manifestation of amplified, autocatalytic processes in the extracellular compartment

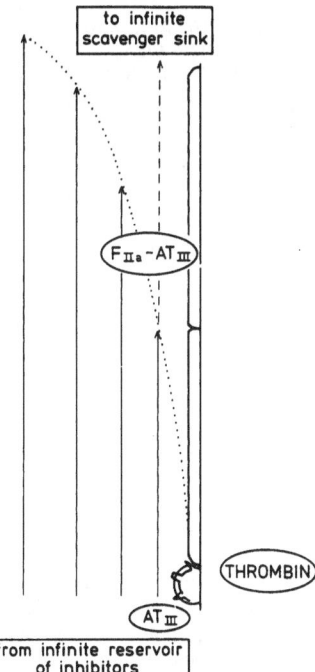

Fig. 1. Schematic representation of the functional coherence of laminar flow of and biochemical reactions in the flowing blood (as examplified in the linear reaction between an activated enzyme (here thrombin) and its inhibitor (here Antithrombin III). Strictly linear convective motion links guarantee that reaction product (here the Antithrombin II – Faktor IIa – Complex) is removed coupling the reaction to an infinite sink for scavenger mechanisms

(intravascular and extravascular) (Fig. 2). In other words: the stability or instability of laminar flow functions as a potent regulator of enzymatic processes incorporating blood cells and plasmatic proenzymes and inhibitor principles *in vivo.*

Mechanical and Chemical "Rectification" in the Circulating Blood and Its Disturbances

Haken [1] has uncovered the operation of "enslaving principles" in (non-biological) dynamic systems; this term represents the subordination of subphases under "director principles" which – due to large scale cooperativity and coherence – greatly amplify the efficacy of energy transfer (e.g. in the synergetic system of Lasers). It goes without saying that quite analogous subordination mechanisms under one dominating attractor process occur abundantly in physiology. Interestingly, we now see that in the extracellular compartment, the coherent operation of the large ensemble of mechanical as well as biochemical subsystems comprising the systemic circulation is subjected to one dominating attractor process (Fig. 3). Since the directed flow of energy (from its arterial reservoir to its sink in the right ventricle) guarantees directionality of all types of convective transport (namely laminar Poiseuille flow in the vessels and unidirectional percolation in the interstitial spaces), it guarantees one type of chemical reaction and *stabilizes* linear reactions between enzymes and inhibitors.

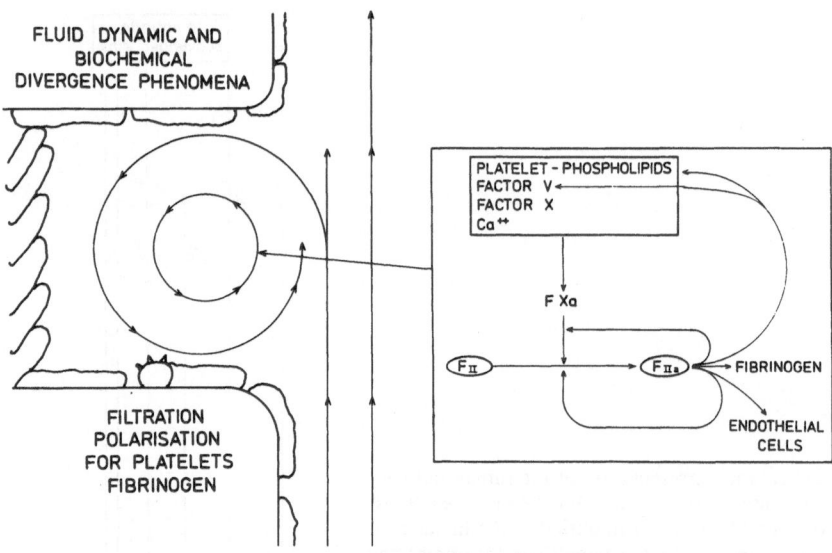

Fig. 2. Schematic representation of the functional coupling between incoherent blood flow and an enzymatically amplified reaction. Unless removed by convective dilution (and binding to its inhibitor), thrombin initiates a multitude of positively fed back reaction loops (e.g. that by activating platelets, factor V and factor X and II). Also, it acts on endothelial cells, by severing their integrity allowing local accumulation of fibrinogen and thrombocytes as reaction partners for chemical reactions and induces a fluid/solid phase transition (due to induction of fibrin-polymerization and platelet aggregation)

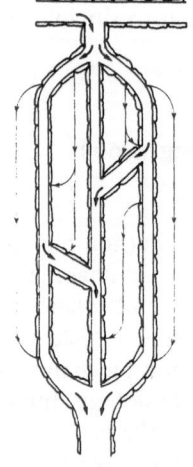

COHERENT CONVECTIVE TRANSPORT PROCESSES
IN THE MICROVASCULAR NETWORKS

CONTROLLED COOPERATIVITY OF

1) Capillary flow rate
2) Cell attendance to capillaries
3) Flow directionality and homogeneity
    of perfusion
4) Reversed osmosis (filtration)
5) Directionality and flow rate of
    interstitial percolation
6) Colloidal osmosis obligatory and
    interstitial scavenger transport

Fig. 3. The concept of rectified microvascular flow: local control of energy flow automatically inducing functional cooperativity between intravascular and transmural (and thence interstitial) flow of blood constituents (see text)

Stable and unstable deterministic *biochemical* processes can occur both in the intracellular and the extracellular compartment; there is, however, a fundamental difference in the enzymatic regulation in the two. While in the closed compartments of cells the reaction rates are subjected to *negative feed back* by intrinsic regulators (e.g. networks of activator-principles, inhibitor-principles, substrate-supply and product-inhibition, see Textbooks of Biochemistry), conversely, in the open extracellular spaces the *site,* the *directionality* and the *reaction rates* of catalyzed processes are almost exclusively regulated by the convective transport regime (v.i.). Once triggered, they are often *positively* fed back. In these, one can differentiate between two extremes and frequent transients between the two:

1. fully rectified linear processes and
2. fully separated, amplified processes. The former are associated with the normal coherent cardiovascular transport processes, the latter with many forms of disturbed, yet maintained but incoherent flow (Fig. 3).

The details of a synergetic concept of the cardiovascular system-control due to "rectification" are outlined in [5], some of the factors listed in Table 1, listing only entirely *passive* mechanisms that all cooperate in "amplifiying" the efficacy of the transport processes in the systemic circulation. For reasons of time and space, only the passive microvascular fluidizing mechanisms (cells rectification and formation of a lubricating plasma layer) and irrigation mechanisms (reversed osmosis at the arteriolar end, colloidal osmosis at the venular end) can be detailed in Fig. 1. There is obligatory synergy between the power associated with intravascular perfusion of microvessels and that of interstitial percolation. Flexible red cells allow the development of long, narrow tubes (diameter 5 μm), the high fluidity of the perfusate allowing a fast flow from the arteriolar end (where mechanical energy is higher than water binding potential of plasmatic colloids) to the venular end, kept at low pressure due the mechanisms effectively voiding the venous capacitance bed. We see that two mechanical processes (modulated by vasomotor influences) provide the high power for rapid capillary perfusion. The extremely high energy dissipation in long narrow tubes links one type of chemical work (forced separation of colloids from their solvent, or "reversed osmosis", conventially called capillary filtration) to its reversal (colloidal osmosis). As the coupled processes of capillary perfusion and interstitial percolation "channel" the flow of energy and matter, the system creates new "dissipative structures", stabilizing not only a mechanical process (interstitial irrigation for nutritional and scavenging functions), but "stabilizing" the directionality of chemical processes.

The latter processes illustrate the obligatory dynamic link between biofluidmechanics and biochemistry: the local catabolite scavenging (vascular, interstitial) links any local "chemical reactor" to an *infinite supply* of buffers and inhibitors, as well as to an *infinitely* large system of catabolite eliminators (lung, kidney) or scanvenging mechanisms (Reticulo-endothelial system and lymphnodes). Since laminar flow inhibits positive feed back, these reactions are of the linear type [3] and follow first order kinetics; we therefore call them "rectified" since the local reaction is linked to the process of laminar flow, thence occurs in a medium on the path from an infinitely large reservoir of inhibitors to an infinitely large sink of scavenging or eliminating mechanisms.

Quite different requirements must be fulfilled in the hemostatic and the host-defense functions of the blood: here, non-linear, positively fed back and reac-

Table 1. Rectifying mechanisms of the cardiovascular system to stabilize blood flow

1. Myocardium:
- Frank-Starling mechanism of the right and left ventricles in complying to changes in preload and afterload
- rectification of flow directionality due to action of all cardiac valves
- mediation of sympathetic and parasympathetic inotropic and chronotropic effects
- active diastolic filling due to elastic and kinetic energies operating in A-V-ring displacement mechanism

2. Large arteries:
- the "Windkessel-function"
- impedance matching due to dilatation in physical exercise
- site of sensor mechanisms for stability of boosted steady state, regular for cardiovascular depressor reflexes

3. Arterioles:
- matching in microvascular conductance and cell attendance to metabolic demands (input regulation)
- matching of microvascular conductance to arterial steady state (myogenic and metabolic output "autoregulation")
- attenuation of pressure and flow pulsatility

4. Exchange capillaries:
- axial RBC alignment
- marginal plasma lubrication
- active control of cytological and plasmatic interactions: electrostatic repulsion between cellular glycocalices (endothelial cells, blood cells) and between cells and plasmatic colloids
- maintenance of flow rate and directionality of reversed osmosis (concentration, performance of chemical work when Pcap > COP) and colloidal-osmosis (performance of osmotic work when Pcap < COP)

5. Interstitial tissue:
- directed percolation and irrigation of pericellular spaces for nutrient and mediator supply
- obligatory link of scavenger input and output

6. Veins:
- venous valve mechanism
- venous tone adaptation to adapt capacity
- site of volume-receptors to match blood volume to systemic capacitance
- obligatory adaptation of cardiac filling (venous output) to microvascular perfusion (venous input)
- obligatory setting of intravascular pressure to atmospheric pressure (zero transmural pressure, ensuring colloidal osmosis in exchange vessels)

tions associated with phase transitions (fluid-solid) are mandatory. The blood components are well suited for this purpose; however, the manifestation of their potential requires local segregation from the coherent motion of blood constituents (Fig. 4). As is detailed in [8], flow separation and the generation of transient "flow reactors" is the most appropriate fashion to allow the progressive self-amplification of enzymatic processes. In the microvascular network, separated flow occurs if there is "non-homogeneous flow", i.e. venular or capillary blockade by various "thixotropic obstacles" (Fig. 2) [6, 11]. If cellular and/or

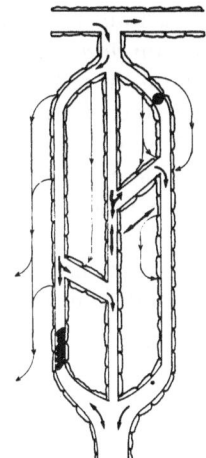

DESTABILIZED MICROCIRCULATION

1) Plugging by blood cells and microemboli (thixotropic occlusion)

2) Compaction stasis
   (thixotropic occlusion)

3) Incoherent perfusion

4) Intermittancy of flow
   (magnitude, direction)

5) Incoherent filtration
   and reabsorption

6) Incoherent interstitial percolation

7) Reduction in exchange area

Fig. 4. The concept of incoherent flow in the "disturbed microcirculation". Blockade of individual segments by "thixotropic obstacles" (plugging granulocytes, compacted blood, microemboli acting exclusively in low flow states [6, 11]) interferes with coherence of intravascular traffic, of flow and exchange. Rectified chemical reactions are impeded, incoherent, catalytically amplified ones are enhanced

molecular reactions of blood elements in permanent stasis (or in erratic to- and for movements) are triggered, separation of the local flow from "coherent flow" in the remaining circulatory bed not just allows, but becomes "conditio sine qua

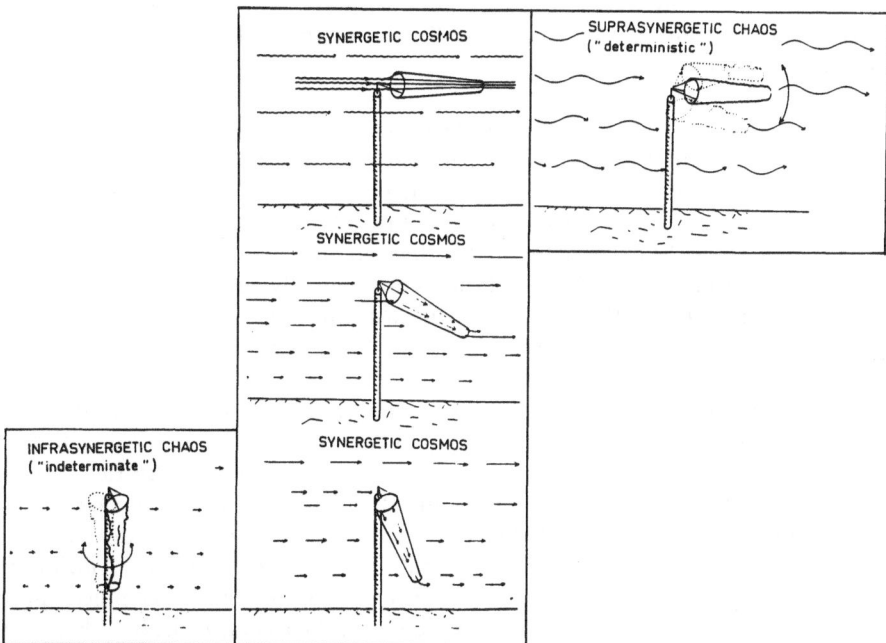

Fig. 5. Functional cooperativity of dynamic systems as examplified by a "windsleeve", in which the continuous flow of energy and matter produces a wide range of synergetic order (see text) bounded by chaotic behavior if the system is not adequately boosted (infrasynergetic or indeterminate chaos) or when it is overpowered (suprasynergetic or deterministic chaos), see text

non" for explosive, self amplified reactions and processes. Whether or not their power is released, therefore depends on *prior* alterations in the fluid-mechanical domain. Any form of flow retardation, in reducing the power of the principle attractor mechanism, allows other attractor processes to come into action: the situation becomes "destabilized". There is an interesting divergence: flow as the mechanical process becomes "indeterminate" (falls into infrasynergetic chaos), biochemical reactions at the same time exploding into the deterministic reactions ("suprasynergetic chaos") (Fig. 5).

Since enzymatically amplified reactions are often associated with reversible rheological phase transitions, i.e. an isothermic change from the fluid to the solid (or quasi-solid) state of aggregation and back, a further destabilizing moment arises. Here, again, the principle of circular causality operates: chemically induced phase transitions to solids or "quasi-solids" destabilize the mechanical process of flow, while at the same time stabilizing the progress of the chemical reactions. Quite often bistable directionality of the flow of energy and matter, associated with the "ebb and tide" of retarded flow near its thermodynamic equilibrium ("indeterminate steady state"). This situation responds in a highly sensitive fashion to "strange attractors", all of which tending to retard flow rates while accelerating chemical reaction rates (and vice versa).

Synergetics of Fluid-Dynamics and Biochemistry: Divergence Phenomena of Flow and Biochemistry in Protracted State of Hypoperfusion

Having shown that nutritional purposes can best be served by the physiological coherence of mechanical and chemical processes in the extracellular compartment, a "conflict of aims" becomes evident. The triggers for hemostatic reactions (mechanical injury and vasoconstriction) and the initial events in host-defense reactions produce "separated flow", i.e. they provide ideal boundary conditions for the manifestation of self-amplifying, enzymatically driven processes. While local destabilization of flow is compatible with life (and essential for survival), generalized and prolonged destabilization of the cardiovascular processes is *not*.

In essence, the colorful spectrum of symptoms of protracted states of hypoperfusion represent two opposing deviations from synergetic order and cooperativity: the mechanical processes "regress" into the realm of "infrasynergetic chaos", the chemical ones "transgress" into that of "suprasynergetic chaos". The indeterminate states of the disturbed microcirculations, subject to the action of "strange attractor processes" that destabilize motion due to local visciidating mechanisms [6, 11], allow the occurrence of a multiplicity of chemical processes[1], a conundrum of causes and consequences. "Circular causality" has to be

---

[1]   The number of mutually interfering processes is endless. Table 2 (taken from a recent review of the author) is by no means comprehensive but illustrates some components of an infinitely tangled multitude of abnormal reactions. The interested readers are referred to other chapters of this book and the literature cited there.

Table 2. Factors reducing microvascular conductance due to abnormal mechanical, cytological and biochemical interactions in disease: reversible and irreversible blood viscidation

1. *Loss of high shear heterophase effects*
    1.1 Abolition of single vessel Fahraeus effect: Loss of dynamic red cell deformation; Irregular red cell screening; Precapillary white cell margination; Abnormally pronounced postcapillary white cell margination
    1.2 Occurrence of low shear heterophase effects
    Fahraeus-Veylens effect white cell margination due to pathological red cell aggregation; Intravascular aggregate sedimentation Fahraeus-effect reversal and compaction stasis
        – Venous occlusion
        – Shift of ratio of pre- to postcapillary resistance: elevation of effective filtration pressure
        – White cell plugging in nutritive capillaries
        – Low capillary conductance
        – Proteolytic damage of endothelial and parenchymal cells
    1.3. Consequences of generalized blood viscidation
    Polycythemia; Leukocytosis; Thrombocytosis; Elevated concentration of acute phase proteins; Hyperfibrinogenemia or macroglobulinemia; Elevated concentration of immunoglobulins (IgG, IgM); Hyper-albuminemia

2. *Consequences of endothelial cell dysfunction*
    2.1 Endothelial swelling: reduced microvascular conductance
    2.2 Endothelial dehiscence
        – Abnormal platelet deposition
        – Abnormal white cell adhesion and emigration
    2.3. Abnormally high basement membrane permeability
        – Local hemoconcentration
        – Filtration-polarization
        – Pathological inhibition of interstitial space (by plasma proteins or proteolytic enzymes)
    2.4. Abnormal interactions between red and white-cells, red cell aggregates and adhesive white cells, red cells and thrombocytes

3. *Consequences of generalized pressure loss in the microvasculature*
    3.1. Less perfect or absent red cell deformation
    3.2. Irregular screening effects producing highly variable composition of RCPM in microvascular bed
    3.3. Enhanced and extended cell-cell and cell-wall contacts
    3.4. Local activation of chemical processes due to lack of convective dilution
        – Proteolytic enzymes (Procoagulatory, Fibrinolytic, Complement system, Kinin system)
        – Oxidative stress
        – Cytolytic and membranolytic processes

4. *Abnormal hydration, osmolarity, and acid-base status of the interstitium*
    4.1. Lactic acidosis
    4.2. Hyperosmolarity
    4.3. Disequilibrium of specific cations (K, Na, Ca ...)
    4.4 Generalized vasorelaxation at rest associated with abnormal RCPM fluidity (erythrocytosclerosis, local hemoconcentration, local white cell accumulation or abnormal ratio of pre- to postcapillary resistance)
    4.5. Abnormal "activation" of leukocytes and thrombocytes (auto- or heterocatalysis)

5. *Abnormal parenchymal metabolism*
    5.1. Glycolysis in response to generalized hypoxia
    5.2. Hypoglycemic derangement of cellular metabolism

assumed, not only among these processes, but among them and the progressive disturbance of nutritional functions.

In long term "low flow states", of course, these reactions are neither restricted to the microvascular nor to the interstitial compartment, as a matter of fact they reach "down" into the intracellular compartments and "up" into the macrovascular one (not to mention the pulmonary circulation and the exchange of blood gases).

In terms of "synergetics", chronical states of hypoperfusion, due to their tendency to break down functional barriers, destabilize both the (large) extracellular and the (small) intracellular "dissipative structures". There is not only enhanced "permeability" of the endothelial lining separating the intravascular from the interstitial spaces, but also a tendency to attenuate the physical and chemical barriers that normally strictly separate intracellular from extracellular processes. Not only overt cytological damage of the parenchymal cells (and associated release of cytosolic and membranal constituents), but discrete electrolytic and pH-abnormalities associated with hypoxic metabolism begin to affect the integrity of the "milieu extérieur" of the parenchymal cells. The consequences are clear: the "boosted steady states" are less distinct, the systems move closer to their respective thermodynamic equilibria (or to "infrasynergetic chaos"). Even when structural defects of boundaries are too small to be detected, functional defects subsequent to spontaneous, unantagonized dissipation processes remove the "essence of synergetic order", namely the mechanical and electrochemical gradients that are normally maintained in meticulous stability throughout life.

At this point, the concept of "circular causality" in chaotic reactions must be introduced. Whether caused by deficiency in supply of energy and matter or by loss of control over its entropy-driven dissipation, "steady states" are "less boosted". This effect alone effectuates the transition from synergetic order to either infrasynergetic or suprasynergetic chaos, for example during the processes taking place if a previously ischemic, biochemically destabilized tissue is reperfused. After breakdown of barriers to ions (especially Ca^{++}), in the absence of high energy phosphate potential and of adequate redox-potential, the oxygen delivered to the disturbed microcirculation is likely to give rise to oxidative damage – rather than to oxidative phosphorylation and thence the replenishment of the intracellular "boosted steady state". The resulting lipid- and proteinoxidation, as well as a host of intracellular calcium mediated alterations certainly represent the epitomy of abnormal transport processes: convective and diffusive transport mechanisms are no longer capable of repairing but rather begin to destroy the "dissipative cellular structures" and thus prevents them from using the delivered oxygen for the restoration of the intracellular energy stores (a topic beyond the scope of the present treatize).

If one focusses on "stability" of synergetic processes – rather than on individual reactions – the striking and far-reaching success of the principle of hemodilution [13, 14] can be explained much more rationally. If simply assuming that it conserves and/or restitutes fluid-mechanical and biochemical coherence and thence physiological cooperativity [6] of all extracellular subsystems, its remarkable safety, its lack of side effects and its efficacy can all be reduced to one action, namely the restoration of "boosted steady states" in the vascular and extravascular compartments, a sine qua non for the restoration of cellular integrity.

The deliberations are certainly biased owing to the past experimental emphasis of the author [5, 6, 11]; microvascular and hemostatic reactions (and their specific rheological components) were primarily discussed so far. Other abnormalities, of course, have analogous effects in "destabilizing" the movement of blood constituents. Suffice it here to mention endothelial defects, all forms of vasoconstriction, and white cell or plugging. These physical reactions have to be viewed also from the biochemical perspective, since all give rise to misplaced proteolytic events, abnormal host-defense reactions and the activation of autacoid systems progressively dominating the extracellular reactions after cell damage [15, 16]. Last but not least, abnormalities of the generalized and local endocrine control had to be left out but seem to prevail (e.g. abnormalities in glucocorticosteroids, catecholamines, histamine, serotonin and the kinin system), as well as malfunctions of the cytokine network. Most importantly, the synergetics of defective filling of the ventricles in diastole has to be considered. As shortly mentioned above, this process thrives not only on the energy stored in the elastic support system of the heart [17], but critically on venous return [18], since the kinetic energy of the blood is essential to perform the work of diastolic filling of the relaxed ventricles.

One is safe in predicting that the conceptional framework provided by research in synergetics and chaos will be put to use more and more in theoretical and practical medicine. Intensive care medicine will appreciate its value only if it can also provide concepts for prevention and therapy. We have reason to believe that this might happen in all therapeutic maneuvers that stabilize the function of the heart and the microcirculation.

Both aims can be achieved by (isovolemic or hypervolemic) hemodilution. In the present author's opinion the clinical efficacy of this procedure cannot possibly be explained by the assumption of its influence on one "reaction" due to reduced "viscosity" [6]. Instead, its *global* effect, its influence on stabilizing the cooperativity of fluid-dynamic and biochemical "processes" must be insinuated to explain its multiple effects [19]. Obviously, macrocirculatory as well as microcirculatory processes must be regarded in order to understand the efficacy of iatrogenically induced hemodilution [6, 11]. Induction of cardiovascular stability [1] and prevention of microvascular chaotic reactions [2] seem to be going hand in hand.

Conclusion

In the conventional paradigmatic system of hemodynamics, acute and protracted forms of "multiorgan failure" are characterized by a multitude of distinct subsystem process abnormalities. The concepts developed in "synergetics" and "chaos theory" for simple dynamic systems can now be applied to networks of complex, interdependent dynamic systems such as they exist in the circulating motion of blood constituents in the cardiovascular and the interstitial bed. This approach requires the integration of the conventional dynamic transport reactions into different energy driven processes. Novel semantics must be applied: the normal circulation is then taken as an oscillating yet stable process in synergetic order, energized phasically by cardiac input of energy and matter. The stability of its oscillation in a "boosted steady state" is kept remote from its thermodynamic equilibrium. This can then be explained by the storage of potential energy in the elastic elements of the "Windkessel vessels" and the kinetic energy of the blood in the venous return as well as by the subtle matching of input and dissipation of energy (acting as the sole "attractor process").

Low flow states are paradigmatic for a *destabilization* of the cardiovascular flow of energy and matter; in the quantitative domain, the cardiac output (often limited by venous return) is inadequate; in the qualitative domain, the strict coherence of subprocesses is lost due to the action of "strange attractor processes". Abnormal hemodynamic, metabolic, proteolytic and oxydative reactions found in circulatory "low flow states" all cooperate in destabilizing the cooperative motion of cell plasma mixtures in the microvascular networks, producing dissociation of perfusion and transcapillary exchange as indeterminate chaotic behavior of the circulatory-, associated with deterministic chaotic behavior of the biochemical processes. "Critical" states of decompensated patients can be classified as "infrasynergetic chaos", different in principle from conventional "chaos reactions" yet intelligible as deviations from synergetic cosmos. The latter can be restored by hemodilution, capable like no other therapeutic regime to conserve and/or restore coherence of mechanical and chemical subsystems.

Didactic Appendix

Semantics and philosophy of "synergetics" and "chaos theory" are so far removed from concepts customary in medicine that the vivid simplicity of a cartoon appears justified, showing the dynamic play of a "wind sleeve" as a "dissipative structure". Its volatile yet stable pattern, reflecting a "boosted steady state", emanates from the "joint efforts" of two phases (air, solids) in processes driven by several energies (gravitational, frictional, elastic). Its stable pattern and orientation lets one understand why the term "dissipative structure" was invented. Moreover, over a wide range of power (kinetic energy of air moving with variable velocities) it properly adapts in a stationary manner. This example of "synergetic order", as well as the fact that it is "framed" by two types of "chaos" is intuitively clear.

If there is very little air flow, there is infrasynergetic (or indeterminate) chaos: the flow of energy is insufficient to "rectify" the sleeve and thus the subsystems cannot cooperate. The motions are erratic, influenced by "strange" attractors processes, i.e. those related to the pressure acting on the *outside* of the sleeve, the folds there, friction in the hinges and at the interface between sleeve ring and pole. The system can neither store nor "amplify" energy. As the wind power reaches a threshold (called "synergetic threshold") dynamic cooperativity of subsystems emanates spontaneously, "catalyzed", as it were, by the appropriate design of the subsystems. The taper of the sleeve is pivotal in ensuring controlled flow of energy:

1. it creates an appropriate outflow impedance and thence allows the system to be "boosted",
2. it "rectifies" the channel by placing the orifice so that it ensures maximum possible uptake of power and
3. when fully straightened out it ensures strictly laminar flow, thence minimizes the frictional energy dissipation, it thence concentrates the energy output and produces the apparent effect of an amplification.

For all these features, strictly passive processes are responsible, all following from principles of minimum energy expenditure, are responsible, jointly producing spontaneous cooperativity, coherence and stability. The reaction to the incident flow of energy is so "reliable", the stability is so robust that such systems can be used to convey information (a typical feature of many, if not all synergetic systems).

As is well known for synergetic systems, there is an upper limit of stability; if the flow of energy (as in an "over-powering" storm) exceeds the capacity of the system, it "explodes" into erratic movements, "wild", unpredictable and jerky movements leading to breakdown of cooperativity, of amplification and of course coherent behavior. Turbulency, intermittency of orientation, elastic vibrations and – as the worst case – mechanical breaks of the sleeve (all classifying as "strange attractors processes") take turns with (often short) periods of order; thence we speak of "deterministic" or "ultrasynergetic" chaos.

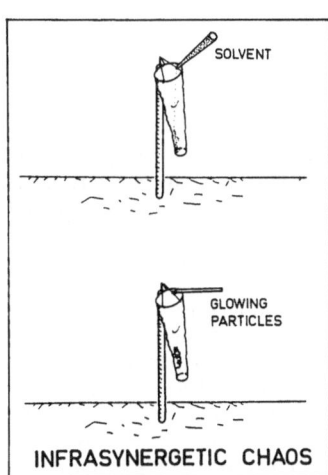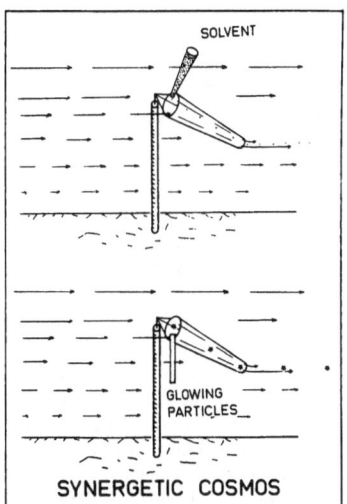

Fig. 6. Schematic representation of the interactions between physical and chemical processes in the wind sleeve as a dynamic system: if in introsynergetic chaos, destructive reactions (dissolution of fabric by "solvent", oxidation by energy rich initiators, "glowing particles") can take place. Subsequent to the action of these processes, the system is less stable. Conversely, if in synergetic order, the reaction rates are suppressed by laminar flow, the reactions are "blown out" rather than "blown on" and the system can survive a temporal "crisis" largely undisturbed

The role of laminar flow in synergetic order, in coherence between mechanical and chemical processes can also be illustrated (Fig. 6): assuming the material of the sleeve to be soluble in an organic solvent, it is plausible that in the synergetic domain neither the addition of the solvent, nor that of glowing particles would have major consequences. Both potential activators (which would induce chemical reaction and or oxydation in the sleeve in its indeterminate state) remain "subliminal". Provided that the synergetic state is associated with strictly laminar flow, the processes of dissolution or of oxydation are "blown out" rather than "blown on" by the wind. Physically this is associated with convective dilution and convective cooling, a process analogous to chemical inhibition. We can extend this little experiment of thought as we assume that in a period of "indeterminate chaos" a chemical reaction would have "damaged" the system (destroyed its "optimal design). Thereafter, the domain of synergetic order would be narrowed down (elevation of the threshold to synergetic, lowering that to chaotic behavior).

The model is closer to the reality of the cardiovascular system than in priori obvious: as a zero'th order approximation, we can take each segment of the vascular tree as a similar "dynamic structure" and the whole vascular network of an ensemble of "powered tubes" put in series and in parallel.

References

1. Haken H (1978) Synergetics. An introduction – nonequilibrium phase transitions and self-organization in physics, chemistry and biology. Springer, Berlin Heidelberg New York
2. Haken H, Haken-Krell M (1989) Entstehung von biologischer Information und Ordnung. Wiss Buchgesellschaft, Darmstadt
3. Prigogine I, Stengers I (1986) Dialog mit der Natur. Neue Wege naturwissenschaftlichen Denkens, 5. Aufl. Piper, München
4. Schuster HG (1981) Deterministic chaos: a strange attractors and chaotic motions of dynamical systems. Rev Mod Phys 53:655–673
5. Schmid-Schönbein H (1990) Synergetics of normal and pathological blood movements in the cardiovascular system. In: Mosora F, Caro C, Baquey CH, Schmid-Schönbein H, Pelissier R, Krause E (eds) Biomechanical transport processes. Plenum Press, New York
6. Schmid-Schönbein H (1990) Blood rheology and oxygen conductance from the alveoli to the mitochondria. In: Fleming JS (ed) Drugs and the delivery of oxygen to tissues. CRC-Press, New York (in press)
7. Arnold VI (1986) Catastrophe theory. Springer, Berlin Heidelberg New York Tokyo
8. Schmid-Schönbein H (1990) Synergetics of fluid-dynamic and biochemical catastrophe reactions in coronary artery thrombosis. In: Bleifeld W, Braunwald WE, Hamm C (eds) Unstable angina. Springer, Berlin Heidelberg New York Tokyo (in press)
9. Schmid-Schönbein H (1990) Biology and rheology of the "acute phase reaction" in chronic degenerative diseases. 5th Eur Conf Clin Hemorheology, Bordeaux 1987 (in press)
10. Göbel W, Perkkiö J, Schmid-Schönbein H (1989) Compaction stasis due to gravitational red cell migration in plastic tubes and mesenteric venules. Virchows Archiv A Pathol Anat 415:243–251
11. Schmid-Schönbein H (1988) Fluid dynamics and hemorheology in vivo: the interactions of hemodynamic parameters and hemorheological "properties" in determining the flow behavior of blood in microvascular networks. In: Lowe GDO (ed) Clinical blood rheology, vol 1. CRC Press, Boca Raton FL, pp 129–219
12. Zwaal RFA, Hemker HC (1986) Blood coagulation. Elsevier, Amsterdam New York Oxford

13. Messmer K, Schmid-Schönbein H (1975) Intentional hemodilution. Karger, Basel
14. Schmid-Schönbein H, Messmer K, Rieger H (1981) Hemodilution and flow improvement. Karger, Basel
15. Schrör K, Sinzinger H, Weidner G, Bräuer H (1984) Prostaglandine and leukotriene bei Endzündung und Schmerz. Albert Roussel Pharma, Wiesbaden
16. Sies H (1985) Oxidative stress. Academic Press, London
17. Krasny R, Köhler J, Kammermeier H (1984) The mechanisms of AV-ring-displacement of the heart. Pflügers Arch 400 (Suppl) Abstr R1
18. Guyton AC (1986) Circulatory shock and physiology of its treatment. Textbook of medical physiology, 7th edn, chapter 8. Saunders, Philadelphia, pp 326–336
19. Goslinga H (1984) Blood viscosity and shock. Springer, Berlin Heidelberg New York Tokyo

Multiple Organ Failure Syndrome: Patterns and Effect of Current Therapy

F. B. Cerra, F. Negro, and S. Eyer

Introduction

The Syndrome of Multiple Organ Failure (MOFS) has been described as the sequential failure of lung, liver and kidney following injury [1–11]. Historically, the MOFS was described as a response pattern following polytrauma [1–7]. Since then, it has been described after a variety of surgical pathologies including: sepsis and septic shock, hypovolemic shock as in ruptured aneurysms, and following persistent inflammation, as in pancreatitis [8–12]. It is also felt to be the most common reason associated with surgical intensive care units (SICU) stays over 5 days and to be the major cause of death in these patients today [12, 13].

Since its description, there has been a tendency in the literature on MOFS to treat it as a single entity, implying a single pathogenesis [1–12]. There have also been a number of advances in the management of the patients believed to be at risk for its development [13]. These advances have occurred in surgical technique, anesthesia technique, and in the advent and development of modern critical care.

In view of these developments, it seems reasonable to ask at least two questions:

1. Is MOFS a single clinical pattern?
2. Has the treatment approach to MOFS altered the outcome of the syndrome?

Determination of the Clinical Patterns of MOFS

Material and Methods

The evaluation was performed over a one year period in the SICU at University Hospitals as part of a protocol approved by the Committee on the Use of Human Subjects in Research at the University of Minnesota. The SICU admits approximately 800 general surgery patients per year for a mean length of stay of 3.8 days. Because the intent of the study was to focus on the subgroup of patients who developed MOFS, and because many of the patients are tertiary referrals who have had their initial surgical and ICU treatment elsewhere, criteria were established for inclusion into the study. The criteria included the following:

1. The presence of a defined event that precipitated the SICU admission at the University Hospital, e.g. septic shock, hemorrhagic shock, or polytrauma.
2. Surgical intervention occurred within 24 hours of the event.
3. The event and the surgery occurred within 24 hours of admission to the SICU at University Hospitals.
4. The patient developed pulmonary failure requiring mechanical ventilation within 5 days of ICU admission.
5. The patient required ICU therapy for more than 5 days.

MOFS was defined in the traditional manner as an event followed by pulmonary failure and liver and/or renal failure that may also have accompanying encephalopathy, coagulopathy, wound failure, and gastrointestinal hemorrhage [4–7]. Renal failure was defined as a progressively rising serum creatinine and/or the initiation of dialysis; liver failure was defined as a progressively rising serum bilirubin together with a progressively falling serum transferrin in the presence of nutritional support, either enteral or parenteral [2, 5, 8, 9].

This methodology provided a pool of 92 patients for analysis. To assess for missed MOFS or mortality prior to the 5 day entrance criteria, a random sample of 50 cases from those not included in the study were analyzed for the presence of MOFS and a mortality outcome. This analysis revealed two mortalities, both from myocardial infarction; and no missed cases of MOFS.

The variables used in the analysis were: ICU mortality, ICU length of stay, age, admission pathology, admission APACHE II score; daily serum bilirubin, creatinine, transferrin, and lactate; daily PaO_2/FiO_2 ratio; and an alkaline phosphatase and SGOT determined every three days.

Data analysis was performed with the techniques of multiple regression and analysis of variance for multiple variables. Significance was tested by two-tail t-test or Z-scores where appropriate. Observed versus expected mortality analysis was done with the Chi-Square method [2]. Significance was defined at the $P < 0.05$ level in all cases.

Results

Ninety-two patients fulfilled the entrance criteria during 1985 and were included in the analysis. The admission pathology is summarized in Table 1. The category of major surgery included pelvic exenteration and GI malignancy with complete extirpation of tumor. The admission sepsis was all abdominal in origin and had a surgically identified source and bacteriology. The bleeding category comprised GI hemorrhage in which cirrhosis and varices were excluded. The transplant patients were primarily renal or pancreas transplants who entered with an infectious complication.

The basic demographic data of survivors and nonsurvivors are presented in Table 2. Patients who expired were older, spent a longer time on a ventilator and a longer time in the SICU. They did not, however, have a longer hospital stay. When time after injury was added as an independent variable, the discriminators of survival were the PaO_2/FiO_2 ratio beginning on Day 1; the serum lactate

Table 1. Admission pathology

Category	Number	MOF
Polytrauma	10	2
Severe sepsis	11	9
Bleeding	23	18
Transplant sepsis	9	7
Cardiac arrest	7	6
Major surgery	30	24
Pancreatitis	2	2
Total	92	68

Table 2. Demographic data and discriminants of survival

Demographic data (mean ± SEM)

	Survived	MOF #1	MOF #2
ICU stay, days	11.0 ± 4.4	21.8 ± 2.3[a]	17.1 ± 1.2[ab]
Hospital stay, days	23.3 ± 2.9	33.2 ± 3.4[a]	27.8 ± 2.0[b]
Ventilator therapy, days	7.5 ± 2.2	19.6 ± 7.8[a]	15.2 ± 1.3[a]
Age, years	49.2 ± 4.4	61.0 ± 4.5[a]	60.3 ± 2.6[a]

[a] $P < 0.05$ to survived
[b] $P < 0.05$ to MOF #1

Discriminators of survival (mean ± SEM)

	ICU day	Survived	Expired
PaO_2/FIO_2	1	311 ± 25	233 ± 14
Lactate (mEq/l)	2	1.1 ± 0.2	3.4 ± 0.7
Bilirubin (mg/dl)	6	2.2 ± 0.6	8.5 ± 2.2
Creatinine (mg/dl)	12	1.9 ± 0.6	3.9 ± 0.3

	MOF #1	MOF #2	MOF #3
Bilirubin (mg/dl)	2.3 ± 1.3 (day 6)	8.2 ± 1.5[a] (day 6)	2.3 ± 1.2[b] (day 12)
Creatinine (mg/dl)	2.2 ± 1.2 (day 10)	4.6 ± 1.7[a] (day 10)	3.4 ± 8.0[a] (day 10)

[a] $P < 0.05$ to MOF #1.
[b] $P < 0.05$ to MOF #1 and 2.

beginning on Day 2; the serum bilirubin beginning on Day 6; and the serum creatinine beginning on Day 12 (Figs. 1–4). The plasma transferrin and serum SGOT and alkaline phosphatase did not discriminate survival from nonsurvival. The transferrin and SGOT progressively fell in all groups throughout the ICU course.

A closer analysis of mortality identified three patterns (Figs. 1–4; Tables 2, 3). The distinctions between these patterns come primarily from the serum bilirubin and creatinine responses, and the type of microbial agent associated with the

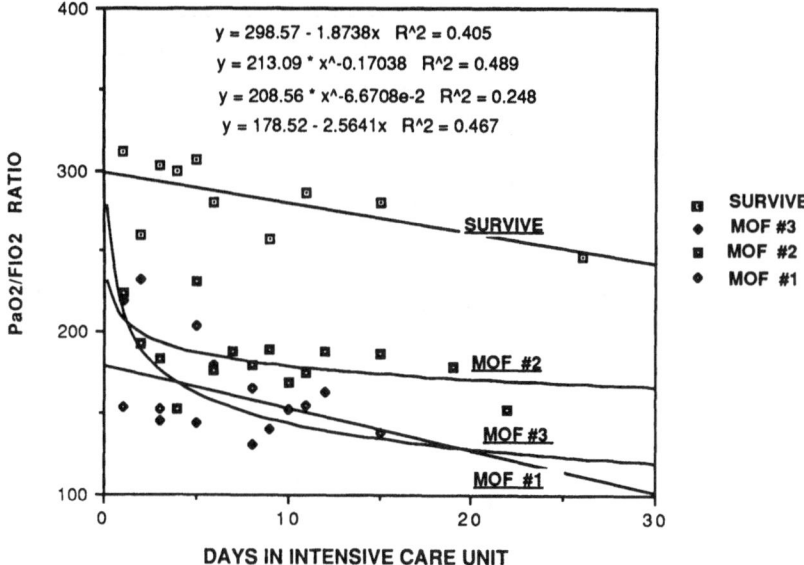

Fig. 1. The PaO$_2$/FiO$_2$ ratio was able to discriminate survivor from nonsurvivor. It was not, however, able to discriminate the nonsurvivor type

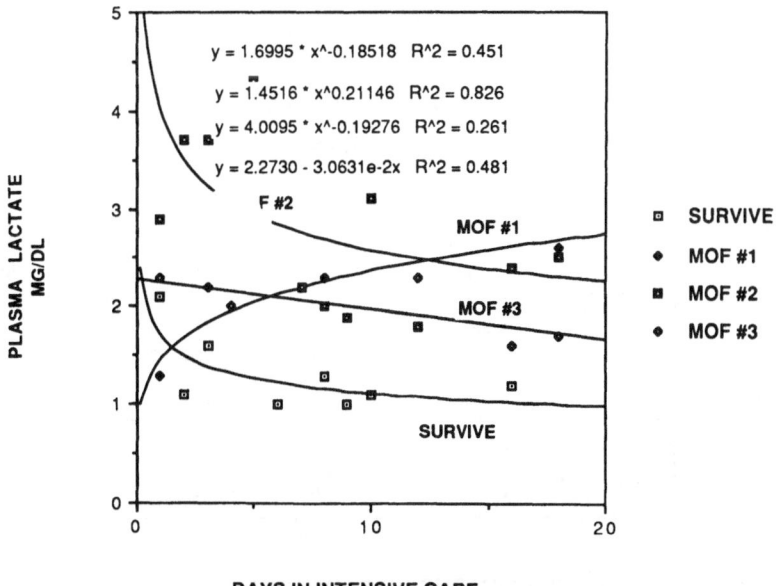

Fig. 2. The plasma lactate was a good discriminator of outcome. It, however, was not able to differentiate the type of death pattern

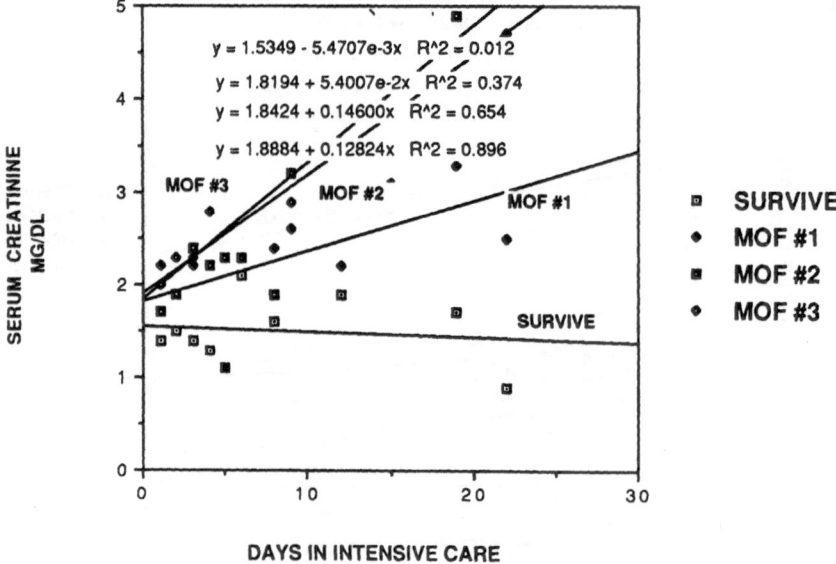

Fig. 3. The time-adjusted serum creatinine was a good discriminator of survival. It was also able to differentiate between the MOF#1 and MOF#2 patterns of response

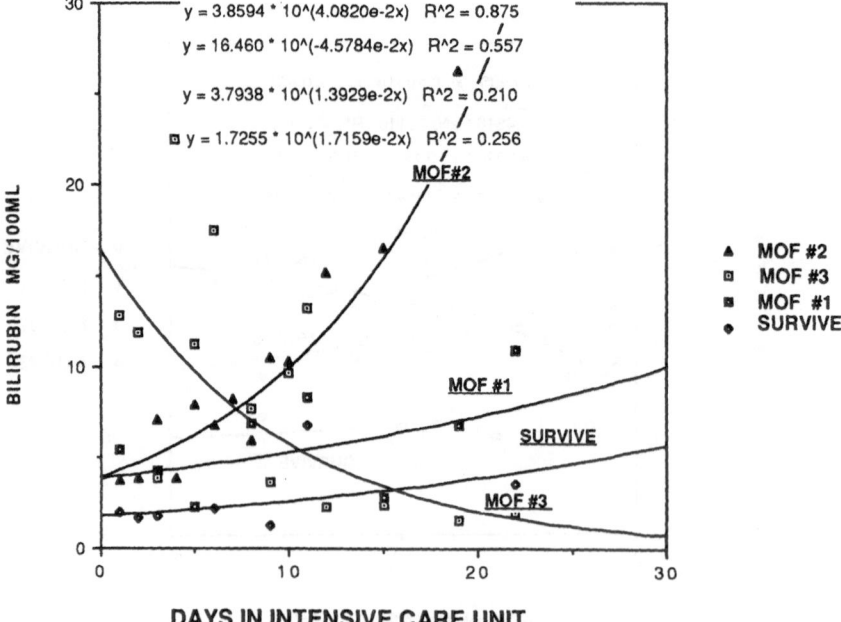

Fig. 4. The time-adjusted serum bilirubin was a good discriminator of survival. It was also the major discriminator between the three patterns of death

Table 3. Relation between MOF and survival

| | Fatalities (N=68) | | | Survivors (N=24) | |
	MOF #1	MOF #2	MOF #3	MOF #2	No MOF
Number of patients	6	46	16	1	23
% of deaths	9	68	23		
% of MOF	12	88			
MOF % die	100	97			
Dialysis	1 (17%)	17 (37%)	3 (19%)		
Recovery of renal function	0	5 (29%)	1 (33%)		

nosocomial infections. In the MOF#3, the serum bilirubin progressively fell to the same level as that of survivors, while the serum creatinine was indistinguishable from the MOF#2 pattern. The MOF#1 pattern was similar to the MOF#2 pattern, but took several days longer to develop and never reached the magnitude of serum bilirubin elevation that was seen in MOF#2. The alkaline phosphatase, SGOT, lactate, and PaO_2/FiO_2 were unable to discriminate between these three death patterns.

The dominant death pattern was MOF#2. However, 23% of deaths was in the MOF#1 pattern. A detailed review of the admission pathology, prior disease status, and therapy did not provide any insight into the origin of these patterns.

Hemodialysis was utilized in a significant percentage of the patients who expired, and in none of those who survived (Table 3). Renal function also returned to the point of requiring no further dialysis in a significant percentage of those patients who subsequently expired. Excluding the dialysis patients from the statistical analysis either before or after recovery of renal function did not change any of the statistical analysis presented.

Table 4 summarizes the septic episodes in each group of patients. No gut decontamination was used in the care of these patients. Systemic antimicrobials were administered according to clinical/laboratory indications in all groups. Sepsis was defined as an observed source with a documented bacteriology in the presence of a hyperdynamic, hypermetabolic state. The patients who expired had an increased number of septic episodes. The number of Gram-septic episodes, however, was not different between survivors and any of the MOF patterns. The number of gram + and fungal infections separated MOF#1 and 2 from Pattern #. Pattern 3 patients were not distinguishable from survivors in the infection patterns.

Evaluation of the Effect of Critical Care on MOFS

Methods

An attempt was made to evaluate the effect of critical care on the occurrence and outcome of MOFS. A more homogeneous patient group was chosen for this

Table 4. Infection episodes acquired after ICU admission

	Total episodes	Gram + episodes	Gram − episodes	Fungus episodes	Virus episodes
Survived	13	3	8	1	1
Died	93	25	30	35	3
Non MOF	7	3	4	0	0
MOF #1					
MOF #2	70	20	22	25	3
	[%]	[%]	[%]	[%]	[%]
Survived		23	62	8	8
Died		27	32	38	3
Non MOF	8	43	57	0	0
MOF #1	17	13	25	63	0
MOF #2	75	29	31	36	4
	Number/ patient	Number/ patient	Number/ patient	Number/ patient	Number/ patient
Survived	0.54	0.13	0.33	0.04	0.04
Died	1.37[a]	0.37[a]	0.44	0.51[a]	0.04
Non MOF	0.43	0.19	0.25	0	0
MOF #1	3.75[a,b]	0.33[a]	0.67	1.67[a,b]	0
MOF #2	1.4[a]	0.40[a]	0.44	0.50[a]	0.06

[a] $P < 0.05$ to survival.
[b] $P < 0.05$ to MOF #2.

evaluation: the polytrauma patients in the SICU at the St Paul Ramsey Hospital. In this unit, a computerized trauma registry has existed since 1975 into which all polytrauma patients are prospectively entered. In 1981, a full-time critical care trained staff-based ICU system with 24 hour physician attendance was implemented.

There were three basic principles in the treatment approach after 1981: source control, resuscitation, and metabolic support. Source control consisted of removal of the cause whenever possible by surgical or medical means and would include such practices as: surgical drainage or removal, early stabilization of fractures and ambulation of the patients, antimicrobial drugs. Resuscitation was done with invasive cardiopulmonary monitoring and adjustment of oxygen content and flow to eliminate flow-dependent oxygen consumption and flow-dependent hyperlactatemia using a combination of volume expansion, systemic resistance unloading and inotropic support. Once resuscitated, monitoring was done to assure that the criteria continue to be met by intermittently reassessing the presence of flow-dependent oxygen consumption and hyperlactatemia and correcting it if it was present. This reassessment occurred on a daily basis until the patient recovered or death ensued. The metabolic support was instituted within 24–48 hours after injury and resuscitation, by either the enteral or parenteral route. The goals were: 30–35 Kcal/kg/day; 1.5–2.0 gm/kg/day of modified amino acids; 3-5 gm/kg/day of glucose; and 0.5 to 1.5 gm/km/day of long chain fatty acid triglyceride depending on clearance capacity. The regimen was adjusted every 5-7 days to maintain nitrogen equilibrium, a BUN of under 110 mg/dl, and an R/Q of under 0.9.

Thus, the design of this evaluation was to compare the mortality before and after the implementation of the management system. The criteria for inclusion into the analysis were:

1. Major polytrauma with acute injury score of 15 or greater;
2. Care initiated and continued at Ramsey;
3. Survival to the initial resuscitation, surgery and the first 48 hours in the SICU;
4. Complete complement of variables used in the analysis.

The primary outcomes were: mortality, MOFS occurrence, and MOFS mortality by both yearly and aggregate comparison. For this analysis, Chi-Square and logistical regression were employed. The other variables analyzed were group comparison variables and included: acute injury score; age; sex; operating surgeon; number, type and pattern of injuries; type of trauma; admission blood pressure; volume replacement and timing of volume replacement; number and types of subsequent surgery; number and types of complications. Chi-Square analysis and logistic regression were used for these comparisons. Significance was set at the $P < 0.05$ level.

Results

For the years 1976-80, there were 432 patients who met analysis criteria, representing 48% of the SICU admissions. For the years 1981-85, there were 409 patients who met analysis criteria, representing 55% of SICU admissions. There were no significant differences between the two groups either by year or in aggregate in any of the above listed group comparison criteria. The gross mortality, however, fell significantly. In the aggregate, it fell from a yearly $19.0 \pm 1.7\%$ for 1976-80 to $11.3 \pm 1.2\%$ in 1981-85 (mean $\pm$ SE). The prevalence of MOFS fell from a yearly mean of 7.2 ± 1.9 for 1976-80 to that of 2.7 ± 1.7 for 1981-85 ($p < 0.05$). There was also a significant reduction in the percentage of patients who developed MOFS and who died: 38.9 ± 3.2 for 1976-80 to $22.8 \pm 3.5\%$ for 1981-85. The MOFS pattern seen was MOF#2. For the remaining deaths, the cause was severe head injury for both periods. Two patients expired from pulmonary emboli in the 1976-80 group; and one patient died from delayed hemorrhage in each of the patient groups.

Discussion

In a heterogeneous patient population of the general surgery SICU, MOFS continues to be the dominant mode of death. Three patterns of MOFS appear to exist primarily differing in the timing of development of renal and hepatic malfunction, at least as reflected in the serum creatinine and bilirubin; and the type of microbial agent associated with the nosocomial infections.

The patients who survived were younger, with less acute lung injury, and without development of renal or hepatic dysfunction. Even though their SICU time was shorter, their overall hospital time was not. This seems to be indicative of the need for rehabilitation services and may reflect the effects of hypermetabolism on the skeletal-muscle mass [15, 16]. Also consistent with this observation is the failure of plasma transferrin levels to discriminate survival. Rather, the levels persistently fell irrespective of the ultimate outcome. Perhaps this observation reflects the presence of a persistent hypermetabolic state [12, 15, 16].

The etiology and pathogenesis of the MOFS remain largely a matter of hypothesis [8]. Three different clinical patterns, however, would be more consistent with several possible mechanisms rather than a single process. Inadequate microcirculatory resuscitation is evolving as a major factor, as is white cell mediated endothelial injury during reperfusion. The hepatic failure phase of the disease is hypothesized to reflect abnormal regulation by the activated Kupffer cell. Likewise, malnutrition is a recognized comorbidity and comortality factor that can be minimized with current nutrition support.

A management system of interested and trained personnel, aggressive source control and metabolic and nutritional support was associated with a reduction in the incidence and mortality risk of MOFS in a setting of young trauma patients who did not have much underlying chronic disease. These latter factors probably account for the difference in outcome of MOFS between the Ramsey and the University Hospitals SICU. Because of the study design, it is not possible to make a determination as to what component of the management system was most responsible for the outcome observed.

Septic episodes remain characteristic of MOFS, particularly Gram + and fungal origins. Gram − etiologies occurred at the same rate in both MOFS and in survivors. In view of the current hypothesis of the gut origin of hypermetabolism and MOFS [17], it might be questioned as to whether this gut failure is a symptom or a cause of the disease process. Either enteral or parenteral nutrition was used in these studies. Recent data indicates that after the first few days, there is no route effect of the nutritional support on outcome from hypermetabolism and MOFS [18]. Recent data on gut decontamination is also suggesting that the nosocomial infection rate can be reduced from enteric organisms, but that the incidence and outcome of MOFS may not be significantly changed [19].

Even though significant advances have been made in the SICU care of patients post-injury, MOFS remains a major cause of morbidity and mortality. Continued research is necessary to better understand the process and to devise better regimens for prevention and management. It is likely that these three patterns of MOFS reflect differing pathogenetic mechanisms. With continued research, better and more specific treatment modalities may result. As an example, white cell antiadherence antibodies administered prior to and during resuscitation to prevent endothelial injury; n-3 polyunsaturated fatty acids administered later in the process to control the activated macrophage.

References

1. McMenany RC, Birkhahn R, Oswald G, et al (1981) Multiple systems organ failure I: The basal state. J Trauma 21:99–114
2. McMenany RC, Birkhahn R, Oswald G, et al (1981) Multiple system organ failure II: The effect of amino acids and glucose. J Trauma 21:228–237
3. Moyer ED, Border JR, Cerra FB, et al (1981) Multiple systems organ failure III: Contrasts in plasma amino acid profiles in trauma-septic patients who subsequently survive and do not survive: Effects of intravenous amino acids. J Trauma 21:263–274
4. Moyer ED, Border JR, Cerra FB, et al (1981) Multiple systems organ failure IV: Imbalances in plasma amino acids associated with exogenous albumin in the trauma-septic patient. J Trauma 21:543–547
5. Moyer ED, Border JR, Cerra FB, et al (1981) Multiple systems organ failure V: Alterations in the plasma proteins as a function of amino acid infusion in the trauma septic patient: Contrasts between survival and death. J Trauma 21:645–649
6. Moyer ED, Border JR, Cerra FB, et al (1981) Multiple systems organ failure VI: Death predictors in the trauma septic state: The most critical determinants. J Trauma 21:862–869
7. Moyer ED, Border JR, Peters D, et al (1981) Multiple systems organ failure VII: Reduction in plasma branched chain amino acids: Correlations with liver failure and amino acid infusion. J Trauma 21:965–970
8. Cerra FB (1987) The multiple organ failure syndrome. In: Gallagher TJ, Shoemaker WC (eds) Critical care: State of the art. Society of Critical Care Medicine, Fullerton, CA, pp 107–128
9. Baue AE (1975) Multiple, progressive or sequential systems failure: A syndrome of the 1970's. Arch Surg 110:779–781
10. Tilney N, Bailey G, Morgan A (1973) Sequential system failure after rupture of abdominal aortic aneurysms. Ann Surg 118:117
11. Pine RW, Wertz MJ, Lennard ES, et al (1983) Determinants of organ malfunction or death in patients with intra-abdominal sepsis. Arch Surg 118:242
12. Cerra FB (1987) Hypermetabolism, organ failure, and metabolic support. Surgery 191:1
13. Madoff RD, Sharpe SM, Fath JJ, et al (1985) Prolonged surgical intensive care. Arch Surg 120:698–702
14. Shoemaker W (1985) Hemodynamic and oxygen transport patterns in septic shock: Physiologic mechanisms and therapeutic implications. In: Sibbald W, Sprung C (eds) Perspectives in sepsis and septic shock. Society of Critial Medicine, Fullerton, CA, pp 203–234
15. Cerra FB, Siegel JH, Wiles JB, et al (1980) Septic autocannibalism: Failure to use exogenous nutritional support. Ann Surg 192:570–581
16. Cerra FB, Siegel JH, Border J, et al (1979) The hepatic failure of sepsis: Cellular versus substrate. Surgery 86:409–422
17. Border J, Hassett J, LaDuca J, et al (1987) The gut origin septic states in blunt multiple trauma (ISS = 40) in the ICU. Ann Surg 206:427–449
18. Cerra FB, McPherson JP, Konstantinides FN, et al (1988) Enteral feeding does not prevent multiple organ failure syndrome (MOFS) after sepsis. Surgery 104:727–733
19. Kever AJH, Rommes JH, Meuessen-Verhage EAE, et al (1988) Prevention of colonization and infection in critically ill patients: A prospective, randomized study. Crit Care Med 16:1087–1094

Selective Gut Decontamination in Ventilated Patients

K. E. Unertl, F.-P. Lenhart, and G. Ruckdeschel

Introduction

Infection has remained a significant cause of morbidity and mortality in critically ill patients despite the discovery of potent antimicrobials and sophisticated
supportive treatment measures. Infections in general ICU occur at rates of 15–20
per 100 patient admissions, thereby exceeding the average rates in general wards
by approximately 3–4 fold [1, 2]. Intubated patients are a subset of patients who
exhibit an extraordinary high risk of developing respiratory infections [3]. Rates
of pneumonia in intubated patients receiving mechanical ventilation are increased about 10 fold compared to patients with no respiratory device so that the
majority of the pneumonias in the ICU occur in patients who are receiving or
have had ventilatory support [3, 4]. Patients with nosocomial infections show
prolonged hospitalization and increased risk of death as compared to their
matched controls [5, 6]. Bacteremias and pneumonias are not only the predominant infections in ICU patients, but are also associated with the highest mortality rate [7]. Crude mortality rates for pneumonias have been reported to be in the
range of 30 to 50% [3, 7]. However the mortality attributable to infection is difficult to assess and varies considerably between various groups. Patients with advanced underlying diseases or multiorgan failure run a very high risk of developing life-threatening infection and are also very likely to die in consequence of
infection. Nevertheless, infection may contribute little to the overall mortality in
these patients since their risk of dying is very high anyway. On the other hand,
patients who do not suffer from serious underlying disease can be expected to
have a relatively low infection risk and also a low mortality rate, but severe infection in these patients may largely influence the outcome [7].

Since therapy of already established infection is still unsatisfactory, methods
of preventing are of great value. For several reasons, the prevention of nosocomial infection in critically ill patients is difficult. Clearly, it is impossible to dis-
pense with life-saving supportive techniques, such as endotracheal tubes, ventilatory assistance, arterial and venous catheters, parenteral nutrition etc. although
these measures in turn increase the risk of infection. In the past, most attempts
have been directed to preventing cross-contamination by hygienic precautions,
e.g. proper hand-washing, decontamination of respiratory therapy equipment,
proper care of intravascular devices etc. [8]. These measures help to control infections by exogenous organisms. However the effect of these measures on the
endemic infection rate is minimal, since endemic infections are frequently

caused by pathogens that derive from the patient's own microflora, which is difficult to control.

Epidemiology of Hospital-Acquired Infections in Ventilated Patients

Most infections in ventilated patients are caused by bacteria, the predominant microorganisms being *enterobacteriaceae, pseudomonadaceae* and *Staphylococcus spp.* Gram-negative bacilli continue to be the most frequent pathogens of respiratory tract infections and urinary tract infections, whereas Staphylococci predominate in infections related to intravascular devices [2]. Many of the infecting pathogens derive from the microbial flora that colonizes the patient's skin and the mucosal surfaces of the alimentary canal.

Healthy individuals live in peaceful co-existence with their oropharyngeal and gastrointestinal microflora. Colonization with potentially pathogenic microorganisms is controlled by numerous factors under physiological conditions. These factors are subsumed under the heading "colonization resistance". They comprise in particular the specific and nonspecific mucosal receptors for bacteria, secretory IgA, gastric juice acidity, intestinal peristalsis, gut-associated lymphoid tissue (GALT), and microbial interference. Owing to the natural resistance to colonization, the stomach and large sections of the small intestine are almost sterile under physiological conditions. The occurrence of Staphylococci is restricted mainly to the naso-oropharynx, whereas gram-negative bacteria are restricted to the colon and the terminal ileum. Apart from *E. coli,* nosocomial gram-negative organisms are only to be detected irregularly and usually in small numbers in the intestinal tract of healthy adults. In contrast, in severely ill patients the alimentary canal is increasingly colonized by nosocomial (mainly gram-negative) pathogens [9]. Critically ill patients have been termed "bacteriologic chameleons" since they easily assume the flora of their medical surroundings owing to their depressed colonization resistance [10].

Bacteria from the intestinal tract can be easily transmitted to other regions of the body. Bacteria may ascend to the stomach and migrate further to the oropharynx and tracheobronchial tree [3]. Fecal bacteria may also be translocated by contact of the hands of the patient or personal to other body sites, including urinary tract, wounds and upper respiratory tract. Correlation between newly colonizing gram-negative bacteria in the oropharynx with those predominating in the intestinal flora has been demonstrated [11]. Also changes in the intestinal flora during hospitalization resulted in changes of the oropharyngeal flora.

The oropharynx develops into an important reservoir of gram-negative bacteria in critically ill patients [12]. Colonization is to be detected in more than 50% of patients within a few days after the beginning of artificial ventilation. Bacterial counts of 10^5/ml are regularly reached or exceeded [13]. A main reason for the colonization of the oropharyngeal mucosa with gram-negative bacteria is their increased adherence to buccal epithelial cells. Studies of bacterial adherence to buccal epithelial cells have shown that binding of gram-negative bacilli is inversely related to the amount of membrane-bound fibronectin, which is markedly reduced in patients with severe disease [4, 14]. Since most respiratory pathogens reach the lung by aspiration of oropharyngeal secretions, oropharyngeal colonization plays a key role in the pathogenesis of gram-negative pneumonia [14].

Gastric overgrowth with gram-negative bacteria may contribute to oropharyngeal and tracheobronchial colonization in ventilated patients and promote respiratory infection [3]. Alterations in the normal acidity of gastric juice are an important prerequisite for proliferation of bacterial microorganisms in gastric juice. High gastric pHs in critically ill patients frequently result from alkalizing stress ulcer prophylaxis, but also from tube feeding [3].

At present, it is impossible to restore the normal colonization defence system in patients with serious illness. The suppression of the potentially pathogenic bacterial flora in the gut and the prevention of acquisition of nosocomial pathogens by use of topical non-absorbable antibiotics hence constitute a promising strategy for prophylaxis of infection.

Selective Decontamination (SDD)

Topical non-absorbable antibiotics have been used for the prevention of colonization and infection in critically ill patients for more than 15 years [15]. In the early 1970s, aerolized polymyxin B, administered into the pharynx and the tracheal tube, was used in patients of a respiratory surgical ICU in an attempt to prevent gram-negative bacillary colonization and infection. Polymyxin B was chosen because it is bactericidal against important gram-negative respiratory pathogens, especially *P. aeruginosa, E. coli* and *Klebsiella spp.* The use of polymyxin B resulted in a significant reduction of colonization and pneumonia rates by *P. aeruginosa*, but the overall rate of pneumonia was not significantly reduced, and infections by organisms intrinsically resistant to polymyxin B remained a significant clinical problem. These results showed that the polymyxins are less than ideal agents due to the limited spectrum of activity and additional agents are needed for broader antimicrobial coverage.

Gentamicin was administered intratracheally in tracheostomized neurosurgical patients by a Belgian study group at the beginning of the 1970s. The observed rates of tracheobronchial colonization and infection decreased, but again undesired changes of the tracheal flora and an increase in the MIC of gram-negative bacilli against gentamicin was seen. Interestingly, the combination of an aminoglycoside with polymyxin B prevented the rise of the MIC to gentamicin, but this strategy was not followed up [16].

Clinical trials in recent years have used non-absorbable antibiotics in a different way for the control of colonization and infection. Depending on the technique which is generally used in granulocytopenic patients, topical antimicrobials were not given to the potential site of infection (e.g. the lower airways) but to the alimentary canal as a principle source of bacterial pathogens. The aim of this strategy is to prevent the first step of many infections in critically ill patients, namely the abnormal colonization of the digestive tract as a result of acquisition and overgrowth with nosocomial pathogens. Combinations of antibiotics are usually given in order to cover the wide spectrum of nosocomial pathogens and in an attempt to decrease the likelihood of antibiotic resistance. A brief initial systemic antibiotic prophylaxis was recommended by some in order to prevent early or incubating infections by pathogens which are already present when the patient is admitted to the ICU.

Clinical Studies

The results of clinical studies that have been published up to now are shown in Fig. 1. All studies show that the microbial flora of the oropharynx and of the gastrointestinal tract is profoundly altered by SDD. As compared to untreated controls, colonization with gram-negative bacteria is substantially reduced within a few days. In general, within three to five days no more than 10% of the treated patients display oropharyngeal colonization with gram-negative bacteria. However, seven to 14 days are required for decolonization of the colon and rectum. SDD is also very effective in preventing acquisition and subsequent colonization with nosocomial gram-negative pathogens. As expected, colonization with intrinsically resistant bacteria (mainly gram-negative cocci and anaerobes) is not affected.

The decreased colonization with potentially pathogenic bacteria resulted in a significant reduction of the overall infection rate in all studies but one. This re-

Reference (No)	Year	Study design	Mode of Application	Drugs and dosage	No. of patients	Primary C	Primary P	Respiratory C	Respiratory P	Sepsis C	Sepsis P	Urinary tract C	Urinary tract P	Wound C	Wound P	Catheter C	Catheter P	Mortality C	Mortality P
Stoutenbeek, C.P. [17]	1984	Prospective with historical control	Topical and systemic	Paste: Polymixin E 2%, Tobramycin 2%, Amphotericin B 2% Oral cavity 4 x daily. Liquid: Polymixin E 100mg, Tobramycin 80mg, Amphotericin 500mg Stomach 4 x daily. Cefotaxim 50mg/kg i.v. 4 x daily	122	0	0	35 p (59)	5 p* (8)	ND		19 p (32)	1 p* (2)	15 p (25)	3 p* (5)	ND		ND.	
Unertl, K. [18]	1987	Prospective randomized	Topical	Liquid: Polymyxin B 50mg, Gentamicin 80mg, Amphotericin B500mg Naso-oro-pharynx stomach 4 x daily	39	0	0	9 p (45)	1 p* (5)	ND		ND		ND		ND		(32)	(28)
Kerver, A.J.H. [19]	1988	Prospective randomized	Topical and systemic	Same procedure as (17)	96	24 (51)	31 (69)	40 i	6 i*	ND		6 i	3 i	7 i	1 i	31 i	22 i	ND	
Ledingham, I McA. [20]	1988	Prospective consecutive	Topical and systemic	Same procedure as (17)	324	114 (71)	131 (80)	18 i	3 i	11 i	8 i	3 i	1 i	2 i	0	ND		(24)	(24)
Konrad, F. [21]	1989	Prospective consecutive	Topical and systemic	Same procedure as (17)	165	16		22 i (42)	5 i* (6)	ND		ND		ND		ND		No significant difference	
Ulrich, C. [22]	1989	Prospective randomized	Topical and systemic	Liquid: Polymixin E 100mg, Norfloxacin 50mg, Amphotericin B 100mg, Trimethoprim 500mg i.v. daily 4 x daily Stomach. Ointment: Polymyxin E 2%, Norfloxacin 2%, Amphotericin B 2% Oral cavity 4 x daily	100	18 p (34,6) 20I	25 p (52) 36I	29 i	7 i	18 i	11 i	26 i	11 i	6 i	4 i	23 i	18 i	28 p (54)	15 p (31)
Brun-Buisson, C. [23]	1989	Prospective incidence	Topical	Liquid: Polymixin E 100mg, Neomycin 1g, Nalidixic acid 1g Stomach 4 x daily Oro-pharynx	122	(28)		26 i (21)		ND		10 i (8)		7 i (5,5)		7 i (5,5)		ND	
[23]	1989	Prospective randomized		Liquid: Povidone Iodine solution Oro-pharynx 3 x daily	85	(33)	(32)	11 i (22)	7 i (19,5)	ND		10 i (20)	2 i (5,5)	3 i (6)	0	1 i (2)	1 i (3)	ND	

Fig. 1. Clinical studies of selective decontamination in relation to infections in critically ill patients. C = Control group; P = prophylaxis group; ND = no data; * = significant difference

duction was above all the result of a 70–90% decline of respiratory infections (Fig. 1). The number of infections in other body sites such as urinary tract, wound, bloodstream/sepsis decreased in most SDD studies. However, the difference from untreated patients was frequently not statistically significant because of the already low incidence of these infections. Whereas there was an appreciable decline in the rate of gram-negative infections, SDD had hardly any effect on infections caused by gram-positive organisms [19, 22]. This lack of efficacy may be explained by the inadequate antimicrobial activity of the antimicrobials commonly used in SDD regimens or the fact that many of the gram-positive pathogens do not derive from the alimentary canal, or both. Recently it has been shown that SDD can also be used successfully for eradication of multiresistant gram-negative strains in the ICU [23]. In this study, in which the antibiotics were exclusively administered gastrointestinally, no reduction of the overall rate of infection could be demonstrated. However, this result does not necessarily contradict other SDD studies. The fall of the overall infection rate under SDD is mainly a result of the decline of gram-negative pneumonias. Since nasopharyngeal decontamination is essential for the prevention of gram-negative pneumonia, the unchanged overall infection rate is possibly explained by the inadequate effect of intestinal decontamination on oropharyngeal colonization. The question as to the relevance of intestinal decolonization in prophylaxis of infections in critically ill patients is then of correspondingly greater importance.

Despite the impressive reduction in the rates of infection in most SDD studies, a significant decrease in the overall mortality as a result of a reduction of fatal nosocomial infections could be attained so far only in a single study [22]. In a further study, a significant reduction of the mortality for the subgroup of trauma patients could be substantiated [20].

Open Questions and Controversies

Despite the increasing number of publications on SDD, several important questions remain still to be answered. These concern for example the selection of patients, the relative significance of systemic antibiotic prophylaxis, the clinical relevance of oropharyngeal as compared to intestinal decontamination, and also the time period of antibiotic prophylaxis. The effect of SDD on mortality and the epidemiological consequences of the selective pressures of SDD are of paramount importance and are thus also crucial for the future clinical role of this regimen.

The Effect of SDD on the Infection-Related Excess Mortality

The effect of SDD on the infection-related mortality is influenced by three factors:

1. the risk of infection of the patients;

2. the extent of reduction in the infection rate by SDD; and
3. the clinical relevance of these infections with regard to the outcome.

In the past, unrealistic assumptions led to exaggerated expectations with regard to the benefit from SDD. In patients who die with an infection a distinction must be made between infection-independent mortality, infection-related mortality and infection-related excess mortality. Pneumonia has the highest mortality associated with nosocomial infections. However, according to more recent estimates, it is to be inferred that two thirds of the deaths associated with pneumonia would also have occurred without infection, so that only up to one third of the deaths can be considered as potentially preventable [4, 7]. If one assumes an average rate of pneumonia in ventilated patients of 20%, an overall mortality of patients with pneumonia of 30%, and a 80% reduction of the incidence of pneumonia by SDD, a sample comprising as many as 500 patients for each branch would be required to demonstrate a difference in mortality with a p < 0,05. This number of cases was not even approximately reached in any of the clinical studies published up to now. All the more it is remarkable that there are obvious indications even now with regard to an improved survival in selected patients. In trauma patients, a significant reduction in mortality has been documented [20]. In patients with a longer stay on the intensive care ward and in patients with mid-range APACHE II score, an improvement of the outcome can also be reckoned with [20].

Selection of Resistant Organisms

The possibility of the emergence of a multiresistant bacterial flora requires careful attention, especially since earlier antibiotic prophylaxis regimens have frequently shown an increase in the number of infections by resistant organisms [15]. However there was also the observation of no rise in resistance despite routine administration of topical antimicrobials for several years [24]. The experiences obtained with SDD in ICU patients also show no increased occurrence of resistant gram-negative organisms. As shown recently, a SDD regimen may even be very useful for eradication of endemic multiresistant *enterobacteriaceae* in the ICU [23].

So far, only in a single study patients were surveyed over a longer time period (30 months) for the emergence of antibiotic resistance [25]. An increase in the rate of resistant organisms to the SDD antimicrobials was not observed. All other studies published on SDD arrive at the same result with regard to the gram-negative pathogens, even it must be conceded that their relevance with regard to the emergence of resistance is restricted because of the relatively short period of observation. In our unit, an increase in the number of resistant pathogens was not seen up to now, despite the continuous use of our SDD regimen in ventilated patients since 1986.

However, it is to be borne in mind that SDD does not affect colonization and related infections by microorganisms intrinsically resistant to the antibiotic regimens (e.g. gram-positive cocci). Colonization by resistant organisms like *coagu-*

lase-negative Staphylococci and *Enterococci* is a relatively frequent finding in patients receiving SDD [13, 21]. It remains to be seen whether the long-term use of SDD will result in an increase of infections with intrinsically resistant gram-positive bacteria. The studies carried out so far on SDD show a preponderance of gram-positive infections, but this is a result of the decline in gram-negative infections [19, 22].

Irrespectively of the application of SDD, infections with gram-positive bacteria appear to increase in severely ill patients. In view of this, special attention must be paid to the selection of intrinsically resistant gram-positive bacteria by this regimen.

Conclusions

Selective decontamination of the pharynx and the gastrointestinal tract with nonabsorbable antibiotics is an interventional strategy which reliably suppresses colonization with gram-negative pathogens in critically ill patients. Consequently, nosocomial infections, in particular gram-negative pneumonias are reduced by SDD. In addition, intestinal decontamination is an effective method to prevent the acquisition of nosocomial multiresistant gram-negative pathogens. Numerous questions, especially the cost/benefit ratio and the effects of long-term application of SDD on the epidemiology of nosocomial infections, require further clarification. Since it can be expected that only selected groups of critically ill patients will benefit from SDD, the general use of this regimen in all seriously ill patients cannot be recommended. Amongst artificially ventilated patients, benefit in terms of a reduced mortality rate has so far been established for trauma patients. Other patients who possibly profit from this strategy are patients with longer unit stay, mid-range APACHE II score, elderly surgical patients as well as patients with ARDS. Controversy surrounds the concept of translocation of intestinal bacteria and of endotoxin as potential mediators of multiorgan failure in critically ill patients and its prevention by SDD. Further studies with an appropriate number of patients and with clearly defined endpoints are required to clarify this and other open questions.

References

1. Chandrasekar PH, Kruse JA, Mathews MF (1986) Nosocomial infection among patients in different types of intensive care units at a city hospital. Crit Care Med 14:508–510
2. Donowitz LG, Wenzel RP, Hoyt JW (1982) High risk of hospital-acquired infection in the ICU patient. Crit Care Med 10:355–357
3. Craven DE, Daschner FD (1989) Nosocomial pneumonia in the intubated patient: role of gastric colonization. Eur J Clin Microbiol Infect Dis 8:40–50
4. Wenzel RP (1989) Hospital-acquired pneumonia: overview of the current state of the art for prevention and control. Eur J Clin Microbiol Infect Dis 8:56–60
5. Freeman J, Rosner BA, McGowan JE Jr (1979) Adverse effects of nosocomial infection. J Infect Dis 140:732–740
6. Craig ChP, Connelly S (1984) Effect of intensive care unit nosocomial pneumonia on duration of stay and mortality. Am J Infect Control 12:233–238

7. Gross PA (1987) Epidemiology of hospital-acquired pneumonia. Semin Respir Infect 2:2–7
8. Weinstein RA, Kabins SA (1981) Strategies for prevention and control of multiple drug-resistant nosocomial infections. Am J Med 70:449–454
9. Le Frock JL, Ellis CA, Weinstein L (1979) The impact of hospitalization on the aerobic fecal microflora. Am J Med Sci 277:269–274
10. Weinstein RA (1989) Selective intestinal decontamination – an infection control measure whose time has come? (editorial) Ann Intern Med 110:853–855
11. Le Frock JL, Ellis CA, Weinstein LA (1979) The relation between aerobic fecal and oropharyngeal microflora in hospitalized patients. Am J Med Sci 277:275–280
12. Johanson WG Jr, Pierce AK, Sanford JP, Thomas GD (1972) Nosocomial respiratory infections with gram-negative bacilli. Ann Intern Med 77:701–706
13. Unertl K, Ruckdeschel G (1987) Maintenance of normal oropharyngeal flora does not prevent colonization and lung infection by gram-negative bacteria in critically ill patients. 27th Interscience Conference on Antibacterial Agents and Chemotherapy, New York (NY) (abstr. no. 1129)
14. Johanson WG Jr (1984) Prevention of respiratory tract infection. Am J Med 69–77
15. Altman FM Jr (1987) Prophylactic strategies for hospitalized patients at risk for pneumonia. Semin Respir Infect 2:74–81
16. Klastersky J, Hensgens C, Noterman J, Monawad E, Meunier-Carpentier F (1975) Endotracheal antibiotics for the prevention of tracheobronchial infections in tracheotomized unconscious patients. A comparative study of gentamicin and aminosidin-polymyxin B combination. Chest 68:302–306
17. Stoutenbeek CP, van Saene HKF, Miranda DR, Zandstra DF (1984) The effect of selective decontamination of the digestive tract on colonisation and infection rate in multiple trauma patients. Intensive Care Med 10:185–192
18. Unertl K, Ruckdeschel G, Selbmann HK, et al (1987) Prevention of colonization and respiratory infections in long-term ventilated patients by local antimicrobial prophylaxis. Intensive Care Med 13:106–113
19. Kerver AJH, Rommes JH, Mevissen-Verhage EAE, et al (1988) Prevention of colonization and infection in critically ill patients: A prospective randomized study. Crit Care Med 16:1087–1093
20. Ledingham IMcA, Alcock AR, Eastaway AT, McDonald JC, McKay IC, Ramsay G (1988) Triple regimen of selective decontamination of the digestive tract, systemic cefotaxime, and microbiological surveillance for prevention of acquired infection in intensive care. Lancet 1:785–790
21. Konrad F, Schwalbe B, Heeg K, et al (1989) Kolonisations-, Pneumoniefrequenz und Resistenzentwicklung bei langzeitbeatmeten Intensivpatienten unter selektiver Dekontamination des Verdauungstraktes. Anaesthesist 38:99–109
22. Ulrich C, Harinck-de Weerd JE, Bakker NC, Jacz K, Doornbos L, de Ridder VA (1989) Selective decontamination of the digestive tract with norfloxacin in the prevention of ICU-acquired infections: a prospective randomized study. Intensive Care Med 15:424–431
23. Brun-Buisson Ch, Legrand P, Rauss A, et al (1989) Intestinal decontamination for control of nosocomial multiresistant gram-negative bacilli. Ann Intern Med 110:873–881
24. Vogel F, Weiner H, Exner M, et al (1981) Prophylaxe und Therapie von Atemwegsinfektionen bei beatmeten Patienten durch intratracheale Antibiotikagabe. Dtsch Med Wochenschr 106:898–903
25. Stoutenbeek CP, van Saene HKF, Zandstra DF (1987) The effect of oral nonabsorbable antibiotics on the emergence of resistant bacteria in patients in an intensive care unit. J Antimicrob Chemother 19:513–520

Adult Respiratory Distress Syndrome (ARDS): A Systemic Disease?

M. Lamy, G. Deby-Dupont, and M. E. Faymonville

Introduction

In 1967, Asbaugh et al. [1] published the first description of an acute pulmonary failure syndrome occurring in 12 patients, associated with a high mortality rate (above 50%), and characterized by dyspnea, tachypnea, cyanosis refractory to oxygen therapy, loss of lung compliance, and diffuse alveolar infiltration visible on X-ray films. This acute lung failure was named adult respiratory distress syndrome (ARDS) a few years later [2]. Since its first description, this syndrome has given rise to much debate about its frequency, its origins, its mortality rate and its treatment, dispute arising essentially because of the lack of an appropriate definition of the syndrome [3–10].

Murray et al. [11] recently proposed to define ARDS as the most severe form of injury to the lung parenchyma, which would be distinguished from mild and moderate forms of lung injury and quantified by an injury score taking into account the chest X-ray data, the degree of hypoxemia, the PEEP value and the lung compliance. They proposed to reserve the name ARDS for the lung failure characterized by an injury score above 2.5, patients with an injury score <2.5 being considered "at risk" for ARDS, suffering from mild to moderate forms of the disease. This extended definition of ARDS also takes into consideration the multiplicity of causes (known or unknown) which are at the origin of the syndrome, and its evolution (from an acute to a chronic phase).

With this extended definition, ARDS can no longer be considered as a lung disease per se, but as a systemic disease occurring in patients after a direct lung injury (pulmonary contusion, pneumonia, pulmonary aspiration, exposure to high partial pressures of oxygen) or an extrathoracic injury (pancreatitis, near-drowning, disseminated intravascular coagulation, multiple long bone fractures, massive trauma, hypertransfusion and sepsis).

ARDS can now be considered:

1. As the first manifestation of a general inflammatory reaction essentially characterized by an accumulation of neutrophils in lung and many other organs, and by the release of a host of mediators.
2. As the local expression of a general permeability defect linked to endothelial damage with extravasation of edema fluid and inflammatory cells.
3. As the most rapidly recognized manifestation of multiple organ system failure (MOSF).

Together with data from the literature, an 8-year study of mediator release in patients with or at risk for ARDS provides us with valuable arguments to sustain this viewpoint.

ARDS: First Manifestation of a General Inflammatory Reaction

Even when ARDS occurs after *direct lung injury,* it can easily become a systemic disease. The local injury triggers alveolar macrophages or damages the components of pulmonary capillary alveolar wall (connective tissue, surfactant, epithelium, endothelium) (Fig. 1). When activated, macrophages undergo a respiratory burst and release oxygen metabolites, numerous mediators (cytokines, prostanoids, leukotrienes, platelet-activating factor (PAF), chemotactic peptides ...) and enzymes which provoke further tissue destruction and the extension of the inflammatory reaction (by attraction and activation of neutrophils, by activation of platelets) with propagation into other body sites distant from the lung [10, 12, 13].

When endothelial cells are damaged, they become activated with a phagocytic function like macrophages, they initiate the complement cascade (by binding of immune complexes) and also produce many mediators, particularly a chemoattractant factor for neutrophils [14], an inhibitor of plasminogen activator and a tissular procoagulant factor, so that endothelial cells are converted into participants in a procoagulant state. The damaged endothelium increases its interaction with neutrophils and enhances their migration through the vascular wall into the

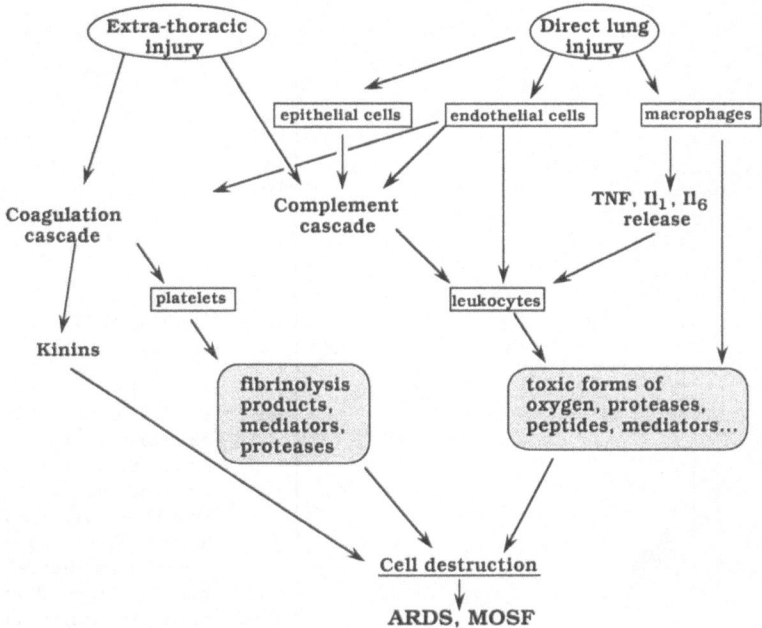

Fig. 1. Role of cells and mediators in the development of ARDS and MOSF

interstitial space [15]. Endothelial cells and macrophages are thus victims and participants in pulmonary injury and serve to extend the inflammatory reaction.

However, this extension can be limited in time and in severity; indeed, many patients quickly show improvement in pulmonary function without clinical signs of extrathoracic inflammation. Figure 2 shows the evolution of the blood concentration of myeloperoxidase (MPO) and trypsin in a patient who developed ARDS 12 hours after lung contusion. MPO, a marker of leukocyte activation [16], is above the normal value (332 ± 96 ng/ml) 12 hours after trauma, but its increase is of short duration with a return to normal after 24 hours. Elastase, another marker of leukocyte activation, shows the same time course with only an early moderate elevation of its blood concentration in the first hours after trauma. No sign of early pancreatic failure (a sign of hypoperfusion) is observable: trypsin (as well as amylase and lipase) is always normal. This patient improved after two days without infection.

When ARDS occurs after *extrathoracic injury,* the development of acute lung failure can be explained by the presence in the blood of a host of mediators (prostanoids, leukotrienes, PAF, vasoactive amines, proteases, active peptides, ...) which are all filtered by the lungs, and by the trapping of platelets, microaggregates and polymorphonuclear leukocytes (PMNL) in pulmonary capillary vasculature [17–21]. The activation of the complement cascade is a common phenomenon in many injuries: wounded and crushed soft tissues release fragments capable of activating complement. This activation triggers the coagulation cas-

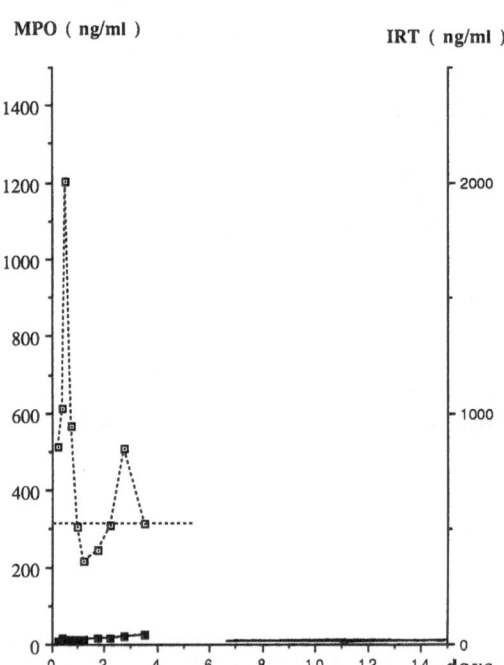

Fig. 2. Evolution of neutrophil myeloperoxidase (MPO: □---□) and immunoreactive trypsin (IRT: ■——■) in a polytrauma patient (women, 62 years) with lung contusion (Injury Severity Score: 2.6). ARDS was present 12 hours after injury. This patient was never infected and rapidly improved. ---Mean normal value for MPO (332 ± 94 ng/ml); —— mean normal value for IRT (32 ± 12 ng/ml)

cade and releases complement fragments (especially C_{5a}) which are chemotactic and activators for PMNL [22]. The coagulation cascade, also directly activated by the primary injury, releases many proteases and mediators, and triggers platelet aggregation with a further release of mediators (TXA_2, serotonin ...) [23-25]. The role of PMNL has been largely recognized as essential in the development of ARDS [13, 26-29]. When activated, they are rapidly sequestered within lung capillaries and undergo a respiratory burst with release of toxic forms of oxygen, proteases and a host of mediators which propagate inflammation [30-32]. However, ARDS can occur in neutropenic patients; in these cases, the main role is likely played by excessive activation of monocytes and macrophages.

In this perspective, ARDS is indeed the first manifestation of a general inflammatory reaction and an evident early marker of extended damage which can affect many other organs. Effros and Mason [33] recently wrote that "studies of "ARDS" represent no more and no less than a study of the phenomena of injury and inflammation in the lung which may differ in some respects from inflammation elsewhere, but no more than likely involve many of the same mechanisms".

ARDS, Local Expression of a General Permeability Defect

Shock states after direct or indirect lung injury are often associated with massive trauma or sepsis, leading to a tissue hypoperfusion to which many organs (such as the pancreas and small intestine) are very sensitive [34-36]. This hypoperfusion triggers a cascade of biochemical events, particularly the slowing or even the arrest of the electron transport chain in mitochondria, the perturbation of oxidative phosphorylation with a drop in ATP production, with as a consequence disorders in the function of the Ca^{2+}-ATP pump, accumulation of Ca^{2+} in cytosol, and ultimately swelling and death of many cells. After reperfusion, oxygen is incompletely reduced and, in the presence of Fe^{2+}, produces toxic excited forms such as the superoxide anion, hydrogen peroxide and hydroxyl radical [34]. Ischemia also leads to the conversion of xanthine dehydrogenase into xanthine oxidase with the production of superoxide anion.

These excited forms of oxygen, together with enzymes and mediators released by the damaged or dying cells, attract and activate macrophages and granulocytes, and injure membranes with as a result a generalized modification of vascular membrane permeability, particularly in the lung where this excessive permeability of capillaries leads to endema with catastrophic consequences on oxygen uptake and delivery. The development of ARDS is thus linked to the activation of different cascades (complement, coagulation ...) and inflammatory cells as well as to problems with vascular permeability, and is accompanied by the release of various mediators which extend the inflammatory reaction.

Fleck et al. [37] in 1985 observed a prompt fall in concentration of some plasma proteins (albumin, transferrin, acute phase proteins) immediately after trauma, which they attributed to the loss of these proteins into the interstitial space due to an increase of microvascular permeability occurring throughout the whole body. Kreuzfelder et al. [38] in 1988 tested the hypothesis of Fleck et al. in trauma patients developing ARDS, and found a temporal relationship between the development of pulmonary edema and the increase in urinary protein concentrations, indicating a systemically increased permeability. Therefore, as Effros and Mason already wrote in 1986, "the edema found in the lungs might simply represent the most obvious and indeed the most serious manifestation of a generalized capillary injury" [33].

ARDS: The Most Rapidly Recognized Manifestation of a Multiple Organ Failure

Other organs are also very sensitive to hypoperfusion which leads to changes of their membrane permeability leading to edema and to organ failure simultaneously with the lung failure, but often with more subtle signs than those in the lung. Observations in animal models and in humans have demonstrated damage to small intestine in hypovolemic shock [35, 36]. The intestinal mucosa, rich in xanthine dehydrogenase, losses its integrity and allows access to the circulation for microorganisms, endotoxin and digestive enzymes. Gram-negative bacteria can be detected in blood two hours after hemorrhagic shock and are still present 48 hours later [35]. This introduction of intestinal bacteria leads to secondary infections (kidneys, lungs, wounds ...) particularly in patients with host defense abnormalities, which often occur in trauma and hemorrhage [39].

The pancreas, a mitochondria rich organ, is very sensitive to hypoperfusion. Experimental studies have shown a rapid and significant drop (more than 70%) in pancreatic blood flow during hypovolemic shock, and histological studies (in man and animals) have shown damage to acinar cells in correlation with the severity, the duration and the cause of shock, with the presence of swollen mitochondria, dilated endoplasmic reticulum, autophagic vacuoles and foci of necrosis [40, 41]. In polytrauma patients, we have demonstrated a pancreatic lesion by the presence in blood of abnormal concentrations of trypsin, amylase and lipase [34, 42, 43]. This enzyme release was biphasic, the first moderate rise occurring 12 to 18 hours after injury (before the onset of lung failure), the second 4 to 6 days after trauma, simultaneously with ARDS and sepsis.

If PMNL are quickly trapped in lung, they are also trapped in numerous other organs, particularly in liver. Mizer et al. [44] in phorbol myristate acetate induced canine ARDS observed an accumulation of PMNL in lung, heart, brain, duodenum, and liver. The number increased 3- to 4-fold in liver parenchyma, with vascular and parenchymal necrosis, as well as thrombosis in hepatic sinusoids. They found structural alterations in the liver in the first six hours after injury, concurrent with lung injury. A common pathway of injury is thus suggested in this animal model of ARDS for lung, liver and other organs, with vascular injury by activated neutrophils as initial event. The importance of hepatic failure has also been recognized by Matuschak and Rinaldo [45, 46], related largely to gut mucosa alterations, due to its strategic situation downstream from gastrointestinal tract.

Recent literature has also underlined the involvement of kidney, heart and brain, and the frequency of sepsis in ARDS patients [47-50]. ARDS is accompanied by 12 to 95% of liver failure, 7 to 30% of gastrointestinal tract or brain failure, 40 to 55% of kidney failure, and 10 to 23% of heart failure [44, 51, 52]. Coagulation cascade and hematopoietic system failures are also frequent. The data of Fleck et al. [37], Kreuzfelder et al. [38] and Mizer et al. [44] suggest a common pathogenetic sequence of events linking the lung injury to the nonpulmonary organ injury by way of general vascular bed damage and neutrophil activation. However, sometimes, the question can be raised as to whether ARDS is primarily a lung disorder that causes nonpulmonary organ failure because of impairment of gas exchange, with secondary decreases in oxygen delivery to peripheral organs, or a more generalized phenomenon of vascular beds more strikingly evident in lung [53].

Figure 3 is an illustration of ARDS occurring together with other organ failure. This patient was admitted in the ICU with multiple fractures (pelvis, ribs) and lung contusion. On day 6, an important activation of leukocytes (MPO: 1450 ng/ml) is observed simultaneously with the development of ARDS and sepsis (leukocyte count: 39 200 cells/mm^3; temperature: 39°C; septic focus in the lung). It is preceded by the presence in blood of abnormal values of trypsin (together with amylase and lipase), markers of pancreatic damage which rise to maximal levels two days later (day 8; IRT value of 2122 ng/ml). Of note, despite the fact that ARDS was still present 14 days after injury and the systemic extension of the disease, the patient survived. At this moment, it is likely that fibrosis has started for several days. From the literature, it is well known that fibrosis is an early phenomenon (Fig. 4) [54, 55]. Endothelial cells, macrophages, leuko-

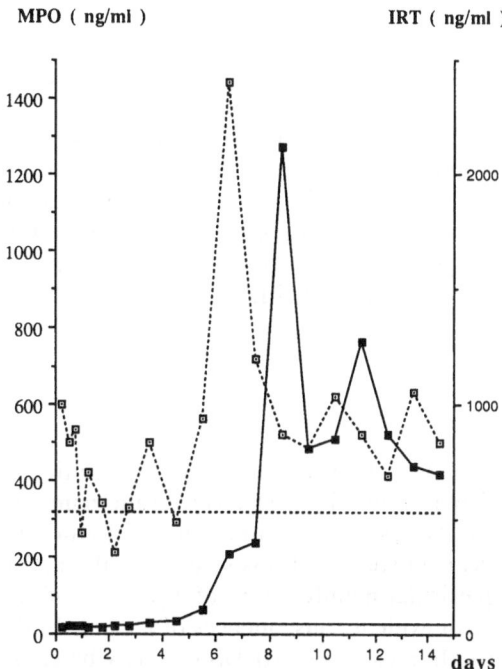

Fig. 3. Evolution of neutrophil myeloperoxidase (MPO: □ - - - □) and immunoreactive trypsin (IRT: ■——■) in a polytrauma patient (man, 47 years) with pelvis and rib fractures (Injury Severity Score: 2.7). This patient developed ARDS and sepsis from day 6. - - - Mean normal value for MPO; —— mean normal value for IRT

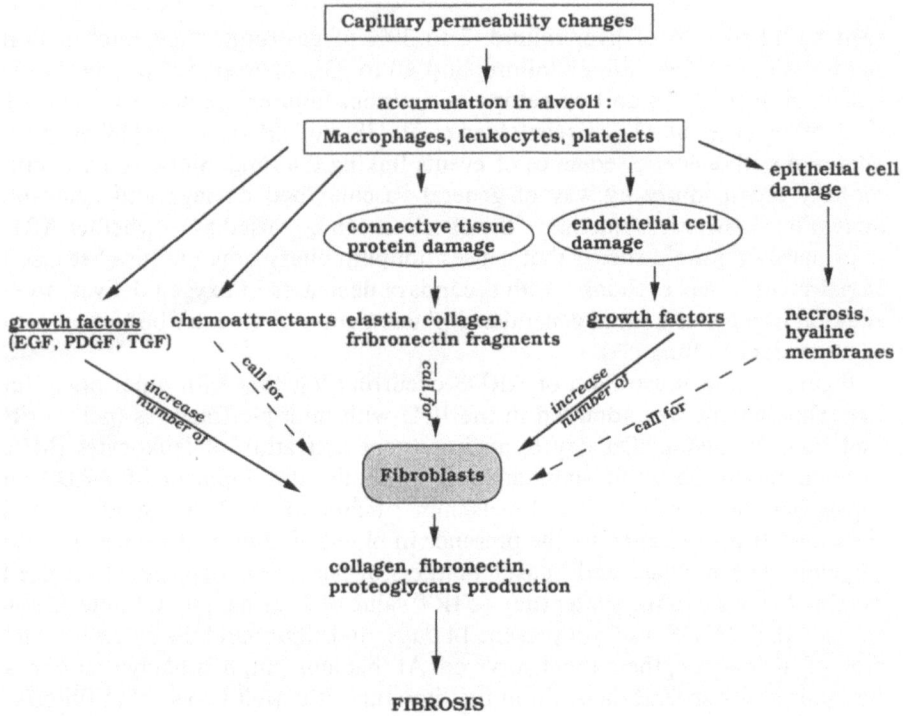

Fig. 4. Fibrosis, later phase of ARDS: mechanisms of attraction and increase of fibroblasts PDGF: platelet derived growth factor; EGF: epidermal growth factor; TGF$_\beta$: transforming growth factor

cytes and platelets that have accumulated in alveoli as a consequence of chemotaxis and increase of vascular permeability; they there release chemoattractive agents and growth factors for fibroblasts. Degraded proteins, hyaline membranes and necrotizing epithelial cells also attract further fibroblasts which when activated produce in excess the proteins of fibrosis. However, when a patient improves and gas exchange returns to normal, the mechanisms of lung repair are triggered by new growth factors leading to a regression of fibrosis and reconstruction of normal lung tissues [56, 57].

Conclusion

1967 was the year of the first description of shock lung, a particular local syndrome which in 1971 received the name of adult respiratory distress syndrome for its ressemblance to infant respiratory distress syndrome. After more than ten years of studies of this syndrome, the new concept has emerged that ARDS is a particular manifestation of a general inflammatory phenomenon and one of the most evident consequences of a whole body modification of vascular permeability. In most cases, ARDS can now be considered as the first manifestation of a multiple organ failure caused by uncontrolled and autodestructive activation of phagocytic cells: all therapeutic approaches must take into account this extended concept of the syndrome.

Acknowledgements: The authors wish to thank the "Fonds National de la Recherche Scientifique", FRSM grant n° 3.4574.89 and the "Fonds Facultaire pour la Recherche Scientifique" for financial assistance. They are also indebted to Mr. G. Hartstein MD for carefull revision of the manuscript and to Mrs N. Bodson for typing.

References

1. Ashbaugh DG, Bigelow DB, Petty TL, Levine VE (1967) Acute respiratory distress syndrome in adults. Lancet 2:319–323
2. Petty TL, Ashbaugh DG (1971) The adult respiratory distress syndrome: clinical features, factors influencing prognosis and principles of management. Chest 70:233–239
3. Fallat RJ, Mielke CH Jr, Rodvien R (1980) Editorial: Adult respiratory distress syndrome and gram-negative sepsis. Arch Intern Med 140:612–613
4. Pepe PE, Potkin RT, Holtman-Reus D, Hudson LD, Carrico CJ (1982) Clinical predictors of the adult respiratory distress syndrome. Am J Surg 144:124–130
5. Kirby RR (1982) The treatment of adult respiratory distress syndrome. Am Rev Respir Dis 1:312–322
6. Fowler AA, Hamman RF, Good JT, et al (1983) Adult respiratory distress syndrome: risk with common predispositions. Ann Intern Med 98:593–597
7. Greene R, Jantsch H, Boggis C, Strauss W, Lowenstein E (1983) Respiratory distress syndrome with new considerations. Radiol Clin North Am 21:699–708
8. Rinaldo JE (1987) The prognosis of the adult respiratory distress syndrome. Inappropriate pessimism? Chest 90:470–471
9. Shale DJ (1987) The adult respiratory distress syndrome: 20 years on. Thorax 442:641–645
10. Putterman C (1988) Adult respiratory distress syndrome: current concepts. Resuscitation 16:91–105
11. Murray JF, Matthay MA, Luce JM, Flick MR (1988) Pulmonary perspectives. An expanded definition of the adult respiratory distress syndrome. Am Rev Respir Dis 138:720–723
12. Rinaldo JE, Roger RM (1982) Adult respiratory distress syndrome: changing concepts of lung injury and repair. N Engl J Med 306:900–909
13. Mallick AA, Ishizaka A, Stephens KE, Hatherill JR, Tazelaar HD, Reffin TA (1989) Multiple organ damage caused by tumor necrosis factor and prevented by prior neutrophil depletion. Chest 95:1114–1120
14. Faber HW, Fairman RP, Millan JE, Rounds S, Glauser FL (1989) Pulmonary response to foreign body microemboli in dogs: release of neutrophil chemoattractant activity by vascular endothelial cells. Am J Respir Cell Mol Biol 1:27–35
15. Martin WJ (1984) Neutrophils kill endothelial cells by a hydrogen-peroxide-dependent pathway: an in vitro model of neutrophil-mediated lung injury. Am Rev Respir Dis 130:209–213
16. Pincemail J, Faymonville ME, Lamy M (1989) Role of neutrophils in critically ill patients: myeloperoxidase, a specific marker of their activation. In: Vincent JL (ed) Update in intensive care and emergency medicine. Springer, Berlin Heidelberg New York Tokyo, pp 24–32
17. Bone R (1986) Adult respiratory distress syndrome. Semin Respir Med 7(S):1–5
18. Heffner JE, Sahn SA, Repine JE (1987) The role of platelets in the adult respiratory distress syndrome. Am Rev Respir Dis 135:482–492
19. Deby-Dupont G, Braun M, Lamy M, et al (1987) Thromboxane and prostacyclin release in adult respiratory distress syndrome. Intensive Care Med 13:167–174

20. Lamy M, Faymonville ME, Adam A, et al (1988) Biochemical changes in patients at risk from the adult respiratory distress syndrome. Does the pancreas play a role? In: Kox W, Bihari D (eds) Shock and the adult respiratory syndrome. Springer, Berlin Heidelberg New York Tokyo, pp 67–77

21. Lamy M, Adam A, Deby-Dupont G, Damas F, Damas P, Faymonville ME (1989) Acute phase proteins and proteases-antiproteases in the inflammatory reaction. In: Bihari DG, Cerra FB (eds) Multiple organ failure. New Horizons III. Fullerton, California, pp 193–216

22. Borg T, Gerdin B, Hallgren R, Modig J (1985) The role of polymorphonuclear leucocytes in the pulmonary dysfunction induced by complement activation. Acta Anaesthesiol Scand 29:231–240

23. Bone RC, Francis PB, Pierce AK (1976) Intravascular coagulation associated with the adult respiratory distress syndrome. Am J Med 61:585–589

24. Saldeen T (1983) Clotting microembolism and inhibition of fibrinolysis in adult respiratory distress. Surg Clin North Am 63:285–304

25. Walshe K, Mackie I, Gallimore M, Machin SJ (1987) Perturbation of the kallikreinkinin system in adult respiratory distress syndrome. Thromb Haemost 58:418

26. Flick MR, Perel A, Staub NC (1979) Increased lung vascular permeability after microemboli in unanesthetized sheep requires circulating leukocytes. Physiologist 22:39–48

27. Powe JE, Short A, Sibbald WJ, Driedger AA (1982) Pulmonary accumulation of polymorphonuclear leukocytes in the adult respiratory distress syndrome. Crit Care Med 10:712–718

28. Hällgren R, Borg T, Venge P, Modig J (1984) Signs of neutrophil and eosinophil activation in adult respiratory distress syndrome. Crit Care Med 12:14–18

29. Rinaldo JE, English D, Levine J, Stiller R, Henson J (1988) Increased intrapulmonary retention of radiolabeled neutrophils in early oxygen toxicity. Am Rev Respir Dis 137:345–352

30. Tate RM, Van Benthuysen KM, Shasby DM, McMurty IF, Repine JE (1982) Oxygen-radical-mediated permeability edema and vasoconstriction in isolated perfused rabbit lungs. Am Rev Respir Dis 126:802–806

31. Weiland JE, Davis B, Holter JF, Mohammed JR, Dorinsky P, Gadek JE (1986) Lung neutrophils in the adult respiratory distress syndrome. Clinical and pathophysiologic significances. Am Rev Respir Dis 133:218–225

32. Whorthen GS, Haslett C, Ress AJ, Gumnay RS, Henson JE, Henson PM (1987) Neutrophil-mediated pulmonary vascular injury. Synergistic effect of trace amounts of lipopolysaccharide and neutrophil stimuli on vascular permeability and neutrophil sequestration in the lung. Am Rev Respir Dis 136:19–28

33. Effros RM, Mason GR (1986) An end to "ARDS". Chest 89:162–163

34. Deby-Dupont G, Faymonville ME, Damas F, Damas P, Lamy M (1988) Shock pancreas. Intense Care News 1:1–6

35. Baker JW, Deitch EA, Berg RD, Specian RD (1988) Hemorrhagic shock induces bacterial translocation from the gut. J Trauma 28:896–906

36. Deitch EA (1988) Does the gut protect or injure patients in the ICU? In: Cerra FB (ed) Perspectives in critical care. Quality Medical Publishing, St Louis, pp 1–31

37. Fleck A, Colley CM, Myers MA (1985) Liver export proteins and trauma. Br Med Bull 41:265–273

38. Kreuzfelder E, Joka T, Keinecke HO, et al (1988) Adult respiratory distress syndrome as a specific manifestation of a general permeability defect in trauma patients. Am Rev Respir Dis 137:95–99

39. Abraham E (1989) Host defense abnormalities after hemorrhage, trauma and burns. Crit Care Med 17:934–939

40. Jones RT, Linhardt GE (1982) Pathology and pathophysiology of the exocrine pancreas in shock. In: Cowley RA, Trump BF (eds) Pathophysiology of shock, anoxia and ischemia. Williams and Wilkins, Baltimore, pp 309–324

41. Hegewald G, Nikulin A, Gmaz-Nikulin E (1985) Ultrastructural changes of the human pancreas in acute shock. Pathol Res Pract 179:610–615

42. Deby-Dupont G, Haas M, Pincemail J, et al (1984) Immunoreactive trypsin in the adult respiratory distress syndrome. Intensive Care Med 10:7–12
43. Lamy M, Faymonville ME, Deby-Dupont G (1987) Shock pancreas: a new entity? In: Vincent JL (ed) Update in intensive care and emergency medicine. Springer, Berlin Heidelberg New York Tokyo, pp 148–154
44. Mizer LA, Weisbrode SE, Dorinsky PM (1989) Neutrophil accumulation and structural changes in nonpulmonary organs after acute lung injury induced by phorbol myristate acetate. Am Rev Respir Dis 139:1017–1026
45. Matuschak GM, Rinaldo JE (1988) Organ interactions in the ARDS during sepsis. Role of the liver in host defense. Chest 94:401–406
46. Matuschak GM, Rinaldo JE, Pinsky MR, Gavaler JS, Van Thiel DH (1987) Effect of end-stage liver failure on the incidence and resolution of the adult respiratory distress syndrome. J Crit Care 2:162–173
47. Bell RC, Coalson JJ, Smith JD, Johanson WG (1983) Multiple organ system failure and infection in adult respiratory distress syndrome. Ann Intern Med 99:293–298
48. Montgomery AB, Stager MA, Carrico J, Hudson LD (1985) Causes of mortality in patients with the adult respiratory distress syndrome. Am Rev Respir Dis 132:485–489
49. Goris RJA, 't Boekhorst TPA, Nuytinck JKS, Grimbere (1985) Multiple-organ failure. Generalized autodestructive inflammation? Arch Surg 120:1109–1115
50. Carrico CJ, Meakins JL, Marshall JC, Fry D, Maier RV (1986) Multiple-organ-failure syndrome. Arch Surg 121:196–208
51. Harris SK, Bone RC, Ruth WE (1977) Gastrointestinal hemorrhage in a respiratory intensive care unit. Chest 72:301–304
52. Kramar S, Khan F, Patel S, Seriff N (1979) Renal failure in the respiratory intensive care unit. Crit Care Med 7:263–266
53. Danek SJ, Lynch JP, Weg JG, Dantzker DR (1980) The dependence of oxygen uptake on oxygen delivery in the adult respiratory distress syndrome. Am Rev Respir Dis 122:387–395
54. Lamy M, Fallat RJ, Koeniger EL, et al (1976) Pathologic features and mechanisms of hypoxemia in adult respiratory distress syndrome. Am Rev Respir Dis 114:267–284
55. Hill JD, Ratliff JL, Parrott JC, et al (1976) Pulmonary pathology in acute respiratory insufficiency: lung biopsy as a diagnosis tool. J Thorac Cardiovasc Surg 71:64–71
56. Knighton DR, Fiegel VD (1989) Growth factors and repair. In: Bihari DG, Cerra FB (eds) Multiple organ failure. New Horizons III. Fullerton, California, pp 371–389
57. Hertz MI, Snyder LS, Harmon KR, Bitterman PB (1989) Repair after acute lung injury: a clinical approach. In: Bihari DG, Cerra FB (eds) Multiple organ failure. New Horizons III. Fullerton, California, pp 217–239

Sepsis and Septic Shock

Foreign Body Infections: From Intravenous Catheters to Hip Prosthesis

M. Herrmann and D. P. Lew

Introduction

The use of foreign bodies to support vital functions (such as intravenous devices) or to replace defective joint functions (such as hip prosthesis) carries a considerable risk of colonization and subsequent infection of the implant, a serious and potentially life-threatening adverse side effect.

Despite differences in design and material of foreign bodies, device-related infections share common pathophysiological features which can be summarized as follows:

(a) A high susceptibility to infection: small numbers of microorganisms, frequently of low pathogenicity (such as *S. epidermidis*), which usually would be eliminated by host's defenses, are capable of inducing a foreign body infection.
(b) A characteristic microflora with a predominance of *S. epidermidis* and *S. aureus,* but also including other pathogens such as fungi and gram-negative organisms.
(c) The persistence of infection despite intensive and prolonged therapy.

It is clear that for most cases (such as intravenous or urinary catheters) the best way to eradicate the infection is to take out the foreign body. However, for infection of permanently implanted material (such as hip prosthesis), the morbidity is particularly important, since, in addition to the antibiotic treatment, one or several surgical interventions are necessary to remove and replace the infected device. This has motivated the search for more conservative treatment strategies, and several reports indicate that eradication of foreign body infection without removal of the device might be possible under specific conditions. Thus, optimal management of such difficult clinical situations requires a detailed analysis of the individual case, the type of material, careful microbiological analysis, and indications (or contraindications) of an antibiotic treatment alone. In this paper, we will discuss some aspects of the pathophysiology, the diagnosis and management of foreign body infections.

Pathophysiology

In order to understand the pathophysiologic events underlying a foreign body infection, it is necessary to characterize three different elements:

1. the foreign surface which induces deposition of host proteins,
2. the colonizing and invading microorganisms, and
3. the local function of neutrophils.

Work in our laboratory during recent years has been focused on the contribution of each of these elements on the pathogenesis of device infection.

1. *Host proteins promote bacterial adhesion to foreign material:* Staphylococci possess specific binding sites recognizing a variety of extracellular matrix proteins. Among these, three proteins have received over the last few years considerable attention: fibronectin, fibrinogen, and laminin. Using a variety of biological and immunological assays, variable amounts of fibronectin and fibrinogen deposited on the surface of foreign material was found [1, 2]. These surface-bound matrix proteins are a prerequisite to mediate adherence of pathogenic Staphylococci to the foreign material [3] and thus to promote initial bacterial colonization.

2. *Characteristics of adherent bacteria:* Recent evidence indicates that fundamental differences exist beween bacteria adherent to surfaces when compared to bacteria present in the fluid phase. A variety of microorganisms, in particular coagulase-negative Staphylococci, develop after prolonged growth on surfaces an amorphous extracellular substance ("slime" or "exopolymers") [4–6]. In vitro studies demonstrate that microorganisms attached to foreign material and exposed to antibiotics in bactericidal concentrations develop tolerance, i.e. a resistance of the bacteria against the lethal effect of the antibiotic [7, 8]. However, whereas the role of "slime" production in the contribution of the virulence of the invading microorganism and the persistence of infection is well established, the in vivo significance of the tolerance of bacteria has still to be shown.

3. *Altered host defense in the vicinity of foreign material – A consequence of neutrophil dysfunction:* When we investigated neutrophils from animals with experimental foreign body infection, we observed that cells recovered from the vicinity of the implant could produce only a weak respiratory burst and had poor bactericidal activity when compared to cells from the blood of these animals. This deficiency was due to prior activation of the neutrophils by the foreign material, similarly to frustrated phagocytosis [9]. Another aspect of neutrophil function on surfaces came from studies with a surface phagocytosis assay: Whereas bactericidal activity of *adherent* neutrophils was poor in protein poor surfaces, it was highly increased in the presence of some matrix proteins such as fibronectin due to recognition of these proteins by specific cell surface receptors present in the membrane of neutrophils. Thus, the nature of proteins deposited over the surface of the foreign body might explain local defects in cellular host defense contributing to the persistance of foreign body infection.

Diagnosis of a Foreign Body Infection

Depending on the localization of the foreign body and the nature of the infecting microorganism, the inflammatory signs can be either masked by the primary affection (which had motivated the implantation of the foreign body), by the surgical intervention, or by the presence of the prosthesis itself. In infections due to certain microorganisms, such as *S. epidermidis, S. viridans,* or fungi, clinical signs of inflammation may lack completely until metastic infection or organ dysfunction develops.

Fever is an important symptom and should always lead to suspicion of infection in a patient with any kind of implanted foreign material. *Pain* may be the only symptom of infection of a joint prosthesis. In particular, constant pain independent of changement of position and responding poorly to antiphlogistic treatment is highly suspect. More specific symptoms correspond to the type of device and include: *Cardiac failure* in a patient with valve prosthesis, *hemorrhage* (gastrointestinal, intra- or retroperitoneal) associated with infection of a vascular graft, *clouded dialysate* and abdominal pain in patients undergoing chronic ambulatory peritoneal hemodialysis, and nonspecific symptoms such as nausea, malaise or *altered sensorium* usually in the absence of meningeal signs in patients with CNS shunt.

The information obtained from radiological examination is often limited due to interference with the foreign material. Plain X-rays can however reveal changes in the position of prosthetic joint components or a periostal reaction. Ultrasound and CT-scan are especially useful to obtain microbiological specimens from the vicinity of the foreign body. Abnormal laboratory findings as leukocytosis or increased sedimentation velocity may be attributed to the postoperative state or underlying disease.

Thus, the diagnosis of a foreign body infection relies on:

1. the information that foreign material is implanted,
2. a careful consideration of clinical symptomatology, physical and laboratory findings, and
3. the careful microbiological analysis of fluids surrounding the foreign body.

Microbiological Findings

As for any severe infection, blood cultures and cultures of suspected liquids or tissues are mandatory before instauration of antibiotic therapy. Blood cultures are particularly important for all endovascular foreign body infections such as intravenous in-lines, prosthetic heart valves, cardiac pacemakers, vascular grafts, and ventriculo-atrial CNS shunts. *S. epidermidis,* usually considered as a contaminant, is highly suspect when isolated several fold from the same site.

Quantitative blood cultures can be performed with the Isolator system and may be useful to compare bacterial numbers drawn via the catheter and from peripheral blood in patients with catheter-related sepsis [10]. Semi-quantitative methods have been proposed for the differentiation of colonization and infection of catheters, since only one initial contaminating microorganism will result in a positive conventional culture of catheters in broth medium [11]. High numbers of microorganisms obtained by aspiration of joint fluid growing on plates is highly suggestive of a joint infection, whereas contaminating organisms grow in small numbers on plates and/or only in broth medium.

Management of a Foreign Body Infection

Surgical Treatment

The principal question after the diagnosis of a foreign body infection is whether the prosthesis may be maintained and the infection cured by antibiotic therapy alone or whether removal of the foreign material is necessary. This decision necessitates a concerted action between the surgeon, the internist, and the infectious disease specialist. An overview of a more general attitude as a function of the type of the device implanted is given in Table 1. However, the final decision has to be made based on the individual case, and a careful follow-up of the patient has to be performed in particular if the prosthesis is maintained.

Some important indications for surgical treatment include:

1. *Fungal disease or particularly resistant microorganisms:* General agreement exists that a foreign body infected by fungi or particularly resistant microorganisms cannot be cured by chemotherapy alone.
2. *Development of heart failure* in patients with prosthetic valve endocarditis. Valve replacement should be seriously considered because of the high mortality in patients with prosthetic valve disease and deteriorating cardiac function [16].
3. *Persistent bacteremia:* Failure of antibiotic therapy to treat foreign device associated bacteremia and/or evidence for recurrent metastatic infection necessitates generally removal of the device.

Table 1. Indications for maintenance or removal of infected devices

---

Maintenance of the device possible[a]
- Implantable intravenous subcutaneous catheters [12]
- Catheters for chronic ambulatory peritoneal dialysis [13]
- Cardiac pacemakers
- Heart valve prosthesis [14]

Removal of the device recommended
- Ventriculo-atrial or -peritoneal CNS shunt [15]

Removal of the device mandatory
- Central-venous catheters causing bacteremia
- Orthopedic prosthesis
- Vascular grafts

---

[a] If the strain is highly susceptible to antibiotics; further contraindications and limitations see text.

Two examples of foreign body infection

1. *Febrile patient with a central venous catheter:* The first step should consist in the search of an infectious focus unrelated to the device (urinary infection, pneumonia, wound infection). Quantitative blood cultures should be obtained percutaneously and via the suspected catheter. Comparison of the number of microorganisms allows sometimes to point out that the catheter is the source of the infection. If blood cultures remain negative and the transcutaneous punction site is not suspect, the catheter may be left in place. Replacement of the catheter is recommended if the patient remains febrile and no other source is detected. Positive blood cultures and/or a suspect site indicate rapid removal of the catheter; insertion of a new catheter in a different site should be performed only after adequate antibiotic therapy has been started.
Implanted catheters with an attached subcutaneous Dacron cuff (Hickman/ Broviac catheters) are not necessarily removed even if causing bacteremia and can be treated successfully in 40-70% of the cases, probably due to the high antibiotic concentrations achieved locally. However, catheters of patients with either signs of an infection of the subcutaneous tunnel, of septic thrombosis of the central vein, or persistance of fever after several days of adequate antibiotic therapy should be removed.

2. *Infection of a joint prosthesis:* Infection of a joint prosthesis, e.g. of the hip, necessitates in almost all instances the complete removal of the foreign material including the bone cement and a large debridement of infected soft tissue and bone. An exception to this rule is the presence of a strain highly susceptible to antimicrobial therapy (such as Streptococci which are highly susceptible to penicillin). In these last cases a cure may be achieved without removal of the foreign material. Many surgeons and infectious disease experts believe that the removal of the infected prosthesis should be followed by several weeks of intravenous therapy and that only after an interval of 3-6 months a new prosthesis should be implanted to decrease the likelihood of reinfection of the new prosthesis. This policy assures a minimal risk of contamination of the definitive prosthesis; however, it is associated with immobilization and severe disability of the extremity.

Antibiotic Therapy

The choice of the initial antibiotic therapy should be ideally made based on a gram stain of the microbiologic specimen. The culture and susceptibility results may indicate subsequent modification of antibiotics. Therapy with bactericidal drugs, possibly in combination, should be administered intravenously for a period of 6 weeks.

1. *Bacteremia associated with an intravenous device:* After removal of the suspect catheter, the initial treatment consists of vancomycin (2·1 g/d) until culture results are obtained, since an increasing percentage of Staphylococci are resistant to methicillin. If the causative strain is sensitive to an antistaphylococ-

cal penicillin, the treatment of choice if flucloxacillin (4·2 g/d). Bacteremias due to *S. epidermidis* in the immunocompetent host and after removal of all foreign material may be treated with IV therapy of shorter duration (about 1–2 weeks). In contrast, even transient *S. aureus* bacteremias carry a considerable risk of metastatic osteomyelitis or endocarditis and therefore, a more prolonged treatment is mandatory. If the catheter has been removed immediately, 2 weeks intravenous therapy are necessary, whereas, if the bacteremia has been more prolonged or if there is any indication of endocarditis or osteomyelitis, 4–6 weeks of intravenous therapy are required.

2. *Infection of a joint prosthesis:* The choice of the initial antibiotic therapy until culture results are obtained is made based on the most frequently encountered microorganisms in this setting. This includes mainly Staphylococci, but gram-negative organisms may as well be responsible for a prosthetic infection. Thus, a reasonable choice may be the combination of an antistaphylococcal penicillin with either an aminoglycoside or with a third generation cephalosporin. If the causative strain is found to be a Staphylococcus, the aminoglycoside may be given initially for the first 2 weeks. Methicillin-resistant Staphylococci require treatment with vancomycin which sometimes may be combined with aminoglycosides and rifampicin. Monitoring of vancomycin serum levels is mandatory, since maximal doses have to be given to assure a good local penetration, and to prevent over-dosing in the case of renal failure.

Concluding Remarks

Due to continuous progress in modern medicine, a further increase in the use of foreign bodies is certain. Control of a variety of foreign body infections will be one of the major tasks of physicians handling nosocomial infections [17]. Despite considerable progress in our understanding of the pathophysiologic events leading to device colonisation and persistant infection, further insights are necessary in order to point out alternative strategies for prevention and treatment of these infections. The development of non-thrombogenic and anti-adhesive materials, of new immunomodulatory substances stimulating the local host defense, and of more potent antibiotics capable to kill adherent bacteria are promising for future research activities. Additional clinical data are necessary to define better risks and benefits of surgical treatment and antibiotic treatment alone or in combination in order to cure these difficult-to-treat infections.

References

1. Vaudaux P, Suzuki R, Waldvogel FA, Morgenthaler JJ, Nydegger UE (1984) Foreign body infection: role of fibronectin as a ligand for the adherence of Staphylococcus aureus. J Infect Dis 149:546–554
2. Vaudaux P, Pittet D, Haeberli A, et al (1989) Host factors selectively increase staphylococcal adherence on inserted catheters: a role for fibronectin and fibrinogen/fibrin. J Infect Dis 160:865–875

3. Herrmann M, Vaudaux PE, Pittet D, et al (1988) Fibronectin, fibrinogen, and laminin act as mediators of adherence of clinical staphylococcal isolates to foreign material. J Infect Dis 158:693–701
4. Christensen GD, Simpson WA, Bisno AL, Beachey EH (1982) Adherence of slime-producing strains of Staphylococcus epidermidis to smooth surfaces. Infect Immun 37:318–326
5. Peters G, Locci R, Pulverer G (1982) Microbial colonization of prosthetic devices. II. Scanning electron microscopy of naturally infected catheters. Zentralbl Bakteriol Parasitenkd Hyg Abt I Orig Reihe B 173:293–299
6. Falcieri E, Vaudaux P, Huggler E, Lew PD, Waldvogel FA (1987) Role of bacterial exopolymers and host factors on adherence and phagocytosis of Staphylococcus aureus in foreign body infection. J Infect Dis 155:524–531
7. Evans RC, Holmes CJ (1987) Effect of vancomycin hydrochloride on Staphylococcus epidermidis biofilm associated with silicone elastomer. Antimicrob Agents Chemother 31:889–894
8. Gristina AG, Jennings RA, Naylor PT, Myrvik QN, Webb LX (1989) Comparative in vitro antibiotic resistance of surface-colonizing coagulase-negative staphylococci. Antimicrob Agents Chemother 33:813–816
9. Zimmerli W, Lew DP, Waldvogel FA (1984) Pathogenesis of foreign body infection: Evidence of a local granulocyte defect. J Clin Invest 73:1191–1200
10. Douard MC, Arlet G, Leverger G, et al (1989) Quantitative blood cultures for diagnosis and management of catheter-related sepsis in leukemic children. 29th Interscience Conference on Antimicrobial Agents and Chemotherapy. Abstract no. 622
11. Maki DG, Weise CE, Sarafin HW (1977) A semiquantitative culture method for identifying intravenous catheter-related infection. N Engl J Med 296:1305–1309
12. Press OW, Ramsey PG, Larson EB, Fefer A, Hickman RO (1984) Hickman catheter infections in patients with malignancies. Medicine 63:189–200
13. Bint AJ, Finch RG, Gokal R, Goldsmith HJ, Juno B, Oliver D (1987) Diagnosis and management of peritonitis in continuous ambulatory peritoneal dialysis. Lancet I:845–848
14. Bisno AL, Dismukes WE, Durack DT, et al (1982) Antimicrobial treatment of infective endocarditis due to viridans streptococci, enterococci, and staphylococci. JAMA 261:1471–1477
15. Bisno AL (1989) Infections of central nervous system shunts. In: Bisno AL, Waldvogel FA (eds) Infections associated with indwelling medical devices. American Society for Microbiology, Washington, DC, pp 93–110
16. Gnann JW, Cobbs CG (1985) Infections of prosthetic valves and intravascular devices. In: Mandell GL, Douglas RG, Bennet JE (eds) Principles and practice of infectious diseases, 2nd edn. Wiley, New York, pp 530–539
17. Maki DG (1989) Risk factors for nosocomial infection in intensive care. 'Devices vs. nature' and goals for the future. Arch Intern Med 149:30–35

The Role of Amino Acid Changes in Septic Encephalopathy*

C. L. Sprung

Introduction

There are several factors which may be important in the altered mental state observed in patients with sepsis. These include a direct central nervous system infection [1-3], endotoxin effects on the brain [4, 5], inadequate perfusion [6, 7], altered metabolism including disturbed plasma and brain amino acid levels [8-17], deranged amino acid transport across the blood brain barrier [15], abnormal levels of neurotransmitters in the brain [8, 16, 17], metabolic disturbances [6], liver insufficiency [8], multiple organ failure [14, 18] or complications of medical therapies.

There are many metabolic causes of an altered sensorium. These include disorders of the liver, kidney, lungs, and pancreas, electrolyte disturbances including sodium, calcium, phosphorus and magnesium, acid-base alterations, hypo and hyperglycemia, hypo and hyperthermia, hypoxemia, exogenous drugs, cofactor deficiencies, and endocrine abnormalities [6, 19-21]. The large majority of these metabolic disturbances can be seen in patients with sepsis [6, 18, 22, 23]. Patients with sepsis often manifest symptoms of encephalopathy including agitation, irritability, lethargy, somnolence, disorientation, confusion, obtundation, stupor and coma [8, 12, 16]. Whether the encephalopathy of sepsis is caused by sepsis alone or is a function of other metabolic etiologies has not been determined. In addition, the exact mental changes that occur in sepsis and their etiology are unclear.

Altered Amino Acid Levels and Encephalopathy in Hepatic Failure

Before addressing the altered metabolism present in sepsis it is useful to review the altered metabolism and its relationship to encephalopathy that has been noted and more fully investigated in hepatic failure. The physiologic principles and many of the findings are similar to those found in sepsis. Patients with liver disease are highly catabolic, have few glycogen stores, are glucose resistant, have decreased ketogenesis and use of fatty acids and have extensive muscle protein

---

* Part of this work was performed during Dr. Sprung's tenure as a Lady Davis Visiting Professor at Hebrew University, Hadassah University Hospital, Department of Anesthesiology, Kiryat Hadassah, P.O. Box 12000, 91120 Jerusalem, Israel.

breakdown [24, 25]. Muscle breakdown results in the release into the circulation of large amounts of various amino acids, with the exception of the branched chain amino acids (BCAA) valine, leucine, and isoleucine, which the muscle can oxidize itself [24]. The liver is the principle or exclusive site for the catabolism of the aromatic amino acids (AAA), phenylalanine, tyrosine and tryptophan and other amino acids including methionine, lysine and threonine [24]. Because the dysfunctioning liver is unable to remove these amino acids from the circulation and because of the increased catabolism of BCAA in the muscle, a characteristic amino acid pattern is found in the blood of experimental animals and patients with hepatic insufficiency and encephalopathy. The picture includes an increase in the plasma levels of tyrosine, phenylalanine and methionine, normal or slightly decreased total plasma tryptophan levels with markedly increased free tryptophan levels, and a decrease in BCAA [9, 25-30]. These changes lead to a decreased BCAA to AAA ratio which has been shown to correlate with encephalopathy [27, 28]. The increased plasma levels of AAA correlate with an increased mortality [27]. The changes in AAA levels may be of greater import in terms of encephalopathy than BCAA levels because cirrhotic patients who develop encephalopathy have changes in their CSF to plasma molar ratios of AAA but little change in the ratios of BCAA and other amino acids [31]. Fischer et al. have shown that the changes in plasma amino acid profiles noted above occur to patients with chronic liver disease when they experience acute exacerbations of encephalopathy [25, 28]. Patients with acute fulminant hepatitis have a different profile with an increase in the plasma levels of all amino acids (especially the AAA and methionine) with the exception of the BCAA which remain normal [25, 28].

The changes in plasma amino acids are believed to be important in amino acid transport, brain concentrations of amino acids, brain neurotransmitters and therefore hepatic encephalopathy [24, 32]. The distorted pattern of essential amino acids in hepatic failure results in changes in amino acid availability to the brain. Unlike capillaries in other organs, the junctions between endothelial cells in the brain are tight, so that free diffusion between cells is difficult and a blood-brain barrier is present. Since the blood-brain transport of large neutral amino acids (including the AAA and BCAA) is mediated by a single, common transport system, the brain concentrations of these amino acids as well as other substances, is closely linked to their rate of transport across the capillary membrane [24, 32, 33]. The entry of tryptophan into the brain, for instance, varies directly with total plasma tryptophan content and inversely with the concentration of the other competing amino acids, particularly the BCAA [34]. This same transport system mediates the efflux of glutamine and other neutral amino acids from the brain [32]. Consequently, increased brain glutamine concentrations may also impair the efflux of neutral amino acids from the brain because of the competition for transport sites [32]. In fact, rises in CSF glutamine levels in cirrhotic patients have been shown to correlate extremely well with the grade of encephalopathy [35]. Therefore, the high plasma concentrations of AAA and low plasma levels of BCAA together with the high brain glutamine levels act in concert to raise brain AAA concentrations [32].

In addition to the effect of competition for the transport system on brain amino acid concentrations, an actual increase in blood-brain neutral amino acid transport activity is found in liver failure [25, 32, 33] which tends to increase the brain AAA even further. It has been demonstrated that brain or CSF levels of the AAA and histidine are increased in hepatic failure whereas the BCAA levels are normal [25, 27, 32]. In dogs with portacaval anastomosis, the appearance of encephalopathy coincides with rises in the CSF concentration of the AAA [29]. In fact infusion of both tryptophan and phenylalanine into awake dogs causes neurologic deterioration which clinically resembles hepatic encephalopathy and culminates in coma [36]. CSF levels of AAA in these animals rise after the infusion to levels observed in experimental hepatic encephalopathy.

The plasma and brain concentrations of the AAA are important factors in the control of the synthesis of brain neurotransmitters [27, 32, 34]. Phenylalanine and tyrosine are precursors of the cerebral neurotransmitters norepinephrine and dopamine as well as other neuroactive substances including phenylethylamine, phenylethanolamine and octopamine [24, 36]. High plasma phenylalanine levels seen in cirrhotic patients may raise brain phenylalanine levels sufficiently to inhibit the rate-limiting enzyme in brain catecholamine synthesis, tyrosine hydroxylase, and suppress the synthesis of norepinephrine and dopamine [24]. Tyrosine which is normally preferentially synthesized to catecholamines is preferentially metabolized to tyramine and subsequently to octopamine when tyrosine accumulates [28]. As noted, tyrosine is increased in hepatic encephalopathy and an excellent correlation between brain tyrosine and octopamine has been demonstrated [28]. Brain norepinephrine and dopamine levels are decreased and brain octopamine levels are increased in hepatic insufficiency perhaps due to these factors [37]. Because the accumulation of octopamine in the brain precedes any accumulation in the blood, it has been suggested that these alterations are secondary to changes within the brain as amines do not penetrate the blood-brain barrier [28, 37]. It is therefore likely that alterations responsible for changes in the synthesis of norepinephrine and octopamine involve their precursors – the AAA [28].

Brain serotonin synthesis, accumulation and turnover is regulated by the brain concentration of its precursor, tryptophan [34]. In cirrhosis, increased brain concentrations of both tryptophan and serotonin have been demonstrated [24, 28, 32]. In addition, enzymatic decarboxylation of the AAA to produce phenylethylamine (from phenylalanine), tyramine (from tyrosine), and tryptamine (from tryptophan) occurs more readily at higher concentrations [36]. Phenylethylamine and tyramine increase the utilization and turnover of catecholamines by promoting synaptic release and inhibiting reuptake [36]. Phenylethylamine and tyramine may themselves be converted into phenylethanolamine and octopamine which can be stored, taken up and released from nerves as weakly acting or "false" neurotransmitters [36]. Increased concentrations of the false neurotransmitters have also been demonstrated in hepatic encephalopathy [28, 29]. Because serotonin-containing neurons are associated with sleep and central catecholamine-containing neurons are associated with arousal, the increased brain concentrations of serotonin and the weak or false transmitters and the decreased levels of catecholamines in hepatic failure may in part explain the observed encephalopathy [24].

Additional support for the hypothesis that the altered amino acid pattern, disturbed transport and changes in brain neurotransmitters are important in the development of hepatic encephalopathy comes from the treatment of experimental animals and patients with hepatic failure with BCAA. BCAA are well tolerated and are associated with a normalization of the plasma amino acid profile as BCAA increase and AAA decrease [27–30]. The change in plasma amino acids coincides with a positive nitrogen balance, a lowering of AAA in the CSF, a normalization of neurotransmitters and an improvement in the encephalopathy [25, 27–30, 36]. Interestingly these changes can be correlated with the dose of BCAA administered [28]. Finally and perhaps most important, recent cooperative studies have demonstrated that mortality can be significantly diminished in patients with hepatic encephalopathy by the use of BCAA [30, 38].

Altered Amino Acid Levels and Encephalopathy in Sepsis

Patients with sepsis have metabolic abnormalities that are similar to those found in patients with hepatic failure and encephalopathy. In fact, identical mechanisms have been postulated for the encephalopathy of sepsis [8, 12, 15–17, 25]. Sepsis is a major catabolic insult which leads to increased muscle breakdown and nitrogen loss [8–10, 13, 22, 23, 39]. This is in part due to modified carbohydrate and fat metabolism. Sepsis accelerates both the oxidation and production of glucose. A diabetic-type glucose tolerance curve with insulin resistance is present and there is decreased ability to oxidize glucose in the periphery [8, 9, 22, 23]. Glycogen stores become depleted and glucose is solely derived by gluconeogenesis when there is no intake [22]. Despite the increased gluconeogenesis, there is decreased free fatty acid availability in sepsis. Hyperinsulinemia causes decreased lipoprotein lipase activity and decreased free fatty acids and ketones leading to further energy deficits [9, 22, 23]. The inability to derive adequate energy from glucose and fat and the development of a peripheral energy deficit, leads to increased breakdown of lean body mass and the oxidation of amino acids, particularly BCAA [9–11, 13, 22, 39]. The oxidation of the BCAA occurs primarily in the muscle. AAA and sulfur-containing amino acids (methionine and cysteine) cannot be utilized by muscle and must be metabolized by the liver.

A distinct plasma amino acid pattern in sepsis and septic encephalopathy has also been demonstrated. The pattern is similar to that seen in hepatic failure and includes increases in the plasma levels of total free amino acids, tyrosine, phenylalanine, tryptophan, methionine and cysteine [8, 10, 12, 22, 25, 40]. In contrast to the patients with hepatic insufficiency, the patients with sepsis have prominent elevations in the sulfur-containing amino acids and the BCAA are normal or low rather than uniformly decreased [8, 12, 25]. Despite these differences, the BCAA to AAA ratio which has been used as a marker for encephalopathy [9, 27, 28] remains low in these septic patients. Some studies, however, have also shown depressed BCAA levels in sepsis [40, 41]. Several investigators believe the changes in plasma amino acid profiles are secondary to the hepatic dysfunction of sepsis [8, 30]. Hepatic abnormalities have been demonstrated in sepsis. Hepatic clearance of indocyanine green dye is impaired within 5 hours of the onset of sepsis [42]. As sepsis continues, involvement of the liver becomes more marked and patients may have varying degrees of hepatic necrosis [9, 10, 18]. Whether the changes in amino acid profiles of septic patients are a function of sepsis itself, hepatic dysfunction, or other causes such as a deficiency of BCAA is unclear.

Various studies of sepsis have shown amino acid patterns to be helpful in predicting survival and mortality [8-12]. Freund et al. noted that survivors have higher levels of plasma BCAA and arginine or alanine whereas the nonsurvivors have higher levels of plasma AAA and sulfur-containing amino acids [8, 12]. AAA and BCAA were also able to discriminate between those patients with and without encephalopathy [12, 40]. In fact amino acid patterns vary with changes in mental functioning. Cerra et al. showed that BCAA are initially low but as death approaches there is an increase in BCAA, AAA, sulfur-containing amino acids, alanine and proline [9-11, 13, 14]. Proline levels correlate with the breakdown of lean body mass and hepatic clearance [11]. We have shown that AAA correlate with Apache II scores and that septic shock patients who die have higher levels of ammonia and sulfur-containing amino acids than those patients who survived.

The abnormal pattern of amino acids in sepsis results in changes in amino acid availability to the brain similar to hepatic failure. Because of competition for the common neutral amino acid blood-brain transport system, an increase in plasma AAA and a decreased BCAA to AAA ratio in sepsis should increase brain AAA. In addition, there is an actual increase in blood-brain neutral amino acid transport activity in sepsis as is seen in hepatic insufficiency [15]. Brain levels of AAA and histidine are increased in sepsis as they are in hepatic failure whereas BCAA levels are increased and not normal as they are in hepatic insufficiency [15-17].

Brain neurotransmitter levels have also been found to be abnormal in sepsis [8, 16, 17]. Freund et al. demonstrated decreased brain levels of both norepinephrine and dopamine in rats with severe sepsis and encephalopathy and increased initial serotonin levels which decrease with severe sepsis [16]. In a later rat study, Freund et al. found increased brain levels of tryptophan, enhanced metabolism of serotonin, and decreased turnover of dopamine resulting in an accumulation of unused dopamine and increased norepinephrine [17]. Increased levels of the false neurotransmitter octopamine and phenylethanolamine have also been noted in patients with sepsis [8]. Obviously, a balance between the above noted neurotransmitters and others such as gamma amino butyric acid and taurine are also important in the development of encephalopathy [16, 17].

Treatment of septic experimental animals and patients with BCAA has also been attempted [8, 17, 43-47]. BCAA have several theoretical and practical benefits to patients with sepsis [25]. First and foremost, BCAA are an energy source which is important in a catabolic, septic patient. BCAA provide a unique source of energy because the oxidation of the first carbon fragment yields high energy phosphate without the requirement of glucose. In fact, the specific type of nutrition provided may be very important in the development and disappearance of encephalopathy. Brain concentrations of neutral amino acids correlate closely with calculated brain-influx rates for amino acids that are variably ingested in the diet [48]. In addition, plasma amino acid levels are usually within a very narrow range as long as hepatic function is normal [49]. With liver injury, however, the specific type of protein given is important in changing both plasma and brain amino acid concentrations [49].

Second, BCAA decrease protein and muscle breakdown and increase protein synthesis [50–53]. The increased protein synthesis is facilitated by a glucose rather than a fat energy source [54]. Patients with hepatic encephalopathy receiving BCAA and hypertonic dextrose have decreases in plasma and CSF tryptophan whereas patients receiving BCAA, hypertonic dextrose and intravenous fat do not have such a decrease in CSF tryptophan levels [30]. Several studies of BCAA in hepatic encephalopathy have demonstrated improvement in encephalopathy when glucose is used as a nonprotein caloric source while no improvement occurs when nonprotein calories are derived from fat [38].

Third, BCAA normalize the plasma amino acid pattern in part by decreasing proteolysis and increasing the use of AAA in the increased protein synthesis [17, 49].

Fourth, BCAA provide the greatest competition for AAA across the blood-brain barrier. By administering BCAA, penetration of AAA to the brain should be prevented and both plasma and brain AAA levels should decrease.

Fifth, BCAA infusions restore brain amino acids and neurotransmitter profiles towards normal [17]. Tyrosine, tryptophan and serotonin levels decrease whereas norepinephrine levels increase [17].

Sixth, BCAA restore immunocompetency. Patients receiving high-dose BCAA have an increase in total lymphocyte count and a return of skin test reactivity [55].

Finally, the theoretically beneficial actions of BCAA on amino acid profiles, blood-brain transport, and neurotransmitters have been shown to translate into reversal of encephalopathy in 5 septic patients [8]. BCAA have been well tolerated in septic patients [8, 43–47].

Studies of BCAA in patients with surgical stress and/or sepsis have revealed conflicting data. Several studies of BCAA have demonstrated improved nitrogen retention [33, 44, 56–58] with one even showing increases in absolute lymphocyte counts and reversal of anergy [44]. Other studies, however, have noted no differences in cumulative nitrogen balance [43, 46, 59]. Several studies evaluating survival showed no beneficial effect of BCAA but all patients survived in one study [43] and the others are from the same group and are only in abstract form [46, 47].

The metabolic derangements and their relationship to encephalopathy have been better formulated for hepatic encephalopathy than for the encephalopathy of sepsis. However, the similarities between hepatic failure and sepsis are striking. These include the catabolic states with proteolysis, altered plasma and brain amino acid profile, deranged blood-brain neutral amino acid transport system, altered brain neurotransmitter levels, similar encephalopathies [16] and hyperdynamic states [9]. These similarities may represent the hepatic dysfunction of sepsis [9, 10] but it is also possible that these alterations represent a common etiology for many of the metabolic encephalopathies [8, 32]. Interestingly, patients with hypercapnia due to chronic respiratory insufficiency have encephalopathy with markedly increased CSF glutamine levels despite normal blood and CSF ammonia concentrations [60]. Patients with pancreatitis may also develop encephalopathy with CSF amino acid aberrations [61]. A deranged blood-brain transport system with increased brain uptake of the neutral amino acids has been demonstrated not only in liver failure and sepsis but also in uremia [16]. Finally, essential amino acids and hypertonic dextrose have been shown to improve survival in patients with acute renal failure [62]. Future studies will define the true importance of amino acid changes in sepsis and septic encephalopathy and whether the manipulation of amino acids can improve the survival of patients with sepsis.

References

1. Diamond IB (1928) Changes in the brain in pyemia and in septicemia. Arch Neurol Psychiatry 20:524–536
2. Anker P, Stroun M (1972) Bacterial ribonucleic acid in the frog brain after a bacterial peritoneal infection. Science 178:621–623
3. Jackson AC, Gilbert JJ, Young GB, Bolton CF (1985) The encephalopathy of sepsis. Can J Neurol Sci 12:303–307
4. Gilles FH, Averill DR, Kerr CS (1977) Neonatal endotoxin encephalopathy. Ann Neurol 2:49–56
5. Mela L (1981) Direct and indirect effects of endotoxin on mitochondrial function. Prog Clin Biol Res 62:15–21
6. Plum F, Posner JB (1980) The diagnosis of stupor and coma, 3rd edn. Davies, Philadelphia, pp 170–303
7. Bolton CF, Young GB (1986) Sepsis and septic shock: Central and peripheral nervous systems. In: Sibbald WJ, Sprung CL (eds) New horizons: perspectives on sepsis and septic shock. Fullerton, CA, Soc Crit Care Med, pp 157–171
8. Freund HR, Ryan JA, Fischer JE (1978) Amino acid derangements in patients with sepsis: Treatment with branched chain amino acid rich infusions. Ann Surg 188:423–430
9. Cerra FB, Siegel JH, Border JR, Wiles J, McMenamy RR (1979) The hepatic failure of sepsis: Cellular versus substrate. Surgery 86:409–422
10. Cerra FB, Siegel JH, Border JR, Peters DM, McMenamy RR (1979) Correlations between metabolic and cardiopulmonary measurements in patients after trauma, general surgery, and sepsis. J Trauma 19:621–629
11. Cerra FB, Caprioli J, Siegel JH, McMenamy RR, Border JR (1979) Proline metabolism in sepsis, cirrhosis and general surgery. The peripheral energy deficit. Ann Surg 190:577–586
12. Freund HR, Atamian S, Holroyde J, Fischer JE (1979) Plasma amino acids as predictors of the severity and outcome of sepsis. Ann Surg 190:571–576
13. Cerra FB, Siegel JH, Coleman B, Border JR, McMenamy RR (1980) Septic autocannibalism. A failure of exogenous nutritional support. Ann Surg 192:570–580
14. Moyer ED, McMenamy RR, Cerra FB, et al (1981) Multiple systems organ failure. III. Contrasts in plasma amino acid profiles in septic trauma patients who subsequently survive and do not survive – Effects of intravenous amino acids. J Trauma 21:263–274
15. Jeppsson B, Freund HR, Gimmon Z, James JH, von Meyenfeldt MF, Fischer JE (1981) Blood-brain barrier derangement in sepsis: Cause of septic encephalopathy? Am J Surg 141:136–142
16. Freund HR, Muggia-Sullam M, Peiser J, Melamed E (1985) Brain neurotransmitter profile is deranged during sepsis and septic encephalopathy in the rat. J Surg Res 38:267–271
17. Freund HR, Muggia-Sullam M, LaFrance R, Holroyde J, Fischer JE (1986) Regional brain amino acid and neurotransmitter derangements during abdominal sepsis and septic encephalopathy in the rat. The effect of amino acid infusions. Arch Surg 121:209–216

18. Coalson JJ (1986) Pathology of sepsis, septic shock and multiple organ failure. In: Sibbald WJ, Sprung CL (eds) New horizons: perspectives on sepsis and septic shock. Fullerton, CA, Soc Crit Care Med, pp 27-59
19. Adams RD, Victor M (1981) Principles of neurology, 2nd edn. McGraw-Hill, New York, pp 231-247
20. Posner JB (1982) General causes of delirium stupor and coma. In: Wyngaarden JB, Smith LH (eds) Cecil textbook of medicine. Saunders, Philadelphia, pp 1914-1920
21. Ropper AH, Martin JB (1983) Derangements in intellect, mood and behavior. In: Petersdorf RG, Adams RD, Braunwald E, et al (eds) Harrison's principles of internal medicine, 10th edn. McGraw-Hill, New York, pp 131-136
22. Forse RA, Kinney JM (1985) The metabolic response to infection. In: Meakins JL (ed) Surgical infection in critical care medicine. Churchill-Livingstone, New York, pp 69-94
23. Cerra FB (1986) Metabolic support of the systemic septic response. In: Sibbald WJ, Sprung CL (eds) New horizons: perspectives on sepsis and septic shock. Fullerton, CA, Soc Crit Care Med, pp 235-256
24. Munro HN, Fernstrom JD, Wurtman RJ (1975) Insulin, plasma amino acid imbalance, and hepatic coma. Lancet 1:772-774
25. Sax HC, Talamini MA, Fischer JE (1986) Clinical use of branched-chain amino acids in liver disease, sepsis, trauma, and burns. Arch Surg 121:358-366
26. Fischer JE, Yoshimura N, Aguirre A, et al (1974) Plasma amino acids in patients with hepatic encephalopathy. Effects of amino acid infusions. Am J Surg 127:40-47
27. Fischer JE, Funovics JM, Aguirre A, et al (1975) The role of plasma amino acids in hepatic encephalopathy. Surgery 78:276-290
28. Fischer JE, Rosen HM, Ebeid AM, James JH, Keane JM, Soeters PB (1976) The effect of normalization of plasma amino acids on hepatic encephalopathy in man. Surgery 80:77-91
29. Smith A, Rossi-Fanelli F, Ziparo V, James JH, Perelle B, Fischer JE (1978) Alterations in plasma and CSF amino acids, amines, and metabolites in hepatic coma. Ann Surg 187:343-350
30. Cerra FB, Cheung NK, Fischer JE, et al (1985) Disease specific amino acid infusion (F080) in hepatic encephalopathy: A prospective, randomized, double-blind, controlled trial. J Parent Enter Nutr 9:288-295
31. Cangiano C, Cascino A, Fiaccadori F, Riggio O, Rossi-Fanelli F, Capocaccia L (1981) Is the blood-brain barrier really intact in portal-systemic encephalopathy? Lancet 1:1367
32. James JH, Jeppsson B, Ziparo V, Fischer JE (1979) Hyperammonemia, plasma amino acid imbalance, and blood-brain amino acid transport: A unified theory of portal-systemic encephalopathy. Lancet 2:772-775
33. James JH, Escourrou J, Fischer JE (1978) Blood-brain neutral amino acid transport activity is increased after portocaval anastomosis. Science 200:1395-1397
34. Fernstrom JD, Wurtman RJ (1972) Brain serotonin content: Physiological regulation by plasma neutral amino acids. Science 178:414-416
35. Hourani BT, Hamlin EM, Reynolds TB (1971) Cerebrospinal fluid glutamine as a measure of hepatic encephalopathy. Arch Intern Med 127:1033-1036
36. Rossi-Fanelli F, Freund H, Krause R, et al (1982) Induction of coma in normal dogs by the infusion of aromatic amino acids and its prevention by the addition of branched chain amino acids. Gastroenterology 83:664-671
37. Dodsworth JM, James JH, Cummings MC, Fischer JE (1974) Depletion of brain norepinephrine in acute hepatic coma. Surgery 75:811-820
38. Fischer JE (1984) Efficacy of branched chain amino acids in the treatment of hepatic encephalopathy. In: Capocaccia L, Fischer JE, Rossi-Finelli F (eds) Hepatic encephalopathy in chronic liver failure. Plenum Press, New York, pp 311-321
39. O'Donnell TF, Clowes GHA, Blackburn GL, Ryan NT, Benotti PN, Miller JD (1976) Proteolysis associated with a deficit of peripheral energy full substrates in septic man. Surgery 80:192-200
40. Sprung CL, Cerra FB, Schein RMH, et al (1989) Amino acid alterations and encephalopathy in the sepsis syndrome. Crit Care Med 17:S54
41. Wannemacher RW Jr (1977) Key role of various individual amino acids in host response to infection. Am J Clin Nutr 30:1269-1280

42. Chaudry JH, Schleck S, Clemens MG (1982) Altered hepatocellular transport. An early change in peritonitis. Arch Surg 117:151-157
43. Bower RH, Muggia-Sullam M, Vallgren S, et al (1986) Branched chain amino acid-enriched solutions in the septic patient. Ann Surg 203:13-20
44. Cerra FB, Mazuski JE, Chute E, et al (1984) Branched chain metabolic support: A prospective, randomized, double-blind trial in surgical stress. Ann Surg 199:286-291
45. Cerra FB, Mazuski JE, Teasley K, et al (1983) Nitrogen retention in critically ill patients is proportional to the branched chain amino acid load. Crit Care Med 11:775-778
46. Van Berlo CLH, von Meyenfeldt MF, Rouflart M, Soeters PB (1985) Does branched chain amino acid enrichment reduce mortality in septic and traumatized patients. Clin Nutr 5:132 (abstract)
47. de Jong KP, von Meyenfeldt MF, Rouflart M, et al (1984) The effect of branched chain amino acids on organ functioning in septic and stressed patients. Clin Nutr 4:71 (abstract)
48. Fernstrom JD, Faller DJ (1978) Neutral amino acids in brain: changes in response to food ingestion. J Neurochem 30:1531-1538
49. Rosen MH, Soeters PB, James JH, et al (1978) Influences of exogenous intake and nitrogen balance on plasma and brain aromatic amino acid concentrations. Metabolism 27:393-404
50. Freund HR, Hoover HC, Atamian S, et al (1979) Infusion of the branched chain amino acids in postoperative patients: anti-catabolic properties. Ann Surg 190:18-23
51. Lindberg BO, Clowes GHA (1981) The effects of hyperalimentation and infused leucine on the amino acid metabolism in sepsis: An experimental study in vivo. Surgery 90:278-290
52. Freund HR, James JH, Fischer JE (1981) Nitrogen-sparing mechanisms of singly administered branched chain amino acids in the injured rat. Surgery 90:237-243
53. Blackburn BR, Moldawer LL, Usui S, Bothe A, O'Keefe SJD, Bistrian BR (1979) Branched chain amino acid administration and metabolism during starvation, injury, and infection. Surgery 86:307-315
54. Gelfand RA, Hendler RS, Sherwin RS (1979) Dietary carbohydrate and metabolism of ingested protein. Lancet 1:65-68
55. Nuwer N, Cerra FB, Shronts EP, et al (1983) Does modified amino acid total parenteral nutrition alter immune-response in high level surgical stress? J Parent Enter Nutr 7:521-524
56. Kern KA, Bower RH, Atamian S, Matarese LE, Ghory MJ, Fischer JE (1982) The effect of a new branched chain-enriched amino acid solution on postoperative catabolism. Surgery 92:780-785
57. Bower RH, Kern KA, Fischer JE (1985) Use of a branched chain amino acid enriched solution in patients unter metabolic stress. Am J Surg 149:266-270
58. Cerra FB, Upson D, Angelico R, et al (1982) Branched chains support postoperative protein synthesis. Surgery 92:192-199
59. Daly JM, Mihranian MH, Kehoe JE, Brennan MF (1983) Effects of post-operative infusions of branched chain amino acids on nitrogen balance and forearm muscle substrate flux. Surgery 94:151-158
60. Jaikin A, Agrest A (1969) Cerebrospinal fluid glutamine concentrations in patients with chronic hypercapnia. Clin Sci 36:11-14
61. Sjaastad O, Gjessing L, Ritland S, Blichfeldt P, Sandres K (1979) Chronic relapsing pancreatitis, encephalopathy with disturbance of consciousness and CSF amino acid aberration. J Neurol 220:83-94
62. Abel RM, Beck CH Jr, Abbott WM, et al (1973) Improved survival from acute renal failure after treatment with intravenous essential L-amino acids and glucose. N Engl J Med 288:695-699

Endotoxins and Gram-negative Septicemia*

S. J. H. van Deventer, A. Sturk, and J. W. ten Cate

Introduction

In approximately 0.39-1.15% of patients admitted to hospitals, gram-negative bacteremia is diagnosed [1, 2]. The large majority of bacteremic patients has clinical characteristics of bacterial infection, most commonly fever, but only a few bacteremic patients will develop the septic syndrome, which can be complicated by hypotension, coagulation activation, increased vascular permeability, and renal failure, and may culminate in a highly lethal syndrome termed multiple organ failure [3]. Although in the past bacteremia was almost considered a gold standard for septicemia, of unselected bacteremic patients only 15% develop clinical symptoms of septicemia [4]. Moreover, it is well established that clinical symptoms of septicemia can develop in patients who have negative blood cultures. These findings may in part be an effect of widespread treatment with antibiotics. More importantly, it has been shown that lipopolysaccharides present in the outer membrane of gram-negative bacteria (endotoxins) can induce many biological phenomena that are observed in septicemia and that endotoxemia may occur in the absence of bacteremia [4-6]. Unfortunately, the clinical criteria for the septic syndrome are rather unspecific, and it remains difficult to make a diagnosis. In this paper we will briefly review evidence, derived from experimental and clinical studies, that endotoxins are of importance in the pathophysiology of septicemia, and we will discuss the usefulness of endotoxin testing in a clinical setting.

Endotoxins

The outer membrane of gram-negative bacteria consists mainly of phospholipids, proteins and lipopolysaccharides. The distribution of these constituents is asymmetrical, and lipopolysaccharides form the main component of the outer section. Bacterial lipopolysaccharides have numerous biological activities, including induction of fever and myocardial depression and activation of the coagulation, fibrinolytic and complement cascades [7-12]. The lipid moiety in lipopolysaccharides known as lipid A, is responsible for these biological effects [13,

* This work was supported in part by a grant from the Nederlandse Organisatie voor Wetenschappelijk onderzoek, s'Gravenhage, The Netherlands.

14]. It is not in the scope of this review to thoroughly discuss molecular interactions that lead to endotoxicity, but it is important to realize that the physical conformation of lipopolysaccharides in the bacterial membrane precludes lipid A exposure. Hence, lipopolysaccharides need to be released from the bacterial membrane in order to exert their biological effects. During incubation with human serum, gram-negative bacteria loose a sizable fraction of their lipopolysaccharides [15]. These lipopolysaccharides form complexes with various serum proteins. One of these proteins, the 60 kDa lipoprotein binding protein (LBP) [16, 17] may be of importance for lipopolysaccharide presentation to macrophages, as it recently has been shown to bind to the CD14 membrane protein [18]. To date however, it is unknown what the physiological role of LBP is and to what extent binding of lipopolysaccharides to LBP is important for activation of macrophages. Finally, ligand binding studies have recently implicated an 80 kDa macrophage protein distinct from CD14 as a functional receptor of lipopolysaccharides [19, 20].

Methods for Determination of Endotoxins in Blood

With the exception of meningococcal septicemia, endotoxin levels in human disease are too low to be detected by physical methods. All currently employed endotoxin assays are bioassays, based on the discovery that lipopolysaccharides specifically induce coagulation of the hemolymph of various horseshoe crabs, which is indicated by the formation of a gel [21]. The original test which employed this principle is widely known as the Limulus gelation assay. Lysates from hemolymph of two horseshoe crabs, Limulus polyphemus and Tachypleus tridentatus, are now commercially available for endotoxin testing. The methodology of endotoxin detection in aqueous fluids such as pharmaceuticals and parenteral nutrition with Limulus or Tachypleus lysates is relatively simple and has widely replaced other bioassays, in particular the rabbit fever assay. In contrast, it has been more difficult to reliably detect endotoxins in blood, in part because levels of circulating endotoxin levels in human disease are low, and in part because of the presence of endotoxin "inhibitors" in blood, which may cause false negative reactions [21]. Although it has been shown that endotoxins in blood bind to several serum proteins as well as lipoproteins [15, 22], the relative importance of these interactions for endotoxin inactivation remains unknown. Nevertheless, several techniques, developed to inactivate endotoxin inhibitors have been proven to enable satisfactory recovery of endotoxins in blood. These techniques include dilution and heat inactivation, and extraction with chloroform or perchloric acid [21, 23-25].

The original endpoint of the Limulus assay was gelation of Limulus lysate, which could be confirmed by inverting the test tube, but it soon became clear that low endotoxin concentrations can cause incomplete gelation. This incited the development of methods to detect changes in the turbidity of Limulus lysate during activation by endotoxins [26-28]. Alternatively, it has been possible to couple chromogenic reactions to the Limulus coagulation assay [29, 30]. In this method the degree of activation of Limulus lysate can be assessed spectrophotometrically. This latter modification of the Limulus gelation assay, known as the chromogenic Limulus test, has been shown to be most useful in the clinical setting.

Endotoxemia in Febrile and Bacteremic Patients

The importance of endotoxemia in human disease states has been investigated in numerous studies. Comparison of these investigations is virtually impossible because of substantial differences in the methodology of endotoxin testing, and variations in study design. We have summarized the findings of 12 studies on endotoxemia in Table 1. Two studies performed in the early 1970s by Levin first demonstrated a correlation between endotoxemia (assessed by a Limulus gelation assay) and septicemia (defined by clinical criteria) [31, 32]. Importantly, these studies showed that gram-negative bacteremia was not invariably accompanied by endotoxemia. Patients who where simultaneously bacteremic and endotoxemic however, had a higher likelihood of hypotension. Subsequent studies initially could not confirm the usefulness of endotoxin testing in a clinical set-

Table 1. Reported sensibilities and specificities of the Limulus assay for bacteremia, septicemia, and death in 12 selected studies

Reference	Gold standard	Study population	Test	Sensibility	Specificity
Levin (1970)	Gram-negative bacteremia	Febrile patients	gel	71%	94%
Levin (1972)	Septic shock	Febrile patients	gel	32%	98%
Das (1973)	Gram-negative infection	Febrile patients	gel	89%	100%
Stumacher (1973)	Gram-negative bacteremia	Bacteremic patients	gel	51%	65%
Fossard (1974)	Gram-negative infection	Surgical patients	gel	95%	65%
Fink (1981)	Septic syndrome	Febrile patients	turb	97%	100%
Fink (1984)	Septic syndrome	Intensive care patients	turb	92%	n.d.
Grundmann (1986)	Septic syndrome	Intensive care patients	gel	81%	n.d.
Hass (1986)	Death	Febrile children (immunocompromized)	chro	45%	80%
Van Deventer (1988)	Septic syndrome	Febrile patients	chro	79%	96%
Van Deventer (1988)	Septic syndrome	Patients with pyelonephritis	chro	79%	95%
Brandtzaeg (1989)	Death	Meningococcal sepsis	chro	86%*	75%*

* levels over 10,000 ng/L.
gel: gelation assay; *turb:* turbidimetric assay; *chro:* chromogenic assay; *n.d.:* not determined.

ting. These results should be cautiously interpreted because of the insensitivity of the endotoxin assays employed, and weaknesses in study design [reviewed in 33]. More recently, using a chromogenic Limulus assay, very high endotoxin levels were detected in meningococcal septicemia [34]. These high levels of endotoxin, up to 10,000 times higher than usually observed in septicemia caused by other gram-negative bacteria, enabled comparison of results of the chromogenic Limulus assay with a physicochemical method for endotoxin detection, and in the limited number of samples that were compared, a good correlation was found between the outcomes of both methods. In another study it was shown that experimental low level endotoxemia in humans could be reliable detected with the chromogenic Limulus assay [11] (Fig. 1). The transient endotoxemia was followed by activation of the common pathway of blood coagulation, transient neutropenia followed by neutrophilia, and release of proteases such as elastase. In conclusion, reliable detection of both high and low level endotoxemia with chromogenic Limulus tests is now feasible.

An important factor in assessing endotoxemia is the timing of the collection of blood samples relative to the development of the septic syndrome. In a study that included all patients that developed fever in a 9 month period in one hospital, endotoxemia was detected in a relatively small subgroup [7]. In these febrile patients endotoxemia proved to be a reliable harbinger of septicemia (sensitivity 79%, specificity 96%). The average time interval between detection of endotoxemia and the development of septicemia was 19.8 hours. Somewhat unexpectedly it was found that most endotoxemic episodes occurred in patients admitted to general wards, many of whom subsequently were transferred to the intensive care department. In contrast, in patients who met criteria for gram-negative septicemia at the time of blood sampling, endotoxemia was not invariably observed. These data may indicate that endotoxemia is transient. Finally, there is reason to believe that models of experimental septicemia, and even acute experimental endotoxemia in humans, may not authentically reflect the pathophysiology of septicemia in critically ill patients, which may be characterized by repeated bouts of transient endotoxemia.

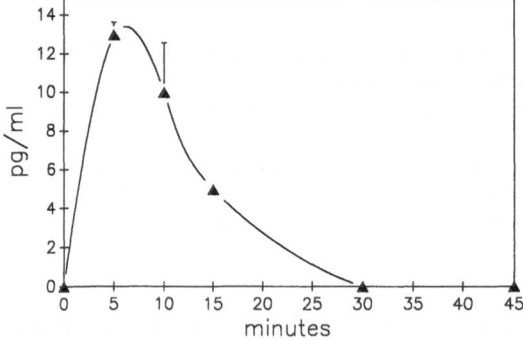

Fig. 1. Kinetics of endotoxemia in healthy volunteers. Six healthy volunteers received a bolus injection of endotoxin (preparation EC-5, 2 ng/kg). Endotoxin levels were measured with a chromogenic Limulus assay. The detection limit of this assay is 3 ng/L. Although in all volunteers comparable endotoxin levels were observed, the biological responses, including release of TNF and IL-6 varied extensively. (From [11])

Endotoxins, Cytokines and Host Defense Responses

Different species, and even different persons, have widely varying responses to endotoxins [11, 35]. These variations in susceptibility seem to be determined by disparities in the responses of host defenses cells, in particular macrophages, as can be measured in terms of release of various cytokines, including interleukin-1, interleukin-6 and tumor necrosis factor [11, 35]. Moreover, endotoxin susceptibility can vary in one individual in the course of a bacterial infection or during endotoxemia. For example, in experimental animals, gram-negative and gram-positive bacterial infections temporarily increase endotoxin susceptibility, whereas *continuous* low level endotoxemia in humans rapidly induces tolerance [reviewed in 36 and 37]. Hence, differences in endotoxin sensitivity, which are in part reflected by variations in cytokine release, determine the biological effects resulting from endotoxemia, and it should therefore come as no surprise, that absolute levels of circulating endotoxins correlate poorly with the severity of septicemia.

Recently, experimental and clinical evidence has accumulated that cytokines are involved in the pathogenesis of septicemia. The most potent stimulus for induction of these cytokines is endotoxin. Indeed, in patients with gram-negative septicemia release of cytokines, in particular TNF and IL-6, has been documented [38, 39]. In view of its biological activities in experimental animals [40], these findings strongly suggest an important role for TNF in the pathogenesis of septicemia. It should be noted however, that release of TNF and IL-6 can also be observed in non-septic critical illness, such as myocardial infarction, renal allograft rejection and uncomplicated surgery [41–43]. To date the importance of TNF release for the subsequent development of septicemia in febrile or bacteremic patients has not been studied, and presently, endotoxemia is the only parameter that has been shown to precede and predict septicemia.

More definitive proof of the importance of endotoxin and various cytokines in the pathogenesis of septicemia in humans will be derived from ongoing clinical studies in which monoclonal antibodies directed to epitopes on lipopolysaccharides or TNF are administered to patients fulfilling clinical criteria for septicemia. If these strategies will prove to be successful, the need for rapid detection of circulating endotoxins will become even more important. Finally, little is known about the kinetics of endotoxemia in septic patients (with the exception of meningococcal septicemia). Preliminary evidence indicates that endotoxemia as well as the release of circulating TNF are transient phenomena. More detailed knowledge of the kinetics of endotoxin and its endogenous mediators will enable development of rational intervention strategies.

References

1. Bryan CS, Reynolds KL, Brenner ER (1983) Analysis of 1,186 episodes of gram-negative bacteremia in non-university hospitals: The effects of antimicrobial therapy. Rev Infect Dis 5:629–632
2. McGowan JE Jr, Barnes MW, Finland M (1975) Bacteremia at the Boston City Hospital: Occurrence and mortality during 12 selected years (1935–1972) with special reference to hospital-acquired cases. J Infect Dis 132:316–320
3. Bell RC, Coalson JJ, Smith JD, Johansen WJ (1983) Multiple organ system failure and infection in adult respiratory distress syndrome. Ann Intern Med 98:593–598
4. Van Deventer SJH, Büller HR, ten Cate JW, Sturk A, Pauw W (1988) Endotoxaemia: An early predictor of septicemia in febrile patients. Lancet 2:605–609
5. Morrison DC, Ulevitch RJ (1978) The effects of bacterial endotoxins on host mediation systems. Am J Pathol 93:527–618
6. Morrison DC, Ryan JC (1987) Endotoxin and disease mechanisms. Ann Rev Med 38:417–432
7. Morrison DC, Kline LF (1977) Activation of the classical and properdin pathways of complement by bacterial lipopolysaccharides (LPS). J Immunol 118:362–368
8. Vukajlovitch SW, Hoffman J, Morrison DC (1987) Activation of human serum complement by bacterial lipopolysaccharides: Structural requirements for antibody dependent activation of the classical and alternative pathways. Mol Immunol 24:319–332
9. Maier RV, Hahnel GB (1984) Microthrombosis during endotoxemia. Potential role of hepatic versus alveolar macrophages. J Surg Res 36:362–370
10. Colucci M, Balconi G, Lorenzet R, et al (1983) Cultured human endothelial cells generate tissue factor in response to endotoxin. J Clin Invest 71:1893–1896
11. Van Deventer SJH, Büller HR, ten Cate JW, Aarden L, Hack E, Sturk A (1990) Experimental endotoxemia in humans. Cytokine release, and activation of the coagulation, complement, and fibrinolytic pathways (submitted)
12. Suffredini AF, Fromm RF, Parker MM, et al (1989) The cardiovascular response of normal humans to the administration of endotoxin. N Engl J Med 321:280–287
13. Galanos C, Lüderitz O, Rietschel ET, Westphal O (1977) Newer aspects of the chemistry and biology of bacterial lipopolysaccharides with special reference to their lipid A component. In: Goodwin TW (ed) International review of biochemistry. Biochemistry of lipids II. University Park Press, Baltimore, vol 14, pp 239–335
14. Galanos C, Lehmann V, Lüderitz O, et al (1984) Endotoxic properties of chemically synthesized lipid A part structures. Comparison of synthetic lipid A precursor and synthetic analogues with biosynthetic lipid A precursor and free lipid A. Eur J Biochem 140:221–227
15. Tesh VL, Morrison DC (1988) The physical-chemical characterization and biological activity of serum released lipopolysaccharides. J Immunol 141:3523–3531
16. Tobias PS, Mathison JC, Ulevitch RJ (1988) A family of lipopolysaccharide binding proteins involved in responses to gram-negative sepsis. J Biol Chem 263:13479–13481
17. Tobias PS, Soldau K, Ulevitch RJ (1989) Identification of a lipid A binding site in the acute phase reactant lipopolysaccharide binding protein. J Biol Chem 264:10867–10871
18. Wright S. Personal communication
19. Lei MG, Morrison DC (1988) Specific endotoxic lipopolysaccharide-binding proteins on murine splenocytes. I. Detection of lipopolysaccharide-binding sites on splenocytes and splenocyte subpopulations. J Immunol 141:996–1005
20. Lei MG, Morrison DC (1988) Specific endotoxic lipopolysaccharide-binding proteins on murine splenocytes. II. Membrane localization and binding characteristics. J Immunol 141:1006–1011
21. Levin J, Tomasulo P, Oser R (1970) Detection of endotoxin in human blood and demonstration of an inhibitor. J Lab Clin Med 75:903–911
22. Tobias PS, McAdam KPJW, Soldau K, Ulevitch RJ (1985) Control of lipopolysaccharide-high density lipoprotein interactions by an acute phase reactant in human serum. Infect Immun 50:73–76
23. Thomas LLM, Sturk A, Kahlé LH, ten Cate JW (1981) Quantitative endotoxin determination in blood with a chromogenic substrate. Clin Chim Acta 11:63–68

24. Tamura H, Obayashi T, Tagaki K (1982) Perchloric acid treatment of human blood for quantitative endotoxin assay using synthetic chromogenic substrate for horseshoe crab clotting enzyme. Thromb Res 27:51–57
25. Obayashi T (1984) Addition of perchloric acid to blood samples for colorimetric Limulus test using chromogenic substrate: Comparison with conventional procedures and clinical application. J Lab Clin Med 104:321–330
26. Cooper JF, Levin J, Wagner JH Jr (1971) Quantitative comparison of in vitro and in vivo methods for the detection of endotoxin. J Lab Clin Med 78:138–148
27. Fink PC, Lehr L, Urbaschek RM (1981) Limulus amebocyte lysate test for endotoxemia: Investigations with a femtogram sensitive spectrophotometric assay. Klin Wochenschr 59:213–218
28. Ditter B, Becker KP, Urbaschek R, Urbaschek B (1983) Quantitativer Endotoxin-Nachweis. Automatisierter kinetischer Limulus-Amoebozyten-Lysate-Mikrotitertest mit Messung probenabhängiger Interferenzen. Drug Res 33:681–800
29. Nakamura S, Morita T, Iwanaga S, Niwa M, Takahashi K (1977) A sensitive substrate for the clotting enzyme in horseshoe crab hemocytes. J Biochem 81:15679
30. Iwanaga S, Morita T, Harada T, et al (1978) Chromogenic substrate for horseshoe crab clotting enzyme. Its application for assay of bacterial endotoxin. Haemostasis 7:183–188
31. Levin J, Poore TE, Zauber NP (1970) Detection of endotoxin in the blood of patients with sepsis due to gram-negative bacteria. N Engl J Med 283:1313–1316
32. Levin J, Poore TE, Young NS (1972) Gram-negative sepsis: Detection of endotoxemia with the Limulustest. Ann Intern Med 76:1–7
33. Van Deventer SJH, Büller HR, Sturk A, ten Cate JW (1990) Predicting septicemia with assays for bacterial lipopolysaccharides (endotoxin) (submitted)
34. Brandtzaeg P, Kierul P, Gaustad P, et al (1989) Plasma endotoxin as a predictor of multiple organ failure and death in systemic meningococcal disease. J Infect Dis 159:195–204
35. Molvig J, Baek L, Christensen P, et al (1988) Endotoxin-stimulated human monocyte secretion of interleukin 1, tumour necrosis factor alpha, and prostaglandin E2 shows stable interindividual differences. Scand J Immunol 27:705–716
36. Galanos C, Freudenberg MA, Matsuura M, Coumbos A (1988) Hypersensitivity to endotoxin and mechanisms of host-response. Prog Clin Biol Res 272:295–308
37. Johnston CA, Greisman SE (1985) Mechanisms of endotoxin tolerance. In: Hinshaw LB (ed) Handbook of endotoxin, vol 2. Elsevier, Amsterdam 85, pp 359–401
38. Waage A, Halstensen A, Espevik T (1987) Association between tumor necrosis factor in serum and fatal outcome in patients with meningococcal disease. Lancet 1:355–357
39. Debets JMH, Kampmeyer R, Van der Linden MPMH, Buurman WA, Van der Linden CJ (1989) Plasma tumor necrosis factor and mortality in critically ill septic patients. Crit Care Med 17:489–494
40. Tracey KJ, Beutler B, Lowry SF, et al (1986) Shock and tissue injury induced by recombinant human cachectin. Science 234:470–474
41. Maury CP, Teppo AM (1987) Raised serum levels of cachectin/tumor necrosis factor alpha in renal allograft rejection. J Exp Med 166:1132–1137
42. Maury CP, Teppo AM (1989) Circulating tumour necrosis factor-alpha (cachectin) in myocardial infarction. J Intern Med 225:333–336
43. Nishimoto N, Yoshizaki K, Tagoh H, et al (1989) Elevation of serum IL-6 prior to acute phase proteins on the inflammation by surgical operation. Clin Immunol Immunopathol 50:313–315

Human and Canine Septic Shock: Studies of Cardiovascular Abnormality, Mediators, and Therapies

C. Natanson and W. D. Hoffman

Introduction

At the National Institutes of Health (NIH), we have conducted clinical and laboratory studies to examine the pathophysiology of the cardiovascular abnormalities in septic shock. We have also developed a canine model that simulates the hemodynamic abnormalities of human septic shock. Results of these and other studies have helped us to understand the mechanisms of septic shock and to evaluate therapies for this highly lethal disorder.

Prevalence of Septic Shock

Septic shock is the most frequent cause of death in intensive care units (ICUs) in the United States [1]. Within the first few days of septic shock, death is frequently caused by refractory hypotension with a low systemic vascular resistance (SVR). In the later stages, death is most frequently caused by sepsis-induced multiple organ system failure syndrome [1]. Even with effective antibiotic therapy, septic shock remains the most prevalent clinical problem in ICUs and a common cause of death.

During the past 50 years, the prevalence of bacterial sepsis has steadily increased. Greater therapeutic use of potent cytotoxic and immunosuppressive drugs, which cause neutropenia or other significant dysfunction on the immune system, have partially led to this increase in septic shock. In addition, increased use of life support systems have placed patients at risk for nosocomial infection. Interestingly, the increased use of broad-spectrum antibiotics has not decreased the incidence of infection but has increased the prevalence of infections caused by resistant microorganisms that are often difficult to eradicate.

Diagnosis

Patients with sepsis or septic shock have diverse symptoms, such as fever, malaise, hypotension, cool extremities with a warm trunk, and chills or rigors. These patients frequently have clinical signs that indicate the source of infection; however, many patients (e.g., the elderly or the immunocompromised) do not have the typical symptoms and signs associated with sepsis, so sepsis shock is often difficult to diagnose. As the disease is so rapidly lethal (40–90% mortality), clinicians should suspect the possibility of septic shock early and treat the disease well before complete diagnostic and clinical information is available [1–3].

Forty % of patients with positive blood cultures will develop septic shock and its accompanying hemodynamic abnormalities [1, 2]. However, in some groups of patients with symptoms indicating a probable diagnosis of septic shock, only about 50% of patients will have positive blood cultures [1, 2]. Patients on antibiotics are less likely than patients not on antibiotics to have positive cultures. Negative cultures may be caused by sampling errors such as false negatives that result from intermittent bacteremia or concurrent antimicrobial therapy. Negative cultures may be caused by bacterial toxins released into the bloodstream without bacteria from the source of infection. Therefore, it is important that clinicians consider the possibility of a diagnosis of septic shock even in patients with negative cultures.

Cardiovascular Abnormality in Septic Shock

Before the 1960s, septic shock was thought to be associated with a decreased cardiac output (CO). In 1965, however, humans with septic shock were shown to have normal or increased CO and low SVR, a finding confirmed in many subsequent studies, which indicated that septic shock was a form of distributive shock. This finding that patients in septic shock had increased or normal CO led to questions about whether septic shock caused myocardial depression [4].

During the 1960s, clinicians began to monitor central venous pressure (CVP) and pulmonary capillary wedge pressure (PCWP) using pulmonary arterial catheters. These hemodynamic measures led to the use of volume resuscitation to treat these patients and to changes in our understanding of septic shock. With adequate preload, patients with septic shock had increased or normal CO. These early studies of patients in septic shock showed them to have a low CO, probably because preload was insufficient.

At the NIH, we study patients in septic shock using serial hemodynamic evaluations. With radionuclide-gated blood pool scans and simultaneous thermodilution pulmonary arterial catheters, we measure systemic pressures, flows, and left ventricular (LV) volumes serially [5, 6]. Data from previous NIH studies show that patients with septic shock develop a significant decrease in LV ejection fraction (EF) within 24 hours of the onset of hypotension (Fig. 1A). This decrease in EF is associated with LV dilation and maintenance of stroke volume (SV) and CO. In survivors, these abnormalities return to normal in seven to ten days. Radionuclide studies of right ventricular (RV) EF also show decreased RVEF and RV dilation. Thus, serial hemodynamic evaluations with radionuclide heart scans reveal a RV and LV dysfunction during sepsis not evident with measures of CO alone. In studies of coronary blood flow, data indicate that sepsis-induced myocardial depression is not caused by an inadequate coronary circulation [7].

Frank-Starling plots also confirm the existence of myocardial depression in septic shock. Patients with septic shock have smaller increases in LV stroke work

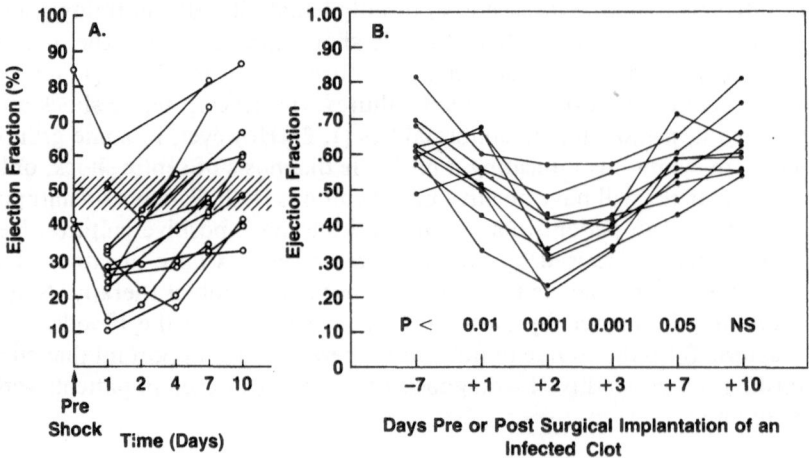

Fig. 1A, B. Serial LVEF vs time in A humans and B dogs with septic shock. Individual EF of patients and dogs are indicated by circles. Lines connect days. The hatched area in Fig. 1A is the normal range. In both Figs. 1A and B, the LVEF profoundly decreases at two to four days and recovers in seven to ten days. (Modified with permission from [21] and [29])

(LVSW) with increases in LV end-diastolic volume (EDV) (produced by volume infusion) than other critically ill patients not in septic shock (Fig. 2A) [5]. Furthermore, when plotting LVSW vs LVEDV for septic shock patients, we found that the curve was downward and to the right, further substantiating the primary LV dysfunction in this disease.

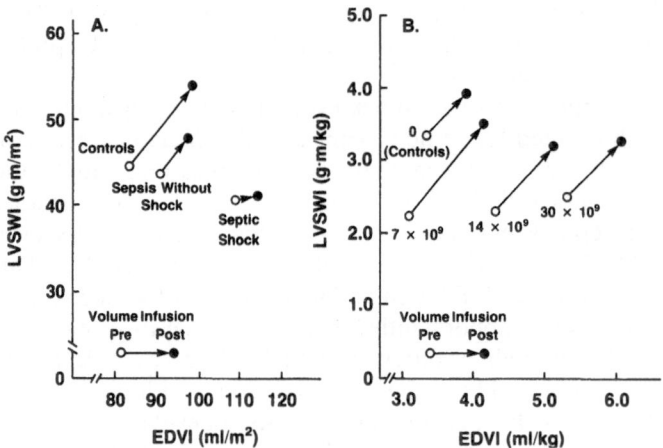

Fig. 2A, B. Frank-Starling Curves of A humans with septic shock (as compared to critically ill controls) and B dogs with septic shock (comparing increasing doses of intraperitoneal bacteria). Mean EDVI and LVSWI are plotted pre- and post-volume infusion. In both Figs. 2A and B, humans and animals with septic shock have Frank-Starling curves downward and to the right, as compared to those of controls. (Modified with permission from [3] and [8])

Interestingly, survivors and nonsurvivors of septic shock have different cardiovascular changes. During the initial phase of sepsis, both survivors and nonsurvivors have increased CO and heart rate (HR), decreased SVR, and normal SV, but later, survivors are more likely than nonsurvivors to have a decreased LVEF with LV dilation [6]. When LVEF is decreased in survivors, the LV dilates to maintain SV and CO via the Frank-Starling mechanism. Even with a low LVEF, nonsurvivors are less likely than survivors to have compensatory LV dilation, and therefore cannot maintain SV. Thus, nonsurvivors depend on increased HR to maintain CO [8], but when HR can no longer maintain CO, death is likely to occur.

Within 24 hours of the onset of hypotension, nonsurvivors (compared to survivors) have significantly more tachycardia, increased CO, and decreased SVR. Therefore, patients maintaining the hyperdynamic state for more than 24 hours have a poor prognosis. In fact, many nonsurvivors have a normal or increased CO immediately before death. In septic shock, most early deaths are caused not by decreased CO but by refractory hypotension from decreased SVR, whereas few early deaths are caused by decreased CO. Consequently, the majority of early deaths caused by septic shock are the result of peripheral vascular abnormality rather than myocardial abnormality [9].

Pathogenesis of Septic Shock

Most non-immunocompromised patients with septic shock have a diagnosable site of infection. Usually, the site of infection is clinically apparent [5, 6]. In contrast, only 50% of septic patients with granulocytopenia have a clinically apparent site of infection. Some investigators hypothesize that these patients may have small, clinically obscure areas of damage that infect the skin, lung, or bowel by releasing microorganisms or leaking toxins into the bloodstream.

The cardiovascular abnormalities and the multiple organ system dysfunction found in septic shock may not be caused directly by microorganisms, but by the release of harmful endogenous substances, such as tumor necrosis factor (TNF) and interleukin-1 (IL-1), in response to exogenous toxins (endotoxins and exotoxins) (Fig. 3). At the NIH, we are currently investigating the complex roles and interactions of exogenous and endogenous substances in producing the abnormalities associated with septic shock. The results of these and other studies have shown that mediators and toxins have an important role in the pathogenesis of septic shock.

Bacterial Factors Mediating Septic Shock

Endotoxin: Endotoxin is a lipopolysaccharide in the outer membrane of gram-negative bacteria [10], which is considered by many to be the primary mediator to induce the cardiovascular abnormalities of septic shock [11]. In a recent NIH study, serial endotoxin levels were measured in ICU patients with probable septic shock. The results of this study showed that endotoxemia correlated with

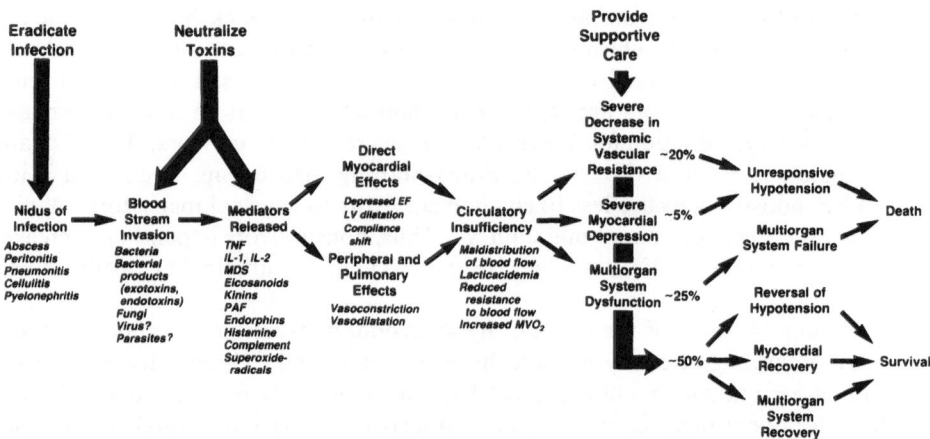

Fig. 3. The pathogenesis of septic shock starting from the nidus of infection and ending in death. Bloodstream invasion of bacteria, fungi, or their toxins induces release of endogenous mediators that have both direct myocardial effects and peripheral circulatory effects. These events lead to circulatory insufficiency in many organ systems and three distinct syndromes that cause death: refractory hypotension caused by a low SVR (approximately 40% of deaths); refractory hypotension from decreased CO (approximately 10% of deaths); and multiple organ system failure (approximately 50% of deaths). (Modified with permission from [13]). Abbreviations: *TNF* (tumor necrosis factor), *IL-1* and *IL-2* (interleukin-1 and -2), *MDS* (myocardial depressant substance), *PAF* (platelet activating factor), *MVO₂* (myocardial oxygen consumption)

measures of disease severity (especially in those patients with positive blood cultures) and that both gram-positive bacteria (without endotoxin) and gram-negative bacteria (with endotoxin) produced the same cardiovascular changes. In another NIH study, endotoxin was given to normal volunteers and found to produce cardiovascular changes similar to those of septic shock [12]. The results of these two studies suggest that endotoxin alone can produce the cardiovascular abnormalities of septic shock and that endotoxin is probably an important pathogenic mediator in some bacterial infections, as the presence of endotoxemia in bacteremic patients with septic shock correlated with death. These results also suggest that endotoxin is not the only mediator of septic shock, as gram-positive bacteria, an organism without endotoxin, produced the same cardiovascular abnormalities of septic shock as those with gram-negative bacteria.

Other Bacterial Toxins: In addition to endotoxin, gram-negative bacteria produce a number of enzymes and other toxins, such as alpha-hemolysin and exotoxin A, may function synergistically with endotoxin to induce septic shock or to induce multiple organ system failure [4, 13].

Gram-positive bacteria, which have no endotoxin, possess common cellular components that have toxic effects and produce exotoxins (e. g., toxic shock syndrome toxin-1), which are pathogenic in a variety of clinical syndromes. Cell wall components, such as peptidoglycans, myramyl dipeptide, and lipoteichoic acids, have also been implicated in septic shock. Several studies have shown that gram-positive bacterial products have toxic effects, indicating an important role for these substances in the pathogenesis of gram-positive septic shock [13].

Host Factors Mediating Septic Shock

Tumor Necrosis Factor: TNF is a 10- to 20-kilodalton protein produced by macrophages, which may also have a role in the pathogenesis of septic shock. When we administered endotoxin to normal human volunteers, it produced measurable circulating TNF within 60 and 90 minutes [14]. In several animal models of septic shock, TNF administration can produce cardiovascular dysfunction, multiple organ system failure, and lethality [15]. Furthermore, animals pretreated with monoclonal or polyclonal antibodies to TNF have been shown to resist infection following challenge with gram-negative bacteria or endotoxin [16, 17]. Therefore, TNF, which may be released in response to circulating endotoxin or viable bacteria, is an important pathogenic mediator in septic shock.

Interleukin-1 and Interleukin-2 (IL-2): Like TNF, IL-1 is produced by macrophages in response to endotoxin or viable microorganisms. IL-1 administration may induce fever and hypotension, decrease SVR, activate T-lymphocytes, and stimulate the release of other lymphokines [18]. When given to rabbits, IL-1 is synergistic to TNF in producing the hemodynamic effects of septic shock [18]. The cyclooxygenase inhibitor, ibuprofen, inhibits the hemodynamic effects induced by IL-1, suggesting that IL-1 works via a prostaglandin pathway.

IL-2 is produced by T-lymphocytes and has been used recently to treat certain human cancers. The IL-2 molecule has been shown to enhance natural killer cell cytotoxicity and to increase cytotoxicity against tumor cells. In a recent study in humans, the hemodynamic effects of IL-2 were evaluated during its use as an antitumor drug. In this study, IL-2 decreased MAP, SVR, and LVEF, and increased CO, HR, and LVEDV [3]. These cardiovascular abnormalities are similar to those produced by human septic shock, suggesting that IL-2 may be an important endogenous mediator of the cardiovascular abnormalities of human septic shock.

Other Mediators: Other substances possibly involved in the pathogenesis of septic shock are complement, myocardial depressant substance (MDS), kinins, endorphins, eicosanoids, platelet activating factor, superoxide radicals, and other lymphokines. In human studies, complement activation has been associated with septic shock and levels of C5a, which have been correlated with decreased SVR in septic shock patients [19]. In other studies, MDS has been found in the sera of patients with septic shock [20]. Furthermore, *in vitro* MDS activity has been correlated with *in vivo* decreased LVEF, LV dilation, and increased circulating lactate. All of these mediators may play a pathogenic role in septic shock, probably interacting in a complex fashion. Thus, additional studies are necessary to determine how these mediators affect the hemodynamic and multiple organ system dysfunction of septic shock.

A Canine Model of Septic Shock

At the NIH, we have developed a canine model that stimulated the pattern of cardiovascular abnormality found in human septic shock. In this animal model, we implant an infected fibrin clot into the peritoneal cavity [21], which causes a slow release of bacteria and toxins, thereby simulating the course of many human bacterial infections. In this model, the cardiovascular function of these dogs is evaluated serially using radionuclide heart scans and thermodilution pulmonary arterial catheters over two to four weeks, the time period when cardiovascular changes occur in human septic shock. Animals are given no intravenous or inhalation anesthesia to prevent any distortion of these cardiovascular changes. Animals are also studied before and after volume infusion, an important therapy in human septic shock. In two to four days of clot implantation, dogs have decreased LVEF (Fig. 1B). With adequate fluid resuscitation, dogs have LV dilation, high CO, and low SVR. In surviving animals, these hemodynamic changes reverse to normal in seven to ten days [22].

With this canine model, we have been able to perform detailed studies of systolic function under controlled circumstances, and have found that the decreased LVEF correlates with decreases in both load-independent and load-dependent measures of myocardial contractility [23]. Frank-Starling plots (a load-dependent measure) and end-systolic volume pressure plots (a load-independent measure) show that decreased LV function corresponds in time course and magnitude to decreased LVEF (Fig. 2B) [21].

Use of this canine model also led to the finding of decreased systolic myocardial function. With adequate fluid resuscitation, however, SV and CO increased or remained normal [21]. This model has helped us understand the discrepancy between decreased systolic function and increased or normal CO, by providing information on LV volume and diastolic function. At 30–40 hours after clot implantation, we found that the LV dilates without increasing pressure, and that LV dilation maintains SV and CO (Fig. 4), which indicates that LV dilation is the appropriate diastolic compensatory response to a sepsis-induced LV systolic abnormality (decreased LVEF). The observation that LV dilation occurs without change in pressure suggests a sepsis-induced compliance change (i.e., increased compliance) [21]. In fact, humans and dogs have a remarkably similar time course and pattern of sepsis-induced systolic and diastolic changes, suggesting a common mammalian hemodynamic response to infection.

Using this canine model, we examined the effects of changing the dose, type, and viability of the bacterial infection on cardiovascular dysfunction and mortality. Increasing the bacterial dose led to corresponding progressive decreases in LVEF and downward shifts on Frank-Starling (Fig. 2B) and end-systolic volume/pressure LV function plots [8]. The highest bacterial dose ultimately caused death. In surviving animals, higher bacterial doses led to progressive LV dilation, but not to decreases in CO. LV dilation was associated with survival and maintenance of SV and CO, suggesting an important diastolic compensation (LV dilation) for sepsis-induced systolic dysfunction. Consequently, dose was found to be an important factor affecting the cardiovascular abnormalities of septic shock.

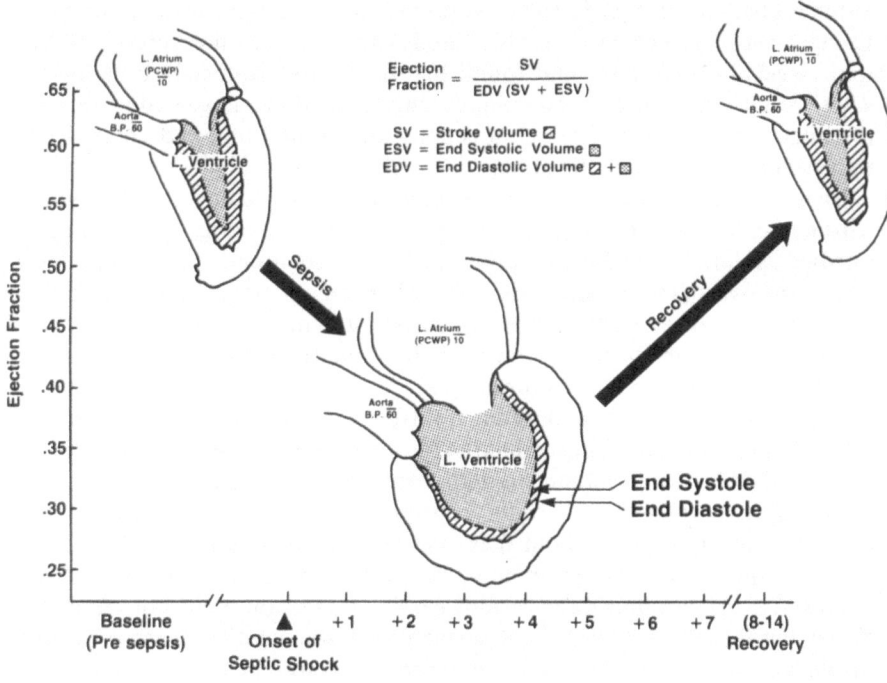

Days Relative to the Onset of Septic Shock

Fig. 4. This figure shows that cardiac output is maintained despite depressed EF during septic shock. The three left ventricles depict the serial changes during septic shock from pre-sepsis (baseline), days two to four of sepsis, and post-sepsis (recovery). The shaded area is the end-systolic volume. The hatched area is the stroke volume. These two areas combined are the end-diastolic volume. On days 2 to 4 of sepsis, the EF decreases, but because the heart is dilated (large EDV), the stroke volume does not change. (Modified with permission from [9])

Changes in bacterial type and viability also affect the cardiovascular response and mortality of patients with septic shock [22]. When comparing the same dose of *Staphylococcus aureus* (serotype 8), *E. coli* (06:H1:K2), and *E. coli* (086:H8), we found that *S. aureus* produced the greatest mortality and hemodynamic dysfunction, whereas *E. coli* (06:H1:K2) produced less lethality and *E. coli* (086:H8) the least mortality and hemodynamic dysfunction. We also compared nonviable and viable bacteria (at the same dose) and found that viable bacteria produced greater lethality and hemodynamic dysfunction. Interestingly, all bacteria produced the same pattern and time course of hemodynamic changes, indicating that septic shock has a final common pathway of injury.

Mediators of Septic Shock: Endotoxin, a lipopolysaccharide in the outer membrane of gram-negative bacteria, has been proposed as a primary pathogenic mediator in all types (bacterial and non-bacterial) of septic shock. To test this hypothesis, we implanted *S. aureus* (a gram-positive organism without endotoxin) in dogs and found that it produced the same cardiovascular changes seen in animals challenged with *E. coli* (a gram-negative organism with endotoxin) [22]. Using a sensitive chromogenic limulus lysate assay, we measured serial endotoxin levels in these dogs and found that *S. aureus* produced no endotoxemia. These results show that not all animals with septic shock have endotoxemia from the infecting bacteria or from endogenous sources and that endotoxin is not the universal mediator of septic shock.

These results led us to examine whether endotoxin alone could produce the cardiovascular changes of septic shock. To answer this question, we implanted purified endotoxin in the intraperitoneal clot and found that it produced the same cardiovascular abnormalities of viable bacterial clots. Therefore, it appears that endotoxin or endotoxemia is not necessary to produce septic shock, but that endotoxin alone is sufficient and probably one of many other bacterial toxins capable of producing this syndrome [22].

In another study, we compared two different *E. coli* strains to determine their effects on endotoxemia and lethality [24]. Dogs received similar doses of either *E. coli* (06:H1:K2), an organism with virulence factors associated with human infection (e.g., hemolysis, serum resistance, and encapsulation), or *E. coli* (086:H8), an organism without these virulence factors. Serum endotoxin levels were measured serially over 28 days. The results of this study showed that both strains of *E. coli* produced the cardiovascular depression typical of human septic shock, but that the *E. coli* strain associated with human disease virulence factors produced greater lethality and more profound and prolonged hemodynamic changes. Interestingly, endotoxin levels were higher in dogs receiving the nonvirulent organism. These data indicate that the virulence factors of some gram-negative bacteria are more important than the level of endotoxemia produced in determining morbidity [24].

Recent studies suggest that the endogenous mediators, such as TNF, IL-1 and IL-2, complement, MDS, eicosanoids, endorphins, platelet activating factor, kinins, and superoxide radicals, which are produced in response to multiple infecting agents, may be mechanisms of the final common pathway of injury in septic shock. In one NIH study, TNF was given intravenously to dogs and found to produce all of the progressive decreases in cardiovascular function normally produced by viable bacteria [25]. In another study, we administered high doses of IL-1 to dogs and found that it produced minimal hemodynamic effects and none of the serial changes seen with viable bacteria or TNF [26]. These two studies indicate that TNF may be one important endogenous mediator of septic shock, but that IL-1 alone cannot produce the characteristic hemodynamic changes of this disease.

Clinical Therapies: Using this canine model, we evaluated the efficacy of cardiovascular support and antibiotic therapy, two conventional treatments for septic shock [27]. All dogs were given a lethal dose of *E. coli* and then one of the following four treatments: antibiotics alone, cardiovascular support alone, combined antibiotics and cardiovascular support, and no therapy (controls). Antibiotic treatment consisted of gentamicin and cefoxitin for ten days. Cardiovascular support consisted of fluid and dopamine titrated to a hemodynamic end point, the same therapy administered to humans in septic shock. Dogs receiving combined therapies had 43% survival, dogs receiving no therapy had 0% survival, and dogs receiving either antibiotics alone or cardiovascular support alone had only 13% survival. Our results also showed that cardiovascular support prolonged survival, giving antibiotics sufficient time to become effective. Thus, cardiovascular support and antibiotic treatment when used together were effective treatment for septic shock, but either therapy when used alone was ineffective.

In another study of clinical therapy, we examined whether plasmapheresis improves survival in septic shock [28]. Plasmapheresis was studied because it was thought to be a possible technique to eliminate toxic mediators of the septic shock syndrome by removing the noncellular blood components. In this study, we implanted lethal doses of bacteria intraperitoneally in dogs treated with fluids and antibiotics. Three study groups were defined: a control group that received no further therapy; a sham pheresis group that had plasmapheresis at 5 h and 24 h post-clot implantation and then had their own infected plasma immediately returned; and a true pheresis group that had plasmapheresis at 5 h and 24 h and then had this volume of plasma replaced with uninfected fresh frozen canine plasma. Surprisingly, the control group and the sham pheresis group had higher survival rates and less hemodynamic depression than the true pheresis group, indicating that plasmapheresis worsened hemodynamics and increased mortality. Therefore, we found that plasmapheresis was more harmful than beneficial in this animal model of septic shock.

References

1. Parrillo JE (1989) Septic shock in humans: Clinical evaluation, pathophysiology, and therapeutic approach. In: Shoemaker WC, Thompson WL, Holbrook PR (eds) Textbook of critical care, 2nd edn. Saunders, Philadelphia, pp 1006–1023
2. McCabe WR, Kreger BE, Johns M (1972) Type-specific and cross-reactive antibodies in gram-negative bacteremia. N Engl J Med 287:261–267
3. Ognibene FP, Rosenberg SA, Lotze M, et al (1988) Interleukin-2 administration causes reversible hemodynamic changes and left ventricular dysfunction similar to those seen in septic shock. Chest 94:750–754
4. MacLean LD, Mulligan WG, McLean APH, et al (1967) Patterns of septic shock in man: A detailed study of 56 patients. Ann Surg 166:543–562
5. Ognibene FP, Parker MM, Natanson C, et al (1988) Depressed left ventricular performance: Response to volume infusion in patients with sepsis and septic shock. Chest 93:903–910
6. Parker MM, Shelhamer JH, Natanson C, et al (1987) Serial cardiovascular variables in survivors and nonsurvivors of human septic shock: Heart rate as an early predictor of prognosis. Crit Care Med 15:923–929
7. Cunnion RE, Schaer GL, Parker MM, et al (1986) The coronary circulation in human septic shock. Circulation 73:637–644
8. Natanson C, Danner RL, Fink MP, et al (1988) Cardiovascular performance with E. coli challenges in a canine model of human sepsis. Am J Physiol 254 (Heart Circ Physiol 23):H558–H569
9. Natanson C, Parrillo JE (1988) Septic shock. Anesth Clin North Am 6:73–85
10. Danner RL, Elin RJ, Hosseini JM, et al (1988) Endotoxin determinations in 100 patients with septic shock. Clin Res 36:453 (abstract)
11. Hinshaw LB, Archer LT, Greenfield LJ, et al (1971) Effects of endotoxin on myocardial hemodynamics, performance, and metabolism. Am J Physiol 221:504–510

12. Suffredini AF, Fromm RE, Parker MM, et al (1989) The cardiovascular response of normal humans to the administration of endotoxin. N Engl J Med 321:280–287

13. Danner RL, Suffredini AF, Natanson C, Parrillo JE (1989) Microbial toxins: Role in the pathogenesis of septic shock and multiple organ failure. In: Bihari DJ, Cerra FB (eds) Multiple organ failure. Soc Crit Care Med, Fullerton, CA, pp 151–191

14. Fromm RE, Suffredini AF, Kovacs JA, et al (1988) Serum tumor necrosis factor response in humans receiving endotoxin. Clin Res 36:372A (abstract)

15. Tracey KJ, Lowry SF, Fahey TJ, et al (1987) Cachectin/tumor necrosis factor induces lethal shock and stress hormone responses in the dog. Surg Gynecol Obstet 164:415–422

16. Beutler B, Cerami A (1986) Cachectin and tumor necrosis factor as two sides of the same biological coin. Nature 320:584–588

17. Tracey KJ, Fong Y, Hesse DG, et al (1987) Anti-cachectin/TNF monoclonal antibodies prevent septic shock during lethal bacteremia. Nature 330:662–664

18. Okusawa S, Gelfand JA, Ikejima T, et al (1988) Interleukin 1 induces a shock-like state in rabbits: Synergism with tumor necrosis factor and the effect of cyclooxygenase inhibition. J Clin Invest 81:1162–1172

19. Ognibene FP, Parker MM, Burch-Whitman C, et al (1988) Neutrophil aggregation activity and septic shock in humans: Neutrophil aggregation by a C5a-like material occurs more frequently than complement component depletion and correlates with depression of systemic vascular resistance. J Crit Care 3:103–111

20. Parrillo JE, Burch C, Shelhamer JH, et al (1985) A circulating myocardial depressant substance in humans with septic shock: Septic shock patients with a reduced ejection fraction have a circulating factor that depresses in vitro myocardial cell performance. J Clin Invest 76:1539–1553

21. Natanson C, Fink MP, Ballantyne HK, et al (1986) Gram-negative bacteremia produces both severe systolic and diastolic cardiac dysfunction in a canine model that simulates human septic shock. J Clin Invest 78:259–270

22. Natanson C, Danner RL, Elin RJ, et al (1989) The role of endotoxemia in cardiovascular dysfunction and mortality: *Escherichia coli* and *Staphylococcus aureus* challenges in a canine model of human septic shock. J Clin Invest 83:243–251

23. Hoffman WD, Natanson C, Danner RL, et al (1987) Load-insensitive and load-sensitive cardiovascular measures are abnormal during septic shock. Clin Res 35:787A (abstract)

24. Hoffman WD, Natanson C, Danner RL, et al (1989) Bacterial organism virulence factors may be more important than endotoxemia in determining cardiovascular dysfunction and mortality in canine septic shock. Clin Res 37:344A (abstract)

25. Natanson C, Eichenholz PW, Danner RL, et al (1989) Endotoxin and tumor necrosis factor challenges in dogs simulate the cardiovascular profile of human septic shock. J Exp Med 169:823–832

26. Natanson C, Eichacker PQ, Hoffman WD, et al (1989) Human recombinant interleukin-1 produced minimal effects on canine cardiovascular function. Clin Res 37:346A (abstract)

27. Natanson C, Danner RL, Akin GL, et al (1988) Antibiotics, fluids and dopamine in a lethal canine model of septic shock: Effects on survival. Clin Res 36:372A (abstract)

28. Natanson C, Hoffman WD, Danner RL, et al (1989) A controlled trial of plasmapheresis fails to improve outcome in an antibiotic treated canine model of human septic shock. Clin Res 37:346A (abstract)

29. Parker MM, Shelhamer JH, Bacharach SL, et al (1984) Profound but reversible myocardial depression in patients with septic shock. Ann Intern Med 100:483–490

Myocardial Dysfunction in Sepsis

H. J. Silverman

Introduction

Sepsis and septic shock remain a major cause of mortality among critically ill patients. Endeavors to discern the underlying pathophysiology have included investigation of the physiologic abnormalities with an eye towards optimal support of the circulation in general and enhancement of oxygen uptake in particular. Due to methodological contraints and conceptual limitations, however, the precise understanding of the hemodynamic abnormalities in sepsis remains elusive and has continued to spark controversy.

The major recognized cardiovascular abnormalities include peripheral vascular dilatation producing hypotension and a microcirculatory defect causing impaired oxygen uptake and oxygen supply dependency.

Recently, investigators have also uncovered the existence of myocardical dysfunction in experimental endotoxic and septic shock, as well as in human septic shock. Acceptance of this belief has followed a tortuous path, because of the high cardiac index (CI) present in most patients and the difficulty of measuring intrinsic cardiac function in the *in vivo* state. Indeed, the CI, as well as other indices of myocardial performance, is sensitive to changes in preload and afterload, and hence, discrimination between abnormal contractility and altered loading conditions is difficult in a shock disorder manifested by alterations in peripheral vascular function. Furthermore, sympatho-adrenal activation, as well as catecholamine release, can enhance myocardial contractility and increase the heart rate to compensate for a decreased stroke volume, thus masking intrinsic myocardial dysfunction. Nonetheless, several different indices of myocardial performance have been used in an attempt to better define cardiac function in endotoxemia and septicemia.

Assessment of Myocardial Function in Animal Studies

Investigators have used ejection phase indices and left ventricular performance curves to demonstrate myocardial dysfunction in several *in vitro* and *in vivo* animal models of endotoxemia [1-3]. Recently, Goldfarb et al. [4] have shown myocardial dysfunction in endotoxemia with end-systolic pressure-diameter measurements, an index of contractility considered by these investigators to be load-independent, although this belief remains controversial [5].

The resulting acute shock state (low CI, high systemic vascular resistance index (SVRI)), however, after the acute administration of large doses of intravenous endotoxin in these animal models, does not consistently reproduce conditions commonly seen in human sepsis (high CI, low SVRI). Hence, the application of observations made in acute endotoxin animal studies to the clinical setting is seriously questioned.

In an effort to replicate the hyperdynamic state of human sepsis, several investigators have developed chronic animal models of septicemia. McDonough et al. [6] developed a model of experimental sepsis by intraperitoneal administration of a pooled fecal inoculum, which produced many of the hemodynamic and metabolic alterations seen in clinical sepsis: fever, tachycardia, mild hypotension, increase in cardiac output and oxygen consumption, and lactic acidemia. Hearts removed from septic rats during this high flow state and perfused *in vitro* using an isolated heart preparation showed a rightward and downward shift in the work function curve, indicative of a severe depression of myocardial function. In a chronically instrumented, awake canine model of hyperdynamic sepsis produced by cecal ligation, Pasque et al. [7] observed in the end-systolic pressure-dimension relationship at 3 and 5 days following cecal ligation.

Finally, Natanson et al. [8] developed a model of hyperdynamic canine sepsis by the implantation of an infected fibrin clot into the peritoneal cavity. Serial determinations of hemodynamics using thermodilution cardiac outputs and radionuclide cineangiography were performed in conscious unsedated animals to determine left ventricular ejection fraction (LVEF) and end-diastolic volumes in the absence of anesthesia effects. Two days post-implantation, there were decreases in LVEF and a downward shift in the ventricular function curve. These results, consistent with a decrease in systolic ventricular performance, was also associated with ventricular dilatation, similar to what was observed in human sepsis by these investigators [9].

Assessment of Myocardial Function in Human Sepsis

Ventricular Function Curves

Several investigators [10–12] have focused on the Frank-Starling relationship as a means to evaluate myocardial function in clinical sepsis. In general, depressed responses to fluid-induced increases in preload, as reflected by the pulmonary artery wedge pressure (PAWP), have been observed. In one investigation [10] 50% of the septic patients exhibited a decrease in the ventricular performance curve in response to fluid loading, whereas in another study [11], only 18 of 40 patients with septic shock exhibited an increase in cardiac output of more than 20%, while 8 patients had decreases in this parameter despite increases in the PAWP. These abnormal responses to fluid administration can be attributed to a decrease in intrinsic myocardial contractility, an increase in impedance to ejection, or a decrease in ventricular compliance [13].

Due to the real possibility of changes in left ventricular compliance during sepsis [14], measurement of end-diastolic volume rather than the PAWP would more accurately reflect left ventricular preload. Hence, Ognibene et al. [12] constructed left ventricular performance curves during volume infusion using serial data from simultaneously obtained thermodilution cardiac output measurements and radionuclide cineangiography to calculate left ventricular end-diastolic volume index (LVEDVI). Left ventricular stroke work index (LVSWI) was used as the measure of ventricular performance. Two patterns of abnormal ventricular performance were observed: some patients exhibited an abnormality in ventricular contractility, as evidenced by failure of the LVSWI to increase despite an increase in LVEDVI; whereas other patients demonstrated a compliance abnormality, as evidenced by a lack of an increase in LVEDVI despite increases in the PAWP after volume infusion. A reduction in LV compliance can be caused by myocardial edema [15], increases in RV end-diastolic volume with subsequent effects on LV distensibility (ventricular interdependence [16]), or high prevolume end-diastolic volumes, which prevents further increases in ventricular dilatation.

Left Ventricular Ejection Fraction

Several investigators have measured LV ejection fraction (LVEF) with radionuclide cineangiography to assess myocardial function in human sepsis. Calvin et al. [17] observed a normal mean LVEF in septic patients without shock; however, 25% of the individual patients had a LVEF less than 0.40.

Parker et al. [9] observed a normal or an elevated CI in 19 of 20 patients with septic shock, but 10 of these patients had moderate or severe depression of LVEF to 40% or less. Paradoxically, survivors had a lower LVEF and a higher LVEDVI compared with nonsurvivors. In survivors, the reduction in LVEF occurred early in sepsis followed by a slow recovery toward normal cardiac function and ventricular size during a 7–10 day period. The authors concluded that myocardial dysfunction may be an early event and that the ability of the left ventricle to dilate may be an adaptive response important in the maintenance of stroke volume and the prevention of pulmonary edema from a high PAWP.

Ellrodt et al. [18] also observed a reduced ejection fraction associated with ventricular dilatation in septic patients, although disparities between survivors and nonsurvivors were not observed.

Mechanisms of Myocardial Dysfunction in Sepsis

Coronary Hypoperfusion

Early investigators [19, 20] hypothesized a role for coronary hypoperfusion in the precipitation of cardiac dysfunction in acute endotoxemia. However, in a hyperdynamic model of gram-negative septicemia, Lange et al. [21] observed depressed heart function despite elevated coronary blood flows.

In human septic shock, Cunion et al. [22] observed coronary flow rates similar to or higher than controls. No evidence of myocardial hypoxia, defined as myocardial lactate production, were observed in the seven patients studied. Similarly, Dhainaut et al. [23] failed to observe myocardial hypoxia in patients with septic shock, except in 6 patients with both low cardiac output and coronary perfusion pressures. These investigations demonstrated that reduced coronary flow and hence, myocardial ischemia may not be a significant cause of myocardial depression in human septic shock. However, the mean ages of the patients in these clinical studies were 45 and 36 years, respectively, and hence, coronary artery disease may not have been prevalent in these patients. Maintenance of mean arterial pressure may be more important in older individuals with coronary artery disease. Raper and Sibbald [24] showed in nonhypotensive sepsis that patients with clinical evidence of coronary artery disease had significant decreases in cardiac output and diastolic ventricular compliance compared with patients without coronary artery disease.

Pulmonary Vascular Resistance

Right ventricular dysfunction secondary to elevations in pulmonary vascular resistance may play a significant role in sepsis-induced heart failure. Several investigators [25, 26] have observed elevations in pulmonary vascular resistance in human sepsis, while recent studies using nuclear angiography have demonstrated decreased RVEF and RV dilatation in patients with septic shock [27, 28]. Significant correlations, however, could not be demonstrated between depressed RVEF and measures of right ventricular afterload, suggesting that elevated pulmonary vascular resistance is not the sole determinant of RV dysfunction.

Nonetheless, presence of RV dilatation raises the possibility of ventricular interdependence: RV compression of the left ventricle causing impaired LV filling and hence, reduction in cardiac output [16]. This effect may contribute to the compliance abnormalities, as well as the abnormal responses to volume infusion reported in clinical studies [10, 11]. Consequently, aggressive volume infusions require careful hemodynamic monitoring.

Regulation of Calcium Transport in Cardiac Muscle

Cardiac contractility is ultimately dependent on the intracellular calcium concentration and hence, alterations in calcium exchange in heart muscle may play a role in myocardial dysfunction in sepsis. Indeed, several investigators [29–31] have demonstrated evidence of altered calcium homeostasis in endotoxic hearts.

The major mechanisms involved in the movement of calcium are illustrated in Fig. 1. In brief, the influx of calcium from the interstitial fluid via slow channels during depolarization of the sarcolemma triggers the release of calcium from the sarcoplasmic reticulum (SR). The resulting increase in free cytosolic calcium binds to a specific calcium receptor protein, troponin C, which causes conformational changes in the tropomyosin and actin-myosin complex leading to a contractile response (systole). Relaxation (diastole) occurs as a result of calcium re-

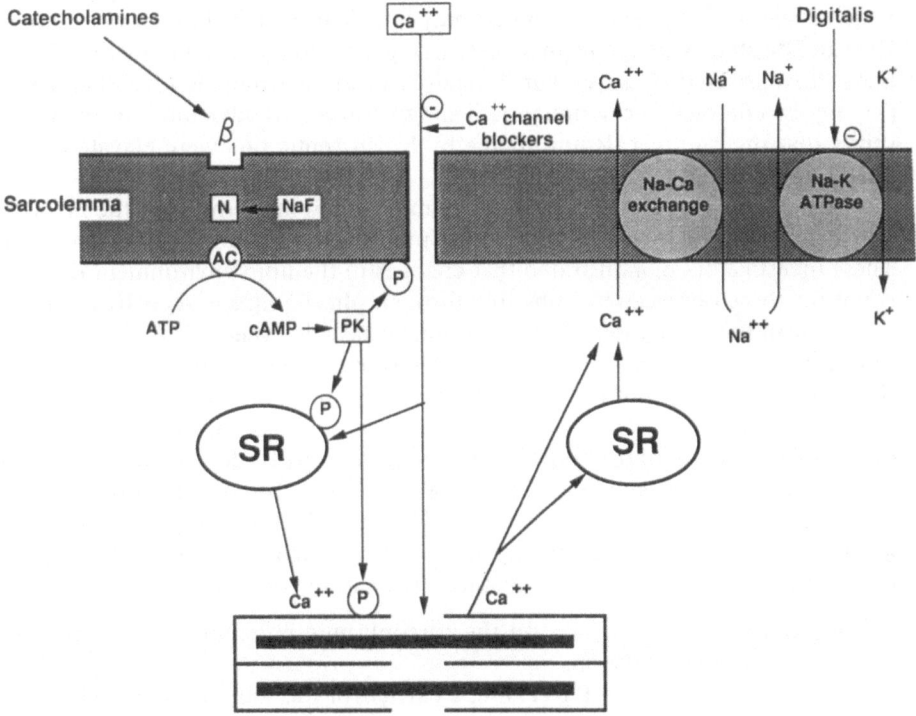

Fig. 1. Mechanisms that potentiate the force of contraction in cardiac muscle. Circulating or neurally released catecholamines stimulate β_1-receptors, which activate adenylate cyclase (AC) via a coupling protein (N). Adenylate cyclase catalyzes the synthesis of cAMP, which activates protein kinase (PK). The active protein kinase phosphorylates proteins (P) in the sarcolemma and sarcoplasmic reticulum, and troponin in the thin filament. The influx of Ca^{++} from the interstitial fluid during excitation triggers the release of Ca^{++} from the sarcoplasmic reticulum (SR). The free cytosolic Ca^{++} activates contraction of the myofilaments (systole). Relaxation (diastole) occurs as a result of uptake of Ca^{++} by the sarcoplasmic reticulum and extrusion of intracellular Ca^{++} by Na^+-Ca^{++} exchange, which is driven by the active transport of Na^+ out of the cell by the Na^+-K^+ pump

uptake by the sarcoplasmic reticulum and extrusion of intracellular calcium by Na-Ca exchange, a passive process driven by the active transport of sodium out of the cell by the Na-K pump.

Calcium homeostasis may be altered in such a way that inadequate calcium is available for contraction and/or removal of cytosolic calcium during diastole is incomplete, thereby causing impaired relaxation and ventricular filling. In the latter case, interventions which decrease calcium entry into the cell would also improve ventricular filling and contractile function.

McDonough et al. [32] demonstrated the complexity of calcium regulation of myocardial function in a hyperdynamic model of experimental sepsis. These investigators showed that myocardial dysfunction was partially improved by increasing calcium delivery with ouabain and also partially alleviated by decreasing calcium influx with the calcium channel blocker, verapamil. The latter observation suggests that calcium overload may impair myocardial function in sepsis. Elevated diastolic calcium from defective sequestration of calcium by the SR has been demonstrated by several investigators in animal models of endotoxemia [33, 34]. In contrast, McDonough [35] showed in a hyperdynamic rat model of sepsis that the rate of calcium uptake by SR in septic rats were elevated compared with control animals.

Alternatively, Liu et al. [36, 37] have demonstrated impairment of the myocardial Na-K pump, as well as the Na-Ca pump after endotoxin administration. These investigators demonstrated that changes in the lipid environment may account for these observations, possibly through phospholipase A_2 activation.

Pivotal in the regulation of calcium homeostasis is cyclic AMP. This ubiquitous intracellular second messenger can substantially alter intracellular calcium flux and thereby the inotropic state. Increases in intracellular cAMP concentration, produced by activation of the membrane-bound enzyme adenylate cyclase or by inhibition of phosphodiesterase, activates cAMP-depentent protein kinases, which are enzymes that phosphorylate other intracellular proteins. Increases in contractility is caused by cAMP-induced phosphorylation of sarcolemma membrane proteins, which opens slow calcium channels leading to greater calcium influx, whereas enhanced relaxation is caused by

1. phosphorylation of ATPase on the sarcoplasmic reticulum, which leads to faster reuptake of calcium,
2. phosphorylation of (Na-K)ATPase, a carrier for the sodium pump, which increases calcium extrusion, or
3. calcium and hence, increased release of calcium.

Catecholamines, through the interaction of cAMP, play a significant role in cardiac contraction and relaxation and therefore, alterations in the β-adrenergic receptor-adenylate cyclase complex may produce impaired myocardial function in sepsis. Indeed, observation of elevated circulating levels of catecholamines and demonstration of a depressed myocardial response to catecholamines in endotoxemia and human septic shock suggest desensitization of β-adrenergic receptors.

Studies from this laboratory have employed an acute model of canine endotoxemia to investigate the effects of endotoxin on the β-adrenergic receptor complex, as well as the precise role of catecholamines in the desensitization process. To distinguish between the effects of endotoxin at the receptor level from those at sites distal to the receptor, lymphocytic β-adrenergic receptor number (measured as binding to [^{125}I]cyanopindolol), as well as NaF- (acting at the nucleotide regulatory protein) stimulated cAMP accumulation was measured.

Table 1 demonstrates the results obtained in animals randomized to three groups: saline vehicle (n = 5), E. coli endotoxin 1.0 mg/kg iv bolus (n = 6), and E. coli endotoxin 1.0 mg/kg after pretreatment with propranolol 1.5 mg/kg iv bolus followed by a continuous infusion 30 μg/kg per min, (n = 5). Five hours after endotoxin injection, lymphocytic β-adrenergic receptor number and NaF-stimulated cAMP accumulation were reduced to 41 ± 6% and 25 ± 7% of baseline values, respectively, which were significantly different from those observed in the control group (both p < 0.01). These changes were associated with a reduced

Table 1. The effects of intravenous endotoxin (1 mg/kg) on lymphocytic beta-adrenergic receptor density (B_{max}) and $NaF(10^{-1}$ M)-stimulated cyclic AMP accumulation in lymphocytes at 5 hours after injection

Treatment	n	B_{max} (fmol/mg protein)		K_d (nM)	
		Baseline	5 Hours	Baseline	5 Hours
Control	5	124±17	180±38 (155±28)	49.8±14.0	49.0±16.2 (95±15)
Endotoxin	5	199±44	84±23 (41± 6)[a,c]	57.6± 7.9	12.8± 3.3 (25± 7)[a]
Endotoxin + Propranolol	4	203±26	259±26 (134±25)	31.0± 6.3	15.1± 7.3 (46±13)[b]

Values are mean ± SEM, numbers in parenthesis refer to mean percent of baseline values. A one-way analysis of variance was performed on these values;
[a] $p < .01$ compared with control;
[b] $p < .02$ compared with control;
[c] $p < .02$ compared with endotoxin + propranolol.

chronotropic response to increasing doses of isoproterenol in the endotoxin group compared with the control group (Fig. 2), suggesting that changes observed on lymphocytic β-adrenergic receptors may be indicative of changes occurring on myocardial tissue. Indeed, reduced β-adrenergic receptor number, as well as altered post-receptor function have been demonstrated in hearts from endotoxin-treated rats [38]. Direct evidence that alterations in lymphocytic β-adrenergic receptors may mirror those on myocardial tissue comes from work performed by Brodde et al. [39], who demonstrated that changes in lymphocytic β₂-adrenergic receptors correlated with changes in myocardial β₁ and β₂-adrenergic receptors in response to non-selective beta-adrenergic agents.

Propranolol pretreatment (Table 1) prevented the endotoxin-induced reduction in β-adrenergic receptor number ($p < 0.02$ compared with the endotoxin group), but not the decrease in NaF-stimulated cAMP accumulation ($p < 0.01$ compared with the control group), suggesting that decreased β-adrenergic receptor number in endotoxic shock is caused by increased plasma levels of circulat-

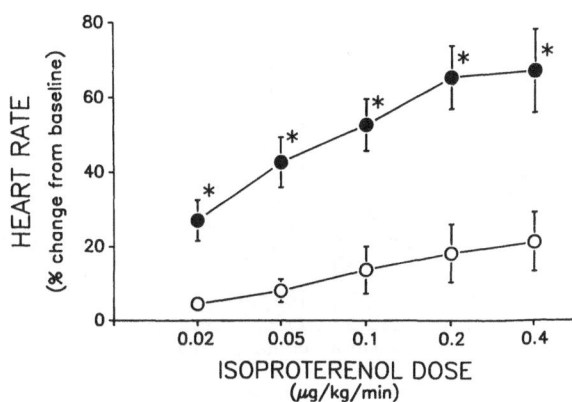

Fig. 2. Heart rate response to an isoproterenol infusion at 5 hours after injection; ●—● control (n=5); o—o endotoxin (n=6); * p<0.05

ing catecholamines, whereas alterations distal to the receptors may be due to other mechanisms, such as activation of protein kinase C [40–42].

Desensitization of β-adrenergic receptors has also been demonstrated in human septic shock [42]. Lymphocytic β-adrenergic receptor function was measured in normal healthy volunteers, non-septic critically ill patients, patients with sepsis, and patients with septic shock. Reduced isoproterenol-stimulated cAMP accumulation was observed in patients with septic shock compared with healthy patients and with critically ill patients without sepsis (Fig. 3). A lesser but significant reduction was also observed in septic patients without shock. NaF-stimulated cAMP accumulation was also significantly depressed in patients with septic shock, but not in patients with sepsis (Fig. 4).

Treatment of Myocardial Dysfunction

A comprehensive discussion of the treatment of myocardial dysfunction is beyond the scope of this chapter, but several recent concepts will be mentioned.

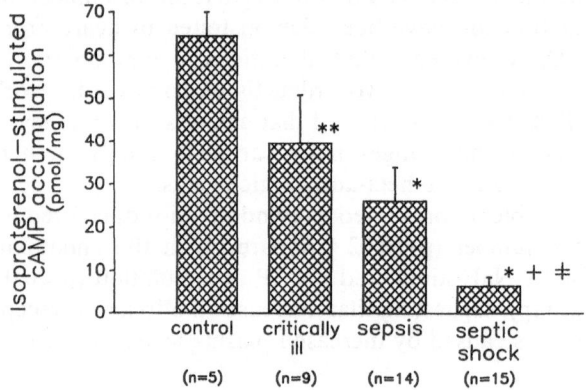

Fig. 3. Isoproterenol-stimulated cAMP accumulation in human lymphocytes; * p < 0.01 vs control, ** p < 0.05 vs control, ⁺ p < 0.05 vs critically ill, ⁺ p < 0.05 vs sepsis

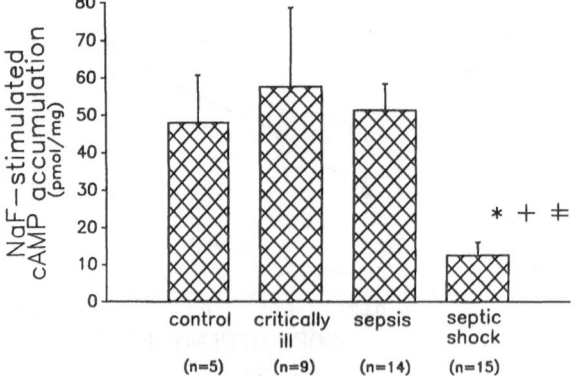

Fig. 4. Sodium fluoride (NaF)-stimulated cAMP accumulation in human lymphocytes; * p < 0.05 vs control, ⁺ p < 0.05 vs critically ill, ⁺ p < 0.01 vs sepsis

Maintenance of an adequate preload is an essential first step in improving myocardial performance. Although recommendations concerning an "optimal PAWP" have been made (e.g. 15 mmHg), careful monitoring is required because increases in filling pressures have been associated with decreases in myocardial performance [10–12]. Furthermore, unexpected large increases in PAWP may occur in patients with decreased myocardial compliance.

After achievement of optimal preload, inotropic support is indicated, regardless of an adequate mean blood pressure, to achieve optimal levels of CI, as well as oxygen delivery (DO_2) and oxygen consumption ($\dot{V}O_2$), in view of the known dependence of $\dot{V}O_2$ on DO_2 in sepsis [43, 44] and the correlation between these values and survival, as demonstrated by Shoemaker et al. [45] in postoperative patients, most of whom had sepsis. Specifically, these investigators observed enhanced survival when CI and DO_2 were maintained above 4.5 L/min·m^2 and 600 ml/min·m^2, respectively.

Dobutamine, an agent with predominant β_1 effects with slight α properties, is probably the preferred inotrope, because it increases cardiac contractility with little chronotropic effect and little or no vasoconstrictor activity [46]. Dosages should probably be maintained below 10 µg/kg/min to avoid increases in heart rate. Further administration of fluids may be required to maximize the CI response to dobutamine due to decreases in preload that occur with this agent [47].

Dopexamine, a dopamine analog, stimulates renal receptors and has potent inotropic effects via activity at β_2-adrenoceptors, but is devoid of α-adrenoreceptor stimulant activity. This agent is probably useful in patients with low cardiac output when inotropic and vasodilatory effects are desirable [48], or when the inotropic effects of dobutamine at β_1-receptors are minimal.

Dopamine has specific dopamine-, non-selective β- and α-adrenergic properties, but its inotropic effects are less compared with dobutamine and unwanted tachycardia occurs at moderate to high doses [46]. Its use, therefore, should probably be restricted at low doses (1–4 µg/kg/min) to selectively improve renal perfusion and urine output, especially when used with norepinephrine [49–51].

Norepinephrine, a potent α-adrenergic and β_1-adrenergic agonist, is recommended to maintain coronary perfusion pressure and thus avoid myocardial ischemia, especially in patients with coronary artery disease. Myocardial oxygen extraction is normally maximal and therefore, increases in myocardial oxygen demand are dependent on increases in coronary blood flow. A complete dependence on β-adrenergic agonists to improve cardiac performance may not adequately increase coronary perfusion; hence, low doses of norepinephrine should be administered (0.5–1.5 µg/kg/min) to maintain mean arterial pressure above 60 mmHg.

Other agents may be administered when the CI response to adrenergic agents are minimal. These include digitalis [52] and amrinone, a phosphodiesterase inhibitor [53]. The efficacy of amrinone may be enhanced if an α-agent (dopamine or norepinephrine) is administered concurrently to counteract amrinone's potent peripheral vasodilating effects.

Prostaglandins (PGE_1 and PGI_2) can also increase cardiac output as well as improve microcirulatory flow. Their exact physiologic effects are probably due to a combination of properties: systemic and pulmonary vasodilatation, inhibition of a myocardial depressant factor, and anti-platelet activity [54].

The role of calcium in the pathophysiology in endotoxemia and sepsis remains controversial. Recently, intracellular calcium overload has been implicated in the development of multiple organ failure [55, 56]. Investigators have observed deleterious effects of calcium administration on survival in endotoxemia [57], whereas calcium channel blocking agents have been observed to improve cardiovascular function and survival in endotoxic shock [58, 59]. Further studies are needed to define the precise role of calcium in septic shock.

Significance of Myocardial Dysfunction

Although the existence of myocardial dysfunction in sepsis is well established, the importance of myocardial dysfunction to mortality in patients with sepsis remains controversial. Parker et al. [9] noted, paradoxically, that a low LVEF was a favorable prognostic sign. Other investigators [18, 60] have observed no differences in other measures of cardiac performance between survivors and nonsurvivors. In contrast, several studies [10, 61] have reported depressed myocardial performance in nonsurvivors compared with survivors.

The presence of a normal CI at the time of death in many patients with sepsis has also prompted several investigators [62] to suggest that a profound peripheral vascular defect is the predominant cause of progressive organ failure and ultimately, death of the patient. But the higher metabolic requirements of the tissues, as well as the oxygen supply dependency that occurs in sepsis require the maintenance of a higher than normal CI (probably greater than $3.5 \, L/min \cdot m^2$) in order to maintain adequate tissue blood flow and oxygenation. In the study performed by Parker et al. [62], the CI was below $3.5 \, L/min \cdot m^2$ in 17 of 29 nonsurvivors of septic shock. Successful treatment, therefore, of patients with sepsis will probably require greater understanding of the myocardial, as well as the peripheral vascular abnormalities that are present in this disease state.

References

1. Hinshaw LB (1979) Myocardial function in endotoxin shock. Circ Shock (suppl) 1:43–51
2. Archer LT (1985) Myocardial dysfunction in endotoxin- and E. coli-induced shock: pathophysiological mechanisms. Circ Shock 15:261–280
3. McDonough KH, Brumfield BA, Lang CH (1986) In vitro myocardial performance after lethal and nonlethal doses of endotoxin. Am J Physiol 250:H240–H246
4. Goldfarb RD, Tambolini W, Wiener SM, Weber PB (1983) Canine left ventricular performance during LD50 endotoxemia. Am J Physiol 244:H370–H377
5. Carabello BA, Spann JF (1984) The uses and limitations of end-systolic indexes of left ventricular function. Circulation 69:1058–1064
6. McDonough KH, Lang CH, Spitzer JJ (1984) Depressed function of isolated hearts from hyperdynamic septic rats. Circ Shock 12:241–251
7. Pasque MK, Van Trigt P, Pellom GL, Freedman BM, Wechsler AS (1988) Assessment of the intrinsic contractile status of the heart during sepsis by myocardial pressure-dimension analysis. Ann Surg 208:110–117

8. Natanson C, Fink MP, Ballantyne HK, MacVittie TJ, Conklin JJ, Parrillo JE (1986) Gram-negative bacteremia produces both severe systolic and diastolic cardiac dysfunction in a canine model that simulates human septic shock. J Clin Invest 78:259-270

9. Parker MM, Shelhamer JH, Bacharach SL, et al (1984) Profound but reversible myocardial depression in patients with septic shock. Ann Intern Med 100:483-490

10. Weisel RD, Vito L, Dennis RC, Valeri CR, Hechtman HB (1977) Myocardial depression during sepsis. Am J Surg 133:512-521

11. Winslow EJ, Loeb HS, Rahimtoola SH, Kamath S, Gunnar RM (1973) Hemodynamic studies and results of therapy in 50 patients with bacteremic shock. Am J Med 54:421-432

12. Ognibene FP, Parker MM, Natanson C, Shelhamer JH, Parrillo JE (1988) Depressed left ventricular performance: response to volume infusion in patients with sepsis and septic shock. Chest 93:903-910

13. Calvin JE, Driedger AA, Sibbald WJ (1981) The hemodynamic effect of rapid fluid infusion in critically ill patients. Surgery 90:61-76

14. Calvin JE, Driedger AA, Sibbald WJ (1981) Does the pulmonary capillary wedge pressure predict left ventricular preload in critically ill patients? Crit Care Med 9:437-443

15. Postel J, Schloerb PR (1977) Cardiac depression in bacteremia. Ann Surg 186:74-82

16. Brinker JA, Weiss I, Lappe DL, et al (1980) Leftward septal displacement during right ventricular loading in man. Circulation 61:626-633

17. Calvin JE, Driedger AA, Sibbald WJ (1981) An assessment of myocardial function in human sepsis utilizing ECG gated cardiac scintigraphy. Chest 38:579-586

18. Ellrodt AG, Riedlinger MS, Kinchi A, et al (1985) Left ventricular performance in septic shock: reversible segmental and global abnormalities. Am Heart J 110:402-409

19. Elkins RC, McCurdy JR, Brown PP, Greenfield LJ (1973) Effects of coronary perfusion on myocardial performance during endotoxin shock. Surg Gynecol Obstet 137:991-996

20. Kleinman WM, Krause SM, Hess ML (1980) Differential subendocardial perfusion and injury during the course of gram-negative endotoxemia. Adv Shock Res 4:139-152

21. Lang CH, Bagby GJ, Ferguson JL, Spitzer JJ (1984) Cardiac output and redistribution of organ blood flow in hypermetabolic sepsis. Am J Physiol 246:R331-R337

22. Cunnion RE, Schaer GL, Parker MM, Natanson C, Parrillo JE (1986) The coronary circulation in human septic shock. Circulation 73:637-644

23. Dhainaut JF, Huyghebaert MF, Monsallier JF, et al (1987) Coronary hemodynamics and myocardial metabolism of lactate, free fatty acids, glucose and ketones in human septic shock. Circulation 75:533-541

24. Raper RF, Sibbald WJ (1988) The effects of coronary artery disease on cardiac function in nonhypotensive sepsis. Chest 94:507-511

25. Clowes GHA, Farrington GH, Zuschneid W, Cossette GR, Sarvis C (1970) Circulating factors in the etiology of pulmonary insufficiency and right ventricular failure accompanying sepsis (peritonitis) Ann Surg 171:663-678

26. Sibbald WJ, Paterson NAM, Holliday RL, et al (1978) Pulmonary hypertension in sepsis. Chest 73:583-591

27. Hoffman MJ, Greenfield LJ, Sugerman HJ, Tatum JL (1983) Unsuspected right ventricular dysfunction in shock and sepsis. Ann Surg 198:307-319

28. Kimchi A, Ellrodt AG, Berman DS, et al (1984) Right ventricular performance in septic shock: a combined radionuclide and hemodynamic study. J Am Coll Cardiol 4:945-951

29. Deaciuc IV, Spitzer JA (1987) Calcium content in liver and heart and its intracellular distribution in liver during endotoxicosis and sepsis in rats. Cell Calcium 8:365-376

30. Levison MA, Tsao TC, Trunkey DD (1984) Myocardial depression. The effect of Ca^{++} and calcium flux during sepsis. Arch Surg 119:803-808

31. Carli A, Auclair M-C, Vernimmen C, Jourdon P (1979) Reversal by calcium of rat heart cell dysfunction induced by human sera in septic shock. Circ Shock 6:147-157

32. McDonough KH, Lang CH, Spitzer JJ (1985) Effect of cardiotropic agents on the myocardial dysfunction of hyperdynamic sepsis. Circ Shock 17:1-19

33. Soulsby EM, Bruni FD, Looney TJ, Hess ML (1974) Influence of endotoxin on myocardial calcium transport and the effect of augmented venous return. Circ Shock 5:23-34

34. Estes JE, Farley PE, Goldfarb RD (1980) Effect of shock on calcium accumulation by cardiac sarcoplasmic reticulum. Adv Shock Res 3:229-237

35. McDonough KH (1988) Calcium uptake by sarcoplasmic reticulum isolated from hearts of septic rats. Circ Shock 25:291-297
36. Liu M-S, Ghosh S (1986) Myocardial sodium pump activity in endotoxin shock. Circ Shock 19:177-184
37. Liu M-S, Xuan Y-T (1986) Mechanisms of endotoxin-induced impairment in Na^+-Ca^{2+} exchange in canine myocardium. Am J Physiol 251:R1078-R1085
38. Shepherd RE, McDonough KH, Burns AH (1986) Mechanism of cardiac dysfunction in hearts from endotoxin-treated rats. Circ Shock 19:371-384
39. Brodde O-E, Becheringh JJ, Michel MC (1987) Human heart beta-adrenoceptors: a fair comparison with lymphocyte beta-adrenoreceptors? TIPS 8:403-407
40. Katada T, Gilman AG, Watanabe Y, Bauer S, Jakobs KH (1985) Protein kinase phosphorylates the inhibitory guanine-nucleotide-binding regulatory component and apparently suppresses its function in hormonal inhibition of adenylate cyclase. Eur J Biochem 151:431-437
41. Wightman PD, Raetz CRH (1984) The activation of protein kinase C by biologically active lipid moieties of lipopolysaccharide. J Biol Chem 259:10048-10052
42. Silverman HJ, Penaranda R, Orens J, Lee N, el-Fakahany EE (1989) Deterioration of the beta-adrenergic receptor complex in human septic shock. Am Rev Respir Dis 135:A351
43. Kaufman BS, Rackow ED, Falk JL (1984) The relationship between oxygen delivery and consumption during fluid resuscitation of hypovolemic and septic shock. Chest 85:336-340
44. Haupt MT, Gilbert RM, Carlson RW (1985) Fluid loading increases oxygen consumption in septic patients with lactic acidosis. Am Rev Respir Dis 131:912-916
45. Shoemaker WC, Appel PL, Kram HB, Waxman K, Lee T-S (1988) Prospective trial of supranormal values of survivors as therapeutic goals in high-risk surgical patients. Chest 94:1176-1186
46. Mueller HS (1986) Catecholamine support of the critically ill cardiac patient: inotropic agents versus vasopressors: α- or β-adrenergic agonists or both? Intensive & Crit Care Digest 5:36-39
47. Vincent J-L, Van der Linden P, Domb M, Blecic S, Azimi G, Bernard A (1987) Dopamine compared with dobutamine in experimental septic shock: Relevance to fluid administration. Anesth Analg 66:565-571
48. Colardyn FC, Vandenbogaerde JF, Vogelaers DP, Verbeke JH (1989) Use of dopexamine hydrochloride in patients with septic shock. Crit Care Med 17:999-1003
49. Schaer GL, Fink MP, Parrillo JE (1985) Norepinephrine alone versus norepinephrine plus low-dose dopamine: Enhanced renal blood flow with combination pressor therapy. Crit Care Med 13:492-496
50. Hesselvik JF, Brokin B (1989) Low dose norepinephrine in patients with septic shock and oliguria: Effects on afterload, urine flow, and oxygen transport. Crit Care Med 17:179-180
51. Desjars P, Pinaud M, Bugnon D, Tasseau F (1989) Norepinephrine therapy has no deleterious renal effects in human septic shock. Crit Care Med 17:426-429
52. Nasraway SA, Rackow EC, Astiz ME, Karras G, Weil MH (1989) Inotropic response to digoxin and dopamine in patients with severe sepsis, cardiac failure, and systemic hypoperfusion. Chest 95:612-615
53. Vincent J-L, Domb M, Van der Linden P, Motte S, de Boelpaepe C, Contempré B, Cantraine F (1988) Amrinone administration in endotoxin shock. Circ Shock 25:75-83
54. Chernow B, Roth BL (1986) Pharmacologic support of the cardiovasculature in septic shock. In: Sibbald WJ, Sprung C (eds) Perspectives on sepsis and septic shock. Soc Crit Care Med, pp 178-202
55. Hulsmann WC, Lamers JMJ, Stam H, et al (1981) Calcium overload in endotoxemia. Life Sci 29:1009-1014
56. Malcolm DS, Holaday JW, Zaloga GP (1988) Calcium and calcium antagonists in shock and ischemia. In: Chernow B (ed) The pharmacoligic approach to the critically ill patient. Williams & Wilkins, Baltimore, pp 889-900
57. Malcolm DS, Zaloga GP, Holaday JW (1989) Calcium administration increases the mortality of endotoxic shock in rats. Crit Care Med 17:900-903

58. Bosson S, Keunzig M, Schwartz SI (1985) Verapamil improves cardiac function and increases survival in canine E. coli endotoxin shock. Circ Shock 16:307–316
59. Lee HC, Lum BKB (1986) Protective action of calcium entry blockers in endotoxic shock. Circ Shock 18:193–203
60. Groeneveld ABJ, Bronsveld W, Thijs LG (1986) Hemodynamic determinants of mortality in human septic shock. Surgery 99:140–152
61. Artucio H, Digenio A, Pereyra M (1989) Left ventricular function during sepsis. Crit Care Med 17:323–327
62. Parker MM, Shelhamer JH, Natanson C, Alling DW, Parrillo JE (1987) Serial cardiovascular variables in survivors and nonsurvivors of human septic shock: Heart rate as an early predictor of prognosis. Crit Care Med 15:923–929

Manipulation of the Immunoinflammatory Cascade in Sepsis: Facts and Perspectives

J. F. Dhainaut, I. Hamy, and B. Schremmer

Introduction

Septic shock continues to be a frequently encountered problem carrying a high mortality [1]. The invading organism interacts with the host to induce a complex array of responses, the initiating event being the release of microbial toxins. These have been divided into two broad classes: exotoxins (products of *Staphylococcus aureus* and *Clostridium perfringens*), and endotoxins (LPS) which originate from the cell wall of gram-negative bacteria. Circulating LPS of bacterial origin continue to have biological effects, even in absence of actively proliferating bacteria.

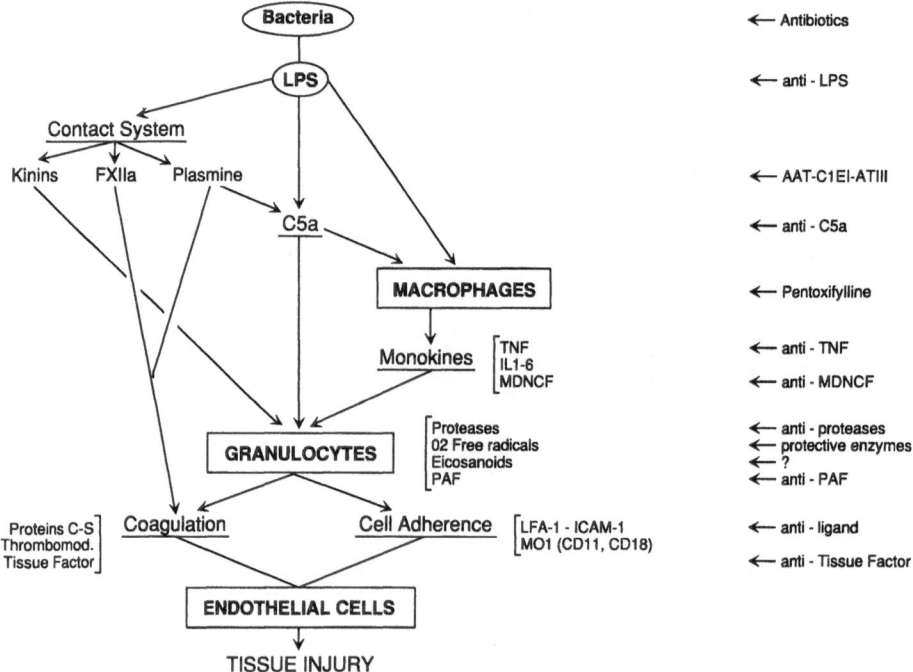

Fig. 1. The immunoinflammatory cascade in sepsis. Abbreviations: AAT = α_1-antitrypsin; C_1E_1 = C1 esterase inhibitor; $ATIII$ = anti-thrombin III; *Thrombo.* = thrombomodulin

Indeed, release of LPS and other bacterial cellular debris, immune complexes, virus... activate various humoral and cellular host defense systems, which include complement, kinin and clotting cascades with activation of various leukocytes (mononuclear phagocytes and granulocytes). These cells, in turn, release several potent mediators, such as tumor necrosis factor (TNF), and will express new cell surface adhesion molecules. The coordinate activation of both humoral and cellular limbs of the immunoinflammatory cascade (Fig. 1) results in an effective defense against infection. However, in many cases, this response becomes exaggerated, causing tissue damage, thereby threatening the host [2, 3]. Despite the development of antibiotics capable of killing a wide variety of gram-negative bacteria, mortality from gram-negative infections remains high (60 to 80%). In fact, with a few notable exceptions such as colistin and polymyxin [4], antibiotics have little effect on the specific effects of LPS, and may even promote the release of LPS from bacteria [5]. Alternative approaches are clearly needed.

In this brief review, we will concentrate on the steps in the cascade for which there exist therapeutic interventions. Antibodies recognizing LPS and the various mediators involved in the cascade, pharmacological agents that inhibit mediator production, recombinant protease inhibitors, as well as protective enzymes and oxygen-derived free radical scavengers have the potential of reducing the severity of the inflammatory response in vivo and improve the outcome of bacterial infections.

Role of the Acute Phase Response in Neutralizing LPS

An important yet confusing aspect of the immunoinflammatory cascade is the so-called non-specific host defense mechanism [3]. It had been known for decades that animals or humans given a single or repetitive doses of LPS become tolerant to the effects of a subsequent challenge. Early studies [6] reported that the reticuloendothelial system was activated and that clearance and/or metabolism of LPS was enhanced. However, blockade of the reticuloendothelial system with thorotrast did not lead to loss of tolerance once acquired [7]. Injection of large amounts of sera from a tolerant animal devoid of LPS antibodies to a nontolerant animal renders it tolerant [8]. Furthermore, sera from patients with fever, bacteremia, or gram-negative shock had a 10-fold greater capacity to induce tolerance to LPS than sera from normal controls [3]. The injection of activated macrophage supernatants and human rIL-1 also induces increased neutralizing activity, suggesting that detoxification of LPS may be controlled by inducible macrophage factors [3]. The mechanism of the detoxification of LPS is incompletely understood. LPS is first disaggregated by a serum component and secondary binds to serum lipoprotein. It seems that the detoxification is related to the presence of a heat-stable esterase associated with LDL, as well as an inducible esterase present in HDL [3].

The clearance and subsequent distribution of LPS from the bloodstream into the body tissues occur in two phases: an initial rapid clearance (minutes) into the reticuloendothelial cells and a slower phase (hours), during which LPS bound to HDL circulates and is taken up by HDL receptors. There is a targeting of LPS to cholesterol-rich tissues such as the adrenal gland [9], a process that may be related to the adrenal damage occasionally observed in fulminant septicemia. Antibody to the O-polysaccharide chain enhances the clearance of both LPS and preformed LPS-liprotein complexes by the liver and spleen and inhibits the binding of LPS to HDL. Cellular processes may also detoxify LPS. Recently, an enzyme has been isolated from human granulocytes that releases the nonhydroxylated fatty acids from the lipid A moiety of LPS [10].

The mechanisms involved are complex and incompletely understood, and it has not yet been possible to take advantage of them clinically.

Antibodies Against LPS

Antisera have been primarily used in the past for the treatment of typhoid, rabies, tetanus, diphteria, and pneumococcal pneumonia. Because there exists a large number of gram-negative organisms serotypes, it is impratical to prepare type-specific antisera to target all possible organisms. Monoclonal antibodies (MoAbs) against LPS are being developed with the aim of preventing or reversing the effects of LPS and facilitating the removal of gram-negative bacteria from bloodstream by the reticuloendothelial system.

The Concept of Anti-Core Glycolipid Antibodies

The structures of several LPS are now completely known. Each LPS-containing bacterial species is distinguished by its so-called "O" or somatic antigens which are repeating oligosaccharide subunits. Connected to this region is the LPS "core", composed of a group of sugars highly conserved across bacterial species and the lipid A biologically the portion most toxic of the LPS molecule.

Several investigators have shown that survival of patients with bacteremia due to various gram-negative bacilli was related to the titers of strain-specific and anti-core glycolipid antibodies present at the onset of bacteremia [11], suggesting that passive immunotherapy by strain-specific as well as anti-core glycolipid antibodies might be of benefit.

The E. coli (J5) and Salmonella minnesota (Re) mutants possess enzyme defects that render them incapable of incorporating the immunodominant oligosaccharide side chains to the core region of the LPS molecule [11]. LPS of these strains have been used to develop polyclonal and MoAbs which have the additional characteristic of being reactive to the antigenic core-lipid A moiety common to most gram-negative bacteria [11]. These MoAbs have now been generated in substantial quantities and clinical trials are underway in the United States [12] and Europe.

However, it should be noted that not all investigators have been able to demonstrate an in vivo protective effect of core-reactive antibodies in animal model of gram-negative sepsis. Ziegler [13], like Baumgartner and Glauser in the following chapter, give an excellent critical review of these studies.

Core Versus Type-Specific Antibodies

The protective effects of type-specific antibodies recognizing the "O" antigens determinants have been convincingly demonstrated, and when directly compared in the same model by the same investigator, the antibodies have been shown to be much more potent than the core-reactive antibodies [14]. These antibodies belong to both IgM and IgG classes and function mainly as opsonins and, at times, bacteriocidins. These observations have been extended to MoAbs [15].

In 1983, Ziegler et al. [16] reported a crucial clinical study of the efficacy of J5 antisera in the treatment of gram-negative sepsis. Because they could not relate protection to titers of the antiserum administrated, regardless of the immune status of the donor, no attempt was made to demonstrate that antibodies to LPS were the active principle in these sera. As noted above, "tolerant" sera contain a number of ill-defined mediators and substances that are apparently capable of neutralizing LPS. Several investigators have shown that LPS immunization can cause a polyclonal type-specific response. Two other human studies using J5 anti-sera prophylactically have not been conclusive. Recently, Baumgartner and Glauser [11] were unable to demonstrate a protective effect of a purified anti-J5 IgG. A clinical trial of purified high titer anti-Re antibodies is underway in Europe. Because low dose type-specific antibodies have been shown to be much more potent than the core-reactive antibodies, and serologic analyses have suggested that only a restricted number of serotypes cause the most serious bacteremias, Larrick [2] has suggested treatment with a cocktail of type-specific MoAB.

LPS-Induced Mediator Release

LPS interacts with both humoral and cellular elements. These include complement, kinin and clotting cascades. LPS and mediators released from the humoral systems act together to activate phagocytes and granulocytes.

Serum Mediators: The Complement, Kinin and Clotting Cascade

Contact activation has only been recently recognized [17]. At least four proteins, coagulation factor XII (Hageman factor), prekallikrein (PKK), high molecular weight kininogen (HMwK) and coagulation factor XI are known to participate in a contact activation. This activation of proenzymes occurs when plasma contacts negatively charged surfaces, leading to a burst of proteolytic activation: kallikrein is generated, bradykinin is released, complement is activated through the first component, the fibrinolytic system is activated through activation of plasminogen, and the intrinsic coagulation cascade is initiated through the action of FXIIa on FXI. Enzymes activated during contact activation are closely regulated by protease inhibitors (C_1-esterase inhibitor, α_2-macroglobulin, α_1-antitrypsin, antithrombin III ...). In septic shock, patients have low concentrations of both contact activation proteins and protease inhibitors, especially in those who died [18].

The plasma kallikrein-kinin system is closely interrelated to other protease systems [19]. Polymorphonuclear leukocytes contain proteases with proteolytic activity directed against coagulation and complement factors. Elastase release from granulocytes was shown in patients with septicemia. α_1-antitrypsin-elastase and α_1-proteinase inhibitor-elastase complexes are increased in these plasma. Plasma kallikrein probably contributes to the neutrophil activation in vivo, since it has been shown in vitro to induce release of elastase from human neutrophils, even in the absence of C5 [20]. In addition, endotoxin leads to the generation of tissue factor, the cofactor of the extrinsic pathway, from endothelial cells and macrophages [21]. These observations underscore the role of plasma proteolysis in the pathophysiology of sepsis.

Several classes of inhibitors have potential as treatment of endotoxemic states [22]. MoAbs have been developed against each protein of the contact system and are currently being tested in animal models of sepsis. Genetically engineered protease inhibitors are another therapeutic possibility. A naturally occurring variant, designated α_1-antitrypsin Pittsburgh, changes the protein from an elastase inhibitor to an extremely potent inactivator of coagulation proteases. In an animal model of septicemia, pretreatment by recombinant α_1-antitrypsin Pittsburgh prolonged survival [21]. Site-directed mutation, resulting in the change of the amino-acid in P2 position to alanine, yields an inhibitor that has a 20-fold greater affinity for kallikrein than thrombin, capable of modulating hypotension experimentally induced by infusion of activated factor XII. Other recombinant or synthetic proteolytic inhibitors are in various stages of development.

Elevated levels of C5a have been associated with sepsis and the development of ARDS [23]. Stevens et al. [24] showed that neutralizing anti-C5a rabbit antibodies protected against a lethal challenge of *E. coli* bacteria. Interference with the coagulation process may block the inflammatory cascade. Both activated protein C [25] and anti-thrombin III [26] have shown excellent results in baboons. Another promising approach is the inhibition of tissue factor with MoAbs [27].

Monokines

Macrophages are known to produce a plethora of mediators following activation. Among the most important released by these cells during endotoxemia are TNF, interleukin-1 (IL-1), interleukin-6 (IL-6), and macrophage-derived neutrophil chemotaxis factor (MDNCF) [28].

TNF appears to play a pivotal role in the orchestration of the inflammatory cascade [29–31]. Tracey et al. [32] demonstrated that a neutralizing murine anti-TNF fragments MoAbs administered to baboons one hour before lethal *E. coli*-challenge protected against shock, but did not prevent multiple organ failure. However, complete protection was conferred by administration of MoAbs two hours before bacterial infusion. A clinical trial of a murine anti-rTNF MoAB is in progress in Europe.

The production of prostaglandins of the E type induced by LPS inhibit the generation of the TNF and IL-1 genes [33]. PGE_2 activates adenyl cyclase, leading to elevated levels of cytoplasmic cAMP. cAMP mediates inhibition of many cell functions. Pharmacologic agents, such as pentoxifylline, that inhibit phosphodiesterase, the enzyme that hydrolyzes cAMP, are now known to protect animals from the deleterious effects of endotoxemia. In addition, pentoxifylline decreases neutrophil adherence and superoxide production [34].

A particularly interesting phenomenon is the marked synergism observed between some cytokines. TNF induces IL-1 transcription and acts with this cytokine in LPS-induced organ injury [35–37]. Interferon (INF) gamma released from T cells stimulates mononuclear phagocytes that release TNF and IL-1 [38, 39]. MDNCF is released from LPS, TNF or IL-1-stimulated monocytes [40]. Inhibition of MDNCF activity with MoAbs has been shown to decrease the elimination of granulocyte influx into foci of inflammation and markedly reduces the magnitude of organ injury.

LPS-Mediated Microvascular Damage

Several pathways and mediators activate endothelial and inflammatory cells (Fig. 1). During this process, these cells express increased number of leukocyte adherence molecules of the CD11–CD18 complex consisting of the LFA-1 and MO-1 molecules. These molecules mediate the ability of leukocytes to adhere to each other and to endothelial cells. The ligand of LFA-1 is the intercellular adhesion molecule, ICAM-1 induced by IL-1 and INF gamma [41, 42]. MoAbs that bind to these molecules inhibit the function of inflammatory cells, and decrease tissue damage.

Tissue damage through activated granulocyte is mainly due to toxic oxygen products, neutral proteases, arachidonic acid metabolites, kinins and platelet activating factor (PAF) [28]. Phospholipids of the endothelial membranes are especially vulnerable to the oxydizing action of free oxygen radicals [43, 44]. This endothelial damage can be blocked either by the substitution of protective enzymes, such as superoxide dismutase and catalase, which are normally present in large concentrations in the cells, or by treatment with the so-called free radical scavengers (N-acetylcystein) [45]. These treatments only attenuate organ injury after endotoxin injection. Probably free radicals are partly involved in the development of organ failure, and cyclooxygenase metabolites and proteinases may also mediate endotoxin-induced injury. Pharmacological interventions in the arachidonic acid cascade have led to contradictory results [46]. It appears, however, that thromboxane contributes to pulmonary hypertension, dilating prostaglandins are beneficial early in septic shock [47], and cyclooxygenase inhibitors are not suitable for therapy [48].

Several other mediators have been implicated in the immunoinflammatory cascade, including endorphins [49, 50] and PAF [51, 52] for which specific receptor antagonists are available. Animal studies have indicated that organic inhibitors of PAF can reverse the vascular effects of LPS. Lastly, despite beneficial effects in attenuating inflammatory reaction in several animal studies [53, 54], corticosteroids have failed to improve the survival of patients with septic shock [55].

Conclusion

Several steps in the immunoinflammatory cascade may be neutralized by MoAbs, or protease inhibitors, or modulated by pharmacologic agents. Because cascades are activated at different periods during sepsis, with consequent immunoregulation and feedbacks, exact timing of administration of agents will probably prove to be important. These new approaches appear promising although limited data is available at the present time as to how effective these will be. MoAbs offer several advantages, but are not without their problems; they are immunogenic and relatively expensive.

References

1. Luce JM (1987) Pathogenesis and management of septic shock. Chest 91:883–888
2. Larrick JW (1989) Antibody inhibition of the immunoinflammatory cascade. J Crit Care 4:211–224
3. Warren HS, Chedid LA (1987) Strategies for treatment of endotoxemia: significance of the acute-phase response. Rev Infect Dis 9:S630–S638
4. Rifkind D (1967) Prevention by polymyxin B of endotoxin lethality in mice. J Bacteriol 93:1463–1464
5. Shenep JL, Morgan KA (1984) Kinetics of endotoxin release during antibiotic therapy for experimental gram-negative bacteria sepsis. J Infect Dis 150:380–388
6. Beeson PB (1947) Tolerance to bacterial pyrogens. II. Role of the reticulo-endothelial system. J Exp Med 86:39–44
7. Greisman SE, Carozza FA Jr, Hills JD (1963) Mechanisms of endotoxin tolerance. I. Relationship between tolerance and reticuloendothelial system phagocytic activity in the rabbit. J Exp Med 117:663–674
8. Freedman HH (1959) Passive transfer of protection against lethality of homologous and heterologous endotoxins. Proc Soc Exp Biol Med 102:504–506
9. Mathison JC, Ulevitch RJ (1979) The clearance, tissue distribution, and cellular localization of intravenously injected LPS in rabbits. J Immunol 123:2133–2143
10. Hall CL, Munford RS (1983) Enzymatic deacylation of the lipid A moiety of Salmonella typhimurium LPS by human neutrophils. Proc Natl Acad Sci USA 80:6671–6675
11. Baumgartner JD, Glauser MP (1987) Controversies in the use of passive immunotherapy for bacterial infections in the critically ill patient. Rev Infect Dis 9:194–205
12. Gorelick K, Jacobs R, Chmel H, et al (1989) Efficacy results of a randomized multicenter trial of E5 antiendotoxin monoclonal antibody in patients with suspected gram-negative sepsis. Abstracts of the 29th ICCAC, p 101 (2)
13. Ziegler EJ (1988) Protective antibody to endotoxin core: The Emperor's new clothes? J Infect Dis 158:286–290
14. McCabe WR, Greely A, DiGenio T, et al (1982) Humoral immunity to type-specific and cross-reactive antigens of gram-negative bacilli. J Infect Dis 128:S284–S289
15. Salles MF, Mandine E, Zalisz R, Guenounou M, Smets P (1989) Protective effects of murine monoclonal antibodies in experimental septicemia: *E. coli* antibodies protect against different serotypes of *E. coli*. J Infect Dis 159:641–647
16. Ziegler EJ, McCutchan JA, Fierer J, et al (1983) Treatment of gram-negative bacteremia and shock with human anti-serum to a mutant *E. coli*. N Engl J Med 37:1225–1230

17. Cochrane GG, Griffin JH (1982) The biochemistry and pathology of the contact system of plasma. In: Kunkel HG, Dixon FJ (eds) Adv immunol, vol 33. Academic Press, New York, pp 241-306
18. Aasen AO (1987) The role of proteolytic enzyme systems with particular emphasis on the plasma kallikrein-kinin system during septicemia and septic shock. In: Vincent JL, Thijs LG (eds) Septic shock. Springer, Berlin Heidelberg New York Tokyo, pp 116-128 (Update in intensive care and emergency medicine, vol. 4)
19. Erdos EG (1976) The kinins. A status report. Biochem Pharmacol 25:1563-1569
20. Wachtfogel YT, Kucich U, James HL, et al (1983) Human plasma kallikrein releases neutrophil elastase during blood coagulation. J Clin Invest 72:1672-1677
21. Colman RW (1989) The role of plasma proteases in septic shock. N Engl J Med 320:1207-1209
22. Van der Starre P, Sinclair D, Damen J (1980) Inhibition of the hypotensive effect of plasma protein solutions by C1 esterase inhibitor. J Thorac Cardiovasc Surg 79:738-741
23. McCabe WR (1973) Serum complement levels in bacteriemia due to gram-negative organisms. N Engl J Med 288:21-23
24. Stevens JH, Shapiro JM, Mihm FG, et al (1986) Effect of anti-C5a antibodies on ARDS in septic primates. J Clin Invest 77:1812-1826
25. Taylor FB Jr, Chang A, Esmon CT, et al (1987) Protein C prevents the coagulopathic and lethal effect of E coli infusion in the baboon. J Clin Invest 79:918-926
26. Vinazzer H (1987) Therapeutic use of antithrombin III in shock and DIC. Symposium on "Newer strategies in the management of thrombotic disorders". Chicago
27. Morrissey JH, Fakhrai H, Edgington TS (1987) Molecular cloning of the cDNA for tissue factor, the cellular receptor for the initiation of the coagulation protease cascade. Cell 50:129-135
28. Schlag G, Redl H (1987) Mediators of sepsis. In: Vincent JL, Thijs LG (eds) Septic shock. Springer, Berlin Heidelberg New York Tokyo, pp 51-73 (Update in intensive care and emergency medicine, vol. 4)
29. Beutler B, Cerami A (1988) The common mediator of shock, cachexia and tumor necrosis. Adv Immunol 42:213-231
30. Michie HR, Spriggs DR, Manogue KR, et al (1988) Tumor necrosis factor and endotoxin induce similar metabolic responses in human beings. Surgery 104:280-286
31. Tracey KJ, Lowry SF, Fahey TJ, et al (1987) Cachectin/TNF induces lethal shock and stress hormone responses in the dog. Surg Gynecol Obstet 164:415-422
32. Tracey KJ, Fong Y, Hesse DG, et al (1987) Anti-cachectin/TNF monoclonal antibodies present septic shock during lethal bacteremia. Nature 330:662-664
33. Kettelhut IC, Fiers W, Goldberg AL (1987) The toxic effect of tumor necrosis factor in vivo and their prevention by cyclooxygenase inhibitors. Proc Natl Acad Sci USA 84:4273-4277
34. Mandell GL (1988) ARDS, neutrophils and pentoxifylline. Am Rev Respir Dis 138:1103-1105
35. Dinarello CA (1984) Interleukin-1 and the pathogenesis of the acute-phase response. N Engl J Med 311:1413-1418
36. Larrick JW, Kunkel SL (1988) The role of tumor necrosis factor and IL-1 in the immunoinflammatory response. Pharmaceutical Res 5:129-139
37. Okusawa S, Gelfand JA, Ikejima T, Connatty RJ, Dinarello CA (1988) Interleukin 1 induces a shock-like state in rabbits: synergism with tumor necrosis factor and the effect of cyclooxygenase inhibition. J Clin Invest 81:1162-1172
38. Girardin E, Grau GE, Dayer JM, Roux-Lombard P, et al (1988) Tumor necrosis factor and interleukin 1 in the serum of children with severe infectious purpura. N Engl J Med 319:397-400
39. Talmadge JE, Bowersox O, Tribble H, Sang He Lee, Shepard M, Liggitt D (1987) Toxicity of TNF is synergistic with gamma-interferon and can be reduced with cyclooxygenase inhibitors. Am J Pathol 128:410-425
40. Matsushima K, Morishita K, Yoshimura T, et al (1988) Molecular cloning of a human monocyte-derived neutrophil chemotactic factor (MDNCF) and the induction of MDNCF mRNA by IL-1 and TNF. J Exp Med 167:1883-1893

41. Makgoba MW, Sanders ME, Luce GE, et al (1988) ICAM-1 is a ligand for LFA-1-dependent adhesion of B, T and myeloid cells. Nature 331:86–88
42. Dustin ML, Rothlein R, Bhan AK, et al (1986) Induction of IL-1 and interferon gamma: tissue distribution, biochemistry and function of a natural adherence molecule (ICAM-1). J Immunol 137:245–253
43. Schoenberg MH (1987) Participation of oxygen free radicals in septic shock. In: Vincent JL, Thijs LG (eds) Septic shock. Springer, Berlin Heidelberg New York Tokyo (Update in intensive care and emergency medicine, vol. 4, pp 108–115)
44. Slater TF (1984) Free radical mechanism in tissue injury. Biochem J 222:1–15
45. Bernard GR, Lucht WD, Niedermeyer ME (1984) Effect of N-acethylcystein on the pulmonary response to endotoxin in the awake sheep and upon in vitro granulocyte function. J Clin Invest 73:1772–1784
46. Oettinger W (1987) Role of prostaglandins and thromboxane. In: Vincent JL, Thijs LG (eds) Septic shock. Springer, Berlin Heidelberg New York Tokyo (Update in intensive care and emergency medicine, vol. 4, pp 89–107)
47. Holcroft JW, Vassar MJ, Weber CJ (1986) Prostaglandin E1 and survival in patients with the adult respiratory distress syndrome. A prospective trial. Ann Surg 203:371–378
48. Ogletree ML, Brigham KL (1979) Indomethacin augments endotoxin induced increased lung vascular permeability in sheep. Am Rev Respir Dis 119:383–389
49. Hinds CJ (1987) Endogenous opioids in shock. In: Vincent JL, Thijs LG (eds) Septic shock. Springer, Berlin Heidelberg New York Tokyo (Update in intensive care and emergency medicine, vol. 4, pp 268–275)
50. Holaday JW, Faden AI (1978) Naloxone reversal of endotoxin hypotension suggests role of endorphins in shock. Nature 275:450–451
51. Parratt JR, Pacitti N (1987) In: Vincent JL, Thijs LG (eds) Septic shock. Springer, Berlin Heidelberg New York Tokyo (Update in intensive care and emergency medicine, vol. 4, pp 74–88)
52. Sun X, Hsueh W (1988) Bowell necrosis induced by tumor necrosis factor in rats is mediated by plateled-activating factor. J Clin Invest 81:1328–1331
53. Waage A (1987) Production and clearance of tumor necrosis factor in rats exposed to endotoxin and dexamethasone. Clin Immunol Immunopath 45:348–355
54. Colardyn F, Vogelaers D (1987) Corticosteroids in patients with septic shock. In: Vincent JL, Thijs LG (eds) Septic shock. Springer, Berlin Heidelberg New York Tokyo, pp 260–267
55. Bone RC, Fischer CJ, Clemmer TP, et al (1987) A controlled clinical trial of high-dose methylprednisolone in the treatment of severe sepsis and septic shock. N Engl J Med 317:653–658

Immunotherapy of Gram-negative Septic Shock

J. D. Baumgartner and M. P. Glauser

Introduction

The mortality associated with gram-negative bacteremia remains in the range of 20–35% [1, 2]. In patients developing gram-negative septic shock (i.e. 20–30% of the patients with gram-negative bacteremia and an unknown percentage of the patients with focal gram-negative infections not associated with detectable bacteremia), fatality ratios may reach 50% or more [3–5]. This finding is attributed to the deleterious effects of the lipopolysaccharide (LPS, also called endotoxin), a component of the outer membrane of gram-negative bacteria. Indeed, antibiotics are unable to prevent the toxic effects of LPS, and may even promote the release of LPS from bacteria. A state of shock may also occur during gram-positive bacterial infections, and unfrequently, during fungal and even viral infections. However, both the incidence of shock complicating infections as well as the mortality observed when shock has developed are higher in gram-negative infections than in gram-positive infections.

Immunotherapy is an approach to improve the outcome from gram-negative infections. Among the various structures of gram-negative bacteria, LPS is extremely immunogenic, and antibodies to LPS demonstrate a better protective potency in vivo than antibodies directed at other antigenic determinants of gram-negative bacteria. We will focus mainly in this review on the present knowledge in the field of passive immunotherapy of gram-negative infections with antibodies to LPS determinants, and we will describe the controversies which have emerged during more than 20 years of active research.

Endotoxin Structure

LPS is composed of three major parts. The innermost part, the *lipid A*, made of fatty acids linked to a diglucosamine, is the structure responsible for the toxic effects of LPS. Attached to the lipid A by a saccharide molecule called 3-deoxy-D-manno-2-octulosonate (KDO) is the *core region*, which is composed of a few sugars, phosphate and ethanolamine. The outer part of LPS, the *side-chains* (O-polysaccharide or O-antigens) consists of repeating units of oligosaccharides, which vary from one gram-negative strain to the other and is responsible for antigenic specificity (serotypes). Several hundreds of serotypes of gram-negative bacteria may be responsible for infections in humans. In contrast, the core-LPS structure (lipid A and core region) is more conserved from one gram-negative strain to another than the side-chains. However, it must be stressed that this structure is also subject to significant inter- and intra-species variability [6–8].

Serotype-Specific Antibodies

Immunization with gram-negative bacilli that possess a complete LPS molecule on their surface induces anti-LPS antibodies directed primarily to the immunodominant, species-specific O-antigens. Studies in animals have shown that these specific antibodies are highly protective against infections caused by the immunizing bacterial strain, but do not afford protection against challenges with strains of other antigenicity. Two approaches have been attempted however to circumvent the problem of the high diversity of serotypes.

The *first approach* is to administer polyvalent purified immunoglobulins. The purified immunoglobulin fraction contains the antibodies present in the pool of plasma from which it is extracted. Intravenous immunoglobulins (IVIG) have a good opsonic activity against various bacteria and have been shown to protect against various infections in animals. Carefully planned clinical trials appear mandatory for exploring the efficacy and the cost-effectiveness of IVIG in bacterial infections. Some studies of the prophylaxis or the treatment of infections in intensive care unit patients or in neonates have suggested a certain efficacy of IVIG [9]. Unfortunately, the results of some of these trials are subject to criticism because of problems in study designs such as non-blinded evaluations, small numbers of cases or insufficient documentation of infections. In addition, the protection was apparent only in some sub-group of patients or in some special types of infections that might have been analyzed separately a posteriori. Currently, the role of IVIG in the management of bacterial infections or septic shock is still controversial [9].

The *second approach* is to focus on infections in which only a few different LPS serotypes exist, such as infections with *Pseudomonas aeruginosa*. *P.aeruginosa*- hyperimmune IVIG preparations have shown good immunologic and opsonic activity in vitro and were protective in animal experiments [10]. However, there have been no reports of clinical trials with such preparations. Recently, murine or human type-specific anti-*P.aeruginosa* monoclonal antibodies of various sub-classes were also shown to be protective in animal models [11]. The administration of a mixture of type-specific monoclonal antibodies is therefore a feasable alternative. However, even if effective, this serotype-specific passive immunotherapy will apply only to a minority of patients with microbiologically documented *P.aeruginosa* infections. Since a delay of 24 to 48 hours is often necessary before the etiologic diagnosis of bacterial infections can be made, a major problem in this tpye of approach is the need for rapid identification of the infecting pathogen.

Core LPS Antibodies

Rough mutants of gram-negative bacilli are characterized by enzymatic deficiencies preventing the attachment of the O-polysaccharide side-chains to the central core LPS. Depending on the type of the lacking enzyme, these mutants expose on their surface various parts of the core region which are hidden on smooth bacteria by the O-side chains. Since the core LPS might share structures which are common to all gram-negative bacilli, a working hypothesis formulated during the sixties was that core LPS antibodies might cross-react between various gram-negative bacteria, and might possibly be protective against a wide range of gram-negative bacteria. The administration of core LPS antibodies is therefore an attractive alternative to the administration of specific antibodies in the management of patients with gram-negative septic shock.

The concept of cross-protection afforded by core LPS antibodies is supported by three lines of arguments: first, by results of experimental studies of passive immunotherapy with antisera from rabbits immunized with rough mutants [12–14]. Second, by retrospective studies in humans which have suggested that high titers of antibodies to core LPS were related with improved survival of patients with gram-negative bacteremia [15, 16]. Third, by prospective clinical trials which have shown that the survival of patients with gram-negative bacteremia was improved in those who received serum of humans immunized with rough mutant of gram-negative bacteria, and that similar serum might prevent gram-negative shock in high risk surgical patients [3, 17]. However, contradictory results have been reported.

In Vitro Studies of Core LPS Antibodies

The concept of cross-protection afforded by antisera to rough mutants implies the existence of antibodies which cross-react with core LPS determinants of smooth gram-negative bacteria (GNB). Even if some chemical analogies can be demonstrated among core regions from different GNB, it remains to be established whether these chemical analogies correspond to common antigenic structures. In addition, covalent linkages of O-side chains to external core sugars are taking place during the synthesis of LPS in the smooth strains. Such linkages may induce conformational changes either leading to differences in antigenic specificities or preventing access of antibodies to the core region. So far, cross-reactions of core LPS antibodies with smooth LPS have not been unequivocally and directly demonstrated. While some groups reported data suggesting that polyclonal [18–22] or monoclonal [23–26] core LPS antibodies might cross-react with smooth strains, other attempts in which purified LPS was used as antigen in direct or indirect hemagglutination tests, complement-dependent hemolysis assays, precipitin tests in agar gel, RIAs, ELISAs, and immunoblot assays have revealed little cross-reactive antibody in antisera to rough mutants [12, 27–29]. With monoclonal antibodies, some cross-reactivity with smooth LPS appeared only after acid hydrolysis, suggesting that the side-chains might restrict the access of antibodies to antigenic sites on the inner core [6, 30–32].

Some of these discrepancies might be explained by the different serologic methods used. Indeed, the difficulties for developing reliable serological methods for measuring core LPS antibodies result from the fact that core LPS structures are hydrophobic, especially lipid A. This hydrophobic nature is responsible for non-specific sticking of immunoglobulins, possibly leading to artefactual apparent cross-reactivity (Heumann D, Baumgartner JD, Jacot-Guillarmod H, Glauser MP. Antibodies to core lipopolysaccharide determinants: absence of cross-reactivity with heterologous lipopolysaccharides. Submitted for publication).

Experimental Models of Protection with Core LPS Antibodies

In addition to the difficulties in demonstrating in vitro cross-reactivity, the mechanisms of the protection attributed to core LPS antibodies have not been established. Indeed, rabbit core LPS antiserum is apparently not bacteriolytic in the presence of complement, it increases only weakly the opsonophagocytosis of gram-negative bacteria and the intravascular clearance of LPS [33, 34]. Therefore, the protection found experimentally by some authors has to be explained by other mechanisms, possibly by neutralization of LPS (i.e. the binding of antibody to LPS would by itself remove the toxicity of the molecule). However, a neutralization of LPS by core LPS antibodies has not been demonstrated until now [35].

The first studies suggesting that antisera directed against rough mutants of GNB might protect against unrelated smooth GNB or endotoxins have been published almost 20 years ago [12-14] and subsequent experiments gave similar results [33, 36-39]. However, the precise epitope(s) of the core LPS and the type of immunoglobulins (IgG, IgM or both) hypothetically involved in cross-protection remain unknown [40]. In addition to the difficulties in defining the mechanisms of protection, controversies have emerged as to the very existence of the cross-protection afforded by antisera to rough mutants. Indeed, several investigators were not able to demonstrate a protective effect of core LPS antisera in animal models of gram-negative sepsis [10, 27, 41-46], while anti-O side-chains antisera were uniformally protective. Similar contradictory results were also found with core LPS monoclonal antibodies. Some authors found cross-protection with anti-lipid A monoclonal antibodies [23, 47] while others found no protection with many antibodies tested [6, 24]. A criticism often raised against the negative studies was that they were made in animal models using high inocula of bacteria or high endotoxin challenge, possibly preventing the demonstration of a protection by core LPS antibodies, which are believed to possess a weaker protective power, although much broader, than homologous antibodies. Using models of endotoxemia or bacteremia in compromised mice with very small challenges, we nevertheless failed to demonstrate a protection with rabbit core LPS antiserum, whereas homologous antisera were protective [46]. In addition, rabbit J5 antiserum did not suppress LPS-induced TNF secretion in mice, whereas the protective homologous antiserum was very effective (Baumgartner JD, Heumann D, Gerain J, Weinbreck P, Grau GE, Glauser MP. Association between in vivo suppression of LPS-induced tumor necrosis factor and protective efficacy of anti-LPS antibodies: Role of O-side-chains-specific compared to core LPS antibodies. Submitted for publication). TNF is a cytokine which is now recognized as a major mediator of the toxicity of LPS. TNF is secreted by macrophages and other cells triggered by LPS. The absence of impact of rabbit J5 antiserum on LPS-induced TNF secretion suggests that core LPS antibodies may not be able to prevent the interactions between LPS and the immune system.

An explanation for contradictory observations resides in the fact that endotoxin contamination of antibody preparations or of antisera to be tested might give false apparent protection. Indeed, as little as 4 ng of LPS/kg of mouse body weight given prophylactically may induce efficiently a state of tolerance in mice, and is protective against lethal challenge with gram-negative bacteria [48, 49]. Since in most of the animal models used for testing the protective power of antibodies, the test preparation is administered before LPS or bacterial challenge, and since antibody preparations are easily contaminated by small amounts of LPS, apparent protection in animal models might have been artefactual due to tolerance induced by minute amounts of LPS contained in the preparations tested.

Retrospective Studies in Humans Relating Outcome from Gram-negative Bacteremias to Core LPS Antibody Levels

In humans, the importance of anti-endotoxin antibodies in the defense against gram-negative infections has been suggested clinically by retrospective studies relating the outcome of patients to titers of core LPS antibodies at the onset of bacteremia due to various gram-negative bacilli [15] or due to *P.aeruginosa* [16]. Two rough strains were used as antigens to detect core LPS antibodies in patients: the Re mutant of *S.minnesota* used by McCabe et al. [15], and the J5 mutant of *E.coli* O111 used by Pollack et al. [16]. Both studies (Table 1) showed that the survival of patients with gram-negative bacteremia was related to their titers of core LPS antibodies measured by indirect hemagglutination or ELISA.

Table 1. Relation of survival to core LPS antibody titers in patients with gram-negative bacteremia

Author [ref.]	Antibody measured (method of detection)	Antibody levels	Survival [%]	P value
McCabe et al.[a] [15]	Anti-Re LPS (indirect HA)	<1:80	40	<0.01
		>1:80	85	
Pollack et al.[b] [16]	Anti-J5 LPS (ELISA)			
	IgG antibody	<10	14	<0.001
		>10	79	
	IgM antibody	<30	44	<0.01
		>30	81	

HA = hemagglutination.
[a] Antibody levels, expressed as titers, were measured in 175 patients with gram-negative bacteremia.
[b] Antibody levels expressed in μg/ml were determined in 43 patients with *P. aeruginosa* bacteremia.

Both IgG and IgM core LPS antibodies were associated with a lower mortality. Although these studies did not demonstrate a causal relationship between high levels of core LPS antibodies and survival, they suggested that core LPS antibodies might play a role in the defense of patients against gram-negative bacteremia.

However, results challenging the role of core LPS antibodies came recently from a study of intravenous immunoglobulins in septic shock patients [50]. During this trial, serum samples have been collected in patients at study entry and antibodies to J5 LPS, to Re LPS and to lipid A were measured [51]. There was no correlation between high levels of any of these antibodies and an improved outcome of the patients (Table 2). The only significant correlation was that non-survivors had a median level of anti-lipid A IgM higher than survivors, a finding which is not supportive for a protective role for anti-lipid A IgM. Therefore, the findings of this prospective study did not confirm the findings of the retrospective studies of McCabe et al. [15] and Pollack et al. [16].

Prospective Clinical Studies with Antiserum for the Prophylaxis or the Treatment of Gram-negative Bacteremia and Septic Shock

Although the observations reported above, both in animals and in humans, remain controversial and do not resolve the questions on the precise mechanisms of cross-protection afforded by antisera to rough mutants, the anticipated benefits in patients were so appealing that clinical studies with antiserum obtained by immunizing volunteers with the rough mutant *E.coli* J5 (J5 antiserum) were empirically started.

In a randomized, double-blind, multicentric study coordinated by E.J. Ziegler, 212 patients with documented gram-negative bacteremia received either J5 antiserum or control serum [3]. The mortality rate was 39% in controls and 22% in recipients of J5 antiserum. In those patients with shock at randomization

Table 2. Relationship between survival and core LPS antibody levels in patients with gram-negative septic shock. (From [51])

Antigens[a]	Immunoglobulin class	Median antibody levels (µg/ml)		
		Survivors (n = 30)	Non-survivors (n = 28)	P value
J5 LPS	IgG	1.8	2.3	NS
	IgM	2.0	1.9	NS
Re LPS	IgG	4.8	6.0	NS
	IgM	0.6	0.5	NS
Lipid A	IgG	<0.5	0.5	NS
	IgM	<0.5	1.0	<0.01

NS = not significant.
[a] Coated on ELISA plates as complexes with high density lipoproteins.

(i.e. patients needing vasopressor therapy for more than 6 hours), the mortality rate was reduced from 77% in controls to 44% in recipients of J5 antiserum (Table 3).

In view of the success of J5 antiserum in treating patients with established gram-negative bacteremia or shock, a randomized double-blind, prophylactic trial in surgical patients at high risk of developing gram-negative infections was performed [17]. The results showed that J5 immune plasma did not prevent the acquisition of new focal gram-negative infections. In contrast, J5 immune plasma seemed to prevent the development of gram-negative septic shock (15 cases in 136 control patients and 6 cases in 126 J5 recipients) and its fatal outcome (9 and 2, respectively) (Table 3). The incidence of shock and death due to gram-positive bacteria or fungi was not different in the 2 study groups.

In the clinical trials reported above, the demonstration of the mechanism responsible for the cross-protection afforded by antiserum to rough mutants has not been convincingly established. Indeed, there was no significant relationship between anti-J5 LPS antibody levels administered to the patients and the improved outcome both in the therapeutic study of J5 antiserum [3] and in the prophylactic study of J5 plasma (personal unpublished data).

The absence of correlation between the protection afforded by J5 antiserum and the levels of anti-J5 LPS antibodies might be explained by the possibility that the antibody responsible for the cross-protection was missed by the serological assays using J5 LPS as antigen. Indeed, the J5 LPS is a complex structure composed of several sugars (including KDO) and lipid A. Thus, it might be that immunization with *E.coli* J5 can elicit a mixture of antibodies directed at different epitopes such as terminal core sugars as well as deeper structures of the lipid A or the lipid A-KDO region. In this hypothesis, antibodies to the terminal core sugars might be predominant and J5-specific, whereas antibodies to lipid A or lipid A-KDO might be less abundant but cross-reactive. To investigate whether the protective factor in J5 antiserum could be antibodies directed at other LPS epitopes, we measured in 70 healthy volunteers the antibody response to J5 LPS,

Table 3. Clinical studies of human J5 antiserum or plasma in the treatment or prevention of gram-negative infections

Study[a] [ref.] (type of preparation)	Control group	J5 group	P value
Therapeutic study [3] (serum)			
Mortality: – all patients	42/109 (39%)	23/103 (22%)	0.011
– patients in shock	30/ 33 (77%)	18/ 41 (44%)	0.003
Prophylactic study [17] (plasma)			
No of septic shocks	15/136	6/126	0.049
No of subsequent deaths	9	2	0.033

[a] See text for the description of the patients studied.

Table 4. Effects of vaccination of humans with *E. coli* J5 on antibodies to LPS. (From [52])

Antigen[a]	Median IgG levels (μg/ml)			Median IgM levels (μg/ml)		
	Pre-immune	Immune	Fold-increase	Pre-immune	Immune	Fold-increase
J5 LPS	4	13	3.25	3	9	3
Re LPS	5	5	1	1	1	1
Lipid A	3	3	1	<0.5	<0.5	1
0111 LPS	<0.5	<0.5	1	1	1	1
Smooth LPS[b]	21	26	1.24	4	4	1

[a] Coated on ELISA plates as complexes with high density lipoproteins.
[b] Mixture of LPS from 7 smooth bacterial strains.

to Re LPS (which is composed only of lipid A and KDO) and to lipid A after vaccination with *E.coli* J5 [52]. We found that J5 vaccine in humans produced only a three-fold median increase in IgG or IgM antibodies to J5 LPS. This modest increase contrast with the several hundred-fold increase observed in rabbits. There was no increase of antibodies to other deeper rough structures (lipid A and Re LPS) (Table 4). In addition, there was also no significant increase in antibodies to smooth structures (LPS from *E.coli* 0111, the parent strain of J5 mutant, and a mixture of LPS from 7 smooth bacterial strains), suggesting that immunization with *E.coli* J5 did not elicit a polyclonal antibody response. Therefore, the protection afforded by J5 antiserum could not be attributed to any of the antibody that we measured.

Prospective Study with Purified Intravenous Immunoglobulins to E.coli J5 for the Treatment of Septic Shock

A randomized, double-blind, prospective, multicenter study was performed to address the issue of the treatment of gram-negative septic shock with a purified intravenous IgG preparation obtained from pooled plasma of volunteers immunized with *E.coli* J5 (J5-IVIG). Patients presenting with established gram-negative septic shock received either standard immunoglobulins (IVIG) (Sandoglobulin) or J5-IVIG. The mortality of gram-negative septic shock was similar in J5-IVIG recipients (15 of 30 patients, i.e. 50%) and in standard IVIG recipients (21 of 41 patients, i.e. 49%) [50]. In addition, no significant difference was observed with regard to the time to reversal of shock and with regard to the duration of survival in ultimately dying patients. Therefore, J5-IVIG was not superior to standard IVIG in reversing gram-negative septic shock or in reducing its mortality. The discrepancy between the success of J5 antiserum in preventing and treating gram-negative septic shock, and the lack of difference between anti-J5 IVIG and standard IVIG, is difficult to explain until more data will be available on the protective factors in J5 antiserum.

Discussion

The discrepancy between the clinical data suggesting that J5 antiserum might afford cross-protection and the failure to experimentally demonstrate the mechanism of protection may have several explanations.

A first explanation is that the antibody responsible for protection might not be accurately measured by the presently available serological methods. Many epitopes are present on J5 or Re LPS, so that the detection of the protective antibodies might be obscured by quantitatively predominant but functionally unimportant antibodies. Additional studies are needed to better understand the fine immunological structure of LPS with the help of monoclonal antibodies. In addition, significant antigenic differences may exist between LPS chemically extracted from bacteria and coated on plastic ELISA plates for the measurement of antibody levels on one hand, and the biological forms of LPS responsible for septic shock on the other hand.

A second explanation is that the factor responsible for the protective effect of J5 antiserum in humans might be of another nature than cross-protective anti-core LPS antibodies. Although a polyclonal response against a wide spectrum of O-antigens may occur non-specifically after a stimulation such as immunization with J5 bacteria, we have found that this possibility was unlikely in volunteers after J5 vaccination [52]. Alternatively, J5 vaccine may increase non specifically some unrecognized acute phase reactants capable of neutralizing LPS or of altering its metabolism, or counteracting the biological effects of humoral or cellular factors released by the stimulation of LPS.

Lastly, it might be that the positive results observed experimentally and clinically are artefactual. Experimentally, many contradictory results have been published. Various artefacts must be carefully avoided. In vitro, the hydrophobic nature of core LPS may be responsible for a non-specific sticking of immunoglobulins during serologic tests, apparently suggesting cross-reactivity. In vivo, a minute contamination with LPS of preparations administered in experimental models might induce very rapidly and efficiently a state of tolerance against subsequent gram-negative infections, thus artificially suggesting cross-protection [48, 49]. In view of the uncertainties associated with the experimental data, the clinical studies remain the cornerstones of this field. However, they too have their limitations. In the Ziegler's study [3], the mortality of patients in septic shock in the control group was 77%, an unusually high value which might be due to the randomization by chance of the most severe cases in this group. In our own study [17], although 262 patients have been analyzed, only 21 developed a gram-negative shock and 11 among them died. Since, as in Ziegler's study, the collective of patients was rather inhomogenous, chance might account for some unnoticed unbalance at randomization. This is to emphasize the need for further studies in this field.

At the time this review has been written, two large-scale multicentric studies of core LPS IgM monoclonal antibodies have been performed in patients with gram-negative bacteremia. The final analysis of the data are still not available. Another study involved purified intravenous immunoglobulins enriched in anti-Re LPS antibodies for the prophylaxis of infections in high-risk surgical patients. This study included about 350 patients and is now completed. The analysis of the results is underway. The fourth study investigated J5 plasma in children with fulminant meningococcemia. This last study utilized plasma prepared from volunteers immunized with a schedule similar to the one used in the three successful clinical studies [3, 17]. The population of patients is however much more homogenous, consisting of children without underlying disease infected with only one type of bacteria. This study has recently been stopped prematurely after about 70 patients because the intermediate analysis did not show an improved outcome in the J5 group and because there were concerns about the risk of transmitting viral diseases through the use of whole plasma in children who have no chronic underlying diseases and are otherwise not transfused. Finally, another trial of J5 plasma is still running in patients after bone marrow grafts (to test whether J5 plasma might reduce the severity of graft versus host disease by decreasing the endotoxin burden). The analysis of these studies with monoclonal and with polyclonal antibodies should become available during the year 1990. They might allow to clarify whether the concept of cross-protection afforded by antibodies to core LPS against gram-negative bacteria is a myth or a reality.

References

1. Kreger BE, Craven DE, Carling PC, McCabe WR (1980) Gram-negative bacteremia. IV. Reevaluation of clinical features and treatment in 612 patients. Am J Med 68:344–355
2. Bryan CS, Reynolds KL, Brenner ER (1983) Analysis of 1186 episodes of gram-negative bacteremia in non-university hospitals: the effects of antimicrobial therapy. Rev Infect Dis 5:629–638
3. Ziegler EJ, McCutchan JA, Fierer J, et al (1982) Treatment of gram-negative bacteremia and shock with human antiserum to a mutant Escherichia coli. N Engl J Med 307:1225–1230
4. Bone RG, Fisher CJ, Clemmer TP (1987) A controlled clinical trial of high-dose methyl-prednisolone in the treatment of severe sepsis and septic shock. N Engl J Med 317:653–658
5. The Veterans Administration Systemic Sepsis Cooperative Study Group (1987) Effect of high-dose glocroticoid therapy on mortality in patients with clinical signs of systemic sepsis. N Engl J Med 317:659–665
6. Pollack M, Chia JKS, Koles NL, Miller M, Guelde G (1989) Specificity and cross-reactivity of monoclonal antibodies reactive with the core and lipid A regions of bacterial lipopolysaccharide. J Infect Dis 159:168–188
7. Fuller NA, Wu MC, Wilkinson RG, Heath EC (1973) The biosynthesis of cell wall lipopolysaccharide in Escherichia coli. VII. Characterization of heterogenous "core" oligosaccharide structures. J Biol Chem 248:7938–7950
8. Jansson PE, Linbdberg AA, Lindberg B, Wollin (1981) Structural studies on the hexose region of the core in lipopolysaccharides from enterobacteraceae. Eur J Biochem 115:571–577
9. Baumgartner JD, Glauser MP (1987) Controversies in the passive immunotherapy of bacterial infections in the critically-ill patients. Rev Infect Dis 9:194–205
10. Pennington JE, Menkes E (1981) Type-specific versus cross-protective vaccination for gram-negative pneumonia. J Infect Dis 144:599–603
11. Pennington JE (1988) Impact of molecular biology on Pseudomonas aeruginosa immunization. J Hosp Inf 11 (Supplement):96–102
12. Chedid L, Parant M, Parant F, Boyer F (1968) A proposed mechanism for natural immunity to enterobacterial pathogens. J Immunol 100:292–301

13. Braude AI, Douglas H (1972) Passive immunization against the local Shwartzman reaction. J Immunol 108:601–610
14. McCabe WR (1972) Immunization with R mutants of *S.minnesota*. I. Protection against challenge with heterologous gram-negative bacilli. J Immunol 108:601–610
15. McCabe WR, Kreger BE, Johns M (1972) Type-specific and cross-reactive antibodies in gram-negative bacteremia. N Engl J Med 287:261–267
16. Pollack M, Huang AI, Prescott RK, et al (1983) Enhanced survival in *Pseudomonas aeruginosa* septicemia associated with high levels of circulating antibody to *Escherichia coli* endotoxin core. J Clin Invest 72:1874–1881
17. Baumgartner JD, Glauser MP, McCutchan JA, et al (1985) Prevention of gram-negative shock and death in surgical patients by prophylactic antibody to endotoxin core glycolipid. Lancet ii:59–63
18. Young LS, Hoffman KR, Stevens P (1975) Core glycolipid of enterobacterianceae: immunofluorescent detection of antigen and antibody. Proc Soc Biol Med 149:389–396
19. Eskenazy M, Konstantinov G, Ivanova R, Strahilov D (1977) Detection by immunofluorescence of common antigenic determinants in unrelated gram-negative bacteria and their lipopolysaccharides. J Infect Dis 135:965–969
20. Baumgartner JD, O'Brien TX, Kirkland TN, Glauser MP, Ziegler EJ (1987) Demonstration of cross-reactive antibodies to smooth gram-negative bacteria in *Escherichia coli* J5 antiserum. J Infect Dis 156:136–143
21. Overbeck BP, Schellekens JFP, Lippe W, Dekker BAT, Verhoef J (1987) Carumonam enhances reactivity of *Escherichia coli* with mono- and polyclonal antisera to rough mutant *Escherichia coli* J5. J Clin Microbiol 156:136–143
22. McCallus DE, Norcross NL (1987) Antibody specific for *Escherichia coli* J5 crossreacts to various degrees with an *Escherichia coli* clinical isolates grown for different lengths of time. Infect Immun 55:1042–1046
23. Dunn DL, Bogard WC, Cerra FB (1985) Efficacy of type-specific and cross-reactive murine monoclonal antibodies directed against endotoxin during experimental sepsis. Surgery 98:283–289
24. Minner KM, Manyak CL, Williams E (1986) Characterization of murine monoclonal antibodies to *Escherichia coli* J5. Infect Immun 52:56–62
25. Mutharia LM, Crockford G, Bogard CJr, Hancock REW (1984) Monoclonal antibodies specific for *Escherichia coli* J5 lipopolysaccharide: Cross-reaction with other gram-negative bacterial species. Infect Immun 45:631–636
26. Nelles MJ, Niswander CA (1984) Mouse monoclonal antibodies reactive with J5 lipopolysaccharide exhibit extensive serological cross-reactivity with a variety of gram-negative bacteria. Infect Immun 46:677–681
27. Ng AK, Chen CLH, Chang CM, Nowotny A (1976) Relationship of structure to function in bacterial endotoxins: serologically cross-reactive components and their effect on protection of mice against some gram-negative infections. J Gen Microbiol 94:107–116
28. Siber GR, Kania SA, Warren HS (1985) Cross reactivity of rabbit antibodies to lipopolysaccharide of *Escherichia coli* and other gram-negative bacteria. J Infect Dis 152:954–964
29. Schwartzer TA, Alcid DV, Numsuwan V, Gocke DJ (1989) Immunochemical specificity of human antibodies to lipopolysaccharide from the J5 rough mutant of *Escherichia coli* O111:B4. J Infect Dis 159:35–42
30. Gigliotti F, Shenep JL (1985) Failure of monoclonal antibodies to core glycolipid to bind intact strains of *Escherichia coli*. J Infect Dis 151:1005–1011
31. Pollack M, Raubitschek AA, Larrick JW (1987) Human monoclonal antibodies that recognize conserved epitopes in the core-lipid A region lipopolysaccharides. J Clin Invest 79:1421–1430
32. Shenep JL, Gigliotti F, Davis DS, Hildner WK (1987) Reactivity of antibodies to core glycolipid with gram-negative bacteria. Rev Infect Dis 9 (Suppl):S639–S643
33. Ziegler EJ, Douglas H, Sherman JE, Davis CE, Braude AI (1973) Treatment of *E. coli* and *Klebsiella bacteremia* in agranulocytic animals with antiserum to a UDP-Gal epimerase-deficient mutant. J Immunol 111:433–438
34. Young LS, Stevens P, Ingram J (1975) Functional role of antibody against "core" glycolipid of enterobacteriaceae. J Clin Invest 56:850–861

35. Chia JKS, Pollack M, Guelde G, Koles NL, Miller M, Evans ME (1989) Lipopolysaccharide (LPS)-reactive monoclonal antibodies fail to inhibit LPS-induced tumor necrosis factor secretion by mouse-derived macrophages. J Infect Dis 159:872–880

36. Ziegler EJ, McCutchan JA, Douglas H, Braude AI (1975) Prevention of lethal pseudomonas bacteremia with epimerase-deficient E.coli antiserum. Trans Assoc Am Physicians 88:101–118

37. Johns M, Skehill A, McCabe WR (1983) Immunization with rough mutants of Salmonella minnesota. IV. Protection by antisera to O and rough antigens against endotoxin. J Infect Dis 147:57–67

38. Sakulramrung R, Domingue GJ (1985) Cross-reactive immunoprotective antibodies to Escherichia coli O111 rough mutant J5. J Infect Dis 151:995–1104

39. McCabe WR, DeMaria AJr, Berberich H, Johns MA (1988) Immunization with rough mutants of Salmonella minnesota: Protective activity of IgM and IgG antibody to the R595 (Re chemotype) mutant. J Infect Dis 158:291–300

40. Baumgartner JD, Wu MM, Glauser MP (1989) Interpretation of data regarding the protection afforded by serum, IgG or IgM antibodies after immunization with the rough mutant R595 of Salmonella minnesota. J Infect Dis 160:347–348

41. Hodgin LA, Drews J (1976) Effect of active and passive immunizations with lipid A and Salmonella minnesota Re 595 on gram-negative infections in mice. Infection 4:5–10

42. Greisman SE, DuBuy JB, Woodward CL (1978) Experimental gram-negative bacterial sepsis: reevaluation of the ability of rough mutant antisera to protect mice. Proc Soc Biol Med 158:482–490

43. Peter G, Chernow M, Keating MH, Ryff JC, Zinner SH (1982) Limited protective effect of rough mutant antisera in murine Escherichia coli bacteremia. Infection 10:228–232

44. Trautmann M, Hahn H (1985) Antiserum against Escherichia coli J5: A re-evaluation of its in vitro and in vivo activity against heterologous gram-negative bacteria. Infection 13:140–145

45. Greisman SE, Johnston CA (1987) Failure of antisera to J5 and R595 rough mutants to reduce endotoxemic lethality. J Infect Dis 157:54–64

46. Weinbreck P, Baumgartner JD, Cometta A, Heumann D, Glauser MP (1988) Failure of passive immunization with rabbit antiserum to E.coli J5 in bacteremia and endotoxemic lethality in mice. Abstract 622. In: Program and Abstracts of the 28th Interscience Conference on Antimicrobial Agents and Chemotherapy, Los Angeles. Am Soc for Microbiology, Washington, pp 218

47. Teng NNH, Kaplan HS, Hebert JM (1985) Protection against gram-negative bacteremia and endotoxemia with human monoclonal IgM antibodies. Proc Natl Sci USA 82:1790–1794

48. Woods JP, Black JR, Barritt DS, Connell TD, Cannon JG (1987) Resistance to meningococcemia apparently conferred by anti-H.8 monoclonal antibody is due to contaminating endotoxin and not to specific immunoprotection. Infect Immun 55:1927–1928

49. Chong KT, Huston M (1987) Implications of endotoxin contamination in the evaluation of antibodies to lipopolysaccharides in a murine model of gram-negative sepsis. J Infect Dis 156:713–719

50. Calandra T, Glauser MP, Schellekens J, Verhoef J, the Swiss-Dutch J5 Immunoglobulin Study Group (1988) Treatment of gram-negative septic shock with human IgG antibody to Escherichia coli J5: A prospective, double-blind, randomized study. J Infect Dis 158:312–319

51. Baumgartner JD, Heumann D, Calandra T, Glauser MP, and the Swiss-Dutch J5 study group (1989) Antibodies to core LPS in patients with gram-negative septic shock: Absence of correlation with outcome. In: Program and Abstracts of the 29th Interscience Conference on Antimicrobial Agents and Chemotherapy, Houston. Am Soc for Microbiology, Washington, pp 175

52. Baumgartner JD, Heumann D, Glauser MP (1988) Effects of vaccination of humans with E.coli J5 bacteria on antibodies to core LPS and immunoglobulin levels. Abstract 200. In: Program and Abstracts of the 28th Interscience Conference on Antimicrobial Agents and Chemotherapy, Los Angeles. Am Soc for Microbiology, Washington, pp 145

Therapy of Septic Shock: New Strategies

R. C. Bone and R. C. Brown

Introduction

The high frequency and often devastating consequences of sepsis make it a major cause of death from infection in the United States today [1]. Although bacteremia may be asymptomatic, it too often comes to clinical attention as an acute catastrophic event recognized by a characteristic constellation of signs and symptoms. Indeed, the term sepsis implies bacteremia coupled with a host response to the circulating microorganisms. Factors that determine the presence or absence of clinical symptoms are largely unknown, though they are of obvious importance in the therapy of bacteremic patients. Conversely, several clinical and laboratory features of bacteremic patients mitigate for or against survival and the development of a particularly devastating manifestation of sepsis, the adult respiratory distress syndrome (ARDS). This review will discuss risk factors, incidence, and prognostic indicators of sepsis and septic ARDS, and conclude with a brief review of two controversial aspects of therapy for septic lung injury: corticosteroids and prophylactic positive end expiratory pressure (PEEP).

Clinical Manifestations of Sepsis

Manifestations of bacteremia are diverse in their range and representation in individual patients (Table 1). Skin lesions such as septic bulla, Janeway lesions, Roth spots, and others may be observed [2]. Fever and chills, thought to be pa-

Table 1. Clinical manifestation of bacteremia

Fever or hypothermia
Chills
Skin lesions
Altered mental status
Organ dysfunction
- Kidney
- Gastrointestinal
- Lung
- Cardiovascular

thophysiologically dependent upon the production of endogenous pyrogen (interleukin 1), frequently are present. Altered mental status may be observed and may, in fact, be the first manifestation of sepsis in elderly patients. Decreasing urine output, which may be associated with peripheral edema, is a reflection of inadequate perfusion and, more ominously, early renal failure [2]. Also, the gastrointestinal, pulmonary, and cardiovascular systems frequently show evidence of dysfunction in the presence of bacteremia [3]. Dysfunction of each of these organ systems is prognostically important, since mortality rate is well correlated to the number of organ systems injured [4]. Early dysfunction involving the cardiovascular system, however, is the single most reliable predictor of early death in endotoxemia [5] and is the most frequent immediate cause of death in septic patients in the first 24 hours.

Laboratory abnormalities may be helpful in the evaluation of bacteremic patients (Table 2). Arterial blood gases obtained early in the course of bacteremia are likely to reflect respiratory alkalosis secondary to stimulation of central respiratory centers. If cardiovascular compensation is inadequate to maintain vital organ perfusion, lactic acidosis will supervene. Hypoxemia may be present, though abnormal arterial-alveolar oxygen ratios or gradients are earlier indicators of pulmonary dysfunction. Coagulation abnormalities, most commonly thrombocytopenia with or without other evidence of disseminated intravascular coagulation, are frequently observed [6]. Granulocytosis with predominance of immature forms, or granulocytopenia and falling white blood cell counts are

Table 2. Clinical abnormalities associated with bacteremia

Arterial blood gases
- Respiratory alkalosis → metabolic (lactic) acidosis
- Increased alveolar-arterial oxygen gradient
Coagulation abnormalities
Granulocytosis/granulocytopenia
Complement system activation

Table 3. Definition of sepsis

Serious infection is evidenced by two or more of the following:
- Core temperature >39°C or <35°C
- Neutrophil count >12,000 µl or <3000/µl or >20% immature forms
- One positive blood culture for a commonly accepted pathogen
- A known or suspected source for systemic infection (such as the urinary tract) from which a recognized pathogen has been cultured
- Gross pus in an enclosed space
Systemic response is evidenced by one of the following:
- Unexplained arterial hypotension
- Systemic vascular resistance (SVR) <800 dynes/sec·cm^{-5}
- Unexplained metabolic acidosis (base deficit >5 mEq/L)

suggestive of bacteremia. Patients with gram-negative bacteremia may have evidence of complement system activation [7].

Many investigators find it helpful to define a subset of bacteremic patients whose clinical features portend poorer prognosis. The term sepsis or septic syndrome implies that a patient has good evidence of a serious infection and a systemic response to that infection (Table 3). Criteria for definition of a serious infection include such factors as hyperthermia or hypothermia, granulocytosis or granulocytopenia, positive blood culture for a recognized pathogen, or gross pus in an enclosed space. Systemic response to infection is implied by the presence of clinical manifestations, such as otherwise unexplained arterial hypotension, low systemic vascular resistance, or metabolic acidosis. While most patients who are bacteremic and febrile but lack other manifestations of sepsis do well, the mortality rate for patients with cardiovascular collapse, even when the site of infection is known and appropriate antibiotics are given, is between 50 and 70% [6, 8]. Interestingly, treatment in an ICU does not appear to alter the outcome of pneumococcal bacteremia once shock is established [9]. Thus, a more specific definition of sepsis may guide us toward the features of sepsis that can be used to predict outcome.

Sepsis Syndrome

The sepsis syndrome can be defined in terms of the systemic response to sepsis expressed as tachycardia, fever or hypothermia, tachypnea, and evidence of inadequate organ perfusion or organ dysfunction. More specifically, it can be defined as hypothermia (T < 96°F), fever (T > 101°F), tachycardia (> 90 bpm), tachypnea (> 20 respirations/min), clinical suspicion of infection, and evidence of inadequate organ perfusion or function expressed as poor or altered cerebral function, hypoxemia ($PaO_2 < 75$ mmHg), elevated plasma lactate, or oliguria (urine output < 30 ml/hr or < 0.5 ml/kg body weight per hour) [10]. When sepsis syndrome is accompanied by hypotension unresponsive to fluid therapy it is referred to as septic shock. Although the exact incidence is not known, 70 000–300 000 cases of sepsis are estimated to occur in the United States each year [11]. Shock develops in approximately 40% of these patients and adversely affects survival [6]. A number of recent innovations in medical practice may have actually increased the likelihood of sepsis and septic shock [11]. These innovations include aggressive oncologic chemotherapy, corticosteroid or immunosuppressive therapy for organ transplantation or inflammatory diseases, increasing survival of patients predisposed to sepsis, and more frequent use of invasive medical procedures [11, 12].

Patients with the sepsis syndrome (n = 191) were prospectively evaluated and comprised the placebo group of a multicenter trial of methylprednisolone in sepsis syndrome and septic shock [10]. Forty-five % of the patients were found to be bacteremic; 31% were in septic shock (sepsis syndrome plus systolic blood pressure < 90 mmHg or decreased from baseline systolic blood pressure > 40 mmHg) at study entry. An additional 24% of the patients developed shock after admission, with 70% doing so within 24 hours of study entry; shock reversal occurred with a frequency of 73%. Twenty-five % of the patients developed ARDS. Mortality for patients with sepsis syndrome who did not develop shock was 13%. Mortality for the groups of patients with shock at admission and shock subsequent to admission was 27.5% and 43.2%, respectively. Forty-seven % of bacteremic patients developed shock after study admission compared to 29.6% of non-bacteremic patients ($p < 0.05$). Other than development of shock, there were no significant differences between the bacteremic and non-bacteremic patients. Also, the outcomes for patients with gram-negative and gram-positive bacteremias did not differ significantly.

Prognostic Indicators in Sepsis

A large series of bacteremic patients reported by Kreger and McCabe detailed the clinical features and effects of antibiotic therapy in 612 patients with gram-negative bacteremia over a 10-year period [6]. For purposes of evaluation, patients were classified according to their underlying illness as being rapidly fatal, ultimately fatal, or nonfatal. Historical features that were associated with increased mortality in patients in any of the underlying disease categories are listed in Table 4. Factors that also were examined but did not materially affect the outcome of bacteremia included race, gender, and the coexistence of neoplastic diseases. The majority of factors listed in Table 4 impair the immune response of the host, and may be postulated to influence survival by this mechanism.

The single best clinical indicator of sepsis and poor outcome was the presence of shock. Shock occurred in 44% of the patients evaluated in this study; fatality in patients with shock was 47%, in contrast to mortality of 7% in patients who did not manifest shock. These data are in close accordance with those of Winslow [8], who noted that 64% of patients with septic shock from gram-positive or gram-negative bacteremia died. Additional clinical factors in Kreger's patients that were associated with the development of shock were age >65 years; antecedent corticosteroid, antimetabolite, or antibiotic therapy; azotemia; and congestive heart failure [6]. In a prospective study of serial cardiopulmonary variables in patients with septic shock, Abraham reported that arterial hypotension was precipitated by a drop of the cardiac index from the high levels classically described in "warm" sepsis to normal ranges [13]. These data suggested to the

Table 4. Pre-existing factors that adversely influence the outcome of sepsis. (From [6])

Antecedent antibiotics
Antecedent antimetabolites
Antecedent corticosteroids
Azotemia
Congestive heart failure
Diabetes mellitus
Nosocomial infection

investigators that loss of cardiac compensation for low systemic vascular resistance was the immediate cause of the hypotensive crisis.

Winslow et al. have reported that arterial lactic acid levels are higher in septic patients who died than in those who survived, though the overlap was too great to make this a test of prognostic significance in any individual patient [8]. The clinical and laboratory features associated with increased mortality in sepsis are listed in Table 5.

Additional laboratory tests that are reported to be abnormal in patients with sepsis are the levels of cyclo-oxygenase metabolites thromboxane B_2 and 6-keto-prostaglandin $F_{1\alpha}$ [14, 15], plasma fibronectin, and angiotensin-converting enzyme. Thromboxane B_2 is a metabolite of thromboxane A_2, a vasoconstrictive and platelet aggregatory lipid. Similarly, 6-keto-$PGF_{1\alpha}$ is a stable metabolite of prostacyclin, a vasodilatory and antiaggregatory metabolite of arachidonic acid metabolism. Although the mean levels of these metabolites were higher in non-surviving than in surviving patients, the separation of values was insufficient to allow this test to be applied prognostically. Angiotensin-converting enzyme (ACE) is a carboxypeptidase that converts angiotensin 1 to angiotensin 2 and is found in highest concentrations in lung capillary endothelial cells. Endothelial cell injury causes release of angiotensin-converting enzyme into the blood, the level of which is reported to be correlated to severity of lung injury [16]. Severe sepsis is associated with a decrease in plasma fibronectin, a non-immunologic opsonin that facilitates removal of degradation products by the reticuloendothelial cell system [17]. Plasma fibronectin levels are touted as a prognostic indicator in sepsis. Each of these tests is of limited value in an individual patient, since the overlap with control patient populations remains significant.

For nearly 10 years, it has been recognized that high titers of antibody to a core lipopolysaccharide shared by most gram-negative bacteria protects patients against the development of shock and death [18]. More recently, levels of circulating antibodies to *Escherichia coli* endotoxin core were shown to correlate well to enhanced survival in patients with *Pseudomonas aeruginosa* septicemia [19]. These observations suggested that immunization against this common core antigen may be protective against cardiovascular changes associated with septicemia. Active immunization of sheep using the core glycolipid fraction of a J5 *E. coli* mutant is effective in reducing the pulmonary hypertension and the decrease in cardiac output and alveolar-arterial oxygen gradient that is secondary to gram-negative endotoxemia [20]. Passive immunization is also effective in this model, though protection is incomplete. Passive administration of antiserum raised in

---

Table 5. Clinical and laboratory features that adversely influence survival in sepsis

Shock
Lactic acidosis
Elevated blood levels of cyclo-oxygenase metabolites
Subtherapeutic levels of antibiotics
Low levels of circulating antibodies to a common core lipopolysaccharide antigen of gram-
negative bacteria

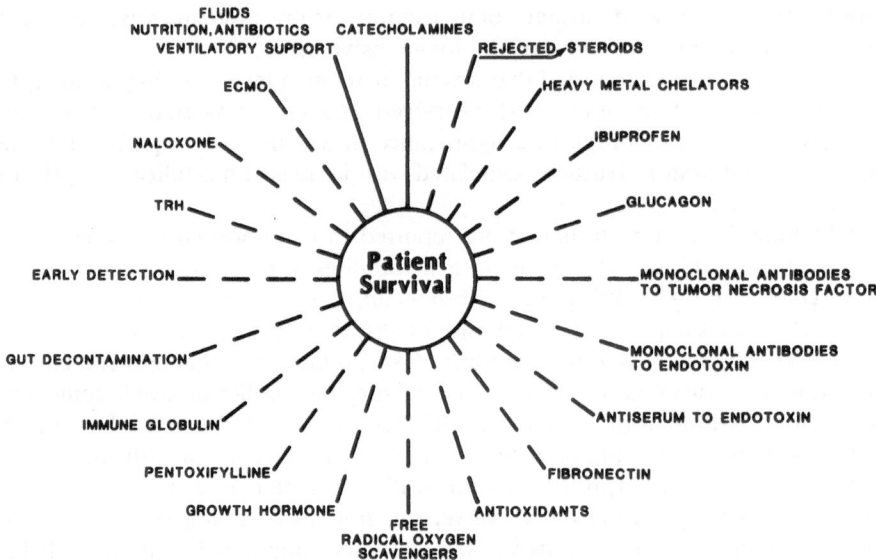

Fig. 1. Conventional and proposed treatment of septic shock and multi organ failure

normal human volunteers against a mutant *E. coli* is reported to reduce mortality and death due to gram-negative bacteremia [21]. These results were reinforced by the observation that administration of plasma rich in antilipopolysaccharide immunoglobulin B provided a survival advantage to gynecologic patients with septic shock [22]. Since these two studies were unblinded and suboptimally controlled, however, verification of these results will be critically important.

Kreger and McCabe's study [6] clearly demonstrated that early and appropriate antibiotic therapy is highly effective in reducing mortality secondary to gram-negative bacteremia. In all categories of patients, initial selection of appropriate antibiotic therapy improved outcome. Furthermore, this advantage extended to patients who had already entered into a shock state. These results have been extended by Moore et al., who found that administration of sufficient doses of aminoglycosides to achieve therapeutic levels reduced the mortality rate relative to patients similarly treated but in whom subtherapeutic levels of aminoglycosides were detected [23]. These data underscore the importance of delivering to patients judiciously chosen antibiotics in adequate doses as early as sepsis is suspected. New treatments are now being defined and evaluated in animal models and multicenter studies. A graphic example of potential agents for therapeutic use in septic shock is shown in Fig. 1

References

1. McCabe WR (1973) Gram negative bacteremia: Disease-a-month. Chicago, Year Book Medical Publishers
2. Sheagren JH (1986) Shock syndromes related to sepsis. Cecil Textbook of Medicine. Saunders, Philadelphia, pp 1473–1477
3. McCabe WR, Treadwell TL, Maria AD (1983) Pathophysiology of bacteremia. Am J Med 75:7–18
4. National Heart, Lung, and Blood Institute (1979) Extracorporeal support for respiratory insufficiency: Collaborative study. National Heart, Lung, and Blood Institute, Washington, DC
5. Goldfarb RD, Tambolini W, Wiener SM, et al (1983) Canine left ventricular performance during LD50 endotoxemia. Am J Physiol 244:H370–H377
6. Kreger BEW, Craven DE, McCabe WR (1980) Gram-negative bacteremia: IV. Re-evaluation of clinical features and treatment in 612 patients. Am J Med 68:344–355
7. McCabe WR (1973) Serum complement levels in bacteremia due to gram negative organisms. N Engl J Med 288:21–23
8. Winslow EJ, Loeb HS, Rahimtoola SH, et al (1973) Hemodynamic studies and results of therapy in 50 patients with bacteremic shock. Am J Med 54:421–432
9. Hook EW, Horton CA, Schaberg DR (1983) Failure of intensive care unit support to influence mortality from pneumococcal bacteremia. J Am Med Assoc 249:1055–1057
10. Bone RC, Fisher CJ, Clemmer TP, et al (1989) The sepsis syndrome: a valid clinical entity. Crit Care Med 17:389–393
11. Parker MM, Parillo JE (1983) Hemodynamics and pathogenesis. J Am Med Assoc 250:3324–3327
12. Shubin H, Weil MH (1976) Bacterial shock. J Am Med Assoc 235:421–424
13. Abraham E, Shoemaker WC, Bland RD, et al (1983) Plasma fibronectin in medical ICU patients. Crit Care Med 11:799–803
14. Halushka PV, Reines HD, Barrow SE, et al (1985) Elevated 6-keto-prostaglandin F1a in patients in septic shock. Crit Care Med 13:451–453
15. Reines HD, Cook JA, Halushka PV, et al (1982) Plasma thromboxane concentrations are raised in patients dying with septic shock. Lancet 2:174–175
16. Fourrier F, Chopin C, Wallaert B, et al (1985) Compared evolution of plasma fibronectin and angio-converting enzyme levels in septic ARDS. Chest 87:191–195
17. O'Connell MT, Becker DM, Steele BW, et al (1984) Plasma fibronectin in medical ICU patients. Crit Care Med 12:479–482
18. Zinner SH, McCabe WR (1976) Effects of IgM and IgG antibody in patients with bacteremia due to gram-negative bacilli. J Infect Dis 133:37–45
19. Pollack M, Huang AI, Prescott RK, et al (1984) Enhanced survival in pseudomonas aeruginosa septicemia associated with high levels of circulating antibody to *E. coli* endotoxin core. J Clin Invest 72:1874–1881
20. Girotti MJ, Menkes E, MacDonald JWD, et al (1984) Effects of immunization on cardiopulmonary alterations of gram-negative endotoxemia. J Appl Physiol 56:582–589
21. Ziegler EJ, McCutchan JA, Fierer J, et al (1982) Treatment of gram-negative bacteremia and shock with human antiserum to a mutant *E. coli*. N Engl J Med 307:1225–1230
22. Lachman E, Pitsoe SB, Gaffin SL (1984) Anti-lipopolysaccharide immunotherapy in management of septic shock of obstetric and gynecological origin. Lancet 1:981–983
23. Moore RD, Smith CR, Lietman PS (1984) The association of aminoglycoside plasma levels with mortality in patients with gram-negative bacteremia. J Infect Dis 149:443–448

Acute Respiratory Failure

The Influence of Mixed Venous PO_2 on Arterial Oxygenation

D. R. Dantzker

Theoretical Considerations

Each functional gas exchanging unit of the lung serves as a tonometer into which inspired air and mixed venous blood are added at rates equal to their individual alveolar ventilation ($\dot{V}A$) and blood flow ($\dot{Q}$). The resultant PO_2 of the end-capillary blood leaving each of these lung units ($PeCO_2$) depends on the inspired PO_2, the PO_2 of the mixed venous blood ($P\bar{v}O_2$), the ability of the blood and gas phases to equilibrate and the ventilation-perfusion ratio ($\dot{V}A/\dot{Q}$). Since the arterial PO_2 (PaO_2) is the blood flow weighted mean of the $PeCO_2$'s of all these units, an alteration of any of these factors will lead to a change in the PaO_2. Four mechanisms of abnormal gas exchange, hypoventilation, impaired diffusion, shunt and ventilation-perfusion inequality, are usually invoked to explain alterations in the arterial blood gases. These are each due to an abnormality of the respiratory system. However, an alteration of the $P\bar{v}O_2$ can sometimes have as significant an impact on arterial oxygenation as any pulmonary mechanism. Since a changing $P\bar{v}O_2$ is indicative of an entirely different spectrum of potential clinical problems, requiring differing therapeutic interventions, it is important that it is also be considered as a potential etiology of a changing PaO_2. This chapter will briefly review the evidence for the importance of the $P\bar{v}O_2$ in contributing to clinical abnormalities of gas exchange.

The extent to which the $PeCO_2$ is altered by a change of the $P\bar{v}O_2$ depends on the $\dot{V}A/\dot{Q}$ of the unit [1]. In the case of shunt, any change in the $P\bar{v}O_2$ is obviously translated directly to the end-capillary blood without modification. For ventilated units, the impact will be greatest for lung units with low $\dot{V}A/\dot{Q}$ (< 1.0) and negligible for those with high $\dot{V}A/\dot{Q}$ (> 10.0) as shown in Fig. 1.

The resultant effect of a change in $P\bar{v}O_2$ on PaO_2 will depend on the overall $\dot{V}A/\dot{Q}$ distribution in the lung. It will be absent in a totally homogeneous lung (only a theoretical occurrence since mild $\dot{V}A/\dot{Q}$ inequality exists even in the most normal lung) and greatest in the presence of significant $\dot{V}A/\dot{Q}$ inequality and shunt. The theoretical impact of a changing $P\bar{v}O_2$ on PaO_2 was clearly pointed by Kelman et al. [2] and West [3] and it has subsequently been shown to play an important role in patients with a variety of acute and chronic cardiopulmonary disorders.

Figure 2 is a theoretical model which allows us to see, in simple terms, the impact that an alteration in $P\bar{v}O_2$ might have on the PaO_2 in a lung with a normal degree of $\dot{V}A/\dot{Q}$ inequality, one with the amount of $\dot{V}A/\dot{Q}$ inequality com-

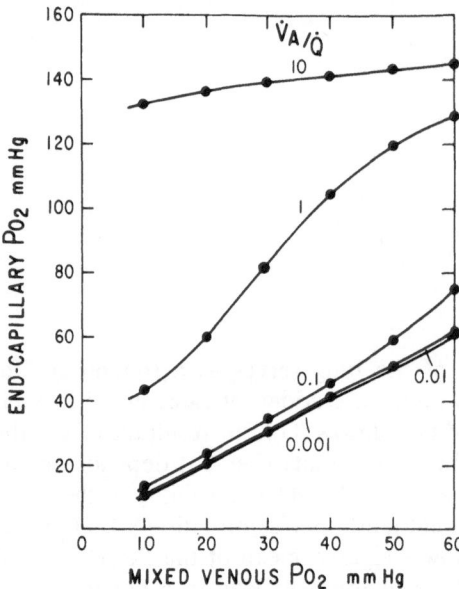

Fig. 1. The effect of changing the mixed venous PO_2 on the end-capillary PO_2 of lung units with varying ventilation-perfusion ratios ($\dot{V}A/\dot{Q}$). The impact on the end-capillary PO_2 is greatest for lung units with VA/Q of less than 1.0 and diminishes as the $\dot{V}A/\dot{Q}$ increases above 1.0. (From [1] with permission)

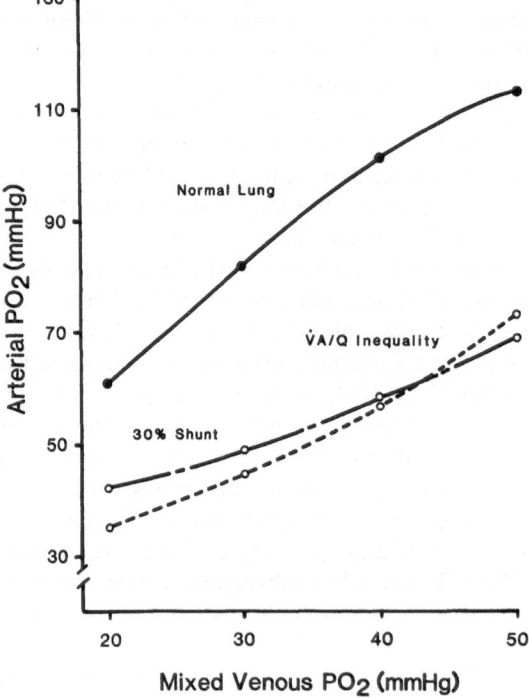

Fig. 2. The effect of a change of mixed venous PO_2 on the arterial PO_2 in a theoretical lung with a normal $\dot{V}A/\dot{Q}$ distribution (solid line), significant $\dot{V}A/\dot{Q}$ inequality (dashed line), and a 30% shunt. (From [21])

monly found in someone with significant chronic obstructive pulmonary disease and in someone with a moderate amount of intrapulmonary shunting. For the purpose of this exercise, the total $\dot{V}A$ and $\dot{Q}$ were kept constant and O$_2$ consumption ($\dot{V}O_2$) was increased to lower the $P\bar{v}O_2$. While this is clearly an unlikely clinical situation, a low $P\bar{v}O_2$ does result when there is a disparity between O$_2$ availability and O$_2$ utilization. In all three settings, the fall in $P\bar{v}O_2$ is accompanied by a similar fall in PaO$_2$.

Clinical Implications

Obstructive Lung Disease

The mechanisms of abnormal gas exchange in many forms of obstructive lung disease have been well characterized [4–6]. $\dot{V}A/\dot{Q}$ inequality is the predominant abnormality in all forms of obstructive lung disease although shunting has also been described in patients with cystic fibrosis and when respiratory failure complicates chronic obstructive pulmonary disease (COPD). Mithoefer et al. were the first to point out the importance of mixed venous oxygenation as a determinant of the arterial PO$_2$ in patients with COPD [7]. They observed that for equal degrees of abnormal gas exchange, as estimated by the venous admixture, the resultant PaO$_2$ depended heavily on the patient's cardiac output and hemoglobin through the influence these factors had on the $P\bar{v}O_2$. A similar impact of the $P\bar{v}O_2$ has been reported in young adults with cystic fibrosis [6]. Young patients with asthma have been shown to have a relatively well preserved PaO$_2$ despite significant $\dot{V}A/\dot{Q}$ inequality which has been explained, in part, by their ability to maintain a high cardiac output and thus a higher than normal $P\bar{v}O_2$ [5]. Following bronchodilator therapy, asthmatics often have a worsening of the $\dot{V}A/\dot{Q}$ inequality but only a minor fall in PaO$_2$, once again due to a concomitant rise in cardiac output [5].

Pulmonary Edema

The major abnormality of pulmonary gas exchange in both cardiac [8] and noncardiac [9] (ARDS) pulmonary edema is the presence of intrapulmonary shunting. Patients with mild congestive heart failure have predominantly low $\dot{V}A/\dot{Q}$ units rather than shunt [10]. As such, one might expect arterial oxygenation in these patients to be quite vulnerable to factors that alter $P\bar{v}O_2$. When this was studied in post myocardial infarction patients, the degree of hypoxemia correlated with the degree of heart failure, but not the amount of shunt, indicating the modulating role of cardiac output on the PaO$_2$ [8].

Pulmonary Vascular Disease

The abnormal gas exchange in patients with acute pulmonary embolism results from a combination of $\dot{V}A/\dot{Q}$ inequality, intrapulmonary and intracardiac shunt and diffusion impairment [11, 12]. However, the effect of these pulmonary abnormalities on arterial oxygenation are amplified by a low $P\bar{v}O_2$ which is commonly present. In one recent series of patients studied after acute pulmonary embolism, it was estimated that only 1 of 10 patients would have had significant hypoxemia if their $P\bar{v}O_2$ had been normal [11]. Thus the widened A-a gradient invariably seen following pulmonary embolism probably overestimates the degree of vascular obstruction. Because of this, changes in the PaO_2 which occur subsequent to an embolic episode are as likely to represent alterations in cardiovascular function as they are to signal a change in the degree of vascular obstruction.

Patients with chronic pulmonary vascular occlusive disease, which in developed countries is most likely to be due to recurrent unresolved pulmonary emboli or primary pulmonary hypertension, have only mild to moderate $\dot{V}A/\dot{Q}$ inequality and small amounts of shunting despite the marked degree of hypoxemia which is often seen [13]. As with acute pulmonary vascular occlusion, the amplifying factor is a low cardiac output and concomitant reduction in the $P\bar{v}O_2$. Treatment of the pulmonary hypertension in these patient with vasodilators, routinely increases the degree of $\dot{V}A/\dot{Q}$ inequality but rarely causes an accentuation of the hypoxemia because of the coincident improvement in cardiac output [14].

Exercise

Exercise is perhaps the most commonly encountered situation in which the $P\bar{v}O_2$ plays an important role in determining the PaO_2. The increased metabolic requirements of the muscles play a significant stress on gas exchange. Cardiac output increases coincident with the onset of exercise to provide the increased O_2 required for energy production as well as to supply the necessary increase in substrate and to remove the excess heat which is produced. However, while cardiac output may increase, to as much as 4 to 5 times baseline values at peak exercise, it is not sufficient to provide for the increased O_2 requirements which may reach greater then 10 times the resting value [15]. Thus the fraction of the delivered O_2 which is extracted by the tissues must also increase and the O_2 extraction ratio which is about 0.33 at rest may increase to greater than 0.80 at maximum exercise levels. This increase occurs very early in a progressive exercise study. The resultant widening of the arterial-venous O_2 difference leads to sharp drops in the $P\bar{v}O_2$ and if all other factors remained unchanged would lead to a fall in the PaO_2 as shown in Fig. 2. However, in addition to the increase in cardiac output, minute ventilation increases, proportionally greater than cardiac output, such that the mean $\dot{V}A/\dot{Q}$ may increase 3 to 5 times the baseline value at peak exercise [16]. As pointed out earlier, the impact of a falling $P\bar{v}O_2$ on $PeCO_2$ depends on the $\dot{V}A/\dot{Q}$ of the lung unit and it decreases as the ratio exceeds 1.0. The effect of increasing the overall $\dot{V}A/\dot{Q}$ on the impact of a falling of $P\bar{v}O_2$ is shown for the three previously discussed lung models in Fig. 3. For each case, the effect of decreasing the $P\bar{v}O_2$ has been recalculated at three different levels of minute ventilation and thus at increasing overall $\dot{V}A/\dot{Q}$ ratios consistent with those seen during mild to moderate levels of exercise.

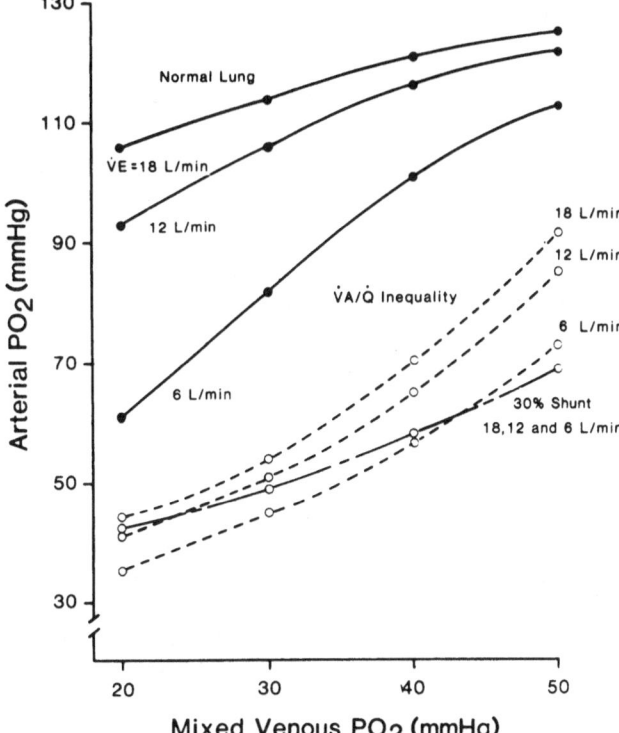

Fig. 3. The effect of increasing minute ventilation on the relationship between mixed venous PO₂ and arterial PO₂. The conditions are the same as those in Fig. 2. Increasing minute ventilation is quite effective in improving the hypoxemia in normal lungs, but much less effective when significant ventilation-perfusion inequality or shunt is present. (From [21])

In the case of the normal lung, the increase in minute ventilation can almost abolish entirely the effect of the fall in $P\bar{v}O_2$, preventing the hypoxemia which would otherwise occur. This is similar to the predictions of Gledhill et al. who calculated, in their normal subjects, that a shift in the mean $\dot{V}A/\dot{Q}$ from 0.92 at rest to 3.2 during exercise prevented the sharp drop in PaO_2 which would have otherwise occurred [17]. The situation in patients with cardiopulmonary disease, however, is quite different. Whereas normal subjects maintain a relatively unchanged PaO_2 during exercise, despite a mild increase in $\dot{V}A/\dot{Q}$ inequality and falling $P\bar{v}O_2$, exertional hypoxemia is common in many forms of pulmonary and pulmonary vascular disease. Patients have significant $\dot{V}A/\dot{Q}$ inequality to begin with and their ability to augment minute ventilation and/or cardiac output is often impaired. It was initially suggested that the fall in PaO_2 during exercise was due to a worsening of the $\dot{V}A/\dot{Q}$ inequality. However, when actual measurements of the $\dot{V}A/\dot{Q}$ distribution were made, it became apparent that, at least at the modest levels of exercise that most of these patients were able to accomplish, there were no significant changes in the degree of $\dot{V}A/\dot{Q}$ inequality found. This has now been demonstrated in patients with COPD [18], cystic fibrosis [6], interstitial lung disease [19] and chronic obliterative pulmonary vascular disease [20].

With the exception of interstitial lung disease, where a small portion of the worsening hypoxemia appears to be due to a failure of complete alveolar end-

Table 1

	PaO$_2$ (mmHg)	PaCO$_2$ (mmHg)	P$\bar{v}$O$_2$ (mmHg)	Cardiac Output (L/min)	Minute Ventilation (L/min)	O$_2$ Consumption (ml/min)	Mean $\dot{V}/\dot{Q}$	log S.D.
Obliterative pulmonary vascular disease								
Rest	64	31	32	4.9	8.5	243	153	0.53
Exercise	56	30	23	7.5	29.6	586	3.91	0.45
Rest vs exercise	p < 0.05	NS	p < 0.001	p < 0.001	p < 0.01	p < 0.001	p < 0.001	NS
Chronic obstructive pulmonary disease								
Rest	76[a]	56	38	4.3	7.4	231	0.76	0.73
Exercise	63[a]	62	32	9.0	15.2	672	0.78	0.73
Rest vs exercise	p < 0.04	p < 0.02	p < 0.01	p < 0.02	p < 0.01	p < 0.01	NS	NS

[a] Many patients were breathing an increased fractional concentration of O$_2$.
NS = not significant.

capillary equilibration (i.e. abnormal diffusion), the basis for the increased hypoxemia in each case due to was the impact of the falling P$\bar{v}$O$_2$ on the end-capillary PO$_2$ of the low $\dot{V}A/\dot{Q}$ units and the shunt. The data from two of the studies are shown in Table 1. This contrasts patients with chronic pulmonary vascular occlusion who had mild $\dot{V}A/\dot{Q}$ inequality and no ventilatory impairment but severe limitation of cardiac function, with patients with severe COPD who had marked $\dot{V}A/\dot{Q}$ inequality and severe ventilatory limitation, a more normal cardiac response to low level exercise, but severe ventilatory limitation. In both cases, there was a fall in PaO$_2$ with very mild exercise, but no increase in the degree of ventilation-perfusion inequality as defined by the log SD of the perfusion distribution. In addition, there was no evidence for diffusion impairment. The cause of the exercise hypoxemia in the patients with pulmonary vascular disease was explained by the sharp fall in P$\bar{v}$O$_2$ which could not be compensated by even the exaggerated ventilatory response to exercise characteristically seen in these patients. The patients with COPD had an added contribution to their exercise hypoxemia due to an insufficient ventilatory response to even this mild degree of exercise. This resulted in no increase in the mean $\dot{V}A/\dot{Q}$ and further increase in PaCO$_2$.

Many patients with lung disease demonstrate no change in PaO$_2$ with exercise or in some cases, even an increased PaO$_2$. Based on the above observations, this must result from an improvement in their $\dot{V}A/\dot{Q}$ distribution of sufficient magnitude to offset the invariable fall in P$\bar{v}$O$_2$.

References

1. West JB (1977) Ventilation-perfusion relationships. Am Rev Respir Dis 116:919–943
2. Kelman GR, Nunn JF, Prys-Roberts C, Greenbaum R (1967) The influence of cardiac output on arterial oxygenation: A theoretical study. Br J Anaesth 39:450–457
3. West JB (1969) Ventilation-perfusion inequality and overall gas exchange in computer models of the lung. Respir Physiol 7:88–110

4. Wagner PD, Dantzker DR, Dueck R, et al (1977) Ventilation-perfusion inequality in chronic obstructive pulmonary disease. J Clin Invest 59:203–209
5. Wagner PD, Dantzker DR, Iacovoni VE, et al (1978) Ventilation-perfusion inequality in asymptomatic asthma. Am Rev Respir Dis 118:511–516
6. Dantzker DR, Paten GA, Bower JS (1982) Gas exchange at rest and during exercise in adults with cystic fibrosis. Am Rev Respir Dis 125:400–405
7. Mithoefer JC, Ramirez C, Cook W (1978) The effect of mixed venous oxygenation on arterial blood in chronic obstructive pulmonary disease. Am Rev Respir Dis 117:259–264
8. Wagner PD, Dantzker DR, Tornabene VW, et al (1976) Effects of ventilation-perfusion inequality on arterial PO$_2$ following acute myocardial infarction. Clin Res 24:110A
9. Dantzker DR, Brook CJ, Dehart P, et al (1979) Ventilation-perfusion distributions in the adult respiratory distress syndrome. Am Rev Respir Dis 120:1039–1052
10. Bencowitz HZ, LeWinter MM, Wagner PD (1984) Effect of sodium nitroprusside on ventilation-perfusion mismatching in heart failure. JACC 918–922
11. Manier G, Castaing Y, Guenard H (1985) Determinants of hypoxemia during the acute phase of pulmonary embolism in humans. Am Rev Respir Dis 132:332–338
12. Huet Y, Lemaire F, Brun-Buisson C, et al (1985) Hypoxemia in acute pulmonary embolism. Chest 88:829–836
13. Dantzker DR, Bower JS (1979) Mechanisms of gas exchange abnormality in patients with chronic obliterative pulmonary vascular disease. J Clin Invest 64:1050–1056
14. Dantzker DR, Bower JS (1981) Pulmonary vascular tone improves V$_A$/Q matching in obliterative pulmonary hypertension. J Appl Physiol 51:607–612
15. Ekblom B, Astrand P, Saltin B, Stenberg J, Wallstrom B (1968) Effect of training on circulator response to exercise. J Appl Physiol 24:518–528
16. Hammond MD, Gale GE, Kapitan KS, Ries A, Wagner PD (1986) Pulmonary gas exchange in humans during exercise at sea level. J Appl Physiol 60:1590–1598
17. Gledhill N, Froese AB, Dempsey JA (1977) Ventilation to perfusion distribution during exercise. In: Dempsey JA, Reed CE (eds) Muscular exercise and the lung. University of Wisconsin Press, Madison, pp 325–343
18. Dantzker DR, D'Alonzo GE (1986) The effect of exercise on pulmonary gas exchange in patients with severe chronic obstructive pulmonary disease. Am Rev Respir Dis 134:1135–1139
19. Wagner PD (1977) Ventilation-perfusion inequality and gas exchange during exercise in lung disease. In: Dempsey JA, Reed CE (eds) Muscular exercise and the lung. University of Wisconsin Press, Madison, USA
20. Dantzker DR, D'Alonzo GE, Bower JS, Popat K, Crevey BJ (1984) Pulmonary gas exchange during exercise in patients with chronic obliterative pulmonary hypertension. Am Rev Respir Dis 130:412–416
21. Dantzker DR (1983) The influence of cardiovascular function of gas exchange. Clin Chest Med 4:149–159

Determination of Lung-Ventilation and Perfusion by Isotope Technique

G. Hedenstierna and L. Tokics

Introduction

The assessment of regional lung ventilation and perfusion is of importance in the diagnosis of pulmonary emboli, the functional evaluation prior to lung resection, the grading of functional impairment in chronic obstructive and restrictive lung disease, mucociliary dysfunction, and in experimental and clinical research. With an increasing knowledge of the nonuniform distribution of ventilation and perfusion, and of other morphological and functional variables, assessment of regional lung function is becoming increasingly important. This paper will give a short historical background, analyze methodological problems in advanced gamma-camera technique, and present data in anesthetized man.

Historical Background

In 1955, Knipping et al. used for the first time radioactive gas (volatile methyl iodide labelled with iodine-131) for the study of regional ventilation and blood flow [1]. Radioactivity in various parts of the lung was measured with external counters. In this way, they were able to detect regional differences in ventilation caused by local disease. West and Dollery [2] demonstrated regional differences in blood flow, using oxygen-15, a short-lived cyclotron-produced isotope. This isotope is inhaled in the form of carbon dioxide, and the rate at which it is removed from a region of the lung during breath-holding is a measure of local blood flow. Ball and co-workers [3] showed that blood flow as well as ventilation could be measured using reactor-produced xenon-133. The use of more long-lived radioactive substances made the isotope technique generally available.

Taplin et al. [4] introduced radioactive macroaggregates for the assessment of the distribution of lung blood flow. Initially measurements were made of albumin labeled with iodine-131, but technetium-99m is superior because of shorter half-life and lower energy which gives a better counting efficiency. Regional ventilation was assessed by inhalation of radioactive gas, xenon-133, or later on, krypton-85. The latter isotope has a more suitable energy level but its short half-life (13 s) requires its on-site production by means of a rubidium generator [5]. During the 1970s, the inhalation of isotope-labelled particles and the recording of their deposition in the bronchial tree have been increasingly used for the study of ventilation distribution [6, 7].

The imaging of the isotope activity within the lung has also shown considerable development. In the very first method of measuring regional ventilation, 16 counters were positioned over the posterior aspects of the chest [8], although much fewer counters have been used in most succeeding studies. An alternative solution is the moving of pairs of counters over each lung (scanning technique) [9]. This requires very stable conditions and precludes an analysis of dynamic events. These techniques have in most laboratories been replaced by the gamma camera, a large sodium iodide crystal, the gamma rays being focused by a series of parallel holes in a lead collimator [10]. By arranging series of photo multipliers behind the crystal, the position and intensity of the scintillations can be indicated as a two-dimensional display.

It is possible to reconstruct a three-dimensional distribution of the isotope activity, or a two-dimensional display perpendicular to the gamma camera, by counting the activity while the gamma camera is moving around the body (the camera stops briefly at different angles for the measurement of activities). Since the gamma rays are emitted as single photons, the technique is called single photon emission computed tomography (SPECT). Nuclides which emit positrons make possible another technique, coincidence counting. When the positron anihilates with an electron, two gamma rays are given off in exactly opposite directions. If the thorax is surrounded by a ring of many small crystals, the simultaneous detection of the two gamma rays give positional information. This technique, positron emission tomography (PET) enables the same spatial imaging as SPECT, but has the advantage of making possible detection of fast events, whereas SPECT only allows an analysis of static situations (or the "freezing" of a dynamic event). The PET-technique is, however, hampered by a large and heavy equipment and a need of a cyclotron-produced short-lived isotopes [7, 11].

Present Research Situation

Since the demonstration of an increasing ventilation and blood flow down the lung, from top to bottom, the clinical use of the gamma camera has mainly been confined to the detection of pulmonary emboli, by obtaining two-dimensional views of the lungs. Not until recently a new interest has emerged in the analysis of regional ventilation and blood flow. This is because of an accumulating evidence of a non-uniform distribution of ventilation and blood flow also in the non-gravitational planes, i.e. in the medial-lateral and cranial-caudal directions in a supine subject. A suspicion of a non-gravitational inhomogeneity of the perfusion distribution was raised by some studies during the 1970s in anesthetized dogs. Thus there was more perfusion in the middle of the lung and less in the periphery during conventional mechanical ventilation [12], and a redistribution of blood flow towards the lateral and basal borders during ventilation with positive end-expiratory pressure (PEEP), with the animal in the supine position [13]. Radioactively labelled microspheres were used and the lung was taken out, cut into small pieces and the activity measured in a well. Distortion of the lung from its in vivo shape could therefore not be ruled out. Recent reports on the perfusion distribution in awake healthy man, using SPECT, also suggest a certain maximum blood flow in the middle of the lung [14], although different results and opinions have also been presented [15]. Hakim et al. [16] have suggested that the decreasing blood flow towards the periphery of the lung is due to an increasing distance of the pulmonary arterial vessels, creating an increasing resistance to blood flow. Their results were obtained in animal preparations and need to be reproduced in humans. Also, knowledge of the normal distribution of ventilation and blood flow in the anesthetized and mechanically ventilated supine man is required before studies in the intensive care patient. In the following sections, the techniques and results of measuring the spatial distribution of ventilation and blood flow in anesthetized, mechanically ventilated, lung healthy men are presented.

Human Study

Methods and Procedure

We used transaxial SPECT with the tomographed volume viewed around the perimeter (360°C) from 64 projections. The lungs were defined as all tissue that was perfused and/or ventilated, as judged from the distribution of intravenously injected human macro-aggregated albumin (MAA) and an inhaled aerosol, each labelled with different isotopes. The emitted radioactivity was detected with a gamma camera (Maxi Camera 400T, General Electric), equipped with a medium energy collimator. Data were processed by a computer with dedicated software (PDP/11, SPETS and Gamma-11, Digital Equipment Corp.). Two radionuclides with different gamma energies were used, indium-113m and technetium-99m. The aerosol was generated by a nebulizer (UltraVent, Mallinckrodt Inc.) producing droplets with a median mass aerodynamic diameter of 0.5–0.6 μm. Computerized x-ray tomography (CT) was performed on a Siemens Somatom-2. Scan time was 5s at 115 mAs and 125 kV. Slice thickness was 8 mm.

The patients were catheterized in the awake state with a thermistor-tipped pulmonary artery (Swan-Ganz) catheter and a brachial or radial artery catheter. Cardiac output was determined in triplicate by thermodilution technique.

Anesthesia was induced with thiopentone (3–5 mg/kg BW) and fentanyl (0.1–0.2 mg), followed by maintenance with halothane (0.6–1.3%) in oxygen:nitrogen (2:3) and pancuronium bromide in iterative doses for muscular relaxation. All patients were intubated by a tracheal tube. The patients were ventilated with a Servo Ventilator 900C (Siemens Elema) at a rate of 12 breaths/min and tidal volume adjusted to an end-tidal CO_2 concentration of 4%.

The patients were examined in the awake state by CT. Initially a frontal scout-view of their trunk was obtained to position a caudal transverse scan just above the diaphragm, and another scan 5 cm cranial to the first one. The patients were then anesthetized and 15 min later another two CT scans were performed at the same levels relative to the spine. The SPECT-procedure was confined to anesthesia and started with the inhalation with the isotope-tagged aerosol. When sufficient activity had been deposited in the lungs (4–6000 counts/s), MAA labeled with the other isotope, was injected. In some patients indium-133m was inhaled and technetium-99m injected and vice versa. This was because the number of counts from technetium-99m should exceed the number from indium-133m by a factor 5 as indium is seen in the technetium window. By switching the isotopes we could choose whether to obtain the best resolution in the ventilation or the perfusion images without exceeding the permitted dose. Typically 45 000 and 210000 counts were collected in each projection during 20 s from indium-113m and technetium-99m, respectively. The approval by the Ethics Committee of Huddinge Hospital restricted the total dose of radiation to a dose-equivalent of 1 mSv.

The inhalation of isotope-tagged aerosol in the anesthetized and paralyzed patient was accomplished by connecting the nebulizer to the inspiratory limb of the respiratory tubings of the ventilator. By using pressure-controlled ventilation, end-inspiratory pressure and end-tidal carbon dioxide concentration were kept at the same level during as before inhalation, although an additional flow from the nebulizer of 10 l/min was introduced into the respiratory tubings.

Calculations

Both isotopes were tomographed simultaneously and the counts were stored in two 64×64 matrices. Two sets of transverse scans were reconstructed, one for ventilation and the other for perfusion. Before making any calculations on the SPECT data we subtracted a background, which was individually determined in each patient. We measured the transverse horizontal diameter (supine subjects) within the thorax on the CT scans and subtracted a background from all volume elements (voxels) of the SPECT scans so that the diameters of the SPECT scans were equal to the diameters on the corresponding CT scans. The background subtracted amounted to about 20% of the maximum value of any voxel. Each voxel was then assigned a value for ventilation and perfusion according to the ratio of its count rate to total count rate. On the CT scans the amount of atelectasis appearing during anesthesia was calculated with planimetry.

Results

During anesthesia there were marked gradients of ventilation and perfusion in the 3 orthogonal directions, especially in the direction parallel to gravity (Fig. 1). Ventilation was distributed to ventral parts of the lung and perfusion to dorsal parts in the supine subject. In transverse SPECT scans near the diaphragm there were several patients in whom ventilation, but no blood flow could be seen in ventral parts (Figs. 1, 2). Conversely, in dorsal parts blood flow dominated over ventilation and in the bottom regions there was no ventilation at all, creating an area with shunt. These shunt areas corresponded to atelectatic areas detected by CT, favoring the hypothesis that dependent atelectasis is the main cause of shunt during anesthesia. There were also gradients of ventilation and perfusion in the two horizontal directions (cranial-caudal and lateral-medial directions). In

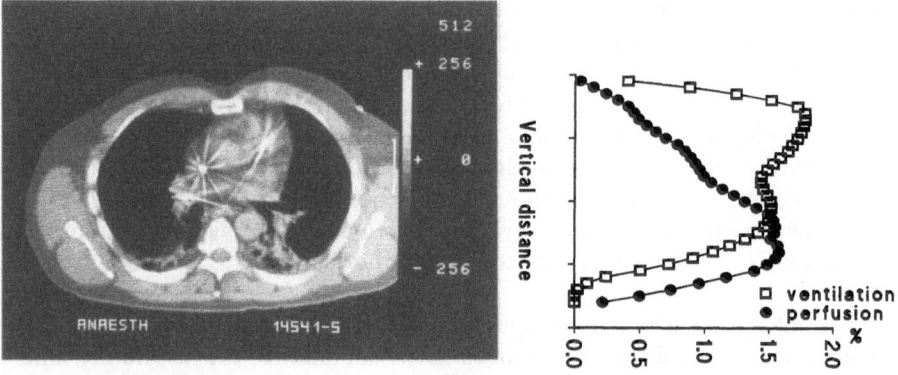

Fig. 1. A transverse CT scan of the caudal lung region, and the corresponding vertical distribution of ventilation and perfusion (from the SPECT) in an anesthetized patient (in percentage of minute ventilation and cardiac output, respectively). Note the large atelectasis in dependent lung regions, and the lack of ventilation but the abundance of blood flow corresponding to the atelectatic region. Note also the marked domination of ventilation over perfusion in non-dependent lung regions

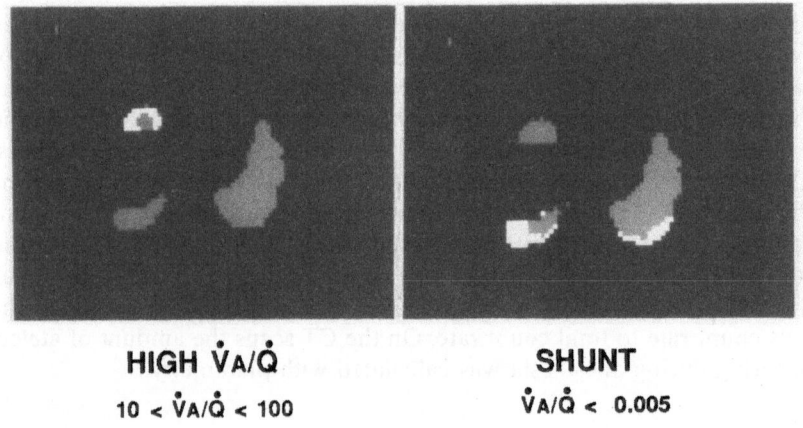

Fig. 2. Transverse SPECT scans during anesthesia showing lung tissue which is perfused and/or ventilated. The scan level is through the right hemidiaphragm so that only the ventral and dorsal costodiaphragmatic regions of the right lung are seen, together with a complete view of the basal part of the left lung. In the left panel, lung regions with blood flow but no ventilation (shunt) are indicated in white, and in the right panel, lung regions which are very well ventilated but poorly perfused (ventilation-perfusion ratio 10) are indicated in white

both directions there was a maximum of the distributions in the middle of the lung, but, as opposed to the vertical direction, the distributions of ventilation and perfusion were similar. Thus, the non-gravitational ventilation and perfusion inhomogeneities produced no clear ventilation/perfusion mismatch (Fig. 3).

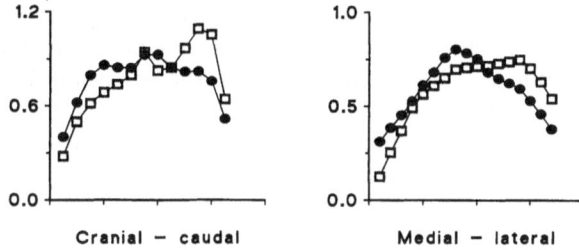

Fig. 3. Horizontal distribution of ventilation (□—□) and perfusion (●—●) in cranial-caudal and medial-lateral directions in an anesthetized subject. Data have been obtained from a single row of voxels going through the central parts of the lung in the sagittal and transverse planes, respectively. Ventilation and blood flow are given in arbitrary units

Discussion

Methodological problems: Ethical constraints made it impossible to test the reproducibility of the method in this setting. The validity of measurements of lung perfusion using SPECT have previously been evaluated in animals [17]. The distribution of perfusion in the reconstructed SPECT scans was similar to the distribution obtained by direct imaging of the corresponding slices of dried lung placed upon the gamma camera. The administration of an isotope by aerosol has not been evaluated by similar direct techniques. Large droplets may impact in the airways where flow is turbulent, although most of this problem can be overcome by using small-sized, monodispersed aerosols [18–20]. A further improvement in the assessment of the ventilation distribution may be a technique based on the combustion of a carbon-rod which has been labeled with technetium-99m [21]. The particle size is less than 0.2 μ and the behavior of the particulate should thus be close to a gas (Technegas).

Previous studies have indicated a reduced ventilation in the dependent lung in the lateral postion during anesthesia by the separate recording of ventilation of each lung by means of a double lumen tube [22, 23], and by frontal or lateral imaging of isotope distributions [24, 25].

Using the SPECT technique, we were able to obtain a very detailed pattern of the ventilation distribution from top to bottom of the lung (frontal-dorsal direction). Thus, the maximum ventilation in the upper third of the lung and the absence of ventilation in the bottom of the lung are observations not previously obtained in anesthetized man. With the SPECT technique, the vertical distribution of perfusion can also be analyzed in detail. Thus, as a major feature, blood flow increased down the lung, in similar with what has been reported earlier [24, 26]. However, the present technique gave further details. Thus the uppermost lung regions were more or less unperfused, corresponding to a zone I [27]. This required the simultaneous recording of ventilation distribution, to make possible the detection of non-perfused lung-tissue (with the perfusion scan alone, this information would have passed undetected). The maximum perfusion was in the lower third of the lung, but in the bottom a decrease in perfusion could be detected, corresponding to a zone IV. Also, the use of macroaggregates for detecting blood flow made it possible to discover perfused and collapsed, non-venti-lated lung tissue. This would not have been possible by the infusion of a gas like xenon which will give a view of the perfusion distribution in air-filled lung re-gions only.

The non-gravitational, cranial-caudal and medial-lateral, perfusion distribu-tions were similar to the distributions reported by some authors in awake, supine man [14, 16] and anesthetized supine dogs [17], with a maximum in the middle of the lung. Hakim et al. have proposed this to be due to regional differences in vascular resistance due to the length of the vessels [16]. Since ventilation is dis-tributed in a similar fashion with a maximum in the middle of the lung, one might suspect a mechanism that acts also on the bronchial tree. However, that regional differences in peripheral airway resistance would produce non-gravita-tional ventilation inhomogeneity is difficult to believe. Another mechanism than the length of vessels and airways may therefore be looked for.

Clinical usefulness: The value of SPECT lies in the better resolution and possibil-ity of reconstruction ventilation and perfusion distribution in all three planes. By this means, a local cause of shunting in the lungs (e.g. mucus plugging, aspira-tion) can be detected. The inhomogeneous distribution of densities in the ARDS – lung, as analyzed by CT scanning [28] also calls for studies on the ventilation and perfusion distributions during this life-threatening disease. The size of zone I, producing a dead space-like effect, and zone IV, which in fact partly compen-sates for impeded or eliminated ventilation in dependent regions, need to be studied during various diseases and therapeutic interventions. SPECT is the technique that offers such possibilities.

References

1. Knipping HW, Bolt W, Venrath H, Valentin H, Endler P (1955) Eine neue Methode zur Prüfung der Herz- und Lungenfunktion. Dtsch Med Wochschr 80:1146–1147
2. West JB, Dollery CT (1960) Distribution of blood flow and ventilation-perfusion ratio in the lung, measured with radioactive CO. J Appl Physiol 15:405–410
3. Ball WC Jr, Stewart PB, Newsham LGS, Bates DV (1962) Regional pulmonary function studied with xenon. J Clin Invest 41:519–531
4. Taplin GV, Johnson DE, Dore EK, Kaplan HS (1964) Lung photoscans with macroaggre-gates of human serum radioalbumin. Experimental basis and initial clinical trials. Health Phys 10:1219–1227
5. Fazio F, Jones T (1975) Assessment of regional ventilation by continuous inhalation of radioactive Krypton-81m. Br Med J 2:673–675
6. Pircher FJ, Temple JR, Kirsch WJ, Reeves RJ (1965) Distribution of pulmonary ventilation determined by radioisotope scanning. Am J Roent 94:807–814
7. Hales CA, Gibbons R, Burnham C, Kazemi H (1976) Determinants of regional distribution of a bolus inhaled from residual volume. J Appl Physiol 41:400–408
8. Knipping HV, Bolt W, Valentin H, Venrath H, Endler P (1957) Regionale Funktionsanalyse in der Kreislauf- und Lungen-Klinik mit der Hilfe der Isotopenthoracographie und der selektiven Angiographie der Lungengefäße. München Med Wochenschr 99:1, 3
9. Dollery CT, Gilliam PM (1963) The distribution of blood and gas within the lungs mea-sured by scanning after administration of Xenon 133. Thorax 18:316–325
10. Anger HO (1963) Gamma-ray and positron scintillation camera. Nucleomics UCLA 21:56–65

11. Anger HO (1967) Radioisotope cameras. In: Hine GJ (ed) Instrumentation in nuclear medicine, vol 1. Academic Press, New York, p 486
12. Greenleaf JF, Ritman EL, Sass DJ, Wood EH (1974) Spatial distribution of pulmonary blood flow in dogs in left decubitus position. Am J Physiol 227:230-244
13. Hedenstierna G, White FC, Wagner PD (1979) Spatial distribution of pulmonary blood flow in the dog with PEEP ventilation. Am Physiol Soc 938-946
14. Orphanidou D, Hughes JMB, Meyers MJ, Al-Suhali A-R, Henderson B (1986) Tomography of regional ventilation and perfusion using krypton-81m in normal subjects and asthmatic patients. Thorax 41:542-551
15. Nicolaysen G, Shepard J, Onizuka M, Tanita T, Hattner RS, Staub NC (1987) No gravity-independent gradient of blood flow distribution in dog lung. Am Physiol Soc 540-545
16. Hakim TS, Lisbona R, Dean GW (1987) Graviaty-independent inequality in pulmonary blood flow in humans. J Appl Physiol 62:1114-1121
17. Hakim TS, Dean GW, Lisbona R (1988) Effect of body posture on spatial distribution of pulmonary blood flow. J Appl Physiol 64:1160-1170
18. Hayes M, Taplin GV, Chopra SK, Knox DE, Elam D (1979) Improved radioaerosol administration system for routine inhalation lung imaging. Radiology 131:256-258
19. Rizk NW, Luce JM, Hoeffel JM, Price DC, Murray JF (1984) Site of deposition and factors affecting clearance of aerosolized solute from canine lungs. Am Physiol Soc 56:723-729
20. Wollmer P, Eriksson L, Andersson A-C (1985) Clinical assessment of a commercial delivery system for aerosol ventilations scanning by comparison with krypton-81m. J Nuclear Techn 13:2:63-67
21. Burch WM, Sullivan PJ, Lomas FE, Evans VA, McLaren CJ, Arnot RN (1986) Lung ventilation studies with technetium-99m Pseudogas. J Nucl Med 27:842-846
22. Rehder K, Hatch DJ, Sessler A, Fowler WS (1972) The function of each lung of anesthetized and paralyzed man during mechanical ventilation. Anesthesiology 37:16-26
23. Bindslev L, Santesson J, Hedenstierna G (1981) Distribution of inspired gas to each lung in anesthetized human subjects. Acta Anesthesiol Scand 25:297-302
24. Hulands GH, Greene R, Iliff LD, Nunn JF (1970) Influence of anesthesia on the regional distribution of perfusion and ventilation in the lung. Clin Sci 38:451-460
25. Rehder K, Sessler AD, Rodarte JR (1977) Regional intrapulmonary gas distribution in awake and anesthetized-paralyzed man. J Appl Physiol 42:391-402
26. Landmark SJ, Knopp TJ, Rehder K, Sessler AD (1977) Regional pulmonary perfusion and V/Q in awake and anesthetized-paralyzed man. J Appl Physiol 43:993-1000
27. Hughes JMB, Glazier JB, Maloney JE, West JB (1968) Effect of lung volume on the distribution of pulmonary blood flow in man. Resp Physiol 4:58-72
28. Gattinoni L, Mascheroni D, Torresin A, et al (1986) Morphological response to positive end-expiratory pressure in acute respiratory failure. Computerized tomography study. Intensive Care Med 12:137-142

Measurement of Alveolar-Capillary Permeability

A. J. Byrne and I. K. Farquhar

Introduction

Since the Adult Respiratory Distress Syndrome (ARDS) was described over 20 years ago [1], a considerable volume of literature has accumulated on the pathophysiology of this fascinating condition [2], but no specific test or marker for its diagnosis has become universally accepted. The diagnosis depends upon a predisposing cause (pulmonary or non-pulmonary) with clinical signs, such as hypoxemia, tachypnea, evidence of decreased lung compliance, and pulmonary infiltrates on chest roentgenography (CXR) [3, 4]. Such diagnostic criteria exclude left ventricular failure and chronic lung disease, which implies that ARDS cannot coexist with these conditions.

Recently it has been suggested that ARDS may not be a distinct pathophysiological entity, but may represent the extreme end of a spectrum of severity of acute lung injury [5, 6]. Early diagnosis of ARDS may allow more effective management [7] and schemes to predict ARDS have been described [8, 9]. There is obviously a need for a 'Gold Standard' to aid diagnosis and treatment in ARDS, but for any marker to become widely accepted it should have the following features: selectivity, sensitivity, safety, index of severity, minimally invasive, repeatability, quick and easy to perform, and economy.

Increased alveolar-capillary permeability to water and solutes is the cardinal feature of ARDS [10], and measurements of the consequent flux of water, protein and smaller molecules have been used as markers for diagnosis and evaluation of treatment. This chapter aims to review methods that have been used to measure alveolar-capillary permeability, which are applicable to the intensive care environment. A brief description of the physiology of pulmonary edema is included.

Anatomy and Physiology of the Alveolar-Capillary Barrier

The alveolar-capillary barrier separates the air in the alveoli from the blood in the pulmonary microcirculation. Capillaries lie in an asymmetrical manner in the alveolar walls, to give a thin membrane (less than 0.5 μm) on one side where the endothelium and epithelium share a common basement membrane, and a thicker barrier on the other side. The interstitial space is bounded by the separated basement membranes of the endothelial and epithelial cells [11]. A monomolecular layer of surfactant lines the alveoli. The intercellular junctions between epithelial cells are 'tighter' (less permeable) than between endothelial cells.

The modified Starling equation [12] describes the fluid flux (Q_f) across the pulmonary endothelium (Fig. 1):

$$Q_f = K_f \cdot ([P_{mv} - P_{pmv}] - \sigma[\pi_{mv} - \pi_{pmv}])$$

The filtration coefficient (K_f) is a measure of hydraulic conductance across the whole pulmonary microvasculature. The direction and rate of fluid flux, Q_f, depends upon the balance of hydrostatic and colloid osmotic pressures (COP). The difference between microvascular pressure [P_{mv}] and perimicrovascular pressure [P_{pmv}] = ΔP, and the difference between microvascular COP [π_{mv}] less perimicrovascular COP [π_{pmv}] = $\Delta\pi$. When ΔP is $>\Delta\pi$ then fluid is extravasated and if ΔP is $<\Delta\pi$ then fluid is reabsorbed (reverse filtration). The reflection coefficient (σ) is a measure of permeability of the membrane to a molecule. When equal to 1, the membrane is totally impermeable, and when equal to 0 it is totally permeable and offers no barrier. For albumin, the reflection coefficient of the pulmonary endothelium is approximately 0.6 [13].

Although this equation predicts a constant flow of protein and water into the lung interstitium, the tendency to accumulation of extravascular lung water (EVLW) is minimized by anti-edema safety factors:

1. Lymphatic drainage of the interstitium (Q_l) has a large reserve capacity (approximately $10 \times$ baseline flow).
2. As the hydrostatic pressure (P_{mv}) rises, water will enter the interstitium and cause a corresponding rise P_{pmv}. This tends to decrease the hydrostatic pressure gradient, ΔP.
3. Water entering the interstitium will dilute its protein content, thus reducing π_{pmv} and increasing the COP gradient, $\Delta\pi$.

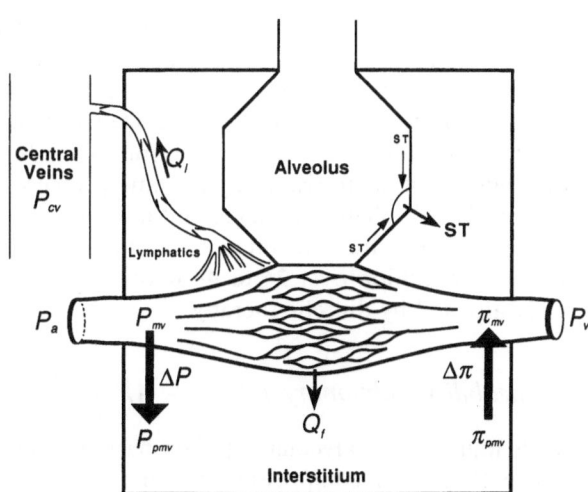

Fig. 1. Diagram of alveolar-capillary barrier

Recent experimental work has suggested that the rate of transvascular fluid flux at any hydrostatic pressure is constant and proportional to P_{mv} [14]. This implies that lymphatic drainage is the most important protection against increases in EVLW.

The alveolar side of the barrier has approximately one tenth of the permeability of the endothelium, and is virtually impermeable to all but the smallest molecules. This disparity in permeability is related to the difference in the pore size of the junctions between epithelial cells and of junctions between endothelial cells (0.46–1.0 nm versus 4.0–5.8 nm). The epithelial basement membrane has a significant fixed, negative electrostatic charge which would tend to repel albumin which is anionic at body pH [15]. Some controversy exists about the role of surfactant. Hills has suggested that it acts as a water repellant; the surface tension (ST) forcing water to collect as convex droplets at the pleated angles of the alveoli [16]. This water is then pumped by hydrostatic forces (ST) into the interstitium. Depletion of surfactant has been shown to increase alveolar permeability markedly [17].

Cardiogenic Pulmonary Edema

The critical hydrostatic pressure, P_{crit}, at which transvascular fluid flux occurs, depends upon the balance of hydrostatic and osmotic forces:

$$P_{crit} = \sigma(\pi_{mv} - \pi_{pmv})$$

Assuming, $\sigma = 0.6$ for albumin, then $P_{crit} \approx 10$ mmHg.

At hydrostatic pressures below 10 mmHg (Fig. 2a), fluid reabsorption will occur (reverse filtration). With pressures above 10 mmHg, fluid flux will increase in a linear manner, but will be compensated for by an increase in lymph drainage, Q_l (homeostasis). When maximal lymph drainage is reached (Q_{lmax}), any further increase in hydrostatic pressure will result in accumulation of EVLW (edema). In normal lungs, this occurs at a hydrostatic pressure of approximately 18 mmHg. Increasing EVLW will inhibit the alveolar pump mechanism progressively leading to alveolar flooding, and clinically evident pulmonary edema.

There are two important clinical consequences of the above. Firstly, any fall in serum albumin concentration will reduce COP and lower P_{crit}. This results in a lower hydrostatic pressure threshold for edema formation. Secondly, the edema that follows an acute rise in hydrostatic pressure, as occurs in heart failure, is resolved by lymphatic drainage, and not by reversal of fluid flux, provided the hydrostatic pressure is maintained above P_{crit} (≈ 10 mmHg). This accounts for the slow resolution over 24 to 48 hours of pulmonary edema which is not directly affected by diuretic therapy.

Permeability Pulmonary Edema – ARDS

Acute injury to the alveolar-capillary barrier results in increased permeability to protein [18], which comprises a spectrum of severity [19]. The increasing permea-

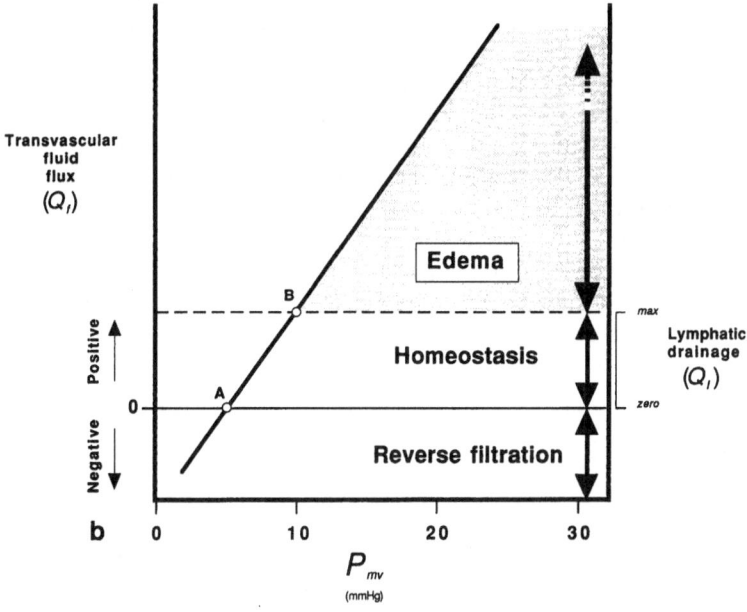

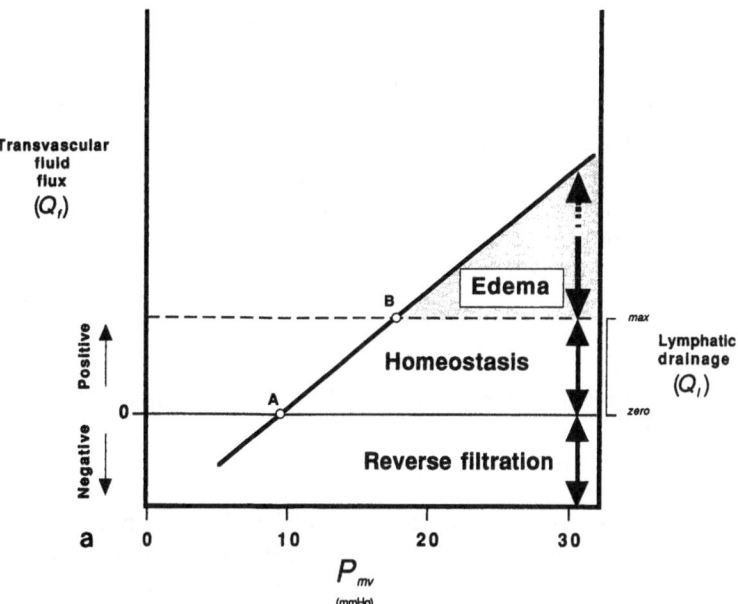

Fig. 2a, b. Diagrammatic representation of relationship between transvascular fluid flux and P_{mv} with **a** normal permeability and **b** increased permeability.
$A = P_{crit}$, $B = P_{mv}$ at which edema formation occurs

bility of the endothelium, as characterized by a decrease in reflection coefficient, σ, towards zero, is associated with a corresponding increase in filtration coefficient, K_f, and fluid flux [20] (Fig. 2b). The cardinal difference between cardiogenic and permeability pulmonary edema is the protein content of the edema fluid [10]. When alveolar pulmonary edema occurs, the edema fluid suctioned from the airway has the same constituents as interstitial fluid, and, therefore lung lymph [20]. The protein content of cardiogenic edema is low with a lymph/plasma (L/P) ratio of less than 0.5. In permeability pulmonary edema the L/P ratio approaches unity, and is characteristically greater than 0.7 [21].

The acute lung injury of ARDS is associated with depletion of surfactant which may be due to a combination of factors. There may be a direct effect on the surfactant-producing type II pneumocytes, or surfactant may be denatured by proteins or other large molecules which leak into the alveoli [22].

Vascular Pressure Measurement – Relevance to Edema Formation

Pulmonary capillary wedge pressure (PCWP) is generally assumed to be a measure of P_{mv}, because pulmonary vascular resistance (PVR) is normally low. With increasing PVR, as occurs in ARDS, there is not only an increase in the gradient of pressure along the pulmonary circulation, but also a change in the distribution of resistance between the venous (P_v) and arterial (P_a) sides. A complex relationship between PCWP and P_{mv}, therefore, exists. It has been shown that analysis of the pressure waveform seen on inflation of the balloon of a pulmonary flotation catheter can give a better estimation of P_{mv} than PCWP. On inflation there is a fall in pressure from P_a to P_v. As the rate of fall slows, an inflection point is seen; this approximates to P_{mv} [23].

Lung lymphatics drain into the central venous system, and elevation of central venous pressure (P_{cv}) will increase the lymph-duct outflow pressure and decrease lymph flow. Rises in P_{cv} have no effect when fluid flux, Q_f, is normal, but both cardiogenic edema and permeability edema will be worsened if the P_{cv} is allowed to rise [24].

Measurement of Alveolar-Capillary Permeability

EVLW Estimation

The various methods of estimation of EVLW have been recently reviewed [25]. Permeability pulmonary edema has been shown to give a greater accumulation of EVLW at lower hydrostatic pressures than cardiogenic edema [26], but this measurement cannot directly differentiate between the two causes of edema. Measurements of protein accumulation in the lung interstitium are, therefore, more specific in characterizing the type and time course of the edema formation.

Measurement of Alveolar Permeability

The alveolar membrane offers a barrier to hydrophilic molecules at the intercellular junctions. Increased permeability occurs with damage to the epithelium, and this can be measured as the increased vascular uptake of small molecules when inhaled as aerosols. As the molecules are small, it is assumed that the endothelium is freely permeable to them. Early methods for measuring alveolar permeability have been reviewed [27], but the measurement of the pulmonary clearance of inhaled technetium-99m-labeled diethylenetriamine pentaacetate (^{99m}Tc-DTPA) has become established clinically.

^{99m}Tc-DTPA is an inert, γ-emitting molecule with a short half-life (6 hours) and small molecular weight (492 daltons). When given as an aerosol, its clearance from the lung can be measured either by a gamma camera, or by externally placed scintillation counter(s). A semi-logarithmic plot of lung activity with time gives a monoexponential decline for which the half-life ($T_{1/2}$) or the clearance rate constant in $\%min^{-1}$ (k) can be calculated. Cigarette smoking [27], high inspired oxygen concentrations (50%) [28], and lung disease [29, 30] have all been shown to significantly increase lung clearance of this tracer. Chronic obstructive pulmonary disease (COPD), however, does not appear to alter alveolar permeability as measured by ^{99m}Tc-DTPA clearance [29]. This method can discriminate between cardiogenic and permeability pulmonary edema [31], and it has been proposed as an adjunct to identifying patients at risk from ARDS [32]. Studies of normal control subjects show a wide variation, which may reflect differences in

Table 1. Summary of human ^{99m}Tc-DTPA permeability studies – derived from quoted references

Subject group	(No. of subjects)	k±SEM (%/min)	Subject group	(No. of subjects)	k±SEM (%/min)	Ref.
Normal	(16)	0.9±0.1	Smokers	(23)	2.9±0.4	[27]
Normal	(7)	1.6±0.2	Idiopathic pulmonary fibrosis	(5 of 5)	4.2±0.3	[29]
			Sarcoidosis	(4 of 8)		
			Pneumoconiosis	(2 of 5)		
Normal	(9)	1.2±0.2	Sarcoidosis	(8 of 14)	2.8±0.6	[30]
Normal[a]	(13)	0.8±0.1	ARDS (no PEEP)	(9)	5.1±0.7	[31]
Normal[b]	(11)	1.3±0.2	ARDS (with PEEP)	(5)	6.8±1.0	
			Cardiogenic pulmonary edema	(6)	2.9±0.5	
Normal	(6)	0.9±0.1	Smokers	(6)	1.8±0.3	[33]
Normal	(7)	1.2±0.1	Smokers	(7)	3.6±0.8	[34]
			ARDS	(12)	5.2±0.9	

[a] Posterior, upright position.
[b] Interior, supine position.

detector type or position of patient and detector [31] (Table 1). Any institution using this method would therefore need to define its own normal range.

The application of positive end-expiratory pressure (PEEP) affects ^{99m}Tc-DTPA clearance [33], and a recent study [34] comparing this technique with a method for estimating protein flux (vide infra) in ARDS patients, concluded that the latter was more specific. The extreme sensitivity of the radioaerosol method renders it unable to separate smokers from those with preexisting lung disease or ARDS patients. Part of this lack of specificity may be due to the difficulty in delivering the aerosol uniformly throughout the lung in a disease process characterized by alveolar flooding, and ventilation-perfusion abnormalities [31].

Recent experimental work has suggested that ^{99m}Tc-DTPA clearance may be increased in surfactant depletion [17], which occurs in premature infants with acute hyaline membrane disease [35]. Resolution of the defect does not, however, predict the developement of bronchopulmonary dysplasia [36].

Measurement of Pulmonary Endothelial Permeability

Two basic approaches to the measurement of increased endothelial permeability to protein in sepsis and ARDS have been investigated:

Measurement of radiolabeled protein accumulation in bronchoalveolar secretion (BAS) – ^{131}Iodine-labeled human serum albumin (^{131}I-HSA) given intravenously has been shown to accumulate in BAS, and can differentiate between cardiogenic and permeability pulmonary edema [37]. This technique has been used to investigate the effect of high-dose corticosteroid therapy in septic ARDS, where 14 of 19 patients responded with a significant decrease in permeability. The 5 nonresponders had higher shunt fractions and pulmonary artery pressures than the responders [38]. The great methodological problems in collecting BAS with the inherent errors involved make this method less sensitive and more invasive than external scintillation counting (vide infra).

Measurement of radiolabeled protein accumulation in the lung measured by external counting (single-isotope method) – autologous albumin radiolabeled with a γ-emitting isotope (^{99m}Tc or ^{131}I) will accumulate in the lungs of ARDS patients when given intravenously [39]. This can be measured by external counting over the lungs and heart; where an increasing ratio of lung/heart counts indicates accumulation of albumin in the lungs. Counting using a gamma camera with computer is not applicable for most intensive care units because of the bulk and cost of the equipment. The results from using a portable radiation probe detector with counter have been shown to be as accurate as those using a gamma camera [40], but the sensitivity and specificity of single isotope techniques has recently been questioned [41].

Measurement of radiolabeled protein accumulation in the lung measured by external counting (double-isotope method) – counts from radiolabeled protein arise from both intravascular and extravascular sources. Changes in pulmonary blood flow or blood volume will therefore affect the counts arising from the lung, and consequently the lung/heart ratio. This can be corrected for by simultaneously labeling an intravascular marker, such as red blood cells (RBC), with a suitable isotope ([99mTc]). The lung/heart ratio of counts from the ^{131}I-HSA is divided by the lung/heart ratio of counts from the ^{99m}Tc-RBC, and this is plotted against time to give an index of albumin leak. This Albumin Leak Index has been shown, in an animal model, to be both specific for permeability edema when compared with cardiogenic edema, and sensitive to graded levels of experimentally-induced lung injury [41].

More recently, Basran et al. [42] have described a modified version of a double-isotope technique [43] which involves *in vivo* labeling of the plasma protein, transferrin with indium-113m, and RBC with technetium-99m. External counting is performed with a portable probe detector over the right upper lung and cardiac blood pool. The difference in the energy values of the gamma rays of the two radionuclides allows simultaneous counting (Fig. 3).

Lung/heart ratios for [113m]In-transferrin are divided by lung/heart ratios for ^{99m}Tc-RBC, and the resulting plot against time yields a slope which is the Plasma Protein Accumulation Index (PPAI) (Fig. 4). This technique permits easy bedside monitoring for periods up to nine hours, and lends itself to the monitoring of drug therapy [44]. Recent experimental work in pigs has confirmed that this technique detects plasma protein leakage in lung injury of differing degrees,

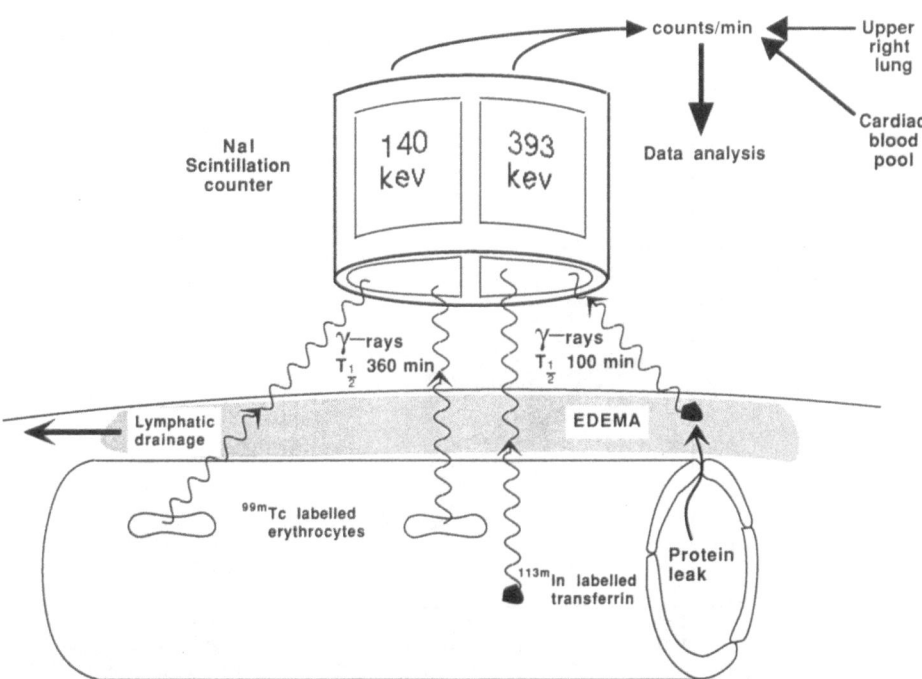

Fig. 3. Diagram showing the theory of lung vascular permeability monitoring using a double-isotope technique

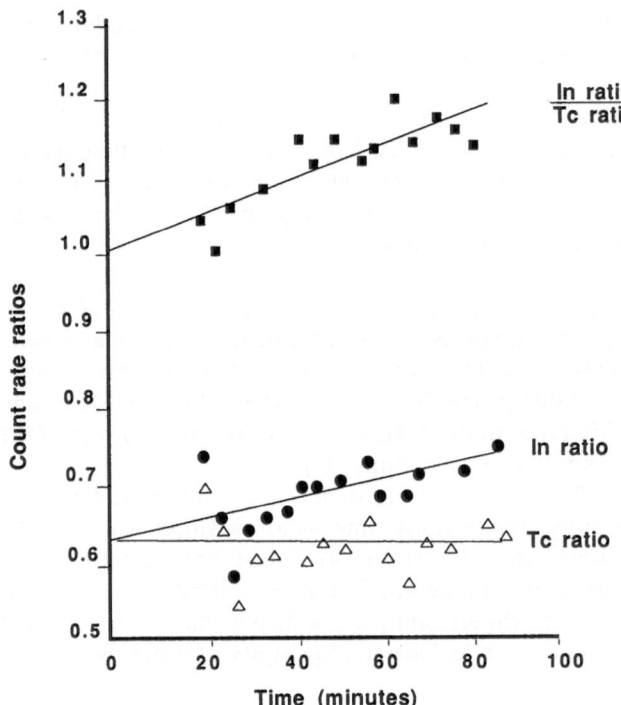

Fig. 4. Example of a lung vascular permeability study in a patient with ARDS. The PPA index (slope of In ratio/Tc ratio plot against time) of 2.5×10^{-3} min^{-1} is above the normal range ($< 0.5 \times 10^{-3}$ min^{-1}). (From [42])

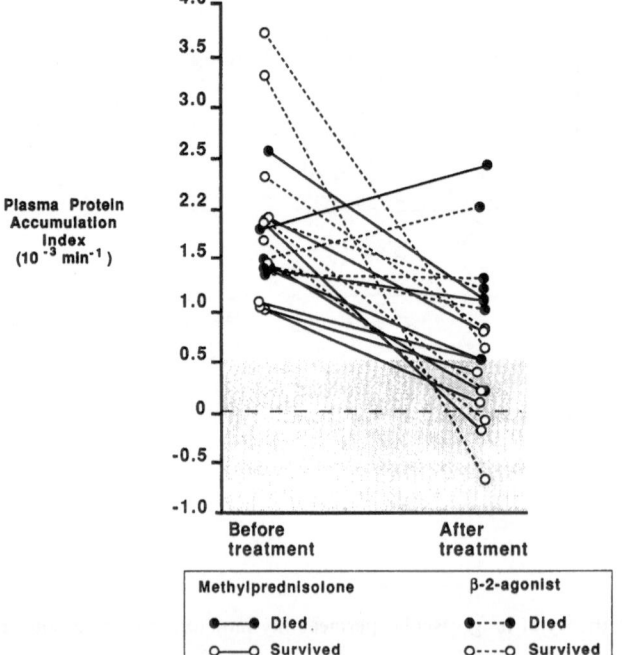

Fig. 5. Survival of ARDS-patients following either methylprednisolone or terbutaline. The interrupted line indicates the range of normal PPA index. (From [46, 47] with permission)

and correlates with changes in functional residual capacity, lung compliance and arterial PO_2 [45].

The effect of a pulse-dose of methylprednisolone [46] or a short infusion of the β-agonist terbutaline [47] has been investigated in ARDS patients using this technique. Response to either of these agents correlated with survival (Fig. 5).

Conclusions

The double-isotope technique (^{113m}In-transferrin & ^{99m}TC-RBC) with portable probe detector fulfils most of the criteria of acceptability for intensive care use. The technique involves in vivo radiolabeling with readily available radiopharmaceuticals. It is therefore minimally invasive and relatively cheap. The short half-lives of the radionuclides, along with the low radiation dose (0.5 mGy) allows repeated investigations, even on a daily basis [42].

ARDS comprises a broad spectrum of lung injury which is accompanied by an increased lung vascular permeability to protein. The severity and time course of the increased permeability is variable, and its identification and measurement does not always correlate with the diagnosis of ARDS made solely on clinical criteria [48]. The adoption of the 'umbrella' term ARDS probably covers many different pathophysiological processes which cannot be diagnosed by one simple test or marker. In conclusion, the double-isotope technique can quantify the increased pulmonary permeability to protein in acute lung injury, and is a useful tool for investigating potential treatments.

References

1. Ashbaugh DG, Bigelow DB, Petty TL, Levine BE (1967) Acute respiratory distress in adults. Lancet 2:319–323
2. Editorial (1986) Adult respiratory distress syndrome. Lancet 1:301–302
3. Petty TL, Fowler AA (1982) Another look at ARDS. Chest 82:98–104
4. Shale DJ (1987) The adult respiratory distress syndrome – 20 years on. Thorax 42:641–645
5. Rocker GM, Wiseman MS, Pearson D, Shale DJ (1989) Diagnostic criteria for adult respiratory distress syndrome: time for reappraisal. Lancet 1:120–123
6. Rocker GM, Wiseman MS, Pearson D, Shale DJ (1988) Neutrophil degranulation and increased pulmonary capillary permeability following oesophagectomy: a model of early lung injury in man. Br J Surg 75:883–886
7. Weigelt JA (1987) Current concepts in the management of the adult respiratory distress syndrome. World J Surg 11:161–166
8. Pepe PE, Potkin RT, Reus DH, Hudson LD, Carrico CJ (1982) Clinical predictors of the adult respiratory distress syndrome. Am J Surg 144:124–130
9. Weigelt JA, Snyder WH III, Mitchell RA (1981) Early indentification of patients prone to develop adult respiratory distress syndrome. Am J Surg 142:687–691
10. Fein A, Grossman RF, Jones JG, et al (1979) The value of edema fluid protein measurement in patients with pulmonary edema. Am J Med 67:32–38
11. Weibel ER (1984) The pathway for oxygen: structure and function in the mammalian respiratory system. Harvard University Press, Cambridge, Massachusetts
12. Staub NC (1974) Pulmonary edema. Physiol Rev 54:678–811

13. Taylor AE, Gaar KA (1970) Estimation of equivalent pore radii of pulmonary capillary and alveolar membranes. Am J Physiol 218:1133–1140

14. Richardson WN, Bilan D, Hoppensack M, Oppenheimer L (1987) Fast-phase transvascular fluid flux and the Fahreus effect. J Appl Physiol 62:1513–1520

15. Barrowcliffe MP, Jones JG (1987) Solute permeability of the alveolar capillary barrier. Thorax 42:1–10

16. Hills BA (1981) What is the true role of surfactant in the lung? Thorax 36:1–4

17. Evander E, Wollmer P, Jonson B, Lachmann B (1987) Pulmonary clearance of inhaled 99m Tc-DTPA: effects of surfactant depletion by lung lavage. J Appl Physiol 62:1611–1614

18. Anderson RR, Holliday RL, Driedger AA, Sibbald WJ (1979) Documentation of pulmonary capillary permeability in the adult respiratory distress syndrome accompanying human sepsis. Am Rev Resp Dis 119:869–877

19. Sibbald WJ, Driedger AA, Wells GA, Koval JJ (1983) Clinical correlates of the spectrum of lung microvascular injury in human noncardiac edema. Crit Care Med 11:70–78

20. Weiner F, Carlson RW, Pur VK, Weil MH (1983) Mathematical model to study fluid and protein transfer in pulmonary edema in man. Crit Care Med 11:132–141

21. Sibbald WJ, Cunningham DR, Chin DN (1983) Non-cardiac or cardiac pulmonary edema? A practical approach to clinical differentiation in critically ill patients. Chest 84:452–461

22. Jones JG, Somerville ID (1989) Lung surfactant: composition, physiology and replacement therapy. In: Kaufman L (ed) Anaesthesia review 6. Churchill Livingstone, London, pp 185–202

23. Holloway H, Perry M, Downey J, Parker J, Taylor A (1983) Estimation of effective pulmonary capillary pressure in intact lungs. J Appl Physiol 54:846–851

24. Allen SJ, Drake RE, Williams JP, Laine GA, Gabel JC (1987) Recent advances in pulmonary edema. Crit Care Med 15:963–970

25. Staub NC (1986) Clinical use of lung water measurements – Report of a workshop. Chest 90:588–594

26. Sibbald WJ, Warshawski FJ, Short AK, Harris J, Lefcoe MS, Holliday RL (1983) Clinical studies of measuring extravascular lung water by the thermal dye technique in critically ill patients. Chest 83:725–731

27. Jones JG, Minty BD, Royston D (1982) The physiology of leaky lungs. Br J Anaesth 54:705–721

28. Griffith DE, Holden WE, Morris JF, Min LK, Krishnamurthy T (1986) Effects of common therapeutic concentrations of oxygen on lung clearance of ^{99m}Tc DTPA and bronchoalveolar lavage albumin concentration. Am Rev Respir Dis 134:233–237

29. Rinderknecht J, Shapiro L, Krauthammer M, et al (1980) Accelerated clearance of small solutes from the lungs in interstitial lung disease. Am Rev Respir Dis 121:105–117

30. Jacobs MP, Baughman RP, Hughes J, Fernandes-Ulloa M (1985) Radioaerosol lung clearance in patients with active pulmonary sarcoidosis. Am Rev Respir Dis 131:687–689

31. Mason GR, Effros RM, Uszler JM, Mena I (1985) Small solute clearance from the lungs of patients with cardiogenic and noncardiogenic pulmonary edema. Chest 88:327–334

32. Tennenberg SD, Jacobs MP, Solomkin JS, Ehlers NA, Hurst JM (1987) Increased pulmonary alveolar-capillary permeability in patients at risk for the adult respiratory distress syndrome. Crit Care Med 15:289–293

33. Nolop KB, Braude S, Hughes JMB, Royston D (1985) The effect of PEEP on epithelial and endothelial solute flux in smokers and non-smokers. Am Rev Respir Dis 131:A403

34. Braude S, Nolop KB, Hughes JMB, Barnes PJ, Royston D (1986) Comparison of lung vascular and epithelial permeability indices in the adult respiratory distress syndrome. Am Rev Respir Dis 133:1002–1005

35. Jeffries AL, Coates G, O'Brodovich H (1984) Pulmonary epithelial permeability in hyaline-membrane disease. N Engl Med 311:1075–1080

36. O'Brodovich H, Coates G (1988) Pulmonary clearance of ^{99m}Tc-DTPA in infants who subsequently develop bronchopulmonary dysplasia. Am Rev Respir Dis 137:210–212

37. Anderson RR, Holliday RL, Driedger AA, Lefcoe M, Reid R, Sibbald WJ (1979) Documentation of pulmonary capillary permeability in the adult respiratory distress syndrome accompanying sepsis. Am Rev Respir Dis 119:869–877

38. Sibbald WJ, Anderson RR, Reid B, Holliday RL, Driedger AA (1981) Alveolo-capillary permeability in human septic ARDS. Effect of high-dose corticosteroid therapy. Chest 79:133–142
39. Tatum JL, Burke TS, Sugerman HJ, Strash AM, Hirsch JI, Fratkin MJ (1982) Computerised scintigraphic technique for the evalution of adult respiratory distress syndrome: initial clinical trials. Radiology 143:237–241
40. Spicer KM, Reines DH, Frey GD (1986) Diagnosis of adult respiratory distress syndrome with Tc-99m human serum albumin and portable probe. Crit Care Med 14:669–676
41. Dauber IM, Pluss WT, VanGrondelle A, Trow RS, Weil JV (1985) Specificity and sensitivity of noninvasive measurement of pulmonary vascular protein leak. J Appl Physiol 59:564–574
42. Basran GS, Byrne AJ, Hardy JG (1985) A noninvasive technique for measuring lung vascular permeability in man. Nucl Med Commun 6:3–10
43. Gorin AB, Kohler J, DeNardo G (1980) Noninvasive measurement of pulmonary transvascular protein flux in normal man. J Clin Invest 66:869–877
44. Basran GS, Hardy JG (1988) Monitoring pulmonary vascular permeability using radiolabeled transferrin. J Thorac Imag 3:28–35
45. Wetterberg T, Svensjo E, Larsson A, Sigurdsson G, Wagner G, Willen H (1989) Acute lung injury monitored with radiolabeled transferrin and lung volume measurements. Acta Anaesthesiol Scand 33:359–368
46. Basran GS, Byrne AJ, Hardy JG (1986) The effect of methylprednisolone on the pulmonary accumulation of transferrin in the adult respiratory distress syndrome. Eur J Respir Dis 68:336–341
47. Basran GS, Hardy JG, Woo SP, Ramasubramanian R, Byrne AJ (1986) Beta-2-adrenoceptor agonists as inhibitors of lung vascular permeability to radiolabeled transferrin in the adult respiratory distress syndrome in man. Eur J Nucl Med 12:381–384
48. Rocker GM, Pearson D, Stephens M, Shale DJ (1988) An assessment of a double-isotope method for detection of transferrin accumulation in the lungs of patients with widespread pulmonary infiltrates. Clin Sci 75:47–52

Host Defense Mechanisms in Acute Lung Injury – Smoke Inhalation in Fire Victims

C. G. Gemmell, J. Kinsella, and C. J. Clark

Introduction

The mortality rate amongst fire victims is increasing in the United Kingdom [1] with pulmonary complications becoming the major cause of death, especially since wound sepsis in the burned patient can be effectively treated. Inhalation of smoke arising from the combustion of man-made polystyrene foam-containing furniture is the main cause for these pulmonary complications [2, 3]. It has already been shown that chronic exposure to cigarette smoke and industrial pollutants can impair pulmonary cellular defense mechanisms and it has been suggested that smoke inhalation may act similarly, and thereby increase susceptibility to infection. Alternatively, patients may develop a clinical picture resembling adult respiratory distress syndrome (ARDS) in which lung injury may be due to the release of inflammatory mediators including highly reactive oxygen radicals from phagocytic cells.

Cellular Changes in Lung Compartment

Whilst there is an enormous amount of literature on burns injury, there is a conspicuous gap in the literature on smoke inhalation injury, especially the changes in the lung compartment. Bronchoalveolar lavage (BAL) offers a direct approach in studying some of the pathophysiological changes that occur in the lungs of burned patients [2, 4, 5]. These changes include an influx of neutrophils into the lungs and an increase in total cell yields from BAL fluid in these patients (Table 1). Patients with smoke inhalation, and especially those with burns injury as well, have a moderate increase in total cell yields but not significantly so during the early period.

Patients who were lavaged a second time (from the opposite lung) showed significant increases in their total cell yields, compared to their initial lavages ($p < 0.005$). The increase is almost completely due to an influx of neutrophils into the lungs. This influx soon changes the cell profile in BAL fluid of these patients so that there is a reciprocal rise and fall in the proportions of neutrophils and macrophages respectively. Even in the first 24 hours the proportion of neutrophils becomes significantly higher in patients with smoke inhalation alone ($p < 0.002$) and in those with combined injury ($p < 0.002$) than in control subjects. The proportion of macrophages becomes significantly lower in smoke inhalation

Table 1. Bronchoalveolar lavage fluid analysis

Cell type	Smoking controls (n = 18)	Burns alone (n = 15)	Smoke alone (n = 10)	Smoke + burns (n = 17)
Macrophages				
Mature	1.37 (0.92–2.72)	2.45 (0.84–4.60)	1.6 (1.21–3.50)	4.16 (0.49–20.00)*
Immature	0	0	0.10 (0–0.18)	3.75 (0.14–11.90)
Polymorphonuclear leukocytes	0.14 (0.01–0.44)	0.02 (0–0.11)	0.46 (0.04–1.59)*	0.38 (0–3.00)*
Total	1.47 (1.00–3.20)	2.18 (0.80–5.50)	2.27 (1.89–4.16)*	8.17 (1.13–34.20)**

* Median (interquartile range) cells $\cdot 10^5$/ml.
Significant difference compared with controls: * $p < 0.05$ and ** $p < 0.01$ (U test).

only ($p < 0.001$) and smoke plus burns ($p < 0.002$), when compared with control subjects. Patients with burns only do not show any increase in neutrophil population. After the first 24 hours this situation progresses further so that the cell profiles in repeat BAL samples from the same patients with or without smoke inhalation show an even greater rise and fall in the proportions of neutrophils and macrophages respectively ($p < 0.01$), (Figs. 1 and 2).

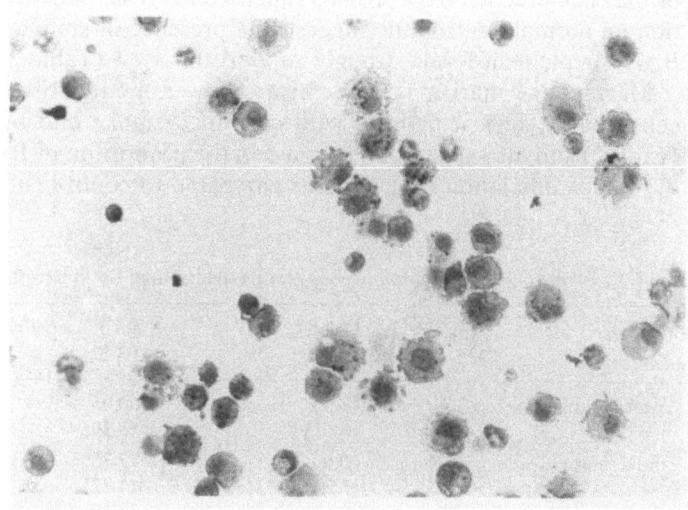

Fig. 1. BAL cells from a patient with smoke inhalation injury on admission to hospital – Leishman staining; magnification × 400

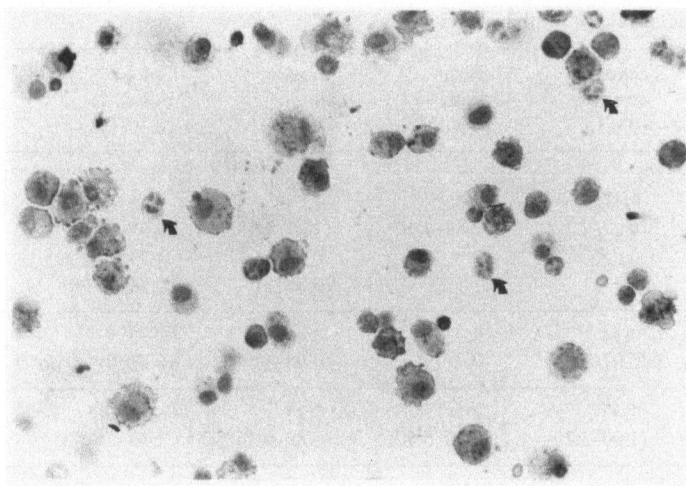

Fig. 2. BAL cells from same patient as in Fig. 1 but taken 24 hours after admission – Leishman staining; magnification × 400; ⇢ = PMN.

This accumulation of neutrophils may be due to:

(a) to the release of macrophage products such as neutrophil chemotactic factor known to be released by activated macrophages [6]
(b) products of complement activation or
(c) LTB_4.

Such factors have been shown to attract neutrophils into the lungs. Measurement of the chemotactic effect of BAL supernatants from patients with smoke inhalation on normal neutrophils suggests the presence of similar factors and data on BAL complement levels strongly support this view (Table 2).

Macrophage marker measurements show a modest rise in $UCHM_1$-positive cells (monocytes) in patients with combined smoke and burn injury ($p < 0.02$) (Table 3) and also suggest an increase in the proportion of RFD_9-positive cells in the smoke inhalation only patients compared to control subjects ($p < 0.02$). The

Table 2. Percentage of macrophage subgroups determined by macrophage markers

Marker	Mean%	(SEM) positive for:	
	RFD_7	RFD_9	$UCHM_1$
Control subjects	43.05	60.05	0.99
(n = 12)	(6.61)	(5.59)	(0.40)
Smoke alone	40.00	77.75*	3.64
(n = 9)	(5.36)	(1.72)	(1.40)
Smoke and burns	44.5	67.85	5.26*
(n = 14)	(5.78)	(4.75)	(1.43)

* $p < 0.02$.

Table 3. Levels of complement activation products in BAL fluid in smoke inhalation injury

	Units/L BAL fluid			µg/L BAL fluid	
	$C1s$-C-Inh	$C3_{-p}$	$C5b_{-9}$	$C5a$	$C3a$
Control subjects	138.5 (499)	76.9 (277.3)	0 (0)	1.72 (0.9)	10.71 (4.97)
(n = 14)	0 (138.5)	0 (76.9)	0 (0)	1.60 (0.24)	9.8 (1.33)
Smoke alone	300 (669.7)	0 (0)	237.5 (477.9)	1.62 (1.06)	19.37 (10.5)
	0 (236.8)	0 (0)	0 (168.9)	1.50 (0.37)	23.2 (3.5)
(n = 8)	NS	NS	NS	NS	NS
Smoke + burns	3327 (4197.4)	560 (653.5)	411.1 (816.2)	2.53 (2.21)	98.84 (172.05)
	2500 (1399.1)	250 (206.6)	0 (272.1)	1.75 (0.70)	34.6 (54.4)
(n = 10)	$P < 0.05$	NS	NS	NS	NS

NS = not significant.

importance of this finding can only be conjectural because the function of the various subgroups of macrophages defined by these markers is not yet known. RFD$_9$-positive cells are tangible macrophages with wide distribution in the body. It is interesting that these studies did not show any significant change in RFD$_7$-positive cells which are supposed to be mature macrophages.

Functional Changes in Macrophages

Measurement of chemotaxis of alveolar macrophages from patients with smoke inhalation showed increased unstimulated and stimulated migration towards the various chemotaxins. Patients with smoke inhalation alone showed only a trend but it was clear that patients with combined injury demonstrated highly significant differences in migration compared to control subjects (Table 3).

The finding of increased migration of macrophages from patients with smoke inhalation may be due to the presence of a new population of macrophages as suggested by increased RFD$_9$-positive cells moving into the alveoli and capable of expressing various receptors for chemotactic agents such as C_{5a}. Alternatively this could be due to stimulation of the resident macrophages by a phagocytic load (smoke debris Fig. 1a), resulting in their activation and expression of receptors for chemotactic factors previously internalized.

Our findings contrast with those of others [4] who reported significantly lower alveolar macrophage chemotaxis from a group of seven patients with smoke inhalation. Their BAL cell profile consisted of a high proportion of neutrophils (35%) which in our experience physically interferes with the migration of macrophages. BAL cell profiles in our patients consisted mainly of macrophages (86%) and only 11% neutrophils.

The chemiluminescence of alveolar macrophages obtained from lavage fluid of patients with smoke inhalation injury, smoke/burns injury has also been compared to that of a cohort of patients with cutaneous burns only or to cigarette smokers. *In toto* the subjects comprised 42 fire victims admitted to our hospital and 18 control patients attending for diagnostic bronchoscopy. Ten of the fire victims had clinical [2] and biochemical (blood carboxyhemoglobin concentration corrected to estimate smoke exposure) evidence of smoke inhalation, but no cutaneous burns. Fifteen of the fire victims had cutaneous burns only; 16 had combined smoke and cutaneous burns injury. The controls were smokers but who had no active infection, inflammation or neoplastic process on clinical examination, bronchoscopy or follow-up.

The results were highly skewed. Spontaneous chemiluminescence (no particulate stimulus) was similar in cells from patients with cutaneous burns alone and controls (Fig. 3a). Chemiluminescence stimulated by opsonised *Staphylococcus aureus* cells was also similar (Fig. 3b). Cells from patients with smoke inhalation only showed similar spontaneous chemiluminescence to control subjects but a significantly increased response to stimulation. The patients with combined injury had a significant increase in spontaneous and stimulated chemiluminscence compared with controls [7]. The stimulated response in the combined injuries group was significantly less than that of the smoke inhalation only group, suggesting that the preactivation of oxidative metabolism of the macrophages had reduced their capacity to respond to a further bacterial stimulus. This might have important implications with respect to host susceptibility to bacterial infection.

On this basis phagocytic ingestion of opsonised *S. aureus* was monitored in each group of patients. In each case the efficacy of phagocytic ingestion was assessed according to whether:

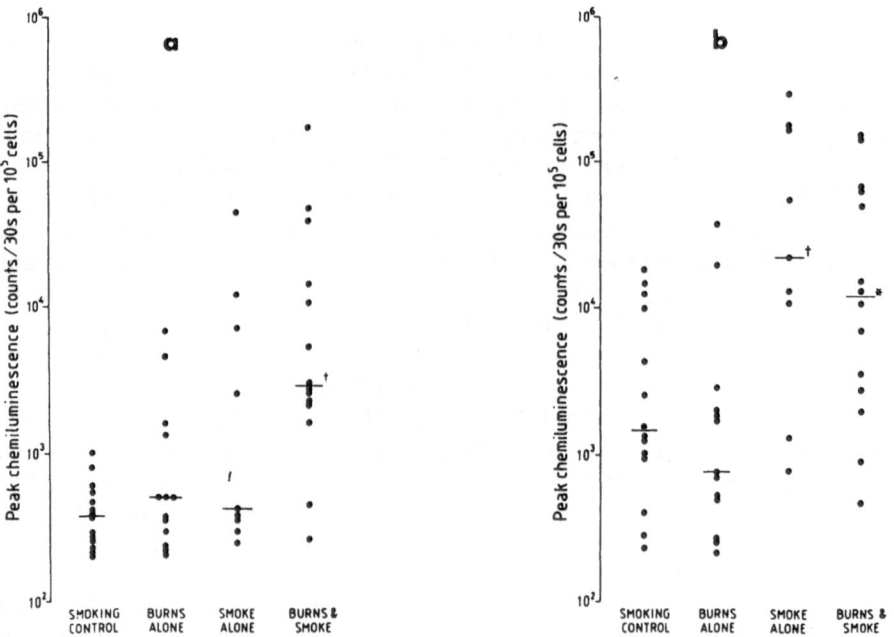

Fig. 3a, b. Chemiluminescence of alveolar macrophages in smoke inhalation and burns injury patients. **a** Spontaneous chemiluminescence; **b** stimulated chemiluminescence

(a) $\leq 25\%$ of the target bacteria were ingested (Status 1)

(b) 25–50% of the target bacteria were ingested (Status 2) and

(c) $> 50\%$ of the target bacteria were ingested (Status 3).

There is evidence that phagocytic efficacy is impaired in patients with combined injury compared to those with smoke inhalation only. This difference was seen whether or not the patients had been exposed to low or high levels of smoke ($\leq 25\%$ and $\leq 50\%$ blood carboxyhemoglobin respectively). At carboxyhemoglobin levels of $\leq 25\%$, macrophages from a greater number of patients (4/10) with combined injury displayed phagocyte efficacy Status 2 compared to that of smoke injury only (1/10). Similarly at carboxyhemoglobin levels of $\leq 50\%$ macrophages from 7/10 patients with combined injury displayed phagocytic Status 1 compared to only 2/10 with smoke inhalation alone [8]. Control subjects (cigarette smokers) usually possess macrophages belonging to Status 2 or 3.

The picture that emerges in patients with smoke inhalation is that of an accumulation of neutrophils in the lung compartment and activation of alveolar macrophages. This phenomenon is accentuated in patients with burns and smoke inhalation and is quantitatively different from that of simple "depression" of systemic immune functions described in burns only. A number of studies have shown decreased chemotaxis in peripheral polymorphonuclear leukocytes and monocytes in burned patients [9–11]. We have not been able to compare peripheral blood cell function in this respect with alveolar macrophages in our patients. In addition, phagocytic killing of bacteria was reduced five days post-burn and these changes were most marked in patients who ultimately died of microbial sepsis.

Humoral Changes

Serum opsonin levels in patients with severe burn injury are also decreased immediately after the burn occurs but returns to normal by the fourth to fourteenth day post-burn [12]. Serum levels of IgG, properdin and C_3 whilst initially low, returned to normal values by the ninth day. Factor B levels rose rapidly during the first three weeks after injury to more than twice the normal levels. Serum levels of C reactive protein are raised and fibronectin levels decreased in patients with smoke inhalation injury.

BAL fluid from patients with smoke inhalation and burn injury contained higher levels of complement components C_{1r}, C_{1s} and Factor H. They also showed lower levels of C3 than control subjects along with higher levels of C3-P suggesting consumption of C3 with activation of the alternative pathway. Although the difference in the levels of C3-P between patients with smoke inhalation alone and those with combined injury was not significant, examination of raw data is very revealing. In smoke inhalation only none of 10 samples examined (from 8 patients) showed detectable levels of C3-P; in combined injury patients, 5 samples (5 patients) out of 13 samples (9 patients) showed detectable levels of this complement product. Four out of five of these latter patients died. Furthermore, patients with both smoke inhalation and burns showed significant activation of the classical pathway as shown by the levels of C_{1s}-C_{Inh} complex. Does this apparent activation of both the alternative and classical pathways of complement play a key role in promoting further pathophysiological changes in patients with combined smoke inhalation and burns injury with a subsequent high mortality?

Data on levels of antiproteases are not available from patients with smoke inhalation and burns. It is not unreasonable, however, to speculate that loss of serum factors known to occur through burn wounds in these patients may include antiproteases. This would render the lungs of these patients more vulnerable to the injurious effects of neutrophils [13, 14]. Such reduced antiprotease activity has been noted in patients with ARDS. Furthermore, and perhaps more importantly, the presence of products of complement activation such as C5a would lead to the release of proteolytic enzymes, resulting in further complement activation. Thus a vicious cycle which results in lung damage is set in motion.

In smoke inhalation injury, alveolar macrophage activation is perhaps sufficient to recruit neutrophils to the lung compartment. The presence of additional burns injury allows complement activation due to tissue damage leading to further neutrophil sequestration in the lungs. The consequent increase in permeability allows exudation of complement components into the lungs which are cleaved and activated by neutrophil proteases. In severe cutaneous burn injury, intravascular complement activation may be the starting point of the cycle. On

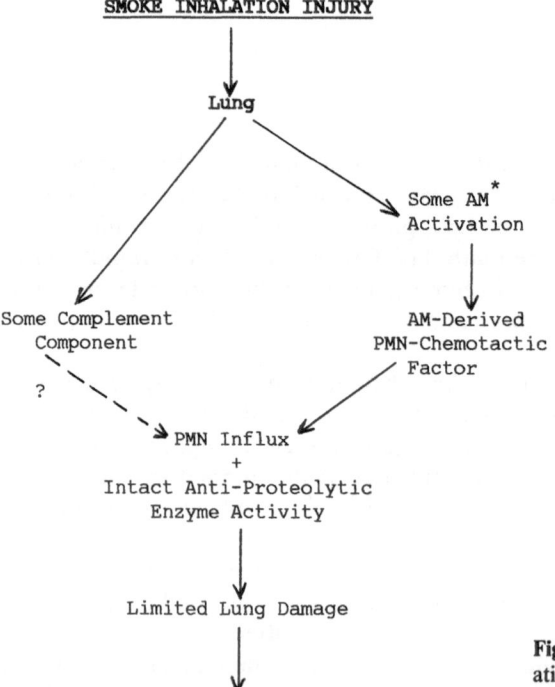

Fig. 4. Consequences of smoke inhalation injury. AM* = alveolar macrophage

this basis it is possible to put forward an hypothesis in lung injury in these conditions (Fig. 4). With such a possible sequence of events possible the potential use of antioxidants in ameliorating lung damage in patients with smoke inhalation injury becomes relevant.

References

1. United Kingdom fire statistics (1986) HM Stationary Office London (1988)
2. Clark CJ, Reid WH, Gilmour WH, Campbell D (1986) Mortality probability in victims of fire trauma: revised equation to include inhalation injury. Br Med J 292:1303–1305
3. Thompson PB, Herndon DN, Traber DL, Abston S (1986) Effect on mortality of inhalation injury. J Trauma 26:163–165
4. Demarest GB, Hudson LD, Altman LC (1979) Impaired alveolar macrophage chemotaxis in patients with acute smoke inhalation. Am Rev Resp Dis 119:279–286
5. Riyami BMS, Tree R, Kinsella J, et al (1990) Changes in alveolar macrophage, monocyte and neutrophil cell profiles after smoke inhalation injury. J Clin Path (in press)
6. Hunninghake GM, Gadek JG, Fales HM, Crystal RG (1980) Human alveolar macrophage derived chemotactic factor for neutrophils. J Clin Invest 66:473–483
7. Clark CJ, Pollock AJ, Reid WH, Campbell D, Gemmell CG (1988) Role of pulmonary alveolar macrophage activation in acute lung injury after burns and smoke inhalation. Lancet 2:872–874
8. Gemmell CG, Pollock AJ, McMillan F, Clark CJ, Reid WH, Campbell D (1987) Structural and functional changes in alveolar macrophages following the exposure of fire victims to smoke. Eur J Clin Invest 17:321
9. Fikrig SM, Karl SC, Suntharalingam K (1977) Neutrophil chemotaxis in patients with burns. Ann Surg 186:746–748
10. Warden GD, Mason AD, Pruitt BA (1974) Evaluation of leukocyte chemotaxis in vitro in thermally injured patients. J Clin Invest 54:1001–1004
11. Altmann LC, Furukawa CT, Klebanoff SJ (1977) Depressed mononuclear leukocyte chemotaxis in thermally injured patients. J Immunol 119:199–205
12. Alexander JW, Moncrief JA (1966) Alteration of the immune response following severe thermal injury. Arch Surg 93:75–88
13. Johnson KT, Ward PA (1981) Role of oxygen metabolites in immune complex injury of lung. J Immunol 126:2365–2369
14. Ward PA (1986) Host-defence mechanisms responsible for lung injury. J Allergy Clin Immunol 58:373–378

Respiratory Changes Induced by Upper Abdominal and Cardiac Surgery

F. Clergue and J. L. Pansard

Introduction

Thoracic and upper abdominal surgery are known to be associated with a high incidence of pulmonary atelectasis and pulmonary infections. After upper abdominal surgery, pulmonary complications occur in 30 to 75% of patients, depending on the criteria defining these complications, on the nature and the duration of the surgical procedure, and on postoperative therapeutic management. Most of the alterations of the respiratory system are specific of these types of surgery, since they do not appear in peripheral surgery, and develop during the first postoperative day [1]. Some of these respiratory impairments are already present as soon as the patient emerges from anesthesia, some are not present during the recovery period and appear progressively during the first postoperative day.

Respiratory Changes After Upper Abdominal Surgery

A *restrictive syndrome* is usually observed as soon as the patients emerge from anesthesia. Vital capacity and FEV_1 decrease by approximately 60% of preoperative values after upper abdominal surgery and by 40% after lower abdominal surgery. This restrictive syndrome is immediately maximal, then progressively recovers over one to three weeks.

Another alteration in lung function is a *decrease in functional residual capacity* (FRC). FRC is known to decrease by 500 ml in adults during general anesthesia. However, Ali et al. [2] have shown that during the immediate postoperative period (4 and 10 hours after the end of surgery), FRC, measured by the helium dilution method, is not different from its preoperative value. It is only 16 hours after the end of surgery that the decrease in FRC becomes significant. This decrease becomes maximal at the end of the first postoperative day, reaching 70% of the preoperative value. Then, in the absence of further complications, FRC returns progressively to its preoperative level within 1 to 2 weeks.

This delayed decrease in FRC suggests that anesthesia is probably poorly involved in the postoperative decrease in FRC.

Hypoxemia is another typical feature of the postoperative period of upper abdominal surgery [1]. Decreases in PaO_2 usually strictly follow changes in FRC.

Changes in the *pattern of breathing* are also observed during the postoperative period. If minute-ventilation usually remains unchanged after surgery, patients breathe with a smaller tidal volume and at a higher respiratory rate than preoperatively. Postoperative pain has frequently been suggested to be responsible for this rapid and shallow breathing. Actually, it has been shown that this breathing pattern persists even after complete pain relief using opiate analgesia, suggesting that other mechanisms may be involved in this breathing mode [3].

Postoperative Diaphragmatic Dysfunction

Several studies have recently pointed out the possible responsibility of a *diaphragmatic dysfunction* on the postoperative respiratory changes observed after upper abdominal surgery.

Description of Postoperative Diaphragmatic Dysfunction

A decrease in diaphragmatic activity was first speculated to be responsible for postoperative respiratory dysfunction by W. Pasteur in 1914. However, it is only recently that several studies tried to demonstrate the responsibility of diaphragmatic dysfunction in postoperative respiratory changes. In 1973, Tahir et al. [4] observed with fluoroscopy a reduction in the course of the diaphragm during tidal breathing after abdominal surgery.

In 1983, Ford et al. [5] studied the consequences of a cholecystectomy on diaphragmatic function. The first technique used to assess the relative contribution of the diaphragm during tidal breathing analyzed the changes in transdiaphragmatic pressure swings (Pdi) or in the ratio of gastric pressure over esophageal or transdiaphragmatic pressures (Pgas/Pes or Pgas/Pdi). The diaphragmatic function was also assessed by the analysis of the changes in the external abdominal dimensions, since an increase in the diameter or in the circumference of the abdomen is usually associated with the diaphragmatic contraction during inspiration. In this study, a decrease in diaphragmatic function was observed after surgery. During the immediate postoperative period, the pattern of breathing, which was predominantly abdominal preoperatively, was shifted to a predominantly thoracic breathing. These changes were observed during the immediate postoperative period, 2 and 4 hours after the end of surgery, and returned close to the preoperative values 24 hours after surgery.

In another study, Simonneau et al. [6] reported the postoperative changes in diaphragmatic function in 5 patients after an elective upper abdominal surgery. In this study, diaphragmatic function was assessed by three different methods: changes in transdiaphragmatic pressure swings, changes in the circumferences of thorax and abdomen, and displacement of the diaphragm over the range of vital capacity using an ultra-sound technique. All these indirect indices of diaphragmatic function were shown to be markedly decreased on the first postoperative day. In some of these patiens, a paradoxical inward motion of the abdomen was shown during inspiration. All these alterations returned progressively to normal during the 7 postoperative days. It was also important to note that an efficient pain relief, achieved by an epidural administration of 150 γ of fentanyl, had no effect on diaphragmatic dysfunction.

Mechanisms of Postoperative Diaphragmatic Dysfunction

Different mechanisms have been speculated to explain this postoperative diaphragmatic dysfunction. A remaining effect of *anesthesia* might have been involved in the genesis of the diaphragmatic impairment. In an experimental study, Road et al. [7] demonstrated that no change in diaphragmatic function was observed when dogs were only anesthetized, while a diaphragmatic impairment was observed when a cholecystectomy was associated. No change in diaphragmatic function was observed after lower abdominal surgery.

A direct effect of the *surgical trauma on the diaphragm* was ruled out by Dureuil et al. [8]. In 5 patients undergoing upper abdominal surgery, diaphragmatic contractility was assessed by changes in the ratio of gastric pressure swings over transdiaphragmatic pressure swings (Pgas/Pdi), while both phrenic nerves were electrically stimulated on the neck. Four hours after surgery, no change in diaphragmatic contractility was noted. This suggested that postoperative diaphragmatic dysfunction was more probably resulting from a *reflex inhibition of phrenic nerve output*, induced by the surgical trauma.

Previous reports have already described similar respiratory reflexes, such as an inhibition or a stimulation of respiration induced by a mechanical stimulation of either abdominal viscera, or intercostal and abdominal muscle proprioceptor afferents. Some of these afferents are conducted by medullary pathways, while others travel through the vagus or the phrenic nerves. In a recent study, Ford et al. [9] showed in spontaneously breathing dogs, that a mechanical stimulation of the gallbladder was immediately associated with a fall of tidal volume and with a decrease in phrenic nerve output. The short interval between the gallbladder stimulation and the decrease in diaphragmatic contraction led to conclude that the mechanism involved was a neural reflex. Since similar results were obtained after vagotomy, this suggested that most of the afferents of this inhibitory reflex were not traveling by the vagus nerve [9].

In humans, Mankikian et al. [10] showed that a thoracic epidural block, with local anesthetics (bupivacaine 0.5%), could restore diaphragmatic function on the first postoperative day following upper abdominal surgery. The epidural block also induced an increase in tidal volume, which returned to the preoperative values, and a decrease in respiratory rate.

Different respiratory effects can be assumed to be associated with the thoracic epidural block. It may interrupt both the afferent inputs originating from the abdominal viscera and from the abdominal and chest wall, and the efferent outputs reaching the abdominal and intercostal muscles.

The improvement in diaphragmatic function induced by the epidural block could be a consequence of the blockade of the afferent pathway, interrupting an inhibitory reflex. However, the different indices used to assess diaphragmatic function are all influenced by variations in abdominal muscle activity. Both gastric pressure and abdominal dimensions are not specific of diaphragmatic activity. They are markedly influenced by a contraction of abdominal muscles, which increase gastric and transdiaphragmatic pressures, and decrease abdominal dimensions. Mankikian et al. [10] pointed out the difficulty of analyzing diaphragmatic function indices, i.e. gastric pressure swings and abdominal dimension changes during the postoperative period in the presence of active contractions of abdominal muscles.

Duggan and Drummond [11] recently showed that the activity of abdominal muscles increases markedly during the postoperative period of upper abdominal surgery. During inspiration, they noted a 3 to 5 fold increase in the activity of these muscles, as compared with preoperative condition. But, the major change was observed during expiration, with a progressive increase in EMG activity of these muscles, followed by an abrupt decrease at the onset of the following inspiration (Fig. 1). This pattern of breathing could falsely be interpreted as an abdominal paradoxical breathing cycle, and mimic a decrease in diaphragmatic activity. Therefore, it could be speculated that the motor block of 0.5% epidural bupivacaine, by cutting off the activity of abdominal muscles, just eliminated the interference due to the abdominal muscles contraction on the indices of diaphragmatic activity, rather than it changed the real activity of the diaphragm.

To solve this question, Pansard et al. [12] repeated the study, adding the recording of diaphragmatic EMG activity, using electrodes inserted intraoperatively into the diaphragm. They showed that epidural bupivacaine is associated with an increase in diaphragmatic EMG activity, strongly suggesting that the hypothesis of a reflex inhibition of diaphragmatic activity is at least partly involved in the postoperative respiratory dysfunction. However, the contraction of abdominal muscles may also play a major role in the postoperative decrease in FRC and in the development of postoperative respiratory complications.

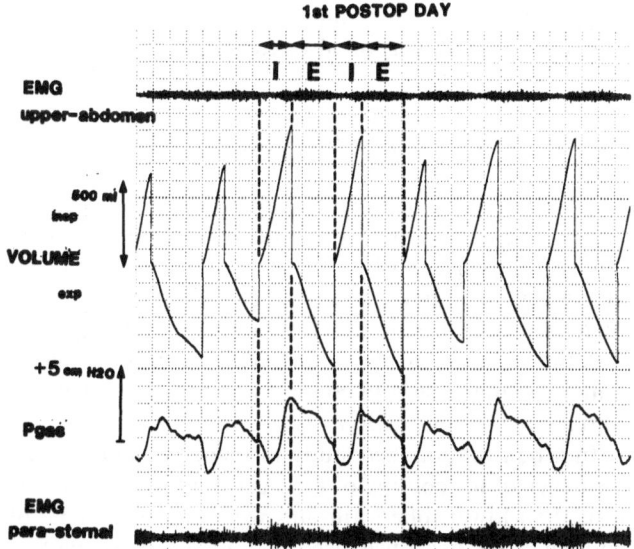

Fig. 1. Recording performed in a patient on the first postoperative day following upper abdominal surgery of simultaneous changes in the EMG of the abdominal muscles, of inspired and expired volume, of gastric pressure (Pgas), and of the EMG of the para-sternal muscles. Note the abrupt fall in gastric pressure at the onset of inspiration, corresponding to the relaxation of the abdominal muscles

Respiratory Changes After Thoracic and Cardiac Surgery

Pulmonary complications represent a frequent event after thoracic and cardiac surgery. In patients undergoing thoracic surgery for lung cancer, the operative mortality rate ranges from 2.1% to 12.4%, the first factor involved in this mortality being the pulmonary complications. In cardiac surgery, the incidence of pulmonary complications is much lower than in thoracic surgery. Postoperative pneumonias are observed in 0.6% of patients undergoing coronary bypass surgery (CABG) [13]. However, pulmonary complications still are the second factor increasing the length of hospital stay, after wound infection.

The respiratory changes which occur during the postoperative period of thoracic surgery are similar to those described after upper abdominal surgery, while somewhat less important. Vital capacity and FEV_1 decrease by 40–50%. FRC decreases by 20–30%, and hypoxemia is also observed during the first postoperative days when the patients do not receive supplemental O_2. As for upper abdominal surgery, the same factors have been speculated to explain these respiratory changes.

After *thoracic surgery* for pulmonary resection, Maeda et al. [14] recently studied the changes in diaphragmatic function during the postoperative period. During the first postoperative days, they observed a decrease in the maximal strength of the diaphragm and in the ratio of gastric over transdiaphragmatic pressure swings (Pgas/Pdi). Of the 20 patients studied, the lowest diaphragmatic functions were observed in the 4 patients who developed postoperative respiratory failure requiring prolonged mechanical ventilation. These data suggest that thoracic surgery is responsible for a postoperative diaphragmatic dysfunction.

In *cardiac surgery,* left lower lobe atelectasis are reported to be present in 86–90% of patients during the immediate postoperative period. While the factors involved in the respiratory complications of upper abdominal surgery may also be responsible for the respiratory changes observed after thoracic and cardiac surgery, cardiac surgery may be associated with specific complications, related either to the extracorporeal circulation or to the cardiac cooling.

Phrenic Nerve Injury After Cardiac Surgery

The left phrenic nerve, which is positioned between the pericardium and the left pleura, is exposed to an intraoperative hypothermic injury during the period of cold cardioplegia during cardiopulmonary bypass surgery. In dogs, Dureuil et al. [15] demonstrated that *topical cooling of the phrenic nerve* could induce a complete block of phrenic nerve conduction and emphasized the importance of the duration of the topical cooling. While a rapid recovery was demonstrated after a 5 min cooling, a 30 min cooling was associated with a prolonged impairment of phrenic nerve conduction.

In a non-randomized study in man, Benjamin et al. [16] showed the possible influence of ice cooling of the heart on the development of postoperative atelectasis. Left lower lobe infiltrates were present in 65% of patients, when a topical cooling of the heart was used, and in 30% of patients in the absence of ice cooling. The excursion of the left hemidiaphragm was shown to be decreased in 69% of patients with left lower lobe infiltrates, suggesting the possible responsibility of an impaired diaphragmatic function on the development of atelectasis.

Estenne et al. [17] studied 12 patients before and 8 to 13 days after CABG. After surgery, vital capacity was decreased by 20% and FRC by 9.5%. The conduction times of the right and left phrenic nerves and the ratio of the EMG activity of left and right hemidiaphragms were unchanged after surgery in 11 of the 12 patients. These authors concluded that phrenic-diaphragm dysfunction is rarely involved in the postoperative loss of lung volume. However, this study was performed during the second postoperative week, when most of the postoperative alterations in respiratory function have recovered.

In order to establish the relationship between intraoperative cold cardioplegia and phrenic nerve injury, Wilcox et al. [18] measured the phrenic conduction time during phrenic nerve stimulation in 57 patients before and after cardiac surgery. They found a postoperative abnormality in phrenic nerve function in 5 patients, while left lower lobe atelectasis were present in 50 of 57 patients. These authors concluded that transient phrenic nerve injury was unlikely the explanation for the almost routine development of left lower lobe atelectasis. The other intraoperative factors they found to be more frequently associated with postoperative atelectasis were the intraoperative opening of the pleural space, the duration of surgery, the number of grafts, the low body temperature, and the lack of use of a polystyrene pad to protect the phrenic nerve from intrapericardial ice.

Diaphragmatic Function After Cardiac Surgery

Since it could be speculated that the same mechanisms of respiratory dysfunction could develop after cardiac surgery than after upper abdominal surgery, we recently studied the postoperative changes in diaphragmatic function in 8 patients undergoing cardiac surgery. The different measurements were performed the day before surgery, and on the first and fifth postoperative days.

On the first postoperative day, after extubation, a change in the pattern of breathing was observed in all patients, when compared with preoperative condition. A significant decrease in tidal volume and a higher respiratory rate were noted. Breathing was predominantly thoracic postoperatively, with a significant decrease in the abdominal contribution to tidal breathing, while swings in gastric pressure were significantly decreased (Fig. 2). These findings were similar to those previously observed after upper abdominal surgery. Furthermore, while some diaphragmatic activity was still observed on gastric pressure tracings or on diaphragmatic EMG recordings in some patients, abdominal muscles had a phasic contraction starting before the end of inspiration, lasting during expiration, and followed by an abrupt relaxation at the onset of the following inspiration.

These changes were similar to those previously described after upper abdominal surgery [10, 11]. In this study, no paradoxical inward displacement of the abdominal wall was observed during inspiration, suggesting that the expansion

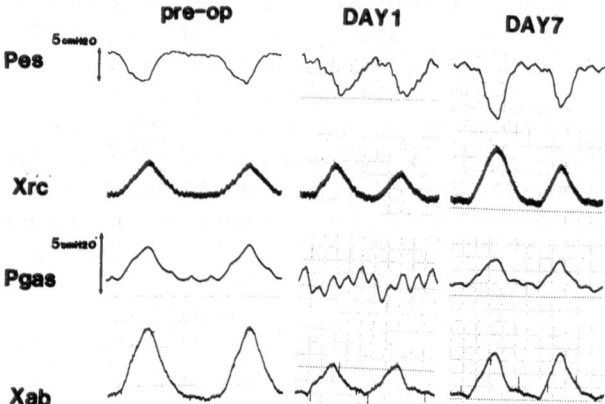

Fig. 2. Simultaneous recording of changes in esophageal (Pes) and gastric pressure (Pgas), and in rib cage (Xrc) and abdomen (Xab) external dimensions, measured by respiratory inductance plethysmography, in a patient before cardiac surgery (pre-op), and on the first and the seventh postoperative day. Note the change in Pgas on the first postoperative day

of the abdominal wall at the beginning of inspiration was the consequence of a sudden relaxation of the abdominal muscles. This was further confirmed by the abrupt fall in gastric pressure during the first part of inspiration. Five days after cardiac surgery, all these abnormalities has not yet returned to the preoperative values. This study shows that identical respiratory changes are induced by both upper abdominal and cardiac surgery.

Conclusion

These new developments in the understanding of postoperative respiratory changes do not yet lead to clear clinical conclusions concerning the management of these patients during the postoperative period. If upper abdominal, thoracic and cardiac surgery probably decrease diaphragmatic activity during the postoperative period, the role played by the contraction of the abdominal muscles has still to be clarified. If a contraction of the abdominal muscles has already been reported to be induced by a decrease in FRC, the use of these expiratory muscles can also contribute to the decrease in FRC.

Postoperative physiotherapy is the major therapeutic maneuver that has clearly been shown to decrease the incidence of postoperative pulmonary complications. Several recent studies have shown that the different maneuvers that can be performed, deep breathing exercises, intermittent positive pressure breathing, or incentive spirometry are associated with similar favorable results [19]. If postoperative pain probably is not the main determinant in the development of postoperative complications, pain relief, by allowing postoperative physiotherapy to be more efficient, should be more frequently offered in association with an active program of physiotherapy, when patients can be monitored carefully. In the choice of postoperative analgesia, the use of local anesthetics administered epidurally has been shown to increase diaphragmatic activity, and will have to be carefully compared to the other methods of analgesia.

References

1. Craig DB (1983) Postoperative recovery of pulmonary function. Anesth Analg 60:46–52
2. Ali J, Weisel RD, Layng AB, Kripke BJ, Hechtman HB (1974) Consequences of postoperative alteration in respiratory mechanics. Am J Surg 128:376–382
3. Clergue F, Montembault C, Despierres O, Ghesquiere F, Harari A, Viars P (1984) Respiratory effects of intrathecal morphine after upper abdominal surgery. Anesthesiology 61:677–685
4. Tahir AA, George RB, Weill H, Adriani J (1973) Effects of abdominal surgery upon diaphragm function and regional ventilation. Int Surg 58:337–340
5. Ford GT, Whitelaw WA, Rosenal TW, Cruse PJ, Guenter CA (1983) Diaphragm function after upper abdominal surgery in humans. Am Rev Respir Dis 127:431–436
6. Simonneau G, Vivien A, Sartene R, et al (1983) Diaphragmatic dysfunction induced by upper abdominal surgery. Am Rev Respir Dis 128:899–903
7. Road JD, Burgess KD, Whitelaw WA, Ford GT (1984) Diaphragm function and respiratory response after upper abdominal surgery in dogs. J Appl Physiol 57:576–582
8. Dureuil B, Viires N, Cantineau JP, Aubier M, Desmonts JM (1986) Diaphragmatic contractility after upper abdominal surgery. J Appl Physiol 61:1775–1780
9. Ford GT, Grant DA, Rideout KS, Davison JS, Whitelaw WA (1988) Inhibition of breathing associated with gallbladder stimulation in dogs. J Appl Physiol 65:72–79
10. Mankikian B, Cantineau JP, Bertrand M, Kieffer E, Sartene R, Viars P (1988) Improvement of diaphragmatic function by a thoracic extradural block after upper abdominal surgery. Anesthesiology 68:379—386
11. Duggan J, Drummond GB (1987) Activity of lower intercostal and abdominal muscle after upper abdominal surgery. Anesth Analg 66:852–855
12. Pansard JL, Philip Y, Bahnini A, et al (1987) Effects of thoracic extradural block on diaphragmatic activity after upper abdominal surgery. Anesthesiology 67:A537 (Abstract)
13. Weintraub WS, Jones EL, Craver J, Guyton R, Cohen C (1989) Determinants of prolonged length of hospital stay after coronary bypass surgery. Circulation 80:276–284
14. Maeda H, Nakahara K, Ohno K, Kido T, Ikeda M, Kawashima Y (1988) Diaphragm function after pulmonary resection. Am Rev Respir Dis 137:678–681
15. Dureuil B, Viires N, Pariente R, Desmonts JM, Aubier M (1987) Effects of phrenic nerve cooling on diaphragmatic function. J Appl Physiol 63:1763–1769
16. Benjamin JJ, Cascade PN, Rubenfire M, Wajszczuk W, Kerin NZ (1982) Left lower lobe atelectasis and consolidation following cardiac surgery: the effect of topical cooling on the phrenic nerve. Radiology 142:11–14
17. Estenne M, Yernault JC, De Smet JM, De Troyer A (1985) Phrenic and diaphragm function after coronary artery bypass grafting. Thorax 40:293–299
18. Wilcox P, Baile EM, Hards J, et al (1988) Phrenic nerve function and its relationship to atelectasis after coronary artery bypass surgery. Chest 93:693–698
19. Celli BR, Rodriguez KS, Snider GL (1984) A controlled trial of intermittent positive pressure breathing, incentive spirometry, and deep breathing exercises in preventing pulmonary complications after abdominal surgery. Am Rev Respir Dis 130:12–15

Respiratory Support

Diaphragm Pacing

W. Vincken and H. De Boeck

Introduction

Diaphragm pacing (DP) represents a perfect hybrid between artificial and spontaneous ventilation. Using external and internally implanted components, the pacemaker delivers an electrical current to the phrenic nerve, thus provoking diaphragmatic muscle contraction and a natural negative-pressure breath in patients otherwise incapable of sustaining spontaneous ventilation by using their diaphragms.

That ventilation can be sustained by electrical stimulation of the phrenic nerves, was first reported by Sarnoff et al. in 1948 [1]. However, initiating in 1964 Glenn et al. [2], have the merit to have developed a partially implantable phrenic nerve pacemaker for long-term ventilatory assistance employed for the first time in patients with central alveolar hypoventilation in 1970 [3] and in quadriplegic patients with respiratory muscle paralysis in 1972 [4]. Today, about 700 diaphragm pacemakers providing partial or full ventilatory support have been employed worldwide in adult and, since the last decade, also in pediatric patients.

Diaphragm Pacing System

The most widely available system manufactured by Avery Laboratories Inc. (Farmingdale, New York) is described here. Other systems are available, such as the Atrostim Pekka model (Atrotech, Tampere, Finland), generally using the same principles as the Avery system.

The diaphragm pacemaker consists of external and internal components. The external battery-powered transmitter emits a radiofrequency (2.05 MHz) signal which is conducted via an insulated cable to a circular antenna taped to the skin overlying the subcutaneous pocket wherein the receiver has been implanted. The radiofrequency signal is transmitted transcutaneously to the subcutaneous receiver which, coupled to an anode disc, demodulates and converts the signal into an electric current consisting of a series (pulse train) of 150 μsec impulses spaced 40 to 140 ms apart. The pulse train is conveyed via an insulated leadwire to a monopolar or bipolar electrode implanted around the phrenic nerve. Monopolar electrodes are easier to implant and unlike bipolar electrodes, do not completely surround the nerve. They, hence, are less likely to cause nerve damage due to perineural fibrosis interfering with nerve blood supply. Bipolar electrodes should only be used if the patient already has another electrical stimulator implanted, e.g., a demand cardiac pacemaker.

The external transmitter contains the adjustable controls of the various pacing parameters. Depending on the pacing schedule, the duration of the pulse train, or inspiratory time (Ti), is set at 1.3–2 seconds and its repetition rate, or respiratory rate (RR), at 8–15/min. The stimulus frequency, or number of pulses in the pulse train per second, is set at 7–25 Hz, determining a pulse interval (PI) of 40–140 ms. The current amplitude of the first pulse in the train is set at the threshold amplitude. This threshold is determined under fluoroscopy of the diaphragm in the supine position and equals the minimal current amplitude at which a beginning of diaphragmatic contraction can be observed. The threshold current amplitude usually is 60% of or 1–2 mA below the current amplitude necessary for maximal diaphragmatic contraction [5, 6]. The current amplitude of the last pulse in the train is set at the minimal value which produces maximal diaphragmatic excursion under fluoroscopy. The amplitude of the intervening pulses in the pulse train progressively increases from the threshold to the last pulse, thus providing a gentle, smooth recruitment of all available diaphragmatic motor units.

Surgical Technique

The pacing electrode is implanted under strict aseptic conditions on the phrenic nerve in its cervical or thoracic course [6, 7]. Despite its greater complexity, the thoracic approach is preferred except in those patients in whom thoracotomy represents an excessive surgical risk or is rendered difficult by prior pleural disease. In a majority of individuals, at least one accessory branch of the phrenic nerve, arising from the third cervical through the first thoracic spinal segment, joins the main phrenic nerve below the thoracic inlet [8]. Electrode implantation on the cervical course of the phrenic nerve, hence, may not recruit all available diaphragmatic motor units, a risk which is avoided by the thoracic approach.

The thorax is entered via a 15 cm long axillary incision in the third intercostal space or an anterior incision in the second interspace. The nerve is located along its mediastinal course and its viability is retested using a nerve test probe. The electrode is anchored to the surrounding tissue behind the nerve 5 to 10 cm above the heart to prevent the occurrence of cardiac arrhythmias while pacing, i.e., where the nerve crosses the superior vena cava on the right side and the aortic arch on the left. From the electrode, a leadwire is passed to the extrathoracic subcutaneous pocket, which necessitates a second skin incision at the lower anterior rib cage and accommodates the receiver, the anode disc and the excess wire placed in a teflon bag. Prior to and after closing, the system is checked using a sterile antenna. A pleural drain is left in place for the next 2–3 days. Bilateral systems are implanted in 2 sessions, 7 to 14 days apart.

Indications and Contra-Indications

The main indication for DP consists of ventilator-dependent patients with chronic respiratory insufficiency due to interruption of neural pathways connecting the brain stem respiratory centers to the phrenic motoneurons. Patients with an irreversible and complete high-cervical cord lesion (usually a traumatic transsection) above the C_3-C_5 level where the lower phrenic motoneurons are located present a quadriplegia with paralysis of all respiratory muscles except the accessory neck muscles. Their phrenic motoneurons and axons which constitute the phrenic nerve are, however, intact, viable and hence amenable to pacing. By contrast, patients with lower spinal cord lesions are not candidates for DP. In those with lesions at the C_3-C_5 level, most phrenic motoneurons are damaged and their axons cannot conduct externally applied electrical impulses. In those with lesions below the C_5 level, the phrenic motoneurons are not disconnected from the brain stem respiratory centers and, although intercostal and abdominal respiratory muscles are paralyzed, their diaphragms are capable of sustaining spontaneous breathing. Hence, it is extremely important in quadriplegic patients to accurately localize the level of the spinal cord lesion. For this purpose electrophysiological techniques must be used since the level of spinal cord damage not always corresponds to the level of radiologically visible vertebral damage.

Another important indication for DP is inadequate central respiratory drive due to central alveolar hypoventilation (CAH) or Ondine's curse [9]. This condition is characterized by impaired automatic, but maintained voluntary control of respiration with markedly reduced or absent ventilatory responses to chemical stimuli [10]. Hypoventilation with hypercapnia and hypoxemia occur during sleep, but improve while awake (when the patient voluntarily adjusts ventilation) or with artificial ventilation. Both congenital [11, 12] and acquired forms have been reported, but only rarely have underlying medullary lesions been demonstrated. Because patients with CAH have no primary pulmonary, thoracic or neuromuscular disorders, both adults [3, 13] and infants [11, 12] can and have been treated with DP, especially during sleep.

Mandatory for successful application of DP is that the phrenic neuromuscular apparatus from the phrenic motoneuron to the diaphragm muscle fiber be intact, viable and well-functioning. Diaphragmatic weakness or paralysis resulting from disease in any part along this axis are formal contra-indications to DP: spinal cord lesions at the C_3-C_5 level, disorders of anterior horn cells (poliomyelitis, amyotrophic lateral sclerosis), of the phrenic nerve itself (neuropathy, traumatic section), of the myoneural junction (myasthenia gravis) or of the diaphragm muscle (myopathy, myotonic dystrophy) are not amenable to electrical stimulation of the phrenic nerve.

Severe underlying obstructive or restrictive intra- or extrapulmonary disease also constitute a contra-indication, since DP can only provide adequate ventilation in the presence of sufficiently normal functioning lung and chest wall.

Other considerations in selecting patients for DP include the patient's age and life-expectancy, his or his family members' ability to understand and properly use the device and the availability of adequate follow-up care and professional assistance. In patients with traumatic spinal cord lesions and respiratory paralysis, spontaneous recovery of sufficient diaphragm function to sustain adequate spontaneous ventilation may occur up to 9 months after the accident. Hence, DP usually should not be considered before sufficient time has elapsed to ensure that the lesion is irreversible. This, however, may be difficult and we have observed a quadriplegic patient with recovery of spontaneous daytime ventilation 23 months after traumatic cervical cord transsection and 6 months after initiation of DP.

Preoperative Screening

The preoperative selection of a candidate for DP is based on the unequivocal demonstration of an intact and viable phrenic neuromuscular apparatus. In patients with CAH this is done during voluntary spontaneous breathing. In patients with respiratory muscle paralysis, absence of electrical and mechanical activity of the diaphragm during spontaneous efforts and normal or near-normal diaphragm contraction during transcutaneous electrical stimulation (TES) of the phrenic nerve in the neck must be demonstrated.

TES uses a train of 1 ms pulses of 1 to 15 mA current delivered transcutaneously to the phrenic nerve, carefully located behind the lateral border of the sternocleidomastoid muscle, 2 to 4 cm above the clavicula, anterior to the scalenus anticus muscle. During TES, excitation of the ipsilateral diaphragm muscle is detected using surface EMG electrodes placed in the eight intercostal space at the anterior and posterior axillary lines. Phrenic nerve conduction time (PNCT) or the interval between application of the stimulus in the neck and the onset of the diaphragm muscle action potential should be shorter than 14 ms in adult, normal-sized patients. Normal PNCT in adults ranges from 7.5 to 10 ms (mean $\pm$ SD: 8.4 $\pm$ 0.8 ms) [14] and is shorter in children, in whom it ranges from 2.7 to 7.8 ms, depending on age and, hence, size [15].

Apart from an adequate electrical response, the ipsilateral diaphragm muscle must also exhibit a sufficient mechanical response to TES of the phrenic nerve. This electromechanical coupling can be observed in the supine patient using different methods, i.e., a brisk outward movement of the anterior abdominal wall at visual inspection, a brisk caudad excursion of at least 5 cm of the diaphragm contour at fluoroscopy, and generation of sufficient transdiaphragmatic pressure (Pdi) or the difference between gastric (Pg) and esophageal (Pes) pressure measured with balloon catheters placed in the stomach and esophagus.

Pacing Schedule

To allow for healing of the surgical wounds and resorption of periphrenic edema, pacing is not started before 2 weeks have elapsed since the last operation. Pacing should be introduced very carefully and progressively, especially in quadriplegic patients. These patients have been on a mechanical ventilator for several months prior to the start of DP, and their diaphragms have undergone disuse atrophy. Too rapid introduction of high-current electrical stimulation for too long pacing periods may cause diaphragm fatigue and, as has been shown in animal experiments, even irreversible muscle fiber damage [5, 16]. To avoid this, initial pacing should aim at progressive reconditioning of the diaphragm, using both short repetitive training pacing periods and carefully selected settings of pacemaker parameters.

The first day pacing periods of 1–3 min/hour during the daytime are interrupted by periods of rest on the mechanical ventilator for the rest of the hour. When diaphragm fatigue does not occur (detected as a more than 25% decrease in tidal volume (V_T) or an increase in end-tidal PCO_2 at the end of the pacing period), the pacing periods are prolonged daily by 1–3 min/hour. Once pacing periods of 30 min/hour are achieved (usually after 14 days), they can be prolonged by 5 min increments each day or two, but intervening resting periods of equal duration should always be provided. When pacing applied continuously for 12 hours does not result in diaphragm fatigue, the resting periods are gradually shortened until full-time pacing is achieved (usually after 3 to 8 months).

Recommended pacemaker settings have changed continuously since its introduction in clinical practice. Earlier recommendations included unilateral alternating pacing using submaximal current amplitudes, relatively high stimulus frequencies (25–30 Hz), hence short PI (33–40 ms), and RR of 15–17/min [17]. Subsequently, it was shown that lower RR and stimulus frequencies minimized the electrical charge to the phrenic nerve and lowered the risk for diaphragm fatigue [5]. The most recent recommendations include simultaneous bilateral pacing at slow RR (7–10/min), using low stimulation frequencies (7–11 Hz), hence, prolonged PI (90–140 ms), delivered during Ti of 1.3 s [18]. Such a pacing schedule may not provide sufficient V_T or minute ventilation at the start of pacing, when higher stimulus frequencies may be required to augment V_T. However, except in instances of spasm, quadriplegic patients usually have low ventilatory requirements, being continuously at rest. The aim should always be to attain the recommended pacing schedule, allowing for deviations tailored to the individual requirements of the patient. Evidence has been provided that low-frequency stimulation of the phrenic nerve not only hypertrophies and strengthens the diaphragm but also converts its muscle fibers from fast-twitch ones to slow-twitch, fatigue-resistent fibers rich in oxidative enzymes [18–20].

Failure of Pacing and Precautions

Decreased efficiency or complete failure of DP may result from several factors related to either pacemaker malfunction [21] or to the patient. The most frequent cause of internal component malfunction is receiver failure, usually due to fluid infiltration through the silicone rubber coating. More rarely, electrode wire or wire insulation breakage (in mobile children with CAH), electrode displacement, mechanical or ischemic nerve injury (more often due to bipolar than monopolar electrodes) and infection at the implant sites have been noticed. Before suspecting the implanted equipment, the adequacy of external components should be checked: battery exhaustion, antenna breakage (most commonly at

the connector sites), transmitter failure or faulty settings must be excluded. Patient-related factors that may reduce adequacy of DP are excessive use of drugs
interfering with neuromuscular transmission (e.g., aminoglycoside antibiotics,
muscle relaxants, sedatives or respiratory depressants), intercurrent diseases that
modify respiratory mechanics and/or increase ventilatory demands (e.g., infections, in particular of the respiratory tract) and diaphragmatic fatigue (due to
improper pacemaker settings). The efficiency of DP may depend on body posture: while DP may provide adequate ventilation in the supine quadriplegic,
changing to the sitting position may require higher pacemaker settings [22] or an
abdominal binder to augment V_T.

A back-up mechanical ventilator should always be available to replace DP in
case pacing fails and the patient should be trained to sustain spontaneous ventilation using the accessory neck muscles or glossopharyngeal breathing [23]. The
tracheostomy may be reduced in size and plugged during DP, but should be
maintained for several reasons: to provide quick access to the airway in case of
pacing failure; to facilitate suctioning of respiratory secretions (DP does not
restore expiratory muscle function and efficient coughing); and to bypass upper
airway obstruction occurring during sleep at the level of the oropharynx in
some patients with CAH [24] or at the level of the vocal cords in some quadriplegic patients [25].

The pacemaker does not contain an apnea alarm function and may interfere
with demand cardiac pacemakers [26], especially if monopolar electrodes are
used. Magnetic resonance imaging and shock wave lithotrypsy are contra-indi-
cated. Finally, the patient must learn to coordinate swallowing with the imposed paced inspirations to avoid aspiration of food or liquids.

Advantages of DP

As compared to conventional positive pressure mechanical ventilation, DP offers several advantages. Since inspiration occurs through the normal route of
breathing instead of via a tracheostomy, the inspired air is better conditioned
(humidified, heathed and filtered), and the risk of lower respiratory tract infection, an otherwise frequent and threatening complication in quadriplegic patients, is significantly reduced. Likewise, since expiratory flow occurs through
the larynx, phonation and speech and, hence, the patient's social contact
markedly improve. During DP, the patient speeks during expiration, whose duration is longer than inspiration, whereas the mechanically ventilated patient
can only phonate during the shorter Ti using a fenestrated and/or uncuffed tracheostomy tube, allowing an inspiratory air leak towards the vocal cords. Devoid of the more cumbersome and noisy mechanical ventilator, which also
creates a psychological barrier, the patient's autonomy is improved, allowing
discharge from the hospital and return to the home setting. There, his/her mobility is improved since less equipment has to be attached to the wheelchair
when leaving home. Apart from these benefits, we have shown that DP, as compared to positive pressure ventilation, improves gas exchange and arterial oxy-

genation, by interfering less with venous return in quadriplegic patients who, because of autonomic dysfunction have increased venous capacitance and relative hypovolemia [27].

Conclusion

Diaphragm pacing offers an effective alternative for long-term ventilatory support of carefully selected patients with CAH or quadriplegia due to high cervical cord lesions. Viability of the entire phrenic neuromuscular axis is an essential prerequisite for successful DP and has to be unequivocally demonstrated by preoperative electrophrenic stimulation. The implantation of the pacemaker's internal components should rely in the hands of an experienced surgeon. Postoperatively, careful setting of the pacemaker controls with frequent reevaluation are necessary to avoid diaphragmatic fatigue and to enhance diaphragm reconditioning to a fatigue-resistant muscle type. Setting up a clinical program for DP necessitates a multidisciplinary team capable not only of correct application of the technique but also of permanent stand-by in case of pacing failure. Because of this, and the relative paucity of indications for DP, the technique should, in our opinion, remain centralized to specialized-care hospitals whereto candidates for DP can be converged. Improved gas exchange, psychosocial contact and reintegration in the home setting are undeniable advantages of DP. From the manufacturer, improvements in the pacemaker apparatus, in particular the subcutaneous receiver, are needed.

References

1. Sarnoff SJ, Hardenberg E, Whittenberger JL (1948) Electro-phrenic respiration. Am J Physiol 155:1-9
2. Glenn WWL, Hageman JH, Mauro A, et al (1964) Electrical stimulation of excitable tissue by radiofrequency transmission. Ann Surg 160:338
3. Glenn WWL, Holcomb WG, Gee JBL, et al (1970) Central hypoventilation: long term ventilatory assistance by radiofrequency electrophrenic respiration. Ann Surg 172:755-773
4. Glenn WWL, Holcomb WG, McLaughlin AJ, et al (1972) Total ventilatory support in a quadriplegic patient with radio-frequency electrophrenic respiration. N Engl J Med 286:513-516
5. Oda T, Glenn WWL, Fukuda Y, et al (1981) Evaluation of electrical parameters for diaphragm pacing: An experimental study. J Surg Res 30:142-153
6. Glenn WWL, Hogan JF, Phelps ML (1980) Ventilatory support of the quadriplegic patient with respiratory paralysis by diaphragm pacing. Surg Clin North Am 60:1055-1078
7. Ilbawi MN, Idriss FS, Hunt CE, et al (1985) Diaphragm pacing in infants: techniques and results. Ann Thorac Surg 40:323-329
8. Kelley WO (1950) Phrenic nerve paralysis. Special consideration of the accessory phrenic nerve. J Thorac Surg 19:923-928
9. Severinghaus JW, Mitchell RA (1962) Ondine's curse - failure of the respiratory center while awake. Clin Res 10:122
10. Farmer WC, Glenn WWL, Gee JBL (1978) Alveolar hypoventilation syndrome. Studies of ventilatory control in patients selected for diaphragm pacing. Am J Med 64:39-49

11. Mellins RB, Balfour HH Jr, Turino GM, et al (1970) Failure of automatic control of ventilation (Ondine's curse). Report of an infant born with this syndrome and review of the literature. Medicine 49:487–504
12. Yasuma F, Nomura H, Sotobata I, et al (1987) Congential central alveolar hypoventilation (Ondine's Curse): a case report and review of the literature. Eur J Pediatr 146:81–83
13. Judson JP, Glenn WWL (1968) Radio-frequency electrophrenic respiration. Long-term application to a patient with primary hypoventilation. JAMA 203:1033–1037
14. Shaw RK, Glenn WWL, Hogan JF, et al (1980) Electrophysiological evaluation of phrenic nerve function in candidates for diaphragm pacing. J Neurosurg 53:345–354
15. Brouillette RT, Ilbawi MN, Hunt CE (1983) Phrenic nerve pacing in infants: a review of experience and report on the usefulness of phrenic nerve stimulation studies. J Pediatr 102:32–39
16. Ciesielski TE, Fukuda Y, Glenn WWL, et al (1983) Response of the diaphragm muscle to stimulation of the phrenic nerve, a histochemical and ultrastructural study. J Neurosurg 58:92–100
17. Glenn WWL, Holcomb WG, Hogan JF, et al (1973) Diaphragm pacing by radio-frequency transmission in the treatment of chronic ventilatory insufficiency. J Thorac Cardiovasc Surg 66:505–520
18. Glenn WWL, Hogan JF, Loke JSO, et al (1984) Ventilatory support by pacing of the conditioned diaphragm in quadriplegia. N Engl J Med 310:1150–1155
19. Salmons S, Gale DR, Sreter FA (1978) Ultrastructural aspects of the transformation of muscle fiber type by long-term stimulation: changes in Z discs and mitochondria. J Anat 127:17–31
20. Salmons S, Henriksson J (1981) The adaptive response of skeletal muscle to increased use. Muscle Nerve 4:94–105
21. Weese-Mayer DE, Morrow AS, Brouillette RT, et al (1989) Diaphragm pacing in infants and children. A life-table analysis of implanted components. Am Rev Respir Dis 139:974–979
22. Danon J, Druz WS, Goldberg NB, et al (1979) Function of the isolated paced diaphragm and the cervical accessory muscles in C1 quadriplegics. Am Rev Respir Dis 119:909–919
23. Montero JC, Feldman DJ, Montero D (1967) Effects of glossopharyngeal breathing on respiratory function after cervical cord transsection. Arch Phys Med Rehab 48:650–653
24. Glenn WWL, Gee JBL, Cole DR, et al (1978) Combined central alveolar hypoventilation and upper airway obstruction. Treatment by tracheostomy and diaphragm pacing. Am J Med 64:50–60
25. Scharf SM, Feldman NT, Goldman MD, et al (1978) Vocal cord closure. A cause of upper airway obstruction during controlled ventilation. Am Rev Respir Dis 117:391–397
26. Wicks JD, Davison R, Belic N (1978) Malfunction of a demand pacemaker caused by phrenic nerve stimulation. Chest 74:303–305
27. Vincken W, Corne L (1987) Improved arterial oxygenation by diaphragmatic pacing in quadriplegia. Crit Care Med 15:872–873

Pressure Release Ventilation

J.-J. Rouby

Introduction

Pressure release ventilation is a new mode of ventilatory support in which intermittent PEEP release provides mechanical assistance to alveolar ventilation. It differs from intermittent positive pressure ventilation and inspiratory pressure support as far as pressure changes throughout the respiratory cycle: during these two modes, either a preset tidal volume or a preset inspiratory pressure are delivered by the ventilator to the patient and, as a consequence, airway pressure increases during the inspiratory phase; during pressure release ventilation, passive exhalation of the respiratory system follows PEEP release and is associated with a marked decrease in airway pressure, the pressure re-increasing during the next expiration. Because of the limitation of the increase in peak airway pressure during pressure release ventilation, the risk of pulmonary barotrauma is theoretically reduced.

There are two different types of pressure release ventilation:

1. Airway Pressure Release Ventilation (APRV), initially proposed by Downs in the United States [1], throughout which entire alveolar ventilation is ensured by preset periodical PEEP releases.
2. Intermittent Mandatory Pressure Release Ventilation (IMPRV), advocated by our group, in which the patient's alveolar ventilation is partially assisted by a PEEP release applied every 2, 3, 4, 5 or 6 spontaneous breaths, the patient being connected to a mechanical ventilator. This ventilatory mode is now provided by mechanical ventilators which offer the possibility of associating a small pressure support level ($\leqslant 5$ cmH$_2$O) in order to antagonize the extra-work of breathing due to the endotracheal tube and the ventilatory circuits [2].

Airway Pressure Release Ventilation

As shown in Fig. 1, APRV can be delivered using a modified oxygen-powered ventury CPAP system. Two additional valves have been added on the expiratory circuit: a second threshold resistor valve and a release valve connected to a timer. According to the position of the release valve, expiration can occur either through the first PEEP valve (high PEEP, release valve closed), or through the

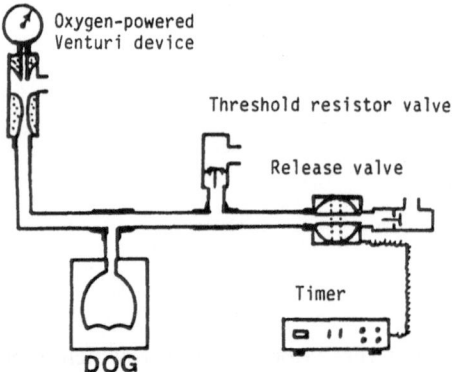

Oxygen-powered
Venturi device

Threshold resistor valves

Release valve

Timer

Fig. 1. Airway pressure release ventilation system. (From [8])

DOG

second PEEP valve (low PEEP, release valve open). The frequency of PEEP release can be modified through a timer. APRV was shown to ensure normal alveolar ventilation in paralyzed dogs under general anesthesia [3]. In animals without acute respiratory failure, the PEEP was released from 8 cmH$_2$O to zero, 20 times per minute. In animals with oleic acid lung injury, the PEEP was released from 15–20 cmH$_2$O to 5 cmH$_2$O, 20 times per minute. When compared with continuous positive pressure ventilation, APRV was associated with a significant reduction in peak airway pressure, although both ventilatory modes were compared at the same level of mean airway pressure. Since high peak airway pressure seems to be involved in mechanical ventilation-induced lung damage [4–6], APRV could contribute to decrease the incidence of pulmonary barotrauma. In contrast, there is no difference between APRV and conventional ventilation in terms of hemodynamics: arterial pressure, heart rate, cardiac output and cardiac filling pressures are identical when both ventilatory modes are compared at the same level of mean airway pressure [3, 7].

It is also possible to superimpose APRV on patient's or animal's spontaneous breathing activity [7, 8]. If 20 APRV breaths per minute are insufficient to prevent spontaneous ventilatory efforts, high PEEP is increased to obtain a larger airway pressure release gradient, and consequently, a higher tidal volume [8]. The APRV rate is then reduced to maintain an airway pressure release time shorter than one-half of the respiratory cycle. However, since spontaneous respiratory rate can markedly vary with time, the APRV rate has to be frequently adjusted in order to avoid discoordination between PEEP release and spontaneous respiratory activity. In such conditions, spontaneous breathing activity is partially assisted by intermittent PEEP releases. In anesthetized animals with drug-induced respiratory depression in whom the use of CPAP is constantly associated with alveolar hypoventilation and hypercarbia, APRV enables a normalization of alveolar ventilation without increasing peak airway pressure [8]. It must be pointed out that intermittent PEEP release does not alter arterial oxygenation in presence of acute respiratory failure [8].

Intermittent Mandatory Pressure Release Ventilation (IMPRV)

Technical Aspects

In contrast to APRV, the PEEP release frequency depends on patient's spontaneous respiratory frequency during IMPRV (Fig. 2). The patient is connected to
a normal conventional mechanical ventilator which can provide IMPRV. Inspiratory efforts are detected through a trigger; the sensitivity of which can be set
from -0.5 cmH$_2$O to -3 cmH$_2$O. Once the spontaneous inspiratory activity is
detected by the ventilator, then PEEP can be released every 2, 3, 4, 5 or 6 spontaneous respiratory cycles. To avoid discoordination between patient's spontaneous breaths and PEEP releases, PEEP should be released only during expiration.

There is already one commercially available ventilator which provides IM-
PRV: the CESAR ventilator (Air liquide, CFPO, France). In this ventilator, the
PEEP valve, which is completely original technologically-speaking, is connected
to a central microprocessor which periodically gives the PEEP release order
(Fig. 3). The following parameters can be set on the ventilator: the superior

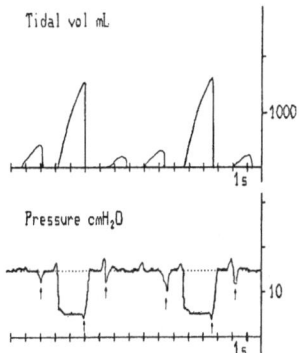

Fig. 2. Simultaneous recording of expired tidal volume and
airway pressure in a patient under Intermittent Mandatory
Pressure Release Ventilation (CESAR ventilator, Air liquide, CFPO, France). PEEP is released from 15 to 5
cmH$_2$O every 2 spontaneous respiratory cycles. The patient's "spontaneous tidal volumes" are around 200 ml,
whereas the "assisted tidal volumes" associated with intermittent PEEP release are around 1500 ml. The minute ventilation is of 15 l·min^{-1} and the PaCO$_2$ is of 38 mmHg.
Arrows indicate patient's spontaneous inspiratory efforts.
The trigger sensitivity is set at -1.5 cmH$_2$O

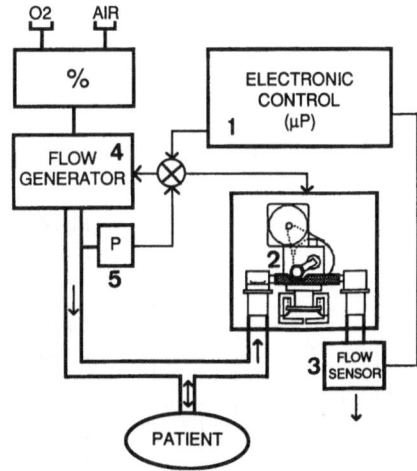

Fig. 3. Simplified schema of the CESAR ventilator. (1) Central microprocessor commanding
the different functions of the ventilator (2) expiratory valve connected to the microprocessor
(3) Flow sensor (hot wire) measuring gas flow
and tidal volume (4) Flow generator delivering
a maximum instantaneous inspiratory flow of
180 l/min (5) Differential pressure transducer
regulating pressure within ventilatory circuits
and connected through the microprocessor to
the flow generator (pressure support function)

PEEP level, the amount of PEEP release and the PEEP release frequency. In addition, the trigger level can be varied from minus 0.5 cmH_2O to minus 3 cmH_2O and a pressure support of 5 cmH_2O can be superimposed to antagonize the extra-work of breathing due to the respiratory circuits [2]. Therefore, the CESAR ventilator provides ideal conditions for IMPRV. One advantage of this new ventilatory mode is that ventilatory assistance depends on the patient's spontaneous respiratory rate: the more rapid the patient's respiratory frequency, the more frequent the PEEP release and the greater the ventilatory assistance. Another advantage of the CESAR ventilator is that it offers the possibility of combining pressure support and IMPRV. Since the patient is intubated or tracheostomized and connected to the respiratory circuits of the ventilator, then an extra-work of breathing has to be generated to overcome the gas flow resistance within the connecting tubes. It has been recently shown [2] that the administration of an inspiratory pressure support level of 5 cmH_2O could suppress the additional work of breathing and, therefore, prevent fatigue and increase patient's confort (Fig. 4). It must be pointed out that the patient's connection to a ventilator provides the possibility of continuously monitoring tidal volume, airway pressure, gas flow and respiratory frequency. In the CESAR ventilator, these useful respiratory parameters are continuously displayed on a monitoring screen and each 72 hour parameter trend can be reviewed.

Pathophysiology

During pressure release ventilation, tidal volume varies from one respiratory cycle to another. PEEP release, which always occurs during expiration in IMPRV, is followed by a marked increase in the expired tidal volume (Figs. 2 and 4) due to the sudden reduction of lung volume. During the next expiration, lung volume is re-established at the precedent level without any phenomenon of gas trapping, via an increase in the PEEP level. During pressure release ventilation, functional residual capacity changes according to PEEP changes (Fig. 5).

It is important to differentiate "spontaneous tidal volumes" generated by the patient's spontaneous breathing activity at the superior PEEP level, from "as-

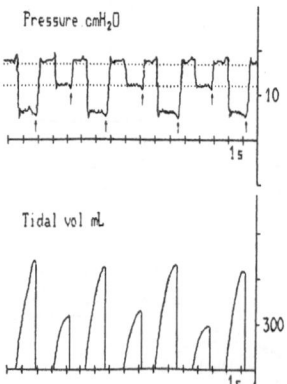

Fig. 4. Simultaneous recording of airway pressure and expired tidal volume in a patient under Intermittent Mandatory Pressure Release Ventilation using an inspiratory pressure support of 5 cmH_2O (CESAR ventilator, Air liquide, CFPO, France). PEEP is released from 12 to 5 cmH_2O every 2 spontaneous respiratory cycles. The patient's "spontaneous tidal volumes" are around 300 ml, whereas the "assisted tidal volumes" associated with intermittent PEEP release are around 600 ml. Arrows indicate patient's spontaneous inspiratory efforts. The trigger sensitivity is set at -0.5 cmH_2O

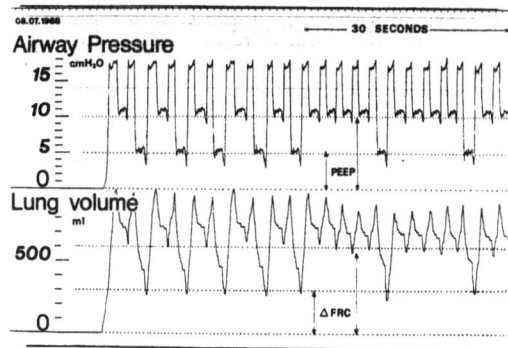

Fig. 5. Simultaneous changes in airway pressure and lung volume in a patient under Intermittent Mandatory Pressure Ventilation (CESAR Ventilator). PEEP is released from 11 to 5 cmH$_2$O and an inspiratory pressure support of 6 cmH$_2$O is used. First, PEEP is released every 2 spontaneous respiratory cycles and then, every 5 spontaneous respiratory cycles. Increase in lung volume above apneic functional residual capacity (ΔFRC) oscillates with PEEP release from 300 ml to 600 ml. ΔFRC changes are not modified by decreasing the rate of PEEP release

sisted tidal volumes" generated by the PEEP release. "Spontaneous tidal volume" increases with the pressure support level and the patient's spontaneous inspiratory activity, and decreases when static respiratory compliance is reduced [9]. "Assisted tidal volume" is influenced by the amount of PEEP release, the patient's spontaneous inspiratory activity and the static respiratory compliance. For a given respiratory compliance, the greater the amount of PEEP release, the greater the "assisted tidal volume". For a given amount of PEEP release, the "assisted tidal volume" increases when the preceding patient's inspiratory effort increases. Because of the variability of patient's spontaneous inspiratory activity, "spontaneous" as well as "assisted tidal volumes" vary from one cycle to another although airway pressure remains remarkably constant. Since in clinical practice, esophageal pressure, which indirectly reflects spontaneous inspiratory activity, is not routinely monitored, the presence or the absence of tidal volume

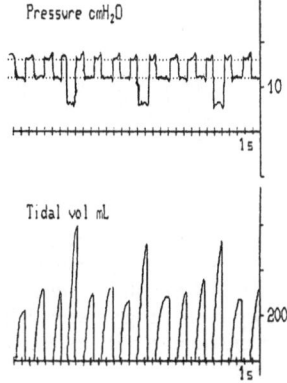

Fig. 6. Simultaneous recording of airway pressure and expired tidal volume in a patient under Intermittent Mandatory Pressure Release Ventilation (CESAR ventilator, PEEP release from 12 to 5 cmH$_2$O every 4 spontaneous respiratory cycles, trigger sensitivity -0.5 cmH$_2$O, inspiratory pressure support level of 5 cmH$_2$O). Patient's "spontaneous tidal volumes" vary from 250 ml to 400 ml, and "assisted tidal volumes" are respectively of 600 ml, 510 ml and 560 ml. These volume changes result from changes in transpulmonary pressure. Since airway pressure does not change from one respiratory cycle to another, expired volumes variability indicates changes in spontaneous inspiratory activity that can be evidenced by measuring changes in esophageal pressure during inspiration

changes with time, provides information concerning the patient's spontaneous breathing activity (Fig. 6).

When compared to pressure support ventilation, IMPRV enables a significant decrease in peak airway pressure, which never exceeds the superior PEEP level [10]. In contrast, respiratory frequency is lower during pressure support ventilation (Fig. 7), possibly because this ventilatory mode markedly reduces patient's work of breathing [11].

Respiratory effects of changing PEEP release frequency depend on the patient's initial clinical status: in non sedated patients, able to produce efficient spontaneous breathing, the decrease in PEEP release frequency induces an in-

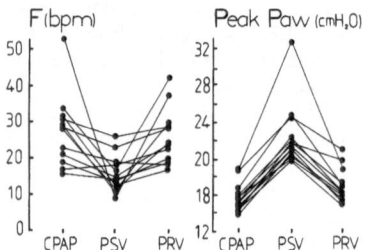

Fig. 7. Comparative effects on respiratory frequency (F) and peak airway pressure (Peak Paw) of CPAP, pressure support ventilation (PSV) and Intermittent Mandatory Pressure Release Ventilation (PRV) in 12 critically ill patients with mild acute respiratory failure. The 3 ventilatory modes are administered randomly to each patient during a one hour period and using the same level of mean airway pressure (12 cmH$_2$O). In each individual, Intermittent Mandatory Pressure Release Ventilation and CPAP are associated with peak airway pressure reduction and increased respiratory rate when compared with pressure support ventilation. (From [10])

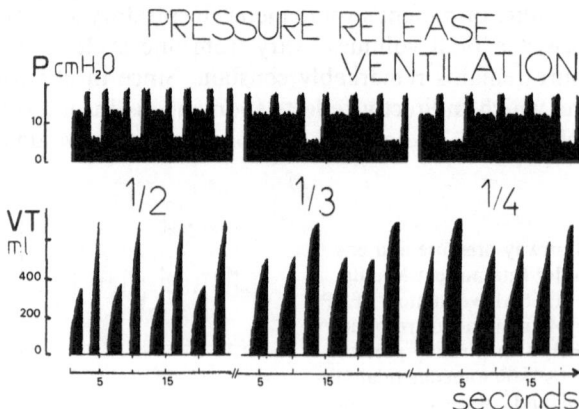

Fig. 8. Effects on airway pressure (P) and tidal volume (VT) of decreasing PEEP release frequency in a non-sedated patient during Intermittent Mandatory Pressure Release Ventilation (CESAR Ventilation, PEEP release from 12 to 4 cmH$_2$O every 2, 3 and 4 spontaneous respiratory cycles, trigger sensitivity -0.5 cmH$_2$O, inspiratory pressure support of 5 cmH$_2$O). The decrease in PEEP release frequency induces an increase in patient's "spontaneous tidal volumes"

crease in patient's "spontaneous tidal volume", whereas minute ventilation and alveolar ventilation remain unchanged (Fig. 8); in contrast, in patients with central respiratory depression or chest wall mechanical impairment, the reduction in PEEP release frequency is associated with a decrease in minute ventilation, leading to alveolar hypoventilation and hypercarbia.

Clinical Indications

Pressure release ventilation can be applied to paralyzed patients – APRV – or to spontaneously breathing patients – IMPRV –. The application of PEEP release to a spontaneously breathing patient requires several technical conditions. First, PEEP release should always be synchronized with patient's expiration, to avoid abrupt changes in airway pressure during an inspiratory effort which creates a feeling of disconfort. Second, this ventilatory mode should be integrated in a conventional ventilator in order to monitor usual respiratory parameters. Third, the PEEP level should be automatically changed according to the patient's respiratory frequency; therefore, the PEEP valve conception should be modified to enable a connection with the microprocessor commanding the ventilator. Fourth, because IMPRV is a ventilatory mode during which a patient connected to a ventilator spontaneously breathes, the possibility of adding a small amount of pressure support should exist. Finally, as with any ventilatory mode, alarms should be present on main respiratory parameters such as respiratory frequency, tidal volume, peak airway pressure and minute ventilation. There is already one ventilator commercially available which satisfies these conditions: the CESAR ventilator (Air liquide, CFPO, France).

What could be the clinical indications of pressure release ventilation? The next paragraph is based on the results of several studies completed in the Department of Anesthesiology of La Pitié Hospital in Paris over a 2 year period. While this article was being written, all these studies were under peer review in different international journals so that no reference can be given except in an abstract form [10, 11].

1. In paralyzed patients, APRV is associated with a reduction in peak airway pressure when compared with conventional positive pressure ventilation [7]. No difference was to be found in any of the other hemodynamic and respiratory parameters. The advantage of APRV in paralyzed patients appears limited to its effect on peak airway pressure.
2. In spontaneously-breathing patient with mild acute respiratory failure, but without central respiratory depression or mechanical chest wall impairment, we found that CPAP and IMPRV gave identical results on all hemodynamic and respiratory parameters. When compared with pressure support ventilation, both CPAP and IMPRV were associated with increased respiratory frequency and lower peak airway pressure (Fig. 7). In this population of patients, when switching CPAP for IMPRV, minute ventilation and respiratory rate did not change. A significant reduction in "spontaneous tidal volume" occurred, suggesting that a significant part of the patient's alveolar ventilation

was supported by PEEP release (Fig. 9). Therefore, in this category of critically ill patients, the advantage of IMPRV over CPAP is not clinically obvious. In critically ill patients with circulatory shock and/or severe acute respiratory failure, IMPRV is most often not clinically tolerated: a very high respiratory rate persists, despite the maximum PEEP release frequency (one PEEP release every 2 spontaneous breaths), and, the patient becomes progressively exhausted. One possibility then, is to sedate the patient in order to decrease the respiratory rate and to maintain IMPRV as long as the patient is still able to trigger the flow.

3. Pressure release ventilation does offer significant advantages in patients with mechanical chest wall impairment or drug induced central respiratory depression. In such situations, CPAP invariably results in insufficient alveolar ventilation leading to increased respiratory rate and hypercarbia and imposing continuous positive pressure ventilation. Pressure release ventilation enables the continuation of spontaneous ventilatory mode, by partially assisting alveolar ventilation through PEEP release. As long as the patient is able to trigger inspiratory flow, IMPRV ensures adequate gas exchange, without increasing peak airway pressure.

   - One of the main indications of IMPRV concerns agitated patients with acute respiratory failure in whom the administration of narcotics or benzodiazepines is necessary. Even when using large doses of respiratory depressant agents, the vast majority of critically ill patients maintain a certain

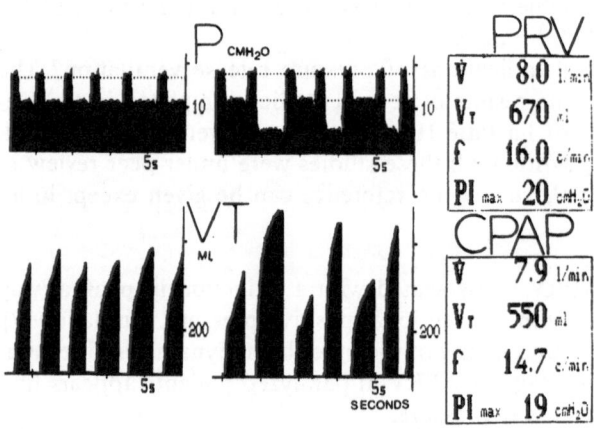

Fig. 9. Comparative effects of CPAP and Intermittent Mandatory Pressure Release Ventilation (PRV) on airway pressure (P) and expired tidal volume (VT) in a non-sedated critically ill patient with mild acute respiratory failure (CESAR ventilator, inspiratory pressure of 5 cmH_2O during both modes, mean airway pressure of 10 cmH_2O during both modes). Minute Ventilation ($\dot{V}$), respiratory frequency (F) and peak airway pressure (PI max) are similar in both modes. During Intermittent Mandatory Pressure Release Ventilation (PEEP release from 12 to 5 cmH_2O every 2 spontaneous respiratory cycles, trigger sensitivity − 1 cmH_2O), "assisted tidal volume" is around 670 ml, and "spontaneous tidal volumes" are around 400 ml, much less than tidal volumes during CPAP which vary between 500 and 600 ml. Because of the PEEP release induced ventilatory assistance, the patient reduces his own contribution to minute ventilation

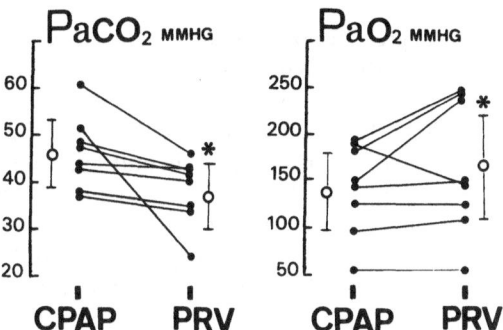

Fig. 10. Comparative effects on $PaCO_2$ and PaO_2 (FIO_2 0.6) of CPAP and Intermittent Mandatory Pressure Release Ventilation (PRV) in 8 critically ill patients with acute respiratory failure and receiving intravenous narcotics because of agitation. All patients are ventilated with a CESAR ventilator and both ventilatory modes are compared at the same level of mean airway pressure (12 cmH_2O) and using a trigger sensitivity of -0.5 cmH_2O and an inspiratory pressure support of 5 cmH_2O. Under CPAP, 6 patients have a $PaCO_2$ above 40 mmHg. In each individual, Intermittent Mandatory Pressure Release Ventilation (PEEP release every 2 spontaneous respiratory cycles) decreases $PaCO_2$. Simultaneously PaO_2 increases in 7 of the 8 patients ($p < 0.05$)

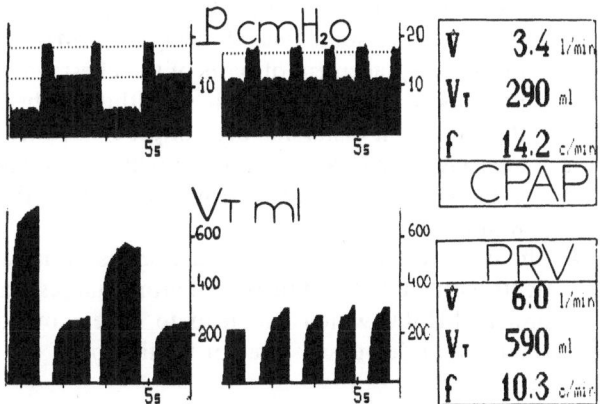

Fig. 11. Comparative effects of CPAP and Intermittent Mandatory Pressure Release Ventilation (PRV) on airway pressure (P) and expired tidal volume (V_T) in a critically ill patient with acute respiratory failure receiving a continuous intravenous infusion of Fentanyl (2500 mcg/24 h) for agitation. The patient is ventilated using a CESAR ventilator. Both ventilatory modes are compared at the same level of mean airway pressure (12 cmH_2O) using a trigger sensitivity of -0.5 cmH_2O and an inspiratory pressure support of 5 cmH_2O. CPAP is associated with a low minute ventilation ($\dot{V}$), with an expired tidal volume of 290 ml, with a respiratory frequency of 14 bpm and a $PaCO_2$ of 61 mmHg. Intermittent Mandatory Pressure Release Ventilation (PEEP release from 12 to 4 cmH_2O every 2 spontaneous respiratory cycles) increases minute ventilation to 6/min, slightly reduces respiratory frequency from 14 to 10 bpm, whereas patient's "spontaneous tidal volume" remains low, around 300 ml. The marked increase in minute ventilation, only related to "assisted tidal volume" (around 600 ml), enables a decrease in $PaCO_2$ from 61 mmHg to 45 mmHg

degree of spontaneous inspiratory activity and are able to trigger inspiratory flow. When using CPAP, patient's tidal volume is too low, respiratory frequency remains in the normal range and $PaCO_2$ increases. As shown in Fig. 10, the use of IMPRV normalizes $PaCO_2$. Similar results have also been shown in experimental anesthetized dogs with acute respiratory failure [8]. As demonstrated in Fig. 11, the marked increase in tidal volume which results from PEEP release enables an increase in minute ventilation, whereas patient's "spontaneous tidal volume" remains low during CPAP and IMPRV. Finally, IMPRV in critically ill patients receiving potent respiratory depressant agents, enables the continuation of spontaneous respiratory mode and the maintenance of mean airway pressure, without increasing peak airway pressure as in pressure support ventilation or continuous positive pressure ventilation.

- Another indication of IMPRV is represented by critically ill patients with acute respiratory failure and mechanical chest wall impairment. Tetraplegic patients with persisting diaphragmatic activity, patients with peripheral neuromuscular disease and postoperative patients with marked reduction in lung volumes secondary to large thoracoabdominal incisions, are unable to achieve adequate tidal volumes under CPAP although they have persisting spontaneous inspiratory activity. Hypercarbia, high respiratory rate and fatigue rapidly occur under CPAP. IMPRV, by assisting alveolar ventilation through intermittent PEEP releases, normalizes $PaCO_2$ and respiratory rate without increasing peak airway pressure.

- We also have some data showing that IMPRV can reverse the paradoxical inward displacement of parts of the chest wall observed in multiple trauma patients with mobile flail chest. Although the reasons for the correction of the chest wall distorsion are not yet clear, IMPRV appears as an interesting alternative ventilatory mode for patients with mobile flail chest and also for patients with cervical cord injury showing thoracoabdominal paradoxical wall motion.

4. The contraindications of pressure release ventilation are those of PEEP. Patients with COPD and increased bronchial resistance develop instrinsic PEEP under IMPRV which can lead to severe overdistention, pulmonary barotrauma and decreased alveolar ventilation.

References

1. Downs JB, Stock MC (1987) Airway pressure release ventilation: a new concept in ventilatory support. Crit Care Med 15:459-461
2. Brochard L, Rua F, Lorino H, Lemaire F, Harf A (1988) The extra-work of breathing due to the endotracheal tube is abolished during inspiratory pressure support breathing. Am Rev Respir Dis 137:A64
3. Stock MC, Downs JB, Deborah A, Frolicher BS (1987) Airway pressure release ventilation. Crit Care Med 15:462-466
4. Parker JC, Townsley MI, Rippe B, Taylor AE, Thigpen J (1984) Increased microvascular permeability in dog lungs due to high peak airway pressures. J Appl Physiol 57:1809-1816

5. Dreyfuss D, Basset G, Soler P, Soumon G (1985) Intermittent positive-pressure hyperventilation with high inflation pressures produces pulmonary microvascular injury in rats. Am Rev Respir Dis 132:880–884

6. Kolobow T, Moretti MP, Fumagalli R, et al (1988) Severe impairment in lung function induced by peak airway pressure during mechanical ventilation. Am Rev Respir Dis 135:312–315

7. Garner W, Downs JB, Stock C, Rasanen J (1988) Airway pressure release ventilation (APRV). A human trial. Chest 94:779–781

8. Rasanen J, Downs JB, Stock MC (1988) Cardiovascular effects of conventional positive pressure ventilation and airway pressure release ventilation. Chest 93:911–915

9. Rouby JJ, Jawish D, Andreev A, Arthaud M, Viars P (1989) Déterminants du volume courant en aide inspiratoire. Ann Fr Anesth Rean 8:R253

10. Jawish D, Rouby JJ, Andreev A, Arthaud M, Poete P, Viars P (1989) Aide inspiratoire, ventilation spontanée avec pression expiratoire positive et ventilation spontanée avec pression positive variable: une étude comparative randomisée. Ann Fr Anesth Rean 8:R255

11. Brochard L, Harf A, Lorino H, Lemaire F (1989) Inspiratory pressure support prevents diaphragmatic fatigue during weaning from mechanical ventilation. Am Rev Resp Dis 139:513–521

Tracheobronchial Suctions During Mechanical Ventilation

A. Tenaillon

Introduction

Tracheobronchial suctions are routinely carried out by nurses and are essential for ventilated patients. Each intensive care unit empirically determines its own procedure without any evaluation. Universal guidelines have not been defined. Analyzing complications, we will try to clarify the safest suction techniques.

Five problems will be discussed: tracheobronchial trauma, ineffectiveness, hypoxemia, cardiac dysrhythmias and nosocomial infections.

Tracheobronchial Trauma

During mechanical ventilation, epithelial erosions with petechias, linear ulcerations or local hemorrhages are frequently observed under broncho-fibroscopy [1]. These lesions may be entirely due to the suction catheter rubbing during its installation, but a drawing in of the mucosa has been also experimentally demonstrated with some suction catheters at high vacuum level [1]. The interruption of the vacuum has been advocated to avoid these hazards by promptly relieving invagination of the mucosa in the eyes of the catheter [2]. It has also been suggested that the basic design of catheters be changed to minimize mucosal contact, by the addition of side holes to the end hole or the adjonction of a distal bead [1]. The usefulness of these devices is however controversial [3]. In our experience, suction-induced tracheobronchial lesions do not seem to be severe with end hole catheters and short interrupted aspiration. We did not find any difference between two levels of subatmospheric pressure (-200 cmH$_2$O vs -700 cmH$_2$O); in both groups of patients previous tracheobronchial lesions resolved at the same time [4].

So, apart from catheters with only one side hole, all the other catheters are equivalent regarding tracheobronchial trauma; distal bead catheters seem potentially better but they are more expensive. Nevertheless, whatever the catheter, the most important precaution is to introduce the suction catheter gently and not too far into the airways [5].

Aspiration Inefficiency

The aim of tracheobronchial suction is to periodically clean the airways from their secretions and to avoid atelectasis, nosocomial bronchopulmonary infections and endotracheal tube obstruction. The efficiency of bronchial tree toilet is difficult to evaluate. Suction catheters are able to reach central airways. The peripheral airways toilet depends from cough, mucociliary clearance, secretion viscosity and flow. All these parameters lead to the drainage into the central airways. We have not found in the medical literature any systematic evaluation of the relationship between aspirations and bronchopulmonary complications. However, it appears in some patients that bronchopneumonia or atelectasis can be caused by inefficient suctions.

One question is whether these problems are linked to the suction procedure or to the secretion quality? It has been demonstrated that it is better to suction patients only when needed rather than to do it systematically at a constant interval. Suction is needed when crakles are heard, when the patient is coughing or when respiratory pressures increase [6]. We have proved that a high vacuum level (-700 cmH$_2$O) was more efficient than a lower one (-200 cmH$_2$O) and that an intermediate level (-400 cmH$_2$O) is probably sufficient [4]. Strong hydration of the patients, beta 2 agonists, Mesna or equivalent drugs, tracheal instillations of saline or bicarbonate serum have all been suggested to improve secretion drainage [7].

Another question is whether it is necessary to push the suction catheter beyond the carena in the right or left bronchial tree.

For about 80% of the patients, routine suction only reaches one side of the bronchial tree, usually the right one. This is true whatever the endotracheal tube used (tracheostomy canula, oral or nasal tube) [5, 8, 9]. Maneuvers such as right or left rotation of the head, use of curved catheter do not significantly influence the catheter position [5, 8, 9]. We have recently shown in a group of 24 patients that pulmonary nosocomial complications were not linked to the tracheobronchial suctions but only to the absence of cough for more than 48 hours [5]. Therefore it is probably unnecessary and even dangerous to push the suction catheter beyond the carena in ventilated patients when cough is present especially if clapping is regularly performed. In case of right or left atelectasis, bronchofibroscopy would be more efficient than blind suctions.

The second goal of tracheobronchial suctioning is to keep the endotracheal tube lumen clear. Total tube occlusion is a severe but quickly recognized complication which occurs seldom. However, partial occlusions are common and hardly diagnosed without systematic endotracheal tube fibroscopy and/or longitudinal section of the tube after extubation.

We have analyzed about 200 endotracheal tubes in several studies. In 62%, deposits inside the tube induced occlusion of more than 50% of the tube lumen; only 20% were totally secretion free. These plugs usually appeared after a few days but sometimes already within 8 hours [4]. These results were not modified by increasing gas humidity (Fischer Paeckel heated humidifier) nor by the use of heat and moisture exchanger [10] (Pall BB 2215) or high vacuum levels, but they were partially improved by Mesna aerosol (6/24 h). As a result we designed a new brush protected catheter to avoid partial or even total tube occlusions [11]. Used twice a day, this new device allowed us to reduce tracheal tube occlusion to 10% of the lumen in 36 patients ventilated during 18 ± 4 days.

Suction-Induced Hypoxemia

Many investigators have reported a marked decrease in PaO_2 during endotracheal suctioning. Serious arrhythmias and even fatal cardiac arrest can be observed in mechanically ventilated patients with severe hypoxemia. This PaO_2 decrease is attributed to the interruption of mechanical ventilation, and consequently of high oxygen mixture delivery and fall of FRC when PEEP was necessary. However, some authors have incriminated the suction maneuver itself through a large FRC decrease and even suction-induced atelectasis [12]. In 6 patients we recently studied the changes in FRC during the complete suction procedure. Whatever the level of subatmospheric pressure, when the suction catheter diameter was inferior to half to the tracheal tube lumen and the suction time under 15 seconds [13], there was no FRC decrease during the suction itself and the PaO_2 fall was only due to the short weaning of the ventilator [14]. We also proved that suction induced hypoxemia could be prevented by conducting aspiration without removing mechanical ventilation [14]. Many other techniques have been proposed for many years to reduce this hypoxemia, including manual or artificial hyperinflations before and after suctioning; higher FiO_2 for a short time before and after suction; oxygen administration through a special double lumen suction catheter [15, 16] or a special endotracheal tube; high frequency jet ventilation [17] and upholding of mechanical ventilation during the entire aspiration procedure [18, 20]. The most efficient techniques must be able to maintain pulmonary volume and high FiO_2; the easiest is the on ventilator suctioning method.

Cardiac Dysrhythmias

Endotracheal suctioning can be complicated by bradycardia, hypotension and even cardiac arrest [21, 22]. These phenomena may preclude adequate suction of airways secretions. They occur in general in severe hypoxemic patients and/or in patients with neurological disorders such as high cervical spinal cord transsection. Bradycardia appears to be due to a vagal reflex induced by suction and largely favored by hypoxemia. These dysrhythmias can be prevented by ensuring adequate oxygenation during suctioning and/or by using nebulized or parenteral atropine before suction [21, 22].

Suctioning-Induced Infections

The real role of tracheobronchial suction in the development of nosocomial pulmonary infections has not been clearly defined. However, the many in and out maneuvers of the suction catheter through the tracheobronchial tree represent a risk of contamination. Indeed the catheter is driven through at least two septic zones: the T-piece of the respiratory circuit and the endotracheal tube, both contaminated by patients' germs. It is well known that the rubbing of a catheter on a mucosa can cause bacteremia. Moreover suction tracheobronchial lesions can favor local infections. Such septic risks have to be minimized by rigorously aseptic techniques: sterile disposable suction catheters, introduction via sterile gloves or special protecting package. A multiple use suction catheter in a closed circuit system has also been proposed [23].

Conclusions

Several recommandations can be made to reduce the risks associated with tracheobronchial aspiration:

- Suction should be performed only when crackles are heard;
- The material should include disposable sterile suction catheter, 0.6 size ratio with endotracheal tube lumen, sterile package for the installation devices with an end-hole and possibly an end-bead;
- T-piece can be used with a special valve allowing suction during ventilation;
- The tip of the catheter should be located just above the carena;
- Subatmospheric pressure used should be between 300 and 400 cmH$_2$O;
- The suction should be short lasting less than 15 seconds. The total maneuver should not exceed 30 seconds; it can be repeated after 5 or 8 min;
- The endotracheal tube should be cleaned by a special brush twice a day;
- The use of Mesna or identical products 4 to 6 times per day can be considered except in asthmatic patients.

References

1. Sackner MA, Landa JF, Greeneltch N, Robinson MJ (1973) Pathogenesis and prevention of tracheobronchial damage with suction procedures. Chest 64:284–290
2. Ogburn-Russel L (1987) The effect of continuous and intermittent suctioning on the tracheal mucosa of dogs. Heart Lung 16:338
3. Jung RC, Gottlieb LS (1976) Comparison of tracheobronchial suction catheters in human. Chest 69:179–182
4. Tenaillon A, Perrin-Gachadoat D, Burdin M, Salmona JP, Chahbenderian J (1985) Incidence sur la perméabilité des sondes d'intubation et sur l'état de la muqueuse trachéale du degré d'aspiration chez les malades sous ventilation mécanique. Rean Soins Intens Med Urg 1:259
5. Lherm T, Tenaillon A, Boiteau R, Burdin M, Perrin-Gachadoat D (1988) Positionnement des sondes d'aspiration et conséquences pulmonaires en cas d'intubation naso-trachéale. Rean Soins Intens Med Urg 4:383
6. Knipper J (1984) The evaluation of adventicious sounds as an indicator of the need for tracheal suctionning. Heart Lung 13:292–293
7. Hanley MW, Rudd T, Butler J (1978) What happens to intratracheal saline instillations? Am Rev Respir Dis 117:124

8. Kirimli B, King JE, Pfaeffle HH (1970) Evaluation of tracheobronchial suction techniques. J Thor Cardiovasc Surg 59:340–344
9. Scott AA, Sandham G, Rebuck AS (1977) Selective tracheobronchial aspiration. Thorax 32:346–348
10. Tenaillon A, Cholley G, Boiteau R, Perrin-Gachadoat D, Burdin M (1988) Filtre échangeur de chaleur et d'humidité versus humidificateur chauffant en ventilation mécanique prolongée. Rean Soins Intens Med Urg 5:3–10
11. Boiteau R, Tenaillon A, Perrin-Gachadoat D, Burdin M, Gosgnach M (1988) Etude d'un dispositif permettant de prévenir l'obstruction des sondes d'intubation. Rean Soins Intens Med Urg 4:382
12. Messadi AA, Brochard L, Mollet JL, Vasile N, Harf A, Lemaire F (1988) Modification du volume pulmonaire, induite par l'aspiration trachéale. Etude tomodensitométrique. Rean Soins Intens Med Urg 4:483
13. Rindfleisch SH, Tyler ML (1983) Duration of suctioning: an important variable. Respir Care 28:457–459
14. Froissart M, Boiteau R, Tenaillon A, et al (1988) Etude de la désaturation et de son mécanisme pendant les aspirations trachéales. Rean Soins Intens Med Urg 4:283
15. Kelly RE, Yao FSF, Artusio JF (1987) Prevention of suction-induced hypoxemia by simultaneous oxygen insufflation. Crit Care Med 15:874–875
16. Bodai BI, Walson CB, Briggs S, Goldstein M (1987) A clinical evaluation of an oxygen insufflation/suction catheter. Heart Lung 16:39–46
17. Guntupalli K, Sladen A, Klain M (1984) High-frequency jet ventilation and tracheobronchial suctioning. Crit Care Med 12:791–792
18. Bodai BI (1982) A means of suctioning without cardiopulmonary depression. Heart Lung 11:172–207
19. Brown SE, Stansbury DW, Merril EJ, Linden GS, Light RW (1983) Prevention of suctioning-related arterial oxygen desaturation; comparison of off-ventilator and on-ventilator suctioning. Chest 83:621–627
20. Craig KC, Benson MS, Pierson DJ (1984) Prevention of arterial oxygen desaturation during closed-airway endotracheal suction: effect of ventilator mode. Respir Care 29:1013–1018
21. Mathias CJ (1976) Bradycardia and cardiac arrest during tracheal suction; mechanism in tetraplegic patients. Eur J Intens Care Med 2:147–156
22. Winston SJ, Gravelyn TR, Sitrin RG (1987) Prevention of bradycardic responses to endotracheal suctioning by prior administration of nebulized atropine. Crit Care Med 15:1009–1011
23. Ritz R, Scott LR, Coyle MB, Pierson DJ (1986) Contamination of a multiple-use suction catheter in a closed-circuit system compared to contamination of a disposable, single-use suction catheter. Respir Care 31:1086–1091

High-Frequency Ventilation

J.-J. Rouby

Introduction

There are three different types of high-frequency ventilation (HFV): high-frequency oscillation (HFO), high-frequency positive pressure ventilation (HEPPV) and high-frequency jet ventilation (HFJV). HFO has been extensively studied by the physiologists but still remains an experimental method of mechanical ventilation. Up to now, only HFPPV and HFJV have received defined clinical applications and occupy a specific place in the wide range of ventilatory support techniques available for anesthesia and critical care. When compared with conventional techniques, their main advantages lie in the fact that they enable adequate gas exchange using small tidal volumes close to the patient's dead space volume. In the anesthetized patient, this enables a reduction of movements in the operating field and facilitates surgical working conditions. In the critically ill, this enables reduction in peak airway pressure and in the deleterious hemodynamic effects resulting from the increase in intrathoracic pressure. As long as certain technical conditions are respected, such as adequate warming and humidification of the gas mixture delivered to the patient, then HFPPV and HFJV offer an attractive alternative to conventional ventilation in a limited number of indications.

Technical Aspects

HFPPV and HFJV, which are very similar, deliver small tidal volumes (between 1 and 5 ml/kg) at high frequencies (between 60 and 400/min) and require a specific ventilator characterized by a reduced internal volume and non-compliant ventilatory circuits. The use of a conventional ventilator to provide HFV invariably results in an insufficient tidal volume delivered to the patient due to the gas compression within the internal volume of the ventilator. In HFPPV, a technique developed by Sjöstrand in Sweden in the mid seventies, a pneumatic valve interrupts a gas flow of air and oxygen supplied to the ventilator at a constant driving pressure. Inspired gases are delivered to the patient through conventional connectors attached to the endotracheal tube, and expiration passively occurs through an expiratory valve. Tidal volume decreases with respiratory frequency and increases with inspiratory/expiratory (I/E) ratio and is equal to the volume delivered by the ventilator (there is no entrainment). Respiratory frequencies ranging from 60 to 100 breaths/min and tidal volumes between 1.5 and 5 ml/kg can be used. HFJV, a technique developed by Klain and Smith in the USA in the early eighties, differs from HFPPV in two aspects: first, driving pressure of gases is higher and can be modulated; second, inspired gases are delivered to the patient through different injection systems which produce gas entrainment. Because HFJV is much more widely used than HFPPV, the HFJV system will be described here in detail.

Circuit for High-Frequency Jet Ventilation

As shown in Fig. 1, air and oxygen are supplied to the jet ventilator under a high pressure (4 atmospheres) and are mixed in a blender where there is a pressure drop of about 1 atmosphere (Atm). Therefore, the driving pressure of gases arriving at the jet ventilator is around 3 Atm. Gases are then pulsed either by a pneumatic valve or by an electronically controlled solenoid valve in a non-compliant connecting tube fixed to the injection system. There is a 0.5 Atm pressure loss within the ventilatory circuits and, therefore, the operating pressure in the connecting tube is around 2.5 Atm. Inside the ventilator there is a second stage pressure regulator, which enables smooth control of driving pressure, and consequently of operating pressure, from its maximal value to zero. Because most of the injection systems accelerate gases and produce gas entrainment, the tidal volume delivered to the patient (VT) is equal to the jet gas volume delivered by the ventilator (Vjet) plus the entrained volume (E):

$$V_T \ (ml) = Vjet + E$$

Therefore, most of the HFJV circuits include an open circuit which provides warmed and humidified gases for entrainment. This additional circuit connected to the injection system via a three-way swivel adapter should be able to deliver a maximal flow of 30 l/min at the same FiO_2 as the gases delivered by the ventilator.

Finally, a safe jet ventilator should:

– provide a range of respiratory frequencies between 0 and 400/min;
– enable changes in I/E ratio independent of respiratory frequency;
– display the minute ventilation, the jet gas volume delivered by the ventilator and the operating pressure;
– include a system for monitoring mean airway pressure;
– include low and high pressure alarm systems.

Humidification and Warming of Gases Delivered to the Patient

If HFJV is to be administered to a patient for more than two hours, then adequate warming and humidification of the gas mixture is critical. A good number of the failures attributed to HFJV itself are in fact failures in the humidification

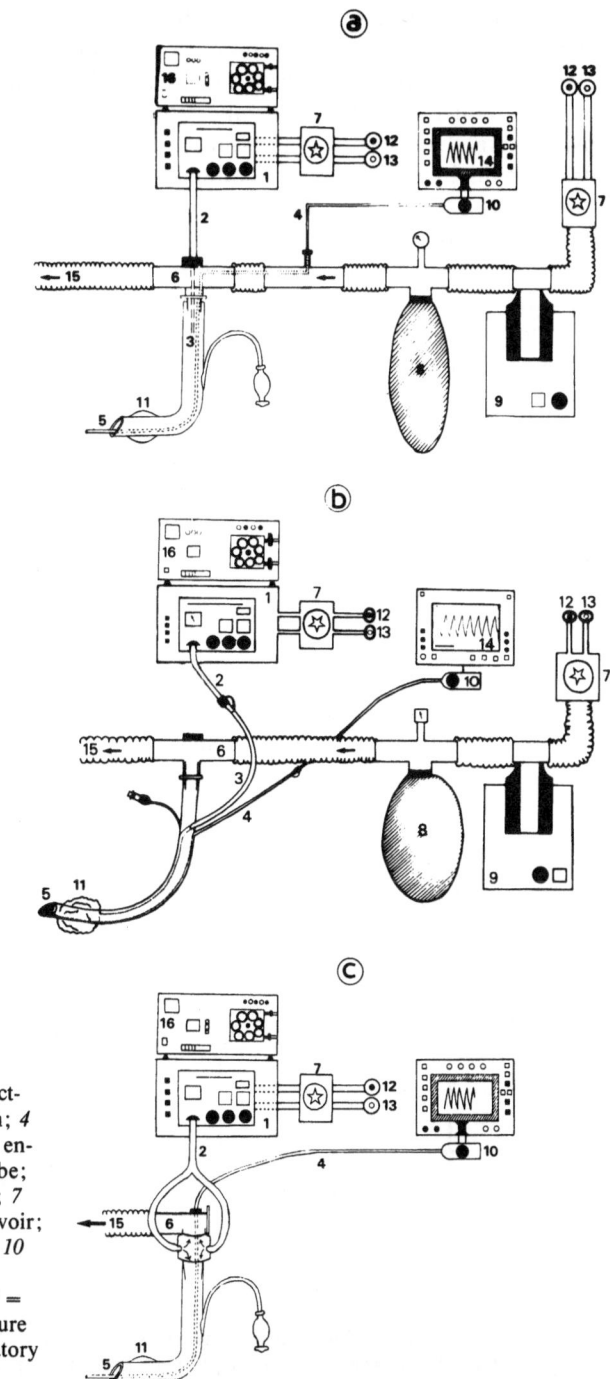

1 = jet ventilator; 2 = connecting tube; 3 = injection system; 4
= intratracheal catheter; 5 = endotracheal or tracheostomy tube;
6 = three-way swivel adapter; 7
= blender; 8 = balloon reservoir;
9 = conventional humidifier; 10
= pressure transducer; 11 =
cuff; 12 = oxygen supply; 13 =
air supply; 14 = airway pressure
monitoring; 15 = open expiratory
line; 16 = jet humidifier

Fig. 1. a Injection system using an injection cannula. **b** Injection system using the jetting channel of a special endotracheal tube. **c** Injection system not associated with gas entrainment

system. The first rule is to avoid „home-made systems" and to recognize the complexity of the problem. The most difficult problem is to provide adequate warming of the gases. As shown in Fig. 2, along the injection system there is a marked reduction in pressure: operating pressure is between 1 and 2.5 Atm (35 psi), whereas mean airway pressure is around just a few cmH₂O. This pressure drop results in a marked gas cooling within the trachea. Therefore, the temperature of gases within the connecting tube has to be above 60°C in order to reach a temperature of 37°C within the trachea. In fact, the only way to achieve adequate warming and humidification of the gases during HFJV is to use a hot vaporizer. A continuous infusion rate of distilled water is vaporised at 100°C and delivered to the connecting tube during each expiratory phase. Electrical resistances imbedded in the connecting tube wall avoid gas cooling and condensation so that gas temperature at the entry of the injection system will remain above 60°C. As during conventional ventilation, 44 mg of water must be added to each liter of dry gas delivered by the ventilator to reach 100% relative humidity. The quantity of water ($\dot{Q}_{H_2O}$ in ml/hour) which should provide the vaporizer depends on the minute ventilation delivered by the ventilator ($\dot{V}$ in liters/minute) [1]:

$$\dot{Q}_{H_2O} = 2.64\dot{V}_{H_2O}$$

Consequently, any changes in ventilatory settings should be associated with a corresponding change in the rate of humidification. Warming and humidification of the additional gases are achieved by a conventional humidifier. Most of

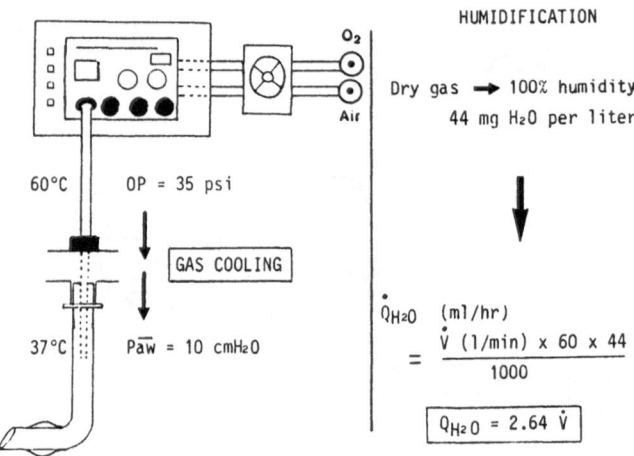

Fig. 2. Humidification and warming of the gases delivered to the patient during HFJV. On the left part of the figure the decrease in pressure and in temperature is shown. The operating pressure (OP) within the connecting tube is of 35 psi and the mean airway pressure is 10 cmH₂O. This pressure drop induces a decrease in the temperature from 60°C to 37°C. On the right part of the figure is shown the quantity of water ($\dot{Q}_{H_2O}$) required to humidify a dry gas delivered at a flow of $\dot{V}$

the jet ventilators commercially available are not equipped for adequate warming and humidification of the gases delivered to the patient. The Acutronic ventilator is equipped with a particularly reliable and efficient heater and humidifier which has been proved clinically safe for long-period HFJV.

The Different Methods of Injection

Injection systems using injector cannulas: This type of injection uses short injector cannulas, 4 to 5 cm in length, with varying internal diameters. As shown in Fig. 1a, a rigid (metallic) injector cannula can be inserted into a three-way swivel adapter fixed to the tracheostomy or the endotracheal tube. A semi-rigid, specially constructed injector cannula can also be percutaneously inserted into the trachea under local anesthesia. This type of injection, which is used for laryngeal and vocal cord surgery and in emergency situations when endotracheal intubation is impossible, requires complete permeability of the upper airways and solid fixation to avoid accidental displacement. When decreasing the internal diameter of the injection cannula, the tidal volume and the HFJV induced PEEP effect decrease, reducing CO_2 elimination and mean airway pressure [2].

Injection systems using a special jet endotracheal tube: This type of injection requires the presence of a Hi-Lo jet Tm endotracheal tube (NCC, Division Mallinckrodt, Argyle) characterized by the existence of 2 additional channels (Fig. 1b): the jet insufflation channel, ending 6 cm before the distal tip of the endotracheal tube and the airway pressure-monitoring channel. This type of injection is one of the most convenient in providing HFJV. The connection between the ventilator and the jet insufflation channel is souple, permitting movements of the patient's head. Suctioning without interrupting HFJV is possible, rendering this dangerous maneuver particularly safe in hypoxemic patients. The distal site of injection close to the carina has two important consequences: first, the anatomical dead space is reduced and second, gas entrainment decreases, representing only 25% of tidal volume. When compared to injection systems using injector cannulas, this type of injection tends to decrease tidal volume and "PEEP effect" while maintaining the same level of CO_2 elimination [2].

Injection systems using intratracheal and intrabronchial catheters: This type of injection, which requires small internal diameter catheters positioned within the tracheobronchial tree, is used for laryngeal surgery, bronchoscopies, laryngoscopies, tracheal and bronchial surgery. The catheter can be positioned either using oral and nasal approaches or using a percutaneous transtracheal route. It can also be passed through a conventional endotracheal tube or solidarized to a flexible fiberoptic bronchoscope. When using a rigid bronchoscope, a special additional metallic channel fixed on the external wall is used for injection [3]. Because the length (>30 cm) and the small internal diameter (<2 mm) of these catheters markedly increase resistance to gas flow, a high driving pressure (>3 Atm) is most often necessary to deliver an adequate tidal volume to the patient.

Injection systems suppressing gas entrainment: As shown in Fig. 1c, this type of injection requires a specially-constructed intermediary piece characterized by two orifices facing each other, by which means the injection is performed. Absence of entrainment markedly simplifies the minute ventilation monitoring, since the tidal volume is equal to the jet gas volume which is generally displayed on the front panel of the ventilator. This type of injection is frequently used when HFJV is combined with conventional ventilation.

Effects on Lung Volume and Pressures. Mean Airway Pressure Monitoring

It is important to keep in mind that HFV is a positive pressure ventilation. Because of expiratory flow limitation, all types of HFV induce a "PEEP effect" whose intensity depends on factors related to the ventilatory settings and to the patient himself. As shown in Fig. 3, HFJV increases functional residual capacity and mean volume (around which the lungs oxillate). The "PEEP effect" increases with I/E ratio, driving pressure and, to a lesser degree, with respiratory frequency [4]. At fixed ventilatory settings the higher the respiratory compliance, the greater the "PEEP effect". In other words, patients with normal or elevated respiratory compliance can be markedly overdistented by using inadequate ventilatory settings – I/E ratio > 0.43 and driving pressures > 2 bars –, whereas patients with acute respiratory failure and reduced respiratory compliance can benefit from the "PEEP effect" [5].

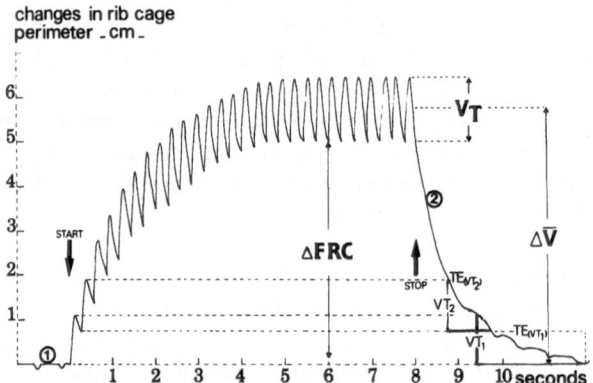

Fig. 3. Recording of changes in rib cage perimeter – equivalent to changes in lung volume – induced during a short period of HFJV in an anesthetized patient. Left and right arrows indicate the starting and finishing times of HFJV. Ventilatory settings used are frequency 200/min, I/E ratio 0.43 and driving pressure 2.2 Atm. ΔFRC = increase in functional residual capacity; $\Delta\bar{V}$ = mean pulmonary volume above apneic functional residual capacity; V_T = tidal volume; V_{T1} = first V_T; V_{T2} = second V_T; TE (V_{T1}) spontaneous relaxation time of V_{T1}; TE (V_{T2}) = spontaneous relaxation time of V_{T2} ① baseline corresponding to apneic functional residual capacity (with cardiac artefacts); ② passive exhalation curve with cardiac artefacts in its inferior section. (From [4] with permission)

Is there a simple respiratory parameter to monitor which accurately reflects the "PEEP effect"? If the case is negative, then HFV would certainly appear as an unpredictable and unsafe technique. Lung volume changes cannot be easily monitored in clinical practice. Mean airway pressure, which is the pressure corresponding to the mean lung volume above apneic functional residual capacity, is easy to measure. During HFPPV and HFJV it has been shown that mean airway pressure is a good reflect of mean alveolar pressure (Fig. 4). In other words, there is no gradient between the pressure measured in the upper airways and in the distal airways [5, 6], so that HFJV induced increase in mean lung volume can be inferred from mean airway pressure according to the static respiratory compliance. Consequently, the continuous monitoring of mean airway pressure appears mandatory when high driving pressures or elevated I/E ratio are used. Unfortunately, this does not apply to HFO. Because the expiratory phase is active, some distal bronchi collapse during expiration, creating a pressure gradient between proximal and distal airways, and consequently, mean airway pressure no longer reflects mean alveolar pressure. Finally, the monitoring of mean airway pressure is one of the principal elements of safety during HFPPV and HFJV. In order to avoid an artefact of negative pressure due to gas entrainment, airway pressure should be measured in the trachea at least 5 cm below injection site [7]. In patients with normal lungs, mean airway pressure should never exceed 5 cmH$_2$O. In patients with acute respiratory failure, there is a strong relationship between the increase in mean airway pressure and improvement in arterial oxygenation [4]. The addition of a PEEP valve on the expiratory circuit is not necessary and contributes to a decrease in alveolar ventilation [8].

What are the mechanisms of CO$_2$ elimination during HFV? In patients with normal respiratory function, normocapnia is obtained with tidal volumes of 2 ml/kg, i.e., tidal volumes close to dead space volume. This clearly suggests that other mechanisms than convection, such as augmented dispersion and pendeluft, play a role in gas transport during HFV. In contrast, in patients with diseased lungs, normocapnia requires higher tidal volumes around 3 ml/kg, probably because acute respiratory failure is frequently associated with increased physiological dead space.

Factors influencing the different components of tidal volume are well known [4]. The jet gas volume delivered by the ventilator increases with I/E ratio and driving pressure, and decreases with respiratory frequency. Entrainment increases with driving pressure and decreases with I/E ratio and frequency. When the injection system produces gas entrainment, tidal volume increases with driv-

Fig. 4. Relationship between mean alveolar pressure and mean airway pressure in 15 critically ill patients with acute respiratory failure ventilated with HFJV. Changes in airway pressure are induced by increasing I/E ratio. For each patient, three different I/E ratios are used: 0.25, 0.43 and 0.67. The dark line is the identity line. (From [5] with permission)

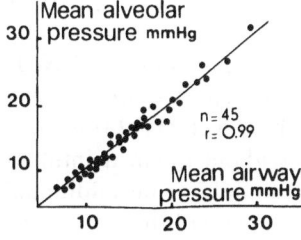

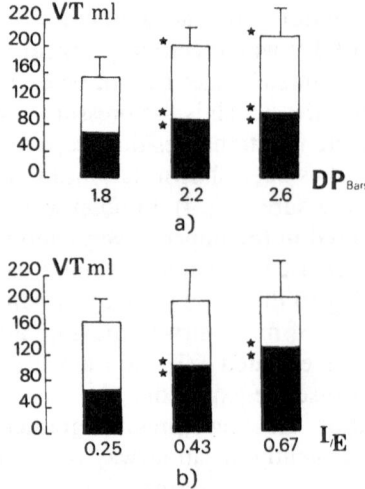

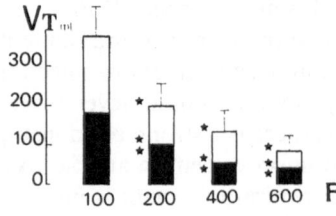

Fig. 5. Effect of increasing driving pressure (DP), I/E ratio and frequency (F) on tidal volume (V_T), jet gas volume delivered by the ventilator (■) and entrainment (□) in 15 critically ill patients under HFJV using an injector cannula fixed to the proximal tip of the endotracheal tube (mean ± SD, * $p < 0.05$ compared with control value). (From [4] with permission)

ing pressure, decreases with respiratory frequency and does not change with I/E ratio (Fig. 5). When the injection system is not associated with gas entrainment, tidal volume is equal to the jet gas volume delivered by the ventilator.

Clinical Indications of High-Frequency Positive Pressure Ventilation and High-Frequency Jet Ventilation

HFPPV and HFJV have been used in almost all types of surgery and acute respiratory failures with no apparent decisive advantage. However, in a limited number of indications, their superiority over conventional methods of ventilation has been clearly established [9].

Indications in Anesthesia

(a) Situations in which HFV enables patients to be ventilated by means of small-diameter injection systems.
ENT surgery, bronchoscopies, laryngoscopies, laser surgery can be performed without tracheal intubation, using either a percutaneous transtracheal injector cannula or an additional jetting channel fixed to the fiberoptic bronchoscope. Surgery of the upper airways, such as tracheal reconstruction or bronchial resec-

tion (Fig. 6) can be performed using catheters passed through the endotracheal tube [10]. Measurement of mean airway pressure is not possible and CO_2 elimination can be monitored using transcutaneous PCO_2.

(b) Surgical resection of aneurysms involving the thoracic descending aorta and requiring a left thoracic incision with retraction and collapse of the left lung.
To avoid life-threatening intraoperative deterioration of arterial oxygenation, administration of CPAP to the left lung through the left channel of the Carlens

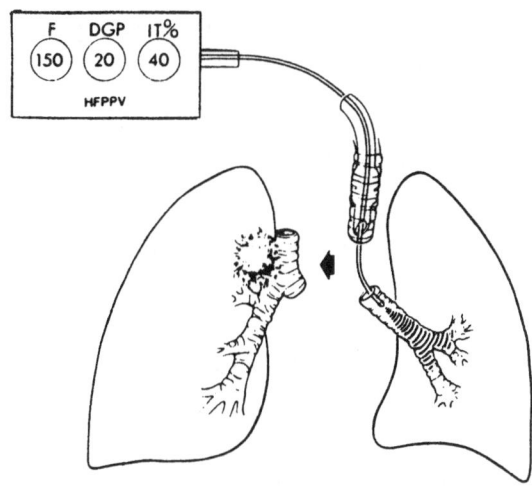

Fig. 6. HFV system used for right sleeve pneumonectomy with squamous cell carcinoma of the right upper lobe involving the tracheobronchial angle. A frequency of 150 bpm, a driving gas pressure of 20 psi and an inspiratory time of 40% are used. The high frequency ventilator is connected to a catheter passed through the endotracheal tube and placed inside the left main bronchus. (From [10])

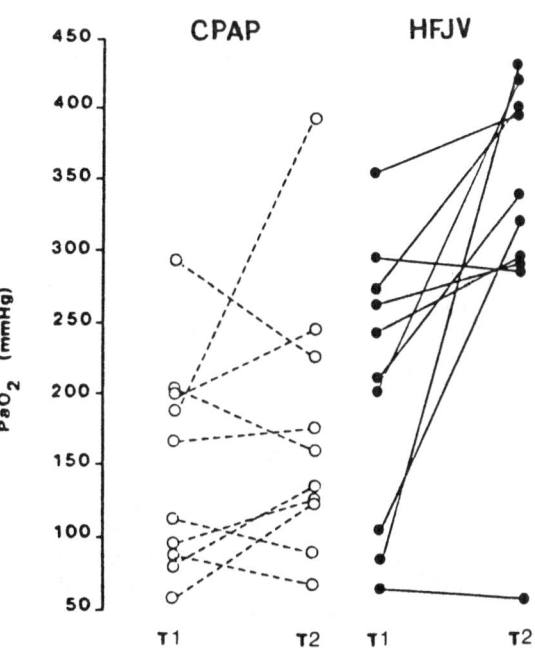

Fig. 7. Changes in PaO_2 ($FIO_2 = 1$) observed in patients undergoing surgical resection of aortic aneurysms involving the thoracic descending aorta. Each patient being in the right lateral decubitus position, a left thoracotomy is performed and the left lung is collapsed in order to facilitate surgical access to the aorta. In T_1, conventional mechanical ventilation is applied to the right lung, the left lung being non ventilated. In T_2, either CPAP or HFJV are applied to the left lung at a mean airway pressure of 10 cmH$_2$O. The improvement in arterial oxygenation is highly significant in the HFJV group whereas the effect of CPAP is unconstant and unpredictable. (From [12])

tube is generally recommended. However, this type of one-lung ventilation is not always effective in avoiding severe hypoxemia. HFJV applied to the left lung while conventional ventilation is maintained on the right lung, appears much more efficient in terms of gas exchange (Fig. 7). In fact, HFJV enables collapsed alveoli to be recruited rapidly, whereas CPAP induced alveolar recruitement is slower and passive. To avoid left lung overdistension which could alter surgical working conditions, mean airway pressure should not exceed 10 cmH$_2$O.

(c) Situations in which movements of the operating field can be suppressed by HFV.
- Vocal cord surgery [11]: By using a percutaneous transtracheal injection cannula and by selecting adequate ventilatory settings, the operating field remains completely free and the vocal cords are kept immobile, thus providing ideal surgical working conditions for microsurgery.
- Lithotripsy: The use of HFJV during extracorporeal shock-wave lithotripsy dramatically minimizes stone movement, reduces the number and intensity of the required shock-waves and enables the use of fewer electrodes. Single breath measurement of end-tidal PCO$_2$ provides satisfactory monitor for CO$_2$ elimination in partially submerged patients.

Indications in Critical Care

(a) Emergency situations during which tracheal intubation is impossible.
The insertion of a transtracheal injector cannula is life-saving for the patient. It must be emphasized that minimal permeability of the upper airways should persist to avoid pulmonary overdistension.

(b) Acute respiratory failure with circulatory shock.
HFV represents an interesting alternative to conventional ventilation with PEEP in patients with acute respiratory failure and circulatory shock (Fig. 8): arterial pressure and cardiac output are found to be higher in HFV conditions when both techniques are compared at the same level of mean airway pressure and

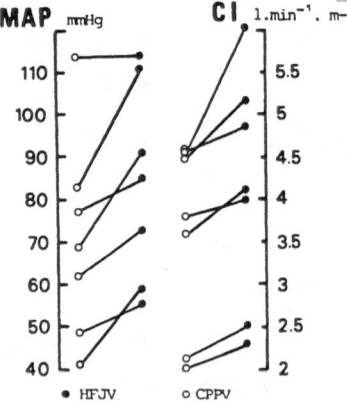

Fig. 8. Comparative effects of continuous positive pressure ventilation (CPPV) and HFJV on arterial pressure (MAP) and cardiac index (CI) in 7 patients with respiratory failure and circulatory shock. Both ventilatory modes are compared at the same level of mean airway pressure and alveolar ventilation. (From [12])

alveolar ventilation [12]. HFV appears to better respect regulatory mechanisms of arterial pressure, possibly by less stimulating pulmonary stretch receptors which normally alter the efficiency of baroreflex regulation of arterial pressure [13].

(c) Acute ventricular failure.
The administration of small tidal volumes at high frequencies provides the possibility of increasing intrathoracic pressure selectively during systole by synchronizing HFV on the ECG. In cardiac patients with low cardiac output, synchronous HFJV markedly improves cardiac index and left ventricular function, when compared to intermittent positive pressure ventilation [14]. This beneficial effect results from a decrease in left ventricular afterload produced by the elevation of intrathoracic pressure during left ventricular ejection (Fig. 9).

(d) Bronchopleural fistulas with large airleak flows.
HFV is indicated in presence of a massive bronchopleural fistula, when conventional ventilation fails to provide adequate gas exchange. It must always be kept

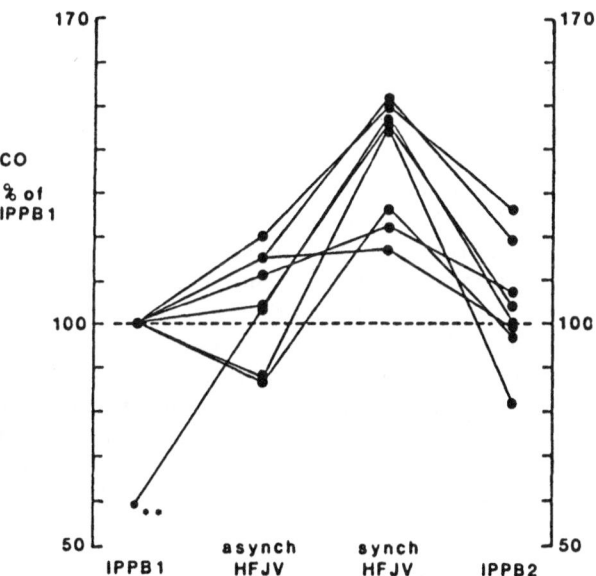

Fig. 9. Effects of intermittent positive pressure ventilation (IPPB) and HFJV on cardiac output (CO) in 8 patients with severe congestive cardiomyopathy who were candidates for cardiac transplantation. After induction of anesthesia and before surgical incision, CO was measured at the end of 5-min periods of stabilization during 4 sequential steps: 1) Intermittent positive pressure ventilation (IPPB$_1$) using a tidal volume of 10 ml/kg and a frequency of 15 bpm; 2) and 3) HFJV (Acutronic MK 800 ventilator) delivered either asynchronously with the heart rate (asynch HFJV) or synchronously with each ventricular systole (synch HFJV); 4) Intermittent positive pressure ventilation (IPPB$_2$). HFJV delivered synchronously with cardiac cycle increases cardiac output significantly more than asynchronously delivered HFJV or IPPB delivered either before or after runs of HFJV. (From [14])

in mind that mean airway pressure is the main determinant for both arterial oxygenation and air leak flow [15]. When a large bronchopleural fistula complicates an acute pulmonary disease, severe hypoxemia with CO_2 retention occurs during conventional ventilation because the major part of the tidal volume is lost through the bronchopleural fistula and because PEEP cannot be maintained throughout expiration. During HFV, the short expiratory time prevents the lungs from returning to their resting FRC between each ventilatory cycle, thus facilitating alveolar recruitment and increasing mean airway pressure. At this stage, the price to pay for the improvement in gas exchange is an increase in airleak flow. Subsequently, and only if parenchymal pulmonary lesions regress with treatment, mean airway pressure can be diminished progressively, thus enabling a gradual decrease in airleak flow. When a large bronchopleural fistula complicates upper airways surgery in the absence of pulmonary lesions, HFV provides the possibility of using low mean airway pressure and, therefore, of decreasing airleak flow. It must be emphasized that the airleak flow can be decreased only when HFV can ensure adequate gas exchange at a mean airway pressure lower than that of conventional ventilation.

(e) Tracheal lesions secondary to trauma, tracheostomy or prolonged intubation.
When a tracheal lesion complicating tracheostomy, prolonged intubation or trauma has been surgically repaired and requires mechanical ventilation with a deflated cuff, HFV is superior to conventional ventilation in providing adequate gas exchange. HFV is particularly beneficial in the treatment of tracheal rupture, tracheomalacia [16] and tracheoesophageal fistula [17].

(f) Severe acute respiratory failure with elevated peak airway pressure (> 50 cmH₂O) and reduced respiratory compliance can benefit from a combination of HFV and conventional ventilation.
This promising technique, although not yet evaluated in a large series of patients, can markedly improve arterial oxygenation without increasing airway pressures. A combination of 8 tidal volumes of 4 ml/kg (using an inspiratory time below 10% to avoid elevated peak airway pressure) with HFV, markedly improves arterial oxygenation without surpassing a mean airway pressure of 10 cmH_2O. Since pulmonary barotrauma is directly influenced by the level of peak airway pressure within healthy regions of the diseased lung, this combined ventilation appears as a safer method of ventilatory support.

Contra-Indications to High-Frequency Ventilation

Because of the risk of pulmonary overdistension, HFV is contraindicated in presence of chronic obstructive pulmonary disease and status asthmaticus. In unilateral lung disease, HFV applied to both lungs results in overdistension of the non-diseased lung, with deterioration of gas exchange and hemodynamic instability.

References

1. Doyle HJ, Napolitano AE, Lippman HR, et al (1984) Different humidification systems for high-frequency jet ventilation. Crit Care Med 12:815-819
2. Benhamou D, Ecoffey C, Rouby JJ, Spielvogel C, Viars P (1987) High-frequency jet ventilation: the influence of different methods of injection on respiratory parameters. Br J Anaesth 59:1257-1264
3. Vourc'h G, Fischler M, Michon F, Melchior JC, Seigneur F (1983) High-frequency jet ventilation vs manual jet ventilation during bronchoscopy in patients with tracheo-bronchial stenosis. Br J Anesth 55:969-972
4. Rouby JJ, Simonneau G, Benhamou D, et al (1985) Factors influencing pulmonary volumes and CO_2 elimination during high-frequency jet ventilation. Anesthesiology 63:473-482
5. Rouby JJ, Fusciardi J, Bourgain JL, Viars P (1983) High-frequency jet ventilation in postoperative respiratory failure: determinants of oxygenation. Anesthesiology 59:281-287
6. Perez Fontan JJ, Heldt GP, Gregory GA (1986) Mean airway pressure and mean alveolar pressure during high-frequency jet ventilation in rabbits. J Appl Physiol 61:456-463
7. Brichant JF, Rouby JJ, Viars P (1986) Intermittent positive pressure ventilation with either positive end-expiratory pressure or high frequency jet ventilation (HFJV) or HFJV alone in human acute respiratory failure. Anesth Analg 65:1135-1142
8. Mal H, Rouby JJ, Benhamou D, Viars P (1986) High-frequency jet ventilation in acute respiratory failure: which ventilatory settings? Br J Anaesth 58:18-23
9. Rouby JJ, Viars P (1989) Clinical use of high frequency ventilation. Acta Anaesthesiol Scand 33 (suppl 90):134-139
10. El-baz N, Jensik R, Faber LP, Faro RS (1982) One-lung high-frequency ventilation for tracheoplasty and bronchoplasty: a new technique. Ann Thorac Surg 34:564-571
11. Klain M, Smith B (1977) High-frequency percutaneous transtracheal jet ventilation. Crit Care Med 5:280-287
12. Fusciardi J, Rouby JJ, Barakat T, Mal H, Godet G, Viars P (1986) Hemodynamic effects of high-frequency jet ventilation in patients with and without circulatory shock. Anesthesiology 65:485-491
13. Rouby JJ, Houissa M, Brichant JF, et al (1987) Effects of high-frequency jet ventilation on arterial baroreflex regulation of heart rate. J Appl Physiol 63:2216-2222
14. Pinsky MR, Marquez J, Martin D, Klain M (1987) Ventricular assist by cardiac cycle-specific increases in intrathoracic pressures. Chest 91:709-715
15. Albeda SM, Hansen-Flaschen JH, Taylor E, Lanken PN, Wollmann H (1985) Evaluation of high-frequency jet ventilation in patients with bronchopleural fistulas by quantitation of the airleak. Anesthesiology 63:551-554
16. Smith GA, Castresana MR, Mandel SD (1983) Ventilatory management of tracheomalacia utilizing high-frequency jet ventilation. Anesth Analg 62:538-539
17. Oliver A, Orlowski J (1985) A double-crossover study comparing conventional ventilation with high-frequency ventilation in a patient with tracheosophageal fistula. Resuscitation 12:225-231

Patients' Experiences of Mechanical Ventilation

H. Haljamäe, I. Bergbom-Engberg, and B. Hallenberg

Introduction

Modern intensive care means maximum application of modern technology and invasive diagnostic procedures in a hospital setting requiring the greatest expenditure of nursing staff [1, 2]. The ICU environment is no doubt frightening and stress-evoking for the critically ill patient due to its hectic pace where physical needs are often paramount and psychological needs secondary, if noted at all [3]. This means that the ICU patient confronts a more intensive barrage of stressors than other categories of patients, and is less emotionally resilient and thus less able to adapt to these stressors [2]. The result may be that the patient initially experiences a psychological distress characterized by anxiety, depression, confusion, fear, or anger in response to the illness and hospitalization [4], while later cognitive, affective, and perceptual functions become disturbed. At that stage the patient experiences a phenomenon referred to as „ICU psychosis" or „ICU syndrome" [5, 8]. The etiology is probably multifactorial including both pathophysiological disturbances caused by the medical condition and various nursing care activities in the busy ICU environment [9]. Cerebral hypoxia as well as analgesic and sedative drugs may influence the ability of the critically ill patient to interpret adequately various types of stimuli [8, 10] in a nursing situation characterized by repeated disturbances upsetting the ability of the patient to relax and rest [9, 11, 12].

The critically ill intubated patient needing ventilatory support is in an even more difficult situation due to the inability to communicate verbally. The ability to interact with the surrounding environment is furthermore restricted by all the pieces of equipment typing the patient to the bed and perhaps also by heavy sedation or even therapeutic paralysis [13]. Dependence on machines and medical staff is consequently a necessary reality for critically ill respiratory treated patients.

Patients' Recall of Respirator Treatment

Recent studies show that only about 50% of respirator treated patients remember the period of mechanical ventilation when interviewed more than 2 months later [14–17]. Factors influencing the recall of the respirator therapy are age, sex, the severity of the medical condition, and the duration of the respirator treatment.

More young individuals, especially females, remember having been mechanically ventilated. Patients being unconscious when admitted to the ICU and trauma patients with head injuries usually belong to the non-recaller group [16]. The duration of the respirator treatment seems an important factor since in our own studies [14–17] the awareness of the treatment was found poor (<40%) in patients respirator treated for internal medical diseases for less than 1 to 2 days as compared to patients treated for more than 11 days (>70%). Jones et al. [18] have similarily found that only 30% of patients ventilator treated for about 15 hours recalled the treatment.

The ability to recall the treatment will also be influenced by the regimens used for sedation during the respirator therapy. In many ICUs the aim seems to be to keep most patients so well sedated that they are more or less detached from the ICU environment [19]. In our ICU setting a lighter level of sedation is usually preferred and unpublished data indicate that even the use of regional techniques for postoperative pain treatment combined with light sedation in surgical patients in need of postoperative ventilatory support does not include any major drawbacks out of psychological point of view for the patients. The creation of an emotionally supportive environment based on proper nursing interventions may be as efficient for minimizing the psychological stress load on the patient as heavy sedation routines [4].

Information about the respirator treatment to e.g. elective surgical patients prior to the actual therapeutic situation does not seem to influence the recall of the treatment [16]. An explanation for this could be that many of the agents used for general anaesthesia may influence mental function and the memory process for a prolonged period of time [20–22] and thereby also the awareness of the treatment [16]. In the preoperative period the patient may also experience considerable frustration when facing the necessity of anesthesia and surgery for a major surgical condition. This may induce perceptional and cognitive mental barriers influencing the ability to understand and interpret almost any given information [23], including that given about the respirator treatment. Even if available data on patients' experiences of respirator treatment do not clearly demonstrate that preinformation about the treatment reduces the incidence of unpleasant and frustrating psychological experiences [15–17] we still consider it of major importance to give such information whenever possible.

Experiences of Discomforts

Most patients who remember having been respirator treated claim, even up to 4 years later, still to recall the situation as unpleasant and stress-evoking [17]. The underlying medical illness or trauma condition will certainly have psychological effects but the respirator treatment includes additional physical as well as psychological stressors. Discomforts experienced by mechanically ventilated patients are in order of frequency summarized in Table 1.

As can be seen from the table, almost 50% of respirator treated patients seem to find the situation so unpleasant and frightening that anxiety and/or fear, or in 30% of the patients, even agony and/or panic are experienced [17]. In Table 2,

Table 1. Discomforts experienced during respirator treatment in order of frequency

Complaint	% of patients
Anxiety/fear	47
Not able to talk	46
Secretion	39
Pain	36
Difficulties in sleeping	35
Agony/panic	30
Suctioning	30
Insecurity	29
Nightmares	26
Extubation/decannulation	20
Synchronization problems	18
Difficulties in resuming spontaneous breathing	11

Table 2. Relationships between different emotional or somatic experiences and various nursing care activities in connection with respirator treatment (based on level of significance for Pearson correlation coefficients)

	Secretion	Synchronization	Suctioning	Extubation	Breathing spontaneously
Anxiety/fear	−	+ +	−	−	+ +
Agony/panic	−	+ +	+	−	+ +
Nightmares	−	−	−	−	−
Difficulties in sleeping	−	+	+	−	−
Insecurity	−	+ + +	−	−	+
Pain	−	−	−	−	−

the relationships between different emotional or somatic experiences on one hand and various respirator treatment related nursing care activities on the other are shown.

Airway related nursing care activities such as suctioning of secretion seem to be experienced as unpleasant by the respirator patient and may make it difficult for the patient to rest and sleep but strong emotional reactions such as anxiety/fear or agony/panic are only occationally induced [15, 17].

The dominating stressor for the patient during the respirator treatment is synchronization difficulties (Table 2). Synchronization problems after suctioning may be experienced as feelings of being suffocated by getting no or too much air. In patients with borderline arterial oxygen tension it is obvious that suctioning of secretions may cause cerebral hypoxia if the procedure is not kept short enough [24]. An oxygen debt can thus explain why it so often is difficult for patients to readapt to the breathing pattern of the respirator after suctioning and the reported correlations between suctioning, synchronization and severe emotional reactions [17]. Cardiac arrhythmias induced by the suctioning could be an additional stress-evoking factor. Arrhythmias are as such probably experienced as unpleasant by the patient but they may, due to circulatory effects, also further impair cerebral oxygenation. Prevention of hypoxia and cardiac arrhythmias (e.g. bradycardia) by proper preoxygenation routines and perhaps also by endotracheal nebulization of anticholinergics is therefore of importance for avoidance of severe emotional reactions to occur in respirator treated patients [17, 25, 26].

The second most stress-evoking situation for the respirator treated patient seems to be to resume spontaneous breathing (Table 2). The administration of sedative and analgesic drugs is usually reduced during the weaning period prior to extubation or decannulation. This could be one reason why patients feel more anxious and afraid since they become aware of the fact that a failure to resume spontaneous breathing will mean an additional period of mechanical ventilation. During the weaning process the patients usually also have to breathe spontaneously through the rather narrow endotracheal tube, which requires an increased breathing effort [27]. The adaptive capacity of patients in connection with the weaning process could furthermore be influenced by circulatory readjustments and a risk for acute left ventricular dysfunction due to mobilization of retained water from the tissues when the positive pressure type of ventilation is ended [28]. It is therefore of major importance to pay special attention to the psychological status of the respirator patient during the weaning period and to create an as emotionally supportive nursing environment as possible.

Nursing Care Related Factors and Feelings of Security/Insecurity

Nursing care and equipment related reasons for feelings of security and insecurity given by more than 150 respirator treated patients [15] are summarized in order of frequency in Table 3.

The most important factor in the ICU environment for feelings of security seems to be the presence of a nurse at the bedside who the respirator patient feels that he/she can trust. Patients claiming to have felt insecure during the treatment similarly refer to lack of trust in the nursing staff as one of the more important reasons. Nursing staff members that the patients claim to feel confidence and trust in are those who seem professional, i.e. those giving the patient the impression that they know what they are doing all the time and who always

Table 3. Some nursing care and respirator equipment related reasons for feelings of security and insecurity of mechanically ventilated patients

Security	Insecurity
1. Presence of nurse that can be trusted	1. Fear of equipment failure
2. Presence of relatives	2. Lack of trust in the nursing staff
3. Information before nursing activities	3. Communication difficulties
	4. Not able to distinguish between what is real/ unreal

inform and explain various nursing care related activities. Thereby the patient gets a feeling that the nurse really cares since a personal relationship is created. The presence of such a nurse may increase the patients' own feelings of control and thereby also the feeling of security [29]. The same mechanism may explain why the presence of relatives is considered supporting and stress-alleviating by the patients.

The importance of psychological preparation for the respirator patient is obvious since many patients refer to information before nursing activities as an important factor for feelings of security and claim that the experience of distress, anxiety and pain thereby is reduced [15]. The inability of patients to trust the technical equipment seems in most cases also related to temporary minor technical dysfunction that is not properly explained to the patient. It is rather easy to realize that a patient, knowing that his/her life is dependent on the function of the technical equipment, feels insecure if an acute equipment dysfunction is not properly explained and adequate reassurance given. Quite often repeated information and reassurance about nursing care activities and the safety of the technical equipment has to be given since the ability of the respirator patient to distinguish between what is real or unreal is impaired due to the medical condition and effects of the pain treatment and sedation routines used.

Restricted interaction with the surrounding environment increases anxiety and makes the respirator patient feel insecure. Verbal expression is impossible for patients requiring mechanical ventilation. The result may be that the patient feels isolated and unable to control the situation. Our studies [14–17] indicate that almost 50% of the patients recalling the treatment considered the inability to talk and to communicate a major problem (Table 1). It is therefore important that modern oral and non-oral communication options are made available for intubated patients so that this reason for frustration and feeling of isolation can be alleviated as much as possible [30].

Conclusions

About 50% of respirator treated patients seem to recall the treatment situation and claim to have experienced it mainly as unpleasant and stress-evoking resulting in feelings such as anxiety/fear or even agony/panic. The main reasons for such emotional reactions are synchronization difficulties during the treatment and the stressful weaning period. Important stress-alleviating factors are the presence of a nurse that the patient feels trust in, repeated information about nursing activities and the reliability of the techniqual equipment, proper prevention of hypoxic episodes in connection with suctioning of secretions, and the establishment of an acceptable method of communication. Proper regimens for analgesia, sedation and anxiolysis are necessary but light sedation routines combined with regional techniques for analgesia, when appropriate, may be more stress-alleviating than heavy sedation techniques, since the former approach allows the maintenance of a supporting psychological contact with the nursing environment.

References

1. Benzer H, Mutz N, Pauser G (1983) Psychological sequelae of intensive care. Intern Anaesthesiol Clin 21:169-180
2. MacKellaig JM (1987) A study of the psychological effects of intensive care with particular emphasis on patients in isolation. Intens Care Nurs 2:176-185
3. Gaudinski MA (1977) Psychological considerations with patients on respirators, aviation, space environment. Med 48:71-73
4. Belitz J (1983) Minimizing the psychological complications of patients who require mechanical ventilation. Crit Care Nurse 3:42-46
5. Layne OL, Yudofsky SC (1971) Postoperative psychosis in cardiotomy patients. The role of organic and psychiatric factors. N Engl J Med 284:518-520
6. Ashworth P (1979) Sensory input and alterated consciousness. Nursing 8:350-353
7. Fisher ME, Moxham PA (1984) ICU syndrome. Crit Care Nurse 4:39-46
8. McGonigal KS (1986) The importance of sleep and the sensory environment to critically ill patients. Intens Care Nurs 2:73-83
9. Ballard KS (1981) Identification of environmental stressors for patients in a surgical intensive care unit. Issues Mental Health Nurs 3:89-108
10. Holland J, Sgroi SM, Marwit SJ, Solkoff N (1973) The ICU syndrome: Fact and fancy. Psychiatry Med 4:241-249
11. Bentley S, Murphy F, Dudley H (1977) Perceived noise in surgical wards and an intensive care area: An objective analysis. Br Med J 2:1503-1506
12. Redding JS, Hargest TS, Minsky SH (1977) How noisy is intensive care? Crit Care Med 5:275-276
13. Parker MM, Schubert W, Shelhamer JH, Parillo JE (1984) Perceptions of a critically ill patient experiencing therapeutic paralysis in an ICU. Crit Care Med 12:69-71
14. Bergbom-Engberg I, Hallenberg B, Wickström I, Haljamäe H (1988) A retrospective study of patients' recall of respirator treatment (1): Study design and basic findings. Intens Care Nurs 4:56-61
15. Bergbom-Engberg I, Haljamäe H (1988) A retrospective study of patients' recall of respirator treatment (2): Nursing care factors and feelings of security/insecurity. Intens Care Nurs 4:95-101
16. Bergbom-Engberg I, Haljamäe H (1989) Patients experiences during respirator treatment – Reason for intermittent positive-pressure ventilation treatment and patient awareness in the intensive care unit. Crit Care Med 17:22-25
17. Bergbom-Engberg I, Haljamäe H (1989) Assessment of patients' experience of discomforts during respirator therapy. Crit Care Med 17:1068-1072
18. Jones J, Hoggart B, Withey J, Donaghue K, Ellis BV (1979) What the patients say: A study of reactions to an intensive care unit. Intensive Care Med 5:89-92
19. Merriman HM (1981) The techniques used to sedate ventilated patients. A survey of methods used in 34 ICUs in Great Britain. Intensive Care Med 7:217-224
20. Bruce DL, Bach MJ, Arbit J (1974) Trace anesthetic effects on perceptional cognitive, and motor skills. Anesthesiology 40:453-458
21. Davison LA, Steinhelber JC, Eger II EI, Stevens WC (1975) Psychological effects of halothane and isoflurane anesthesia. Anesthesiology 43:313-324
22. Flatt JR, Birrell PC, Hobbes A (1984) Effects of anaesthesia on some aspects of mental functioning of surgical patients. Anaesth Intens Care 12:315-324
23. Ley P (1982) Giving information to patients. In: Eiser JR (ed) Social psychology and behavioral science. Wiley & Sons, New York, pp 339-373
24. Boutros AR (1970) Arterial oxygenation during and after endotracheal suctioning in the apneic patient. Anesthesiology 32:114-118
25. Kelly RE, Yao S-SF, Artrusio JF Jr (1987) Prevention of suction-induced hypoxemia by simultaneous oxygen insufflation. Crit Care Med 15:874-875
26. Winston SJ, Gravelyn TR, Sitrin RG (1987) Prevention of bradycardiac responses to endotracheal suctioning by prior administration of nebulized atropine. Crit Care Med 15:1009-1011

27. Shapiro M, Wilson RK, Casar G, Bloom K, Teague RD (1986) Work of breathing through different sized endotracheal tubes. Crit Care Med 14:1028–1031
28. Lemaire F, Teboul J-L, Cinotti L, et al (1988) Acute left ventricular dysfunction during unsuccessful weaning from mechanical ventilation. Anesthesiology 69:171–179
29. Ashworth P (1987) The needs of the critically ill patient. Intens Care Nurs 3:182–190
30. Honsinger MJ, Yorkston KM, Dowden PA (1987) Communication options for intubated patients. Respiratory Management May/June: 45–52

Respiratory Mechanics

Respiratory Mechanics in Chronic Obstructive Pulmonary Disease

G. Iotti and A. Braschi

Introduction

Endotracheal intubation, mechanical ventilation, and lack of collaboration are different frequent factors complicating the study of ICU patient by the conventional approach of pulmonary function laboratories.

Nevertheless, looking at the problem of respiratory mechanics evaluation under a different perspective, it can be seen that the close connection between patient and ventilator can even be an advantage. Indeed, a modern mechanical ventilator is able to accurately control pressure, flow rate and volume applied to the respiratory system, which can be very helpful to perform measurements of respiratory mechanics. Moreover, the apparatus is continuously collecting physiological signals from the respiratory system, like airway pressure and airflow. These signals are used both for feedbacks to the system operating mechanical ventilation and for monitoring purposes. Unfortunately the monitoring capability of mechanical ventilators has never been fully exploited, being conceived to satisfy safety requirements more than assessment of pulmonary function. Automatic acquisition of respiratory mechanics indexes is generally poor and inaccurate. For these reasons, while waiting for more advanced monitoring systems, the study of respiratory mechanics generally still requires additional equipment, manual maneuvers and bothersome measurements and calculations.

The evaluation of respiratory mechanics in chronic obstructive pulmonary disease (COPD) patients in acute respiratory failure (ARF) is particularly interesting, since the assessment of the magnitude of the different loads on ventilation can allow more rational titration of both pharmacological and mechanical therapies. This is particularly important during the process of weaning from mechanical ventilation, which is probably the most difficult and delicate phase of treatment.

Elastic Load: AutoPEEP

In quietly breathing normal subjects, the end-expiratory lung volume (EELV) corresponds to the relaxed equilibrium volume, and end-expiratory alveolar pressure (P_{alv}) is balanced with airway opening pressure (P_{awo}). On the contrary, COPD patients in ARF commonly present dynamic hyperinflation of the respiratory system [1, 7, 9]. This means that at the end of exhalation, i.e. when either the patient or the ventilator starts a new respiratory cycle, EELV and end-expiratory P_{alv} are still higher than resting volume and Pawo respectively.

As a general rule, dynamic hyperinflation is due to an imbalance between the expiratory time and the time necessary for full exhalation to equilibrium [5]. In COPD patients, the latter is greatly increased due to high lung compliance and, most of all, to increased airway resistance and expiratory flow limitation. On the other hand, COPD patients in ARF exhibit a reduction of the expiratory time due to increase of respiratory frequency and T_i/T_{tot}, which further contributes to dynamic hyperinflation.

Dynamic hyperinflation can be detected by observation of persistent expiratory flow at the end of the expiratory time during controlled ventilation, and at the beginning of the inspiratory effort during spontaneous or assisted breathing [4, 11]. Nevertheless, full assessment for diagnostic and prognostic purposes, and eventually for prediction of successful weaning, requires a quantification of this phenomenon.

Dynamic hyperinflation can be quantified in terms of volume, as dynamic increase of EELV above resting volume, $\delta EELV_{dyn}$. This parameter can be easily evaluated in mechanically ventilated, paralyzed patients by analysis of a passive expiratory spirogram. After a standard mechanical inflation, the patient is allowed to fully exhale to the end-expiratory P_{awo} that is being used, i.e. atmospheric pressure or PEEP. $\delta EELV_{dyn}$ is equal to the exhaled volume minus the tidal volume (V_t). When PEEP is used, a passive spirogram also allows us to evaluate static hyperinflation due to PEEP, $\delta EELV_{st}$. After completing exhalation to PEEP, this is withdrawn and the patient is allowed to fully exhale into the atmosphere. $\delta EELV_{st}$ is the extra volume measured by the spirometer. These measurements probably underestimate pulmonary hyperinflation, mainly because of the long time sometimes required by these maneuvers, with volume loss due to oxygen absorption by the lungs [2]. Nevertheless, such a quantification of hyperinflation could give an idea of the difficulties that the inspiratory muscles have to face because of shorter initial length, geometric disadvantage, and the opposing action of the elastic recoil of the thorax.

Nonetheless, the mechanical disadvantage due to dynamic hyperinflation is probably better quantified in terms of pressure, as difference between P_{alv} and P_{awo} at the end of expiration. This parameter, known as AutoPEEP or intrinsic PEEP ($PEEP_i$), is the end-expiratory elastic recoil pressure of the respiratory system. It represents an elastic threshold load that the inspiratory muscles have to overcome, to obtain and maintain inspiration [5, 7].

During controlled ventilation, AutoPEEP can be measured in paralyzed patients by an airway occlusion maneuver performed exactly at the end of the expiratory time [10, 11]. The abrupt interruption of the expiratory flow creates a static condition, in which P_{awo} reflects the elastic recoil pressure of the respiratory system. In case of dynamic hyperinflation, a pressure increase is seen, followed by a plateau. AutoPEEP is measured as the difference between this plateau pressure and end-expiratory P_{awo}, i.e. atmospheric pressure or PEEP. Some ventilators are provided with a special function to perform end-expiratory occlusion. Otherwise, this can be obtained by simply adding a one-way valve into the inspiratory limb of the patient circuit (Figs. 1, 2, and 3). By disconnecting the inspiratory limb of the circuit from the ventilator during an expiratory time, the

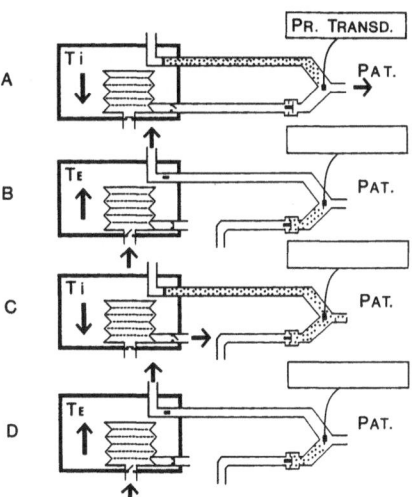

Fig. 1. End-expiratory occlusion during controlled ventilation. A one-way valve is inserted into the inspiratory limb of the patient circuit. *A:* Inspiratory time (Ti): standard inflation is performed. *B:* During the expiratory time (Te) the inspiratory limb is disconnected from the ventilator; exhalation takes place as usually. *C:* End-expiratory occlusion obtained by the combined action of the ventilator expiratory valve and the one-way valve, which seals the inspiratory limb. *D:* Exhalation continues towards resting volume

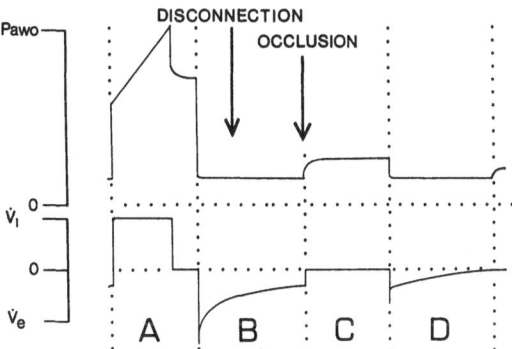

Fig. 2. End-expiratory occlusion during controlled ventilation. (For *A, B, C,* and *D* see Fig. 1)

expiratory valve of the ventilator will operate an end-expiratory occlusion that will be maintained for the duration of an inspiratory time. AutoPEEP during controlled ventilation can be measured even without performing occlusion maneuvers, but simultaneous recording of pressure and airflow at the airway opening is necessary [10]. Indirect measurements have also been proposed, for continuous monitoring of this parameter [3, 8].

By means of the occlusion method, AutoPEEP can be measured in intubated patients also during spontaneous or assisted breathing [1, 6]. After occlusion, a depression of P_{awo} is seen, corresponding to an inspiratory effort occluded at EELV. This is followed by a pressure increase above its end-expiratory value, up to a plateau corresponding to inspiratory muscle relaxation (Fig. 4.) For a reliable measurement, expiratory muscle relaxation must be verified. Moreover, since the degree of dynamic hyperinflation during these modes of ventilation may vary from cycle to cycle, several measurements should be averaged. The maneuver can be performed either by means of the occlusion facilities of specifically equipped ventilators, or by using a device provided with two one-way valves and

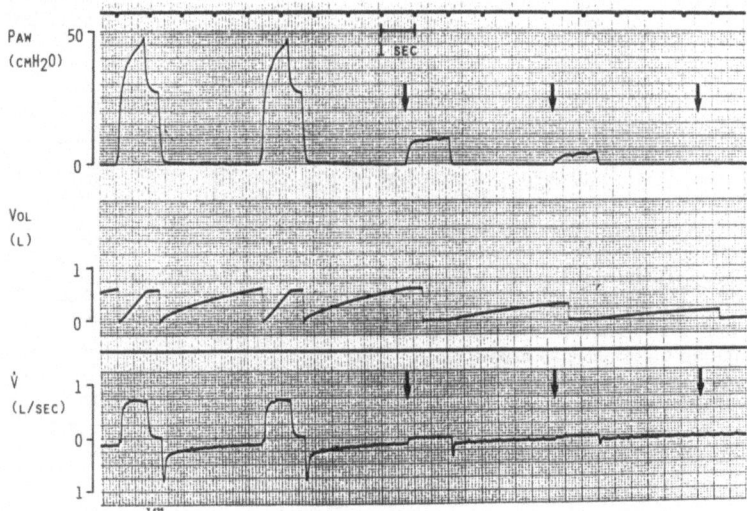

Fig. 3. Recording of airway opening pressure (P_{aw}), spirogram (Vol) and airflow ($\dot{V}$) in a COPD patient during controlled mechanical ventilation. An end-expiratory occlusion (first arrow) unmasks dynamic hyperinflation and allows AutoPEEP measurement

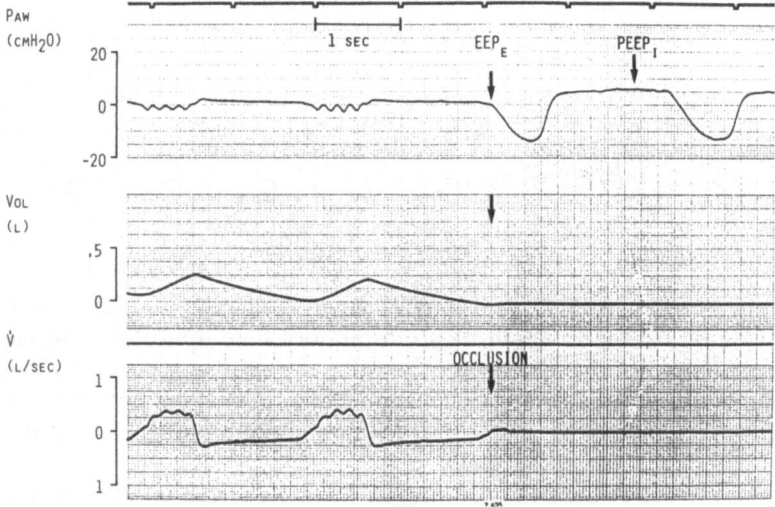

Fig. 4. Recording of airway opening pressure (P_{aw}), spirogram (Vol) and airflow ($\dot{V}$) in a COPD patient during spontaneous breathing. An end-expiratory occlusion unmasks dynamic hyperinflation and allows AutoPEEP measurement. EEP_E: end-expiratory airway opening pressure. $PEEP_I$: end-expiratory intrapulmonary pressure

two occlusion balloons. As an alternative to occlusion, AutoPEEP can be measured on a breath-by-breath basis by simultaneous recording of esophageal pressure and airflow at the airway opening [4].

Elastic Load: Compliance

Total compliance (C_{rs}) is a measurement which expresses the ease with which the respiratory system can be distended. While AutoPEEP defines the threshold load of inspiration, C_{rs} defines the elastic load of tidal ventilation. Though the entire pressure/volume relationship of the respiratory system can be studied [2], generally C_{rs} evaluation is limited to the range in which tidal ventilation takes place. C_{rs} measurement has a reasonable interest in COPD patients. Generally this parameter is abnormally high in basal conditions, while lower values are frequently seen during ARF.

A problem to be considered first is the correct evaluation of V_t, which should be measured at the airway opening. If the measurement is carried out at the expiratory port of the ventilator, the value must be adjusted by substraction of the volume stored in compressible and compliant circuit elements (V_s). During controlled ventilation, V_s can be calculated from circuit compression factor (F_{cc}), end-inspiratory pause pressure (P_{plat}) and PEEP:

$$V_s = F_{cc} \cdot (P_{plat} - PEEP)$$

If dynamic hyperinflation can be ruled out, controlled ventilation offers optimal conditions for an easy and reliable calculation of quasistatic C_{rs}, provided that the patient is relaxed and an end-inspiratory no-flow pause is employed. In fact P_{plat} reflects the elastic recoil pressure of the respiratory system after an inflation corresponding to the V_t, while the elastic recoil pressure before inflation is assumed to be equal to the end-expiratory P_{awo}. The following equation, which is used by the monitoring system of most of ventilators, can thus be obtained:

$$C_{rs} = \frac{V_t}{P_{plat} - PEEP}$$

Nevertheless, when applied to COPD patients in ARF generally presenting important dynamic hyperinflation, this method causes gross underestimation of C_{rs} [10]. Corrections must be introduced, concerning either the effective end-expiratory P_{alv}, or the effective volume related to the pressure difference that is being considered. The measurement of AutoPEEP offers the simplest, and probably the more accurate correction, by replacing the term PEEP with (PEEP+Auto-PEEP) [10]:

$$C_{rs} = \frac{V_t}{P_{plat} - (PEEP + AutoPEEP)}$$

With this correction the pressure/volume relationship is explored within the range of tidal ventilation. Other possible corrections require the measurement of $\delta EELV_{dyn}$ and $\delta EELV_{st}$ and examine a wider range of the same relationship:

$$C_{rs} = \frac{\delta EELV_{dyn} + V_t}{P_{plat} - PEEP}$$

$$C_{rs} = \frac{\delta EELV_{stat} + \delta EELV_{dyn} + V_t}{P_{plat}}$$

During controlled ventilation with constant inspiratory flowrate, an alternative method can be considered, which is independent of the effect of dynamic hyperinflation and does not require any end-inspiratory pause [9]. The method is based on the identification of P_{awo} at the onset of inflation (P_0), which is obtained by back extrapolating the linear tract of the ramp of P_{awo} to flow onset. If inspiratory resistance is assumed constant, the change of recoil pressure corresponding to V_t can be evaluated as peak P_{awo} (P_{peak}) minus P_0, thus obtaining the following equation:

$$C_{rs} = \frac{V_t}{P_{peak} - P_0}$$

Unfortunately this calculation provides inaccurate results whenever the assumption of inspiratory resistance constancy is false. Nonetheless, observation of the profile of P_{awo} during constant flow inflation can provide interesting information [4]. Indeed, the pressure time tracing under these conditions corresponds to a pressure volume tracing. Particularly, if the upper part of the curve is characterized by an increase of the slope, this is probably due to decreasing compliance and means that the respiratory system is overdistended. Figure 5 shows the different points of a P_{awo} recording to be considered for C_{rs} calculation.

Resistive Load: Airway Resistance

Airway resistance (R_{aw}) is the major source of frictional resistance, and is characteristically increased in COPD patients. R_{aw} is defined as the ratio of the pressure gradient between the extremities of the airway (which are the opening and the alveoli) to the resulting flowrate. R_{aw} measurement involves several problems. The ratio between driving pressure and flowrate is not constant under con-

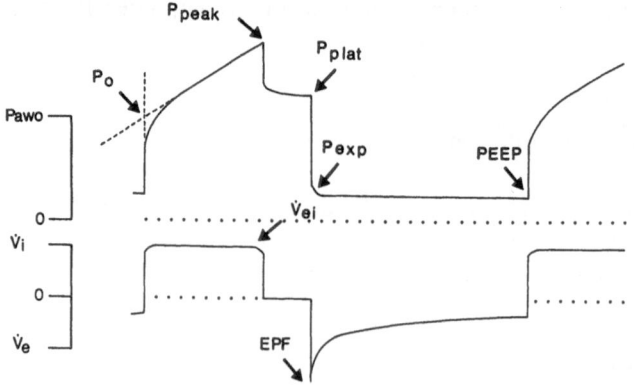

Fig. 5. Recording of airway opening pressure (P_{awo}) and airflow ($\dot{V}_i$: inspiratory flow; $\dot{V}_e$: expiratory flow) during controlled mechanical ventilation with constant inspiratory flowrate

ditions of turbulent flow, as in the case of breathing. When using P_{awo} as pressure at the external extremity of the airway, R_{aw} includes the resistance of the artificial airway, which may be different to that of natural airway by-passed by the endotracheal tube. When data are calculated by ventilator monitors, the resistance of a part of the patient circuit may also be included, according to the point of pressure measurement. Finally, if expiratory airway collapse and flow limitation take place, the evaluation of expiratory resistance may be misleading. For all these reasons, a value of R_{aw} must be correctly interpreted. Especially, the finding of increased R_{aw} gives no information about the reason for and the location of airway obstruction.

The conditions for an easy and reliable measurement of R_{aw} are met during controlled ventilation, when an end-inspiratory pause is used. Besides P_{awo} and flowrate, the other term necessary for R_{aw} calculation is P_{alv}. This can be evaluated at the airway opening after occlusion, provided that patient is relaxed and sufficient time is given to allow for pressure equilibration. The occlusion can be accomplished at any point of the respiratory cycle, but the more convenient approach is the employ of an end-inspiratory pause. Inspiratory R_{aw} is thus calculated at end-inspiration from P_{peak}, P_{plat} and end-inspiratory flowrate ($\dot{V}_{ei}$) [12]:

$$\text{Inspiratory } R_{aw} = \frac{P_{peak} - P_{plat}}{\dot{V}_{ei}}$$

In the same way, expiratory R_{aw} can be calculated at the onset of exhalation from P_{plat}, expiratory P_{awo} (P_{exp}) and expiratory peak flowrate (EPF):

$$\text{Expiratory } R_{aw} = \frac{P_{plat} - P_{exp}}{EPF}$$

If AutoPEEP has been measured, it is also possible to calculate R_{aw} at the onset of inflation [12] and at the end of exhalation. Figure 5 shows some points of a tracing of P_{awo} and airflow to be considered for R_{aw} calculation.

As an alternative approach, if C_{rs} is known, expiratory R_{aw} can be calculated from an analysis of the passive expiratory spirogram [12].

References

1. Fleury B, Murciano D, Talamo C, Aubier M, Pariente R, Milic-Emili J (1985) Work of breathing in patients with chronic obstructive pulmonary disease in acute respiratory failure. Am Rev Respir Dis 131:822–827
2. Gattinoni L, Mascheroni D, Basilico E, Foti G, Pesenti A, Avalli L (1987) Volume/pressure curve of total respiratory system in paralysed patients: artifacts and correction factors. Intensive Care Med 13:19–25
3. Jonson B, Nordström L, Olsson SG, Akerback D (1975) Monitoring of ventilation and lung mechanics during automatic ventilation. A new device. Bull Physiopath Resp 11:729–743
4. Marini JJ (1988) Monitoring during mechanical ventilation. Clin Chest Med 9:73–100
5. Marini JJ (1989) Should PEEP be used in airflow obstruction? Am Rev Respir Dis 140: 1–3

6. Murciano D, Aubier M, Bussi S, Derenne JP, Pariente R, Milic-Emili J (1982) Comparison of esophageal, tracheal, and mouth occlusion pressure in patients with chronic obstructive pulmonary disease during acute respiratory failure. Am Rev Respir Dis 126:837-841
7. Milic-Emili J, Gottfried SB, Rossi A (1987) Dynamic hyperinflation: intrinsic PEEP and its ramifications in patients with respiratory failure. In: Vincent JL (ed) Update in intensive care and emergency medicine vol 3. Update 1987. Springer, Berlin Heidelberg New York Tokyo, pp 192-198
8. Rodi G, Sala Gallini G, Braschi A, Iotti G, Emmi V, Rossi C (1989) Nouvelle méthode d'évaluation indirecte de l'Auto-PEEP en ventilation controlée. Rean Soins Intens Med Urg 5:459 (abstr)
9. Rossi A, Gottfried SB, Higgs BD, Zocchi L, Grassino A, Milic-Emili J (1985) Respiratory mechanics in mechanically ventilated patients with respiratory failure. J Appl Physiol 58:1849-1858
10. Rossi A, Gottfried SB, Zocchi L et al (1985) Measurement of static compliance of the total respiratory system in patients with acute respiratory failure during mechanical ventilation. The effect of instrinsic pulmonary end-expiratory pressure. Am Rev Respir Dis 131:672-677
11. Truwit JD, Marini JJ (1988) Evaluation of thoracic mechanics in the ventilated patient. Part 1: primary measurements. J Crit Care 3:199-213
12. Truwit JD, Marini JJ (1988) Evaluation of thoracic mechanics in the ventilated patient. Part II: applied mechanics. J Crit Care 3:199-213

Lung Mechanics in ARDS

A. Pesenti, P. Pelosi, and L. Gattinoni

Introduction

Alterations of the mechanical properties of the respiratory system are so constant in adult respiratory distress syndrome (ARDS) to be considered an integral part of its definition [1].

Modern ventilators often incorporate continuous monitoring of "respiratory mechanics", thus making a considerable amount of data and informations available in daily clinical practice. However, a detailed and systematic analysis of respiratory mechanics in ARDS is difficult, mainly because of the nonuniformity of methods and conditions of measurements.

We propose a tentative view of lung mechanics, which, far from attempting to be exhaustive, integrates some morphological data (computerized tomography) with functional studies (gas exchange and hemodynamics). We will follow a train of reasoning stemming from an oversimplification: the lung in ARDS is non-homogeneously diseased, and zones which appear almost normal coexist with zones of consolidation, edema, or atelectasis.

ARDS: The Non-homogeneous Lung

Microvascular injury and lung edema are probably the initial events in ARDS. These phenomena are diffuse and probably ubiquitous to the entire lung parenchima. Available data however indicate that following this initial phase the lung is no longer homogeneous, and individual lung zones could arbitrarily be assigned to at least two types, the ones (almost) "healthy", the other "diseased" [2].

Gas exchange studies support this view: by using the multiple inert gas technique, Dantzker [3] first reported the presence of areas of normal-high ventilation/perfusion ratio together with true shunt, defined as the truly non ventilated compartment. By contrast, the hypoventilated (low ventilation/perfusion ratio) compartment was only marginally represented: hence the ARDS lung is non-homogeneous, and discontinuous.

Computerized tomography (CT) scan studies of the lung provide the morphological counterpart of these gas exchange data: radiological densities (areas of the lung containing little or no gas) are patchy, while regions of normal radiographic appearance are preserved [4]. By appropriate methods it is possible to compute the amount of normally aerated lung tissue, as well as the amount of tissue appearing as dense and non aerated. Densities tend to be located in the most dependent regions of the lung (i.e. in the dorsal lung if the patient lies supine) [5].

Pulmonary mechanics also are consonant with this view of the lung as non-homogeneous, and will be the subject of the following discussion.

Lung Volumes

A striking reduction in lung volumes (Table 1), namely functional residual capacity (FRC), has been one of the first quantitative observations in ARDS [6, 7].

Most methods of measurements are adaptations of gas dilution techniques (helium dilution or nitrogen washout). Trapped gas cannot be measured: hence these methods provide a measure (rather accurate indeed, if there are no leaks in the system) of the volume of gas contained in airspaces open to the airways under the conditions of measurements.

True chest volume or total intrathoracic volume (including gas, solid and liquid) may be provided by alternative measurements (like strain gauges, magnetometers, inductive plethysmographs, etc). Total intrathoracic volume appears to be quite similar to normal, both in experimental [8] and clinical settings.

In our own study, the chest transverse CT scan section of normal subjects breathing spontaneously (209.6 ± 40.6 cm^2) was not different from the transverse section of anesthetized and paralyzed ARDS patients at PEEP of 5 cmH$_2$O (209.1 ± 41.9 cm^2). These data are consistent with the concept that fluid (or consolidation) dislodges the gas out of the airspaces. It is then possible to conclude that the dimensions of the lung remain approximately constant: strictly speaking, not the lung volume but the gas volume is decreased.

Areas of the lung become occupied by fluid or inflammatory cells and debris, either interstitial or intraalveolar: lung weight, measured in vivo by CT scan quantitative analysis, increases substantially, up to three to four times the normal

Table 1. Selected lung mechanics data in normal subjects and in ARDS patients

	TSLC [ml/cmH$_2$O]	Lung weight [g]	Gas volume [ml]
Normal patients	65.0 ± 20.1 (n=21)	974 ± 220 (n=8)	2562 ± 553 (n=8)
ARF patients	42.2 ± 18.4 (n=20)	2590 ± 1201 (n=22)	1173 ± 553 (n=22)

TSLC = measured in paralyzed patients by super-syringe at 8–10 ml/kg bw inflation; *Lung weight* = measured by CT scan at end-expiration. Normals spontaneously breathing (PEEP 0 cmH$_2$O). ARDS patients paralyzed, at PEEP 5 cmH$_2$O; *Gas volume* = measured by helium dilution. Normals at FRC during spontaneous breathing. ARDS patients at end-expiration, paralyzed, PEEP 5 cmH$_2$O.

[9], (Table 1): ARDS lungs are the heaviest seen in the practice of pathology [10]. It is possible to demonstrate a significant positive correlation between the lung gas volume, as measured by the helium dilution method, and the amount of normally inflated tissue (measured by CT scan) [11]. Moreover, the efficiency of gas exchange decreases when the amount of densities increases [9].

We have reported a positive regression between mean pulmonary artery pressure and the excess weight of the lung [9]. We can speculate that the increased mean pulmonary artery pressure causes an increased edema formation in the diseased lung, but one cannot exclude that lung edema itself, via vascular compression, may in turn cause a further increase in pulmonary artery pressure.

The increased weight of the lung may offer the explanation for the preferential dependent location of lung densities at the CT scan: the dependent regions will have to bear the pressure of the heavy upper structures and the normal top to bottom density gradient will be exaggerated to complete collapse of the bottom zone.

Compliances of the Respiratory System

We define as compliance of the respiratory system the change in lung volume obtained by a unit change of airway pressure. The compliance of the respiratory system includes two compliances in series: the lung and the chest wall. The individual measurement of each of the two components requires the measure of the intrapleural pressure, which in the clinical setting is very rarely available. The use of esophageal pressure as an indicator of intrapleural pressure has some limitations [12]. Practical reasons therefore make the respiratory system compliance more commonly used than lung compliance. A reduced compliance of the respiratory system is an hallmark of ARDS (Table 1).

The usage has accepted the definition of total static lung compliance (TSLC) as the ratio between a standardized inflation volume (e.g. 10 ml/kg bw) and the pressure correspondingly generated [13]. TSLC however is not a lung compliance, but the compliance of the respiratory system (lung + chest wall). In ventilated patient methods to measure compliances fall into two major categories [12]: the first (dynamic compliance) includes the effect of inspiratory resistance and is based on the ratio between tidal volume and the difference: (peak inspiratory pressure) – (end expiratory pressure). If a sufficiently long end-inspiratory pause is used the dynamic component is eliminated and this compliance is called "quasi-static". Care should be taken to avoid the underestimate of end expiratory pressure caused by the AutoPEEP phenomenon [14], especially when high tidal volumes, high respiratory frequencies and/or long inspiratory times (inverted ratio ventilation) are used.

This approach explores compliance in the actual tidal volume range only, and the obtained figures may change depending upon the PEEP level and the tidal volume in use. Indeed, Suter et al. [15] could identify in ARDS patients a PEEP level at which compliance was maximal, and recommended this as the level of best PEEP for the individual patient.

The other approach requires a long inspiratory-expiratory maneuver, done in steps or at very low flows (1 l/min) to obtain, in the anesthetized paralyzed patient, a true static pressure volume (PV) loop. As we will soon discuss, the PV loop offers several informations: we should nevertheless keep in mind that this is an entirely artefactual maneuver, that little has to do with the actual ventilation and tidal volume in use at the time of measurement. It represents however a tool of proven diagnostic [16], prognostic [17] and even therapeutic [18] value.

Since the PV curve measurement requires an almost apneic period, adequate corrections for gas exchange and temperature equilibration during the maneuver are mandatory [19]. As expected from the data of quasi-static compliance the PV curve is often non-linear, both in the inspiratory and in the expiratory limb. In this case it is possible to identify a "knee" at a certain value of pressure where the slope shows a definite change. A proposed explanation for the phenomenon is the following: during inspiration, when pressure reaches a certain critical value, a sizable number of previously collapsed alveoli, suddenly open up, increasing the compliance of the system (critical opening pressure). During deflation, at a pressure generally lower than the opening one, those same alveoli collapse, decreasing the compliance (closing pressure).

The phenomenon is generally called recruitment, and constitutes one of the suggested bases for the rational use and selection of PEEP [20, 21]. The ratio between the slope of the PV curve in its initial inspiratory portion and the subsequent slope once the pressure is higher than the "knee" provides a quantitative appraisal of recruitment [13]. The presence of recruitment can be inferred, based on changes induced by changes in PEEP, also from gas exchange and morphological data. In this respect Matamis et al. [22] reported a correlation between chest Xrays and the PV curve. CT scan provides the morphological evidence of recruitment by PEEP, and it is possible to demonstrate and measure recruitment in terms of mass of tissue normally aerated [13]. It may be concluded indeed that compliance is an indirect measure of the amount of tissue participating in ventilation (i.e. normally aerated).

Although the concept of maximizing recruitment in selecting PEEP is entirely acceptable and becoming part of the common practice, a caution is however necessary in interpreting the data. In fact a PV curve may be curvilinear even if no recruitment is taking place, while an apparently straight PV curve might mask a substantial recruitment phenomenon (Fig. 1). Moreover, we still do not know whether PEEP should be selected on the basis of the opening pressure (i.e. higher than the knee in the inflation limb), or higher than the closing pressure (i.e higher than the expiratory knee).

Mean airway pressure (Paw) rather than PEEP has been advocated in many instances as the major determinant of oxygenation. To optimize recruitment a choice is proposed between PEEP and Paw. Experimental studies by Kolton et al. [23] concluded that constant airway pressure throughout the ventilatory cycle (as with high frequency ventilation) is preferable to the phasic pressure pattern associated with continuous positive pressure ventilation. In selecting a PEEP value higher than the "knee" it is possible to prevent alveolar collapse during expiration, and achieve, for the same Paw, a better gas exchange than the one warranted at a PEEP lower than the recruiting pressure [24].

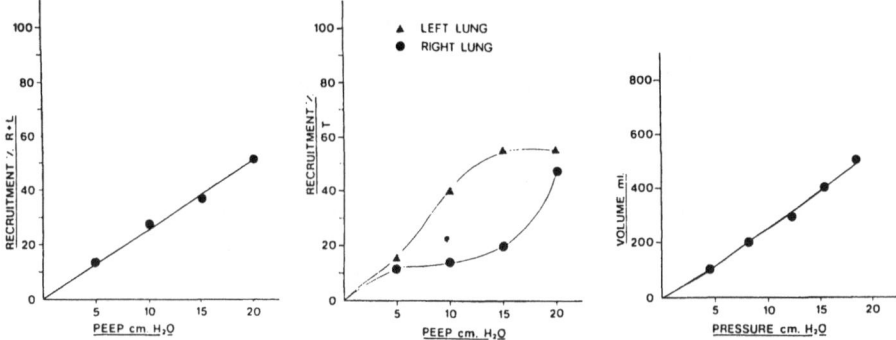

Fig. 1. Left: Percent recruitment of the lungs (right lung + left lung) as a function of PEEP. Percent recruitment has been computed from the CT scan as a proportion of the maximal recruitment observed at 45 cmH$_2$O pressure. Center: Percent recruitment of the left and right lung separately. In this individual case the left lung recruits up to 15 cmH$_2$O, while the right one recruits maximally between 15 and 20 cmH$_2$O. Right: The combined effect of the two lungs plus the chest wall results in an almost straight inspiratory PV curve. The recruitment is continuous, and no inflection point is identified

Recruitment and Central Hemodynamics

PEEP selection based on PV curve opening pressure may offer important hemodynamics advantages: Brun-Buisson et al. [25] demonstrated that cardiac output remains stable when PEEP is applied in patients exhibiting recruitment. When sizable recruitment is not evident cardiac output decreases for increasing levels of PEEP.

In our CT scan studies we could demonstrate that a pulmonary artery pressure increase induced by PEEP was present only in those subjects presenting very little or no recruitment. In contrast those patients with sizable recruitment did not exhibit any increase in pulmonary artery pressure [5].

Thoracic Compliance and Chest Wall Compliance

The use of the PV curve in clinical practice assumes that changes in the respiratory system compliance reflect mainly changes in lung compliance, denying substantial changes in the mechanical characteristics of the chest wall. Jardin et al. [26] have demonstrated that in a population of critically ill patients whose total respiratory system compliance (TSLC) was decreased, chest wall compliance was, even if not reaching statistical significance, lower than in subjects with normal TSLC.

Changes in chest wall compliance could be determined by many different factors that may be important in the individual patient: between these we should consider the changes in intraabdominal pressure and the edema of the chest wall (ARDS patients have usually a rather high central venous pressure and tend to accumulate fluids in the body, mainly because they need positive pressure ventilation).

Finally, we should consider the concept of specific lung compliance, as applicable to ARDS patients. The ratio compliance/FRC is claimed to indicate the intrinsic mechanical properties of the lung parenchima, in an attempt to standardize compliance to the size of the ventilated lung. In CT scan studies specific compliance was computed as compliance divided by the amount of normally aerated tissue present in the lung. This computation gave values not different from the ones found in normal subjects, suggesting that the residual healthy regions of the lung maintained normal mechanical properties [13].

This concept however should be mitigated by the consideration that the small residual healthy lung is contained in a chest of normal capacity and compliance, giving rise to an apparently higher specific compliance of the chest wall-lung system. This is so, because in standardizing the compliance of the respiratory system to the FRC of the residual "healthy" lung, we standardize the chest wall component to this same reduced volume, while at the opposite the chest wall has maintained an almost normal volume. The smaller the ventilated lung, the higher will be the specific compliance of the system.

In conclusion the residual "healthy" lung in ARDS could be seen as a small lung contained in a normal, disproportionately big, and compliant, chest.

Resistances to Airflow

Pulmonary resistances appear to be increased in ARDS [27, 28]: this may be due to a reduction of the airway caliber, but also to a reduced number of airways leading to ventilated alveoli, since airway resistances are arranged in series.

Inspiratory resistances may be divided into their ohmic flow resistive component and an additional impedance due mainly to time constant inequalities within the lung. The later is specifically increased in ARDS as compared to cardiogenic pulmonary edema, thus further substantiating the concept of a non-homogeneous lung in ARDS.

Conclusions

We have discussed some aspects of the mechanical properties of the respiratory system in ARDS, in view of the evidence offered by functional and morphological studies. The bulk of data and methods relative to lung mechanics has been produced in the era of controlled mechanical ventilation in sedated, paralyzed patients.

More recent trends in therapy appear to privilege partial ventilatory support and the maintenance of spontaneous breathing: since lung mechanics are the major determinants of respiratory work, and this in turn defines the limits of spontaneous breathing, a frequent assessment of the patient respiratory mechanics becomes more and more important for the successful individualization of ventilatory therapy.

An effort to update methods and technologies from the paralyzed to the spontaneously breathing patient will be most fruitful.

References

1. Petty TL, Asbaugh DG (1971) The adult respiratory distress syndrome. Clinical features, factors influencing prognosis and principles of management. Chest 60:233-239
2. Gattinoni L, Pesenti A (1987) ARDS: the non-homogeneous lung; facts and hypotesis. Intensive Crit Care Dig 6:1-4
3. Dantzker DR, Brook CJ, Dehart P, Lynch JP, Weg JG (1979) Ventilation - perfusion distributions in the adult respiratory distress syndrome. Am Rev Respir Dis 120:1039-1052
4. Manuder RJ, Shuman WP, McHugh JW, Marglin SI, Butler J (1986) Preservation of normal lung regions in the adult respiratory distress syndrome. Analysis by computed tomography. JAMA 255:2463-2465
5. Gattinoni L, Pesenti A, Baglioni S, Vitale G, Rivolta M, Pelosi P (1988) Inflammatory pulmonary edema and positive end-expiratory pressure: correlations between imaging and physiologic studies. J Thorac Imag 3:59-64
6. Ramachandran PR, Fairley HB (1970) Changes in functional residual capacity during respiratory failure. Can Anesth Soc J 17:359-369
7. Suter PM, Schlobohm RM (1974) Determination of functional residual capacity during mechanical ventilation. Anesthesiology 41:605-607
8. Slutsky AS, Scharf SM, Brown R, Ingram RH Jr (1980) The effect of oleic acid induced pulmonary edema on pulmonary and chest wall mechanics in dogs. Am Rev Respir Dis 121:91-99
9. Gattinoni L, Pesenti A, Bombino M, et al (1988) Relationships between lung computed tomographic density, gas exchange and PEEP in acute respiratory failure. Anesthesiology 69:824-832
10. Teplitz C (1976) The core pathobiology and integrated medical science of adult acute respiratory insufficiency. Surg Clin North Am 56:1091-1135
11. Gattinoni L, Pesenti A, Torresin A, et al (1986) Adult respiratory distress syndrome profiles by computed tomography. J Thorac Imag 1:25-30
12. Suter PM (1985) Assessment of respiratory mechanics in ARDS. In: Zapol WM, Falke KJ (eds) Acute respiratory failure. Dekker, New York Basel, pp 507-519
13. Gattinoni L, Pesenti A, Avalli L, Rossi F, Bombino M (1987) Pressure-volume curve of total respiratory system in acute respiratory failure. Computed tomographic scan study. Am Rev Respir Dis 136:730-736
14. Rossi A, Gottfried SB, Zocchi L, et al (1985) Measurement of static compliance of the total respiratory system in patients with acute respiratory failure during mechanical ventilation. The effect of "intrinsic PEEP". Am Rev Respir Dis 131:672-677
15. Suter PM, Fairley HB, Isenberg MD (1975) Optimum end-expiratory airway pressure in patients with acute respiratory failure. N Engl J Med 292:284-289
16. Bone RC (1976) Diagnosis of causes for acute respiratory distress by pressure volume curves. Chest 70:740-746
17. Mancebo J, Benito S, Martin M, Net A (1988) Value of static pulmonary compliance in predicting mortality in patients with acute respiratory failure. Intensive Care Med 14:110-114
18. Gattinoni L, Pesenti A, Caspani ML, et al (1984) The role of total static lung compliance in the management of severe ARDS unresponsive to conventional treatment. Intensive Care Med 10:121-126
19. Gattinoni L, Mascheroni D, Basilico E, Foti G, Pesenti A, Avalli L (1987) Volume/pressure curve of total respiratory system in paralyzed patients: artefacts and correction factors. Intensive Care Med 13:19-25
20. Lemaire F, Harf A, Simmoneau G, Matamis D, Rivara D, Atlan G (1981) Echanges gazeux, courbe statique pression-volume et ventilation en pression positive de fin d'expiration. Etude dans seize cas d'insuffisance respiratoire aiguë de l'adulte. Ann Anesth Franc 5:435-441
21. Holzapfel L, Robert D, Perrin F, Blanc PL, Palmier B, Guerin C (1983) Static pressure-volume curves and effect of positive end-expiratory pressure on gas exchange in adult respiratory distress syndrome. Crit Care Med 11:591-596

22. Matamis D, Lemaire F, Harf A, Brun-Buisson C, Ansquer JC, Atlan G (1984) Total respiratory pressure-volume curves in the adult respiratory distress syndrome. Chest 86:58-66
23. Kolton M, Cattran CB, Kent G, et al (1982) Oxygenation during high frequency-ventilation in two models of lung injury. Anesth Analg 61:323-327
24. Pesenti A, Marcolin R, Prato P, Borelli M, Riboni A, Gattinoni L (1985) Mean airway pressure vs positive end-expiratory pressure during mechanical ventilation. Crit Care Med 13:34-37
25. Brun-Buisson C, Abrouk F, Ben Lakhal S, Lemaire F (1987) Reduction of venous admixture with PEEP during human ARF. Respective role of alveolar recruitment vs decrease in blood flow. Am Rev Respir Dis 135(S):A6
26. Jardin F, Genevray B, Brun-Ney D, Bourdarias JP (1985) Influence of lung and chest wall compliance on transmission of airway pressure to the pleural space in critically ill patients. Chest 88:653-658
27. Broseghini C, Brandolese R, Poggi R, et al (1988) Respiratory mechanics during the first day of mechanical ventilation in patients with pulmonary edema and chronic airway obstruction. Am Rev Respir Dis 138:355-361
28. Bernasconi M, Ploysongsang Y, Gottfried SB, Milic-Emili J, Rossi A (1988) Respiratory compliance and resistance in mechanically ventilated patients with acute respiratory failure. Intensive Care Med 14:547-553

Work of Breathing During Mechanical Ventilation

J. J. Marini

Quantifying the Work of Breathing

Indices of Muscle Metabolism

Oxygen Consumption: The quantification of breathing effort can be approached in three different but related ways. The first is to measure the O_2 consumption difference resulting from the application or removal of a breathing stress, attributing the difference in total oxygen consumption ($\Delta \dot{V}O_2$) to the activity of the respiratory pump [1]. In theory, this method has the advantage of quantifying effort at the basic level of cellular metabolism. Because the breathing effort involves muscular activity not strictly associated with useful chest movement, the $\Delta \dot{V}O_2$ technique helps account for the grossly inefficient nature of the ventilatory musculature that often characterizes critical illness. Unfortunately, it also includes a component related to the energy expended by nonrespiratory tissues as well as a component related to the expiratory work of breathing. However theoretically attractive, this methodology has several major drawbacks for clinical practice. First, the energy cost of breathing normally constitutes such a small fraction of the total body O_2 requirement that precise measurement may not be easy [2]. This inherent problem of signal detection is multiplied in the clinical setting by the need to use supplemental oxygen. High inspired fractions of O_2 provided at an elevated minute ventilation may be required to support the patient suffering an oxygenation crisis. As a result, large volumes of O_2 are inspired and expired with every breath. By comparison, even total body O_2 consumption is quite small. Therefore, the O_2 sensor applied to the inspired and expired gas must be extremely accurate to prevent large percentage errors from occurring [3]. Equipment that bases the O_2 consumption estimate on volumetric measurements may circumvent some of these problems, but has not yet been thoroughly evaluated.

Stability, both of the patient (regarding total body O_2 consumption) and of the inspiratory gas composition (regarding FiO_2) must be excellent, or large errors will be introduced [3]. Computation of $\dot{V}O_2$ from the product of cardiac output and the O_2 content difference between arterial and mixed venous blood (CaO_2–$C\bar{v}O_2$) is easily accomplished, but fraught with error. Although conceptually attractive, this technique is subject to multiplicative arithmetic errors of inherently imprecise measurements (cardiac output, CaO_2, $C\bar{v}O_2$), in addition to transient imbalances between arterial and venous blood at the time of sampling. Perhaps the most serious indictment of either technique for sequential estimation of ventilatory effort is that repeated measurements are both time-consuming and require an active intervention in the ventilatory status.

Electromyography: The integrated electromyogram (EMG) provides an indirect but continuous indication of the tension and metabolic activity of the muscle it monitors. For any specific patient, there appears to be a close relationship between the magnitude of the integrated electromyogram signal and the respiratory muscle uptake of oxygen [4]. Unfortunately, raw EMG measurements cannot be compared across different patients, because EMG amplitude varies widely from person to person, dependent on electrical conductivity. Furthermore, tracking the activity of any single muscle group may not faithfully reflect the total activity of all respiratory muscles taken together. Finally, the diaphragmatic EMG is difficult to record in many patients without semi-invasive techniques. I therefore consider electromyography to be a valuable tool for research, but not yet for clinical application to the respiratory problems of ventilated patients.

Measures of External Mechanical Work

Estimating the Work of a Spontaneous Cycle: From a practical standpoint, ventilatory effort is more conveniently indexed from measurements of the pressures and flows generated by the respiratory musculature, as reflected by the external mechanical work of breathing (WB = $\int P\dot{V}dt$) [5]. External work is done when a pressure gradient (the transstructural pressure, P_{TS}) moves a passive structure (e.g., the lung) through a volume change (the time integral of air flow, $\int\dot{V}dt$).

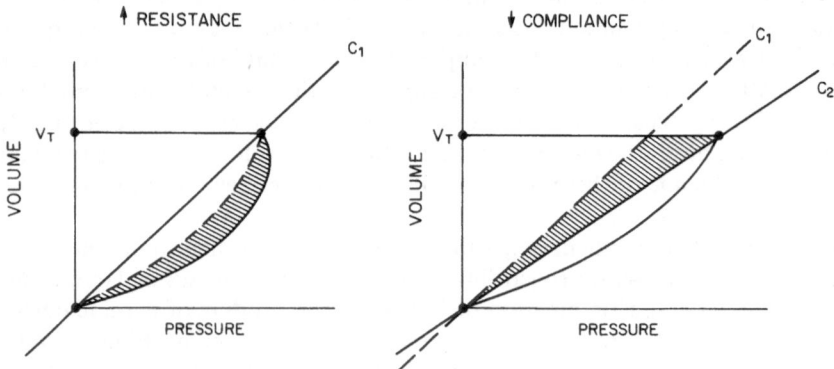

Fig. 1. Measuring the inspiratory work of breathing from a plot of distending pressure (horizontal axis) against inspired volume. C1 and C2 refer to conditions of normal and reduced compliance, respectively. In the left figure, the unshaded area enclosed by the three heavy dots and dashed line quantifies the workload under basal conditions. The shaded areas indicate the increments of work needed under conditions of high resistance (left panel) or decreased compliance (right panel) conditions

When the passive thorax is expanded by positive pressure, as during controlled mechanical ventilation, the airway is pressurized, a volume change occurs, and the machine performs work on the system [6]. Note that exhalation is normally passive, so that the mechanical work of breathing is of most interest during the inspiratory half cycle. The P_{TS} applied across the entire thorax during inspiration is the airway pressure minus atmospheric pressure. If we are just interested in the work done across the lung, the relevant P_{TS} is airway pressure minus intrapleural pressure, whereas, for the passive chest wall, the relevant pressure difference is pleural pressure minus atmospheric pressure. These pressure-volume (work) integrals can be computed electronically by integrating the product of P_{TS} and flow over the inspiratory period. This product can also be computed graphically by plotting cumulated inspired volume versus P_{TS}, and quantifying the area enclosed by the relevant portion of the resulting figure (Fig. 1).

The lung is an inherently passive structure that moves equally well, whether inflated by negative intrathoracic pressure or by positive pressure applied at the airway opening. If an estimate of pleural pressure is available (for example, esophageal pressure), the work done across the lung can be easily measured in either case. However, during *spontaneous* breathing such an analysis fails to quantify the work done in moving the chest wall. The pressure that moves the chest wall is generated deep within the muscles themselves and is consequently inaccessible to measurement. (Negative intrapleural pressure *opposes* chest expansion and therefore does not act to displace the chest wall outward). For this reason, indirect methods must be used in quantifying the work done in thoracic cage inflation during spontaneous breathing. The most common technique, undoubtedly imprecise, is to measure the work of inflating the passive chest wall during voluntary relaxation, sedation, or neuromuscular paralysis, assuming that a similar value applies during active contraction [7]. The total work done across the entire system is obtained by adding this estimate to the measured value for work done across the lungs.

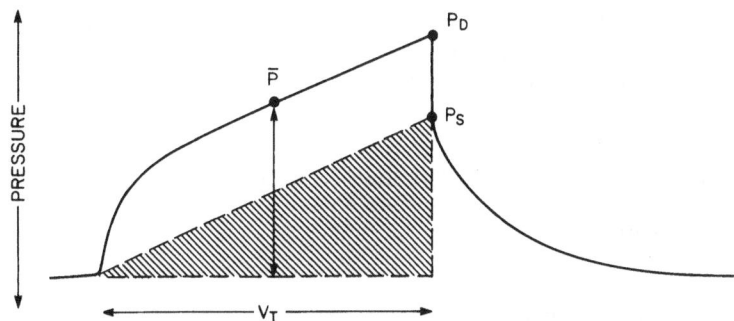

Fig. 2. Tracing of airway pressure against inspired volume during controlled inflation of a passive subject under constant flow conditions. Designated points refer to the pressures that correspond to peak dynamic (P_D), peak static (P_S), and mean ($\bar{P}$) values. P reflects the work done per liter of ventilation. The shaded area corresponds to inspiratory work done against elastic impedance of the lung and chest wall, whereas the unshaded area reflects work done against frictional impedance

When a passive patient is ventilated with positive pressure delivered at a constant flow rate, the airway pressure-volume curve closely resembles a trapezoid (Fig. 2). Under these specific conditions, time is a linear analogue of volume, so that the airway pressure measured at mid cycle ($\bar{P}$), multiplied by the tidal volume, yields work. $\bar{P}$ estimates the work performed per liter of ventilation by the machine at the selected values of tidal volume and inspiratory flow. One Joule of work is done when a volume of one liter moves against a pressure gradient of 10 cmH$_2$O. (For example, if the pressure at mid cycle were 25 cmH$_2$O, the work per liter of ventilation would be 2.5 Joules per liter.) The airway pressure tracing can be easily recorded at the bedside using the standard transducer and strip-chart recording apparatus normally employed for pulmonary arterial pressure measurement. However, to avoid infection or gas embolism, the transducer must be dedicated exclusively to this purpose. A simpler, if less accurate, method is to estimate the airway pressure at mid cycle from the difference in peak dynamic (PD) and peak static (PS) pressures developed under passive, constant flow conditions [6]. The expression (PD − ½PS) yields a rough estimate of P. When dynamic hyperinflation produces AutoPEEP, the expression becomes P ≈ PD − − ½(PS − AP). Such estimates of WB would be reasonably accurate for the values of tidal volume and flow delivered by the mechanical ventilator, but are not valid indicators of P for the tidal volumes (VT) and flows ($\dot{V}$) of the spontaneously breathing patient with greatly different parameters. For accuracy, the patient must be inflated passively by the mechanical ventilator at a tidal volume and flow rate that reflect the average values of these parameters seen during spontaneous ventilation. Such matching of VT and $\dot{V}$ is often difficult to accomplish at the bedside without deep sedation or neuromuscular paralysis.

The mean inflation pressure, $\bar{P}$ – the work per liter of ventilation, can also be expressed in terms of measured resistance, compliance, tidal volume, and mean inspiratory time (Ti) according to a modification of the "equation of motion" formulated by Otis: P = R(VT/Ti) + VT/2C + AutoPEEP. Ti can be determined directly from a strip tracing of airway pressure. It must be clearly understood that "P" in this expression is the mean distending pressure of the system, i.e., the *difference* between the pressures on either side of the structure in question, or P_{TS}. For example, P is equal to P_{aw} when the entire respiratory system is considered, but P = (P_{aw}-P_{pl}) when just the lung is of interest. The expression

Table 1. Measures of inspiratory effort during the breathing cycle

Metabolism-based measures
– O$_2$ consumption
– Electromyography

Measures of external work
– Spontaneous breathing
– – Equation of motion: P = R(Vt/Ti) + VT/2C + AutoPEEP
– – Pressure-volume area (Lung only)
– Mechanical ventilation
– – Passive: P during constant flow
– – Active: P V area difference for passive and machine assisted cycles

given above is valid both for passive inflation and for active breathing. However, when it is used to estimate the work of spontaneous breathing, care must be taken that R, C, Ti, and VT refer to the spontaneous values (Table 1).

Summary of Techniques to Estimate Mechanical Work During Spontaneous Breathing: We therefore have several means for estimating the external mechanical work performed during spontaneous breathing in the clinical setting. The work of lung inflation can be measured directly from a plot of esophageal pressure and inspired volume during unassisted breathing, with the work of chest wall inflation estimated from values published in the literature. During passive inflation, the mechanical work required to expand the entire thorax can also be measured – without the need for an esophageal catheter – from a plot of airway pressure and volume. Finally, when inspiratory flow is constant, the work per liter of ventilation, $\bar{P}$, can be estimated from mid-cycle airway pressure. $\bar{P}$ can be directly measured from a strip chart record of airway pressure. It can also be estimated from peak dynamic and static pressure values or from the measured components of the modified equation of motion. Any method of estimating spontaneous work from airway pressure data is only valid if flows and tidal volumes mimic spontaneous values and if inflation proceeds passively. Furthermore, it must be kept in mind constantly that these mechanical measures are very indirect indicators of underlying metabolic activity of the muscle itself and may bear no consistent relationship to the sense of dyspnea unless related to maximal ability to perform work.

Estimating the Work of a Triggered (Volume-Assisted) Machine Cycle: Mechanical support for ventilation is usually intended to reduce or eliminate breathing effort. However, typical volume-preset machine cycles differ markedly from spontaneous tidal breaths. Ventilators are usually set to deliver flows and tidal volumes that far exceed the spontaneous values [8]. Furthermore, the flow contour of the delivered breath differs from the natural pattern, in that its waveform follows a stereotypic pattern and remains invariant from cycle to cycle. Substantial delay may also be incurred before full machine support is achieved. (It may not be surprising, therefore, that the patient often fails to quickly terminate the inspiratory effort that initiates a machine cycle, especially when dyspneic) [7, 8].

The inspiratory work of breathing performed during ventilator-aided breaths can be estimated by comparing the machine work done during active and passive cycles [7, 8]. Provided that inspiratory flow rate and tidal volume are held constant, the difference in *machine* work between assisted and controlled cycles estimates the patient's contribution to chest inflation during active effort (Fig. 3).

Determinants of the Work of Breathing

Spontaneous Cycles

As suggested by the equation of motion already discussed, the key determinants of the work of breathing per liter of ventilation are just those that determine the

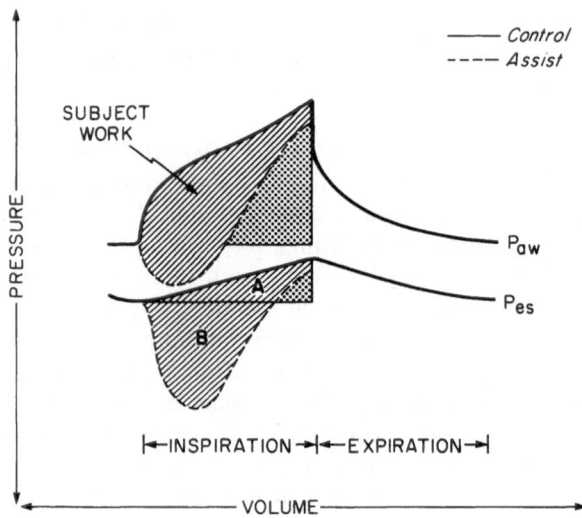

Fig. 3. Calculation of the patient's inspiratory mechanical work of breathing during a triggered machine cycle from pressure-volume information (schematic). The area difference between airway (Paw) or esophageal (Pes) pressure-volume tracings obtained under control and assist conditions (cross-hatched) indicates the subject's work per breath. The stippled regions represent machine work done during the assisted cycle to inflate the entire thorax (Paw × V curve) or the chest wall alone (Pes × V curve). Areas A and B estimate the work done by the patient to help inflate the chest wall and lung/external circuit, respectively. (From [24] with permission)

mean inflation pressure P̄: tidal volume, mean inspiratory flow rate (VT/Ti), the impedance characteristics of the chest (R and C), and AutoPEEP. The total work per breath (W_b) is the product of P̄ and the size of the breath, VT, whereas the total work per unit time is determined by the product of W_b and minute ventilation.

The clinical circumstances that determine the primary components of the work equation are those that influence the impedance of the chest, the rate of inspiratory airflow, and the depth of breathing. Thus, unless counterbalanced by another component of the equation of motion, pathologic conditions that increase resistance (bronchospasm, retained secretions, external loads), elastance (lung edema, pleural effusion, lung or chest wall restrictive disease), inspiratory flow rate, or VT (high $\dot{V}_E$ requirement) will increase the ventilatory workload. Note that $\dot{V}_E$ is doubly important to patient effort, influencing both work per liter of ventilation and the minute ventilation itself.

Ventilator-Assisted Cycles

Apart from muscle strength, ventilatory drive is the key determinant of how much work is done by the patient during volume preset, machine-assisted cycle [8]. Drive is of central importance because the machine is sufficiently powerful to perform the entire work of chest inflation – were the patient able to relax immediately after initiating the cycle. Because they influence drive, minute ventilation requirement ($\dot{V}_E$) and breathing discomfort are both important indirect determinants of the patient's effort. It is interesting to note that the impedance to inflation (chest compliance and airway resistance) does not significantly influence the amount of work performed by the patient during a volume preset machine cycle, so long as the inspiratory flow delivered from the machine exceeds the patient's spontaneous inspiratory flow demand. When delivered flows are sufficient, resistance changes that occur within the patient's airway or in the machine circuitry are met by increased pressure output from the ventilator, not by patient effort.

Having emphasized that ventilatory drive is the single most important determinant of the work performed by the patient during a machine-aided cycle, it follows that manipulation of machine settings can impressively influence the patient's work component. The trigger sensitivity setting is one of these [7]. The less sensitive the machine's activation threshold, the more work will be done per liter of ventilation during the inspiratory cycle. The development of AutoPEEP diminishes the *effective* triggering sensitivity, because positive end-expiratory alveolar pressure must first be counterbalanced to initiate inspiratory flow [9]. As already noted, the inspiratory flow setting of the ventilator can also make an important difference when flow is set lower than the patient's spontaneous need. Under these circumstances, the resistance of the patient and the machine circuit, as well as the compliance of the thorax, reemerge as important determinants of how much work is performed by the patient [8].

On theoretical grounds, any factor that augments the output of the ventilatory center may influence the work of breathing. Variations in VT, flow profile, and positive end-expiratory pressure (PEEP) level may be important to the extent that they influence ventilatory drive. PEEP may also influence the work output of the patient when associated chest distention weakens the ability of the inspiratory muscles to perform external work. Note that in this instance, a metabolic analysis (Δ VO$_2$) and a mechanical analysis ($\int$Vdt) of effort could lead to opposite conclusions regarding the impact of PEEP on patient *effort!* Conversely, PEEP could also reduce both work output and the patient's effort, depending on the activity of the expiratory muscles. If expiratory muscle activity prevents PEEP from recruiting lung volume, PEEP or continuous positive airway pressure (CPAP) may help to ventilate the lungs during the inspiratory cycle as the system recoils outward toward the equilbrium position of the system [10]. In this way, "work sharing" may occur as the expiratory muscles temporarily use PEEP as a counterspring against which to store energy in exhalation, for release at the outset of the inspiratory phase.

Importance of the Work of Breathing During Mechanical Ventilation

During spontaneous ventilation, the oxygen cost of breathing appears to be quite high in patients who require mechanical support. One study of patients with acute respiratory failure indicated that the oxygen cost of spontaneous breathing averaged approximately 25% of total body oxygen consumption, with occasional patients expending several times this amount in the breathing effort. Such requirements represent at least a tenfold increase over the normal resting value. When such ventilatory burdens are alleviated from a patient with congestive heart failure, additional oxygen is freed for delivery to other vital organ systems (provided that overall oxygen delivery remains unchanged). Experimental studies of animals placed into circulatory shock by pericardial tamponade seem to confirm this, indicating a survival advantage for those who receive mechanical ventilation [11]. The cardiac stress that accompanies reassumption of the breathing workload is a frequent reason for patients with COPD and congestive heart failure to fail attempts at machine withdrawal [12]. Thus, it appears that when tissue oxygenation is compromised, mechanical ventilatory support may help to improve the overall matchup of oxygen delivery and demand.

Another major reason to be concerned about the work of breathing experienced by patients during mechanical ventilation is that it could impose a burden sufficient to invoke dyspnea or agitation, as well as prevent recovery from muscle fatigue [13]. In such instances, reducing the inspiratory work of breathing during mechanical ventilation could be necessary for expedient removal of machine support. At the present time, it is unclear to what extent the work of initiating the ventilatory cycle contributes to ventilator dependence. However, from recent studies of active breathing efforts during mechanical ventilation, it seems likely that the level of muscle activity is at least sufficient to prevent disuse atrophy of ventilatory musculature [7].

Although the external mechanical work accomplished by the patient is easily measured, it must be borne in mind that it correlates imprecisely with ventilation-associated oxygen consumption (VO$_2$r). These two values are interrelated via the expression: $W = VO_2r \times \varepsilon$, where ε is the efficiency of converting consumed oxygen to useful mechanical work. Just as the stroke work performed by the heart is improved by reducing its afterload, so, too, does the work output of the ventilatory pump depend on its impedance for any given level of pressure development. Because the afterload impedance forced by the ventilatory pump is crucial in determining the external work actually accomplished by pressure development, – external work itself may not reflect the tension developed by the muscle fibers in a straightforward way, particularly when loading conditions

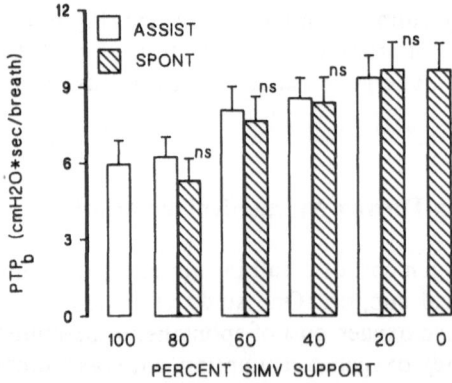

Fig. 4. Inspiratory pressure time product per breath (PTP$_b$) developed by patients with acute respiratory failure for assisted cycles (open bars) and spontaneous breathing cycles (cross-hatched bars) during SIMV. Note that the PTP$_b$ varied little for loaded (spontaneous) and unloaded (assisted) cycles at any specified level of machine support. (The *work* accomplished per breath, however, was greater for the unloaded machine-aided cycles)

vary (as during synchronized intermittent mandatory ventilation [SIMV]). At the bedside, the product of the pressure developed by the muscles and the time over which it is generated (the pressure time product), is clearly a preferable (if still imperfect) index of effort under conditions of changing afterload [14] (e.g. during SIMV, Fig. 4).

Reducing the Work of Breathing During Mechanical Ventilation

Breathing cycles during mechanical ventilation are of two essential types: spontaneous and machine-aided. The inspiratory work required for a spontaneous breath is influenced by the impedance for chest inflation and by the breathing pattern, as reflected in the depth, rate, and configuration of the pressure waveform. The added work imposed by the external apparatus to which the patient is connected has attracted a great deal of recent attention [15]. An endotracheal tube presents resistance to gas flow in direct proportion to its length, and when flow is laminar in inverse proportion to the fourth power of its radius. Even in a constant flow laboratory experiment the resistance of standard endotracheal tubes may exceed the total resistance of the normal respiratory system [16]. Resistance increases dramatically when rapid flow moves through tubes of narrow diameter. Thus, a first approach to minimizing the work of breathing is to ensure that the endotracheal tube is of adequate diameter and free of intraluminal kinks, constrictions, and adherent secretions. Resistance measured in vivo is often much higher than that measured in vitro [17]. Nasotracheal tubes present greater resistance than do orotracheal tubes or tracheostomy tubes and are therefore less desirable when the goal is to minimize patient work of breathing. The use of pressure support can help to offset the effort needed to overcome tube resistance (3–7 cmH$_2$O are usually applied for this purpose, depending on the flow demand). (CPAP can perform a similar function, if expiratory muscle activity forces the system below its equilibrium position, thus giving an inspiratory boost release).

Although it is common knowledge that endotracheal tubes present an important source of flow resistance, many practitioners remain unaware that the valving systems of the machinery they employ also affect the ease with which spontaneous breaths can be drawn through the circuit. Some demand-valve systems for delivering CPAP are slowly responsive and/or impose considerable resistance to ventilation once flow is established. Demand-valve resistance impacts the work of breathing during spontaneous cycles and during assisted machine cycles when the inspiratory flow demanded exceeds the set rate of flow delivery [7]. As a general rule, continuous-flow systems seem less resistive than demand-flow systems, but there is considerable variance from manufacturer to manufacturer of ventilator equipment. Similar problems impact the expiratory work of breathing [18]. The mushroom and scissor valves that gate exhalation offer considerable flow resistance, especially when PEEP is applied, adding to the total respiratory burden. For all of these reasons, many patients tolerate extubation more easily than low-level intermittent mandatory ventilation.

The mode chosen for ventilation support greatly influences the breathing workload. When all patient effort is silenced, the patient performs no respiratory work. Conversely, during CPAP breathing, each cycle is powered by spontaneous effort. When well-adjusted, assisted mechanical ventilation (AMV) is the least energy consumptive of the modes that allow the patient to control the onset of the breathing cycle. Under normal circumstances, AMV appears to be about 25 to 50% as energy costly as fully spontaneous breathing, but the percentage can increase greatly during vigorous breathing. During SIMV, the lowest levels of machine support are associated with the greatest breathing efforts.

What specific measures should be taken to minimize WB during mechanical ventilation (Table 2) The airway should be kept free of excess secretions. Secretions both obstruct the bronchial lumen and cause increased turbulence, thereby raising the pressure differential needed to drive flow. Such factors are almost inconsequential when the airway lumen is of normal size, but markedly increase airway resistance in patients with endogenous airway obstruction or those breathing through a narrow tube lumen. The patient should be positioned in such a way that elastance of the chest wall is minimized, i.e., sitting upright rather than supine, so that the hydrostatic forces of abdominal weight do not press on the underside of the diaphragm, thereby loading inspiration. Three to 5 cmH$_2$O of PEEP should be added in most supine patients to overcome positional losses in lung volume and tissue compliance [19]. If there is a component of reactive airways disease, bronchodilators should be used liberally, and modest doses of glucocorticoids may be helpful. Diuretics can be used to minimize the amount of lung water and improve lung compliance, especially in the setting of cardiogenic pulmonary edema. Large air pockets and fluid collections should be drained from the pleural space.

If the goal is to minimize the respiratory workload, while allowing the patient to retain control of $\dot{V}_E$, then AMV is usually the most appropriate ventilatory mode. Trigger sensitivity should be minimized and inspiratory flow rate should be set at a level that exceeds the peak inspiratory flow demand of the patient – as a rule of thumb – about 4 times the $\dot{V}_E$ requirement and generally in the range of 60 to 80 L per minute. Adding low levels of PEEP to patients with AutoPEEP can improve effective triggering sensitivity in patients who experience dynamic airway compression during tidal exhalation [9]. Above all, the patient should be made comfortable. For some patients, this may mean adjusting the VT and peak inspiratory flow rate so that the inspiratory cycle lengths of the patient and ma-

Table 2. Reducing WB during mechanical ventilation

$\downarrow$ V$_E$	Correct acidosis, fever, agitation, excessive deadspace
$\downarrow$ Impedance	R: Address bronchospasm, secretions, endotracheal tube, inspiratory flow C: Administer diuretics, drain pleural space, position optimally, add CPAP

$\downarrow$ Dyspnea	Improve patient-ventilator interactions
	    Change to different ventilator mode
	    Match inspiratory cycle length and rate of delivered flow to inspiratory flow demand
	    Improve trigger sensitivity

chine are synchronized. Such matching minimizes dyspnea and the attendant work. For this reason, pressure support ventilation may be preferable to an equivalent level of SIMV in some patients [20].

The single most important factor determining the patient's workload is the V_E requirement. Whatever steps can be taken to reduce $\dot{V}_E$ (e.g. reduction in CO_2 output or physiologic deadspace, reduction in ventilatory drive) have a clear and immediate impact on total work. (This is particularly true in patients prone to develop dynamic hyperinflation and AutoPEEP). Any metabolic influence that increases CO_2 production is to be avoided. Specifically, the patient should be kept from becoming agitated or febrile, shivering, seizures, and myoclonus must be prevented. Analgesics, antipyretics, or sedatives may be needed to reduce agitation, drive, and workload. Although adequate nutrition is essential, patients must not be overfed or supported on a diet based primarily on carbohydrates. CO_2 production may increase in both of these circumstances. Deadspace can be minimized by shortening the length of tubing between the ventilatory Y-piece and the endotracheal tube, by avoiding hypertension, overdiuresis, pulmonary embolism, and excessive PEEP.

In my own practice, I have often encouraged compensatory bicarbonate retention to allow $PaCO_2$ to increase without incurring acidemia. In this way, V_E can be reduced, without effecting metabolic output CaO_2; each tidal exhalation vents a greater volume of the CO_2 generated by metabolic processes. Currently however, I am more cautious about adopting this strategy, since elevating $PaCO_2$ may simultaneously impair muscle function – at least when hypercarbia develops acutely [21]. When judiciously applied, PEEP may improve lung compliance and dilate airways in response to lung volume recruitment, thereby reducing W_b. Yet, hyperinflation must be avoided, because overdistention places the inspiratory musculature at a mechanical disadvantage, thereby reducing the efficiency of the muscular pump in accomplishing external work. PEEP may also increase deadspace and V_E.

There should be special awareness of the potential problems of the patient with decompensated airflow obstruction (CAO). In these patients especially, panic reactions must be avoided. During periods of increased anxiety, higher $\dot{V}_E$ requirements may lead to dynamic hyperinflation, weakness, discoordinate (inefficient) breathing, and hemodynamic compromise. In the setting of CAO, reducing the V_E requirement as well as the severity of airflow obstruction are two key goals. Many such patients have positive pressure continuously at the alveolar level, even when it is not applied intentionally. Not only does the resulting hyperinflation mechanically disadvantage the respiratory muscles, but also the associated AutoPEEP effect increases the work of breathing and blunts the effective triggering sensitivity of the machine both during machine assisted and spontaneous cycles [9, 22]. To initiate inspiratory flow in the presence of AutoPEEP, expiratory flow must first be stopped by counterbalancing the alveolar recoiling pressure. This not only adds to the inspiratory work during spontaneous cycles, but also increases the pressure deflection needed to activate a machine-assisted cycle. The effective triggering sensitivity becomes the set value plus the level of AutoPEEP. This level may be minimized by reducing $\dot{V}_E$ requirement and by improving airflow obstruction. Some recent experimental data indicate that low levels of PEEP purposely added to the machine circuit may help to offset the inspiratory work requirement of AutoPEEP, without markedly increasing end-inspiratory pressures. For optimal benefit, however, the patient must have Auto-PEEP on the basis of dynamic airway compression during tidal exhalation. This technique, although rational from a physiologic viewpoint, is still undergoing clinical evaluation.

Workload Compensation

Because the ability to wean a patient from a mechanical ventilator depends upon restoration of balance between ventilatory demand and capability, it is important to attack both problems simultaneously. Muscle bulk should be improved by a nutritional program geared to maintain positive nitrogen balance. Whenever possible, the patient should be placed in a supported, upright posture. Muscle strength and endurance are optimized by achieving the levels of hemoglobin, arterial oxygen tension, cardiac output, and electrolytes vital to neuromuscular performance. Other measures are more controversial. Experimentally, theophylline and beta-adrenergic agents appear to marginally increase diaphragmatic contractility, whereas acute CO_2 retention has the opposite effect [21].

Few would argue that respiratory effort should be minimized during the initial phase of machine support for ventilatory failure. However, soon thereafter many physicians withdraw support to the point of tolerance, hoping to keep the respiratory system exercising and strong. Ironically, adequate rest may be essential to sleep quality and recovery from fatigue [23].

References

1. Cherniack RM (1959) The oxygen consumption and efficiency of the respiratory muscles in health and emphysema. J Clin Invest 38:494–499
2. Otis AB (1964) The work of breathing. In: Feen WO, Rahn H (eds) Handbook of physiology (Section 3, Vol 1). American Physiological Society, Washington DC, pp 463–476
3. Browning JA, Linberg SE, Turney SZ, Chodoff P (1982) The effects of a fluctuating FIO_2, on metabolic measurements in mechanically ventilated patients. Crit Care Med 10:82–85
4. Bigland-Ritchie B, Woods JJ (1984) Changes in muscle contractile properties and neural control during human muscular fatigue. Muscle Nerve 7:691–699
5. McGregor M, Becklake M (1961) The relationship of oxygen cost of breathing to respiratory mechanical work and respiratory force. J Clin Invest 40:971–980
6. Marini JJ, Rodriguez RM, Lamb VJ (1986) Bedside estimation of the inspiratory work of breathing during mechanical ventilation. Chest 89:56–63
7. Marini JJ, Capps JS, Culver BH (1985) The inspiratory work of breathing during assisted mechanical ventilation. Chest 87:612–618
8. Marini JJ, Rodriguez RM, Lamb VJ (1986) The inspiratory workload of patient-initiated mechanical ventilation. Am Rev Respir Dis 134:902–909
9. Smith TC, Marini JJ (1988) Impact of PEEP on lung mechanics and work of breathing in severe airflow obstruction. J Appl Physiol 65(4):1488–1499
10. Martin JG, Shore S, Engel LA (1982) Effect of continuous positive airway pressure on respiratory mechanics and pattern of breathing in induced asthma. Am Rev Respir Dis 126:812–817

11. Aubier M, Trippenbach T, Roussos Ch (1981) Respiratory muscle fatigue during cardiogenic shock. J Appl Physiol 51:499–508
12. Lemaire F, Teboul JL, Cinotti L, et al (1988) Acute left ventricular dysfunction during unsuccessful weaning from mechanical ventilation. Anesthesiology 69:171–179
13. Marini JJ (1986) The physiologic determinants of ventilator dependence. Respir Care 31(4):271–282
14. Marini JJ, Smith TC, Lamb VJ (1988) External work output and force generating during synchronized intermittent mechanical ventilation. Am Rev Respir Dis 138:1169–1179
15. Marini JJ (1987) The role of inspiratory circuit in the work of breathing during mechanical ventilation. Respiratory Care 32(6):419–430
16. Gottfried SB, Rossi A, Higgs BD, et al (1985) Noninvasive determination of respiratory system mechanics during mechanical ventilation for acute respiratory failure. Am Rev Respir Dis 131:414–420
17. Wright PE, Marini JJ, Bernard GR (1981) In vitro versus in vivo comparison of endotracheal tube airflow resistance. Am Rev Respir Dis 140:10–16
18. Marini JJ, Kirk W, Culver BH (1985) Flow resistance of the exhalation valves and PEEP devices used in mechanical ventilation. Am Rev Respir Dis 131:850–854
19. Marini JJ, Tyler ML, Hudson LD, Davis BS, Huseby JS (1984) Influence of head-dependent positions on lung volume and oxygen saturation in chronic airflow obstruction. Am Rev Respir Dis 129:101–105
20. MacIntyre NR (1986) Respiratory function during pressure support ventilation. Chest 89:677–683
21. Juan G, Calverley P, Talamo C, et al (1984) Effect of carbon dioxide on diaphragmatic function in human beings. N Engl J Med 310:874–879
22. Macklem PT (1984) Hyperinflation. Am Rev Respir Dis 131:1–2
23. Braun NMT, Faulkner J, Hughes RL, Roussos Ch, Sahfal V (1983) When should respiratory muscles be exercised? Chest 84:76–84
24. Marini JJ (1988) Monitoring during mechanical ventilation. Clin Chest Med 9:73–100

Measurement of the Work of Breathing in the Mechanically Ventilated Patient

J. Mancebo

Introduction

Work, in physics, means to apply a force through a distance and in a solid system, work is performed when this force moves its point of application across a determined length. When the physical system is a fluid, work is performed when a pressure changes the volume of the system. The relation is as follows: Work (W) = Pressure (P) × Volume (V) [1–3].

In the respiratory system, the pressure generated by the muscles produces a displacement of gas. Therefore, the work done by the respiratory muscles during the breathing cycles, the work of breathing (WOB), is mathematically expressed as WOB = PdV, that is to say, the area on a pressure-volume diagram. Such diagrams are represented by the tidal volume displacement plotted against the appropriate pressures.

The units of measurement are both the kilogram per meter (Kgm) and the Joule (J), the equivalence being: 1 Kgm = 9.8 J. One Joule represents the energy which is needed to move one liter volume through a 10 cmH_2O pressure gradient. Another equivalence is that of calories (cal) versus Joules, 1 cal being = 4.18 J. Finally, the WOB is sometimes expressed as power or work per unit of time and in such cases the unit is 1 J per second = 1 Watt.

The WOB done by the respiratory muscles is performed against 5 types of forces [1, 3] although only the first two types are really relevant from a clinical point of view.

1. Elastic forces are developed in pulmonary and chest wall tissues when there is a change in volume. The energy necessary to deform the elastic system during inspiration is restituted during expiration by moving the gas without energy cost, when expiration is passive.
2. Resistive forces are offered essentially by the airways to the flow of gas and by the nonelastic deformation of tissue.
3. Inertial forces depend on the mass of tissues and gases, and can be considered as negligible in the calculation of the WOB.
4. Gravitational forces. The effect of gravity is, in practice, included in the measurement of elastic forces.
5. Distorting forces. Distortion of the chest wall is observed in high ventilations such as during exercise and CO_2 induced hyperventilation, and also during resistive breathing. These are specially important when the distribution of vol-

ume change of the respiratory system is abnormal. If the volume distribution is preferential to the rib cage or abdominal compartment, the WOB may be underestimated if this abnormality is not taken into account.

Theory of Measurement

During mechanical ventilation, WOB can be measured from three different pressure gradients, which in turn are the respective relevant transstructural pressures for the different components of the respiratory system: airway pressure (Paw), esophageal (pleural) pressure (Peso), and transpulmonary pressure (Ptp), which is the difference between Paw and Peso.

WOB from Paw and Tidal Volume Loops

Under conditions of passive inflation, the relevant distending pressure for the entire thorax (lung plus chest wall) is Paw, so $W = Paw \, dV$. This area enclosed beneath a plot of Paw against tidal volume (Vt) represents the mechanical work done by the ventilator on the respiratory system during chest inflation. In certain cases it also represents the mechanical work done by the respiratory muscles against the impedance of the ventilator, its demand valve and its circuitry. In such a way the allocation of the WOB between the patient and the ventilator may be varied by patient effort [4–6] (Figs. 1 and 2).

If this inflation is performed in a completely relaxed subject, the measured work is probably of the same magnitude as that done by the respiratory muscles in normal breathing, provided that the breathing pattern of the spontaneously

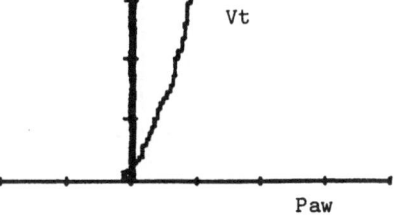

Fig. 1. Airway pressure (Paw)-tidal volume (Vt) loop of a subject passively ventilated with an intermittent positive pressure breathing apparatus. Each mark on the pressure axis represents 10 cmH_2O and each mark on the volume axis represents 200 ml

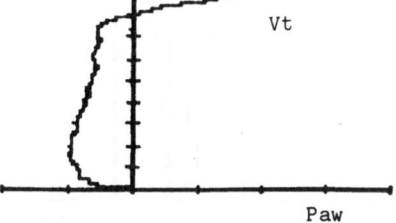

Fig. 2. Airway pressure (Paw)-tidal volume (Vt) loop of the same subject in Fig. 1 but during CO_2-induced hyperventilation. In this example the subject is driving the IPPB apparatus. The marks on the pressure and volume axes represent 10 cmH_2O and 200 ml, respectively

breathing subject is strictly identical to that delivered by the ventilator [5]. However, this method is subject to criticism because the distribution of volume change may be different from that during spontaneous breathing [1].

WOB from Transpulmonary Pressure and Tidal Volume Loops

Ptp represents the distending force for the lung parenchyma. The WOB measured from Ptp-Vt loops is the work necessary to distend the lung, the passive structure of the respiratory system, and reflects the mechanical characteristics of the pulmonary tissue. However, it does not reflect the energy dissipated by the respiratory muscles [7] (Fig. 3).

When measuring the transpulmonary WOB, we are indirectly evaluating lung compliance represented by the elastic work, and the airway resistance and flow-resistive properties in moving lung tissue represented by resistive work. Stiff lungs will require a high elastic work to be distended, and as the flow resistance becomes greater or the airflow more rapid, more resistive work will then be required to overcome the flow-resistive forces.

WOB from Peso and Tidal Volume Loops

The WOB performed by the inspiratory muscles on the entire respiratory system is measured from Peso against Vt loops. However, the isolated changes of Peso do not mean work done by the muscles. The pressures developed by muscles are revealed by the pressure differences developed by the structures between the

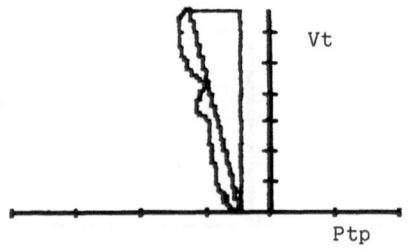

Fig. 3. Transpulmonary pressure (Ptp)-tidal volume (Vt) loop during CO_2-induced hyperventilation. The marks on the pressure and volume axes represent the same increments as in Figs. 1 and 2

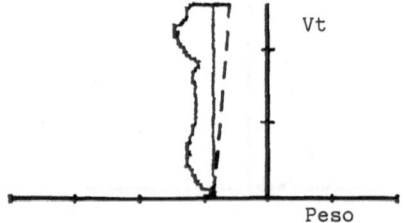

Fig. 4. Campbell diagram showing the esophageal pressure (Peso) and tidal volume (Vt) of a spontaneous inspiration in a normal subject. The broken line represents the static compliance of the relaxed chest wall. The marks in the pressure and volume axes are the same as in previous figures

relaxed and active states. This is illustrated in the diagram which shows pleural pressure as a function of lung volume, the so called Campbell's diagram [8] (Fig. 4).

In Campbell's diagrams we can distinguish three components:

1. The lung volume in the ordinate axis;
2. The static volume-pressure curve of the relaxed chest wall (Pstw), which is represented by the points of Peso obtained during the different lung volumes and when the airways are closed and the muscles are relaxed;
3. The pleural pressure (Peso) developed by the inspiratory muscles during an active inspiration, which is exactly the mirror image of the static volume-pressure curve of the lung, when lung volume is held constant and with open airways at different levels of inflation.

The horizontal distance between the curves Pstw and Peso is the pressure difference between the relaxed and active states due to muscle action, and represents the pressure that the inspiratory muscles must provide to maintain the respiratory system at a given volume with open airways, assuming that there is no distortion of the chest wall [2, 8]. The area between these two curves is the mechanical work done by the muscles during the inspiration and is highly correlated with the energy dissipated by the muscles to allow a volume change in the respiratory system in mechanically ventilated patients [9]. However, the measures of the external WOB do not account for isometric activity or discoordinate contraction by opposing muscle groups [10].

Methodology

In the patient under mechanical ventilation the WOB can be measured at the bedside with equipment which should include the following: a pneumotachograph to measure flow, a flow integrator to calculate volume from the electrically time-integrated flow signal, differential pressure transducers to measure Paw, Peso and Ptp, a recording system, and a plotter in order to draw the plots of pressure against tidal volume. Airway pressure is usually measured between the pneumotachograph and the endotracheal tube. Esophageal pressures are measured from latex balloons attached to polyethylene catheters. The balloons are usually 0.1 mm thick, 8 cm long and about 15 mm in diameter, and are filled with 0.5 mL of air. Appropriate placement of the esophageal balloons should be verified by an occlusion test [11]. With an occluded airway the negative inspiratory deflection on the Paw tracing, measured at the mouth, should be equal to the negative deflection on the Peso tracing.

The surface enclosed beneath the plots of pressure and Vt can be measured by planimetry or electronic integration. Another method consists of using a microprocessor system: the signals of flow and pressure are digitized and sampled by the microprocessor, which computes the inspiratory WOB from the area subtended by the curve of pressure and Vt. The flow signal is used to calculate the

Vt and other breathing pattern parameters such as inspiratory time, expiratory time, total breath duration, mean inspiratory flow and peak inspiratory flow, respiratory rate and minute ventilation.

Methodologic Limitations

Most techniques have their limitations and the technique concerning the measurement of WOB is not an exception to this rule.

Validity of the Peso: The Peso is usually viewed as a good estimate of the pleural pressure and is considered to represent a value which reflects the different regional pleural pressure. The pleural pressure gradient is influenced by gravity, and the Peso can be modified by the weight of the thoracic content, especially when patients lie supine. Due to these shortcomings it is advisable to perform an occlusion test. With an occluded airway the muscular contraction does not induce a volume change and consequently the Ptp (Paw-Ppl) is unaffected, so to consider that Peso is a good estimate of Ppl the ratio of variation of Peso to Paw with closed airways should be close to the unit [11].

Chest Wall Distortion: The evaluation of the WOB is made under the assumption that the respiratory system follows its relaxation pressure-volume curve. However, this is not exactly true in certain situations, such as during exercise or CO_2-induced hyperventilation in which the configuration of the respiratory system for the same pulmonary volume is not equal to that obtained during a relaxed maneuver. To the extent that contraction of the respiratory muscles deforms the respiratory system relative to its relaxed configuration at a given lung volume, the pressure exerted by the muscles is greater than that indicated by the volume-pressure diagram [12]. This implies that any distribution of volume change between the two chest wall pathways, the rib cage and the abdomen, different to that obtained during relaxation results in a distortion of the chest wall from its relaxation characteristics. Therefore, extra work is done by the muscles when the volume change is preferential to the rib cage or abdominal compartment since this produces a distortion in the chest wall [2]. Such distortion is explained by the fact that in these situations there is a decrease in the chest wall compliance and consequently an increase in elastic work. Finally, distortion may occur if there is a deformation of the chest wall itself, such as in certain diseases and during resistive breathing.

Chest Wall Compliance: The value is usually estimated from the theoretical value, about 4% of the forced vital capacity per cmH_2O [13], or 0.2 liters/cmH_2O in an erect man of average size. This value is a straight line, and the volume-pressure relationship of the relaxed chest wall is curvilinear in the uppermost and lowermost extremes of lung volume. Additionally, the measurements are usually made either in supine or the semirecumbent position, a condition in which there may be a slight increase in the compliance of the chest wall as a consequence of gravity when changing from upright to supine position [12].

Chest Wall Resistance: The flow-resistive properties of the chest wall are not usually taken into account when measuring the WOB in spontaneously breathing patients, because the pressure-volume diagrams are referenced to the static characteristics of the chest wall. However, in paralyzed patients under mechanical ventilation the flow-resistive work done on the chest wall may be determined by subtracting the work of the flow resistance of the lung and airways from the total flow resistive work [2].

Compressibility of Gas: This effect may alter the measurement of volume and WOB. The measurement of volumes at the mouth by pneumotachography may underestimate or overestimate the real volume changes in the lung. During mechanical ventilation with high Paw the volume measured at the mouth is higher than the intrapulmonary volume change. Conversely, during spontaneous ventilation with high airway resistances, the volume measured at the mouth is lower than the intrapulmonary volume change [14].

Work Due to AutoPEEP: AutoPEEP means that the alveolar pressure has not decreased at the level of applied PEEP, if any, at the end of exhalation. It often develops in patients with airflow obstruction, with high minute ventilation requirements, and in those with dynamic airway collapse. In these patients AutoPEEP should first be counterbalanced in order to initiate the inspiratory flow, and thus the inspiratory muscles generate a force which is not measured as mechanical work because there is not a volume displacement. However, when measuring the WOB from Campbell's diagrams the amount of AutoPEEP should be taken into account in order to evaluate the total mechanical work performed by the inspiratory muscles [9, 15, 16].

Clinical Utility

The measurement of the mechanical WOB in intensive care patients has several clinical implications. In current practice, some of the pulmonary mechanic parameters which are usually monitored are lung compliance and airway resistance and many critically ill patients have alterations in these parameters. The mechanical WOB is an integrative index of the impedance to chest inflation [5], and its measurement can serve first of all to quantify the work done by the respiratory muscles, with the methodologic limitations which have already been explained.

   In patients recovering from acute respiratory failure and who are still under partial ventilatory support, the mechanical WOB is well correlated with the oxygen consumption of the respiratory muscles, and high levels of WOB, above 8–10 J/min, are associated with electromyographic evidence of diaphragmatic fatigue [9]. The measures of work can be obtained repeatedly, and when used with other parameters such as mouth occlusion pressure at 100 msec, minute ventilation, mean inspiratory flow, or maximum inspiratory pressure, may provide a useful basis to evaluate patients who are difficult to wean from mechanical ventilation [9, 13, 17]. Furthermore, the measures of work may be employed to evaluate the therapeutic effects of certain drugs on the respiratory system [18].

In patients on mechanical ventilation, the mechanically assisted breaths may represent an excessive workload which can tax the ventilatory reserve. For this reason the measurement of WOB is useful as it helps to optimize the machine settings and the type of ventilatory mode [5, 6, 15, 19]. It may additionally allow the clinical evaluation of those patients who present weaning difficulties after prolonged periods of mechanical ventilation. Finally, the measurement of the WOB has been extensively used to evaluate the characteristics of mechanical ventilators, either at the level of the demand valve, the endotracheal tubes, the inspiratory or expiratory circuitry [20–22] and to analyze different forms to provide inspiratory flow and stop inspiration [23, 24].

References

1. Otis AB (1964) The work of breathing. In: Fenn WO, Rahn H (eds) Handbook of physiology, Sect 3, vol I. American Physiological Society, Washington DC, pp 463–476
2. Roussos C (1985) Energetics. In: Roussos C, Macklem PT (eds) The thorax: Part A. Dekker, New York, pp 437–492
3. Roussos C, Campbell EJM (1986) Respiratory muscle energetics. In: Fishman AP, Macklem PT, Mead J (eds) Handbook of physiology. Sect 3, vol III (Mechanics of breathing, Part 2). American Physiological Society, Bethesda, pp 481–509
4. Marini JJ, Capps JS, Culver BH (1985) The inspiratory work of breathing during assisted mechanical ventilation. Chest 87:612–618
5. Marini JJ, Rodriguez M, Lamb V (1986) Bedside estimation of the inspiratory work of breathing during mechanical ventilation. Chest 89:56–60
6. Marini JJ, Rodriguez M, Lamb V (1986) The inspiratory workload of patient-initiated mechanical ventilation. Am Rev Respir Dis 134:902–909
7. Harf A, Atlan G (1975) Travail ventilatoire. Rev Fr Mal Resp 3:795–802
8. Mead J, Smith JC, Loring SH (1985) Volume displacements of the chest wall and their mechanical significance. In: Roussos C, Macklem PT (eds) The thorax: Part A. Dekker, New York, pp 369–392
9. Brochard L, Harf A, Lorino H, Lemaire F (1989) Inspiratory pressure support prevents diaphragmatic fatigue during weaning from mechanical ventilation. Am Rev Respir Dis 139:513–521
10. Truwit JD, Marini JJ (1988) Evaluation of thoracic mechanics in the ventilated patient. Part II: Applied mechanics. J Crit Care 3:199–213
11. Baydur A, Behrakis PK, Zin WA, Jaeger M, Milic-Emili J (1982) A simple method for assessing the validity of the esophageal balloon technique. Am Rev Respir Dis 126:788–791
12. Agostoni E, D'Angelo E (1985) Statics of the chest wall. In: Roussos C, Macklem PT (eds) The thorax: Part A. Dekker, New York, pp 259–295
13. Fleury B, Murciano D, Talamo D, Aubier M, Pariente R, Milic-Emili J (1985) Work of breathing in patients with chronic obstructive pulmonary disease in acute respiratory failure. Am Rev Respir Dis 131:822–827
14. Boyer F, Robert D, Gaussorgues P, Piperno D (1987) Le travail des muscles respiratoires. Définitions et mesures. In: Société de Réanimation de Langue Française (ed) Fonction diaphragmatique. Travail respiratoire. Expansion Scientifique Française, Paris, pp 79–102
15. Smith TC, Marini JJ (1988) Impact of PEEP on lung mechanics and work of breathing in severe airflow obstruction. J Appl Physiol 65:1488–1499
16. Pride NB, Macklem PT (1986) Lung mechanics in disease. In: Fishman AP, Macklem PT, Mead J (eds) Handbook of physiology. Sect 3, vol III (Mechanics of breathing, Part 2). American Physiological Society, Bethesda, pp 659–692

17. Fiastro JF, Habib MP, Shon BY, Campbell SC (1988) Comparison of standard weaning parameters and the mechanical work of breathing in mechanically ventilated patients. Chest 94:232–238
18. Mancebo J, Brochard L, Amaro P, Harf A, Lemaire F (1989) Effect of inhaled bronchodilators on the work of breathing in intubated patients weaning from mechanical ventilation (Abstract). Am Rev Respir Dis 139:A97
19. Sassoon CSH, Mahutte CK, Te TT, Simmons DH, Light RW (1988) Work of breathing and airway occlusion pressure during assist-mode mechanical ventilation. Chest 93:571–576
20. Capps JS, Ritz R, Pierson DJ (1987) An evaluation, in four ventilators, of characteristics that affect work of breathing. Respir Care 32:1017–1024
21. Banner MJ, Downs JB, Kirby RR, Smith RA, Boysen PG, Lampotang S (1988) Effects of expiratory flow resistance on inspiratory work of breathing. Chest 93:795–799
22. Wright PE, Marini JJ, Bernard GR (1989) In vitro versus in vivo comparison of endotracheal tube airflow resistance. Am Rev Respir Dis 140:10–16
23. Beydon L, Chasse M, Harf A, Lemaire F (1988) Inspiratory work of breathing during spontaneous ventilation using demand valves and continuous flow systems. Am Rev Respir Dis 138:300–304
24. Brochard L, Mollo JL, Mancebo J, Amaro P, Lemaire F, Harf A (1989) Comparison of the efficacy of inspiratory pressure support delivered by three ventilators (Abstract). Am Rev Respir Dis 139:A361

PEEP in Mechanically Ventilated COPD Patients

A. Rossi, R. Brandolese, and J. Milic-Emili

Introduction

Mechanical ventilation with positive end-expiratory pressure (PEEP) is a widely used technique to improve pulmonary oxygenation in patients with the adult respiratory distress syndrome (ARDS) [1]. In contrast, the use of PEEP has generally been discouraged in patients with chronic obstructive pulmonary disease (COPD). This is because the degree of hypoxemia is generally mild (and readily improved with supplemental oxygen alone) and also to avoid the risk of barotrauma due to pulmonary hyperinflation. However, recent studies suggest that application of PEEP may be of benefit in COPD patients when used to improve respiratory muscle efficiency during assisted modes of mechanical ventilation or when weaning is being attempted [2].

Intrinsic "PEEP"

The concept of the use of PEEP (or CPAP: continuous positive airway pressure) in patients with acute respiratory failure (ARF) due to exacerbation of COPD can be better understood when considering the abnormalities in respiratory mechanics which occur, particularly the presence of dynamic pulmonary hyperinflation. Because of the increased airflow resistance, the time available for expiration is insufficient for complete exhalation to occur so that the end-expiratory lung volume (EELV) is greater than the elastic equilibrium volume of the respiratory system. Under these circumstances, the elastic recoil pressure at end-expiration (Pel, rs) exceeds the pressure recorded at the airway opening (either PEEP or ZEEP, zero end-expiratory pressure) [3, 4]. This positive end-expiratory Pel, rs has been "auto"-termed or "intrinsic" PEEP (PEEPi) and has a number of important implications [3, 4]. The adverse hemodynamic effects of PEEPi have been discussed elsewhere [3]. In terms of respiratory muscle effort, PEEPi acts as an "inspiratory threshold load" which has to be counterbalanced in order to inflate the lung [2]. During controlled mechanical ventilation, the pressure required to overcome PEEPi is provided by the ventilator [4]. In contrast, during assisted modes of mechanical ventilation, PEEPi must be offset by the patient's inspiratory muscles, which must generate a subatmospheric pressure in the central airways in order to trigger the assisted mechanical breath [2, 5]. This is true not only for conventional assisted mechanical ventilation, but also for other modes of assisted ventilation such as synchronized intermittent mandatory ventilation and pressure support [6].

The dynamic hyperinflation which occurs during mechanical ventilation in COPD patients is in addition to any increase in absolute lung volume to the loss of lung elastic recoil. At high lung volume, the operational length of the inspiratory muscles is reduced and their strength and mechanical efficiency is significantly decreased. Clearly, PEEPi provides a significant burden for the inspiratory muscles, which can severely impair the ability to resume spontaneous ventilation. For example, with ventilatory modes requiring patient effort (e.g. assist-control ventilation and pressure support), PEEPi is added to the "triggering" pressure (generally set at 1–2 cmH$_2$O) so that the total pressure which has to be developed by the inspiratory muscles to initiate the mechanical breath is markedly increased [2, 5]. Obviously, reducing PEEPi will be of benefit.

Role of PEEP

Recent data demonstrate that application of low levels of PEEP can decrease PEEPi and hence the work of breathing during assisted modes of mechanical ventilation [5, 6]. Similarly, constant positive airway pressure (CPAP) is equally effective in reducing inspiratory effort in spontaneously breathing COPD patients being weaned from mechanical ventilation [7].

The ability of PEEP to reduce PEEPi is critically dependent upon the presence of expiratory flow limitation. While it is generally accepted that flow limitation occurs during forced expiration, it is now well recognized to also occur in mechanically ventilated COPD patients [8–10]. In the presence of expiratory flow limitation, an increase in the downstream impedance (e.g. the external application of PEEP) relative to the site of flow limitation should have little effect on the rate of lung emptying until the applied PEEP exceeds a critical level somewhat lower than the initial PEEPi [8, 11].

It should be noted that PEEPi has also been observed in mechanically ventilated patients without COPD [12]. Expiratory flow can be impaired by factors other than air flow limitation, e.g. narrow bore endotracheal tubes, ventilator circuits, and other devices [2, 9, 12]. The resistance of both endotracheal tubes and ventilator circuits is flow dependent and can be as high as 13 cmH$_2$O/L/sec in a common ventilator setting [13]. However, values of PEEPi higher than 5 cmH$_2$O are seldom found in patients without COPD [12]. In the absence of expiratory flow limitation, the application of PEEP through the external ventilator circuit will decrease driving pressure and hence expiratory flow. This will further increase EELV [8, 14].

The role of PEEP in mechanically ventilated COPD patients with acute respiratory failure is to provide support for the inspiratory muscles by offsetting PEEPi, i.e. the inspiratory threshold load [5, 6]. Sufficient clinical information is not yet available to provide exact guideline for the titration of the level of external PEEP in COPD patients. However, pulmonary hyperinflation should not be further enhanced by excessive amount of PEEP. In fact, this will tend to negate the beneficial effect of removing PEEPi by decreasing inspiratory muscle length and force generating capacity. In addition, adverse hemodynamic effects and the risk of barotrauma will be increased [2, 14, 15]. Therefore, application of PEEP requires close monitoring of its effect on lung volume.

Monitoring the Effect of PEEP

This can be accomplished in a number of ways. For example, EELV can be monitored using respiratory inductance plethysmography (Respitrace) [6, 11, 16]. Alternatively, the end-expiatory Pel, rs can be directly determined from the measurement of the difference between the value of the plateau in airway pressure during an end-expiratory occlusion and the pressure recorded at the airway opening at the end of an unoccluded expiration [5, 11]. This maneuver provides a simple way to check whether and to what extend PEEP replaces PEEPi or adds to it, according to the equation:

$$PEEPt = PEEP + PEEPi$$

where PEEPt is the value of the occluded plateau pressure relative to atmosphere (clearly during mechanical ventilation on ZEEP, PEEPt = PEEPi). The end-expiratory occlusion can be performed easily during controlled mechanical ventilation, when the respiratory muscles are relaxed, whereas it can present some problems when the patient's respiratory muscles are active, for example during assisted mechanical ventilation and pressure support, i.e. when a reliable measurement of PEEPi is required during application of increasing levels of external PEEP. However some recent work has shown that PEEPi can be measured by means of the end-expiratory occlusion also when patients are ventilated with the assist mode or pressure support [5, 6]. In this regard, it should be noted that airway occlusion can be readily performed using the end-expiratory hold button of the Servo 900C Siemens ventilator [13]. Both these techniques are noninvasive and are well suited to bedside monitoring during the application of PEEP in mechanically ventilated COPD patients.

Volume-Flow Curves

A useful way to monitor the effects of the application of PEEP on respiratory mechanics in ICU patients is the analysis of the volume/flow (VF) relationship during a relaxed expiration. Under those conditions, exhalation is passively driven by the elastic recoil of the total respiratory system, while flow resistance is the only opposing force. The method was originally used by McIlroy et al. [17] in awake human adults and has been modified and successfully applied for the "single breath" measurement of respiratory mechanics in anesthetized animals [18] and humans [19] and in infants [20]. The "single breath" method assumes that respiratory compliance is constant throughout expiration and that EELV corresponds to Vr. Since this is not always the case in ICU patients with ARF [9], the application of the "single breath" method in such patients is problematic.

However, even simple inspection of the relaxed expiratory VF curves in mechanically ventilated patients can provide useful information [21, 22]. In fact, when PEEPi is absent, the expiratory flow decreases smoothly throughout expiration. By contrast, when EELV is above (i.e. PEEPi is present), the expiratory flow is abruptly terminated by the next mechanical inflation, such that the expiratory VF curve has a characteristic "truncated" appearance (Fig. 1). This particular information could be obtained also from the flow time profile [4, 23], however, the shape of the VF curve is also important. In anesthetized animals, with the upper airway bypassed by a tracheal cannula, the relaxed expiratory VF relationship is linear [18]. In anesthetized humans it tends to be curvilinear, i.e. it exhibits a concavity toward the volume axis which mainly reflects the resistive properties of the endotracheal tubes [19]. In critically ill patients, the VF relationship may be more complex. In the presence of dynamic expiratory flow limitation the VF curve is convex toward the volume axis either throughout expiration or during the late part of it [9, 21]. During mechanical ventilation, COPD patients with ARF in general exhibit an expiratory VF curve which is both "truncated" and convex toward the volume axis. This is indicative of expiratory flow limitation and dynamic pulmonary hyperinflation (Fig. 1). In mechanically ventilated ARDS patients, after sudden removal of PEEP, the expiratory flows in general increase at all lung volumes because of the concomitant increase in expiratory driving pressure and the VF curve is not convex toward the volume axis [22]. By

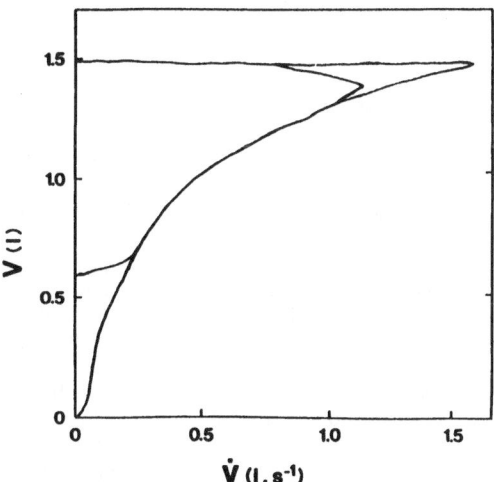

Fig. 1. Relaxed expiratory volume/flow curves in a mechanically ventilated COPD patient with PEEP of 4 cmH$_2$O (smaller loop) and without PEEP (outer loop). With 4 cmH$_2$O of PEEP, the intrinsic PEEP was 7.5 cmH$_2$O. During expiration with PEEP of 4 cmH$_2$O, the volume/flow loop exhibited a characteristic "truncated" appearance due to the onset of the next mechanical inflation before expiration could be completed, i.e., the patient was dynamically hyperinflated. Complete relaxed expiration against atmospheric pressure resulted in a reduction of the end-expiratory lung volume, but during most of expiration the rate of lung emptying was unchanged due to preexisting dynamic expiratory flow limitation, such that removal of PEEP did not affect the effective expiratory driving pressure

contrast, in mechanically ventilated COPD patients the rate of lung emptying remains essentially unchanged after removal of PEEP (Fig. 1). In fact, in the patient of Fig. 1, the applied PEEP (4 cmH$_2$O) was lower than PEEPi (11.5 cmH$_2$O) and did not affect expiration because of dynamic expiratory flow limitation. Thus display of the VF curves during mechanical ventilation provides a simple, though qualitative, way to assess the presence of dynamic hyperinflation ("truncated" end-expiratory flow) and expiratory flow limitation (shape of VF curve) as well as to monitor the effects of applied PEEP on expiratory flow.

Conclusion

In mechanically ventilated patients with PEEPi and dynamic expiratory flow limitation, application of PEEP can be used to support the inspiratory muscles during "triggered" mechanical inflations and weaning, in order to reduce the amount of the inspiratory effort. Although the theory and some experimental data are encouraging, at present time more clinical research is required to investigate the benefits which can be obtained from the use of PEEP in COPD patients. Clearly, pulmonary hyperinflation should not be increased. Therefore, close monitoring of the EELV is needed during application of increasing levels of PEEP. This can be accomplished with some simple and non-invasive techniques, suitable for use at bedside, which have been also discussed in this article.

References

1. Ashbaugh DG, Petty TL (1973) Positive end-expiratory pressure. J Thor Cardiovasc Surgery 65:165–170
2. Milic-Emili J, Gottfried SB, Rossi A (1987) Dynamic hyperinflation: Intrinsic PEEP and its ramifications in patients with respiratory failure. In: Vincent JL (ed) Update in intensive care and emergency medicine, vol 3. Springer, Berlin Heidelberg New York Tokyo, pp 192–198
3. Pepe PE, Marini JJ (1982) Occult positive end-expiratory pressure in mechanically ventilated patients with airflow obstruction. Am Rev Respir Dis 126:166–170
4. Rossi A, Gottfried SB, Zocchi L, et al (1985) Measurement of static compliance of total respiratory system in patients with acute respiratory failure during mechanical ventilation. Am Rev Respir Dis 131:672–678
5. Smith TC, Marini JJ (1988) Impact of PEEP on lung mechanics and work of breathing in severe airflow obstruction. J Appl Physiol 65:1488–1499
6. Calderini E, Petrof BJ, Gottfried SB (1989) Continuous positive airway pressure (CPAP) improves the efficacy of pressure support (PS) ventilation in severe chronic obstructive pulmonary disease (COPD). Am Rev Respir Dis 139:A155
7. Petrof BJ, Legare M, Goldberg P, et al (1990) Continuous airway pressure reduces work of breathing and dyspnea during weaning from mechanical ventilation in severe chronic obstructive pulmonary disease. Am Rev Respir Dis (in press)
8. Gay PC, Rodarte JR, Hubmayr RD (1989) The effects of positive expiratory pressure on isovolume flow and dynamic hyperinflation in patients receiving mechanical ventilation. Am Rev Respir Dis 139:621–626
9. Gottfried SB, Rossi A, Higgs BD, et al (1985) Noninvasive determination of respiratory system mechanics during mechanical ventilation for acute respiratory failure. Am Rev Respir Dis 131:414–420

10. Kimball WR, Leith DE, Robins AG (1982) Dynamic hyperinflation and ventilator dependence in chronic obstructive pulmonary disease. Am Rev Respir Dis 126:991–995
11. Simkovitz P, Brown K, Goldberg P, et al (1987) Interaction between intrinsic and externally applied PEEP during mechanical ventilation. Am Rev Respir Dis 135:A202
12. Broseghini C, Brandolese R, Poggi R, et al (1988) Respiratory mechanics during the first day of mechanical ventilation in patients with pulmonary edema and chronic airway obstruction. Am Rev Respir Dis 138:355–361
13. Broseghini C, Brandolese R, Poggi R, et al (1988) Respiratory resistance and intrinsic positive end-expiratory pressure (PEEPi) in patients with the adult respiratory distress syndrome (ARDS). Eur Respir J 1:726–731
14. Marini JJ (1989) Should PEEP be used in airflow obstruction? Am Rev Respir Dis 140:1–3
15. Tuxen DV (1989) Detrimental effects of positive end-expiratory pressure during controlled mechanical ventilation of patients with severe airflow obstruction. Am Rev Respir Dis 140:5–9
16. Hoffman RA, Ershowsky P, Krieger BF (1989) Determination of auto-PEEP during spontaneous and controlled ventilation by monitoring changes in end-expiratory thoracic gas volume. Chest 3:613–616
17. McIlroy MB, Tierney DF, Nadel JA (1963) A new method for measurement of respiratory compliance and resistance of lungs and thorax. J Appl Physiol 17:424–427
18. Zin WA, Pengelly LD, Milic-Emili J (1982) Single-breath method for measurement of respiratory mechanics in anesthetized animals. J Appl Physiol 52:1266–1277
19. Berhakis PK, Higgs BD, Baydur A, et al (1983) Respiratory mechanics during halothane anesthesia and anesthesia paralysis in humans. J Appl Physiol 55:1085–1092
20. Mortola JP, Milic-Emili J, Nowaraj A, et al (1984) Muscle pressure and flow during expiration in infants. Am Rev Respir Dis 129:49–53
21. Saetta M, Rossi A, Gottfried SB, et al (1985) Expiratory volume-flow relationship during mechanical ventilation in patients with acute respiratory failure. Am Rev Respir Dis 131:A132
22. Dal Vecchio L, Polese G, Poggi R, Rossi A (1989) Intrinsic PEEP in stable COPD patients. Eur Respir J 2
23. Bernasconi M, Brandolese R, Rossi A (1988) Advances in the assessment of respiratory function during mechanical ventilation of patients with acute respiratory failure. Int Care World 5:52–54

Pulmonary Hypertension

Pulmonary Hypertension
in Bronchopulmonary Dysplasia

P. Daoud, F. Beaufils, and J.-F. Hartmann

Introduction

Bronchopulmonary dysplasia (BPD) was first described by Northway et al. in 1967 [1]: it is a sequela of variable duration of the respiratory distress syndrome of the newborn and particularly of the premature, whose lungs are deficient in surfactant at birth. In most cases BPD evolves toward a full normalization of the pulmonary function within a few months to two years. Some patients, however, remain in severe respiratory insufficiency leading to fatal outcome in the absence of prolonged mechanical ventilation and oxygen therapy [2]: most of these patients have pulmonary hypertension.

Already suspected by Northway et al. [1] in BPD patients with clinical and electrical signs of acute right ventricular failure, pulmonary hypertension in BPD was first documented in 1974 by Harrod et al. [3] using pulmonary catheterism. It should now be early recognized through the use of non-invasive techniques such as echo-Doppler techniques [4].

BPD prognosis is worsened by the presence of pulmonary hypertension and is further influenced by the response to oxygen therapy: a quick improvement is the hallmark of predominant arteriolar vasoconstriction [5], whereas a delayed response reflects anatomical reorganization [6, 7], a situation associated with a poorer outcome. However, in contrast to previous reports [6, 7], our experience is that pulmonary hypertension in severe BPD is reversible, when subjected to both prolonged supplemental oxygen therapy and mechanical ventilation, particularly if those measures are implemented at an early time in the course of BPD evolution.

After reviewing the basis of pulmonary hypertension in BPD and its diagnosis we will report our experience in 5 patients with severe BPD and pulmonary hypertension.

Anatomical Basis of Pulmonary Hypertension in BPD

Normal Pre- and Post-natal Lung Growth

At 16 weeks of gestation, all the branches of the tracheobronchial tree, down to the preacinar level, are formed. New branches cannot appear beyond that age. Between 16 and 26 weeks of gestation, respiratory bronchioles and saccules appear. Saccules increase in size and number beyond that date. Post natal growth is caracterized mainly by alveolar multiplication, from the second month to the end of the third year of life: alveoli, during that period, increase from 20 to 300 millions.

The lung vascular bed is subjected to similar developmental stages: at 16 weeks all the preacinar arteries have appeared. Beyond that date, intraacinar arterial multiplication takes place and goes on after birth.

Regarding pulmonary hypertension, the most important phenomenon is arterial maturation, as described by Reid [8]. Maturation is caracterized by a slow transition from a non-muscularized to a muscularized stage. The proportion of non-, partially and fully muscularized arteries is similar in the fetus and in the adult. However, their distribution differs with age: in the fetus, muscularized arteries do not appear beyond the terminal bronchioles, whereas they reach the alveoli in the adult.

Abnormal Development of the Lung Vascular Bed in Severe BPD [9–12]

The arterial wall contains two types of cells which are the precursors of the smooth muscle fibers: the pericytes and the intermediate cells. The latter undergo transformation into smooth muscle fibers under conditions of chronic hypoxia.

In turn, this results in the extension toward the periphery of arterial muscularization. Some areas may even show a reduced lumen diameter [12] or even a full vascular obstruction, resulting in a decrease in the ratio of arterial vessels to lung surface area.

Mechanisms of Pulmonary Hypertension in BPD

Three mechanisms are involved in the appearance of pulmonary hypertension in patients with BPD: a persistent ductus arteriosus, chronic hypoxia and pulmonary hypoplasia.

Patent Ductus Arteriosus (PDA)

PDA is a common complication of respiratory distress syndrome in premature babies and has been implied in BPD genesis. In our opinion, PDA must be closed early by indomethacin or surgery: the high pulmonary blood flow secondary to large PDA is responsible for vascular lesions wich were classified into 6 stages by Heath and Edwards [13], the last of which is associated with irreversible changes in the vascular bed. However, in patients with severe BPD, even a lately diagnosed PDA should be closed, since postnatal lung growth takes place until 3 years of age.

Chronic Hypoxia

Chronic hypoxia as a leading mechanism of pulmonary hypertension has been well established experimentally [14, 15] and clinically in adults with chronic obstructive pulmonary disease (COPD) [16, 17]. Chronic hypoxia is also a major feature in BPD patients [5-7] but may remain unrecognized when occurring only during sleep. Gaultier [18] has documented that children with COPD were more proned to central and obstructive apneas during sleep than controls. In addition, they experienced episodes of paradoxic inward rib cage motion with arterial desaturation.

These features were recognized in one patient who had severe pulmonary hypertension contrasting with the moderate degree of BPD and the lack of desaturation while awake: nocturnal mechanical ventilation was instituted and subnormal pulmonary artery pressures achieved after two years.

Pulmonary Hypoplasia

Various degrees of pulmonary hypoplasia were documented in children born after prolonged rupture of fetal membrane and oligoamnios [19]. The hypoplasia involves both the airways and alveoli and the vascular bed: it could lead to pulmonary hypertension by reducing the total vascular cross-section available for pulmonary blood flow.

Diagnosis of Pulmonary Hypertension

A repeated search of pulmonary hypertension must now be included in the routine management of the BPD patient, particularly when BPD is severe [2]. Although pulmonary catheterism remains the gold standard to establish the diagnosis and quantify the pulmonary hypertension [6, 7, 20], it is an invasive procedure which should be performed only selectively. Prior to catheterism, non-invasive techniques should always be used: they are simple to realize, devoided of side effects and allowing for repeated measurements, i.e. every trimester or every other trimester.

Electrocardiogram (ECG)

As compared to age-matched controls, the ECG shows a right deviation of the QRS axis and an increased R/S ration in V_1 and V_2; the V_1 lead displays a qR aspect and a positive T wave. The R/S ratio is increased in V_1 and V_2 and less than 1 in V_6.

Echo-Doppler Techniques

M-Mode Echography: With pulmonary hypertension the kinetics of the pulmonary valves are changed to a W shaped aspect related to the loss of the diastolic slope and the mesosystolic partial closure of the pulmonary valves. The pulmonary artery trunk is dilated as is the right ventricle in late diastole. The RPEP/RVET ratio is increased above 0.3 and its value related to the severity of the pulmonary hypertension [21]. According to Fouron [4], the higher the RPEP/RVET ratio value the worse the prognosis.

Two-dimensional Echography: Although frequently impaired by the chest distension, 2D-echography brings valuable informations regarding right ventricular volume, septum kinetics and pulmonary artery dilation and guides the pulsed Doppler examination.

Pulsed Doppler: The pulsed Doppler is the non-invasive technique we are most familiar with. The sampling volume of the single gated Doppler is positioned in the pulmonary artery trunk. The analysis of the morphology and the chronology of the velocity curves gives the acceleration time (AcT), from the beginning to the peak of the ejection curve, as well as the right ventricular ejection time (RVET). The AcT/RVET ratio is then computed. Normal values are 119 ± 18 ms for AcT and 0.41 ± 0.03 for the AcT/RVET ratio [22]. In pulmonary hypertension AcT is decreased: since the logarithm of the pulmonary artery pressure is strongly correlated with both AcT and AcT/RVET [23, 24], a reliable measure of the pulmonary hypertension can be achieved with this technique.

Continuous Doppler: It allows measurement of the pulmonary flow regurgitation. By applying the Bernouilli's theorem, pulmonary artery pressure can be obtained [25].

Colored Doppler: Color coding of the regurgitation flow improves its analysis and should enhance the results obtained with continuous wave Doppler. Experience with this technique remains limited.

Non-invasive Pulmonary Artery Pressure Measurements

Non-invasive measurements of pulmonary artery pressure should be performed in all BPD patients. Timing and modalities of these measurements should be tailored to the patient's conditions: the more unstable the patient, the more critical the need to obtain pulmonary artery pressure measurements, since unchecked increases of arterial desaturation and hypercapnia will worsen the pulmonary hypertension. In our opinion those measurements should be done in a sedated patient and obtained under a wide range of FiO_2.

Whenever a reduction of respiratory support is considered, i.e. a decrease of the respirator settings or a partial or full weaning from the respirator, measurements should be obtained before and after changing the conditions in order to

prevent untimely modifications of respiratory support. In addition, pulse oximetry and transcutaneous or end-tidal CO_2 should be obtained at the time of pulmonary pressure determination: the combined analysis of these non-invasive
measurements should improve the selection of the best levels of oxygenation and
mechanical ventilation in patients with severe BPD and pulmonary hypertension.

Prognosis of Severe BPD with Pulmonary Hypertension

Severe BPD with pulmonary hypertension is usually associated with a poor
prognosis [7, 20], particularly when the response to O_2 is decreased [6]. According to Fouron [4], a persistent hypertension beyond the third month of life is
associated with an increased risk of death. For Berman [6], the lack of reactivity
to O_2 implies irreversible pulmonary hypertension. A similar finding was disclosed recently by Goodman [7]: of 10 children who did not normalized their
pulmonary artery pressure with supplemental O_2, five died.

In contrast with these results, we were able to normalize or significantly decrease pulmonary hypertension in 5 patients with severe BPD, following a modification of our management towards long term mechanical ventilation and prolonged oxygen therapy. One patient had been admitted at birth and the other
four between 1 and 27 months of age. All were in acute respiratory failure at
time of admission. Their initial status, once the stabilization was obtained, is
shown in Table 1. All had increased respiratory rate, hypoxia and hypercapnia
while breathing room air. Mean pulmonary artery pressure measured by pulsed
Doppler and/or pulmonary catheterism was 46 ± 13 mmHg (range 38 to 68
mmHg).

Table 1. Follow-up of 5 BPD patients. Data are obtained on room air (unless otherwise specified) and during spontaneous ventilation

Patient	Age (months)	PaO_2	$PaCO_2$	Weight	Length	P_{AP}
1	17	43	40	−2.5 SD	−2.5 SD	68
2	7	40	60	−3.5 SD	−4.5 SD	38
3	24	60	45	−3.5 SD	−2.5 SD	48
4	27	40	44	−1.5 SD	−2.5 SD	40
5	2	45 $FiO_2 = 0.4$	50	−4.5 SD	−4.5 SD	45 $FiO_2 = 0.5$
1	39	80	33	+1.5 SD	Mean	22
2	42	75	37	−1.5 SD	−1.5 SD	24
3	54	>70	34	−1.5 SD	−0.5 SD	20
4	55	70	40	Mean	+1.5 SD	28
5	30	75	40	Mean	Mean	19 $FiO_2 = 0.45$

P_{AP} = Mean pulmonary artery pressure.

Treatment included mechanical ventilation and oxygen therapy along with routine measures such as hypercaloric feeding, respiratory physiotherapy, gastroesophagal reflux treatment and antibiotics when needed. Indications for mechanical ventilation were based on Hartmann criteria [2]; as already stated, one patient disclosed signs of severe alveolar hypoventilation only during sleep. Weaning from mechanical ventilation was always slow and guided by the non-invasive measurements, the growth status and the ability for the patient to maintain previous achievements in the face of a reduced respiratory support.

It appears that pulmonary hypertension in severe BPD patients is not irreversible (Table 1). Despite unsignificant initial O_2 reactivity and delayed treatment, (beyond 3 months of age in 4 of 5 patients), pulmonary artery pressure returned to normal or significantly decreased in all patients.

These results are in agreement with the data obtained in experimental conditions and in adults with COPD. In rats exposed to chronic hypoxia only a return to permanently normoxic conditions results in complete regression of arteriolar hypermuscularization, right ventricular hypertrophy and pulmonary hypertension. Similarly, in adults with COPD undergoing oxygen therapy for 12 to 18 hours a day, improvement in pulmonary artery pressure is directly related to the duration of oxygen therapy [17].

These data only support the need of supplemental O_2. In our opinion, mechanical ventilation offers two major benefits. First, it prevents sleep hypoxia, a critical step towards permanent normoxia. Second, it offers optimal conditions for the patient's growth, and thus for normal postnatal lung growth. Weinstein et al. [26] have shown that oxygen consumption is increased in BPD patients, and Wolfson et al. [27] have related that phenomenon to an increased workload of the respiratory muscles. Similarly, Kurzner et al. [28] have established a negative correlation between the body weight and the oxygen consumption.

Thus, patients with severe BPD appear to spend a high proportion of their caloric intake in their respiratory work at the expense of their body growth. By reversing this trend, mechanical ventilation insures optimal conditions for body and lung growth, including, presumably, the lung vascular bed.

Conclusion

In most series, long term management of patients with severe BPD and pulmonary hypertension is solely based on supplemental oxygen therapy [6, 7]. This may allow for a partial reduction but not for a full normalization of pulmonary hypertension. In addition, growth remains poor in most cases [20].

From our results in five patients with severe BPD and pulmonary hypertension, we suggest that adding prolonged mechanical ventilation to supplemental oxygen therapy may overcome the limitations of oxygen therapy alone by preventing sleep associated arterial desaturation and by improving body and lung growths through a reduction of caloric expenditure in the breathing workload. The total duration of mechanical ventilation, its modalities and the allowance for periods of spontaneous breathing remain controversial issues: they have been clarified by non-invasive measurements of pulmonary artery pressure and blood gases. Further improvements in the management of severe BPD patients should arise, in the near future, from respiratory muscles fatigue studies and monitoring.

Finally, our results suggest that prompt institution of mechanical ventilation in severe BPD may prevent, in a number of cases, the development of pulmonary hypertension.

References

1. Northway WH Jr, Rosan RC, Porter DY (1967) Pulmonary disease following respiratory therapy of hyaline membrane disease. N Engl J Med 276:357–368
2. Hartmann JF, Beaufils F, Vervel C (1987) Facteurs pronostiques dans les formes graves de dysplasies bronchopulmonaires. Arch Fr Pediatr 44:423–431
3. Harrod JR, L'Heureux P, Douglas Wangensteen O, Hunt CO (1974) Long term follow up of severe repiratory distress syndrome treated with IPPB. J Pediatr 84:277–286
4. Fouron JC, Leguennec JC, Villemant D, et al (1980) Value of echocardiography in assessing the outcome of bronchopulmonary dysplasia. Pediatrics 65:529–535
5. Abman SH, Wolfe RR, Accurso FJ, et al (1985) Pulmonary vascular response to oxygen in infants with severe bronchopulmonary dysplasia. Pediatrics 75:80–84
6. Berman W Jr, Katz R, Yabek SM, et al (1982) Evaluation of infants with bronchopulmonary dysplasia using cardiac catheterization. Pediatrics 70:708–712
7. Goodman G, Perkin RM, Anas NG, et al (1988) Pulmonary hypertension in infants with bronchopulmonary dysplasia. J Pediatr 112:67–72
8. Reid LM (1979) The pulmonary circulation: remodeling in growth and disease. Am Rev Respir Dis 119:531–546
9. Bonikos AS, Bensch KG, Northway WH Jr, Adwards DK (1976) Bronchopulmonary dysplasia: the pulmonary pathologic sequel of necrotizing bronchiolitis and pulmonary fibrosis. Hum Pathol 77:643–665
10. Stocker JT (1986) Pathologic features of long standing "healed" bronchopulmonary dysplasia: a study of 28 to 40 months old infants. Human Pathol 17:943–961
11. Thurlbeck WM (1979) Morphologic aspects of bronchopulmonary dysplasia. J Pediatr 95:842–843
12. Reid L (1979) Bronchopulmonary dysplasia pathology. J Pediatr 93:836–840
13. Heath D, Edward JE (1958) The pathology of hypertensive pulmonary vascular disease. Description of 6 grades of structural changes in alveolous arteries with special reference to congenital cardiac defect. Circulation 18:533
14. Kay JM (1980) Effect of intermittent normoxia on chronic hypoxic pulmonary hypertension, right ventricular hypertrophia and polycythemia in rats. Am Rev Respir Dis 121:993–1001
15. Kay JM, Suyama KL, Keane PM (1981) Effect of intermittent normoxia on muscularization of pulmonary arterioles induced by chronic hypoxemia in rats. Am Rev Respir Dis 122:454–459
16. NOTT Group (1980) Continuous or nocturnal oygen therapy in hypoxemic chronic obstructive lung disease. Ann Intern Med 93:391–398
17. Timms RM, Fhaja FU, Williams GW, the NOTT (1985) Hemodynamic response to oxygen therapy in chronic obstructive pulmonary disease. Ann Intern Med 102:29–36
18. Gaultier C, Praud JP, Clement AD, et al (1985) Respiration during sleep in children with COPD. Chest 7:168–173
19. Thibeault DW, Beatty EP, Hall RT, Bowen SK (1985) Neonatal pulmonary hypoplasia with premature rupture of fetal membrane and oligoamnios. J Pediatr 107:73–77
20. Berman W Jr, Katz R, Yabek SM, et al (1986) Long term follow up of bronchopulmonary dysplasia. J Pediatr 109:45–50
21. Hirshfeld S, Meyer R, Schwartz DC, et al (1975) The echographic assessment of pulmonary artery pressure and pulmonary vascular resistance. Circulation 52:642–649

22. Perez D, Azancot A, Lamberti A (1985) Hypertension artérielle pulmonaire chez l'enfant; Evaluation quantitative par échocardiographie-Doppler pulsé. Congrès Français d'Echocardiographie. Paris
23. Kitabake A, Inoue M, Asaq M, et al (1983) Non-invasive evaluation of pulmonary hypertension by a pulsed Doppler technique. Circulation 68:302–309
24. Marchandise B, De Bruyne B, Delaunois L, Kremer R (1987) Non-invasive prediction of pulmonary hypertension in chronic obstructive pulmonary disease by Doppler echocardiography. Chest 91:361–364
25. Masuyama T, Koama K, Kitabake A, et al (1986) Continuous wave Doppler echocardiographic detection of pulmonary regurgitation and its application to non-invasive estimation of pulmonary artery pressure. Circulation 74:484–492
26. Weinstein MR (1981) Oxygen consumption in infants with bronchopulmonary dysplasia. J Pediatr 99:958–961
27. Wolfson MR, Bhutan VK, Shaffer TH, Bowen FW (1984) Mechanics and energetics of breathing helium in infants with bronchopulmonary dysplasia. J Pediatr 104:752–757
28. Kurzner SI, Garg M, Bautista DB, et al (1988) Growth failure in bronchopulmonary dysplasia: Elevated metabolic rates and pulmonary mechanics. J Pediatr 112:73–80

Pulmonary Hypertension in ARDS

M. Leeman

Introduction

The adult respiratory distress syndrome (ARDS) is an acute respiratory failure due to non-hemodynamic pulmonary edema, also called permeability edema. It is a common complication of several critical diseases such as circulatory shock, sepsis and trauma. The clinical picture includes hypoxemia, decreased lung compliance and diffuse bilateral infiltrates on chest roentgenogram. The arterial hypoxemia in ARDS mainly results from intrapulmonary shunt due to perfusion of unventilated lung units.

Pulmonary hypertension is a common hallmark of ARDS and results from an increase in pulmonary vascular resistance (PVR). Its level seems related to the severity of lung injury [1]. However, few data are available on pulmonary vascular pressure/flow relationships in patients with ARDS.

It has been realized in recent years that PVR calculation, as (pulmonary artery pressure minus left atrial pressure) divided by cardiac output, is insufficient to evaluate the functional status of the pulmonary circulation. Indeed, the relationship between pulmonary artery pressure (Ppa) and flow (Q) has been found linear over a physiological range of Q but becomes curvilinear at low Q, so that the extrapolation of the linear part at zero Q has a positive pressure intercept [2]. Consequently, calculated PVR can be misleading because the extrapolated pressure intercept of the Ppa/Q relationship is in many circumstances superior to left atrial pressure. In other words, the linear portion of the (Ppa minus left atrial pressure)/Q relationship does not pass through the origin. Therefore, passive, flow-dependent changes in Ppa along the same Ppa/Q line can result in different calculated PVR (Fig. 1).

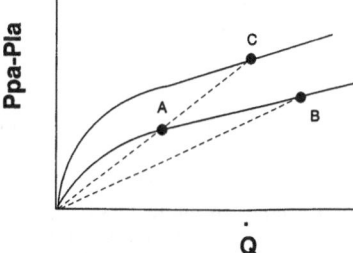

Fig. 1. Two plots of pulmonary artery pressure (Ppa) minus left atrial pressure (Pla)/flow (Q) in the same individual (solid lines). Points A and B present passive changes in pressure along the same relationship, whereas calculated pulmonary vascular resistance (broken lines) decreases. Points A and C indicate active increase in vascular tone, whereas calculated pulmonary vascular resistance is unchanged

According to a recruiting model of the pulmonary circulation incorporating parallel channels with fixed conductances and a distribution of critical closing pressures, the extrapolated pressure intercept of the Ppa/Q relationship represents the effective outflow pressure, which is the greatest of the mean closing pressure or the left atrial pressure [3]. As a consequence, if the mean closing pressure exceeds the apparent outflow pressure (alveolar pressure in zone 2, left atrial pressure in zone 3), it will represent the effective downstream pressure of the pulmonary vasculature and Q will be proportional to the difference between Ppa and the mean closing pressure. Such behavior of the pulmonary circulation has been referred to as a Starling resistor or a vascular waterfall [2, 3]. The slope of the Ppa/Q relationship is influenced by the cross-sectional area of the pulmonary vascular bed and reflects the resistance upstream from the locus of the closing pressure [2].

Few studies have examined the Ppa/Q relationship during ARDS. In ARDS patients with extracorporeal membrane oxygenation, Ppa was minimally modified by large variations in Q produced either by manipulation of a veno-arterial bypass or by isoproterenol infusion [1]. More recently, Ppa/Q relationships have been constructed in intact anesthetized dogs with oleic acid lung injury, an experimental model relevant to clinical ARDS. Q was manipulated by changing venous return, either by opening arterio-venous fistulas or by inflation of an inferior vena cava balloon catheter. As previously described in isolated lung preparations, the Ppa/Q plots were almost linear over the range of Q studied [4–6]. Before oleic acid, the extrapolated pressure intercept approximated left atrial pressure. Oleic acid administration resulted in a parallel shift of the Ppa/Q relationship toward higher pressures. If the Starling resistor model can apply to the pulmonary vasculature, these studies suggest that in lung injury, the closing pressure of the pulmonary vessels increased, exceeded left atrial pressure, became the effective outflow and was responsible for the pulmonary hypertension. It must be pointed out that other recently developed mathematical models of the pulmonary circulation also can predict such parallel shift of the Ppa/Q plots, so that interpretation of slopes and extrapolated pressure intercepts must remain cautious [2].

Pulmonary Hypertension in ARDS

In ARDS, pulmonary hypertension can result from functional as well as several stuctural changes (Table 1).

Table 1. Possible factors contributing to pulmonary hypertension in ARDS

Functional:	pulmonary vasoconstriction
Structural:	thromboemboli
	endothelial swelling
	vascular remodeling
	vascular compression by edema

Intravascular Obliterative Disease

Intravascular occlusion has been described in ARDS patients using bedside balloon occlusion angiography through newly placed pulmonary artery catheters. Pulmonary artery filling defects were found in 19 of 40 patients, regardless of the cause of ARDS. Their presence correlated with the severity of pulmonary hypertension [7]. Non-filling of small pulmonary arteries were associated with thrombotic or non-thrombotic obliterative vascular lesions [7, 8].

Thromboembolism: Capillary microembolism, large microthrombi and macrothrombi were present in 21 of 22 patients who died with ARDS, especially in the early stages of the disease [8]. The presence of macrothrombi found at autopsy correlated with the number of filling defects identified at antemortem angiography. These thrombi were formed of platelets, fibrin, red cells and white cells. In some vessels, the thrombi were recanalized so that blood flow was restored [8].

Endothelial Injury: Detailed ultrastructural observations of the lung's parenchyma in ARDS showed up to 50% reduction in the number of pulmonary capillaries [9]. Swollen endothelial cells with rarefied cytoplasm and dilated endoplasmic reticulum have been found to encroach upon the lumens of the capillaries. Injuried endothelial cells were often adjacent to normal-appearing cells. Some endothelial cells were focally separated from the capillary basement membrane. These changes were similar, regardless of the cause of ARDS. More chronic changes included thickening and reduplication of capillary basement membrane and hypertrophic endothelial cells [8].

Chronic Vascular Remodeling: Many small arteries and intraacinar veins were focally obstructed by eccentric or concentric intimal fibrocellular proliferation that could contribute to the reduction in cross-sectional area. Characteristic findings of late-stage ARDS are tortuous preacinar arteries, stretched and distorded by surrounding parenchymal fibrosis, and nests of dilated capillaries [8].

Morphometric Studies: With increasing duration of ARDS, there was a steady reduction in mean external diameter for partially and fully muscular arteries together with an increase in the concentration of these arteries and in the percentage of their medial thickness, suggesting peripheral extension of smooth muscle into smaller, normally non-muscular pulmonary arteries [10]. For any patient, the pulmonary vascular lesions correlated with the duration of ARDS rather than its cause.

Vascular Compression

The sequence of fluid accumulation in the lung, both in hydrostatic and in permeability edema, proceeds from filling of the interstitium to alveolar flooding. The effects exerted by these two phases have been the subject of many investigations. In a morphometric study in dogs with hydrostatic edema induced by fluid overload or with permeability edema induced by alpha-naphtylthiourea, Michel et al. [11] showed that despite considerable perivascular edema, pulmonary arterial diameter and area were not decreased. Battacharya et al. [12] found in isolated perfused canine lobes with hydrostatic edema, that lobar blood flow did not fall until alveolar flooding occurred. In a dog left caudal lobe preparation, Ali and Wood [13] showed that an equivalent amount of edema, whether induced by oleic acid or by instillation of hypotonic plasma via the airways, produced the same degree of pulmonary blood flow reduction to the affected lobe. Thus, there is now convincing evidence that interstitial edema does not compress pulmonary arteries and that both alveolar and interstitial edema are required to divert blood flow.

Pulmonary Vasoconstriction

Hypoxia or mediator-induced active pulmonary vasoconstriction also can contribute to the pulmonary hypertension in ARDS. Administration of vasodilators such as sodium nitroprusside [1, 14], isoproterenol [1], ketanserin [14], diltiazem [15] and prostaglandin E1 [16] has been shown to decrease PVR in patients with ARDS. In experimental ARDS, numerous vasodilators were also able to reduce calculated PVR. The effects of prostaglandin E1 were studied in intact anesthetized and ventilated dogs with oleic acid lung injury using the Ppa/Q plot approach [6]. The Ppa/Q relationships were linear over the range of Q studied. Oleic acid produced a parallel shift of the Ppa/Q plots to higher Ppa values, indicating pulmonary hypertension. Prostaglandin E1 0.4 $\mu g \cdot kg^{-1} \cdot {}^{min-1}$ intravenously partially reversed the pressor effect of lung injury, as indicated by a decrease in Ppa at each level of Q [6].

Effects of Pulmonary Vascular Tone on Gas Exchange in ARDS

During ARDS, pulmonary hypertension increases right ventricular afterload so that right ventricular dysfunction can occur, resulting in a high mortality rate [1]. Attempts at pharmacological pulmonary vasodilatation may thus appear justified in patients at risk of excessive right ventricular afterload. Moreover, vasodilators have been proposed in the management of ARDS with the aim to increase Q and O_2 delivery to the tissues at lower pulmonary capillary pressure. In dogs with oleic acid lung injury, even a small decrease in a normal pulmonary artery wedge pressure significantly reduced pulmonary edema [17].

However, pulmonary gas exchange usually deteriorate after administration of vasodilators. This has been reported in ARDS patients after sodium nitroprusside [1, 14], isoproterenol [1], diltiazem [15] and prostaglandin E1 [16], and in experimental ARDS after sodium nitroprusside, nitroglycerin, hydralazine, minoxidil and ketanserin. In 6 patients with pulmonary hypertension secondary to ARDS, prostaglandin E1 0.02 to 0.04 $\mu g \cdot kg^{-1} \cdot min^{-1}$ intravenously decreased Ppa and increased Q, indicating reduction in pulmonary vascular tone [16]. After prostaglandin E1, arterial PO_2 decreased by 22% ($P < 0.01$) with no change in mixed venous PO_2 nor in O_2 consumption, and intrapulmonary shunt increased by 52% ($P < 0.01$) with no other modification in the distribution of the ventilation to perfusion ratio as measured using the multiple inert gas elimination technique [16]. Vasodilators can influence gas exchange in ARDS by an increase in pulmonary blood flow or by a decrease in pulmonary vascular tone or by both. An increase in Q may promote vascular recruitment in non-ventilated lung units, increase alveolar edema or blunt hypoxic pulmonary vasoconstriction by increasing mixed venous PO_2. On the other hand, reduced pulmonary vascular tone can impair hypoxic regulation of the distribution of pulmonary perfusion.

While pulmonary vasodilatation aggravates arterial hypoxemia during ARDS, should increased pulmonary vascular tone improve gas exchange? The effects of cyclooxygenase inhibitors have been investigated according to the following reasoning. Impairment of hypoxic pulmonary vasoconstriction, as reported in experimental endotoxin-induced ARDS, could contribute to altered gas exchange. Cyclooxygenase inhibitors have been shown to reduce intrapulmonary

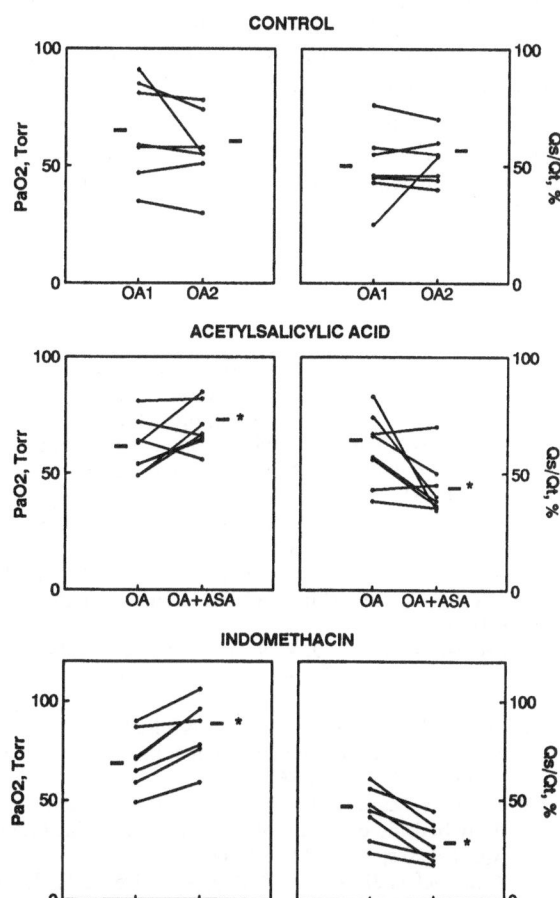

Fig. 2. Individual changes in arterial PO_2 (PaO_2) and in intrapulmonary shunt (Qs/Qt), both measured at similar cardiac output, after placebo (control), acetylsalicylic acid (ASA), and indomethacin (INDO) in dogs with oleic acid (OA) lung injury. *$P < 0.05$

shunt in lobar atelectasis [18], lobar pneumonia [19] and lobar oleic acid injury [20]. The improvement in gas exchange was related to a decrease in perfusion of the hypoxic lobe and an increase in lobar vascular resitance, suggesting enhancement of hypoxic pulmonary vasoconstriction. The effects of acetylsalicylic acid (1 g intravenously) and indomethacin (2 mg$\cdot$kg^{-1} intravenously), two structurally dissimilar cyclooxygenase inhibitors, were investigated in dogs with diffuse bilateral oleic acid pulmonary edema [21]. As described above, oleic acid produced a parallel upward shift of the Ppa/Q relationship. After oleic acid, acetylsalicylic acid and indomethacin further increased Ppa at each level of Q, indicating increased vascular tone. At similar Q, both drugs increased arterial PO$_2$ and reduced intrapulmonary shunt, as measured using a SF6 infusion (Fig. 2). Comparable results have been reported with meclofenamate, another cyclooxygenase inhibitor, also in dogs with oleic acid lung injury [22].

Almitrine is a peripheral chemoreceptor stimulant that has been shown to improve gas exchange and to reduce the mismatching of ventilation to perfusion in patients with chronic obstructive lung disease. When administered in 9 patients with ARDS, almitrine 0.5 mg$\cdot$kg^{-1} intravenously over 30 minutes increased Ppa with no change in Q, ameliorated arterial PO$_2$ and reduced the SF6 intrapulmonary shunt [23]. In dogs with oleic acid pulmonary edema however, almitrine 8 μg$\cdot$kg$^{-1}\cdot$min^{-1} intravenously had no beneficial effect on gas exchange [21]. Such discrepancy could be explained by the dose-dependent action of almitrine on hypoxic pulmonary vasoconstriction [24]. In these experimental and clinical studies, the additional right ventricular afterload imposed by pulmonary vasoconstriction was well tolerated by the right ventricle, since right atrial pressure did not change [21-23].

References

1. Zapol WM, Snider MT, Rie MA, Quinn DA, Fikker M (1985) Pulmonary circulation during adult pulmonary distress syndrome. In: Zapol WM, Falke KJ (eds) Acute respiratory failure, vol 24. Dekker, New York, pp 241-273
2. Mitzner W, Chang HK (1989) Hemodynamics of the pulmonary circulation. In: Chang HK, Paiva M (eds) Respiratory physiology. An analytical approach, vol 40. Dekker, New York, pp 561-631
3. SooHoo SL, Goldberg HS, Graham R, Jasper AC (1987) Zone 2 and zone 3 pulmonary blood flow. J Appl Physiol 62:1982-1988
4. Boiteau P, Ducas J, Schick U, Girling L, Prewitt RM (1986) Pulmonary vascular pressure:flow relationship in canine oleic acid pulmonary edema. Am J Physiol 251:H1163-H1170
5. Leeman M, Closset J, Vachiéry JL, Lejeune P, Mélot C, Naeije R (1989) Sinoaortic deafferentation reduces intrapulmonary shunt in dogs with oleic acid lung injury. J Appl Physiol 67:833-838
6. Leeman M, Lejeune P, Mélot C, Naeije R (1988) Pulmonary vascular pressure:flow plots in canine oleic acid pulmonary edema. Effects of prostaglandin E1 and nitroprusside. Am Rev Respir Dis 138:362-367
7. Greene R, Zapol WM, Snider MT, Reid L, Snow R, O'Connell RS, Novelline RA (1981) Early bedside detection of pulmonary vascular occlusion during acute respiratory failure. Am Rev Respir Dis 124:593-601
8. Tomashefski JF, Davies P, Boggis C, Greene R, Zapol WM, Reid LM (1983) The pulmonary vascular lesions of the adult respiratory distress syndrome. Am J Pathol 112:112-126

9. Bachofen M, Weibel E (1982) Structural alterations of lung parenchyma in the adult respiratory distress syndrome. Clin Chest Med 3:35–56
10. Snow RL, Davies P, Pontoppidan H, Zapol WM, Reid L (1982) Pulmonary vascular remodeling in adult respiratory distress syndrome. Am Rev Respir Dis 126:887–892
11. Michel RP, Zocchi L, Rossi A, et al (1987) Does interstitial lung edema compress airways and arteries? A morphometric study. J Appl Physiol 62:108–115
12. Bhattacharya J, Nakahara K, Staub NC (1980) Effect of edema on pulmonary blood flow in the isolated perfused dog lung lobe. J Appl Physiol 48:444–449
13. Ali J, Wood LDH (1986) Factors affecting perfusion distribution in canine oleic acid pulmonary edema. J Appl Physiol 60:1498–1503
14. Radermacher P, Huet Y, Pluskwa F, Herigault R, Mal H, Teisseire B, Lemaire F (1988) Comparison of ketanserin and sodium nitroprusside in patients with severe ARDS. Anesthesiology 68:152–157
15. Mélot C, Naeije R, Mols P, Hallemans R, Lejeune P, Jaspar N (1987) Pulmonary vascular tone improves gas exchange in the adult respiratory distress syndrome. Am Rev Respir Dis 136:1232–1236
16. Mélot C, Lejeune P, Leeman M, Moraine JJ, Naeije R (1989) Prostaglandin E1 in the adult respiratory distress syndrome. Benefit for pulmonary hypertension and cost for pulmonary gas exchange. Am Rev Respir Dis 139:106–110
17. Prewitt RM, McCarthy J, Wood LDH (1981) Treatment of acute low pressure pulmonary edema in dogs. Relative effects of hydrostatic and oncotic pressure, nitroprusside, and positive end-expiratory pressure. J Clin Invest 67:409–418
18. Garrett RC, Thomas III HM (1983) Meclofenamate uniformly decreases shunt fraction in dogs with lobar atelectasis. J Appl Physiol 54:284–289
19. Light RB (1986) Indomethacin and acetylsalicylic acid reduce intrapulmonary shunt in experimental pneumococcal pneumonia. Am Rev Respir Dis 134:520–525
20. Ali J, Duke K (1987) Does indomethacin affect shunt and its response to PEEP in oleic acid pulmonary edema? J Appl Physiol 62:2187–2192
21. Leeman M, Lejeune P, Hallemans R, Mélot C, Naeije R (1988) Effects of increased pulmonary vascular tone on gas exchange in canine oleic acid pulmonary edema. J Appl Physiol 65:662–668
22. Schulman LL, Lennon PF, Ratner SJ, Enson Y (1988) Meclofenamate enhances blood oxygenation in acute oleic acid lung injury. J Appl Physiol 64:710–718
23. Reyes A, Roca J, Rodriguez-Roisin R, Torres A, Ussetti P, Wagner PD (1988) Effect of almitrine on ventilation-perfusion distribution in adult respiratory distress syndrome. Am Rev Respir Dis 137:1062–1067
24. Nakanishi S, Hiramoto T, Ahmed N, Nishimoto Y (1988) Almitrine enhances in low dose the reactivity of pulmonary vessels to hypoxia. Respir Physiol 74:139–150

Thrombolytic Therapy in Massive Pulmonary Embolism

R. Ritz, G. A. Marbet, and M. von Planta

Introduction

Pulmonary embolism (PE) is a frequent event. In 1975, about 630000 cases of PE were observed in the USA [1]. Without treatment PE carries a mortality rate between 18 and 38% [2], and more than one fifth of patients hospitalized for massive PE die within the first few hours [3]. The threatening load on the right ventricle can be reduced by the early detection of the embolism and the immediate treatment [4, 5]. The primary goals of therapy are on the one hand to prevent an expansion or an early relapse of the PE and on the other hand to eliminate the emboli present in the pulmonary circulation as rapidly and as completely as possible. The secondary goals include the prevention of relapses, chronic pulmonary arterial hypertension and chronic veinous insufficiency.

For the choice of therapy the correct diagnosis and the severity of embolism must be known. For practical purposes the differentiation between massive central and small peripheral PE is useful [6]. In massive PE a more aggressive therapy is mandatory; in addition to heparinization and surgical embolectomy in emergency situations, thrombolytic therapy was introduced in the treatment of massive PE to rapidly unload the right ventricle.

This presentation includes the diagnostic differentiation between massive and small PE, the thrombolytic therapy and the suggested general procedure in patients with massive PE.

Degree of Pulmonary Embolism

For the choice of treatment, i.e. heparinization, thrombolytic agents or surgical embolectomy, the extent of the PE must be estimated. Besides objective angiographic methods [7, 8] Grosser et al. [9] proposed the use of a combined clinical and investigational scoring system, introducing 4 severity degrees of PE (Table 1).

The clinical symptoms in this scoring-system include dyspnea, hyperventilation, chest pain, anxiety, cough, hemoptysis, and syncope.

To differentiate between massive and small PE we recently analyzed 53 patients, admitted to the ICU between 1982 and 1984 [6]. The patients were divided into groups of 34 cases with massive embolism (angiographically documented occlusion $\geq 50\%$ and/or circulatory shock) and 16 cases with small embolism; in

Table 1. Severity degrees of pulmonary embolism. (From [9])

Severity Grade	Hemodynamic disturbance	Art. blood gases	Clinical symptoms
I	Absent	Normal	Short-lasting (secondary small pulm. infarction possible)
II	Mild	Normal	Moderate but persistent (secondary pulm. infarction possible)
III	Moderate	Abnormal	Evident
IV	Severe	Very abnormal	Circulatory shock

3 additional patients the PE was detected only at autopsy. The patient's history and first clinical workup (Table 2), together with special investigations and hemodynamics (Table 3), allowed the differentiation between massive and small embolism.

Patients with massive PE more frequently had a history of dyspnea, syncope, collapse and circulatory arrest, and signs of increased central venous pressure. The more frequent occurrence of chest pain and loud secondary portion of the second heart sound in the patients with small PE could be explained by a possibly less precise examination of the more critically ill patients with massive PE.

ECG signs of right heart strain were more frequent in the patients with massive PE. The measurements of pulmonary artery pressures (Fig. 1) discriminated also well between massive and small embolism.

These results were in agreement with earlier findings of other authors [10]. To define the extent of massive PE, Ohayon et al. [11] used the combination of

Table 2. Frequency of symptoms and clinical findings in patients with massive and small pulmonary embolism. (From [6])

	Massive PE (n = 34)	Small PE (n = 16)
History and symptoms:		
– dyspnea	74%	38%[b]
– circulatory arrest	18%	0%[b]
– collapse	15%	6%[b]
– syncope	12%	6%[b]
– chest pain	56%	69%[a]
– hemoptysis	6%	13%[b]
Physical examination:		
– increased pressure of the jugular vein	64%	14%[b]
– abnormal palpation of the right ventricle	44%	29%
– loud secondary portion of the 2nd heart sound	52%	86%[b]

[a] $p < 0.05$.   [b] $p < 0.01$.

Table 3. ECG and hemodynamics in patients with massive and small pulmonary embolism. (From [6])

	Massive PE (n = 34)	Small PE (n = 16)
ECG:		
– right axis deviation ($\geq 90°$)	9%	0%[b]
– right bundle branch block	52%	22%
– ST-T changes (precordial)	83%	78%[b]
Hemodynamics:		
– heart rate (min^{-1})	112	95[a]
– BPsyst (mmHg)	107	129[b]
– PAPsyst (mmHg)[c]	64	20
– CO (l/min)[c]	4	8

BP = blood pressure, *PAP* = pulmonary artery pressure, *CO* = cardiac output.
[a] $p < 0.05$.   [b] $p < 0.01$.   [c] $n < 10$.

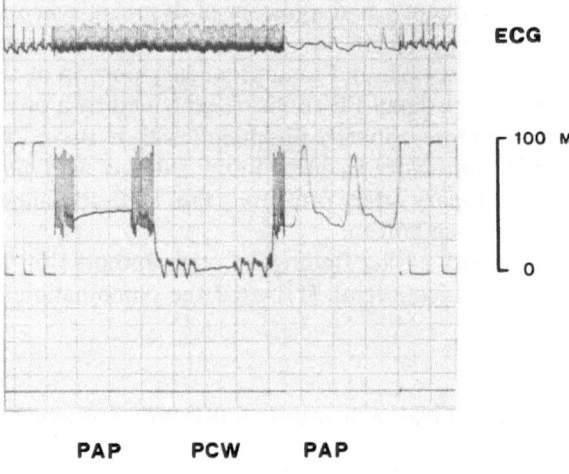

ECG

100 MMHG

0

PAP   PCW   PAP

Fig. 1. Active or primary pulmonary arterial hypertension in a patient (H.G., ♂ 34 y) with massive PE. The extremely high systolic pulmonary artery pressures (PAP) demonstrate precious and repeated embolisations. The normal pulmonary capillary wedge pressure (PCW) excludes a secondary form of pulmonary hypertension, e.g. by backward failure of the left heart

arterial blood gas determinations ($PaO_2 \leq 50$ mmHg, $PaCO_2 \leq 30$ mmHg), elevated pulmonary artery pressures and the angiographic score of Miller et al. [7]. This angiographic method to estimate objectively the extent of PE is in worldwide use, and consists of a scoring system based on filling defects and presence or absence of flow to different zones of each lung (the maximum possible score for flow reduction and involvement of arteries by embolism is 34 points).

Some correlations between hemodynamics and angiographic findings were described by Sasahara et al. [5]. These authors showed that a 25–30% obstruction of the pulmonary vascular bed usually leads to moderate pulmonary hypertension, while an increase of the central venous pressure occurred only with an obstruction of 35% or greater. Cardiac output started to decrease with obstructions of at least 40%. Generally massive PE is defined by an obstruction of the pulmonary vascular bed of at least 48%, corresponding to a Miller-Index of at least 15 points [7]. Thus objective methods to estimate the extent of PE can be used to decide on therapy and to evaluate the effect of treatment.

Thrombolytic Therapy

Our knowledge of fibrinolysis increased substantially in 1933, when Tillet and Garner [12] demonstrated that filtrates of cultures of certain strains of hemolytic *Streptococci* contained a substance capable of inciting rapid fibrinolysis of human plasma clots; this substance was termed streptococcal fibrinolysin. Only in the late 1950s it could be shown that experimentally induced thrombi in the arm veins of human volunteers could be successfully lysed by an infusion of purified streptokinase. This was followed by the production of urokinase, a naturally occurring nonantigenic and nonpyrogenic direct activator of plasminogen made by human kidney cells and excreted into the urine. The first truly quantitative studies on thrombolytic therapy in PE, known as the urokinase-pulmonary embolism trial UPET [4] and urokinase-streptokinase pulmonary embolism trial USPET [13], showed that thrombolytic therapy was more effective in dissolving pulmonary emboli as compared with the spontaneous resolution observed when heparin alone was employed. Equally important was the observation that streptokinase and urokinase were comparable in their lytic effects in vivo.

Today's *rationale* of treating massive PE with thrombolytic agents is mainly based on these studies. In the UPET-study the 12 hours infusion of urokinase showed, compared to heparin, angiographically greater regression of the emboli, scintigraphically better perfusion and faster hemodynamic improvement. In the USPET-study, comparing two different dosage regimens of urokinase and streptokinase with heparin, the reduction of elevated pulmonary artery pressures occurred within 2 hours following the onset of treatment, with its maximum effect after 8 hours. In the follow-up period after one year (86% of the 160 patients, UPET) almost all hemodynamic and angiographic parameters had returned to normal. However, by a more sensitive test, measuring the pulmonary capillary blood volume in 40 patients [14], values returned to normal could only be shown after one year in the patients formerly treated with thrombolytic agents. In contrast, in the heparin treated patients some obstruction persisted because of incomplete resolution; and could eventually lead to pulmonary hypertension and chronic cor pulmonale. The goals in treating massive PE, therefore, include complete resolution of the emboli [5].

Despite the presented short- and long-term advantages of thrombolytic therapy in massive PE the controversy about the risk/benefit ratio continued. The main arguments of the opponents are that the decrease of mortality and recurrency of PE is not proven yet, the rate of complications could be higher and the cost is high [15]. But more recent studies comparing different thrombolytic agents, different dosage regimens and different sites of injection (intravenous versus intrapulmonary), confirmed the known advantages of thrombolysis in massive PE [11, 16, 17]. At the same time one has to expect an increased complication rate by the diagnostic procedures (invasive measurements of hemodynamics and angiography) and an increased incidence of side effects with the thrombolytic agents (bleeding). The frequency of serious bleedings (e.g. hemorrhagic stroke) is about 2% but benign hemorrhages can occur in up to 25% [4, 11, 17]. Initial experiences with the new fibrinolytic agent APSAC (a p-anisoyl derivate of human lys-plasminogen-streptokinase activator complex) confirmed its effectiveness in resolving pulmonary emboli in 10 patients, but two suffered serious bleeding complications. There was also evidence of an unexpected systemic fibrinolytic effect [18]. The first studies using recombinant tissue-type plasminogen activator (rt-PA) in the treatment of massive PE have been published recently [19, 20]; the trial published by Verstraete et al. confirmed the expected resolution of the emboli and the favorable hemodynamic effect; the trial indicated also that the intrapulmonary infusion of rt-PA did not offer a significant benefit over the intravenous route and suggested that a prolonged infusion over 7 hours (100 mg) was superior to a single infusion of 50 mg rt-PA over 2 hours [19].

Despite beneficial effects of thrombolytic therapy on resolution of emboli and of hemodynamic improvement a reduction in mortality has not been clearly demonstrated. In the UPET-study [4] mortality within the two-week study period was 9% in the heparin group and 7% in the urokinase group respectively (not significant); in another group of 67 patients with massive PE treated by urokinase François et al. described an early mortality of 4.5% (during thrombolysis) and an equal mortality of 4.5% after 48 hours [16].

In the UKEP-study [17] 7 out of 129 patients (5%) died during the 48 hours of treatment with two different doses of urokinase. Among the 34 cases in the first rt-PA study, comparing intravenous and intrapulmonary administration, 2 patients died during treatment [19]. Finally, in the most recent study comparing rt-PA and urokinase in treating acute pulmonary embolism [20], 4 of 45 patients died (9%), 2 patients who received rt-PA and 2 who received urokinase.

Thus, no investigator demonstrated so far a statistically significant difference in mortality between patients treated by thrombolysis or heparinization. No difference could be shown by various thrombolytic agents so far. To demonstrate the expected reduction in mortality by thrombolysis a study should probably include several thousands of patients.

Conclusions and Clinical Implications

For the correct treatment of pulmonary embolism (heparinization, thrombolysis or embolectomy) the diagnostic differentiation between small (peripheral) and massive (central) PE is important. This differentiation is possible on the basis of the patient's history and symptoms, physical and special examinations (e.g. ECG, arterial blood gas analysis etc.). With the clinical suspicion of massive PE an angiography should be performed whenever possible. The sensitivity of scintigraphy in PE is inferior [21]. In case of massive PE the hemodynamic measurements will decide between thrombolysis and surgical embolectomy, immediately after angiography and during the later course: whenever circulatory shock appears, we believe that emergency embolectomy is indicated. Our present diagnostic and therapeutic attitude is presented in Fig. 2.

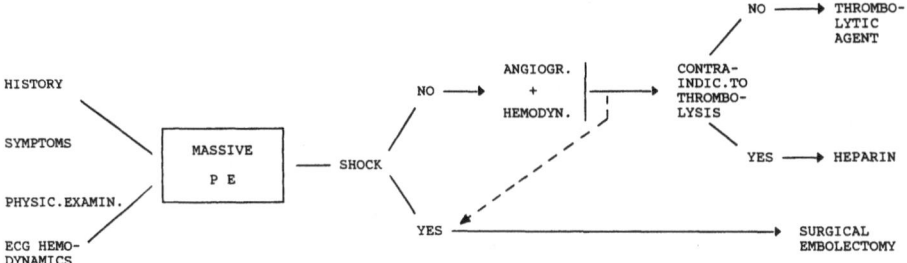

Fig. 2. Diagnostic and therapeutic procedure in patients with massive pulmonary embolism (PE)

Patients with angiographically proven massive PE but without circulatory shock should be treated, in our view, by thrombolysis. For the moment streptokinase or urokinase are used but in the future APSAC, rt-PA or other new agents might be the drugs of choice. The details of the therapeutic procedure, i.e. dosage, administration and duration of the administration of thrombolytic agents and accompanying drugs have been recently described [22].

In view of the encouraging results of thrombolysis with rapid resolution of the emboli, early hemodynamic improvement and a rather low occurrence of side effects, the rationale to treat these patients by thrombolytic agents with the goal of rapidly unloading the threatened right ventricle seems to be justified.

References

1. Rosenow EC, Osmundson PhJ, Brown ML (1981) Pulmonary embolism. Mayo Clin Proc 56:161–178
2. Barrit DW, Jordan SC (1960) Anticoagulant drugs in treatment of pulmonary embolism: controlled trial. Lancet 2:1309–1312
3. Grosser KD (1980) Lungenembolie, Erkennung und differentialtherapeutische Probleme. Internist 21:273–282
4. Sasahara AA, Hyers TM, Cole CM (1973) The urokinase pulmonary embolism trial. A national cooperative study. Circulation 47:(suppl II) 66–72
5. Sasahara AA, Sharma GV, McIntyre KM, Cella G (1986) Le traitement thrombolytique modifie-t-il le pronostic de l'embolie pulmonaire? Haemostasis 16:(suppl 4) 54–61
6. Salzberg A, Ritz R (1987) Massive und kleine Lungenembolie auf der Intensivstation. Schweiz Med Wschr 117:1256–1259
7. Miller GAH, Sutton GC, Kerr IH, Gibson RV, Honey M (1971) Comparison of streptokinase and heparin in treatment of isolated acute massive pulmonary embolism. Br Med J 2:681–684
8. Walsh PN, Greenspan RH, Simon M, Simon AL, Hyres TM, Woosley PC, Cole ChM (1973) An angiographic severity index for pulmonary embolism. Circulation 47:(Suppl II) 101–108
9. Grosser KD, Knoch K (1984) Thromboembolie der Lunge. Intensivmed 21:138–144
10. Artigas A, Bonnin JO, Martinez R, Net A (1980) Hemodynamic response to different degrees of experimentally induced pulmonary vascular obstruction. Intensive Care Med 6:80–81
11. Ohayon J, Colle JP, Tauzin-Fin P, Lorient-Roudaut MF, Besse P (1986) Evolution hémodynamique au cours des fibrinolyses de l'embolie pulmonaire grave. Arch Mal Coeur 79:445–453

12. Tillet WS, Garner RL (1933) The fibrinolytic activity of hemolytic streptococci. J Exp Med 58:485–502
13. Urokinase-Streptokinase Pulmonary Embolism Trial (1974) JAMA 229:1606–1613
14. Sharma GV, Burleson VA, Sasahara AA (1980) Effect of thrombolytic therapy on pulmonary capillary blood volume in patients with pulmonary embolism. N Engl J Med 303:842–845
15. Dalen JE (1980) Controversy: the case against fibrinolytic therapy. J Cardiovasc Med 5:799–813
16. François G, Charbonnier B, Raynaud P, Garnier LF, Griguer P, Brochier M (1986) Traitement de l'embolie pulmonaire aguë par urokinase comparée à l'association plasminogène-urokinase. Arch Mal Coeur 79:435–442
17. The UKEP Study Research Group (1987) The UKEP Study: Multicentre clinical trial on two local regimens of urokinase in massive pulmonary embolism. Europ Heart J 8:2–10
18. Bett JHN, Bunce IH, Cade JF, Concannon AJ, Gallus A, Low J (1987) Initial experience with a new fibrinolytic agent (APSAC) in patients with major pulmonary embolism. Aust NZ J Med 17:77–79
19. Verstraete M, Miller GAH, Bonnameaux H, et al (1988) Intravenous and intrapulmonary recombinant tissue-type plasminogen activator in the treatment of acute massive pulmonary embolism. Circulation 77:353–360
20. Goldhaber SZ, Heit J, Sharma GVRK, et al (1988) Randomised controlled trial of recombinant tissue plasminogen activator versus urokinase in the treatment of acute pulmonary embolism. Lancet 2:293–298
21. Sasahara AA, Sharma G, Barsamian EM, Schoolmann M, Cella G (1983) Pulmonary thrombo-embolism. JAMA 249:2945–2950
22. Marbet GA (1988) Thrombolyse bei akuter massiver Lungenembolie. Schweiz Med Wschr 118:1138–1141

Cardiorespiratory Interactions

J. L. Robotham and M. Takata

Introduction

Cardiorespiratory interactions occur any time there is a change in lung volume and/or intrathoracic pressure (ITP). From this point of view, spontaneous respiration, mechanical ventilation (intermittent positive pressure ventilation, IPPV, or high frequency ventilation), and cardiopulmonary resuscitation (CPR) represent a single coherent physiologic issue. Each reflects a situation in which changes in lung volume and ITP can profoundly influence the cardiovascular system. To understand one completely it is necessary to understand the others.

In chapters in previous editions of this book, the major focus has been on left sided events [1, 2]. In this review we shall focus on right sided events. We shall consider the basic mechanisms affecting blood flow across any vascular compartment or cardiac chamber and then apply these basic mechanisms to understanding systemic venous return and right ventricular (RV) output.

General Principles of Mechanical Interactions

Figure 1 illustrates a model of a compliant vascular compartment with a changing surrounding pressure. Inflow is generated by a constant pressure source and

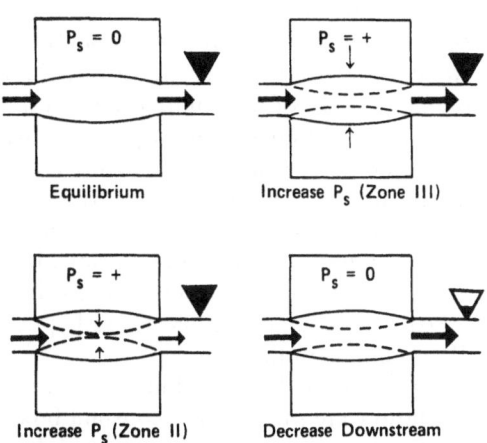

Fig. 1. See text for discussion. (From [50])

reflected by the size of the arrow. The boundaries of the compartment could represent the thorax, abdomen, or an extremity and illustrate the influence of pressure changes around a vascular bed or cardiac chamber.

The vascular bed/cardiac chamber inside the compartment can be given the following characteristics:

1. It will have a pressure-volume relationship (compliance), such that a given volume will exert a given pressure across the wall. This "transmural pressure" is easily calculated as the intravascular minus surrounding box pressure (Ps).
2. There will be a pressure flow relationship (resistance) which allows estimation of an afterload, symbolized by the weight impeding blood leaving the compartment. The true calculation of afterload requires knowledge of not only the resistance, but also the compliance of the outflow vessel and inertance of the fluid and vessel wall.

Let us analyze the transient changes in inflow and outflow with a change in surrounding pressure given a constant pressure source for inflow. When the Ps is acutely increased the transmural pressure must decrease since even if inflow were constant the outflow from the compliant chamber would increase. This transient increase in outflow as Ps is increased is represented by the large arrow as volume is translocated out of this compartment to the next compartment. However, since we have defined the inflow source as being constant pressure not constant flow, the increase in Ps will reduce the gradient for inflow further reducing the vascular volume in the chamber. Using terminology analogous to West's zones of the pulmonary vascular bed [3], a zone III condition exists when the outflow downstream pressure outside the box is higher than the surrounding pressure (e.g. for the abdominal compartment, right atrial pressure is higher than abdominal pressure). A zone II condition exists when Ps is greater than the downstream pressure outside the box (e.g. when abdominal pressure due to ascites is much higher than the downstream right atrial pressure). If the box pressure is increased to produce zone II conditions in which the effective downstream pressure determining flow is Ps, the *dominant* effect now is to *diminish* blood flow out of the compartment and reduce inflow. The vascular pressure in the chamber relative to atmosphere would increase while the *transmural* pressure would decrease (increased Ps, zone II). Hence the increase in box pressure first diminishes the vascular volume by increasing outflow, equivalent to decreasing the effective vascular compliance. Then increases in both back pressure and resistance diminish inflow and outflow. It is clear that opposite changes in outflow are possible with the same increase in box pressure depending on the initial vascular volume, hypervolemia vs hypovolemia, analogous to zone III and zone II conditions in the lung.

Finally in the last panel in Fig. 1, a decrease in vascular volume and increase in outflow are produced at constant box pressure by reducing the afterload. Under these conditions an increase in abdominal pressure as illustrated in the panel immediately above, is equivalent to reducing the resistance (afterload) to systemic venous return to the right atrium in terms of the initial effect on the abdominal compartment's volume and outflow. Thus during spontaneous inspiration, the fall in right atrial pressure relative to atmosphere produced by the decrease in ITP will reduce the "afterload"/downstream pressure for venous return increasing systemic venous return. However, if at the same time diaphragmatic descent markedly increased the abdominal pressure surrounding the large venous compartments in the abdomen, a zone II condition could be produced reducing venous return. One can theoretically predict that under different conditions a spontaneous inspiration could either increase or decrease systemic venous return once not only the respiratory induced changes in intrathoracic pressure but also the abdominal pressure are considered.

Figure 2 schematically uses the same format to illustrate the similarities between decreasing the pressure surrounding a vascular chamber and increasing the afterload/downstream pressure. It should not be surprising that a decrease in box pressure will increase the volume in the vessel or cardiac chamber and thus decrease outflow. This is equivalent to increasing the afterload/downstream pressure which also results in decreasing outflow and increasing vascular volume. For the LV, a fall in ITP or an increase in afterload are mechanically equivalent. For the RV, since both the ventricular chamber and pulmonary artery are surrounded by the same intrathoracic pressure (ignoring for the moment any influence of the pericardium) either an increase or decrease in ITP without a change in lung volume, would not influence the gradient between the two vascular structures. However, considering the systemic vein which fill the RV, a negative ITP increases the gradient for systemic venous return and hence cardiac output. An increase ITP will decrease systemic venous return by raising the downstream pressure for venous inflow, leading to a decreased RV preload and hence cardiac output. This reasoning process should be applicable not only to the normal heart, but also to RV failure, and in the extreme to absent ventricular function, i.e. CPR.

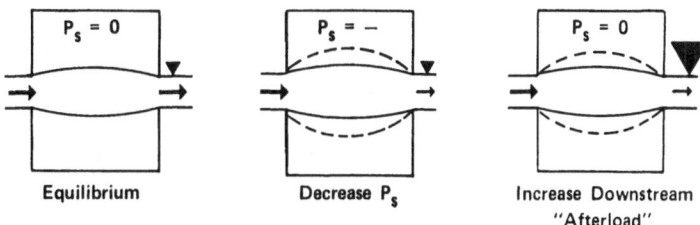

Fig. 2. See text for discussion. (From [50])

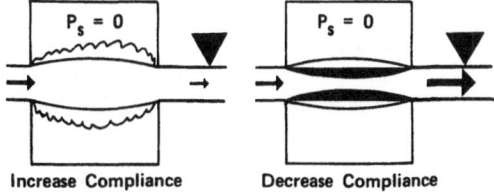

Fig. 3. See text for discussion.
(From [50])

If changes in ITP only influenced the gradient for systemic venous return to, and arterial egress from the thorax, our understanding of the cardiovascular events would be relatively straightforward. However, as illustrated in Fig. 3, independent of changes in box pressure, the vascular volume may also be varied by altering the vascular compartment's compliance. With a constant pressure inflow source, increasing compliance increases the vascular volume, transiently reduces outflow, and then allows increased inflow and outflow through a lower pressure chamber. With the same constant pressure inflow source, decreasing chamber compliance by:

(a) intrinsic stiffening of the walls;
(b) extrinsically pushing on the chamber as occurs if the lungs compress the heart (heart-lung interdependence) [4, 5] or the contralateral ventricle shifts the septum (ventricular interdependence) [6] will raise the chamber pressure, first emptying the chamber by increasing outflow and then reducing inflow due to an increased back pressure, hence reducing steady state outflow.

Thus under conditions of a constant pressure inflow source to a vascular compartment, changes in the surrounding pressure, changes in vascular compliance, and changes in afterload may each independently alter outflow. Since the outflow of one vascular compartment is the inflow for the next vascular compartment, analysis of the next compartment must also include a variable inflow. If we then allow vascular compartments to be linked both in series and in parallel during a spontaneous inspiration as schematically illustrated in Fig. 4, it becomes difficult to predict the net result of a physiologic perturbation which alters inflows, surrounding pressures, compliances and afterload, in multiple compartments, e.g. the abdomen, right heart, the alveolar and extra-alveolar pulmonary vascular beds, the left heart, arterial bed and peripheral venous bed. Despite the complexity, taking one vascular compartment at a time is a logical manner to begin evaluating the whole system.

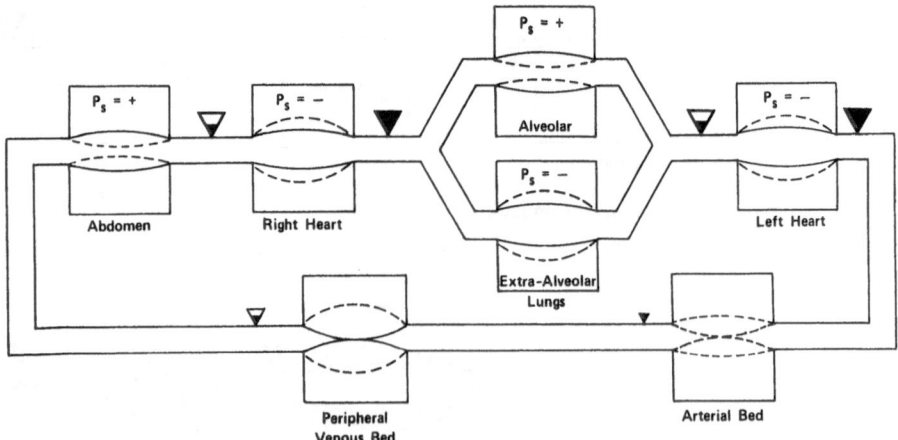

Fig. 4. See text for discussion. (From [50])

Systemic Venous Return

The influence of respiration on systemic venous return remains a dominant factor in cardiopulmonary interactions despite recent emphasis on the effects of respiration on LV performance. Systemic venous return is extremely sensitive to respiratory induced changes in intrathoracic pressure (ITP) during respiration. This is evident in the venous return curve described by Guyton [7, 8] (Fig. 5). By experimentally opening the closed-loop circulatory system at the right atrium (RA) with a right-heart bypass preparation, Guyton plotted the systemic venous return as a function of right atrial pressure (Pra), and showed that characteristics of the venous return curve are determined by the properties of venous compliance and resistance and blood volume. Venous return is exquisitely sensitive to very small increases in Pra, which can be produced by changes in ITP during respiration. Before compensatory reflexes occur, simply raising Pra over 8 mmHg can transiently stop all venous return. The steepness of the normal venous return curve (i.e. gain) suggests why the changes in Pra produced during a single respiratory cycle may produce such large changes in RV stroke volume [9] and why Pinsky could superimpose the changes in RV stroke volume during a single IPPV inspiration on a conventionally determined venous return curve [10]. The normally functioning RV pumps what it receives, maintaining Pra close to zero. Thus with good ventricular function, variation in cardiac output during respiration is determined by changes in systemic venous return.

In contrast with ventricular dysfunction, the influence of respiration on systemic venous may not be the dominant mechanism affecting cardiac output. Changes in ITP will affect not only preload but also afterload. The failing LV

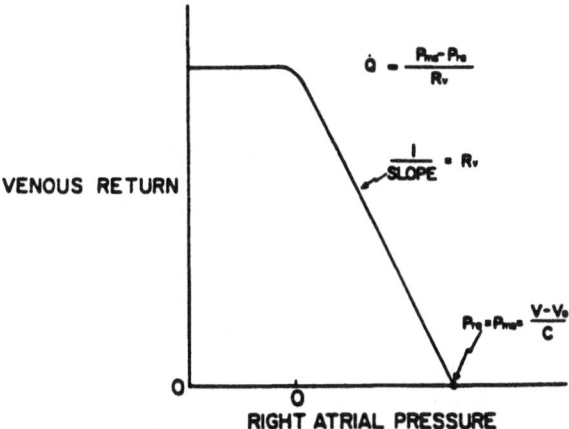

Fig. 5. Schematic representation of a venous return curve assuming a single peripheral venous compartment. Venous return intersects the abscissa at the right atrial pressure (Pra) required to stop all venous return, i.e., Pms, mean systemic pressure. The reciprocal of the slope of the venous return curve equals to the venous resistance (Rv). Maximum venous return occurs with a RA pressure of 0, below which further lowering RA pressure does not increase venous return due to flow limitation. V = total venous blood volume. V_0 = the unstressed blood volume. The difference between $(V-V_0)$ equals the stressed volume. (From [51])

may be dilated and relatively insensitive to further increase in preload, but critically sensitive to changes in afterload. Increasing ITP with LV failure and high systemic venous pressures may have a relatively small effect on decreasing venous return, but a substantial effect on decreasing the afterload for LV ejection [11].

The plateau of the venous return curve demonstrates another characteristic of the venous system, i.e. the flow limitation of the collapsible veins. With the chest open, maximum venous return is reached when Pra falls slightly below atmospheric pressure. Further lowering of Pra to a markedly negative value does not increase venous return due to collapse of the highly compliant vena cava at the junction with the RA. In other words, when the transmural pressure of the vena cava becomes negative, the vena cava collapses and the effective downstream pressure for the venous return is the pressure surrounding the vein (i.e. with the chest open the surrounding ITP=0), not the subatmospheric Pra. This process was originally described by Holt [12], and Duomarco and Rimini [13], and has been analyzed extensively by Permutt et al. with respect to flow of air through the airways [14]. During respiration with the chest closed, this flow limiting condition may also occur but the site of the collapse of the vena cava would be different from the open chest conditions. Since the driving force to lower Pra during respiration is the fall in the ITP, the transmural pressure of the vena cava should always be positive in the thorax. Thus the collapse due to a zero transmural pressure would occur just before the vena cava enters the thorax, where the surrounding pressure in the extrathoracic compartment is more positive than ITP, e.g. on the abdominal side of the diaphragmatic inlet. This has been experimentally demonstrated during respiration [15, 16] using ultrasound to show collapse and flutter of the inferior vena cava (IVC) just inferior to the diaphragm. Therefore, making the ITP markedly negative will not increase the steady state systemic venous return more than when Pra relative to the periphery is zero.

Venous return curves were originally produced with reflex changes blocked [7]. The changes in venous return with acute changes in Pra subsequently have been shown to reflect events occurring during the first 10 sec after an acute perturbation. When Pra is increased acutely relative to the periphery by increasing the ITP, e.g., PEEP, an immediate decrease in venous return is expected. However, when reflexes are intact, approximately 10 sec after an acute perturbation alpha-adrenergic sympathetic activation leads to a compensatory peripheral venoconstriction, which produces a decrease in the compliance of the systemic venous bed, thereby raising the mean systemic pressure and shifting the venous return curve to the right and up. Thus steady-state cardiac output will return toward, but often not to its pre-PEEP values due to the altered venous return curve which results in a increased systemic venous return at a given ventricular function. If the degree of the venoconstriction is not sufficient, plasma volume expansion could increase the systemic venous return by further raising the mean systemic pressure driving venous return. Finally if the increased sympathetic output also raised the inotropic state of the ventricles, venous return would be further enhanced by lower ventricular end-diastolic/atrial pressures. With this information it is clear why adrenergic blockade [17], venodilation, or hemorrhage can lead to precipitous falls in systemic venous return when combined with an increased ITP.

While most studies of ventilation's influence on systemic venous return has focused on changes in ITP affecting Pra, it may well be that respiratory induced changes in extrathoracic intraabdominal pressure (Pab) are equally, if not more important under many conditions. Respiration will produce not only changes in ITP but also in Pab due to the descent of diaphragm. Since the intraabdominal vascular compartment exists directly upstream to the intrathoracic compartment, the effect of respiration on Pab can modulate systemic venous return. If Pab is less than the inferior vena cava (IVC) pressure at the diaphragm level, the abdominal vasculature can be considered in zone III condition analogous to West's model of the pulmonary vascular bed [3, 18]. A transient increase in Pab, as seen during each breath of spontaneous respiration, would express blood out of the abdominal compartment transiently increasing IVC flow into the thorax but tending to impede blood entering from the upstream extraabdominal compartments (i.e. legs). A steady state increase in Pab, as seen during abdominal binding or weaning from mechanical ventilation to spontaneous respiration, would decrease the effective compliance of the abdominal vasculature and shift the venous return curve to the right and up, thereby increasing systemic venous return for a given ventricular function. This phenomenon could account in part for the increase in Pra observed by Lemaire et al. when they attempted to wean patients with LV dysfunction from ventilatory support [19, 20]. The increased preload exacerbated an already precarious situation resulting in acute LV decompensation. In contrast, if Pab exceeds the intraluminal IVC pressure at the entrance to the thorax resulting in a negative transmural pressure at that point (i.e. Pab > Pra), the abdominal vasculature can be considered in a zone II condition. Collapse of IVC and flow-limitation would exist where the IVC enters thorax. A steady state increase in Pab would increase the effective resistance to venous return due to an increase in the effective back pressure to the upstream extraabdominal compartments, thereby decreasing systemic venous return. Under these conditions, every increase in Pab produces an equal increase in abdominal Pivc. This would not change the gradient for venous return from the abdominal vascular compartments (e.g. splanchnic and renal) which experience the same increase in surrounding pressure, but would reduce venous return from the upstream extraabdominal compartments (e.g. the legs).

The concept of abdominal zone conditions may thus explain the apparently conflicting results in the literature with regard to the effects of spontaneous respiration on IVC flow [21–25]. Under hypervolemic conditions with a zone III abdomen, spontaneous inspiration would increase systemic venous return due to a decrease in the ITP and increase in Pab, while under hypovolemic conditions with zone II abdomen, spontaneous inspiration could decrease venous return due to IVC collapse and flow limitation. Thus, analyses of venous return which consider only the respiratory induced changes in ITP without considering the effects of changes in Pab may be seriously flawed. During positive pressure inspiration, ITP must rise above Pab in order for the diaphragm to move caudad. In this case the gradient for systemic venous return must decrease even with a zone III abdomen.

In addition to the effects of respiration on generalized intrathoracic or intraabdominal pressures, the influence of direct mechanical compression of the right heart by the lungs on venous return must also be considered. Brookhart et al. recognized that the lungs can squeeze the heart, reducing systemic venous return and limiting right heart preload [26]. More recent studies [4, 5, 17, 27] have demonstrated that lung inflation may mechanically compress the heart independent of any change in generalized ITP. This mechanism may be very important to understand the hemodynamic events during a wide variety of pathological conditions with elevated lung volume, e.g. pulmonary emphysema, status asthmaticus, or PEEP. These compressive forces are applied to both the left and right hearts, reducing the gradients for both systemic and pulmonary venous return.

In summary, venous return is exquisitely sensitive to small changes in intravascular pressures affecting the gradient for blood flow, making it a major determinant of respiratory induced changes in cardiac output. Changes in venous return can be viewed as resulting from the effects of respiration on a group of compartments within compartments, both in series and in parallel. Each compartment has its own volume, compliance, and resistance, modulated by either the active contraction of respiratory muscles or a mechanical ventilator in addition to secondary reflex or humoral events. Whether phasic or steady-state ventilation changes are considered, the influence of ventilation on venous return must be carefully evaluated before reaching any conclusions about its effect on ventricular function. In many situations, the effect of respiration on the heart is completely secondary to changes in venous return.

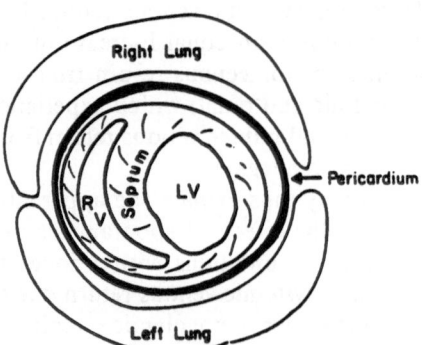

Fig. 6. Schematic representation of the intrathoracic structures that interact during respiration. The right ventricle (RV) is draped over the rounder left ventricle (LV) with the septum between. The muscle fibers of the free walls of both ventricles are in continuity. The pericardium surrounds both ventricles and is in turn surrounded by the lungs. The rib cage, intercostal muscles, diaphragm, and abdominal contents are not shown in this diagram but contribute to the mechanical interactions that the intrathoracic contents experience. A change in any one element may influence the others. (From [52])

Right Ventricular Output

The geometry of the normal RV is very different from the LV. The LV can be considered as an ellipsoid that empties relatively homogeneously during systole [28–30]. The RV is a relatively flat crescent shaped chamber that can be thought of as draped over the septal wall of the LV, its free wall contiguous with the free-wall fibers in the LV (Fig. 6). This anatomic arrangement of a thin-walled RV applied over a thick walled LV provides a number of advantages for the RV. The continuity of the muscle fibers in both free walls allows them to pull together toward a common center of gravity and, thus, essentially assist each other, i.e. act as a common pumping chamber.

The RV normally functions as a low-pressure volume pump. Under normal circumstances, RV ejection may be assisted substantially by LV ejection. Studies in isolated hearts [31–33] have demonstrated that an increased LV volume increases RV developed systolic pressure. In both angiographic and echocardiographic studies of either a normal muscular septum or a prosthetic interventricular septum, rightward motion is seen during systole, consistent with a contribution to RV ejection via this septal motion produced by the higher LV systolic pressure [29, 34–37]. Recent work by Hurford et al. [38] suggests that acutely increasing RV afterload can produce increases in coronary blood flow to the right side of the septum, with little change on the left side of the septum. This suggests that the septum may develop differential mechanical and thus metabolic stresses confined to one side of the septum and thus act as two walls, each responding to the loading conditions of its ipsilateral ventricle. This challenges the conventional notion of the septum as belonging almost exclusively to the thick walled LV. The modulation of the septal contribution to RV systolic function under pathologic conditions has not been established. It is clear however that the loading conditions experienced by the ventricles are a major determinant of the expressed morphology. In the transition from the fetal to the postnatal environment the RV free wall thins rapidly as the pulmonary vascular resistance falls. Under pathologic conditions with a complete transposition of the great vessels, the RV ejecting into the systemic bed is round and thick walled, while the LV ejecting into a low pressure pulmonary bed becomes thin walled and ellipsoid [39]. The influence of chronic lung disease on RV function is an area still in need of much work.

Both ventricles must share a fixed amount of intrapericardial space, the one with the highest pressure shifting the compliant septum toward the other, reducing its compliance and diastolic volume. This interaction is referred to as ventricular interdependence [6, 34]. Studies of this kind suggest that the rapid alterations in RV morphology during the perinatal period could similarly affect RV/LV interactions. Postnatally, if the septum hypertrophies in response to a chronic increase in RV afterload (e.g. secondary to alveolar hypoxia), the degree of diastolic interdependence between the two ventricles decreases [29].

Both clinicians and physiologists agree that under normal conditions, the RV functions superbly as a low-pressure volume pump; however, in the presence of a markedly increased afterload, it is interesting that they may come to different conclusions. Maughan et al. [40] demonstrated in an in vitro system that the RV can function as a pressure pump, generating peak systolic pressures of 80 mm Hg or more for prolonged periods of time. However this is accomplished at the expense of a markedly elevated ventricular end-diastolic pressure, which for the clinician, would signify RV failure. Thus, the clinician is faced with the situation in which a right ventricle may cope with generating an adequate systolic pressure but at the expense of a diastolic pressure producing peripheral edema, ascites, etc. due to a high back pressure in venous return. Respiration may influence RV systolic performance through six mechanisms:

(a) changes in venous return altering preload;
(b) ventricular interdependence altering preload;
(c) reversible hypoxic pulmonary vasoconstriction altering afterload;
(d) fixed anatomic pulmonary vascular disease altering afterload;
(e) mechanical effects resulting from independent changes in ITP and lung volume; and
(f) transmission across the pulmonary bed of LV events altering RV afterlaod.

Any increase in RV preload should modulate RV systolic afterload via the Laplace relationship. Any thinning of the wall will increase the afterload, while if the RV became rounder, the radius of curvature should decrease, diminishing the afterload. Due to the complex geometry of the RV and relatively thin wall, these relationships in the RV are neither well understood nor well studied.

Coronary perfusion of the RV is normally predominantly during systole, the time in the cardiac cycle when the gradient between the aorta and RV is largest. Thus, acute massive increases in both RV systolic and diastolic pressures may limit coronary perfusion and produce RV dysfunction. More chronic pulmonary hypertension with RV remodelling (hypertrophy) leads to coronary flow being predominantly during diastole, analogous to LV coronary flow [41]. The influence of changes in coronary flow on RV function appear to be similar to the relationships established on the left side, but far more detailed studies are necessary, particularly since the incompletely understood influence of resistance and capacitance vessels which may have a profound effect on normal LV perfusion [42], are even less well appreciated in either the normal or remodelled RV.

The Right Ventricle and Positive Pressure Ventilation

While everyone agrees that a negative ITP by increasing systemic venous return will increase RV volume and RV output, there has been controversy over the consequences of a positive IPT produced by IPPV with PEEP. Most studies have found the RV and LV volumes to decrease with PEEP reflecting diminished systemic venous return [43–45]. One clinical study in patients with markedly elevated pulmonary vascular resistances (PVR), reported that further increases in PVR with PEEP can afterload the RV and occasionally dilate the RV [46]. This will shift the septum leftward reducing LV volume. In animal studies, Scharf et al. [47] clearly demonstrated that with the chest open, PEEP increases RV dimensions consistent with an increased RV afterload produced by the increased lung volume. With the chest closed, most animal and human studies have observed decreased RV volumes with the institution of PEEP. Finally, if lung volume increases substantially with PEEP, the lungs can mechanically compress both ventricles, raising end-diastolic pressures [5]. Thus, it may be expected that the combination of increased ITP, lung volume, and pulmonary vascular resistance (PVR) produced by PEEP will raise RA pressure relative to the extrathoracic compartment, reducing the gradient for systemic venous return. However, these factors will have opposite effects on RV volume, increased ITP and lung volume tending to reduce RV volume, while the PEEP induced increase in PVR will tend to increase RV volume.

In summary, RV performance is still poorly understood when compared to knowledge of LV performance. The right heart, however, forms a link in series with the peripheral venous bed, pulmonary vascular bed, and LV and in parallel with the LV, pericardium, and lung parenchyma. Considerable effort is necessary to define its function, particularly in pathologic conditions relevant to the ICU.

Applying these principles to spontaneous respiration, it is clear why airway obstruction, either upper or lower, will adversely affect cardiac function and be particularly deleterious with a compromised LV [11]. First, with hypoventilation, carbon dioxide will increase, imposing a respiratory acidosis leading to cellular dysfunction and increased pulmonary vascular resistance. Secondly, the increased alveolar carbon dioxide will limited the partial pressure that oxygen can develop in the alveolar space leading to hypoxic pulmonary vasoconstriction and increasing right ventricular afterload. Thirdly, the marked increase in respiratory muscle work will produce a metabolic load and oxygen deficit, an increased carbon dioxide and lactate production leading to a combined respiratory and metabolic acidosis which by depressing ventricular contractility further decreases oxygen delivery. If in addition to these adverse conditions, we impose an increased preload, and increased afterload on the LV due to the decrease in ITP [48, 49] it is clear that airway obstruction with spontaneous respiration is the worst possible form of ventilation for the patient in LV failure. If lower airway obstruction is present, lung hyperinflation will increase pulmonary vascular resistance raising RV afterload and any direct compression of the heart by the hyperinflated lungs will diminish venous return.

Conclusion

Interactions between the circulatory and respiratory system continue to challenge the physiologist and clinician. While the focus of interest has been on the left side during the last decade, it is now clear that the next "black box" requiring understanding is on the right side, the systemic veins and the right heart. This chapter is meant to provide some of the basic physiologic principles that have been applied to the right side and illustrate where new studies are needed before a clearer picture can be drawn by the combined efforts of physiologists and clinicians.

Acknowledgements: To Dr. Victor Chernick for permission to extensively adapt significant portions of a review written by the authors for a book edited by R. Mellins and V. Chernick, entitled "Basic Mechanisms of Pediatric Respiratory Disease: Cellular and Integrative" to be published by B. C. Decker, Inc. in 1990. Supported by NIH RO1-HL39138-02.

References

1. Peters J, Robotham JL (1987) Hemodynamic effects of increased intrathoracic pressure. In: Vincent JL, Suter PM (eds) Update in intensive care and emergency medicine, vol. 2 Springer, Berlin Heidelberg New York Tokyo, pp 120-134
2. Peters J (1989) Respiration within the cardiac cycle. In: Vincent JL (ed) Update in intensive care and emergency medicine, vol. 4. Springer, Berlin Heidelberg New York Tokyo, pp 201-218
3. West J, Dollery C, Naimark A (1964) Distribution of blood flow in isolated lung; relation to vascular and alveolar pressures. J Appl Physiol 19:713-724
4. Lloyd TC Jr (1982) Respiratory systems compliance as seen from the cardiac fossa. J Appl Physiol 53:56-62
5. Wallis T, Robotham JL, Compean R, Kindred MK (1983) Mechanical heart-lung interaction with positive end-expiratory pressure. J Appl Physiol 54:1039-1047
6. Bove AA, Santamore WP (1981) Ventricular interdependence. Prog Cardiovasc Dis 23:356-388
7. Guyton AC, Lindsey AW, Abernathy B, Richardson T (1957) Venous return at various right atrial pressures and the normal venous return curve. Am J Physiol 189:609-615
8. Guyton AC, Jones CE, Coleman TG (1973) Circulatory physiology: Cardiac output and its regulation, 2nd edn. WB Saunders, Philadelphia
9. Scharf SM, Brown R, Saunders N, Green LH (1980) Hemodynamic effects of positive pressure inflation. J Appl Physiol 49:124-131
10. Pinsky MR (1984) Instantaneous venous return curves in an intact canine preparation. J Appl Physiol 56:765-771
11. Robotham JL, Scharf S (1983) Effects of positive and negative pressure ventilation on cardiac performance. Clin Chest Med 4:161-187
12. Holt JP (1942) The effect of positive and negative intrathoracic pressure on cardiac output and venous pressure in the dog. Am J Physiol 135:594-603
13. Duomarco JL, Rimini R (1954) Energy and hydraulic gradients along systemic veins. Am J Physiol 178:215-220
14. Permutt S, Riley RL (1963) Hemodynamics of collapsible vessels with tone: the vascular waterfall. J Appl Physiol 18:924-932
15. Natori H, Tamaki S, Dira S (1979) Ultrasonographic evaluation of ventilatory effect on inferior vena caval configuration. Am Rev Respir Dis 120:421-427
16. Smith HJ, Grottum P, Simonsen S (1985) Ultrasonic assessment of abdominal venous return: I. Effect of cardiac action and respiration on mean velocity pattern, cross-sectional area and flow in the inferior vena cava and portal vein. Acta Radiol Diagnosis 26:581-588
17. Scharf SM, Ingram RH (1977) Influence of abdominal pressure and sympathetic vasoconstriction on the cardiovascular response to positive and end-expiratory pressure. Am Rev Respir Dis 116:661-670
18. Wise RA, Robotham JL (1987) Determinants of inferior vena cava (IVC) blood flow with changes in abdominal pressure. Am Rev Respir Dis (Part II) 135:A115
19. Lemaire F, Teboul JL, Cinotti L, et al (1988) Acute left ventricular dysfunction during unsuccessful weaning from mechanical ventilation. Anesthesiology 69:171-179
20. Permutt S (1988) Circulatory effects of weaning from mechanical ventilation: The importance of transdiaphragmatic pressure (editorial). Anesthesiology 69:157-160
21. Alexander RS (1951) Influence of the diaphragm upon portal blood flow and venous return. Am J Physiol 167:738-748

22. Brecher GA, Huba CA (1965) Pulmonary blood flow and venous return during spontaneous respiration. Circ Res 3:210–214
23. Kashtan J, Green JF, Parsons EQ, Holcroft JW (1981) Hemodynamic effect of increased abdominal pressure. J Surg Res 30:249–255
24. Lloyd TC Jr (1983) Effect of inspiration on inferior vena cava blood flow in dogs. J Appl Physiol 55:1701–1708
25. Mixter G (1953) Respiratory augmentation of inferior vena caval flow demonstrated by a low resistance phasic flowmeter. Am J Physiol 172:446–456
26. Brookhart JM, Boyd TE (1947) Local differences in intrathoracic pressure and their relation to cardiac filling pressure in the dog. Am J Physiol 148:434–444
27. Marini JJ, Culver BH, Butler J (1981) Mechanical effect of lung distension with positive pressure or cardiac function. Am Rev Respir Dis 124:382–386
28. Badke FR, Boinay P, Covell JW (1980) Effects of ventricular pacing on regional left ventricular performance in the dog. Am J Physiol 238:H858–H867
29. Little WC, Badke FR, O'Rourke RA (1984) Effect of right ventricular pressure on the end diastolic left ventricular pressure-volume relationship before and after right ventricular pressure overload in dogs without pericardia. Circ Res 54:719–730
30. Walley KR, Grover M, Raff GL, Benge JW, Hannaford B, Glantz SA (1982) Left ventricular dynamic geometry in the intact and open chest dog. Circ Res 50:573–589
31. Oboler AA, Keefe JF, Gaasch WH, Banas JS Jr, Revine HJ (1973) Influence of left ventricular isovolumic pressure upon right ventricular pressure transients. Cardiology 58:32–43
32. Santamore WP, Lynch PR, Heckman JL, Bove AA, Meyer GD (1976) Left ventricular effects on right ventricular developed pressure. J Appl Physiol 41:925–930
33. Santamore WP, Lynch PR, Meier G, Heckman J, Bove AA (1976) Myocardial interaction between the ventricles. J Appl Physiol 41:362–368
34. Little WC, Reeves RC, Arciniegas J, Katholi RE, Rogers EW (1982) Mechanism of abnormal interventricular septal motion during delayed left ventricular activation. Circulation 65:1486–1491
35. Pearlman AS, Clark CE, Henry WL, Morganroth J, Itscortz SB, Epstein SE (1976) Determinants of ventricular septal motion. Influence of relative right and left ventricular size. Circulation 54:83–89
36. Shimazaki Y, Kawashima Y, Mori T, Matsuda H, Kitamura S, Yotota K (1980) Ventricular function of single ventricle after ventricular septation. Circulation 61:653–660
37. Weyman AE, Wann S, Feigenbaum H, Dillon JC (1976) Mechanism of abnormal systal motion in patients with right ventricular volume overload: A cross-sectional echocardiographic study. Circulation 54:179–186
38. Hurford WE, Barlai-Kovach M, Strauss W, Zapol WM, Lowenstein E (1987) Canine biventricular performance during acute progressive pulmonary microembolization: Regional myocardial perfusion and fatty acid uptake. J Crit Care 2:270–281
39. Kidd BSL (1978) Complete transposition of the great arteries. In: Keith JD, Rowe RD, Vlad P (eds) Heart disease in infancy and childhood, 3rd edn. MacMillan, New York, pp 590–611
40. Maughan WL, Shoukas AA, Sagawa K, Weisfeldt ML (1979) Instantaneous pressure volume relationship of the canine right ventricle. Circ Res 44:309–315
41. Murray PA, Baig H, Fishbein MC (1979) Effects of experimental right ventricular hypertrophy on myocardial blood flow in conscious dogs. J Clin Invest 64:421–427
42. Feigl EO (1983) Coronary Physiology. Physiol Rev 63:1–205
43. Cassidy SS, Ramanthan M (1984) Dimensional analysis of the left ventricle during PEEP: relative septal and lateral wall displacements. Am J Physiol 246: (Heart Circ Physiol 14) H792–H805
44. Rankin JS, Olson CO, Arentzence CE, et al (1982) The effect of airway pressure on cardiac function in intact dogs and man. Circulation 66:108–120
45. Santamore PW, Bove AA, Heckman JL (1984) Right and left ventricular pressure-volume response to positive end-expiratory pressure. Am J Physiol 246:H114–H119
46. Dhainaut JF, Devaux JY, Monsallier JF, Brunet F, Villemant D, Huyghebaert MF (1986) Mechanisms of decreased ventricular preload during continuous positive pressure ventilation in ARDS. Chest 90:74–80

47. Scharf SM, Brown R (1982) Influence of the right ventricle on left ventricular function with PEEP. J Appl Physiol 52:254–259
48. Peters J, Kindred MK, Robotham JL (1988) Transient analysis of cardiopulmonary interactions: II. Systolic events. J Appl Physiol 64:1518–1526
49. Peters J, Fraser C, Stuart RS, Baumgartner W, Robotham JL (1989) Negative intrathoracic pressure decreases independently both left ventricular filling and emptying. Am J Physiol (Heart Circ) 257:H120–H131
50. Barash PG, Deutsch S, Tinker J, and the American Society of Anesthesiologists (eds) (1988) How respiration affects circulation. Lippincott, Philadelphia 16:192–196
51. Sylvester JT, Goldberg HS, Permutt S (1983) The role of the vasculature in the regulation of cardiac output. Clin Chest Med 4:111
52. Robotham JL (1984) Hemodynamic events: a physiological approach. In: Montenegro HD (ed) Chronic obstructive pulmonary disease. Churchill Livingstone, New York, p 183

The Role of Ventricular Interaction in Critical Illness

J. E. Calvin

Introduction

Maintenance of normal circulatory homeostasis depends upon an adequate stroke output from both ventricles in response to changes in their respective loading conditions. The anatomical arrangement of both chambers inside the pericardium dictates that the loading conditions of one ventricle can influence the passive filling of the other. Specifically, in both isolated heart preparations and in animal models [1–8], loading the right ventricle with either volume expansion or pulmonary artery constriction shifts the left ventricular (LV) diastolic pressure volume relationship upwards indicating that the ventricle is less distensible. This results in elevated LV filling pressures although LV volumes may be normal or decreased. This observation has served to focus recent attention on the various interactions that exist between both right and left ventricles.

The degree to which systolic and diastolic function of one ventricle can influence the other is a complex interplay of a series interaction, direct interactions mediated by the constraining influence of the pericardium and the position of the septum (the latter of which is influenced by the pressure gradient between both ventricles) and systolic booster effects. The series interaction refers to the fact that the LV input is composed of the right ventricular (RV) output. Should the stroke volume of the right ventricle decrease, LV preload, as measured by LV end-diastolic pressure or LV end-diastolic volume, would also decrease because of decreased pulmonary venous return. This is best demonstrated by analyzing the effects produced by occluding the vena cavae. Such a maneuver first reduces both RV size and output; LV preload and output falls within a few beats [9]. In contrast, a direct ventricular interaction mediated by the pericardium occurs when one or more cardiac chambers dilates sufficiently to both increase total cardiac volume and engage the pericardium. Because of the curvilinear relationship between intrapericardial pressure and volume, intrapericardial pressure increases and imposes an external load upon the heart. A direct interaction mediated by the septum occurs if the difference between LV and RV end-diastolic pressure decreases or reverses (Fig. 1). The septum, behaving much like a compliant membrane, can shift from its normal position curved to the right to a configuration that is curved to the left, thus impairing left ventricular filling [10]. Finally, a systolic "booster" interaction is suggested by experimental evidence that the systolic pressure generation of one ventricle can influence the pressure generation of the other even with preload and afterload controlled [11, 12]. Pre-

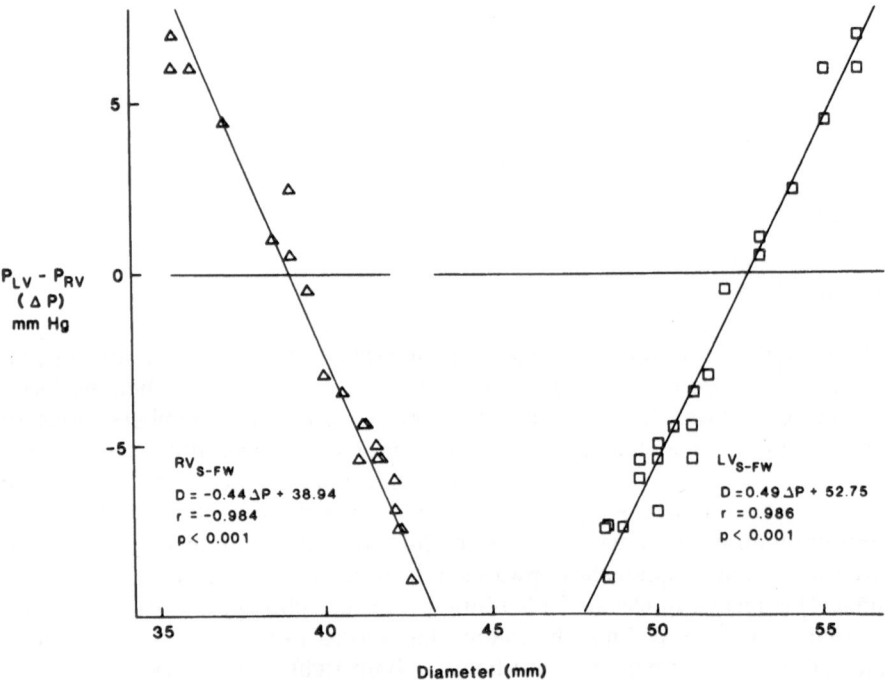

Fig. 1. End-diastolic RV (triangles) and LV (squares) septal to free wall diameters plotted against end-diastolic transseptal pressure gradient for 22 consecutive beats during the onset of pulmonary artery (PA) constriction. As a result of PA constriction, the transseptal pressure gradient decreases and reverses. This is accompanied by an increase in RV septal free wall diameter and a decrease in LV septal free wall diameter. (From [10])

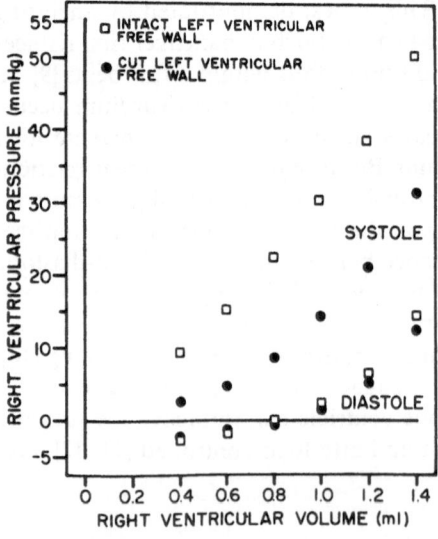

Fig. 2. The influence of cutting the LV free wall on RV isovolumic pressure. This data was obtained from an isolated rabbit heart preparation after cutting the LV free wall. This intervention prevented the left ventricle from generating force during systole and thereby eliminating the contribution of LV free wall to right ventricular developed pressure. (From [2])

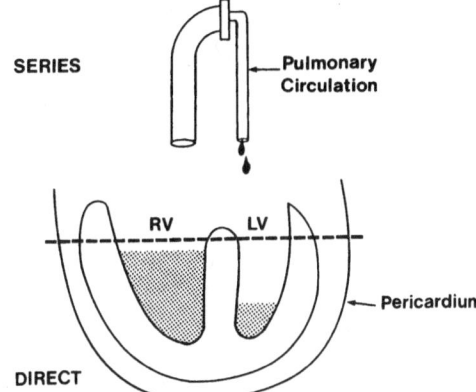

Fig. 3. A schematic diagram depicting the influence of RV pressure overload on series and direct interactions. The left ventricle becomes underfilled because of reduced RV stroke output. This reduction is further enhanced by an increase in intrapericardial pressure and reversal of the transseptal pressure gradient

sumably this is on the basis of shared fibres between the two ventricles (Fig. 2).

In some clinical situations all interactions may occur. For instance, an acute elevation of pulmonary vascular resistance sufficient to cause the right ventricle to fail can depress stroke volume and LV preload by its series effect, increase RV volume and intrapericardial pressure, reverse the transseptal pressure gradient and reduce the systolic booster effects (Fig. 3).

The Effect of a Direct Pericardial Interaction upon Left Ventricular Diastolic Pressure-Volume Relationships

Although it is well accepted that ischemia and hypertrophy can alter LV pressure volume relationships, only recent attention has been paid to external loads, which may cause shifts in LV diastolic pressure-volume relationship. It is now apparent that external loads are indeed important factors, capable of substantially altering ventricular compliance properties. Specifically, the right ventricle through the pericardial interaction can acutely induce shifts of the LV diastolic pressure-volume relationship. Recent studies have emphasized how the right ventricle may influence LV compliance by demonstrating that an upward shift of the LV diastolic pressure-volume curve (i.e., reduced compliance) accompanies RV volume increases at end-diastole (Fig. 4) [1–8, 13]. Although this effect is present with the pericardium open, the coupling is much stronger when it is closed. Ventricular interaction is therefore an important mechanism underlying acute reductions in LV compliance, whether the right ventricle is enlarged due to either pressure or volume overload. Ventricular interaction may also be responsible for some of the improved LV compliance properties observed with the administration of vasoactive medications that reduce volume return to the right ventricle (e.g., nitrates).

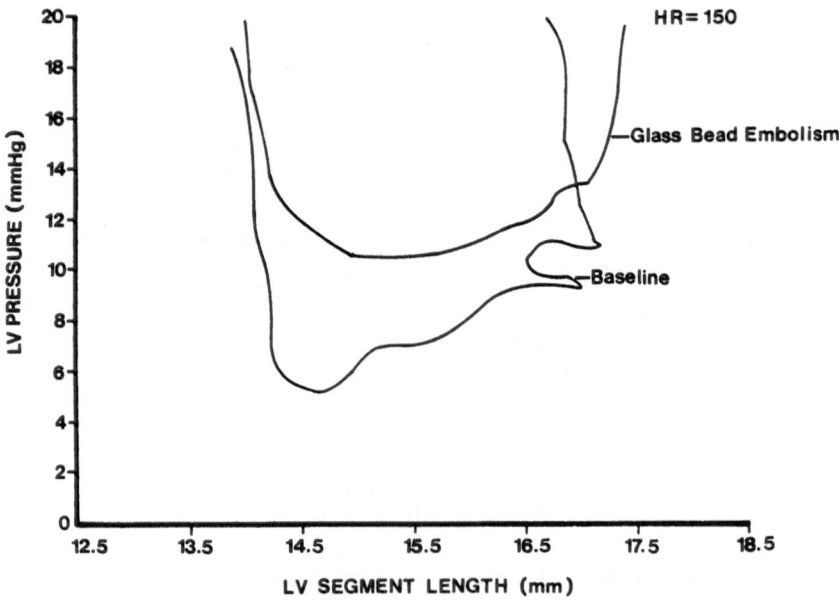

Fig. 4. LV diastolic pressure-segment length relationship during glass bead embolism in a canine model. Preinstrumented dogs were embolized with glass beads sufficient to at least double the mean pulmonary artery pressure. Heart rates were kept constant by pacing. Glass bead embolism resulted in an upward shift in the LV segment length relationship. The pericardium is closed. (From [4])

The Significance of Ventricular Interaction in Normal Physiology

Ventricular interactions have been thought to play a role in the cardiopulmonary response to changes in posture and respiration. Hoffman et al. [14] observed an initial fall in RV stroke volume in dogs tilted from supine to erect position which was then followed by a reduction in LV stroke volume after three beats. Although this is likely to be on the basis of a series interaction, a diastolic interaction could also explain these observed results, in as much as a reduction in RV volume during upright posture could reduce venous return to the right ventricle, reduce intrapericardial pressure and improve LV compliance.

During inspiration, RV end-diastolic volume and stroke volume both increase while LV stroke volume remains constant or decreases. Marked respiratory loading by the Mueller maneuver can cause RV volume increases, shift the septum leftwards and reduce LV compliance. The net effect could decrease LV end-diastolic volume or size [15, 16]. However, one should be careful to remember that increased LV afterload could also partially explain this phenomenon as well as heart lung interactions which could impair ventricular filling by the development of a significant contact pressure between the heart and the lungs.

Observed Ventricular Interdependence in Pathophysiological States

The Role of the Pericardium in Pulsus Paradoxus Produced by Cardiac Tamponade

It is generally accepted that arterial blood pressure can fluctuate with respiration normally. It is well recognized that this fluctuation is more marked with forced inspiratory effort as noted above or pericardial tamponade. Ventricular interaction can explain pulsus paradoxus in cardiac tamponade as well as the Mueller maneuver. The normal reason for the inspiratory fall in blood pressure is a combination of an increase in LV afterload because of the lower intrathoracic pressure and an insufficient increase in venous return to the right ventricle to compensate for the elevated afterload [17]. This latter effect is probably a reflection of the fact that the systemic veins collapse. However, a small selective increase in RV preload is present for at least several beats. Because the two ventricles share pericardial space, and share the septum, two other changes occur as a result: the intrapericardial pressure increases and the transseptal pressure decreases. Normally these changes cause only small oscillation in blood pressure. However, during cardiac tamponade the intrapericardial pressure is already quite high and the venous system is already distended. This increases the interaction between the two ventricles as the constraining barrier of the pericardium is engaged. The respiratory increase in RV preload now encroaches upon LV filling by shifting the septum leftwards (through a decrease in transseptal pressure gradient) and by increasing intrapericardial pressure further. This reduces LV preload more than under normal circumstances. In the face of an elevated LV afterload mismatched to a diminished LV preload, LV stroke volume falls drastically producing the pulsus paradoxus.

Right Ventricular Volume Overload

Hemodynamic abnormalities of LV function have been previously reported in RV volume overload such as atrial septal defect. Hemodynamically, these abnormalities appear to be elevated LV filling pressures and adequate cardiac output at rest or with exercise [2]. Recent echocardiographic studies have determined paradoxical interventricular septal motion in patients with RV pressure overload and volume overload [18, 19] suggesting a transseptal interaction. One recent study has suggested that there is a reduction in LV distensibility in these conditions [20].

Chronic Right Ventricular Pressure Overload

In chronic RV pressure overload, as seen in cor pulmonale, the literature is somewhat mixed. There appears to be a number of studies that support normal LV function [21-23] and a number that support abnormal LV function. In a number of these studies reduced LV ejection fractions [21, 24, 25], LV hypertrophy [26] and elevated filling pressures [27] were observed. A report of Krayen-buehl et al. [28] is noteworthy for it helps to link these apparent contradictions. In 10 women with chronic pulmonary hypertension, they determined that LV end-diastolic pressure was significantly greater and end-diastolic volume significantly smaller in patients with pulmonary hypertension compared to control subjects. They also demonstrated that these patients had abnormal LV geometry and an abnormal septal configuration. These observations, then, suggest that LV dysfunction may be more on the basis of a diastolic abnormality mediated by a direct ventricular interaction.

The Relative Importance of Series Interaction Over Direct Pericardial Interactions During Acute Right Ventricular Pressure Overload

Although all interactions are potentially operational during acute RV pressure overload it has not been well established until recently which interactions are the most important. In an experimental model of acute pulmonary hypertension induced by infusing small glass beads into the pulmonary circulation, we observed that the absence of a pericardium did not prevent the decrease in LV preload and stroke work after glass bead embolism [4]. This suggested to us the predominance of a series interaction over a direct interaction. If the latter were dominant, an open pericardium would have resulted in a smaller decrease in LV preload caused by acute pulmonary hypertension, because the competition between both ventricles for the available space would have been removed. In these studies, LV preload was measured using LV free wall segment length crystals. The end-diastolic length fell to 94% and 96% of baseline values in both open and closed pericardia experiments. Hence, the series interaction appears to dominate, although a direct interaction mediated by the septum may still be present. However, this observation was made with the realization that in this study RV filling pressures, although they had increased by 3 mmHg, were not excessively high when a direct interaction may have had more influence. Similarly, Molaug et al. [29] also found that the pericardium did not restrain the ventricles during selective pressure loading, because as one ventricle dilated, the other shrunk regardless of the presence of the pericardium.

A second observation of ours also supported our hypothesis that a series interaction dominated the direct interaction of the pericardium. Nitroglycerin decreased RV preload (as measured by RV free wall segment length crystal) and shifted the LV pressure-segment length relation downwards (approximately 1 mmHg) in at least 4 of 6 dogs. Although these two effects might have increased LV preload by making more space available within the pericardium and by improving LV diastolic function, they did not. This is most likely because RV stroke volume also fell secondary to decreased RV preload (series effect). The series effects upon stroke volume and biventricular preload outweighed the potential benefits of improved LV diastolic function. Thus, it is apparent that series effects represent the major interaction between both ventricles in as much as flow is concerned. A direct effect or interaction between both ventricles mediated by the pericardium appears to have more influence upon filling pressures.

Ventricular Interaction During Right Ventricular Infarction

RV infarction is clinically characterized by elevated jugular veins, clear chest examination and hypotension. Although not all patients with RV infarction have this clinical triad, RV infarction does constitute an important and reversible cause of cardiogenic shock.

The importance of RV contractility in maintaining cardiac output has been disputed in the past. However, the clinical entity of RV infarction has renewed interest and recently a role for ventricular interaction has been implicated in the pathophysiology of a low cardiac output state in this condition.

In 1982, Goldstein et al. [30] described a canine model of RV infarction produced by ligating the right coronary artery and injecting the distal right coronary with elemental mercury. The infarct, so produced, decreased RV systolic pressure 27%, aortic pressure 29% and cardiac output by 34% with the pericardium intact. In addition, RV transmural pressure, RV end-diastolic size and intrapericardial pressure also increased, ventricular diastolic pressures equalized and LV end-diastolic size and transmural pressure decreased. Opening the pericardium increased ventricular transmural pressures, end-diastolic size, and cardiac output. Therefore, these results suggest that elevated intrapericardial pressure plays a significant role in the pathophysiology of RV infarction by its effect on limiting LV preload.

A study by Goto et al. [31] in one group of open-chest dogs determined that right coronary artery (RCA) occlusion with the pericardium intact reduced aortic flow by approximately 24% and LV septal-lateral dimensions by $8 \pm 5\%$. Other parameters of LV systolic function were normal. In another group of 8 dogs they determined that during RCA occlusion the LV diastolic pressure volume relationship shifted upwards compared to the open pericardial state.

Both of these studies suggest a significant role for ventricular interaction mediated by the pericardium. The role of a transseptal interaction needs further exploration.

Effect of Drugs upon Left Ventricular Diastolic Pressure-Volume Relationships

In patients manifesting reduced LV compliance due to acute myocardial ischemia, both sodium nitroprusside [32] and nitroglycerin [10] have been demonstrated to shift the LV end-diastolic pressure-volume relationship down and to the right and, hence, mediate an improvement in LV compliance. The pericardium appears to be an important modulator of this effect because such shifts are not observed when the pericardium has been surgically removed.

Without this effect on LV end-diastolic pressure-volume relationships (i.e. improved compliance), much of the benefit observed during the use of vasodilators might be effectively counterbalanced by their effects to reduce venous tone and venous return and, therefore, LV preload and stroke volume. However, the concomitant improvement in LV compliance observed with these vasodilators maintains end-diastolic volume while it reduces the end-diastolic pressure. The pres-

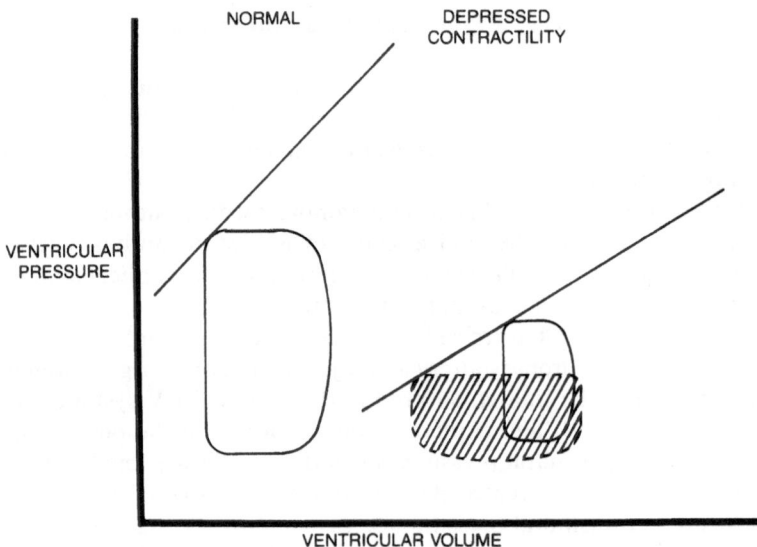

Fig. 5. The influence of vasodilators on ventricular pressure-volume relationships in heart failure. Downward shifting of the pressure-volume relationship results in a reduced filling pressure at a near constant end-diastolic volume which supports maintenance of stroke output

sure-volume loop of a ventricle characterized by depressed contractility is indicated by the solid line in Fig. 5. The effect of a vasodilator, with both afterload-reducing and venodilating effects, is shown by the pressure-volume loop enclosed within the hatched area. In this example, an improvement in LV compliance is characterized as a downward shift of the ventricular diastolic pressure-volume relationship, which thereby maintains end-diastolic volume while end-diastolic pressure falls. The concurrent reduction in afterload results in a lowering of the pressure at which aortic ejection commences and results in the conversion of pressure work to volume work; an increase in SV results while stroke work may not change significantly.

As a result of improved LV compliance, the decrease in end-diastolic pressures (i. e., PCWP) that follows should be accompanied by a reduced $M\dot{V}O_2$. A decrease in the PCWP with vasodilators will also augment those interstitial safety factors responsible for protecting against the development of pulmonary edema. Concurrently, vasodilators reduce LV afterload, which will be associated with improved SV and oxygen transport when end-diastolic volumes are normal to greater than normal before administration.

The Effect of PEEP on Cardiac Function: The Role of Ventricular and Heart/Lung Interactions

Reduced cardiac output with the application of PEEP has been previously variously explained as a consequence of:

1. depressed LV and RV preload;
2. depressed LV contractility and;
3. increased RV afterload [33].

All of these mechanisms have been demonstrated experimentally. Clinically a reduction in ventricular compliance has also been observed with the institution of PEEP which may depress ventricular preload over and above the reduction in venous return. Jardin et al. [34] suggested that the cause of a depression in LV compliance with the use of PEEP was a leftward septal shift consequent upon RV pressure overload, i.e., the concept of direct transseptal ventricular interaction due to a PEEP afterloading effect on the right ventricle.

However, others [3, 35–37] have concluded that PEEP alters LV distensibility by increasing intrapericardial pressures through the external force it applies to the surface of the heart. In a previous study of ours, PEEP was simulated by hyperinflation of the lung in an open chest animal model. Although such a model would be expected to underestimate the PEEP effects, end-expiratory airway pressures of 15 mmHg were maintained. A reduction in both RV and LV size measured by piezoelectric dimension crystals resulted with this degree of positive airway pressure, primarily through a reduction in both RV and LV ventricular septal to free wall dimensions. Despite the reduction in ventricular size, intracavitary pressures were unchanged from control. This observation defined that a primary effect of lung hyperinflation was to reduce ventricular compliance by the lungs physically compressing both ventricles from the outside; there was no evidence that the right ventricle dilated under the effects of the increased RV afterload. Hence, RV dilation could not be responsible for a leftward septal shift.

Using implanted radiopaque markers, Cassidy and Ramanathan [35] also noted that PEEP restricted the outward expansion of the LV lateral wall during diastole; the position of the septum was not displaced by PEEP (Fig. 6). It would therefore appear that PEEP is capable of causing a leftward shift in LV pressure-volume relationships (i.e., reduction in compliance) by altering biventricular geometry because of direct compressive forces exerted on the heart surface with its use.

The effect of PEEP on cardiac performance must integrate heart lung interactions with the observed effects upon biventricular preload and afterload. All these mechanisms can be integrated into a force velocity analysis. Figure 7 demonstrates (left panel) the force-velocity relationship using RV output on the Y-axis and vascular load, as would be measured by the pulmonary input impedance spectra on the X-axis. A reduction in stroke output seen with PEEP is much more than can be accounted for by an increase in afterload alone. Instead of moving from points A to B, in this example, the patient moves to point C because of the combined effects of a reduced RV preload and an increased RV afterload. The only way to restore RV output to normal resting values would be to increase ventricular preload to levels substantially above normal (point D). Hence, increasing transmural pressure to that of the control state may be insufficient to increase RV output because of the increased afterload that the right ventricle encounters with the use of PEEP. In fact, transmural pressures must be

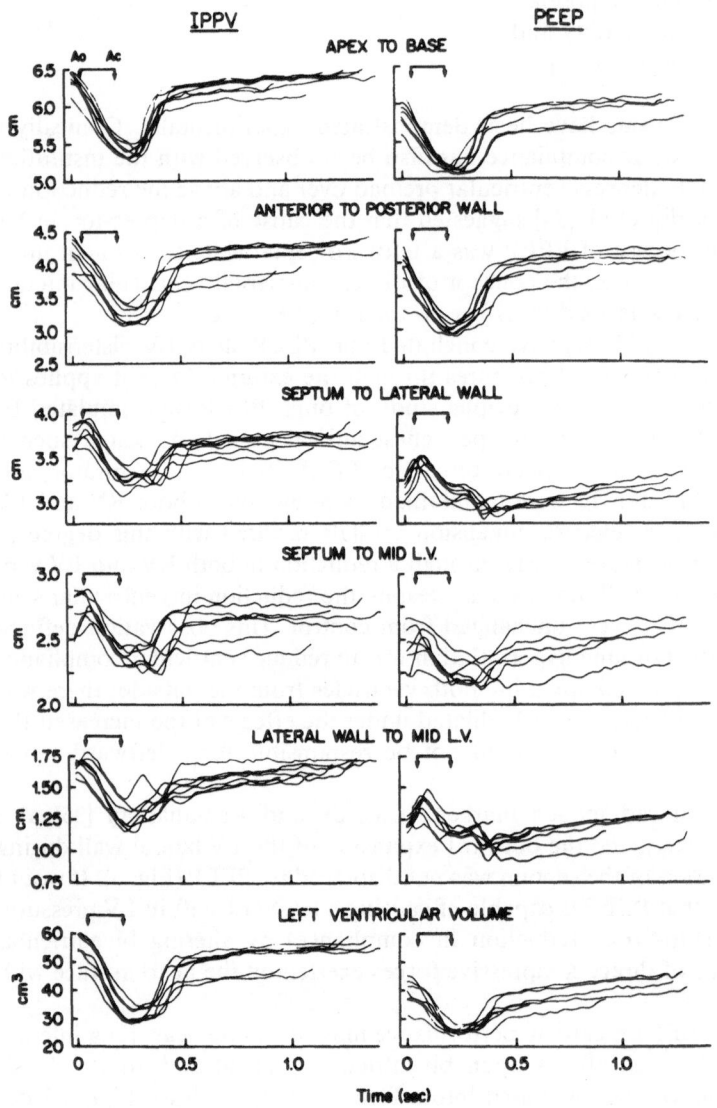

Fig. 6. LV dimensions and volumes plotted throughout one cardiac cycle beginning and ending with an R wave in each dog during intermittent positive pressure ventilation and 10 cm H_2O of PEEP. LV volume falls largely because of inward displacement of the lateral free wall

increased to higher levels found at baseline in order to restore the stroke output to control values.

The effects of PEEP on the left ventricle are somewhat different. PEEP also reduces LV preload because of a reduction in RV stroke output (i.e., a series interaction) as well as by inducing an upward and leftward shift of the diastolic pressure-volume curve (reduced compliance). However, unlike its effects on the

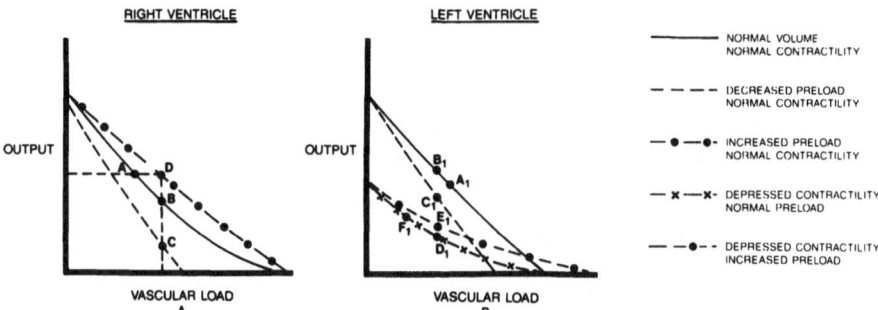

Fig. 7. The influence of PEEP upon ventricular function using force velocity analysis (see text for explanation, reprinted with permission from Textbook of Critical Care Medicine, Saunders)

right ventricle, PEEP reduces rather than increases LV afterload by increasing the intrathoracic pressure [38] (Fig. 7 right panel). A reduction in LV preload with PEEP has less of an effect on forward output because of the concomitant reduction in LV afterload. Hence, the patient moves from points A to C with only a small decrease in LV stroke output ensuing. In cases of LV ventricular failure in which contractility is depressed, the Y-intercept is lower and the slope of the force-velocity relationship is much flatter. Thus, the effect of PEEP on preload is very much abbreviated and its afterload-reducing effects are much more dominant. In this case, the patient would be operating at point E_1 before PEEP administration. The effect of PEEP to concomitantly decrease LV afterload moves the patient to point F_1, resulting in either an unchanged or an increased LV output. This is why PEEP may mediate an improvement in cardiac performance in some patients with LV failure.

References

1. Badke FR (1982) Left ventricular dimensions and function during right ventricular pressure overload. Am J Physiol 242:H611–H618
2. Bove AA, Santamore WP (1981) Ventricular interdependence. Prog Cardiovasc Dis 23:365–388
3. Calvin JE, Baer RW, Glantz SA (1986) Pulmonary injury depresses cardiac systolic function through Starling mechanism. Am J Physiol 251:H722–H733
4. Calvin JE, Langlois S, Garneys G (1988) Ventricular interaction in a canine model of acute pulmonary hypertension and its modulation by vasoactive drugs. J Crit Care 3:43–55
5. Stool EW, Mullins CB, Leshin SJ, et al (1974) Dimensional changes of the left ventricle during acute pulmonary arterial hypertension in dogs. Am J Cardiol 33:868–875
6. Visner MS, Arentzen CE, O'Connor MJ, et al (1983) Alterations in left ventricular three-dimensional dynamic geometry and systolic function during acute right ventricular hypertension in the conscious dog. Circulation 67:353–364
7. Taylor RR, Covell JW, Sonnenblick EH, et al (1967) Dependence of ventricular distensibility on the filling of the opposite ventricle. Am J Physiol 213:711–718
8. Glantz SA, Misbach GA, Moores WY, et al (1977) The pericardium substantially affects the left ventricular diastolic pressure volume relationship in the dog. Circ Res 42:433–441

9. Olsen CO, Tyson GS, Maier GW, et al (1983) Dynamic ventricular interaction in the conscious dog. Circ Res 52:85–104

10. Kingma I, Tyberg JV, Smith ER (1983) Effects of diastolic transseptal pressure gradient on ventricular septal position and motion. Circulation 6:1304–1314

11. Feneley MP, Olsen CO, Glower DD, Rankin JS (1989) Effect of acutely increased right ventricular afterload on work output from the left ventricle in conscious dogs. Circ Res 65:135–145

12. Santamore WP, Lynch PR, Heckman JL, et al (1976) Left ventricular effects on right ventricular developed pressure. J Appl Physiol 41:925–930

13. Lorell BH, Palacios I, Daggett WM, et al (1981) Right ventricular distension and left ventricular compliance. Am J Physiol 240:H87–H97

14. Hoffman JIE, Guz A, Charlier A, et al (1965) Effects of spontaneous respiration, posture and vascular occlusion. J Appl Physiol 20:865

15. Brinker JA, Weiss JL, Lappe DLK, et al (1980) Leftward septal displacement during right ventricular loading in man. Circulation 61:626–633

16. Guzman PA, Maughan WL, Yin FCP, et al (1981) Transseptal pressure gradient with leftward septal displacement during the Mueller manoeuvre in man. Br Heart J 46:657–662

17. McGregor M (1979) Medical intelligence: Pulsus paradoxus. N Engl J Med 301:480–482

18. Weyman AE, Wann S, Feigenbaum H, et al (1976) Mechanism of abnormal septal motion in patients with right ventricular volume overload. Circulation 54:179–186

19. Feneley M, Gavaghan T (1986) Paradoxical and pseudoparadoxical interventricular septal motion in patients with right ventricular volume overload. Circulation 74:230–238

20. Booth DC, Wisenbaugh T, Smith M (1988) Left ventricular distensibility and passive elastic stiffness in atrial septal defect. J Am Coll Cardiol 12:1231–1236

21. Frank MJ, Weisse AB, Moschos CB, et al (1973) Left ventricular function, metabolism and blood flow in chronic cor pulmonale. Circulation 47:798–806

22. Williams JF, Childress RH, Boyd DL, et al (1968) Left ventricular function in patients with chronic obstructive pulmonary disease. J Clin Invest 47:1143–1153

23. Davies H, Ovey HR (1970) Left ventricular function in cor pulmonale. Chest 58:8–14

24. Kline LE, Crawford MH, MacDonald WJ, et al (1977) Noninvasive assessment of left ventricular performance in patients with chronic obstructive pulmonary disease. Chest 72:558–564

25. Steele P, Ellis JR Jr, VanDyke D, et al (1975) Left ventricular ejection fraction in chronic obstructive airways disease. Am J Med 59:21–28

26. Murphy ML, Adamson J, Hutcheson F (1974) Left ventricular hypertrophy in patients with chronic bronchitis and emphysema. Ann Intern Med 81:307–313

27. Unger K, Shaw D, Karliner JS, et al (1975) Evaluation of left ventricular performance in acutely ill patients with chronic obstructive lung disease. Chest 68:135–142

28. Krayenbuehl HP, Turing J, Hess O (1978) Left ventricular function in chronic pulmonary hypertension. Am J Cardiol 41:1150–1158

29. Molaug M, Stokland O, Ilebekk A, et al (1981) Myocardial function of the interventricular septum: Effects of right and left ventricular pressure loading before and after pericardiectomy in dogs. Circ Res 49:52–61

30. Goldstein JA, Vlahakes GJ, Verrier ED, et al (1982) The role of right ventricular systolic dysfunction and elevated intrapericardial pressure in the genesis of low output in experimental right ventricular infarction. Circulation 65:513–522

31. Goto Y, Yamamoto J, Saito M, et al (1985) Effects of right ventricular ischemia on left ventricular geometry and the end-diastolic pressure-volume relationship in the dog. Circulation 72:1104–1114

32. Alderman EL, Glantz SA (1976) Acute hemodynamic interventions shift the diastolic pressure-volume curve in man. Circulation 54:662–671

33. Calvin JE, Kieser TM, Walley VM, Barber G, McPhail NV, Scobie TK (1985) Cardiac mortality/morbidity after vascular surgery: Clinical and pathological correlations. Clin Invest Med 8:A49

34. Jardin F, Farcot JC, Boisante L, et al (1981) Influence of positive end expiratory pressure on left ventricular performance. N Engl J Med 304:387–390

35. Cassidy SS, Ramanatham M (1984) Dimensional analysis of the left ventricle during PEEP: relative septal and lateral wall displacements. Am J Physiol 15:H792–H805
36. Scharf SM, Brown R, Tow DE, et al (1979) Cardiac effects of increased lung volume and decreased pleural pressure in man. J Appl Physiol 42:257–262
37. Robotham JL, Bell RC, Badke FR, et al (1985) Left ventricular geometry during positive end-expiratory pressure in dogs. Crit Care Med 13:617–624
38. Buda AJ, Pinsky MR, Engels NB, et al (1979) Effect of intrathoracic pressure on left ventricular performance. N Engl J Med 301:453–459

Cardiac Dysfunction

The Role of α_1- and α_2-Adrenoceptors in the Regulation of the Cardiovascular System

R. R. Ruffolo Jr. and A. J. Nichols

Introduction

The cardiovascular system is regulated in large part by α-adrenoceptors. The neurotransmitter, noradrenaline (norepinephrine), and the blood-borne hormone, adrenaline (epinephrine), influence cardiovascular function under normal homeostatic conditions and in a variety of pathophysiologic conditions through interaction with α-adrenoceptors in the major effector organs of the cardiovascular system, such as the heart, vasculature and kidney. An understanding of these receptors, in terms of their function, location, and distribution, is of primary importance in treating the critically ill patient inasmuch as many of the drugs available to treat these patients have the capacity to stimulate or block α-adrenoceptors in the cardiovascular system.

α-Adrenoceptors in the Cardiovascular System

α-Adrenoceptor Subclassification

Adrenoceptors may be subdivided into the α-type and β-type [1]. β-Adrenoceptors are selectively activated by adrenaline, noradrenaline and isoprenaline. α-Adrenoceptors are also stimulated by adrenaline and noradrenaline, but are resistant to isoprenaline. β-Adrenoceptors may be subdivided further into the β_1- and β_2-subtypes; isoprenaline and adrenaline stimulate both subtypes, and noradrenaline stimulates only the β_1-subtype. Likewise, α-adrenoceptors have been subdivided into the α_1- and α_2-subtypes, and adrenaline and noradrenaline stimulate both. Although the naturally occurring catecholamines cannot distinguish between α_1- and α_2-adrenoceptors, many synthetic drugs do. Thus, phenylephrine and methoxamine are potent and highly selective α_1-adrenoceptor agonists, whereas clonidine and α-methylnoradrenaline, the latter being the active metabolite of α-methyldopa, are potent and selective α_2-adrenoceptor agonists [2].

Central α-Adrenoceptors

Stimulation of central α_2-adrenoceptors in the ventrolateral medulla induces a reduction in sympathetic outflow to the periphery, manifested as a reduction in arterial blood pressure accompanied by bradycardia. This response has been studied extensively over the past two decades and several comprehensive reviews are available [3–5]. Quantitative structure-activity studies have shown excellent correlation between the α_2-adrenoceptor agonist potency of a series of clonidine analogs, and blood pressure reduction, provided a lipophilicity term is included to correct for penetration through the blood-brain barrier which is required in order to gain access to the site of action within the central nervous system [6].

The characteristic response to intravenous administration of an α_2-adrenoceptor agonist in a normotensive or hypertensive subject is an immediate pressor response, due to stimulation of peripheral arterial postjunctional α_2-adrenoceptors [7]. This pressor response is relatively short-lived, and is followed by a slow decline in arterial blood pressure to levels lower than those observed prior to drug administration. This long-lasting depressor/antihypertensive response is a result of central α_2-adrenoceptor stimulation. Heart rate declines immediately following administration, and continues to be reduced for the duration of the hypotensive response.

The antihypertensive action of α_2-adrenoceptor agonists results from stimulation of postsynaptic α_2-adrenoceptors in the brainstem [8]. Many experiments have been performed in an attempt to locate more precisely the site of action of α_2-adrenoceptor agonists within the brainstem. Although the nucleus tractus solitarius has been often considered as the principal site of action of central α_2-adrenoceptor agonists [3], recent studies using microinjections of clonidine suggest the lateral reticular nucleus in the ventrolateral medulla as a more likely candidate [9]. This nucleus is readily accessible from the ventral surface of the medulla, where α_2-adrenoceptor agonists have been shown to be effective following local application [9].

Central α_2-adrenoceptor stimulation is utilized clinically for antihypertensive therapy. In addition to the directly acting central α_2-adrenoceptor agonists discussed above, α-methyldopa, which has been extensively employed for nearly two decades, is now known to stimulate central α_2-adrenoceptors following metabolic conversion to α-methylnorepinephrine [10], which has much greater α_2-adrenoceptor selectivity than noradrenaline [11]. Following chronic treatment with α-methyldopa in rats, medullary noradrenaline stores are almost completely replaced by α-methylnoradrenaline which is available for interaction with medullary α_2-adrenoceptors to inhibit sympathetic outflow and lower blood pressure.

One important issue associated with antihypertensive therapy with centrally acting α_2-adrenoceptor agonists is the "rebound hypertension" or "withdrawal" phenomenon that often occurs when treatment is abruptly terminated [12]. This phenomenon is characterized by tachycardia and abrupt rises in blood pressure, sometimes to levels greater than that observed before initiation of therapy. Studies in animals have confirmed the presence of a hyper-adrenergic state following abrupt termination of chronic clonidine therapy. Administration of an α_2-adrenoceptor antagonist, such as yohimbine, can also precipitate this withdrawal phenomenon.

The withdrawal phenomenon observed following abrupt cessation of α_2-adrenoceptor agonist therapy bears some similarity to opiate withdrawal [13], and appears to involve overactivity of locus coeruleus neurons [14]. This may represent a rebound phenomenon following chronic suppression of the firing rate of these neurons during chronic antihypertensive treatment. In view of the similarities and possible receptor interactions between α_2-adrenoceptors and opiate receptors, it is not surprising that morphine can suppress, *via* a naloxone sensitive mechanism, some of the cardiovascular rebound effects observed following termination of clonidine infusion in rats [13].

Peripheral Arterial α-Adrenoceptors

Systemic Circulation: It is now widely accepted that arterial vasoconstriction may be mediated by a mixed population of postjunctional vascular α_1- and α_2-adrenoceptors. The physiologic function and/or distribution of these receptors is now beginning to be understood. It appears that in the arterial circulation, postjunctional vascular α-adrenoceptors located at the neuroeffector junction (i.e., junctional receptors) are of the α_1-subtype, while those located away from the neuroeffector junction (i.e., extrajunctional receptors) are of the α_2-subtype [15].

The physiologic role of the postsynaptic junctional arterial α_1-adrenoceptors appears to be in maintaining resting vascular tone. These receptors, which are located in the vicinity of the neuro-vascular junction, would interact with endogenous noradrenaline liberated from sympathetic nerves. In contrast, the extrajunctional α_2-adrenoceptors would not normally interact with liberated noradrenaline since they are located at some distance away from the adrenergic nerve terminal. It has been proposed that the extrajunctional α_2-adrenoceptors may respond to circulating adrenaline liberated from the adrenal gland and acting as a blood-borne hormone [15]. The contribution made by arterial extrajunctional α_2-adrenoceptors to total peripheral vascular resistance may be greater in hypertensive patients than in normotensive patients [16], implying that postjunctional vascular α_2-adrenoceptors may play an important role in pathophysiological states such as hypertension and possibly congestive heart failure, where circulating catecholamine levels are high.

Coronary Circulation: While the precise role of α-adrenoceptor stimulation in the dynamic regulation of coronary blood flow is still unclear, it has been known for some time that following β-adrenoceptor blockade, α-adrenoceptor agonists, or cardiac sympathetic nerve stimulation, can produce coronary artery vasoconstriction leading to an increase in coronary arterial resistance and a decrease in coronary artery blood flow. It has recently been suggested that α_2-adrenoceptors may play a role in the α-adrenoceptor mediated regulation of coronary artery blood flow. In the presence of β-adrenoceptor blockade, intracoronary administration of the selective α_1-adrenoceptor agonist, phenylephrine, and the selective α_2-adrenoceptor agonist, B-HT 933, produce a rapid decrease in coronary artery blood flow, and these effects are blocked by the α_1- and α_2-adrenoceptor agonists, prazosin and rauwolscine, respectively [17]. The reduction in coronary artery blood flow elicited by exogenously administered noradrenaline is antagonized to a greater degree by rauwolscine than by prazosin, indicating a more prominent role of α_2-adrenoceptors in the regulation of coronary artery blood flow [17]. The presence of α_1-adrenoceptors on the large, epicardial coronary arteries has recently been demonstrated [18], while α_2-adrenoceptors appear to be located primarily on the smaller subendocardial resistance vessels of the coronary vascular bed [19].

It has recently been shown that the selective α_2-adrenoceptor antagonist, idazoxan, produces a greater degree of blockade of the coronary vasoconstrictor response to sympathetic nerve stimulation than does the selective α_1-adrenoceptor antagonist, prazosin [19]. Thus, in the coronary circulation, both α-adrenoceptor subtypes mediate vasoconstriction, and the postjunctional vascular α_2-adrenoceptors may be preferentially innervated.

Pulmonary Circulation: Postjunctional vascular α_1- and α_2-adrenoceptors mediate vasoconstriction in the pulmonary circulation of the dog and cat [20, 21]. As such, prazosin and rauwolscine both antagonize the increases in pulmonary perfusion pressure elicited by exogenously administered noradrenaline [20, 21]. Pulmonary pressor responses to endogenous noradrenaline released from sympathetic nerves are antagonized primarily by prazosin, with little or no effect of rauwolscine. It appears, therefore, that endogenous noradrenaline acts primarily on junctional α_1-adrenoceptors in the pulmonary vascular bed of the dog [22].

When pulmonary vascular tone is elevated, even slightly, with a vasoconstrictor agent, responses to the selective α_2-adrenoceptor agonist B-HT 933 are markedly potentiated. Furthermore, the enhanced responsiveness of α_2-adrenoceptors is tone-dependent and highly selective for α_2-adrenoceptors, since responses to the α_1-adrenoceptor agonist, methoxamine, or to angiotensin II are not potentiated by elevating pulmonary vascular tone [22]. The nature of the vasoconstrictor agent used to elevate pulmonary vascular tone does not influence the enhanced α_2-adrenoceptor responsiveness, although the manner in which pulmonary vascular pressure is elevated is critically important. When pulmonary perfusion pressure is elevated by increased pulmonary blood flow as opposed to pulmonary vasoconstriction, responses to α_2-adrenoceptor agonists are not potentiated as they are when vasoconstrictor agents are utilized to elevate pulmonary pressure [22]. This observation indicates that pulmonary vascular smooth muscle tone, and not pulmonary pressure *per se,* is the major determinant of the potentiation in α_2-adrenoceptor responsiveness in the pulmonary vasculature. This selective potentiation of α_2-adrenoceptor-mediated vasoconstriction in the pulmonary circulation under conditions of high pulmonary vascular tone may be relevant to certain pathophysiologic conditions such as congestive heart failure where pulmonary vascular resistance is elevated and circulating catecholamine levels are high. Both of these factors may predispose the patient to a further exacerbation of the elevation in pulmonary vascular resistance by this mechanism involving potentiation in pulmonary vascular α_2-adrenoceptors.

Renal Circulation: The kidneys receive approximately 20% of the cardiac output and make a significant contribution to total systemic vascular resistance. Their dense adrenergic innervation extends to both the afferent and efferent arterioles. Stimulation of the renal nerves, and administration of α-adrenoceptor agonists, produce an increase in renal vascular resistance with redistribution of blood flow from the cortical to the medullary areas. This response is blocked by phenoxybenzamine or phentolamine, indicating the activation of α-adrenoceptors. Studies of the α-adrenoceptor subtype mediating renal vascular responses to exogenously administered agonists suggest an almost exclusive role of postjunctional α_1-adrenoceptors [23].

Mesenteric Circulation: The splanchnic circulation receives approximately 20–25% of the cardiac output, and contains a similar proportion of the blood volume. The major part of the splanchnic blood supply is received by the mesenteric circulation which supplies the small intestine and the upper two thirds of the large intestine *via* the superior mesenteric artery. Consequently, the mesenteric circulation has the potential to play a major role in the determination of total systemic vascular resistance. Sympathetic nerve stimulation and exogenous administration of noradrenaline produce mesenteric arteriolar vasoconstriction *via* activation of α-adrenoceptors [24]. Studies using the *in situ* autoperfused superior mesenteric arterial bed of the rat suggest that predominantly α_1-adrenoceptors are present in the mesenteric vasculature, since vasoconstrictor responses to noradrenaline are blocked exclusively by low doses of prazosin and are relatively unaffected by yohimbine [25].

Cerebral Circulation: The arteries supplying blood to the brain clearly have different pharmacologic characteristics compared to peripheral arteries. A marked decrease in sensitivity to noradrenaline is seen just prior to the entry of the vessel into the subarachnoid space [26]. This point of transition corresponds to the change in embryological origin of the proximal and distal portions of each of these blood vessels.

Although cerebral blood vessels have extensive and active sympathetic innervation, the α-adrenoceptor mediated responses of these vessels to sympathetic nerve stimulation is small compared to peripheral vessels. This may be related either to insensitivity of the α-adrenoceptor, or to reduced α-adrenoceptor number. Nevertheless, there is evidence that the sympathetic nervous system can modulate cerebral blood flow in the conscious animal through and α-adrenoceptor-mediated effect as measured by hypothalamic washout of radioactive xenon in the rabbit [27].

Much information regarding the role of the α-adrenoceptor subtypes in mediating vasoconstriction of cerebral arteries still remain to be elucidated. Nevertheless, at least in certain species including humans, both α_1- and α_2-adrenoceptors can be demonstrated in radioligand binding studies, by vasoconstriction induced by α_1- and α_2-adrenoceptor agonists, and by blockade of the response to the physiologic neurotransmitter, noradrenaline, by selective α_1- and α_2-adrenoceptor antagonists.

Peripheral Venous α-Adrenoceptors

Saphenous Vein: The most commonly studied vein is the canine saphenous vein. De Mey and Vanhoutte [28] first reported the potent vasoconstrictor activity of clonidine in this tissue. Additional studies have shown that highly selective α_2-

adrenoceptor agonists, such as B-HT 920, B-HT 933 and UK 14,304, will produce a vasoconstrictor response that is resistant to antagonism by prazosin and sensitive to blockade by rauwolscine [29]. In the canine saphenous vein, noradrenaline, which can activate both α_1- and α_2-adrenoceptors, appears to activate preferentially the α_2-subtype.

Experiments in isolated human saphenous vein [30] show similar results to those reported for the canine saphenous vein. The response to low concentrations of noradrenaline are essentially unaffected by prazosin, but potently antagonized by yohimbine, suggesting that α_2-adrenoceptors may be more important than α_1-adrenoceptors.

The venous circulation resembles the arterial circulation in that postjunctional vascular α_1- and α_2-adrenoceptors coexist, with each α-adrenoceptor subtype mediating vasoconstriction. However, in contrast to the arterial circulation, postjunctional vascular α_2-adrenoceptors in veins may be preferentially innervated, with postjunctional vascular α_1-adrenoceptors being innervated to a lesser degree and possibly located predominantly extrajunctionally [31].

Pulmonary Vein: Assessment of postjunctional α-adrenoceptor activity in the pulmonary vasculature *in vitro* provides some interesting correlates to what is observed in canine and human saphenous vein. Intralobar pulmonary veins have been reported to contract to the selective α_2-adrenoceptor agonist B-HT 933, and this response is sensitive to inhibition by the selective α_2-adrenoceptor antagonist, rauwolscine [32]. In contrast, intralobar pulmonary arteries are relatively unresponsive to B-HT 933 *in vitro*. These results indicate that postjunctional vascular α_2-adrenoceptors may be preferentially located on the venous side of the pulmonary circulation as also appears to be the case in the peripheral circulation [33].

Hepatic Portal System: A similar situation to that described in the saphenous vein also exists *in vivo* in the intestinal venous circulation. In addition, in the hepatic venous circulation of the cat *in vivo,* blood volume responses to noradrenaline are mediated by postjunctional vascular α_2-adrenoceptors, as is the hepatic venous response to sympathetic nerve stimulation. These results are suggestive of a dominance of α_2- over α_1-adrenoceptors in the hepatic venous circulation, as well as a preferential, if not exclusive, junctional location of vascular α_2-adrenoceptors [34]. Furthermore, α_2-adrenoceptor-mediated responses in the venous circulation appear to be more marked than those in the arterial circulation, consistent with the notion that postjunctional vascular α_2-adrenoceptors may play a more important functional role in venous relative to arterial blood vessels [33].

Other Veins: Most other veins have less of an α_2-adrenoceptor contribution relative to that observed in the saphenous vein. Shoji et al. [35] compared the responsiveness of many canine veins to noradrenaline, phenylephrine and clonidine. The saphenous and cephalic veins have the greatest response to the α_2-adrenoceptor agonist clonidine, followed by the femoral vein. Interestingly, longitudinal, but not helical, strips of portal vein, mesenteric vein and vena cava readily respond to clonidine. Evidence for postjunctional α_2-adrenoceptors in human femoral vein has been obtained by the failure of prazosin to antagonize the response to low concentrations of noradrenaline in this tissue, and by the potent contractile effect observed with guanfacine, a moderately selective α_2-adrenoceptor agonist [36].

Physiologic Significance of Venous α_2-Adrenoceptors: The physiologic significance of venous α_2-adrenoceptors is unclear. *In vivo* studies with α_2-adrenoceptor agonists have failed to demonstrate a significant hemodynamic effect clearly attributable to effects on venous capacitance vessels. It has been suggested that α_2-adrenoceptor mediated venoconstriction can significantly reduce venous capacitance and thereby increase venous return to the heart resulting in an increase in cardiac output. Since venous α_2-adrenoceptors are sensitive to temperature changes [37], and α_2-adrenoceptors are most prominent in the cutaneous veins [31], the venous α_2-adrenoceptor may be involved in blood flow redistribution to optimize the thermoregulatory process.

Myocardial α-Adrenoceptors

The predominant postsynaptic adrenoceptor in the heart is the β_1-adrenoceptor, which mediates a positive inotropic and chronotropic response. However, there are postsynaptic α_1-adrenoceptors in the hearts of most mammalian species, including humans, that mediate a positive inotropic response without notably changing heart rate [38]. The mechanism by which cardiac α_1-adrenoceptors increase force of contraction has not been established, but it appears not to be associated with accumulation of cAMP or stimulation of adenylate cyclase [38]. Rather, it has been demonstrated that α_1-adrenoceptors mediate an increase in phospholipase C activity to increase levels of inositol phosphates. In this respect, α_1-adrenoceptors differ from β_1-adrenoceptors in the myocardium. Other differences between myocardial α_1- and β_1-adrenoceptors are the longer rate of onset and duration of action for α_1-adrenoceptor-mediated inotropic responses. Differences among electrophysiologic actions mediated by α_1- and β_1-adrenoceptors have also been observed. β_1-Adrenoceptor-mediated inotropic responses occur at all rates of contraction, but the effect mediated by α_1-adrenoceptors is most prominent at lower rates.

Renal Tubular α-Adrenoceptors

α-Adrenoceptors in the kidney have been known for many years, and α-adrenergic drugs produce a variety of renal effects. The functions and locations of the renal α-adrenoceptors are now only beginning to be understood. Radioligand binding studies indicate that α_1- and α_2-adrenoceptors coexist in the kidneys of a variety of mammalian species, however the number, proportion, and distribution of each α-adrenoceptor subtype may vary from one species to another.

It is believed that α_1-adrenoceptors predominate in the human renal vasculature and mediate a vasoconstrictor response, thereby modulating renal blood flow (see above). α_2-Adrenoceptors have been identified in the juxtaglomerular and may inhibit renin release. Recently it has been demonstrated that stimulation of renal tubular α_2-adrenoceptors can inhibit the effects of vasopressin on water and sodium excretion [39]. This effect mediated by α_2-adrenoceptors appears to involve inhibition of adenylate cyclase and reductions in cellular cAMP, and may occur at the level of the cortical collecting tubule. The α_2-adrenoceptor-mediated enhancement in sodium and water excretion occurs simultaneously with a decrease in potassium secretion [39]. α-Adrenoceptors, possibly of the α_1-subtype, may enhance sodium and water reabsorption in the proximal convoluted tubules.

The density of renal α_2-adrenoceptors is higher in spontaneously hypertensive and Dahl salt-sensitive hypertensive rats than in their normotensive controls, and high sodium diets may increase α_2-adrenoceptor number even further [40]. Thus, renal α_2-adrenoceptors may be involved in certain forms of genetic hypertension.

Cardiovascular Effects of α-Adrenergic Drugs

Peripheral α-Adrenoceptor Blocking Agents as Antihypertensives: Since vascular tone is mediated predominantly by α-adrenoceptors, it is logical to assume that pharmacologic antagonists of α-adrenoceptors would abate hypertension. Indeed, the α-adrenoceptor antagonists, tolazoline (Priscoline) and phentolamine (Regitine) were introduced as clinical antihypertensive agents many years ago. These competitive α-adrenoceptor antagonists do, in fact, lower blood pressure, but their clinical efficacy has been unaccountably low. One explanation that has been proposed for the ineffectiveness of these agents in hypertension is their ability to potentiate neuronal noradrenaline release by antagonizing prejunctional α_2-adrenoceptors to interrupt the inhibitory negative feed-back loop that regulates neurotransmitter release, thereby increasing synaptic levels of noradrenaline. The elevated levels of noradrenaline in the synaptic cleft may partially overcome the postjunctional α_1-adrenoceptor antagonist effects and thus limit antihypertensive efficacy. This hypothesis has been widely accepted, primarily in light of the increased antihypertensive efficacy observed with prazosin (Minipress), a selective α_1-adrenoceptor antagonist. Since prazosin possesses only weak antagonist activity at presynaptic α_2-adrenoceptors, the neuronal negative feed-back loop remains intact to prevent synaptic concentrations of noradrenaline from becoming elevated [41].

In human forearm, yohimbine, a selective α_2-adrenoceptor antagonist, produces arterial vasodilation and increases blood flow [16]. This finding suggests that at least in this vascular bed, the postsynaptic extrajunctional α_2-adrenoceptor may also play a significant role, along with the junctional α_1-adrenoceptor, in maintaining vascular tone. Vasoconstrictor activity mediated by postsynaptic extrajunctional α_2-adrenoceptors may play more of a role in the hypertensive state, as shown both in animal studies and in clinical studies in which increased vasodilatory activity of yohimbine has been observed in patients with essential hypertension [16].

Circulating catecholamines are known to be elevated in a major subpopulation of patients with essential hypertension, and these high plasma catecholamine levels have been proposed to contribute to the increased vascular resistance characteristic of essential hypertension. The fact that circulating catecholamines appear to be the endogenous agonists for the extrajunctional vascular α_2-adrenoceptors suggests that in this subgroup of patients, postjunctional α_2-adrenoceptors may, in fact, contribute to the elevated peripheral vascular resistance. As such, postjunctional α_2-adrenoceptor blockade may prove to be beneficial in some forms of hypertension.

α-Adrenoceptor Antagonists in Congestive Heart Failure

Vasodilators have assumed a more prominent role in the treatment of congestive heart failure during the past decade. In most patients with congestive heart failure, the optimal vasodilator is one that acts relatively equally on the arterial and venous beds. Sodium nitroprusside does so, but must be administered intravenously. Prazosin, an orally active selective α_1-adrenoceptor antagonist, has been shown to mimic the hemodynamic effects of nitroprusside in congestive heart failure, increasing cardiac output, decreasing left ventricular filling pressure and systemic and pulmonary vascular resistance, and maintaining heart rate [42]. Although acute tolerance has been observed after multiple doses of prazosin over a period of 24–72 h [42], the beneficial effect may return with continued therapy, and long-term clinical trials with prazosin suggest chronic efficacy in patients with congestive heart failure [43]. Prazosin improves symptoms most during exercise.

The factor that correlates best with mortality in patients with heart failure is a high level of circulating catecholamines. Since, as discussed earlier, circulating catecholamines may be the natural substrates for postsynaptic extrajunctional α_2-adrenoceptors in the arterial circulation, and since high plasma catecholamine levels may contribute to the increased total peripheral vascular resistance characteristic of congestive heart failure [44], the evaluation of an α_2-adrenoceptor antagonist in low output cardiac failure is indicated.

References

1. Ruffolo RR (1985) Relative agonist potency as a means of differentiating α-adrenoceptors and α-adrenergic mechanisms. Clin Sci 68 (Suppl 10):9s–14s
2. Ruffolo RR Jr (1983) Structure-activity relationship of α-adrenoceptor agonists. In: Kunos G (ed) Adrenoceptors and catecholamine action – part B. Wiley & Sons, New York, pp 1–50
3. Schmitt H (1971) Action des α-sympathomimétiques sur les structures nerveuses. Actual Pharmacol 24:93–131
4. van Zwieten PA, Thoolen MJMC, Timmermans PBMWM (1983) The pharmacology of centrally acting antihypertensive drugs. Br J Clin Pharmacol 15:455S–462S
5. Ruffolo RR Jr (1984) α-adrenoceptors. Monogr Neural Sci vol 10. Karger, Basel, pp 224–253

6. Ruffolo RR Jr, Nichols AJ, Hieble JP (1988) Functions mediated by α_2-adrenergic receptors. In: Limbird L (ed) The α_2-adrenergic receptors. Humana Press, Clifton, NJ, pp 187–280
7. Onesti G, Schwartz AB, Kim KE (1971) Antihypertensive effect of clonidine. Circ Res 28 (Suppl 2):53–69
8. Schmitt H, Schmitt H (1969) Localization of the hypotensive effect of 2-(2,6-dichlorophenylamino)-2-imidazoline hydrochloride. Eur J Pharmacol 6:8–12
9. Giles TD, Thomas MG, Sander GE, Quiroz AC (1985) Central α-adrenergic agonists in chronic heart failure and ischemic heart disease. J Cardiovasc Pharmacol 7 (Suppl 8):S51–S55
10. van Zwieten PA (1980) Pharmacology of centrally acting hypotensive drugs. Br J Clin Pharmacol 10:13S–20S
11. Ruffolo RR Jr (1984) Stereochemical requirements for activation and blockade of α_1- and α_2-adrenoceptors. Trends Pharmacol Sci 5:160–164
12. Hansson L (1973) Clinical aspects of blood pressure crisis due to withdrawal of centrally acting antihypertensive drugs. Br J Clin Pharmacol 15:485S–489S
13. Thoolen JMC, Timmermans PBMWM, van Zwieten PA (1983) Cardiovascular effects of withdrawal of some centrally acting antihypertensive drugs in the rat. Br J Clin Pharmacol 15:491S–505S
14. Engberg G, Elam M, Svensson TH (1982) Clonidine withdrawal: Activation of brain noradrenergic neurons with specifically reduced α_2-receptor sensitivity. Life Sci 30:235–243
15. Langer SZ, Shepperson NB (1982) Recent developments in vascular smooth muscle pharmacology: the postsynaptic α_2-adrenoceptor. Trends Pharmacol Sci 3:440–444
16. Bolli P, Erne P, Ji BH, Block LH, Kiowski W, Buhler FR (1984) Adrenaline induces vasoconstriction through postjunctional alpha$_2$-adrenoceptors and this response is enhanced in patients with essential hypertension. J Hypertens 2 (Suppl 3):115–118
17. Holtz J, Saeed M, Sommer O, Bassenge E (1982) Norepinephrine constricts the canine coronary bed via postsynaptic α_2-adrenoceptors. Eur J Pharmacol 82:199–202
18. Heusch G, Deussen A, Schipke J, Thamer V (1984) Alpha$_1$- and alpha$_2$-adrenoceptor-mediated vasoconstriction of large and small canine coronary arteries in vivo. J Cardiovasc Pharmacol 6:961–968
19. Kopia GA, Kopaciewicz LJ, Ruffolo RR Jr (1986) α-Adrenoceptor regulation of coronary artery blood flow in normal and stenotic canine coronary arteries. J Pharmacol Exp Ther 239:641–647
20. Shebuski RJ, Fujita T, Ruffolo RR Jr (1986) Evaluation of α_1- and α_2-adrenoceptor-mediated vasoconstriction in the in situ, autoperfused, pulmonary circulation of the anesthetized dog. J Pharmacol Exp Ther 238:217–223
21. Hyman AL, Kadowitz PJ (1985) Evidence for existence of postjunctional α_1- and α_2-adrenoceptors in cat pulmonary vascular bed. Am J Physiol 249:H891–H898
22. Shebuski RJ, Ohlstein EH, Smith JM Jr, Ruffolo RR Jr (1987) Enhanced pulmonary α_2-adrenoceptor responsiveness under conditions of elevated pulmonary vascular tone. J Pharmacol Exp Ther 242:158–165
23. Drew GM, Whiting SB (1979) Evidence for two distinct types of postsynaptic α-adrenoceptor in vascular smooth muscle in vivo. Br J Pharmacol 67:207–215
24. Granger DN, Richardson PDI, Kvietys PR, Mortillaro NA (1980) Intestinal blood flow. Gastroenterology 78:837–863
25. Nichols AJ, Hiley CR (1985) Identification of adrenoceptors and dopamine receptors mediating vascular responses in the superior mesenteric arterial bed of the rat. J Pharm Pharmacol 37:110–115
26. Bevan JA 81979) Sites of transition between functional systemic and cerebral arteries of rabbits occur at embryological junctional sites. Science 204:635–637
27. Rosendorff C, Mitchell G, Scriven DR, Shapiro C (1976) Evidence for a dual innervation affecting local blood flow in the hypothalamus of the conscious rabbit. Circ Res 38:140–145
28. De Mey J, Vanhoutte PM (1981) Uneven distribution of postjunctional α_1- and α_2-like adrenoceptors in canine arterial and venous smooth muscle. Circ Res 48:875–884
29. Ruffolo RR Jr, Zeid RL (1985) Relationship between α-adrenoceptor occupancy and response for the α_1-adrenoceptor agonist, cirazoline, and the α_2-adrenoceptor agonist, B-HT 933, in canine saphenous vein. J Pharmacol Exp Ther 235:636–643

30. Muller-Schweinitzer E (1984) Alpha-adrenoceptors, 5-hydroxytryptamine receptors and the action of dihydroergotamine in human venous preparations obtained during saphenectomy procedures for varicose veins. Naunyn-Schmiedeberg's Arch Pharmacol 327:299–303
31. Flavahan NA, Rimele TJ, Cooke JP, Vanhoutte PM (1984) Characterization of postjunctional α-1 and α-2 adrenoceptors activated by exogenous or nerve-released norepinephrine in the canine saphenous vein. J Pharmacol Exp Ther 230:699–705
32. Ohlstein EH, Horohonich S, Shebuski RJ, Ruffolo RR Jr (1989) Localization and characterization of the canine pulmonary α_2-adrenoceptor. J Pharmacol Exp Ther 248:233–239
33. Ruffolo RR Jr (1985) Distribution and function of peripheral α-adrenoceptors in the cardiovascular system. Pharmacol Biochem Behav 22:827–833
34. Segstro R, Greenway C (1986) α-Receptor subtype mediating sympathetic mobilization of blood from the hepatic venous system in anesthetized cats. J Pharmacol Exp Ther 236:224–226
35. Shoji T, Tsuru H, Shigei T (1983) A regional difference in the distribution of postsynaptic α-adrenoceptor subtypes in canine veins. Naunyn-Schmiedeberg's Arch Pharmacol 324:246–255
36. Glusa E, Markwardt F (1983) Characterization of α_2-adrenoceptors on blood platelets from various species using ^{3}H-yohimbine. Haemostasis 13:96–101
37. Flavahan NA, Vanhoutte PM (1990) The effect of cooling on α_1 and α_2-adrenergic responses in canine saphenous and femoral veins. J Pharmacol Exp Ther (in press)
38. Brodde O-E, Motomura S, Endoh M, Schumann HJ (1978) Lack of correlation between the positive inotropic effect evoked by α-adrenoceptor stimulation and the levels of cyclic AMP and/or cyclic GMP in the isolated ventricle strip of the rabbit. J Mol Cell Cardiol 10:207–219
39. Gellai M, Ruffolo RR Jr (1987) Renal effects of selective α_1 and α_2-adrenoceptor agonists in conscious, normotensive rats. J Pharmacol Exp Ther 240:723–728
40. Pettinger WA, Gandler T, Sanchez A, et al (1982) Dietary sodium and renal α_2-adrenoceptors in Dahl hypertensive rats. Clin Exp Hypertension A4(4&5):819
41. Davey MJ (1980) Relevant features of the pharmacology of prazosin. J Cardiovasc Pharmacol 2 (Suppl 3):S287
42. Arnold SB, Williams RL, Ports TA, Benet LZ, Parmley WW, Chatterjee K (1979) Attenuation of prazosin effect on cardiac output in chronic heart failure. Ann Intern Med 91:345
43. Stanaszek WF, Kellerman D, Brogden RN, Romankiewicz JA (1983) Prazosin update – A review of its pharmacological properties and therapeutic use in hypertension and congestive heart failure. Drugs 25:339–345
44. Ogasawara B, Ogawa K, Hayashi H, Sassa H (1981) Plasma renin activity and plasma concentration of norepinephrine and cyclic nucleotides in heart failure after prazosin. Clin Pharmacol Ther 29:464–469

Ventricular Dysfunction:
Ischemic Versus Non-ischemic

P. Foëx

Introduction

The development of sonomicrometry has made it possible to study ventricular wall motion in great detail. Regional wall motion may be studied in terms of changes in length and changes in tickness, in one or several regions, one or several axes. Changes in diameter may also be determined. In this review, we will examine the normal wall motion in both the right and the left ventricle, the alterations caused by ischemia and the modifications brought about by drug interactions.

What has been learned in experimental studies using this technique is now directly applicable to clinical medicine because advances in echocardiography and cardiac imaging provide us with high definition dynamic pictures of ventricular wall motion.

Sonomicrometry

Sonomicrometry is the standard technique to measure ventricular length or thickness. Introduced by Bugge-Asperheim et al. in 1969, [1], its principle is simple. Pairs of miniature piezoelectric crystals are implanted in the heart. Electrical stimulation of one crystal causes the crystal to vibrate and emit an ultrasound signal. The latter travels through the myocardium at a constant speed of 1.56 mm/μsec. When the signal reaches the other member of the crystal pair, an electric current is generated. The time from activation of the first crystal (the emitter) to that of the second (the receiver) is proportional to the distance between the crystals. The crystals vibrate at 3–6 MHz at a repetition rate of 1 kHz. This rate of stimulation allows the continuous measurement of intercrystal distance throughout the cardiac cycle. This type of measurement is stable, reproducible and accurate over long periods of time.

For length measurements, the alignment of the crystals and their depth in the wall of the left ventricle are critical. Most frequently crystals are inserted at the subendocardium or at midwall for determination of segmental shortening. For studies of myocardial ischemia, crystals are usually implanted at the subendocardium as this portion of the wall is most vulnerable to ischemia [2, 3]. For measurement of wall thickness, crystals are placed at the epicardium and at the

subendocardium. The epicardial crystals may be apposed to the surface or inserted immediately under the epicardium.

In recent years, sonomicrometry has been used not only in experimental animals but in patients undergoing coronary artery surgery in order to monitor regional wall function in areas supplied by coronary grafts.

Normal Left Ventricular Wall Motion

In the normal myocardium segment length decreases while thickness increases
during systole. It has been long recognized that systolic shortening in the left
ventricle is of greater magnitude in the apical than the basal region [4]. Moreover, shortening is of greater magnitude in the short axis than in the long axis. In
the normal myocardium, shortening occurs exclusively during systole. Similarly,
thickening of the wall occurs only during systole (Fig. 1). Interventions that increase the inotropic state of the myocardium increase the extent of wall shortening and thickening while interventions that depress the inotropic state have the
opposite effect. However, it is only recently that a differential effect of negative
inotropic interventions has been described. In an experimental model developed
in order to determine the effects of halothane, nitrous oxide, and the addition of
a calcium antagonist under isoflurane anaesthesia, Diedericks et al. [5] have confirmed that wall motion is more active in the apex than the base of the left ventricle and shown that negative inotropic interventions have a greater effect on
the more dynamic apical region than in the less dynamic basal region. Thus,
differential effects of interventions may occur in the totally normal, well perfused myocardium.

The difference in extent of wall motion may relate to differences in wall tension because of the variable radius of the cavity of the left ventricle, greater near
the base, smaller near the apex. In the basal regions intramural forces are greater
than in the apical region [6] and the changes in force are also greater than in the
apical region. This may reflect a difference in function: the apical region may be
acting as a major volume pump, while the basal region may act as support for
the aortic valve.

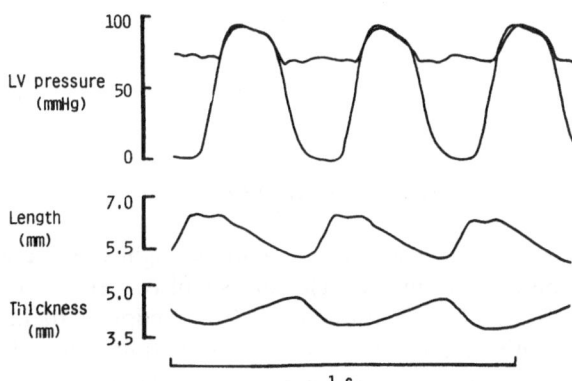

Fig. 1. Recordings of length
and thickness tracings obtained by sonomicrometry, displayed together with aortic and
left ventricular pressure signals

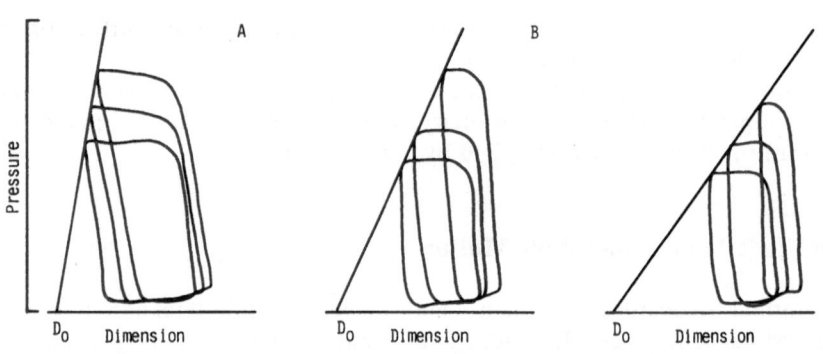

Fig. 2 A–C. Examples of pressure-length relationships obtained by acutely occluding the thoracic aorta. The slope of the end-systolic pressure-length line (ESPLR) is steeper during isoprenaline administration **A,** and flatter during halothane administration **C,** by comparison with the normal inotropic state **B**

As the left ventricle must eject into the high resistance systemic circulation, its contraction is essentially synchronous, though shortening may continue into early diastole in the basal region.

Changes in segmental shortening and in velocity of shortening have been used as indicators of regional contractile function [7]. Similarly, alterations in wall thickening are frequently used as reflecting changes in regional contractile function. However, neither shortening nor thickening can be regarded as true indices of regional contractility as they are also altered by changes in preload and afterload. In order to evaluate true regional myocardial contractility, many authors have used the end-systolic pressure-dimension relationship [8–10] by analogy with the end-systolic pressure-volume relationship described by Suga et al. [11]. The slope of the end-systolic pressure-volume line, obtained by changing left ventricular afterload, increases with positive, while it decreases with negative inotropic interventions. Similarly, in the normally perfused myocardium, the end-systolic pressure-length line becomes steeper with positive, and flatter with negative inotropic interventions (Fig. 2). Recently, it has become increasingly clear that the volume or length at zero pressure (by extrapolation of the end-systolic pressure-volume, or pressure-length line) is not constant [10, 12]. Caution must be exercized in the interpretation of alterations in the end-systolic pressure-dimension relationships as both changes in slope and shifts of the line may occur.

Right Ventricular Wall Motion

At variance with the left ventricle, right ventricular wall motion is not synchronous. The right ventricle consists of two embryologically distinct regions, the inflow and the outflow tracts. Contraction starts in the inflow tract and, in a peristaltic manner reaches the outflow tract. The difference in onset of contraction between inflow and outflow tract may be as long as 50 msec [13]. This delay is reduced by sympathetic stimulation and reflects the slow propagation of the electrical influx in the wall of the right ventricle. This regional differences is not limited to a delay in onset of contraction as contraction starts later and *lasts* longer in the outflow tract. Examination of patterns of wall motion in the right ventricle suggests that the outflow tract may act as a reservoir at the beginning of in flow tract contraction, and as a support for the pulmonary valve apparatus during the early part of diastole. Recent studies suggest that differential effects of interventions such as positive pressure ventilation and pulmonary hypertension exist between inflow and outflow tracts of the right ventricle [14, 15].

Asynchrony of contraction has been demonstrated in the human right ventricle by Chin et al. [16] in a study involving the insertion of markers in transplanted hearts. Out-of-phase right ventricular chords were observed in 33% of transplanted hearts. Inspection of the data suggests that a delay exists, in the human heart, between inflow and outflow tract contraction.

Myocardial Ischemia

Patterns of contraction are disrupted by myocardial ischemia. In a compromized territory, segment length decreases to a much lesser extent than in a normal territory and may even be replaced by lengthening [17, 18]. Similarly, systolic thickening is reduced and may even be replaced by thinning when severe ischemia develops. If systolic shortening is considered alone, progressive ischemia causes a reduction in systolic shortening up to the point where only passive elongation is observed. However, this is an over simplification; more detailed examination of the changes that develop with gradual ischemia reveal that early ischemia is characterized by a reduction in systolic shortening associated with the develop-

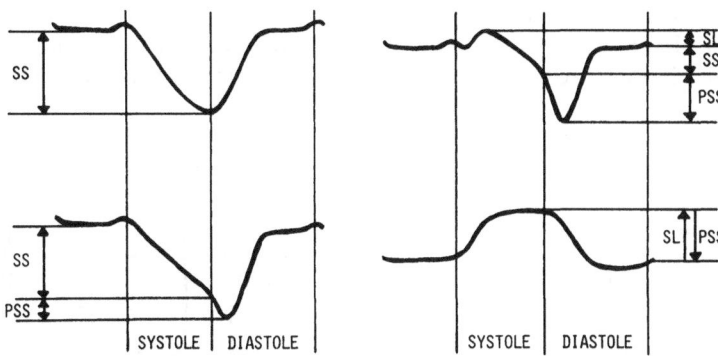

Fig. 3. Examples of changes in wall motion caused by gradual myocardial ischemia. In the normally perfused myocardium, shortening occurs only during systole (A). With mild ischemia, systolic shortening (SS) is decreased and some post-systolic shortening (PSS) is apparent (B). With moderate to severe ischemia, there is systolic lengthening (SL), followed by minimal systolic shortening (SS) and post-systolic shortening (PSS; C). In the totally ischemic myocardium, systolic lengthening (SL) is immediately followed by post-systolic shortening (PSS) and there is no useful shortening during ejection (D)

ment of post-systolic shortening (Fig. 3). As ischemia progresses, some systolic elongation appears followed by systolic and post-systolic shortening. In a totally ischemic segment the change in segment length are due solely to systolic elongation and post-systolic shortening. It must be noted that the total amplitude of wall motion may remain relatively unchanged even though systolic shortening has been abolished.

In conscious dogs reductions of coronary blood flow by as little as 10% may be associated with a detectable reduction in function [19]. However, in the anesthetized animals reductions of coronary blood flow of up to 30% may be associated with apparently normal regional function [20, 21]. Reductions in arterial pressure and heart rate caused by halogenated anesthetics may allow the compromized myocardium to maintain its function by increasing regional oxygen extraction even though coronary flow is reduced.

As segmental shortening is the most frequently used index of regional function, reductions in systolic shortening are considered to be good indicators of changes in myocardial perfusion [2, 7, 19, 22]. Indeed, systolic shortening decreases as ischemia progresses. However, systolic shortening is also reduced by negative inotropic interventions [3, 23], by reductions in preload, and by increases in afterload. Thus reductions in systolic shortening may not be indicative of myocardial ischemia in the presence of negative inotropic interventions.

The pattern of wall motion during brief episodes of complete coronary occlusion differs from those described above during gradual occlusion [24]. With acute occlusion the early change in wall motion is a short period of lengthening followed by shortening which occurs during isovolumic relaxation (Fig. 4). In this case, systolic shortening may remain apparently unchanged over a few beats, even though diastolic wall motion is totally abnormal.

It is increasingly recognized that early markers of ischemia are diastolic wall motion abnormalities. An early diastolic bulge characterizes ischemia caused by the acute occlusion of a coronary artery, while post-systolic shortening is an indicator of gradual ischemia [3, 20, 21, 23]. The reason for this difference may reside in the speed of coronary flow reduction. In the normal myocardium the early increase in coronary flow (isovolumic relaxation) facilitates relaxation of

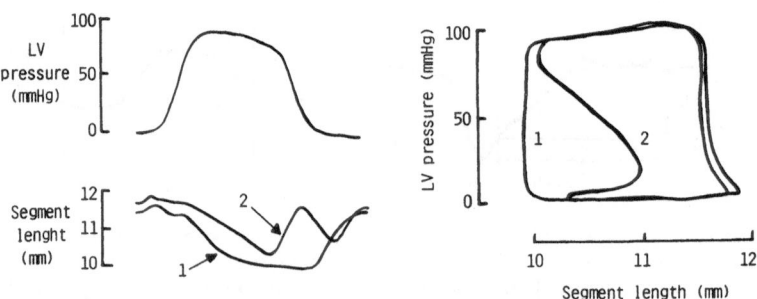

Fig. 4. Acute coronary occlusion causes marked abnormalities of early relaxation (arrow 2) as demonstrated on segment length recordings (left hand panel) and pressure-length loops (right hand panel)

the cardiac fibers. When flow is gradually reduced this facilitation is slowly removed; this may explain the delay in onset of relaxation evidenced by post-systolic shortening. Conversely when flow ceases almost instantly early diastole is totally disrupted. It must be noted that 20 to 30 seconds after acute coronary occlusion the ischemic pattern evolves towards a completely paradoxical wall motion similar to that caused by gradual ischemia (Fig. 3).

The question of the nature of post-systolic shortening is not fully answered. It has been suggested that post-systolic shortening is purely passive and the effect of recoil [25]. As the ischemic segment has been distended by neighbouring segments during systole, it recoils to a smaller length when the normal segments lengthen. On the other hand, post-systolic shortening may be regarded as active: as the ventricular pressure declines rapidly, the ischemic segment is capable of converting chemical energy into mechanical contraction because the load has decreased substantially. As post-systolic shortening has been shown to be a predictor of the extent of recovery of myocardium rendered temporarily ischemic, it is more likely to be an active than a passive phenomenon [26]. Moreover, experiments using voltage-clamped cardiac cells suggest that a long delay before the onset of contraction may be created by the application of positive voltages (Terrar and Victory, personal communication). It is possible that such abnormal conditions exist in the ischemic myocardium, leading to delayed onset of active contraction.

Many studies of the effects of physiological interventions and drugs on myocardium with compromized blood supply have used a model based on a critical coronary stenosis. Critical stenosis is usually defined as the maximum tightening of a micrometer controlled snare which allows regional function to remain normal but abolishes the coronary flow reserve as evidenced by the loss of hyperemic response to a brief coronary occlusion superimposed to the critical stenosis [20, 21, 23].

With such models it can be shown that hypotension (caused by hypovolemia or by agencies which depress myocardial contractility) promotes selectively exaggerated depression of systolic shortening accompanied by the development of post-systolic shortening in areas supplied by a critically constricted coronary artery. Anesthetic agents such as halothane [3, 20, 27] and isoflurane [23] have been shown to have an adverse effect on the compromized myocardium. This selectively exaggerated depression is not due to a specific effect of these agents on the compromized myocardium, it is a consequence of the reduction of the coronary perfusion pressure that attends their administration. As coronary perfusion pressure is the major determinant of flow through a critically constricted coronary artery, diastolic hypotension causes an exaggerated reduction in coronary blood flow. In contrast, narcotics, even in high doses do not reduce arterial pressure, and do not cause selectively exaggerated depression. However, the addition of nitrous oxide may cause significant dysfunction [21]. Calcium antagonists, because they decrease arterial pressure may cause selective depression and dysfunction of myocardium with critically reduced coronary blood flow [28].

Drug-induced Dysfunction

The simultaneous administration of drugs which decrease transmembrane and intracellular calcium fluxes, such as halogenated anesthetic agents (halothane, enflurane, isoflurane) and calcium antagonists (verapamil, diltiazem) may cause significant alterations in left ventricular wall function [29–31]. The main feature of these interactions is the development, in myocardium with normal coronary blood supply, of post-systolic shortening, mostly in the apical region of the left ventricle. As described earlier, post-systolic shortening is usually regarded as a marker for ischemia. However, in the absence of coronary artery stenosis and without massive reductions in coronary perfusion pressure, post-systolic shortening is unlikely to be due to myocardial ischemia and is more likely to represent a delay in the onset of relaxation. Indeed, both delayed onset of contraction and relaxation have been documented with the association isoflurane-verapamil [29]. As calcium antagonists are now known to cause substantial decreases in the velocity of impulse propagation in the left ventricle [32], the delay in onset of contraction may represent a delay in the excitation-contraction coupling; however, other mechanisms may have to be postulated to explain the delay in relaxation. Altered relaxation may reflect cumulative effects of drugs on the dynamic of calcium fluxes. That ischemia is not the cause of this dysfunction is borne out by the absence of alterations in high energy phosphates (measured by magnetic resonance spectroscopy) in response to the addition of verapamil during halothane anesthesia (unpublished observations). Why should the effect predominate in the apical region of the left ventricle is not fully explained. However, it may be a reflection of the differences in wall motion and susceptibility to depression as observed in studies of the non-homogeneity of left ventricular contraction.

Dyssynchrony of function may be caused by ischemia, interactions between inhalational anesthetics and calcium antagonists and also by the association of an inhalational anesthetics and sodium channel blockers such as lidocaine and bupivacaine [32]. It is accompanied by the worsening of global pump function. In this respect drugs that depress myocardial contractility may be considered to depress each single unit and/or modify the regional distribution of onset and offset of contraction.

The observation of dyssynchrony of contraction induced by drugs calls into question the validity of dyssynchrony as a reliable marker of ischemia. As transoesophageal echocardiography gains popularity, observations of wall motion during anesthesia and surgery draw attention to reductions of shortening and dyskinetic patterns which are immediately ascribed to ischemia. As most of the patients with coronary heart disease and/or arterial hypertension receive calcium channel blockers and many are given volatile anesthetics, some of the changes may represent altered calcium fluxes rather than true ischemia.

That non-ischemic dysfunction may occur in man is suggested by a recent study by Leung et al. [33]. Using echocardiography, the authors observed that post-bypass episodes of myocardial dysfunction correlated well with outcome. However, pre-bypass episodes of dysfunction did not correlate with outcome. This may suggest that some episodes of dysfunction (pre-bypass) are not due to ischemia but to interactions between cardiac drugs and anesthetic agents, while others (post-bypass) are clearly indicative of ischemia, hence the correlation with outcome.

Studies of regional wall motion, both in the right and the left ventricle have been, to a significant extent, geared to the evaluation of regional myocardial ischemia. Most of the alterations in wall function observed in animal studies have been ascribed to ischemia because the models were developed to evaluate ischemic dysfunction. More recently, it has become clear that changes in regional function occur outside myocardial ischemia. Reductions in systolic shortening may be due to negative inotropic interventions, not solely to ischemia. Moreover, patterns of dysfunction may develop in the normally perfused myocardium as a result of strong inhibition of calcium or sodium fluxes. Thus, caution should be exercised in the interpretation of alterations in ventricular wall motion.

References

1. Bugge-Asperheim B, Leraand S, Kiil F (1969) Local dimensional changes of the myocardium measured by ultrasonic technique. Scand J Clin Lab Invest 24:361–371
2. Tomoike H, Franklin D, McKown D, Kemper S, Guberek M, Ross J Jr (1978) Regional myocardial dysfunction and hemodynamic abnormalities during strenuous exercise in dogs with limited coronary flow. Circ Res 42:487–496
3. Lowenstein E, Foëx P, Francis CM, Davies WL, Yusuf S, Ryder WA (1981) Regional ischemic ventricular dysfunction in myocardium supplied by a narrow coronary artery with increasing halothane concentration in the dog. Anesthesiology 55:349–359
4. Le Winter MM, Kent RS, Kroener JM, Carew TE, Covell JW (1975) Regional differences in myocardial performance in the left ventricle of the dog. Circ Res 37:191–199
5. Diedericks J, Leone BJ, Foëx P (1989) Regional differences in left ventricular wall motion in the anesthetized dog. Anesthesiology 70:82–90
6. Lunkenheimer PP, Redmann K, Whimster WF, Theissen J, Frieling G, Lunkenheimer A (1988) The problem created by myocardial structure in assessing function. Br J Anaesth 60:25–75
7. Theroux P, Franklin D, Ross J, Kemper WS (1974) Regional myocardial function during acute coronary artery occlusion and its modification by pharmacologic agents in the dog. Circ Res 35:896–908
8. Mahler F, Covell JW, Ross J (1975) Systolic pressure-diameter relations in normal conscious dogs. Cardiovasc Res 9:447–455
9. Kaseda S, Tomoike H, Ogata I, Nakamura M (1985) End-systolic pressure-volume, pressure-length, and stress-strain relations in canine hearts. Am J Physiol 249:H648–H654
10. Foëx P, Francis CM, Cutfield GR, Leone B (1988) The pressure-length loop. Br J Anaesth 60:65S–71S
11. Suga H, Sagawa K, Shoukas AA (1973) Load independence of the instantaneous pressure-volume ratio of the canine left ventricle and effects of epinephrine and heart rate on the ratio. Circ Res 32:314–322
12. Sunagawa K, Maughan WL, Sagawa K (1983) Effect of regional ischemia on the left ventricular end-systolic pressure-volume relationship of isolated canine hearts. Circ Res 52:170–178
13. Raines RA, Le Winter MM, Covell JM (1976) Regional shortening pattern in canine right ventricle. Am J Physiol 231:1395–1400
14. Calvin JE Jr, Baer RW, Glantz SA (1985) Pulmonary artery constriction produces a greater right ventricular dynamic afterload than lung microvascular injury in the open chest dog. Circ Res 56:40–56

15. Santamore WP, Meier GD, Bove AA (1979) Effect of hemodynamic alterations on wall motion in the canine right ventricle. Am J Physiol 236:H254–H262
16. Chin KW, Daughters GT, Alderman EL, Miller DC (1989) Asynergy of right ventricular wall motion in man. J Thorac Cardiovasc Surg 97:104–109
17. Tennant R, Wiggers CJ (1935) The effect of coronary occlusion on myocardial contraction. Am J Physiol 112:351–361
18. Forrester JS, Wyatt HL, Da Luz PL, Tyberg JV, Diamond GA, Swan HJC (1976) Function significance of regional ischemic contraction abnormalities. Circulation 54:64–70
19. Vatner SF (1980) Correlation between acute reduction in myocardial blood flow and function in conscious dogs. Circ Res 47:201–209
20. Francis CM, Foëx P, Lowenstein E, et al (1982) Interaction between regional myocardial ischaemia and left ventricular performance under halothane anaesthesia. Br J Anaesth 54:965–980
21. Philbin DM, Foëx P, Drummond G, Lowenstein E, Ryder WA, Jones LA (1985) Postsystolic shortening of canine left ventricle supplied by a stenotic coronary artery when nitrous oxide is added in the presence of narcotics. Anesthesiology 62:166–174
22. Gallagher KP, Osakada G, Matsuzaki M, Kemper WS, Ross J (1982) Myocardial blood flow and function with critical coronary stenosis in exercising dogs. Am J Physiol 243:H698–H707
23. Priebe H-J, Foëx P (1987) Isoflurane causes regional myocardial dysfunction in dogs with critical coronary artery stenosis. Anesthesiology 66:293–300
24. Doyle RL, Foëx P, Ryder WA, Jones LA (1987) Differences in ischaemic dysfunction following gradual or abrupt coronary occlusion: effect on isovolumic relaxation. Cardiovasc Res 21:507–514
25. Akaishi M, Weintraub WS, Schneider RM, Klein LW, Agarwal JB, Helfont RM (1986) Analysis of systolic bulging. Mechanical characteristics of acutely ischemic myocardium in the conscious dog. Circ Res 58:209–217
26. Brown MA, Norris RM, Tokayama M, White HD (1987) Post-systolic shortening: a marker for early recovery of acutely ischemic myocardium in the dog. Cardiovasc Res 21:703–711
27. Leone BJ, Philbin DM, Lehot J-J, Foëx P, Ryder WA (1988) Gradual or abrupt nitrous oxide administration in a canine model of coronary artery stenosis induces regional myocardial dysfunction that is wordened by halothane. Anesth Analg 67:814–822
28. Leone BJ, Philbin DM, Lehot J-J, Wilkins M, Foëx P, Ryder WA (1988) Intravenous diltiazem worsens regional function in compromised myocardium. Anesth Analg 67:205–210
29. Videcoq M, Arvieux CC, Ramsay JG, et al (1987) The association isoflurane-verapamil causes regional myocardial dysfunction. Anesthesiology 67:635–641
30. Ramsay JG, Cutfield GR, Francis CM, Devlin WH, Foëx P (1986) Halothane-verapamil causes regional myocardial dysfunction in the dog. Br J Anaesth 58:321–326
31. Lehot J-J, Leone BJ, Foëx P (1987) Calcium reverses global and regional myocardial dysfunction caused by the combination verapamil and halothane. Acta Anaesth Scand 31:441–447
32. Leone BJ, Lehot J-J, Runciman WB, et al (1988) Effects of lidocaine and bupivacaine on regional myocardial function and coronary blood flow in anaesthetised dogs. Br J Anaesth 60:671–679
33. Leung JM, O'Kelly B, Browner WS, et al (1989) Prognostic importance of post bypass regional wall-motion abnormalities in patients undergoing coronary artery bypass graft surgery. Anesthesiology 71:16–25

Role of Subendocardial Ischemia in the Pathogenesis of Heart Failure

G. Heyndrickx

Introduction

Heart failure is commonly accompanied by a major defect in myocardial function. The complexity of the structure of the heart explains the many possibilities of abnormal function: anatomical defects, valvular abnormalities, defects in the contractile machinery and reduced O_2 supply all may result in inability of the heart to pump blood to meet the demands of the body. The inability of the pump performance of the heart initially results in compensatory mechanisms such as elevation in filling pressures with pulmonary congestion, followed by decreased cardiac output with general circulatory insufficiency.

The subendocardium is a distinct entity of the left ventricle (LV) and plays an important role for the contractile behavior of the LV in normal conditions as well as in diseased states such as myocardial ischemia and cardiac hypertrophy. The subendocardium or inner half of the LV free wall contributes more to the systolic contraction than does the outer half or subepicardium, while its blood supply is more vulnerable due to the extravascular compressive forces occurring during contraction. Therefore the subendocardium is more readily prone to myocardial ischemia. In order to understand the critical role of the subendocardium for the overall LV function it is important to review some of the basic anatomical and functional characteristics of the cardiac anatomy, as well as the coronary physiology.

Non-uniformity

Anatomical Considerations

The orientation of myocardial fibers in the LV is to be compared to a wicker basket. Loading the ventricle will result not only in changes in fiber length but also in fiber direction. In addition, the LV free wall is built up as a set of fiber shells running in spiral but with the angle of the spiral changing gradually from endocardium to epicardium, resembling an opened japanese fan. No fiber is allowed to move independently but moves as allowed by the adjacent fibres. Except for the papillary muscle and the trabeculae, all fibers are subject to the constraint of the ventricular wall [1].

This heterogeneity in structure has important consequences and allows for a complex pattern of rotational movement whereby expelling the blood is optimalized. This complex anatomy is reflected into important regional contraction differences throughout the LV. Several experimental studies have shown prominent differences in degree and velocity of regional wall thickening and segment length shortening between the superficial layers and the deep layers of the canine LV wall during systole [2, 3]. The greater changes in internal dimensions during contraction appear to result from greater wall thickening and segment shortening in the subendocardium compared to the subepicardium. This non-uniformity of muscular behavior is predictable on the basis of geometric constraint as the myocardium is incompressible. It is however not clear if this reflects an increased active shortening of the subendocardial fibers. This non-uniformity between subendocardium and subepicardium is maintained during inotropic and chronotropic stimulation with no changes in the fractional contribution of inner and outer thickening and shortening.

Metabolic Considerations

The effects of this non-uniformity in regional contractility on the regional metabolism has been addressed by several authors. A number of experiments have indeed shown a significant gradient in venous oxygen saturation across the LV free wall with a progressive decrease in venous oxygen saturation from epi- to endocardium. This observation is in agreement with the many studies in which subepicardial PO_2 was found to be higher than subendocardial PO_2 [4].

Subendocardial glycogen content appears higher while phosphocreatine concentration is probably lower compared with concentration in the subepicardium. A significant gradient however for adenosine triphosphate, lactate or the lactate/pyruvate ratio are not demonstrable in resting conditions.

Regional Myocardial Flow

There is general agreement from the bulk of experimental evidence that myocardial blood flow is not homogenously distributed throughout the LV free wall. A small but significant transmural flow gradient has often been observed with radioactive microspheres. The endo/epi flow ratio of the deposition of microspheres in the normal heart is approximately 1.2 [4].

It is generally acknowledged that the subendocardium has a greater metabolism as well as a higher blood flow compared to the subepicardium. In the normal heart this results in little biochemical differences between inner and outer layers and there is no evidence of hypoxemia or impaired function in the subendocardium. Although some transmural differences appear real, they are small and the subendocardium and subepicardium probably do not differ normally by more than 10–20% in most aspects.

Coronary Circulation

The coronary circulation in contrast to many other vascular beds, is primarily under metabolic control i.e. myocardial perfusion rate varies concordantly with the rate of myocardial metabolism [5]. The coronary circulation distinctively displays a high basal vascular resistance relative to the rate of tissue metabolism. This results in a high coronary extraction of energy yielding substrates as well as oxygen. Despite the close coupling between myocardial flow and metabolism, the regulation of the coronary circulation is extremely complex. Several important regulating mechanisms can be identified.

Driving Pressure

The coronary driving pressure is of paramount importance and is equal to the aortic pressure unless coronary obstruction is present. Due to coronary autoregulation, endocardial flow and function remains constant until mean coronary pressure falls below 40 mmHg [6].

Intramural Pressure

Considerable intramural pressure is generated during systolic contraction and opposes coronary driving pressure. In addition to the intrinsic compression of the myocardial arterioles during contraction, end-diastolic pressure, generated and transmitted from the cavity of the ventricle to the subendocardium adds to the extravascular compressive forces. These cyclic intramyocardial pressure changes explain why maximal coronary blood flow occurs during diastole, at a time of minimal extravascular compression. Interestingly regional myocardial flow distribution is affected differently during systole and diastole with systolic flow perfusing preferentially the subepicardium and diastolic flow perfusing the LV free wall more homogenously [7].

Myogenic Response

The myogenic response of the coronary vascular smooth muscle to transmural pressure differences is responsible for basal coronary tension.

Metabolic Autoregulation

Metabolic autoregulation in response to augmented energy needs is of paramount importance for the regulation of flow and is responsible for the close match observed between changes in oxygen consumption and myocardial flow. Several vasoregulators have been identified of which adenosine is the most popular agent. But other agents, such as oxygen, carbon dioxide, potassium, purines and prostaglandins are also of importance probably through several interactive mechanisms [4].

Autonomic Nervous System

The role of the autonomic nervous system in the regulation of the coronary circulation includes both α-adrenergic mediated coronary vasoconstriction as well as cholinergic and β-adrenergic vasodilation. This neural influences are not only important for the basal coronary vascular tone but autonomic reflexes can prominently contribute to the regulation of the coronary flow response, e.g. increased coronary vasocontrictor tone during exercise. Recent evidence indicates that with exercise the α-adrenergic coronary vasoconstrictor effect is more pronounced in the subepicardial layers than in the subendocardial region of the LV wall, which results in a redistribution of the coronary blood flow through the LV wall in favor of the subendocardium. This observation may answer the paradox as why there is sympathetic coronary vasoconstriction during exercise when myocardial oxygen consumption is greatly augmented and therefore maximal flow required.

Endothelial Cells

Emerging evidence that endothelial cells of the coronary arteries elaborate vasoactive components (EDRF, endothelin) in response to several stimuli indicates that changes in blood flow characteristics and metabolite content of the blood may contribute to basal flow regulation in the coronary bed.

Coronary Flow Reserve

Coronary flow can be increased several fold above resting levels during reactive hyperemia following a transient coronary artery occlusion, as well as during exercise, pacing or after injection of different vasodilating agents (papaverine, dipyridamole). If the stimulus is strong enough, maximal coronary vasodilation will ensue. This flow increment is termed coronary vascular reserve. The maximal flow at any given driving pressure is mainly a function of the total cross sectional area of the coronary resistance vessels [8]. Since maximal flow at any given pressure is not altered, an increase in basal flow, such as with anemia or cardiac hypertrophy will result in a decrease of coronary flow reserve. In situations of coronary obstructive lesions, the arteriolar resistance changes in such a way as to maintain the appropriate relation between myocardial flow and oxygen demand. Progressive stenosis is counteracted by autoregulatory mechanisms so that flow in the segment distal to the stenosis remains unchanged until vasodilator reserve is completely exhausted and flow can no longer increase [9]. From this point on, flow is entirely depended upon driving pressure. The mean driving pressure, in normal conditions, below which flow starts to fall is around 40 mmHg [6].

Cardiac Hypertrophy

Left Ventricular Hypertrophy

Hypertrophy occurs as a compensatory mechanism by which abnormally elevated systolic wall stress is returned towards normal in situations of pressure overload, diastolic volume overload or as a compensatory mechanism in case of regional loss of contractile function. Hypertrophy is characterized by an increase in the cross-sectional area of the myocyte. However, since capillaries do not proliferate, no change in the ratio capillaries to myocyte occurs. Intracapillary distance increases and capillary density is reduced, jeopardizing diffusion at the myocyte level [10].

Animal experiments have shown that resting blood flow as well as oxygen consumption per gram of myocardium is often normal if corrected for heart rate [11, 12]. Since total LV mass is increased, absolute flow to the LV is increased. Transmural blood flow distribution at rest was shown to be altered in cardiac hypertrophy. Inner to outer flow gradient was abolished, not as a result of exhaustion of subendocardial coronary reserve, since flow in this area is able to increase in response to exercise or pharmacologic vasodilation, but rather as a consequence of lowered endocardial stress [12–14]. In hypertensive hypertrophy which results in less severe hypertrophy normal end/epi flow ratio are observed [11]. Myocardial hypertrophy without increased perfusion pressure as occurs in aortic stenosis is associated with impaired minimal coronary vascular resistance [13]. This could be the result of
1. inadequate growth of coronary vasculature during hypertrophy,
2. increased extravascular forces, or
3. combination of both.

Left Ventricular Failure

Once the compensatory mechanisms in LV hypertrophy fail, LV failure occurs, associated with high end-diastolic pressures, exercise intolerance and evidence of pulmonary congestion. At this stage major alterations in subendocardial perfusion are observed. Although resting myocardial blood flow is increased in LV failure due to increased myocardial oxygen consumption associated with higher heart rate and greater wall stress, marked hypoperfusion of the subendocardium is typically noted as well as exhaustion of coronary flow reserve during maximal vasodilation [15]. Histological examination reveals multifocal areas of fibrosis preferentially observed in endocardial regions of hypoperfusion and reduced flow reserve.

Chronotropic and Inotropic Stimulation in Compensated LV Hypertrophy

Baseline LV function as well as the response to sustained β-adrenergic receptor stimulation in animals with compensated severe LV hypertrophy are relatively normal indicating that the hypertrophied LV myocardium functions normally, not only at rest, but also provides a substantial myocardial functional reserve. In contrast, a chronotropic challenge, induced by atrial pacing at more than 200 beats/min resulted in severe systolic and diastolic dysfunction in hypertrophied animals [16]. This reduced response of the hypertrophied LV to chronotropic stress is due to an impairment of myocardial perfusion as a result of decreased diastolic filling period resulting in myocardial ischemia and LV dysfunction. Indeed, although increasing heart rate above 200 beats/min in a model of severe cardiac hypertrophy was met with an increased myocardial blood flow per unit of myocardial mass, the increase in flow was however not evenly distributed throughout the LV free wall, resulting in significant endocardial perfusion abnormalities. Several mechanisms alone or in combination may explain this subendocardial underperfusion:

(a) increased time spent in systole caused selective reduction of blood flow to the subendocardium where perfusion occurs mainly during diastole;
(b) increased extravascular compressive forces mainly from increased LV end-diastolic pressure during pacing are also responsible for selective underperfusion of the subendocardium; and
(c) prolonged isovolumic relaxation could also encroach on diastolic filling time, thereby compromising subendocardial perfusion even more.

During exercise when tachycardia is associated with increased contractility, a similar response pattern in transmural flow distribution was observed in cardiac hypertrophy with a decrease in inner to outer flow ratio to levels significantly less than during normal exercise [12]. From these observation it is clear that the pressure overloaded hypertrophied ventricle may have increased vulnerability to perfusion abnormalities during tachycardia as well as during sympathetic stimulation.

Chronotropic and Inotropic Stimulation in LV Failure

The effects of inotropic stimulation (isoproterenol infusion or exercise) in dogs with LV failure are met with even greater abnormalities in the subendocardial perfusion resulting in decreased endo/epi flow ratio [17, 18]. This subendocardial hypoperfusion occurs at a heart rate elevation which is significantly lower than in compensated LV hypertrophy. The failing heart is thus even more sensitive to tachycardia.

Clinical Studies

Similar observations have been done in patients with LV hypertrophy where basal coronary blood flow was usually found to be normal in absence of obstructive coronary artery disease. Maximal coronary reserve in these patients was tested during chronotropic challenge. Although atrial pacing usually resulted in a normal increase in global myocardial blood flow and oxygen consumption, the production of lactate in a number of patients, suggested some degree of myocardial ischemia, most probably in the subendocardium.

Several investigators have demonstrated in LV hypertrophy, using pharmacological means, an impaired coronary vasodilating capacity [12]. Reactive hyperemic response to a short coronary artery occlusion, applied at the time of surgery for aortic valve replacement in patients with severe aortic stenosis complicated with left ventricular hypertrophy, has been recently studied to evaluate coronary flow reserve. It has been shown that the coronary reactive hyperemic response to a 20 sec left anterior descending coronary artery occlusion, was markedly decreased in contrast to the normal response after 20 sec occlusion of a right ventricular branch of the right coronary artery supplying the normal non hypertrophied right ventricle, indicating that in man severe LV hypertrophy profoundly limits the coronary vasodilation capacity [19]. Similar abnormalities in coronary flow reserve have been observed in patients with volume induced LV hypertrophy (mitral regurgitation, aortic regurgitation).

Coronary reserve in all these cases is limited by functional and anatomical decrements in vascular cross sectional area per increase in myocardial mass.

Myocardial Ischemia

Progressive coronary stenosis tends to reduce perfusion pressure distal to the obstruction. Initially this is compensated for by coronary autoregulation in order to maintain flow constant. The lower limit of endocardial autoregulation was recently shown to be 40 mmHg, below which flow is decreasing proportionally to pressure drop [6]. When coronary blood flow is prevented from increasing during sympathetic stimulation (e.g. exercise) due to coronary artery stenosis, coronary flow fails to increase appropriately in response to metabolic needs and subendocardial blood flow is reduced relative to subepicardial flow, resulting in regional mechanical dysfunction. While there is generally a good correlation between decrease in subendocardial flow and decrease in subendocardial function, this correlation is no longer observed when changes in subepicardial flow are related to changes in subepicardial function [20]. This specific dissociation between reduction in subepicardial flow and reduction in regional subepicardial function results in a more profound overall loss in transmural systolic wall thickening. Several reasons can explain this abnormal flow/function relation in the subepicardium: e.g. regional variations in geometry and wall stress, and tethering influences (see anatomy) and possibly transmural variations in wall stress.

Subendocardial flow reduction resulting in subendocardial ischemia during atrial pacing in an experimental model of two vessel coronary artery stenosis has also been shown to increase myocardial stiffness with an upward shift in LV pressure volume loop [21].

Conclusion

The subendocardium due to its specific anatomical characteristics is more at risk for ischemia whenever transmural myocardial flow distribution becomes altered in situation of epicardial coronary obstructive disease or case of cardiac hypertrophy. During the early phase of the disease process, subendocardial ischemia may only be present during sympathetic stress. Repetitive episodes of subendocardial ischemia as well as progression of underlying disease may ultimately lead to permanent cell damage, multifocal areas of fibrosis, marked hypoperfusion of the subendocardium with exhaustion of subendocardial flow reserve resulting in severe reduction in subendocardial contractile function and loss of overall LV function, culminating in overt heart failure.

References

1. Streeter DD Jr, Hanna WT (1973) Engineering mechanics for successive states in canine left ventricular myocardium. II. Fiber angle and sacomere length. Circ Res 23:656–664
2. Sabbah HN, Marzilli M, Stein PD (1981) The relative role of subendocardium and subepicardium in left ventricular mechanics. Am J Physiol 240:H920–H926
3. Gallagher KP, Osakada G, Matsuzaki M, Miller M, Kemper WS, Ross J Jr (1985) Nonuniformity of inner and outer systolic wall thickening in conscious dogs. Am J Physiol 249:H241–H248
4. Feigl EO (1983) Coronary physiology. Physiol Rev 63:1–205
5. Buckberg GD, Fixler DE, Archie JP, Hoffman JIE (1972) Experimental subendocardial ischemia in dogs with normal coronary arteries. Circ Res 30:67–81
6. Canty JM Jr (1988) Coronary pressure-function and steady-state pressure-flow relation during autoregulation in the anesthetized dog. Circ Res 63:821–836
7. Hess DS, Bache RJ (1976) Transmural distribution of myocardial blood flow during systole in the awake dog. Circ Res 38:5–15
8. Hoffman JIE (1984) Maximal coronary flow and the concept of coronary vascular reserve. Circulation 70:153–159
9. Mosher P, Ross J Jr, McFate PA, Shaw RF (1964) Control of coronary blood flow by an autoregulation mechanism. Circ Res 14:250–259
10. Breisch EA, Houser SR, Carey RA, Spann JF, Bove AA (1980) Myocardial blood flow and capillary density in chronic pressure overload of the feline left ventricle. Cardiovasc Res 14:469–475
11. O'Keefe DO, Hoffman JIE, Cheitlin R, O'Neill MJ, Allard JR, Shapkin E (1978) Coronary blood flow in experimental canine left ventricular hypertrophy. Circ Res 43:43–51
12. Bache JR (1988) Effects of hypertrophy on the coronary circulation. Progr Cardiovasc Dis 30:403–440
13. Bache RJ, Vrobel TR, Arentzen CE, Ring WS (1981) Effect of maximal coronary vasodilation on trasmural myocardial perfusion during tachycardia in dogs with left ventricular hypertrophy. Circ Res 49:742–750
14. Rembert JC, Kleinman RH, Fedor JM, Wechsler AS, Greenfield JC Jr (1978) Myocardial blood flow distribution in concentric left ventricular hypertrophy. J Clin Invest 62:379–386
15. Hittinger L, Shannon RP, Bishop SP, Gelpi R, Vatner SF (1989) Subendomyocardial exhaustion of blood flow reserve and increased fibrosis in conscious dogs with heart failure. Circ Res 65:971–980
16. Fujii AM, Gelpi RJ, Mirsky I, Vatner SF (1988) Systolic and diastolic dysfunction during atrial pacing in conscious dogs with left ventricular hypertrophy. Circ Res 62:462–470

17. Hittinger L, Shannon RP, Kohin S, et al (1990) Isoproterenol induced alterations in myocardial blood flow, systolic and diastolic function in conscious dogs with heart failure. Circulation (in press)
18. Hittinger L, Shannon RP, Kohin S, Manders WT, Kelly P, Vatner SF (1990) Exercise induced subendocardial dysfunction in dogs with left ventricular hypertrophy. Circ Res 66 (in press)
19. Marcus ML, Doty DB, Hiratzka LF, Wright CB, Eastham CL (1982) Decreased coronary reserve. A mechanism for angina pectoris in patients with aortic stenosis and normal coronary arteries. N Engl J Med 307:1362–1367
20. Homans DC, Sublett E, Lindstrom P, Nesbitt T, Bache RJ (1988) Subendocardial and subepicardial wall thickening during ischemia in exercising dogs. Circulation 78:1267–1276
21. Paulus WJ, Grossman W, Serizawa T, Bourdillon PD, Pasipoularides A, Mirsky I (1985) Different effects of two types of ischemia on myocardial systolic and diastolic function. Am J Physiol 248:H719–H728

Management of Severe Heart Failure

T. H. LeJemtel, R. Nisi, and E. H. Sonnenblick

Introduction

When undertaken in the setting of an intensive care unit (ICU), the therapeutic goals for patients suffering from severe heart failure are to immediately increase cardiac output without exacerbating or precipitating myocardial ischemia and to distribute the enhanced cardiac output to the kidneys, heart and brain.

Diagnosis

Severe heart failure is most often diagnosed on the basis of symptoms such as orthopnea and generalized weakness, and physical findings compatible with low cardiac output such as hypotension, depressed urinary output, and fluid accumulation. These symptoms and signs may occur in the course of several clinical entities which include myocardial infarction, post open heart or coronary bypass surgery, sepsis, endocarditis, myocarditis, or idiopathic cardiomyopathy. While the presence of severe heart failure can be clearly established from the data obtained by physical examination, it is eminently desirable to confirm the diagnosis by two-dimensional (2D) Doppler echocardiography [1] followed by right heart catheterization. The information gained by these two techniques are not redundant; to the contrary, they are complimentary. By determining the predominant pathophysiologic mechanism, i.e. valvular regurgitation, systolic or diastolic ventricular dysfunction, right ventricular infarction, pulmonary hypertension, infiltrative processes, these techniques allow us to use the best therapeutic approach for a given case.

2D echocardiography permits measurement of left atrial size and right and left ventricular dimensions in systole and diastole, and thus enables us to derive global and segmental indices of ventricular function such as ejection fraction and fraction shortening. 2D echocardiography is the method of choice to detect pericardial effusion and pericardial tamponade. It also allows measurement of left ventricular wall thickness, systolic wall thickening, and possibly the presence of abnormal deposits like in amyloidosis. Lastly, 2D echocardiography can detect the presence of calcified, poorly mobile valves, flail mitral or aortic leaflets, vegetations, atrial clot, especially protruding into the left ventricle, as well as ventricular or atrial septal defects.

Doppler cardiography can semi-quantitatively measure the amount of valvular regurgitation, the importance of septal shunt, and when tricuspid regurgitation is present, gives an estimate of pulmonary artery pressure. Doppler cardiography can give directional changes in forward aortic stroke volume during therapeutic interventions, and can give a rough estimate of diastolic function.

Right heart catheterization should then be performed using an inflatable balloon-tipped, flow-directed catheter [2] unless fragile right-sided vegetations, severe thrombocytopenia or severe abnormalities in clotting mechanisms are present. Pulmonary capillary wedge pressure should be attempted unless severe pulmonary hypertension is present. In the absence of excessive tachycardia, i. e. heart rate > 120 beats/min, or substantial aortic regurgitation, pulmonary capillary wedge pressure reflects left ventricular filling pressure. Forward stroke volume, which can easily be measured by thermodilution, is fairly accurate in the absence of tricuspid regurgitation. If tricuspid regurgitation is present, directional changes in forward cardiac output can be derived from measurements of pulmonary artery oxygen saturation [3]. Determination of left ventricular filling pressure is essential to rule out the possibility of low output state related to relative hypovolemia. The presence of hypovolemia contraindicates the use of diuretics, and can be reversed by the administration of fluids. Moreover, right heart catheterization can confirm the presence of pericardial tamponade by demonstrating equalization of right and left ventricular filling pressures and the square root size of the right ventricular diastolic pressure. By repeated measurement of oxygen saturation at different sites, right heart catheterization can confirm the presence of an atrial or ventricular septal shunt.

The hemodynamic profile of a patient with severe heart failure who is admitted to our ICU most often includes hypotension and a low output state related to left ventricular systolic dysfunction, as evidenced by a substantially reduced forward stroke volume and an elevated left ventricular filling pressure. However, occasionally a precise pathophysiologic mechanism is responsible for the low output state, and urgent correction of this abnormality is needed. In the event of cardiac tamponade, pericardiocentesis should be rapidly performed. Similarly, when acute mitral or aortic regurgitation complicates the course of myocardial infarction or endocarditis, valve repair or replacement is obviously the intervention of choice. However, the low output state can persist or even increase in the hours that follow correction of the mechanical abnormality. Acute left ventricular dilatation, which is possibly related to sudden subendocardial ischemia, may develop within minutes following pericardiocentesis. The low output state associated with valvular diseases may not be immediately relieved by mitral or aortic valve replacement. In such instances, the therapeutic approach to the low output state becomes less specific and, overall, is similar to that associated with depressed systolic left ventricular function developing in the context of an acute myocardial infarction, severe sepsis or post coronary artery bypass surgery.

Treatment

Two pharmacologic approaches have been advocated to increase left ventricular performance, and more specifically, forward stroke volume in patients with a low cardiac output due to depressed ventricular function.

Vasodilating Agents

Arterial vasodilators predominantly increase forward stroke volume by reducing cardiac afterload [4, 5]. This is particularly beneficial in patients with a very depressed systolic ventricular function whose hearts are particularly affected by changes in the loading conditions [6–10]. Vasodilators have the advantage of reducing myocardial oxygen requirements [11–14], and thus, are unlikely to create or worsen myocardial ischemia unless coronary perfusion pressure is markedly reduced and autoregulation is lost in the coronary vasculature. A fall in systemic arterial pressure is indeed the main disadvantage of arterial vasodilators, and thus limits their use in patients whose systemic arterial pressure is already borderline. Another limitation to their use is the increase in renin levels [15, 16], which is most often observed with non-specific arterial vasodilators. The increase in renin levels may result in worsening of renal function, leading to a decrease in total sodium urinary excretion [17] in patients who are not concomitantly treated with angiotensin converting enzyme (ACE) inhibitors.

When left ventricular filling pressure is already elevated, i.e. > 18 mmHg, ACE inhibitors are most often well tolerated in patients with low output state and hypotension. However, at very advanced stages of the disease process [18], when cardiogenic shock or near cardiogenic shock is present, inhibition of the production of angiotensin II may lead to severe hypotension [19, 20] and renal shut down, and thus ACE inhibitors should be administered with great caution. In addition, since most ACE inhibitors are excreted by the kidneys, the frequency of administration of these agents should be adjusted to the renal function, which is frequently reduced in these patients. In view of the impressive clinical regional and systemic hemodynamic benefits produced by ACE inhibitors [21–23], this pharmacologic intervention is, in our opinion, always justified despite its potential side effects. The initiation of therapy with ACE inhibitors can be made safer by concomitant administration of a positive inotropic agent.

Vasodilators which act predominantly on the capacitance vessels, like nitroglycerin, are particularly useful in patients with low output state when the amount of functional mitral regurgitation is severe, i.e. regurgitation fraction > 20% [24]. The increase in forward stroke volume produced by nitroglycerin closely correlated with the reduction in mitral regurgitant volume. Although the exact mechanism by which nitroglycerin reduces mitral regurgitation is incompletely understood, it is likely that reduction in left atrial size and left ventricular remodelling leading to better working geometry plays an important role. Continuous administration of intravenous nitroglycerin results in tachyphylaxis, which reduces the efficacy of this drug [25, 26]. An ACE inhibitor which, like nitroglycerin, substantially reduces left ventricular filling pressure may be particularly beneficial in this context.

Inotropic Agents

The second pharmacologic approach aimed at improving ventricular performance involves the use of positive inotropic agents. Their use, as far as hypotension is concerned, is considerably safer than that of arterial vasodilators. The major risk of positive inotropic agents is inducement or exacerbation of myocardial ischemia. By producing an excessive increase in heart rate and enhancing myocardial contractility, positive inotropic agents may raise myocardial oxygen requirements above the levels permitted by fixed coronary obstructions in patients with low output due to ischemic heart disease. Despite this risk, the use of synthetically derived catecholamines, i.e. dobutamine, has gained wide acceptance for the treatment of low output state associated with systemic hypotension [27]. Indeed, when carefully titrated, dobutamine tends to reduce heart rate and left ventricular filling pressure [28], thereby decreasing ventricular wall tension and increasing the time to perfusion in diastole. This, in turn, tends to offset the detrimental effects of increasing myocardial contractility in myocardial oxygen requirements [29]. Intravenous administration of dobutamine is initiated at an infusion rate of 2–3 μg/kg/min, and slowly titrated up every 15 minutes according to the clinical and hemodynamic responses. An increase in heart rate of 10–15% represents a contraindication to further increase the rate of infusion. A fall in systemic arterial pressure may contraindicate the titration up of dobutamine in some patients who then have a dismal prognosis. In these patients, intra-aortic counterpulsation balloon or temporary left ventricular assist devices should be rapidly used it a surgical intervention, i.e. valvular replacement, coronary bypass surgery, left ventricular aneurystectomy or cardiac transplant, is contemplated. Otherwise, maintaining systemic arterial blood pressure >80 mmHg with the use of pressor agents, like norepinephrine or high doses of dopamine, may lead to a vicious cycle of worsening renal function, peripheral constriction leading to further ventricular dysfunction, and eventually death. A less well-known adverse effect of dobutamine is the development of hypertension which is observed mostly in patients who were formerly hypertensive. Despite the well reported down regulation of β_1-adrenergic receptors in patients with chronic congestive heart failure [30–32], dobutamine consistently exerts hemodynamic benefits in this clinical situation. An attenuation of these benefits may be observed at times [33], although new tachyphylaxis very rarely occurs. When the precarious hemodynamic state of these patients has been stabilized, continuing or initiating ACE inhibition can be done safely and leads to further improvement. The inverse procedure, which consists of initiating ACE inhibition prior to positive inotropic support, in our opinion, carries a higher incidence of adverse reactions. Since dobutamine does not preferentially dilate the renal vasculature, concomitant administration of dopamine, at a dose which only stimulates the dopaminergic receptors in the renal artery, has the advantage of increasing renal perfusion and improving renal function [34–36]. Administration of dopamine is often prolonged after that of dobutamine, and may help the weaning off of dobutamine. The discontinuation of dobutamine should not be abrupt, since this may lead to a rebound phenomenon with clinical and hemodynamic deterioration, but gradually tapered at a rate of 1–3 μg/kg/min every 3 hours. At least one-third of patients referred for dobutamine dependency to our institution can be weaned from this drug when a slow down titration schedule is used.

A recently developed class of cardioactive agents, the specific type III phosphodiesterase (PDE) inhibitors, improve left ventricular performance by combining potent vasodilating actions to a moderate positive inotropic effect in patients with severe heart failure. Amrinone (Inocor), which is only available in parenteral form, is the prototype of this new class of agents [37, 38]. Due to its moderate inotropic effect and potent veno- and arterial dilating action [39], amrinone has the advantage of improving cardiac output and reducing diastolic filling pressures without increasing myocardial oxygen requirements [40]. Consequently, amrinone is of particular interest in patients with low output and hypotension due to ischemic cardiomyopathy.

Another potentially promising therapeutic application of specific type III PDE inhibitors is their co-joint administration with dobutamine [41–45]. This therpeutic combination produces greater increases in myocardial contractility and cardiac output than either drug alone. It has the advantage of permitting a lower dose of dobutamine, therefore reducing the risks of inducing excessive tachycardia and/or myocardial ischemia. This therapeutic combination has been offered as a bridge to cardiac transplantation, and may circumvent the use of left ventricular assist devices.

Amrinone, in view of its positive inotropic effects, presumably does not reduce systemic arterial pressure as much as pure arterial dilators. In patients with low cardiac output, the half-life of amrinone is of several hours [46]. Therefore, it does have the therapeutic flexibility of dobutamine which has a half-life of only several minutes. Long-term intravenous administration of amrinone may cause thrombocytopenia [46], which may require down titration or discontinuation of the drug. This class of agents appears particularly suited for short-term use [47], as long-term efficacy and safety have been increasingly questioned [48, 49].

Diastolic Dysfunction

Lastly, it is important to recognize that severe heart failure and particularly acute pulmonary edema are not always related to left ventricular systolic dysfunction [50–52]. Approximately half the patients admitted to our ICU with acute pulmonary edema have a normal systolic function when evaluated within 48 hours of the acute event. While acute myocardial ischemia, leading to transient systolic dysfunction [53] or ventricular arrhythmias, resulting in a low cardiac output, cannot be ruled out with certitude, it is likely that in at least a subset of patients the temporary impairment in low output state is related to an impairment of the left ventricular filling. This clinical syndrome is frequently observed in hypertensive patients in their sixties [54, 55]. The treatment of this syndrome totally differs from that of patients with severe systolic ventricular dysfunction. The administration of positive inotropic agents can only lead to excessive tachycardia and myocardial ischemia. Potent loop diuretics should be used with caution since these patients are not as fluid overloaded as those with chronic congestive heart failure. Intravenous nitroglycerin may be of benefit, but if beneficial should be rapidly down titrated to avoid excessive reduction in left ventricular filling pressure. When the acute pulmonary edema does not respond to conventional measures, early mechanical ventilation may be the most judicious way to break the vicious cycle of subendocardial ischemia, poor left ventricular filling, inadequate cardiac output, poor diaphragmatic muscle perfusion, lead to hypoxia and further worsening of the respiratory status.

References

1. Aquirre FV, Pearson AC, Lewen MK, McCluskey M, Labowitz AJ (1989) Usefulness of Doppler echocardiography in the diagnosis of congestive heart failure. Am J Cardiol 63:1098–1103
2. Swan HJC, Ganz W, Forrester JS, et al (1970) Catheterization of the heart in man with the use of a flow directed balloon-tipped catheter. N Engl J Med 283:447–451
3. Rubin SA, Siemienczuk D, Nathan MD, Pranse J, Swan HJC (1982) Accuracy of cardiac output, oxygen uptake, and arteriovenous difference at rest, during exercise, and after vasodilator therapy in patients with severe chronic heart failure. Am J Cardiol 50:973–978
4. Cohen JN, Mathew JK, Franciosa JA, et al (1974) Chronic vasodilator therapy in the management of cardiac shock and intractable left ventricular failure. Ann Intern Med 81:777–781
5. Chatterjee K, Parmley WW, Ganz W, et al (1973) Hemodynamic and metabolic responses to vasodilator therapy in acute myocardial infarction. Circulation 48:1183–1187
6. Kirk ES, LeJemtel TH, Nelson GR, et al (1978) Mechanisms of beneficial effects of vasodilators and inotropic stimulation in the experimental failing ischemic heart. Am J Med 65:189–194
7. Kovowitz C, Parmley WW, Donoso R, et al (1971) Effects of isometric exercise on cardiac performance: the grip test. Circulation 44:994–999
8. Strobeck JE, Ross J Jr (1985) Afterload mismatch in the failing heart. Heart Failure 1:84
9. Cohn JN (1973) Vasodilator therapy for heart failure: the influence of impedance on left ventricular performance. Circulation 48:5–11
10. Ross J Jr, Braunwald E (1964) The study of left ventricular function in man by increasing resistance to ventricular ejection with angiotensin. Circulation 29:739–745
11. Daly P, Rouleau JL, Cousineau D, et al (1984) Acute effects of captopril in the coronary circulation of patients with angina and hypertension. Am J Med 76:111–115
12. Mettauer B, Rouleau JL, Daly P (1986) The effects of captopril on the coronary circulation and myocardial metabolism of patients with coronary artery disease. Postgrad Med J 62 (Suppl 1):54
13. Daly P, Mettauer B, Rouleau JL, et al (1985) Lack of reflex increase in myocardial sympathetic tone after captopril: protein antianginal effect. Circulation 71:317–323
14. Magrini F, Reggiani P, Branzi G, et al (1989) Effects of angiotensin converting enzyme inhibition on coronary blood flow. In: Sonnenblick EH, Laragh JH, Lesch M (eds) New frontiers in cardiovascular therapy: focus on angiotensin converting enzyme inhibitors. Excerpta Medica: Princeton p 298
15. Stern L, Henry DP, Weinberger MH (1981) Increase in plasma norepinephrine during prazosin therapy for congestive heart failure. Am J Med 70:825–830
16. Manthey J, Dietz R, Leinberger H, et al (1980) Vasodilator therapy in heart failure: limited by activation of vasoconstrictor mechanisms? Circulation 62 (Suppl 3):259 (abstr)
17. Schrier RW (1988) Pathogenesis of sodium and water retention in high output and low output cardiac failure, nephrotic syndrome, cirrhosis and pregnancy. N Engl J Med 319:1065–1069
18. Packer M, Medina N, Yushak M (1984) Relation between serum sodium concentration and the hemodynamic and clinical responses to converting enzyme inhibition with captopril in heart failure. J Am Coll Cardiol 3:1035–1040
19. Errington ML, Rocha E, Silva M Jr (1974) The role of vasopressin and angiotensin in the development of irreversible shock. J Physiol 242:119
20. Abboud FM, Heistad DE, Mark AL, et al (1976) Reflex control of the peripheral circulation. Prog Cardiovasc Dis 18:371–385

21. LeJemtel TH, Maskin CS, Mancini D, et al (1985) Systemic and regional hemodynamic effects of captopril and milrinone administered alone and concomitantly in patients with heart failure. Circulation 72:364-369

22. Captopril Multicenter Research Group (1983) A placebo-controlled trial of captopril in refractory chronic congestive heart failure. J Am Coll Cardiol 2:755-760

23. The Consensus Trial Study Group (1987) Effects of enalapril on mortality in severe congestive heart failure: Results of the Cooperative North Scandinavian Enalapril Survival Study (CONSENSUS). N Engl J Med 316:1429-1432

24. Keren G, Katz S, Strom J, et al (1988) Non-invasive quantification of mitral regurgitation in dilated cardiomyopathy: correlation of two Doppler echocardiographic methods. Am Heart J 116:758-762

25. Zelis RT, Mason DT (1969) Demonstration of nitrate tolerance attenuation of the venomotor response to nitroglycerin by the chronic administration of isosorbide dinitrate. Circulation 39-40 (Suppl 3):211-215

26. Needleman P, Johnson EM Jr (1973) Mechanisms of tolerance development to organic nitrates. J Pharmacol Exp Ther 184:709-713

27. Sonnenblick EH, Frishman WH, LeJemtel TH (1979) Dobutamine: A new synthetic cardioactive sympathetic amine. N Engl J Med 300:17-20

28. Kupper W, Waller D, Haurath P, et al (1982) Hemodynamic and cardiac metabolic effects of inotropic stimulation with dobutamine in patients with coronary artery disease. Eur Heart J 3:29-33

29. Tuttle RR, Pollock GD, Todd G, et al (1977) The effect of debutamine on cardiac oxygen balance, regional blood flow, and infarction severity after coronary artery narrowing in dogs. Circ Res 41:357 (abstr)

30. Colucci WS, Alexander W, Williams GH, et al (1981) Decreased lymphocyte β-adrenergic receptor density in patients with heart failure and tolerance to the β-adrenergic agonist pirbuterol. N Engl J Med 305:185-189

31. Bristow MR, Ginsburg R, Minobe W, et al (1982) Decreased catecholamine sensitivity and β-adrenergic receptor density in failing human hearts. N Engl J Med 307:205-209

32. Bristow MR, Hershberger RE, Post JD, et al (1989) β_1 and β_2-adrenergic receptor-mediated adenylate cyclase stimulation in non-failing and failing human ventricular myocardium. Mol Pharmacol 35:295-305

33. Unverferth DV, Blanford M, Kates RE, et al (1980) Tolerance to dobutamine after a 72 hour continuous infusion. Am J Med 69:762-769

34. Allwood MJ, Ginsburg J (1964) Peripheral vascular and other effects of dopamine in man. Clin Sci 27:271-277

35. Goldberg LI (1972) Cardiovascular and renal actions of dopamine: potential clinical applications. Pharmacol Rev 24:1-15

36. Maskin CS, Ocken S, Chadwick B, LeJemtel TH (1985) Comparative systemic and renal effects of dopamine and angiotensin converting enzyme inhibition with enalaprilat in heart failure. Circulation 72:364-369

37. Alousi AA, Farah AE, Lesher GY, et al (1979) Cardiotonic activity of amrinone - WIN 40680, (5-amino-3,4'-bipyridine-6{1H}-one). Circ Res 45:666 (abstr)

38. LeJemtel TH, Keung E, Sonnenblick EH, et al (1979) Amrinone: A new non-glycosidic, non-adrenergic cardiotonic agent effective in the treatment of intractable myocardial failure in man. Circulation 59:1098-1104

39. Millard RW, Dube G, Grupp G, et al (1980) Direct vasodilator and positive inotropic action of amrinone. J Mol Cell Cardiol 12:647-655

40. Jentzer JH, LeJemtel TH, Sonnenblick EH, Kirk ES (1981) Beneficial effect of amrinone on myocardial oxygen consumption during acute left ventricular failure in dogs. Am J Cardiol 48:75-81

41. Rall TW, West TC (1963) The potential of cardiac inotropic responses to norepinephrine by theophylline. J Pharmacol Exp Ther 139:269-274

42. Alousi AA, Stanhus GP, Stuart JC, et al (1983) Characterization of the cardiotonic effects of milrinone, a new and potent cardiac bipyridine on isolated tissues from several animal species. J Cardiovasc Pharmacol 5:804-809

43. Gage J, Rutman H, Lucido D, et al (1986) Additive effects of dobutamine and amrinone on myocardial contractility and ventricular performance in patients with severe heart failure. Circulation 74:367-371
44. Feldman MD, Copelas L, Gwathmey JK, et al (1987) Deficient production of cyclic AMP: Pharmacologic evidence of an important cause of contractile dysfunction in patients with end-stage heart failure. Circulation 75:331-338
45. Colucci WS, Denniss AR, Leatherman GF, et al (1988) Intracoronary infusion of dobutamine to patients with and without severe congestive heart failure: Dose response relationships, correlation with circulating catecholamines, and effects of phosphodiesterase inhibition. J Clin Invest 81:1103-1109
46. Clinical Experience with Amrinone (1982) Overall summary for NDA Amendment, Sterling Winthrop Research Institute, Rennsselaer, New York
47. Anderson JL, Baim DS, Fein SA, et al (1987) Efficacy and safety of sustained (48 hour) intravenous infusions of milrinone in patients with severe congestive heart failure: A multicenter study. J Am Coll Cardiol 9:711-714
48. Maskin CS, Forman R, Klein NA, et al (1982) Long-term amrinone therapy in patients with severe heart failure. Am J Med 72:113-118
49. LeJemtel TH, Sonnenblick EH (1984) Should the failing heart be stimulated? N Engl J Med 310:1384
50. Dougherty AH, Naccarelli GU, Gray EL, et al (1984) Congestive heart failure with normal systolic function. Am J Cardiol 54:778-783
51. Soufer R, Wohlgelemter D, Vita NA, et al (1985) Intact systolic left ventricular function in clinical congestive heart failure. Am J Cardiol 55:1032-1036
52. Plehn JF, Lotuin A, Apstein CS (1987) Life-threatening pulmonary oedema due to left ventricular diastolic dysfunction. Circulation 76 (Suppl IV):411 (abstr)
53. Amsterdam EA (1973) Function of the hypoxic myocardium: experimental and clinical aspects. Am J Cardiol 32:461-467
54. Fouad FM, Tarazi RC, Gallagher JH, et al (1980) Abnormal left ventricular relaxation in hypertensive subjects. Clin Sci 59 (Suppl 6):411S
55. Topol EJ, Traill TA, Fortuin NJ (1985) Hypertensive hypertrophic cardiomyopathy of the elderly. N Engl J Med 312:277-280

Cardiac Arrhythmias in Patients Treated with Antiarrhythmic Agents

H. Löllgen, U. Fahrenkrog, and R. Bausch

Introduction

Prevention of sudden cardiac death by treatment with antiarrhythmic agents has failed to show significant effects. Using different drugs, no improvement in survival could be demonstrated. Some authors were able to demonstrate improved survival in small groups of patients thoroughly investigated using a battery of tests like ambulatory ECG, electrophysiological and exercise testing [1].

In contrast, wide use of antiarrhythmic therapy and quantitative Holter monitoring revealed that antiarrhythmic drugs may aggravate arrhythmias. Though adverse effects of antiarrhythmic drugs are known since several decades, it was only recently that the clinical significance of arrhythmogenic antiarrhythmics [2] or arrhythmogenesis [3–5] has been appreciated. Recently published results of the CAST study highlight the clinical significance of proarrhythmic effects of class Ic antiarrhythmic drugs. Proarrhythmia in general means that a given arrhythmia is worsened by antiarrhythmic agents.

Based on several own case reports, this review deals with

- definition, criteria, pathophysiology, incidence;
- and therapy of proarrhythmia due to antiarrhythmic agents.

Definition

There is no general agreement on the definition of proarrhythmia [5–7]. Morganroth et al. [6] defined proarrhythmia by a more than threefold increase in frequency of baseline premature ventricular beats (PVB) with more than 100 PVB/ hour present at baseline, or a 10-fold increase when the baseline frequency was less than 100 PVB/hour. More generally, proarrhythmia can be defined as the onset of ventricular arrhythmia of a higher degree or exacerbation of ventricular arrhythmia due to drug therapy. New onset of sustained or non-sustained ventricular tachycardia not identified previously, first occurrence of torsades de pointes, sudden death of cardiac arrest respectively, after starting antiarrhythmic therapy may also be accepted as an arrhythmogenic effect (Table 1) [8]. Nomenclature, types, and criteria for proarrhythmia are given in Table 2.

Table 1. Definitions of proarrhythmia. (From [8])

Increase in VPB frequency Baseline frequency (average VPBs/hour)	Increase required to declare proarrhythmia (average VPBs/ hour)
10	10×
30	7×
100	4×
300	3×
1000	2×

Increase in nonsustained ventricular tachycardia (VT) Baseline frequency (episodes of VT/day)	Frequency required to declare proarrhythmia
<5	≥50 episodes/day
≥5	Increase of >10×

New sustained VT
New torsades de pointes VT

VPB = ventricular premature beat.

Table 2. Definition and types of proarrhythmia. (From [7])

Arrhythmogenesis – creation of arrhythmia by any cause
  Proarrhythmia – drug-induced (primarily by antiarrhythmic drugs) arrhythmogenesis
    Provocation of arrhythmia: creation by drugs of a new arrhythmia
    Aggravation of arrhythmia: worsening by drugs of a previously documented arrhythmia

Bradyarrhythmias
  Sinus node dysfunction
  Atrioventricular block
Tachyarrhythmias
  Supraventricular tachyarrhythmias
  Ventricular tachyarrhythmias
Torsades de pointes with QT prolongation
New onset of sustained, uniform ventricular tachycardia (conversion of nonsustained ventricular tachycardia to sustained ventricular tachycardia)
New, multiform, sustained ventricular tachycardia without QT prolongation
Increased frequency of ventricular premature complexes or repetitive forms
Responses to programmed electrical stimulation
  conversion of nonsustained to sustained ventricular tachycardia
  increased rate of ventricular tachycardia
  initiation of ventricular tachycardia with fewer premature stimuli

Performing invasive electrophysiological studies, initiation of an arrhythmia by a lesser stimuli, change of non-sustained to sustained tachycardia or a faster rate of ventricular tachycardia indicates an arrhythmogenic response [9].

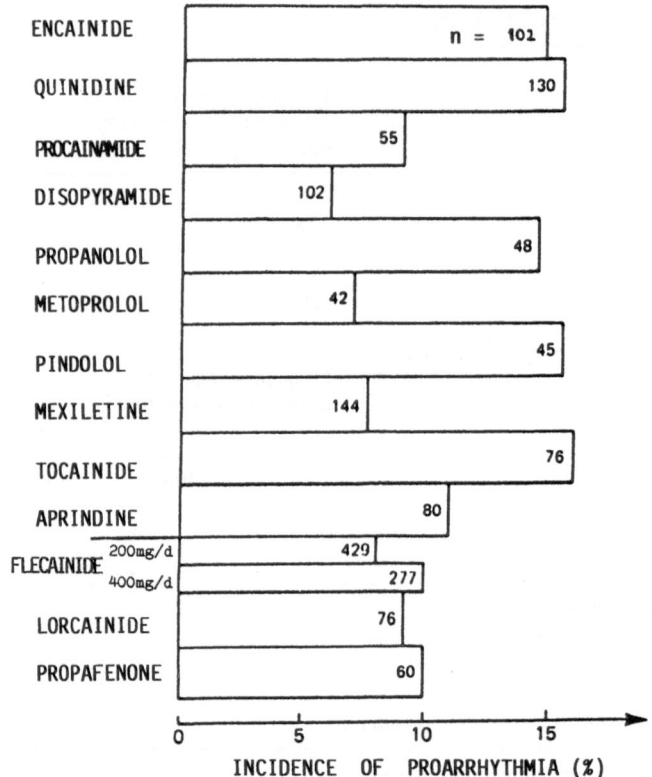

Fig. 1. Incidence of ventricular proar-rhythmia. The overall incidence is about 9%. (From [15])

Incidence

Frequency of proarrhythmic effects varies from 2 to 20% (Fig. 1). This variation partly depends on the definition of proarrhythmia. During electrophysiological testing (EPS), aggravation occurred in 9% [10]. In general, worsening of arrhythmia is more frequently observed during EPS than during Holter monitoring. With the latter method, proarrhythmia is observed up to 18% [2, 10].

Aggravation does occur with almost all antiarrhythmic agents but seems more frequent with class Ic drugs. Cardiac arrest due to adverse effects of antiarrhythmic drugs has also been described for almost all of the drugs with special respect to quinidine and disopyramide. The most severe proarrhythmic effect was observed early after beginning of therapy in many observations [2–4] and often was initiated by atypical ventricular tachycardia or torsade de pointes. Furthermore, increased QT-interval is often associated with torsade de pointes [4, 11].

Mechanisms of Proarrhythmia

Antiarrhythmic drugs interplay with abnormal impulse conduction and initiation. The proarrhythmic effects are assumed to enhance normal or abnormal

Table 3. Promoting factors of proarrhythmia. (From [5])

I. Class Ia: Long QT
- Susceptible heart (congenital, acquired)
- Ischemic heart disease
- Cardiomyopathy
- Hypokalemia, hypomagnesemia
- Slow heart rate
- Low protein diet

II. Class Ic : Incessant sinusoidal ventricular tachycardia
- Previous sustained ventricular tachycardia
- Scarred heart with low ejection fraction
- High drug concentration (?)

automaticity or to favor early or late after-depolarization. This in turn triggers sustained rhythmic activity. In addition, antiarrhythmic agents may interfere with the reentry circle by slowing conduction velocity and changes of refractoriness. Some more promoting factors are shown in Table 3. Furthermore, antiarrhythmic agents modify those factors playing a role in spontaneous induced arrhythmias such as arrhythmic substrate, triggers, and modulating factors [9].

Proarrhythmia may also be favored by toxic serum drug concentrations or drug interference (e. g. amiodarone – digoxin), by electrolyte disturbances and by changes of the autonomic nervous system. This holds true especially for the lengthened QT-interval during therapy or due to inborn long QT-syndrome.

In most cases of sudden cardiac arrest or arrhythmia aggravation by antiarrhythmic drugs, idiosynchratic response is the most likely underlying mechanism with patients having normal or low serum drug levels. In this situation, aggravation leads to a prolonged QT-interval and facilitates reentry ventricular tachycardia.

Proarrhythmia and concomitant QT-prolongation often is associated with torsades de pointes or atypical ventricular tachycardia. This tachycardia is characterized by somewhat widened QRS complexes with changing amplitude twisting around the isoelectric line. The rate is about 200 to 250 bpm. Lengthened QT interval is normally seen with the occurrence of torsades de pointes. The underlying mechanism is similar to those mentioned above, torsades de pointes mostly are related to reentry. Torsades de pointes is of higher incidence during proarrhythmia induced by quinidine, disopyramide or procainamide, but also occurs with drugs such as ajmalin, sotalol, lorcainide and other agents but with a lesser incidence with class Ib antiarrhythmics which normally shorten the QT interval.

The QT interval should not increase beyond 450 to 500 ms (heart rate corrected) or beyond 120% of normal values [3, 4, 11].

Torsade de pointes sometimes are associated with hypokalemia, e.g. in patients receiving diuretic therapy.

Current data do not allow identification of patients who are threatened by torsade de pointes undergoing antiarrhythmic therapy. However, recommendations for preventions are given in Table 4. Following these recommendations,

Table 4. Preventive measures of proarrhythmia

- Antiarrhythmic drug therapy only if indicated
- Correction of electrolyte disturbances,
          of ischemia, of left heart failure
- Initiation of antiarrhythmic drug therapy in hospital
- Control ECG one hour after 1st dosage of the drug
- Control ECG within one week after start of antiarrhythmic therapy
- Instruction of patients to report on dizziness or syncope
- *Discontinue antiarrhythmic drug therapy* IF
     QT > 120% or QT_c > 500 ms
     QRS >125% of pretreatment duration

---

proarrhythmia cannot be totally prevented, however, some patients who are likely to develop proarrhythmia, can be detected early.

Besides true arrhythmogenesis and facilitation of the manifest arrhythmia, unmasking of a latent substrate may also be involved in occurrence of new arrhythmia after starting antiarrhythmic drug therapy. Unmasking means the development of new arrhythmia on the basis of a "quiet" arrhythmia substrate such as preexcitation syndromes [9].

Therapy of Arrhythmias Induced by Antiarrhythmic Agents

Proarrhythmia can be a serious therapeutic problems. Ventricular tachycardia induced by antiarrhythmic agents sometimes are very resistant to conventional therapy and often require repeated cardioversion or defibrillation. Cardiac arrest is not unusual in this setting. The therapeutic approach is summarized in Table 5.

The first step is discontinuation of the offending drug. If cardiac arrest is present, CPR according to standard guidelines should be rapidly started. Defibrillation or cardioversion, also following standard guidelines, is recommended to stop ventricular tachycardia. Often, repeated defibrillations are necessary. In this

Table 5. Therapy of acute ventricular arrhythmia due to proarrhythmia

---

- Discontinue antiarrhythmic drug
- CPR if necessary
- Defibrillation if necessary
- Long QT / Torsade de pointes: $MgSO_4$ (25%) 1-2 mg iv
          (or 8-24 mEq $MgSO_4$ iv, repeat if necessary)
- Overdrive suppresssion: Heart rate > 100 bqm by
          transvenous pacemaker of isoproterenol
             - Consider atropine
- Potassium iv
             - Consider class I_B agents (lidocaine, mexiletine, tocainide)
             - Consider β-blockers (iv)

---

setting, overdrive suppression should be performed by means of transvenous pacemaker stimulation.

Overdrive can also be done by intravenous infusion of isoproterenol which in addition shortens repolarization. This may be useful if QT prolongation is present.

Atropine may also be given for overdrive suppression but care has to be taken to prevent overshooting of sympathetic drive thus favoring ventricular fibrillation.

Torsades de Pointes and QT Prolongation

Magnesium sulfate is the first line therapy for ventricular tachycardia with QT prolongation and for torsade de pointes. Substitution of potassium should be performed even if serum potassium level is in the normal range. If the arrhythmia is resistant to these approaches, antiarrhythmic drugs which shorten the action potential may be used such as lidocaine, mexiletine or tocainide. However, arrhythmia suppression is not very likely to obtain with these drugs in proarrhythmia. Beta-receptor blocking drugs, especially propanolol may be tried, amiodarone in proarrhythmia with short QT interval is still investigational.

Especially in torsade de pointes and QT prolongation and aggravated arrhythmias, overdrive suppression by means of pacemaker therapy is effective and helpful to overcome the period of increased vulnerability and electrical instability.

Prevention of Proarrhythmia

Arrhythmogenesis does occur in a certain percentage during antiarrhythmic therapy and may lead to life-threatening situations in some patients. No reliable predictors are known to date, thus prevention has to be strongly recommended (Table 4).

First, indications of antiarrhythmic therapy have to be very strict. Initiation of antiarrhythmic therapy with type Ia/Ic or III antiarrhythmics should be performed in an inpatient setting only. One hour after first dosage of the drug in question, ECG should be controlled with measurement of QT interval, one more ECG has to be recorded within one week of initiated therapy. The antiarrhythmic agent should be discontinued if QT interval increases beyond 120% or 500 ms (QTc) or if QRS complete is widened more than 25%. In the latter case, antiarrhythmic drug can be continued if the drug it the only effective agent and antiarrhythmic therapy is strongly indicated.

Ambulatory ECG is to be obtained after drug administration to assess efficacy or proarrhythmia. Electrolytes abnormalities have to be corrected, ischemic events even the silent ones should be suppressed, left ventricular failure has to be treated. Patients should be instructed to immediately report any signs of dizziness or syncope. In some patients, provocative electrophysiologic testing is required to determine the possible susceptibility of proarrhythmia, especially if proarrhythmia has been known in that patient.

References

1. Graboys TB, Lown B, Podrid PJ, DeSilva RA (1982) Long term survival of patients with malignant ventricular arrhythmias treated with antiarrhythmic drugs. Am J Cardiol 50:437–443
2. Velebit V, Podrid PJ, Lown B, Graboys TB (1982) Aggravation and provocation of ventricular arrhythmias by antiarrhythmic drugs. Circulation 65:886–894
3. Löllgen H, Hust MH, Nitsche K, Wollschläger H, Bonzel T, Just H (1983) Arrhythmogene Antiarrhythmika (arrhythmogenic antiarrhythmics) Cardiology 70:129–137
4. Löllgen H, Hust MH, Nitsche K (1986) Lebensbedrohliche Komplikationen durch Antiarrhythmika. Intensivmed 23:193–200
5. Horowitz LN, Zipes DP (eds) (1987) A symposium: perspectives on proarrhythmia. Am J Cardiol 59:1E–56E
6. Morganroth J (1987) Risk factors for the development of proarrhythmic events. Am J Cardiol 59:32E–37E
7. Horowitz LN, Zipes DP, Bigger JT, et al (1987) Proarrhythmia, arrhythmogenesis or aggravation of arrhythmia – a status report. Am J Cardiol 59:54E–56E
8. CAPS Investigators (1986) The cardiac arrhythmia pilot study (CAPS) Am J Cardiol 57:91–97
9. Brugada P, Wellens HJJ (1988) Arrhythmogenesis of antiarrhythmic drugs Am J Cardiol 61:1108–1111
10. Podrid PJ, Lampert S, Graboys TB, Blatt CM, Lown B (1987) Aggravation of arrhythmia by antiarrhythmic drugs – incidence and predictors. Am J Cardiol 59:38E–44E
11. Zipes DP (1987) Proarrhythmic effects of antiarrhythmic drugs. Am J Cardiol 59:26E–31E
12. Tzivoni D, Keren A, Cohen AM et al (1984) Magnesium therapy for torsades de pointes. Am J Cardiol 53:528–530
13. Iseri LT, Freed J, Bures AR (1975) Magnesium deficiency and cardiac disorders. Am J Med 59:837–846
14. Delhumeau A (1985) Effects antiarrhythmiques des sels magnesium. Presse Med 11:629–632
15. Seipel L (1989) Therapie der ventrikulären Extrasystolie. Dtsch Med Wschr 114:1571–1575

Complications After Cardiac Surgery

Myocardial Preservation During Cardiac Surgery

W. Flameng

Introduction

Global myocardial ischemia has been the subject of many studies in the field of cardiac surgery, and there is still an ongoing quest for ideal myocardial protective techniques [1]. During prolonged periods of global ischemia myocardial injury can be substantially delayed by hypothermia and cardioplegia [2], but there is no doubt that without timely reperfusion these "protected" globally ischemic hearts would die. Although hypothermia and cardioplegia offer adequate protection during many routine cardiac intervention [3, 4], more extended periods of aortic cross-clamping are still associated with an increased incidence of postoperative low cardiac output and lethal outcome. Another attracting topic for the cardiac surgeons is the prolonged organ preservation for transplantation. Donor heart preservation, i.e. cold storage after cardioplegic arrest, is limited at present to 3 to 4 hours in order to avoid postoperative low cardiac output.

Pathways Leading to Ischemic Cell Death and Possible Modifications by Calcium Antagonists

Although changes to the myocardial tissue induced by ischemia have been intensively studied in the past, the cause of the transition from reversible to irreversible or lethal injury has never been established. Nevertheless, potential causes of irreversibility can be recognized when studying the major features of ischemia. Within a few seconds after onset of ischemia, mitochondrial oxidative phosphorylation stops. This results in a drop of high-energy phosphate production and in an accumulation of catabolites. Creatine phosphate is almost completely depleted within the first 3 min of ischemia, while ATP decreases to about 35% of control by 15 min and to less than 10% by 40 min. A drop in high-energy phosphates is probably the trigger for a sequence of events leading to cell death. At first, energy-dependent membrane ion-pump function decreases and disturbs cell volume regulation. Malfunction of the Na^+, K^+ ATPase induces intracellular accumulation of Na^+ and cell swelling. An enhanced exchange between Na^+ and Ca^{2+} in turn induces an increase in cytosolic Ca^{2+}. Cytosolic Ca^{2+} is further increased by an impaired extrusion of Ca^{2+} via the energy-dependent Mg^{2+}, Ca^{2+} ATPase. Cytosolic Ca^{2+} can also be augmented by a deficiency of calcium sequestration in the sarcoplasmatic reticulum (SR) when the SR calcium pump (Ca^{2+}-activated magnesium ATPase) is inhibited. Such an accumulation and redistribution of intracellular Ca^{2+} has detrimental consequences for the myocyte: mitochondria starts accumulating Ca^{2+} instead of producing ATP; Ca^{2+} activates phospholipases and proteases, which in turn will destroy phospholipid bilayers and proteins. At this stage, rupture of the sarcolemma will occur and will, mainly in the presence of reperfusion, initiate a massive pathologic Ca^{2+} influx. This is the hallmark of irreversibility: massive Ca^{2+} accumulation by the mitochondria will destroy its function and induce irreversible hypercontraction of the myofibrils. Sarcolemmal rupture is also initiated by other mechanisms in the ischemic cell. Accumulation of acylcarnitine and acylCoA occurs, and these agents act as detergents on the membranes. Formation of free radicals may be induced by the increased catabolism of high-energy phosphates. Hypoxanthine, one of the final catabolites of ATP, is oxidized to xanthine and uric acid by the xanthine oxidase reaction. During ischemia, inosine and hypoxanthine rapidly accumulate and, especially when reperfusion is established, the xanthine oxidase reaction might produce and excessive load of superoxide anion. This ion is particularly toxic and produces membrane destruction.

Cardioplegia

Although the pathophysiology of the ischemic process is complex, it is necessary to figure out the triggering mechanism initiating the cascade of reactions leading to irreversible ischemic cell damage and death. Scientists have largely agreed that the limiting factor for reversibility of pure global ischemia is a critical loss of high energy phosphates [5].

If the reversibility of pure global ischemia is energetically limited, the most efficient method to improve the tolerance to ischemia is to switch off, in a reversible way, the main energy consuming system i.e. the contractile mechanism. There is a variety of possibilities to arrest a heart artificially [2]. They can be divided into three main categories:

1. potassium arrest;
2. combined potassium and magnesium arrest;
3. arrest by sodium reduction to near intracellular concentration with simultaneously corresponding minimization of calcium.

These three approaches have been used widely to arrest the heart for routine cardiac surgery. The first is used in many American centers. A representative example is the N. I. H. cardioplegic solution. The second method is widely studied by the group of Hearse in England and a representative example is the St. Thomas' Hospital cardioplegia. The third method originates from the work of Bretschneider in West Germany and resulted in the so-called Bretschneider cardioplegia. All these cardioplegic solutions were tested by our group on their ability to preserve high energy phosphate levels in the human myocardium during routine cardiac surgery procedures and were found to be effective during

1–2 h of cardioplegic arrest [3, 4, 6, 7]. Functional outcome of these hearts was excellent.

Although the formulation of cardioplegic solutions differs greatly, there is general agreement as to the mechanism underlying this action.

Three basic principles of effective cardioplegic protection of the myocardium can be defined:

(a) energy conservation through chemical induction of rapid and complete diastolic arrest;
(b) slowing of the metabolic rate and degradative processes through coincidental use of hypothermia;
(c) prevention or reversal of certain unfavorable ischemia-induced changes with various protective agents.

First Principle of Cardioplegic Protection: Energy Conservation

Although myocardial ischemia itself induces a rapid and dramatic reduction in contractility, residual mechanical activity may persist for some time. Also ventricular fibrillation will occur rapidly and both mechanisms will drain the heart of vital and limited supplies of cellular energy that otherwise might be used for the preservation of cellular integrity.

The most effective method to prolonge the ischemic tolerance of the heart is to switch off the main consumer of energy – the contractile system – by artificial arrest of the heart.

The three methods of cardioplegia described above were able to conserve myocardial high energy phosphate for at least some time. As compared to normothermic ischemic arrest of the heart myocardial tissue ATP content remained much longer at a normal level using cardioplegia. In case of simple ischemic arrest, ATP content was already significantly decreased within one hour (Fig. 1).

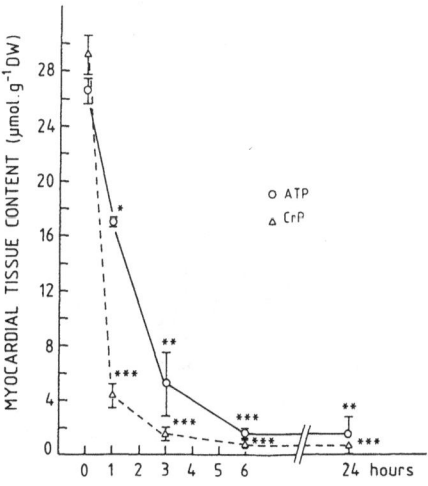

Fig. 1. High energy phosphates breakdown after normothermic excision of the heart followed by cold storage. Mean values (±SEM) of ATP and CrP are presented. * p < 0.05 versus control; ** p < 0.01 versus control; *** p < 0.001 versus control

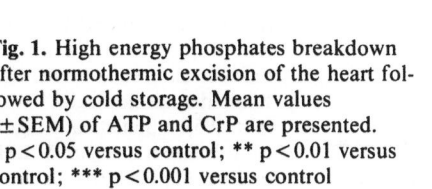

When the heart is arrested with the combination potassium-magnesium (St. Thomas' Hospital solution), ATP content decreased significantly only after 3 h (Fig. 2). When the heart is arrested using only potassium (N. I. H. solution) such a significant decrease is found after a delay of 4 h, and when the heart was arrested with low sodium, low calcium (Bretschneider solution) the ATP content remained in the normal range for 5 h. Because all hearts, including those excised after ischemic arrest, were stored cold at the same temperatures, the ATP-sparing effect must be due to the immediate diastolic arrest of the heart.

A variety of agents or interventions, besides potassium and magnesium loading or calcium depletion, can be used to initiate total diastolic arrest rapidly. Theoretically agents like acetylcholine, neostigmine and tetrodotoxin can be used for the same purpose. The question however remains how reversible the effects of these drugs are. Potassium is probably the safest to the interventions used because most other agents have a narrow range of optimal and safe dosage. The optimal potassium concentration was assessed in a range of 5 to 35 mEq/L utilizing a high energy phosphate index [6]. The ATP moiety is best preserved during ischemia and reperfusion at 15 mEq/L (>5 mEq/liter). The lower dose may not provide persistent depolarization and permit microfibrillation, even in the presence of hypothermia. On the other hand, an extreme dosage of potassium as found in the original Melrose solution (245 mEq/L) is harmful, probably because of the accompanying high hypertonicity caused by the high citrate level. The optimal dose of potassium is 15 to 25 mEq/L when it is used as depolarizing agent in a cardioplegic solution.

Magnesium has been shown to be a highly effective component of protective infusates, which can be additive to hypothermia and other agents [6]. Magne-

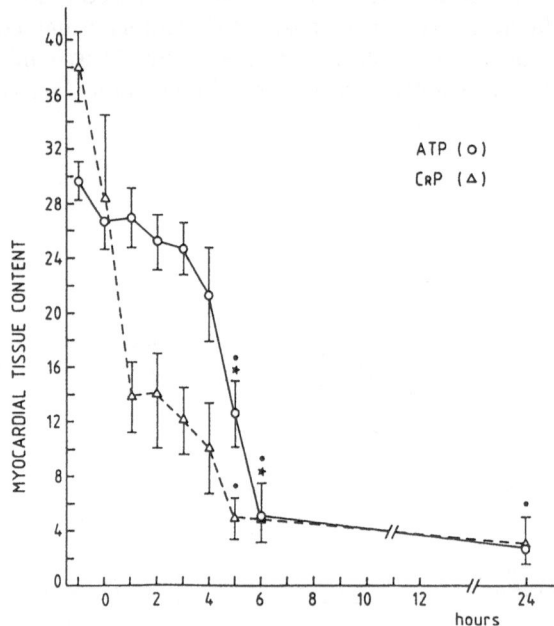

Fig. 2. Effect of single dose St. Thomas' cardioplegia followed by 24 hours of cold storage (0.5 °C) on ATP and CrP content of the myocardium. * Significant difference versus Bretschneider cardioplegia (p < 0.05). * Statistically significant difference versus N. I. H. or I cardioplegia (p < 0.05)

sium and potassium are the most abundant intracellular cations. Magnesium forms a complex with ATP to act as a substrate for enzymatic reactions underlying muscle contraction and relaxation and a cofactor for energy transferring reactions, oxidation, synthesis and transport. In ischemia, with the decrease in ATP, there is an increase in ionized magnesium and a loss of magnesium and potassium to the extracellular space. Hearse et al [6] demonstrated that the increased concentration of cytosolic ionized calcium that occurs with reperfusion can be alleviated by magnesium at a dose of 16 mmol/L in a detailed dose-response study (0 to 50 mmol/L). Hearse believes that magnesium is protective at the extracellular site for the following reasons:

1. reduction of trans-sacrolemmal magnesium gradient;
2. reduction of potassium efflux and calcium influx during ischemia; and
3. reduction of the incidence of dysrhythmias.

On the other hand, the pure potassium arrest (N.I.H. solution) offered a better myocardial preservation than potassium plus magnesium arrest (St. Thomas' Hospital solution) and the buffering capacity of the N.I.H. solution is not different from that of St. Thomas' Hospital solution. Therefore the inferior preservation with a potassium-magnesium arrest suggests an adverse effect of magnesium itself on preservation, although magnesium has the potential to improve the energetic protection of an ischemic heart due to its "calcium antagonistic" effect on the contractile system. Also other authors have shown that preservation of the heart with St. Thomas' Hospital solution was unsatisfying and Gebhard suggested a yet unnoticed adverse effect of magnesium "which can be detected under the given extreme condition of ischemic stress, temperature shifts and myocardial wash-out" [8].

Reduction of sodium and mainly Ca^{2+} in a cardioplegic solution (the so-called Ca^{2+}-free cardioplegia) renders a potential danger to the myocardium. It is known that Ca^{2+}-free perfusion of the heart induces the development of a "calcium-paradox" when the heart is reperfused with a Ca^{2+}-containing solutions [9]. Extracellular Ca^{2+} may fulfill three functions of importance to the myocytes. The first function is that of a source for cellular influx and accumulation. Because Ca^{2+} influx and consequent contraction is against the basic principle of cardioplegia, a great reduction of Ca^{2+}, if not complete or nearly complete exclusion can be advocated. A second function of extracellular Ca^{2+} affects the physical character of the plasma membrane, as Ca^{2+} appears to be a major factor controlling lipid fluidity and permeability. There might be some reason to assume that, since hypothermia induces a less fluid state in membrane lipids, less extracellular Ca^{2+} is needed to obtain optimal membrane fluidity and permeability at a low temperature. However, the optimal requirements for extracellular Ca^{2+} with the respect to membrane biophysics in cardioplegia and cardiac preservation remain to be established. The third function of extracellular Ca^{2+} is that of a factor maintaining the integrity of the cell membrane complex. It is this function of extracellular Ca^{2+} which should be considered carefully when a Ca^{2+}-free cardioplegia is propagated because of the potential hazard of inducing irreversible membrane damage by the Ca^{2+} paradox mechanism. When the heart is perfused with a Ca^{2+}-free solution under normothermic condition for a certain period of time and then reperfused with a Ca^{2+} containing medium irreversible myocardial damage occurs suddenly. The pathophysiology of this Ca^{2+}-paradox phenomenon is complex and involves the destruction of the cell membrane system. However, it was shown that hypothermia prevents this deleterious effect of a Ca^{2+} paradox [10]. Therefore, no real argument against the use of a Ca^{2+} free solution is found. Moreover, it was clearly shown that damage to the myocardium caused by a Ca^{2+}-free perfusion occurs at a far more advanced stage of Ca^{2+}-free perfusion when a sodium-poor solution is used. This protective action of low sodium against the Ca^{2+} paradox can be explained by a delay in Ca^{2+} removal from an essential membrane site during Ca^{2+}-free perfusion.

Second Principle of Cardioplegia: Hypothermia

Toward the end of the 19th century, Van't Hoff (1884) and Arrhenius (1889) studied the thermal coefficient for chemical processes. Van't Hoff found that the velocity of various organic reactions diminished by a factor of 2 for every 10°C reduction in temperature and introduced the concept of Q10 to describe these relationships. Arrhenius however, found that although biochemical reactions exhibited exponential decreases in velocity in relation to decrease in absolute temperature, this relationship does not always yield a Q10 of 2. Empirically, Arrhenius developed equations which state that there is a linear relationship between the logarithm of the rate of chemical process and the reciprocal of absolute temperature (which for a given reaction has come to be known as its Arrhenius plot), and that the activation energy of these processes can be estimated indirectly through the measurement of their velocities at different temperatures. Generally, chemical reactions that depend upon a high energy of activation have higher Q10 values (above 2 or 3) than reactions with low activation energies. Different Q10 characteristics between biochemical and biophysical reactions lead to a heterogenous cooling response between different cellular processes, and between organs. Cellular energy processes such as phosphorylation may decline rapidly, whereas diffusion of ions, metabolites and water may be reduced to a lesser extent.

The heterogeneity of cellular response to hypothermia is further compounded by the phenomenon of lipoprotein phase transitions. According to the Singer-Nicholson fluid-mosaic model of membrane structure, plasma membranes and intracellular membranes are composed of a classic bilayer, in which protein elements are embedded. In normothermia, the proteins exist predominantly in a fluid state, permitting a high degree of freedom for conformational changes of membrane-bound protein and enzyme complexes to occur. As cooling progress, membrane lipids undergo a phase transition from their dynamic fluid state to a more highly ordered gel state characterized by closer packing of phospholipid molecules, increase in bilayer thickness, and reduction in mobility of membrane protein and enzyme complexes. One important consequence of membrane phase transitions is the reduction of permeability for molecular transport. There is a steep increase in the activation energy of membrane bound reactions in hypothermia. Such reactions therefore may show a dramatically decreased rate of activity, expressed as a break in the linearity of their Arrhenius plots. Lipid phase transitions and their associated metabolic consequences may largely determine the lower limits for organ function during hypothermia. Even at 4°C metabolic processes are very slowly operative.

The Third Principle of Cardioplegia: Counter Balance of Ischemia-induced Changes

As mentioned in the introduction, myocardial ischemia initiates a continuum of progressively more serious cellular changes which, unless halted, will lead to cell death and tissue necrosis. The dominant feature of ischemic injury is energy depletion and this can be counteracted in part by the first and the second principles of cardioplegia. There are however, numerous other related and unrelated changes that arise as a consequence of ischemia: unfavorable redistribution of ions, leakage of metabolites and cofactors, loss of cell volume control, physical disruption of cellular and subcellular structures, loss of control of biochemical pathways etc. Numerous 'anti-ischemic' interventions have been suggested to reduce or delay these critical changes, including steroids to stabilize membranes of subcellular particles such as lysosomes, glucose and insulin to support and stimulate anaerobic energy production, oxygen to stimulate aerobic and anaerobic metabolism, mannitol to counteract all edema and various agents, again including mannitol, to scavenge or inhibit active oxygen intermediates such as the superoxide and hydroxyl-free radicals. Most of these pharmacological interventions do not significantly improve the preservation of the myocardium, none of them could significantly improve long-term preservation. Therefore we believe that their contribution is small and their use as additives to a preservation technique is still controversial.

Whole blood and intracellular fluid constitute a mixture of CO_2-bicarbonate and proteins buffers. Acting under conditions where exchange of CO_2-bicarbonate conjugate acid-base pair is only from 12 to 20% of the buffer value attributable to protein. Hence protein is the predominant buffer both in whole blood and cytoplasm and the effect of temperature on protein buffering largely determines the response of pH and PCO_2. Of the 20 genetically coded aminoacids constituting all proteins, one, histidine, is the focus of acid-base regulation. Histidine's side chain imidazole ring has unpaired electrons that can bind a proton and thus cause the imidazole ring to bear a positive charge. However, the affinity of histidine's imidazole ring for protons is relatively weak such that in vivo roughly only half the imidazole rings bear the positive charge, and the remainder are unchanged. Only histidine's imidazole R-groups binds a proton reversibly over the physiological pH range of 6–8. Hence it is this group, well represented in all proteins that is the principal buffer of the cell. Because the act of binding a proton converts an uncharged histidine imidazole side chain into a positively changed group, proton binding not only alters the net protein charge, but it also alters charge-charge interactions on the surface of the protein. Interactions between charges on the surface of the protein importantly affect the conformation of the protein and the association of sub-units. Moreover, histidine imidazoles also play a key role at the active site of many enzymes where their protonation state directly affects activity. Hence supplying a protein with protons simultaneously promotes proton binding and buffering, alters the net charge on the protein, affects the conformation of the protein and alters enzymatic function. Thus control of protein function via adjustment of the fraction of histidine imidazole groups bearing a proton is the central objective of acid-base regulation.

Because the first principle of cardioplegia i.e. diastolic arrest, can be achieved using either potassium, potassium plus magnesium or low sodium low calcium solutions, an additional gain of energetic protection can only be reached by increasing the buffer capacity of the ischemic heart. The margin in which the buffer capacity of the myocardium can artificially be increased is principally limited, because the extracellular space of the heart takes more than 20 to 25%. Consequently, the gain in buffer capacity per kilogram of tissue in no case reaches more than one-fifth to one-fourth of the buffer capacity per liter of cardioplegic solution. Presupposing a non-bicarbonate buffer capacity of the myocardium between 25 and 40 mmol/kg and pH unit and pK value of 6.5 of the buffer system, one needs a 150 to 180 mmol solution of the buffer per liter to double the buffer capacity of the myocardium. These calculations make clear that an effective artificial buffering of the myocardium, for osmotic reasons, can only be realized in combination with low sodium and low calcium cardioplegia. The amino-acid histidine is currently the only buffer substance that largely complies with the condition just mentioned.

Intermittent Reperfusion

In an attempt to limit the period of myocardial ischemia by cross clamping of the aorta, intermittent reperfusion of the coronary vessels by release of the aortic clamp can be performed. This technique also referred to as 'intermittent aortic cross clamping' can be used mainly in aortocoronary bypass grafting because this operation does not require an aortotomy. It is usually combined with general hypothermia up to 25°C.

In a recent study however, we could demonstrate that this technique is inferior to cardioplegic arrest in terms of preservation of high energy phosphates [4].

Pharmacological Protection of the Myocardium

Most popular drugs used for myocardial protection are calcium antagonists.

How can Ca^{2+} antagonists modify these pathways leading to ischemic cell death? Ca^{2+} overload is the final and lethal feature preceding cell death. Within this concept, drugs that are able to prevent this Ca^{2+} overload are potentially protective and can be called "calcium overload blockers". This by no means implies that these drugs have to prevent pathologic Ca^{2+}-influx when they are administered not prior to, but together with, reperfusion. Poole-Wilson for example showed clearly that verapamil, administered together with reperfusion in the ischemic ventricular septum preparation, could not prevent massive Ca^{2+} accumulation in the postischemic myocardial tissue [11]. There is however, abundant evidence that this calcium entry blocker, when given prior to ischemia, prevents Ca^{2+} overload and cell death after reperfusion [12]. Calcium antagonists act as Ca^{2+} overload blockers in the ischemic and postischemic myocardium when the heart is pretreated with these agents. They do so by blocking the pathways leading to Ca^{2+} overload at two different levels: inhibition of ATP breakdown and stabilization of the plasma membrane. Both mechanisms, the ATP-sparing effect and membrane stabilization, are not necessarily of the same importance and the predominance of one of these interactions seems to be related to the specific type of calcium antagonist used. For example, verapamil, nifedipine and diltiazem mainly act via the ATP-sparing effect [12] and also but less via a membrane stabilizing effect [13]. Lidoflazine on the other hand has a predominantly protective effect on the plasma membrane and has little effect on ATP breakdown [14]. Both types of drugs, however, clearly prevent postischemic calcium overload and cell death when used as a pretreatment [12, 15].

Myocardial Protective Effects of Calcium Antagonists: Clinical Studies

Clark was the first to report a well-documented clinical study on the cardioprotective effects of nifedipine during surgically induced global myocardial ischemia in 90 patients [16]. Nifedipine or placebo was added to the cardioplegic solution. The cristalloid cardioplegic solution was hyperkalemic, hypoatriemic, alkalotic and hyperosmotic. The nifedipine concentration ranged from 100–300 µg/l such that the total dose for each patient was in the range of 1.0 to 2.0 µg/g of estimated weight. The study showed an improved left ventricular performance (left ventricular minute work index) immediately after weaning from cardiopulmonary bypass and a lower incidence of myocardial injury as assessed by myocardial pyrophosphate scans. However, the use of nifedipine had no effect on the incidence of acute low cardiac output syndrome or death.

We studied the protective effects of nifedipine as an adjunct to St. Thomas' Hospital cardioplegia, not only in terms of functional and clinical outcome but also in relation to nucleotide metabolism [17]. Thus, both studies provide evidence for the protective properties of the calcium entry blocker nifedipine in the clinical setting. However, more large-scale double-blind placebo-controlled randomized clinical studies are needed to investigate the final goal: improvement of clinical outcome after extensive cardiac surgery. No other study than the two presented above, although placebo-controlled and randomized, contained a patient population that was large enough to allow valid conclusions on differences in clinical outcome.

In another randomized clinical study we assessed the protective properties of another calcium antagonist, lidoflazine [14]. This study differed from the above-mentioned nifedipine studies in two respects. First, this study included only aortocoronary bypass operations which were performed using intermittent aortic cross-claming at 28 °C. Second, lidoflazine was administered intravenously prior to installation of cardiopulmonary bypass.

Table 1. Mortality rate after coronary artery bypass surgery in 1200 consecutive patients after lidoflazine pretreatment (1 mg/kg) + IXC − 28 °C

Cardiac:	Myocardial infarction	4	(0.33%)
	Heart failure	2	(0.17%)
	Unknown	2	(0.17%)
Non-cardiac:		5	(0.42%)
Total:		13	(1.09%)

Encouraged by the results of this study we now use lidoflazine 1.0 mg/kg as a pretreatment routinely in our institution. We reviewed the last 1200 consecutive cases in terms of clinical outcome and obtained excellent results. These results are presented in Table 1. Although we are well aware that these results are of little scientific value we feel that they are worthwhile to report. They show that the drug is safe and that an extremely low incidence of postoperative low cardiac output syndrome can be achieved with this technique.

References

1. McGoon DC (1985) The ongoing quest for ideal myocardial protection. J Thorac Cardiovasc Surg 89:639–653
2. Engelman RM, Levitsky S (1982) Textbook of clinical cardioplegia. Futura Publishing, London, England
3. Flameng W, Borgers M, Daenen W, et al (1981) St. Thomas' Hospital cardioplegia versus topical cooling: ultrastructural and biochemical studies in humans. Ann Thorac Surg 31:339–346
4. Flameng W, Van der Vusse GJ, De Meyere R, et al (1984) Intermittent aortic cross clamping versus St. Thomas' Hospital cardioplegia in extensive aorta-coronary bypass grafting. A randomized study. J Thorac Cardiovasc Surg 88:164–173
5. Bretschneider HJ (1964) Überlebenszeit und Wiederbelebungszeit eines Herzens bei Normo- und Hypothermie. Verh Dtsch Ges Kreislaufforsch 30:11–34
6. Hearse DJ, Braimbridge MV, Jynge P (1981) Protection of the ischemic myocardium: Cardioplegia. Raven Press, New York
7. Bretschneider HJ, Gebhard MM, Preusse CJ (1981) Reviewing the pros and cons of myocardial preservation within cardiac surgery. In: Longmore DB (ed) Towards safer cardiac surgery. MTP Press, Lancaster, England, pp 21–53
8. Gebhard MM, Bretschneider HJ, Gersing E, Schnabel PA, Preusse CJ (1987) Bretschneider histidine-buffered cardioplegic solution: concept, application and efficiency. In: Roberts AJ (ed) Myocardial protection - cardiac surgery. Dekker, New York Basel, pp 95–119
9. Ruigrok TJC, Burgerdijk FJA, Zimmerman ANE (1975) The calcium paradox. A reaffinition. Eur J Cardiol 3:54–63
10. Holland CE Jr, Olson RE (1975) Prevention by hypothermia of paradoxial calcium necrosis in cardiac muscle. J Mol Cell Cardiol 7:917–928
11. Bourdellon PD, Poole-Wilson PA (1982) The effects of verapamil k, quiescence and cardioplegia on calcium exchange and mechanical function in ischemic rabbit myocardium. Circ Res 50:360–368
12. Nayler WG, Ferrari R, Williams A (1980) Protective effect of pretreatment with verapamil, nifedipine and propranolol on mitochondrial function in the ischemic and reperfused myocardium. Am J Cardiol 46:242–248
13. Baker JE, Hearse DJ (1983) Slow calcium channel blockers and the calcium paradox: comparative studies in the rat with seven drugs. J Mol Cell Cardiol 15:475–485

14. Flameng W, Borgers M, Van der Vusse GJ, et al (1983) Cardioprotective effects of lidoflazine in extensive aortocoronary bypass grafting. J Thorac Cardiovasc Surg 5:758-768
15. Flameng W, Daenen W, Borgers M, et al (1981) Cardio protective effects of lidoflazine during 1 hour normothermic global ischemia. Circulation 64:796-807
16. Clark RE, Ferguson TB, Marbarger JP (1981) The first American clinical trial of nifedipine in cardioplegia. J Thorac Cardiovasc Surg 82:848-859
17. Flameng W, De Meyere R, Daenen W, et al (1986) Nifedipine as an adjunct to St. Thomas' hospital cardioplegia. A double-blind, placebo-controlled, randomized clinical trial. J Thorac Cardiovasc Surg 91:723-731

Prevention of the Postperfusion Syndrome After Cardiopulmonary Bypass

C. P. Stoutenbeek and H. M. Oudemans-van Straaten

Introduction

The postoperative period following cardiopulmonary bypass (CPB) is often complicated by a clinical picture resembling septic shock. Most frequently it occurs in a mild form characterized by hyperthermia, marked peripheral vasoconstriction, hypotension, a normal or high cardiac output with a low peripheral vascular resistance.

Although these symptoms resolve spontaneously within 12–24 hours, intensive hemodynamic monitoring and medical treatment consisting of volume infusion and inotropic support is required. Some patients, however, develop a full-blown "postperfusion syndrome" with an increased capillary permeability and severe hypotension leading to multiple organ dysfunction [1, 2]. The lungs most frequently manifest perfusion related injury. Clinically the predominating symptom is noncardiogenic pulmonary edema ('pump lung') resulting in arterial hypoxemia. The histological changes show engorgement of the pulmonary vascular bed, micro-atelectasis and interstitial and alveolar hemorrhage [2]. Renal insufficiency, neurologic changes and hemorrhagic diathesis are other signs of the postperfusion syndrome. The symptoms are often not recognized until a few hours after CPB, when the patient has arrived in the ICU. The treatment includes high-doses of epinephrine and α-adrenergic agents such as phenylephrine to maintain an adequate peripheral vascular resistance. A large volume of blood and fluid may be required to maintain optimal preload as a result of a generalized loss of capillary integrity. Intraaortic counterpulsation (IABP) is sometimes necessary to support the circulation. Pharmacological doses of steroids are recommended by some authors to decrease the inflammatory response and to stop the leak of proteinaceous fluids into the interstitial space.

Etiology

Etiologic factors that have been implicated in the development of the postperfusion syndrome include the activation of the humoral cascades of complement, kallikrein, coagulation and fibrinolysis by the extracorporeal circuit, white blood cell (WBC) trapping in the lungs, release of oxygen-free radicals and protamine reactions. The generally accepted etiology of the postperfusion syndrome is a noninfectious 'whole body inflammatory response' directed against materials of the extracorporeal circuit [1]. The attention has been focussed primarily on complement activation by the extracorporeal circuit and specifically by the bubble oxygenator. However, other explanations are more likely.

During CPB considerable amounts of endotoxin have been found in the blood of patients [3, 4]. The highest values were observed shortly after release of the aortic crossclamp. The concentration then decayed to the baseline level 45 to 75 min after termination of bypass. The mean rise in endotoxin concentration 5 to 15 min after release of the crossclamp was 0.428 ng/ml above baseline level [3]. The duration of CPB clearly influenced the rise of endotoxin level. Kharazmi et al. showed that the rise in endotoxin parallelled with a drop in leukocyte count in all patients, due to leukocyte activation and trapping in the lung. All patients had an elevated temperature postoperatively [5]. The endotoxin found in the patients' blood is most likely derived from the gut. Previous studies have shown that CPB can lead to ischemic damage to organs perfused by the splanchnic circulation e.g. pancreatitis [6].

The hypothesis that the intestinal organs become ischemic during CPB, is supported by a recent study by Fiddian-Green. He determined the pH in the gastric wall by means of a Tonomitor, as a measure of gastric perfusion, in 85 patients undergoing elective cardiac surgery [7]. Inadequate gastric perfusion or ischemia was found in 42 patients (49%). Gastric mucosal ischemia usually appeared during cardiopulmonary bypass or shortly after release of the aortic crossclamp. Most episodes lasted about one hour. Eight patients (9.4%) developed life-threatening complications within 72 h of their operations; five patients died. All 8 complications and all deaths occurred in the patients in whom stomach wall acidosis during the operation was found. The postoperative complications included acute myocardial failure, pulmonary failure and acute pancreatitis [7, 8]. The low (non-pulsatile) flow during CPB and the release of endogenous vasoconstrictors, hypothermia and hyperoxemia may all contribute to splanchnic ischemia.

In a recent collaborative study with Wildevuur et al. in patients undergoing CABG we were able to demonstrate a significant rise in the levels of tumor necrosis factor (TNF), leukotriene B4 and tissue-plasminogen activator after release of the aortic crossclamp, reaching a maximum 30 min after CPB. During CPB the levels of TNF were not elevated [9]. These data are in agreement with the endotoxin-studies suggesting that the release of the aortic crossclamp is the luxating moment. As the aortic crossclamp is released several changes occur simultaneously: first, the ischemic heart and lungs are reperfused, the blood is rewarmed and biochemical processes are initiated and finally the heart will restore pulsatile flow. In animal experiments it has been shown that most of the mucosal injury produced by ischemia occurs at the time of reperfusion and is mediated by oxygen-free radicals [10]. We hypothesize that reperfusion of the ischemic intestinal organs increases the permeability of the mucosa with subsequent absorption of endotoxin, which is known to be a potent stimulus of TNF and other cytokines. TNF is probably the most important mediator of the septic shock like clinical syndrome seen after CPB.

Prevention

In several studies the influence of high doses of corticosteroids on the postperfusion syndrome has been evaluated, with conflicting results. Corticosteroids are reported to affect complement activation [11]. No consistent clinical effects of corticosteroids on circulation [12–14] and pulmonary function [2, 15] are found. These differences might be explained by the different types of corticosteroids being investigated (dexamethasone or methylprednisolone), by the different doses used or by the fact that the observations were made at different moments in relation to CPB [2, 12–15]. Since the peak levels of endotoxin and inflammatory mediators occur towards the end of CPB, the clinical symptoms are most prominent a few hours after CPB and disappear within 12–24 hours. Niazi et al. [14] evaluated the effect of methylprednisolone (30 mg/kg) and of dexamethasone (6 mg/kg) versus a placebo on the hemodynamic changes, up to 6 h after administration. From our observations it appears that the major hemodynamic changes generally arise after this period. Enderby et al. [15] studied the effects of methylprednisolone administered before bypass on the lung function. He assessed the lung function preoperatively, 48 h after the operation, and one week after the operation and found no significant differences. Unfortunately, the first 24 h after the operation in which major changes are seen in pulmonary function has not been studied by them. Miranda et al. [12] found a highly significant effect of dexamethasone administered pre-bypass on the hemodynamic situation in the early postoperative period. However, in this study the mean CPB-time was very long (3 hours) compared to the present standards.

We have undertaken a double-blind randomized placebo-controlled study comparing dexamethasone (1 mg/kg), methylprednisolone (30 mg/kg) and prednisolone (50 mg), on the postoperative hemodynamic situation. We tried to correlate the clinical findings with the effect of corticosteroids on the inflammatory mediators during and after CPB. Twelve patients received dexamethasone, 11 patients methylprednisolone, 11 patients prednisolone and 10 patients received placebo, at induction of anesthesia. No significant difference was found in the levels of activated complement between placebo and steroid-treated patients, which confirms the findings of Boscoe et al. [11]. Dexamethasone completely prevented the rise in TNF. In some of the methylprednisolone-treated patients, however, elevated TNF-levels were found. Dexamethasone suppressed the release of leukotriene B4 after declamping more effectively than methylprednisolone or prednisolone. In the placebo-treated group TNF was still significantly increased on the first post-operative day. The leukocyte and thrombocyte numbers were significantly higher in the dexamethasone and methylprednisolone treated patients than in the placebo-group, which probably reflects the prevention of leukocyte and thrombocyte trapping [9]. The postperfusion syndrome could be completely prevented by dexamethasone and methylprednisolone but not by the low dose prednisolone. Patients treated with a high dose of steroids developed no hyperthermia, had a significant higher blood pressure, a better peripheral circulation, required less intravenous fluids and less cardiotonic medication in the immediate postoperative period and had a significantly shorter stay in the ICU. The oxygenation was better in the dexamethasone-treated patients than in the other groups. However, after 12 hours this difference had completely disappeared. Apart from a slight increase in serum glucose levels, no side effects were observed. In particular no increased incidence of postoperative infections or delayed wound healing was observed.

This study suggests that a relatively low dose of 1 mg/kg dexamethasone is equally effective or superior to 30 mg/kg methylprednisolone to prevent postperfusion phenomena [16]. Complement activation is apparently not the main mediator of the postperfusion syndrome, since in the dexamethasone and methylprednisolone-treated patients the clinical symptoms disappeared, whereas the activated complement levels were increased. The principal mechanism seems to be absorption of endotoxin from the ischemic gut with subsequent activation of TNF and other cytokines. When this hypothesis is correct, preventive measures should be directed to prevent gut ischemia during CPB. Intestinal vasodilating agents such as α-blockers, ACE-inhibitors, ketanserin or dopamine, administered before and during bypass might be effective to prevent gut ischemia. Xanthine-oxidase inhibitors (allopurinol) might attenuate the reperfusion damage of the ischemic mucosa [10]. Other preventive measures could be directed against absorption of endotoxin from the gut. Since most of the endotoxin in the gut is derived from aerobic gram-negative bacilli selective decontamination of the gut might be of benefit. In healthy volunteers the intestinal endotoxin content could be reduced with 90% by selective decontamination [17]. Monoclonal antibodies against TNF, administered at termination of bypass might be effective.

As the scope of cardiac surgery extends to older patients with more complex lesions, the probability of experiencing clinical manifestations of perfusion-related damage increases. Further research to prevent these postperfusion phenomena is indicated.

References

1. Westaby S (1987) Organ dysfunction after cardiopulmonary bypass. A systemic inflammatory reaction by the extracorporeal circuit. Intensive Care Med 13:89–95
2. Maggart M, Stewart S (1987) The mechanisms and management of non-cardiogenic pulmonary edema following cardiopulmonary bypass. Ann Thorac Surg 43:231–236
3. Rocke DA, Gaffin SL, Wells MT, Koen Y, Brock-Utine JG (1987) Endotoxaemia associated with cardiopulmonary bypass. J Thorac Cardiovasc Surg 93:832–837
4. Andersen LW, Beak L, Degn H, Lehd J, Krasnik M, Rasmussen JP (1987) Presence of circulating endotoxins during cardiac operations. J Thorac Cardiovasc Surg 93:115–119
5. Kharazmi A, Andersen LW, Beak L, Valerius NH, Laub M, Rasmussen JP (1989) Endotoxemia and enhanced generation of oxygen radicals by neutrophils from patients undergoing cardiopulmonary bypass. J Thorac Cardiovasc Surg 98:381–385
6. Feiner H (1976) Pancreatitis after cardiac surgery: a morphological study. Am J Surg 131:684–688
7. Fiddian-Green RG, Baker S (1987) Predictive value of the stomach wall pH for complications after cardiac operations: comparison with other monitoring. Crit Care Med 15:153–156
8. Fiddian-Green RG (1989) Studies in splanchnic ischemia and multiple organ failure. In: Marston A, Bulkely GB, Fiddian-Green RG, Haglund UH (eds) Splanchnic ischemia and multiple organ failure, 1st edn. Edward Arnold, pp 349–363

9. Jansen NJG, van Oeveren W, Chang Njoek Joen M, et al. The effect on different doses of corticosteroids on the reperfusion phenomena in cardiopulmonary bypass (submitted for publication)
10. Grisham MB, Granger DN (1989) Free radicals: reactive metabolites of oxygen as mediators of post-ischemia reperfusion injury. In: Marston A, Bulkely GB, Fiddian-Green RG, Haglund UH (eds) Splanchnic ischemia and multiple organ failure, 1st edn. Edward Arnold, pp 135–145
11. Boscoe MJ, Yewdall VMA, Thompson MA, Cameron JS (1983) Complement activation during cardiopulmonary bypass: quantitative study of effects of methylprednisolone and pulsatile flow. Br Med J 287:1747–1750
12. Miranda DR, Stoutenbeek CP, Karliczek G, Rating W (1982) Effects of dexamethasone on the early postoperative course after coronary artery bypass surgery. Thorac Cardiovasc Surgeon 30:21–27
13. Coraim FI, Laufer G, Ilias W, Wollenek G, Wolner E (1987) Release of myocardial depressant factor during cardiopulmonary bypass: influence of corticosteroids (methylprednisolone) and protease inhibitor (aprotinine). Proc Clin Biol Res 236A:611–620
14. Niazi Z, Flodin Ph, Joyce L, Smith J, Mauer H, Lillehei RC (1979) Effects of glucosteroids in patients undergoing coronary artery bypass surgery. Chest 76:262–268
15. Enderby DH, Boylett A, Parker DJ (1979) Methylprednisolone and lung-function after cardiopulmonary bypass. Thorax 34:720–725
16. van den Broek L, Oudemans-van Straaten HM, Stoutenbeek CP. Prevention of the postperfusion syndrome following cardiopulmonary bypass by different types and doses of corticosteroids (submitted)
17. van Saene JJM, Stoutenbeek CP, van Saene HKF (1989) Significant reduction of fecal endotoxin pool by oral polymyxin E and tobramycin in human volunteers. In: van Saene HKF, Stoutenbeek CP, Lawin P, MacLedingham I (eds) Update in intensive care and emergency medicine, vol 7. Springer, Berlin Heidelberg New York Tokyo, pp 128–134

Management of Heart Failure After Cardiac Surgery

M. Goenen, L. Jacquet, and M. Van Dyck

Introduction

Perioperative heart failure still remains the most common complication after open heart surgery, despite major progress in preserving perioperative myocardial function, improving intraoperative myocardial protection and adapting treatment by a better understanding of the mechanism of myocardial dysfunction. Improvements in medical treatment and angioplasty have changed referral patterns for coronary artery bypass graft (CABG) or valve replacements and also have increased the number of high-risk patients submitted to surgery (elderly patients, reoperations, emergency revascularization for refractory ischemia [1]. Left ventricular ejection fraction and left main coronary stenosis have become less significant predictors for mortality and morbidity.

If the morbidity has not changed over the years (1–2% in stable angina and 4–7% in the high-risk patients), perioperative morbidity has increased. In the high-risk patients, the incidence of perioperative morbidity ranges from 10 to 20%. Myocardial infarction and low output occur in almost 5 to 10% of those patients. Further improvements include better preoperative medical management to reduce the extent of ischemia and alternative techniques of myocardial protection.

The future strategies should be directed to avoid perioperative heart failure, earlier detect the reason for ongoing myocardial deterioration and optimize treatment to satisfy the metabolic needs and to restore the myocardial contractile reserve.

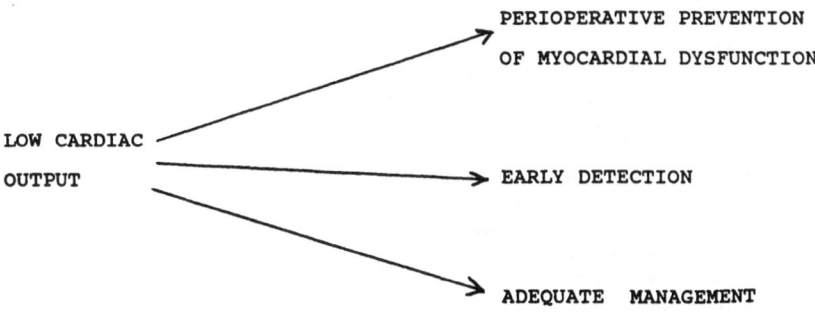

Fig. 1. Strategy for perioperative low output

Therefore, three different aspects may be concerned: prevention, diagnosis and management of heart failure (Fig. 1).

Prevention of Low Output (Table 1)

Careful screening of preoperative heart failure and aggressive therapy with intravenous nitroglycerin and/or β-blockers immediately before CABG remain essential to avoid recurrent ischemic attacks and thereby prevent postoperative low output. Pre-bypass ischemia is significantly related to perioperative myocardial infarction, reperfusion injury and postoperative myocardial low output [3]

Recommendation to prevent pre-bypass deterioration of the myocardial function may include:

1. Maintenance of full anti-anginal therapy,
2. Optimal sedation to avoid stress and anxiety,
3. Avoidance of anemia,
4. Preoperative hemodynamic monitoring and optimal management by administration of intravenous nitroglycerin and incremental doses of β-blocking agents,
5. Use of intra-aortic balloon pumping in patients with refractory anginal attacks or with postmyocardial infarction complications such as septal rupture or mitral insufficiency,
6. Immediately preoperative ECG-recording and CK-MB determination to detect a fresh myocardial infarction.

Intraoperative risk for myocardial function deterioration may be related to inadequate myocardial protection, and reperfusion injury (stunned myocardium), incomplete repair of the lesions, and inappropriate maneuver to emerge from bypass.

Table 1. Major causes of perioperative heart failure

1) Preoperative myocardial dysfunction.
2) Intraoperative global ischemia induced myocardial dysfunction (reperfusion injury, stunned myocardium).
3) Intraoperative myocardial infarction.
4) Incomplete cardiac repair.
5) Early postoperative myocardial infarction.
6) Preload and afterload mismatch.
7) Arrhythmias and conduction disorders.
8) Decreased contractility due to:
   – metabolic disorders
   – hypoxemia, anemia,
   – electrolytes abnormalities.
9) Decreased myocardial compliance:
   – heart compression or tamponade by increased intrathoracic pressure or hemorrhage.

Alternative techniques to the classic cold potassic cardioplegia for myocardial protection may better preserve cardiac reserve: cardioplegia with warm induction, terminal warm cardioplegic infusion and addition of substrates Krebs-cycle intermediates or calcium antagonists.

A high flow/high pressure [4] and a retrograde/antegrade cardioplegic infusion [5] may provide a more homogeneous flow distribution and myocardial cooling, particularly in the jeopardized myocardium. In a in vitro model, reperfusion with leukocyte-depleted blood has shown excellent myocardial function after long-term preservation [6].

During emergence from cardiopulmonary bypass, the anesthetist and the surgeon should avoid overdistention of right or left ventricle, correct electrolytic and metabolic disorders, optimize cardiac rhythm and conduction and assist the heart until adequate rewarming. The use of inotropic stimulants during early reperfusion should be avoided, since contractile work may aggravate any ischemic injury and delay recovery of myocardial function [7].

Early Diagnosis of Myocardial Dysfunction

Classically, the diagnosis of low output states is based on clinical findings, metabolic parameters and hemodynamic monitoring. However, these indirect indicators of cardiac failure are insufficient to early diagnose myocardial dysfunction and to recognize the causing factors.

More recently, new diagnostic methods have been available, including:
- transesophageal echocardiography (TEE);
- continuous mixed venous O_2-saturation monitoring ($S\bar{v}O_2$);
- coronary sinus measurements of venous O_2 saturation, lactic acid and CPK-MB production;
- right ventricular volume and ejection fraction determinations means a modified Swan-Ganz catheter.

Anesthetic agents, vasoactive drugs, myocardial ischemia, surgical events and changes in preload and afterload are all factors that can profoundly affect perioperative cardiovascular function. Besides the diagnosis of septal rupture, valvular dysfunction, pericardial effusion and aortic dissection, 2D-TEE intraoperative monitoring may provide continuous assessment of systolic and diastolic function of both ventricles: segment wall motion abnormalities as evidence of ischemia, changes in ventricular interdependence (abnormal septal motion), function and dimensions by volume loading, infusion of vasoactive drugs or changes in intrathoracic pressure (PEEP ventilation, pneumothorax). Nevertheless, in view of high costs and technical constraints, 2D-TEE cannot be considered as a routine monitoring in the postoperative ICU, but constitutes a useful method in selected high-risk patients [8, 9].

Continuous monitoring of $S\bar{v}O_2$ is not justified in low-risk patients but can be useful in high-risk patients with perioperative myocardial dysfunction. $S\bar{v}O_2$ may detect early metabolic and hemodynamic changes (inadequate cardiac output) and monitor the therapeutic response.

If the classical perioperative hemodynamic monitoring reflects myocardial function, no current methods are available to accurately detect intramyocardial metabolic changes, ischemic and reperfusion injuries, or extension of ischemia due to aggressive inotropic stimulation. Determinations of coronary sinus flow and some metabolic changes may present an approach to diagnose myocardial suffering and monitor therapy but the technical difficulties to insert the catheter into the coronary sinus make it inappropriate for routine postoperative use.

Management of Postoperative Low Output

Postoperative heart failure may result from [9]:

- reversible myocardial damage due to perioperative global ischemia-induced myocardial dysfunction (so-called "stunned myocardium" which may last for several days before recovery) [10],
- irreversible or partially reversible damage due to preoperative myocardial dysfunction, underlying cardiac disease, preoperative acute myocardial necrosis, incomplete cardiac repair.

Both may be worsened by several factors, including:

1. postoperative impaired myocardial perfusion, because of low arterial pressure, increased filling pressures, decreased myocardial perfusion gradient, short coronary perfusion time, ventricular hypertrophy, residual coronary stenosis,
2. metabolic and electrolytes abnormalities as hypoglycemia, hyperkalemia, hypoxemia, acidosis, alkalosis, increased O_2 consumption as by shivering,
3. arrhythmias and conduction disorders,
4. cardiac tamponade,
5. post-bypass endocrine disorders: increased secretion of norepinephrine, aldosterone, ADH, activation of renin angiotensin,
6. hypovolemia,
7. misuse of cardiodepressive drugs.

In the postoperative course, the intensivist is confronted with various hemodynamic signs of low output.

1. *Low filling and systemic arterial pressure and low output* reflect an hypovolemic state easily reversed by adequate volume loading.
2. *Low filling pressures and low systemic resistance with normal to increased cardiac output* is often seen in patients with combined preoperative nitrate and calcium antagonist therapy. Those patients are not in shock, but warm, pink and with repleted veins. Instead of further volume loading, incremental doses of norepinephrine seems to be more indicated.
3. *High pulmonary resistance and right atrial pressure* are more common in pediatric surgery, preoperative pulmonary artery disease and increased intrathoracic pressure. Decrease of intrathoracic pressure (no PEEP, pneumothorax

drainage) and administration of "more selective" pulmonary vascular vasodilators such as prostaglandins or inodilators (phosphodiesterase inhibitors or isoprenaline) may have beneficial effects in the pediatric population [11].

4. *High filling pressure and normal output* are related either to beginning cardiac compression, moderate heart failure or atrio-ventricular valvular dysfunction. Echocardiography is the appropriate method for differential diagnosis and in absence of a mechanical cause, preload reduction is achieved by vasodilators, like nitroglycerin and restoration of a normal A-V sequence.

5. *High filling pressures, low output and increased afterload* are commun phenomena during shivering, awakening, pain and agitation, concomitant to a failing heart. Early diagnosis and management should avoid further deterioration of the myocardial function. Treatment includes correction of all aforementioned factors and intravenous administration of vasodilators such as sodium nitroprusside, provided that arterial pressure is adequate.

6. *Low output syndrome* is characterized clinically by pallor, cold extremities, low urine output, weak pulse, and hemodynamically by high filling pressures, inadequate output and systemic hypotension, bradycardia or tachycardia, and subsequently by metabolic disorders, as result of poor tissue perfusion (lactic acidosis, liver and renal dysfunctions). Differential diagnosis may be achieved by the clinical status, hemodynamic pattern, radiological and echocardiographic findings.

7. *Cardiac tamponade* is suspected by tachycardia, elevated right ventricular filling pressure, low output and systemic hypotension, and mainly confirmed by chest X ray and echocardiography, decrease in chest drainage and finally poor response to inotropic drugs. Emergency thoracotomy is the treatment of choice.

8. *Cardiogenic shock.* Three different modalities of treatment may be concerned:

8.1. *Prompt reoperation:* in instances of acute tamponade, probability of graft occlusion or residual stenosis, or incomplete repair. Major ST-T changes, sudden increase in left ventricular filling pressure and occurrence of dysrythmias are good evidence for graft occlusion or coronary spasm. The latter may occur at any time in the postoperative period [12] and may be reversed by intravenous bolus of nitrates or intravenous or sublingual calcium channel blockers. In a doubtful situation, early reoperation is preferred to rule out a graft kinking, occlusion or a thrombus in the end-arteriectomized vessel. Malfunctioning prosthetic valves or residual outflow tract obstruction may constitute another indication for reoperation.

8.2. *Medical therapy:*

   - *Optimal volume loading:* with the restriction due to the discrepancy between pressure and volume, the optimal filling pressure may differ from patient to patient, from pathology to pathology. In low compliant hearts (cardiac tamponade, ischemia, fibrosis), filling pressures up to 18–20 mm Hg may be indicated, whereas in high compliance (ventricular dilatation, valvular incompetence), lower filling pressures suffice. Judicious use of vasodilating agents may reduce excessive filling without significant drop in arterial blood pressure.

- *Correction of metabolic disorders:*
  Both acidosis and alkalosis are known to influence the action of sympa-thomimetic drugs. So epinephrine increases cardiac output at normal pH, but cardiac output decreases under conditions of severe acidosis or alka-losis. The positive inotropic effects of dobutamine and dopamine are less pronounced in alkalosis; isoproterenol is less affected by acid-base imbal-ance [13]. Excessive hemodilution may lead to decreased O_2-transport, when the impaired heart is unable to compensate by a increase in cardiac output, resulting in hypotension and blunting the pressure reponse to al-pha-adrenergic stimulation [14].
- *Control of heart rate and rhythm* possibly by A-V pacing [15].
- *Enhanced myocardial contractility* by inotropic stimulation can be consid-ered: (a) catecholamines; (b) phophodiesterase inhibitors (PDE); (c) glu-cose-insulin-potassium mixtures; (d) triiodothyronine (T3).

Sympathomimetic drugs like epinephrine, dopamine, dobutamine and iso-proterenol are currently used in perioperative low output and their mecha-nism of action, common doses and side-effects well defined.

Due to their inodilating properties, PDE inhibitors are particularly indi-cated in case of moderate heart failure, high filling pressures and elevated pulmonary artery resistance. In severe cardiogenic shock, PDE-inhibitors have potentiating effects on adrenergic drugs [16].

More recently, the efficacy of metabolic support with glucose-insulin-po-tassium has been demonstrated for left ventricular failure after CABG [17].

Low T3 syndrome is common early after cardiopulmonary bypass (CPB) and an inotropic effect of T3 has been clearly demonstrated in pigs un-dergoing 2–3 hours of myocardial ischemia while being supported by CPB. This was confirmed in patients with extreme low output states after cardiac surgery [18].

These 2 latter forms of therapy need further investigations.

8.3. *Mechanical assistance:*

- *The intraaortic balloon counterpulsation* is still the most commonly used method to assist circulation, when medical therapy fails. The major indi-cations include preoperative control of recurrent ischemic attacks, septal rupture after myocardial infarction, intra-operative assistance to come off bypass and postoperative low output states, refractory to optimal medical therapy. In our opinion, the pump should be used early before excessive administration of catecholamines. Nevertheless, complications are com-mon and suggest a cautious use [19].
- *Left (LVAD), right (RVAD) or biventricular assist devices:*
  If some reports have shown a good long-term survival without subsequent heart transplantation [20], others in turn have restricted its use to potential candidates for heart transplantation because of poor long-term recovery [21]. This discrepancy may result from various factors such as early versus delayed use, degree of severity of cardiogenic shock and associated path-ologies. As with the intraaortic balloon pump, the devices should be used

in the early course of cardiogenic shock and not after a prolonged trial of high doses of catecholamines, exhausting the poor cardiac reserve.

– *Total artificial heart and heart transplantation:*
Shortage of available donors makes emergency heart transplantation mainly impossible. A natural trend to use older organs (over 50 years) in older patients or as bridge to conventional transplantation seems a logical approach. Perspectives for artificial organs or animal grafts are still far away, because remaining major unresolved problems.

Conclusions

After open heart surgery, low cardiac output remains the most common and serious complication. Despite major progress in prevention and treatment, new drugs and mechanical assistance, further investigations are necessary to avoid or to manage low output states: reduction of preoperative ischemia, better myocardial protection, earlier detection of perioperative myocardial suffering and reperfusion injury, myocardial metabolic monitoring, early mechanical assistance versus inotropic agents and finally use of artificial hearts, old donor hearts or animal grafts.

References

1. Christakis GT, Ivanov J, Weisel RD, Birnbaum PL, David TE, Salerno TA (1989) The changing pattern of coronary bypass surgery. Circulation (Suppl) 88, 3, I:151–161
2. Teoh KH, Christakis GT, Weisel RD, et al (1986) Accelerated myocardial metabolic recovery with terminal warm cardioplegia (hot shot). J Thorac Cardiovasc Surg 91:888–895
3. Slogoff S, Keats A (1985) Does perioperative myocardial ischemia lead to postoperative myocardial infarction? Anesthesiology 62:107–114
4. Molina JE, Galliani CA, Einzig ST, Bianco R, Rasmussen TH, Clarck R (1989) Physical and mechanical effects of cardioplegic injection of flow distribution and myocardial damage in hearts with normal coronary arteries. J Thorac Cardiovasc Surg 97:870–877
5. Partington MT, Acar CH, Buckberg GD, Julia P, Kofsky ER, Bugyi HI (1989) Studies of retrograde cardioplegia. I. Capillary blood flow distribution to myocardium supplied by open and occluded arteries. II. Advantages of antegrade/retrograde cardioplegia to optimize distribution in jeopardized myocardium. J Thorac Cardiovasc Surg 97:605–622
6. Breda MA, Drinkwater DC, Laks H, et al (1989) Prevention of reperfusion injury in the neonatal heart with leucocyte-depleted blood. J Thorac Cardiovasc Surg 97:654–665
7. Miller DL, Analouci AR, Wahlstrom SK, Visner MS, Wallace RB (1989) Dobutamine deteriorates recovery from myocardial stunning. Circulation (Suppl) 80:(Abstr) 976
8. Cahalan MK (1989) Transesophageal echocardiography is the "gold standard" for detection of myocardial ischemia. In: Mc Closkey G, Barash PG (eds) Transesophageal echocardiography is not the "gold standard" for detection of myocadial ischemia. J Cardiothorac Anesth 3:369–374
9. Visser CA, Koolen JJ, van Wezel HB, Dunning AJ (1988) Transesophageal echocardiography: technique and clinical application. J Cardiothorac Anesth 2:74–91
10. Braunwald E, Kloner RA (1982) The stunned myocardium: prolonged postischemic ventricular dysfunction. Circulation 66:1146–1149
11. Goenen M, Jacquet L, Durand Y (1988) Heart failure after open heart surgery. In: Perret C, Vincent JL (eds) Update in intensive care and emergency medicine, vol 6. Springer, Berlin Heidelberg New York Tokyo, pp 124–163

12. Addonzio VP, Harken AH, Goldberg S (1983) Postoperative coronary vasospasm. Cardiovasc Clin 14:111-121
13. Kaplan JA, Guffin AV, Yin A (1988) The effects of metabolic acidosis and alkalosis on the response to sympathomimetic drugs in dogs. J Cardiothorac Anesth 2:481-487
14. Estafanous FG, Sheng Z, Pedrinelli R, Azmy SS, Tarazi RC (1987) Hemodilution affects the pressor response to norepinephrine. J Cardiovasc Anesth 1:36-41
15. Trankina MF, White RD (1989) Perioperative cardiac pacing using an atrioventricular pacing pulmonary artery catheter. J Cardiovasc Anesth 3:154-162
16. Goenen M (1989) Historical perspectives and update of amrinone. J Cardiothorac Anesth (in press)
17. Coleman GM, Gradinac S, Taegtmeyer H, Sweeney M, Frazier OH (1989) Efficacy of metabolic support with glucose-insulin-K^+ for LV-pump failure after aorto-coronary bypass surgery. Circulation (Suppl) I:91-96
18. Novitzky D, Human PA, Cooper DKC (1988) Effect of triiodothyronine (T3) on myocardial high energy phosphates and lactate after ischemia and cardiopulmonary bypass. An experimental study in baboons. J Thorac Cardiovasc Surg 96:600-607
19. Goldberger M, Tabak SW, Shak PK (1986) Clinical experience with intra-aortic balloon counterpulsation in 112 consecutive patients. Am Heart J 111:497-502
20. Kanter KR, Ruzevich SA, Pennincton DG, McBride LR, Swartz MT, Willman VL (1988) Follow-up of survivors of mechanical circulatory support. J Thorac Cardiovasc Surg 96:72-80
21. Starnes VA, Oyer PE, Portner PM, et al (1988) Isolated left ventricular assist as bridge to cardiac transplantation. J Thorac Cardiovasc Surg 96:62-71

Diagnosing Myocardial Ischemia in the Operation Room*

S. Reiz, P. Hohner, and S. Häggmark

Introduction

Myocardial ischemia is a frequently observed in patients with coronary artery disease (CAD) subjected to cardiac or major non-cardiac surgical procedures [1–10]. However, its incidence varies widely (Tables 1, 2). This can be attributed to differences in study populations, study protocols and methods used for detection of ischemia.

It has been suggested that myocardial ischemic events in the prebypass period of coronary artery surgery would increase the risk for postoperative myocardial infarction [3, 4]. Interestingly, only about 50% of intraoperative ischemic events

Table 1. Incidence of pre-bypass myocardial ischemia in CABG

	[n]	Incidence [%] Pre-induction	Total	Mode of detection
Wilkinson et al. (1981)	26	27	62	2-lead ECG, lactate
Lieberman et al. (1983)	30	NA	67	2-lead ECG
Slogoff and Keats (1985)	1023	18	37	2-lead ECG
Slogoff and Keats (1986)	495	26	55	2-lead ECG

NA, not available.

Table 2. Incidence of myocardial ischemia in vascular and other noncardiac surgery

	[n]	Incidence [%] Pre-induction	Total	Mode of detection
Roy et al. (1979)	29	NA	38	Multi-lead ECG
Coriat et al. (1982)	50	NA	39	V5 ECG
Reiz et al. (1989)	112	18	86	12-lead ECG, lactate, wall function

NA, not available.

* Supported by grants from the Swedish National Heart and Lung Foundation.

were associated with hemodynamic aberrations. Recently, parts of these results have been refuted [10]. In this study, new post-bypass segmental left ventricular dysfunction (as detected by 2-D transesophageal echocardiography, 2-D Echo), but not pre-bypass myocardial ischemia correlated with adverse cardiac outcome.

There are only preliminary data on perioperative myocardial ischemia in relation to postoperative myocardial infarction or other major postoperative cardiac morbidity in patients with CAD undergoing major non-cardiac surgery [9]. However, such patients should not have a lower incidence of myocardial ischemia intraoperatively, and possibly be at greater risk for adverse cardiac outcome than those who have been subjected to coronary revascularization. All logic therefore suggests that it is important to carefully monitor patients with suspected or known CAD for myocardial ischemia in the intra- and postoperative periods to minimize the risk of adverse cardiac outcome. The aim of this chapter is to review the various techniques employed to detect myocardial ischemia in patients during non-cardiac surgery. In addition, the value of hemodynamic indices of myocardial oxygenation in relation to myocardial ischemia detected by these techniques will be discussed.

Metabolic Diagnosis of Ischemia

Production of lactate in a territory of the myocardium deprived of oxygen is the gold standard for identifying myocardial ischemia. More infrequently, myocardial release of inosine or hypoxanthine [11] have been used to indicate ischemia. These are all techniques which require cannulation of an artery and the coronary sinus with subsequent sampling of blood at the time of suspected ischemia. Lactate can be analyzed in the operating room using rapid enzymatic techniques [12], whereas inosine and hypoxanthine require time-consuming preparation of the blood and sophisticated analysis technology.

Lactate is used as substrate by the heart. In case of insufficient oxygenation it will be produced by the myocytes. This may result in a higher lactate concentration in coronary venous compared to arterial blood, e.g. lactate production (or negative lactate extraction).

Several factors may explain why lactate production is not observed despite obvious ischemia detected by other methods. First, the ischemic territory may be too small to offset a sufficient increase in coronary venous lactate concentration. Second, flow through the ischemic territory may be reduced to a degree where the washout of lactate is so low that it does not contribute to any significant rise in coronary venous lactate concentration. Finally, the coronary venous sampling catheter may be positioned distally to the outflow vein from the ischemic territory. In order to avoid right atrial admixture when sampling blood in the coronary sinus, the sampling catheter orifice should be placed at least 2 cm inside the vein. In many patients this excludes the ability to sample blood from territories perfused by the right coronary artery and the posterior interventricular artery. These areas of the myocardium are drained by veins entering the coronary sinus immediately inside its right atrial orifice and are therefore not included in the sampling. The use of hypoxanthine as a marker of ischemia may overcome the first of the three anatomical problems and, in case of some flow through the ischemic territory, also the second one. However, ischemia in the territory drained by the right coronary vein and the posterior interventricular vein will usually not be detected by any metabolic technique.

Our estimate from studies comparing different techniques is that only ¼ to ⅓ of regional ischemic events occurring during anesthesia are associated with myocardial lactate production [7]. In addition, the concordance between lactate production and other techniques to detect ischemia seems to be poor. This is going to be further discussed below.

Electrocardiography

Scalar Electrocardiography

Scalar electrocardiography with analysis of ST-segment depression or elevation is by far the most commonly employed technique to detect myocardial ischemia in the operating room. Although the specificity of ST-segment deviations for myocardial ischemia probably is high, the sensitivity is very variable. In this respect, a number of factors are of importance: 1. electrode placement, electrode quality and skin preparation; 2. bandwidth and calibration of the ECG signal; 3. number of leads monitored and, in particular which leads are monitored; 4. display of the ECG signal (oscilloscope, computerized ST-analysis, paper recording); 5. degree of preexisting ST abnormality.

As a general rule, the longer the distance between the electrodes and the better the skin preparation and electrode quality, the more easily is the ST-segment deviation detected on an oscilloscope. Standard oscilloscopes incorporate a low-frequency filter to minimize the influence of the electrocautery and other electrical interference. Too often, the ECG signal has not been calibrated. Therefore, changes of the raw ECG signal ST-segments around the diagnostic deviation of 0.1 mV may be distorted or blunted and, thus, go by undetected. Display of the ECG on paper via high bandwidth amplifiers may markedly increase the sensitivity of ECG ischemia monitoring compared to the standard operating room oscilloscope technique.

The V5 lead has been reported to detect about 85% of ST-segment abnormalities recorded by the 12-lead ECG [13]. A combination of leads II, V4 and V5 detects 96% of new ST-segment abnormalities observed on the 12-lead ECG [14]. This does, however, not imply that a 12-lead ECG has a 100% sensitivity to detect ischemia which migh be detected by electrocardiographic techniques. The posterior wall, which can be monitored by ECG from the esophagus or by vector cardiographic technique is not sampled by the standard 12-lead ECG. In addition, septal ischemia does not offset ST-segment changes, but rather causes a decrease in QRS-amplitude and, generally speaking, ischemia of the right ventricle is not sensitively detected by the 12-lead ECG.

Over the last couple of years, most major manufacturers of monitoring equipment have developed computerized systems which include on-line ST-segment analysis of more than one lead and trend function [15]. These systems eliminate the need for continuously running recorders and eliminate the low sensitivity resulting from inattention to the oscilloscope ECG and difficulty in remembering the degree of preexisting ST-segment abnormality. It is interesting to note, however, that not a single study from the peri-operative period comparing this technology to the standard 12-lead ECG displayed on paper has been published. Preliminary data indicate that two- and three-lead automated ST-segment analyzers detect about 70% of abnormalities on a seven-lead system comprising V5 and the six standard extremity leads [16].

It appears as if the degree of ST-segment depression on the preoperative standard 12-lead ECG is a useful predictor of peri- and postoperative myocardial ischemia as detected by the same modality (Table 3).

Even more importantly, the negative predictive power of the preoperative ECG in this respect is close to 100% [17]. Nevertheless, a number of problems remain to be clarified in future research aimed at defining the importance of new ST- and other ECG abnormalities occurring during anesthesia. First, is the degree of ST-segment deviation proportional to the territory of ischemic myocardium and, if so, what is its relation to outcome in other populations than the coronary surgical? Second, what is the importance and prognostic value of new ST-segment deviation in the face of preexisting ST-depression? Is for instance a new depression of 0.1 mV from the isoelectric line in a patient with a previously normal ECG equally important as a comparable change in a patient with preexisting ST-depression? Third, what is the importance of QRS-changes and which is the correlation between these and ST-changes? Data in the cardiology literature suggest that the degree of ST-depression should be corrected for QRS amplitude changes [18]. Fourth, is there any correlation between ischemic time, magnitude of ischemia as measured by the degree of ST-depression and adverse cardiac outcome? Finally, the prognostic importance of other ECG abnormalities, hitherto not regarded as indicative of ischemia, such as new T-wave inversions, sudden onset of nodal rhythm, and multiple premature ventricular contractions has to be considered.

Table 3. Relations between degree of pre-existing ST depression and intraoperative ischemia by 12-lead ECG (n = 119)

ST-segments in awake ECG	Intraop. ST depr. ≥ 0.1 mV		
	No	Yes	Sum
Normal	35	3	38
Depr. < 0.1 mV	52	8	60
Depr. > 0.1 mV	9	12	21
Sum	96	23	119
CHI-2(2) = 24	p = 0.001***		

Vector-Cardiography

Over 30 years ago, Frank [19] devised a new system for recording of electrical activity from the heart, vector-cardiography. This system gives spatial information of the electrocardial events and consists of three leads with the following characteristics: 1. The three leads should be mutually perpendicular and each parallel to one of the rectilinear co-ordinate axes of the body; 2. the three leads should be of equal amplitude from a vectorial standpoint; and 3. the lead vectors should retain the same magnitude and direction for all points where cardiac electromotive forces are generated.

Vector-cardiographic leads which meet conditions (1) and (2) are referred to as orthogonal leads. If, in addition, such leads also meet condition (3) they are called corrected orthogonal leads. The electrode locations as described by Frank are outlined in Fig. 1.

The ventricular depolarization generates potentials which produce an electrical field in the surrounding tissues extending to the body surface. At a given moment of the cardiac cycle, all instantaneous electrical components of this field can be summed and condensed to one vector, which is defined by its spatial magnitude and direction. If the heart is assumed to be a point generator, vectors sequentially obtained during the QRS interval can be projected from this single point as dipoles. The complex surface potential distribution of the electrocardial activity is reduced to three orthogonal components which can be projected and recorded along three perpendicular axes in the vector-cardiogram (X, Y and Z). By plotting these projections the spatial electrocardial forces can be graphically presented in three co-ordinate systems, the frontal, horizontal and sagital planes. Loops of the electrocardial planes can be constructed and for each loop a resulting vector can be calculated. Finally, the direction and magnitude of the spatial vector can be calculated by a pythagorean formula from the three plane vectors. Modern computer technology has made it possible to display the loops and vectors continuously and to obtain trend information displaying their changes within seconds (Fig. 2) [20].

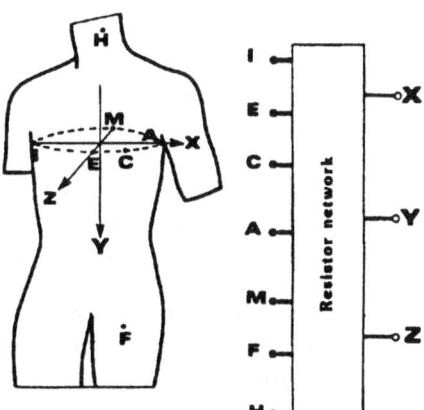

Fig. 1. The vector-cardiographic leads according to Frank [19]

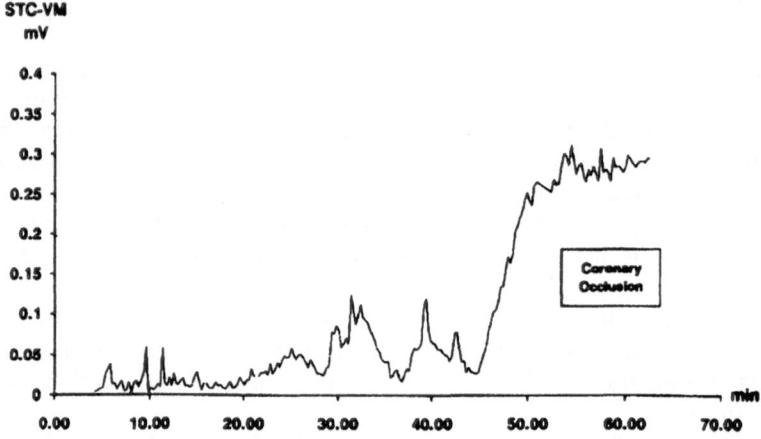

Fig. 2. Change in ST vector magnitude (STC-VM) following acute left anterior coronary artery occlusion 45 min into percutaneous coronary angioplasty. Peaks in STC-VM between 30 and 45 min denote ischemia induced by guide wire manipulations in the coronary artery. The plateau around 0.3 mV suggests an infarction process. This was confirmed at emergency coronary surgery immediately following the detection of the complication

Recent studies demonstrate that the ST-vector shift correlates closely to myocardium at risk during an experimental infarction process and that the QRS-vector shift well predicts the final infarct size [21]. In patients, the QRS-vector shift agrees well with infarct size estimated from myocardial enzymes [22].

Preliminary observations in studies performed with vector-cardiography during anesthesia and surgery suggest that this technique is more sensitive than the 12-lead ECG. Compared with techniques used to indicate ischemia by wall motion abnormality such as transesophageal 2-D Echo, vector-cardiography appears more sensitive and considerably more specific (see further below).

Ventricular Wall Function

Experimentally, there is strong evidence that myocardial ischemia leads to abnormal wall function and stunning of the ischemic territory [23, 24]. Such changes are thought to occur before or in the absence of other abnormalities indicating ischemia [25]. It does not, however, imply that all new wall motion abnormality is the consequence of ischemia. Interestingly, there is only one study reporting the incidence of new wall motion abnormality during anesthesia in patients without CAD [26]. In this study, one of 25 ASA I patients demonstrated new anterior wall motion abnormality during induction and endotracheal intubation. Since there is no gold standard for ischemia which can be used clinically, and since we lack clinical studies in which ischemia has been deliberately produced, the specificity of new wall motion abnormality for ischemia has yet to be defined.

There are several reasons why new wall motion abnormality could occur without any relation to ischemia in the territory contracting abnormally. For instance, an area of the myocardium which has suffered a previous non-transmural myocardial infarction may contract normally at normal ventricular loading conditions. When load increases on the ventricle and/or heart rate rises, this territory may display an abnormal contraction pattern without being ischemic. Videcoq et al. [27] found wall motion abnormalities in the presumed absence of myocardial ischemia when a calcium channel blocker was administered to dogs receiving isoflurane. They attributed this to a delayed onset of cardiac contraction. Similar results have been reported after intracoronary injection of nifedipine in man [28]. It is highly likely that any technique using ventricular wall motion as a gold standard for myocardial ischemia may overestimate its true incidence.

Two techniques for detection of abnormal wall function have been applied to patients in the operating room. These are echocardiography and cardiokymography.

Echocardiography

M-mode echocardiography was introduced over 10 years ago as a simple technique to document changes in left ventricular diameter during anesthesia [29]. The development of transesophageal 2-D Echo (TEE) has markedly increased the ability to assess left ventricular (LV) contraction pattern compared with the M-mode technique. For the purpose of studying regional LV function, the TEE transducer is placed in the distal part of the esophagus, thus displaying a cross section of the left ventricle at the level of the insertion of the papillary muscles. This position of the probe allows recording of the regional contraction pattern and the degree of systolic wall thickening of the anterior, lateral, and posterior LV walls, as well as of the interventricular septum. Akinesia and dyskinesia are easily detected and both intra- and interobserver variability as regards these abnormalities are low [30]. Hypokinesia and, in particular, impairment of systolic wall thickening are not easily detected and are subject to major disagreement between independent observers [30]. A stand-alone system for display of several cine-loops simultaneously is essential for the use of the TEE technique for on-line diagnosis of hypokinesia and wall thinning. Such a system allowed comparison of suspected abnormalities with a control loop and also improved accuracy of assessment of the degree of abnormal contraction within each cardiac cycle. In addition to the previously mentioned factors, a change of the position of the heart within the thoracic cavity, various maneuvers such as sternotomy, opening of the pericardium, and positive pressure ventilation, or an altered position of the transducer in the esophagus, may affect the ability to reliably diagnose myocardial ischemia by this technique.

It is evident that new hypokinesia and abnormal systolic wall thickening is usually detected during retrospective analysis of the TEE tapes. Such changes are more common than akinesia and dyskinesia [30]. This indicates that the high sensitivity of TEE in detecting myocardial ischemia hitherto reported is of little importance for the anesthesiologist in the operation room who needs on-line information for his decision-making. It is possible that future computerized systems with automated on-line analysis of several cine-loops will provide instant information when new regional wall function impairment occurs. In this context, it is indeed interesting that the lack of treatment of patients with intraoperative ischemia diagnosed retrospectively as new wall motion abnormality by TEE has not resulted in increased cardiac morbidity [31].

Cardiokymography

Cardiokymography (CKG) was originally developed to improve the sensitivity of the exercise test for the diagnosis of CAD [32–34]. It uses a 5-cm diameter transducer strapped to the chest over the anterior LV wall. The transducer induces an electromagnetic field which can penetrate totally through the body. Motion within this field causes a change in effective capacitance and frequency of oscillation. The change in frequency is converted into a change in voltage proportional to the original motion. It is displayed with the ECG signal on a recorder to allow estimation of the ventricular ejection period. The CKG is highly focal and therefore ignores motions which are not perpendicular to and directly under the coil. It is evident that respiration interferes with the recording of the LV contractions. Samples therefore have to be taken during apnea at end-expiration. Surgical manipulation is another obvious cause of baseline drift and signal interference.

The validation of the ability of the CKG to record anterior LV wall motion has been performed under numerous experimental and clinical conditions [32–36]. The combination of 12-lead ECG and CKG during exercise has the same sensitivity and specificity as the non-quantitative thallium scintigraphic stress test for the diagnosis of CAD verified by coronary angiography [37, 38]. Compared with the normal, systolic inward motion (type I), CKG abnormality is

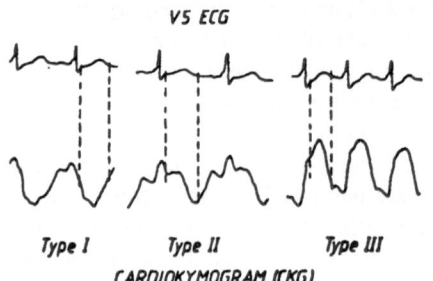

Fig. 3. V5 ECG (top) and CKG (bottom) recorded simultaneously during tracheal intubation of a patient with coronary artery disease. Before intubation there is a normal systolic inward motion (Type I). Within seconds of insertion of the laryngoscope, a partial early systolic outward motion (Type II) is recorded without ECG changes. Two min later the CKG demonstrates total outward motion during systole (Type III). At this time the ECG is still not diagnostic of ischemia. Hatched lines denote the ejection period. (From [7])

graded as type II (partial systolic outward motion) or type III (total systolic outward motion) [34] (Fig. 3).

There are only a few studies which have documented the incidence of new wall motion abnormality during anesthesia by CKG. Bellows et al. [36] studied patients during induction of anesthesia for CABG. Their CKGs were compared with those recorded in a control group of ASA class I patients anesthetized for dental extractions. In the latter group, one of the 25 patients displayed a new CKG abnormality. In comparison, eight of 25 patients with CAD had evidence of new wall motion abnormality during the induction. Only one of these patients had simultaneous ST-segment depression exceeding 0.1 mV on the ECG.

Häggmark et al. [7] recorded the CKG in 53 vascular surgical patients at defined perioperative intervals; preinduction, periinduction, prior to skin incision and 10 and 30 min after the start of abdominal surgery. They documented 89 ischemic episodes in 39 of the 53 patients. Seventy-four episodes were diagnosed by a new abnormal CKG. They also recorded the V5 ECG and measured myocardial lactate extraction at the same intervals. In this study, CKG abnormality was significantly more common than ischemia, as indicated by the other two techniques.

Despite the obvious advantage of high "sensitivity" and low cost, the CKG technique has several drawbacks compared with the TEE. It only allows analysis of the contraction pattern in the anterior LV wall, it is subjected to interference from respiratory movements and surgical manipulations and it cannot be used during cardiothoracic surgery. Finally, as with TEE, new wall motion abnormalities diagnosed retrospectively and, thus untreated at the time they occurred, have not been shown to lead to increased postoperative cardiac morbidity.

Hemodynamic Indices of Myocardial Ischemia

It has been suggested that the rate-pressure product (RPP = SAP × HR) should be a valid index for myocardial ischemia. RPP correlates with myocardial oxygen consumption in the exercising patient [39], whereas these variables agree poorly during anesthesia [40]. In addition, the worst possible combination of hemodynamic aberrations, hypotension and tachycardia [2] (see below) results in a normal RPP. A hemodynamic ischemia risk index, the pressure-rate ratio (P/R = MAP/HR), which would be more logical during anesthesia, has been proposed by Buffington [41]. In experimental studies in dogs with a fixed coronary artery stenosis, he was able to demonstrate a close correlation between ischemia in the territory supplied by the stenosed artery and a P/R < 1. Since a majority of coronary artery stenoses in humans are eccentric, incorporating an elastic vascular wall element, it is possible that this ischemia risk index does not always have the same high predictive value.

Kaplan and Wells [42] suggested that an elevation of the pulmonary capillary wedge pressure (PCWP) associated with abnormal wave from (A-C or V-waves) was a more sensitive index of myocardial ischemia undergoing CABG than the V5 ECG ST-segment depression. The agreement between an elevated PCWP combined with abnormal pressure wave form and ischemia diagnosed by other methods was confirmed in vascular surgical patients by Häggmark et al. [7]. However, it did not appear as if this hemodynamic index of ischemia was more sensitive than ECG. An increase of PCWP by 8 mmHg or more in the absence of an abnormal wave form coincided with ischemia, as detected by any of the other technique (ECG, lactate metabolism, and wall function) alone or in combination, in about 50% of observations. A similar inability of an isolated elevation of the PCWP to predict ischemia was demonstrated by Lieberman et al. [2] in patients undergoing CABG. In comparison, vascular patients who demonstrated an increase of PCWP by 8 mmHg or more, associated with abnormal PCWP wave form, had a 92% likelihood of being ischemic. However, only 13% of all PCWP measurements and 21% of all ischemic events were associated with an abnormal wave form. Thus, the value of the pulmonary artery catheter for the diagnosis of ischemia is limited. Häggmark et al. [7] also analyzed changes in stroke volume in relation to myocardial ischemia and could not find that this index of ventricular pump function sensitively could discriminate between ischemic and non-ischemic events.

Comparison of Different Techniques Used to Diagnose Ischemia

Only a few research groups have performed studies aimed at comparing the "sensitivity" of various techniques used to detect myocardial ischemia in the operating room. As may be realized from the above discussion, there is no gold standard for ischemia that can be used clinically. Consequently, these studies do not give us an indication as to the degree of sensitivity of these techniques, but rather the frequency by which they demonstrate abnormalities suggestive of ischemia when applied simultaneously in the same patients.

Wilkinson et al. [1] studied the patterns of ischemia during halothane or morphine anesthesia for CABG. They found that ST-segment depressions were not statistically more common than simultaneously measured myocardial lactate production. In contrast, Reiz et al. [43], who studied vascular surgical patients subjected to isoflurane anesthesia found only one of 21 patients with lactate production compared with 11 simultaneous ECG abnormalities suggesting ischemia.

Lowenstein and Reiz [44] compared the V5 ECG with myocardial lactate extraction in vascular surgical patients with CAD and in patients without CAD. Only one of 35 intraoperative samples from patients without CAD demonstrated a greater than 50% decline in myocardial lactate extraction from awake values and none was associated with new ECG abnormalities. Compared with the awake control measurements, mean myocardial lactate extraction for the group was not altered by anesthesia. At the time when patients with CAD displayed new perioperative ST-segment depressions, myocardial lactate extraction had decreased by 50% or more in 92% of measurements. Lactate production was, however, present in only 29% of the ischemic events as displayed by the ECG. When ischemia was not evident from the ECG, myocardial lactate extractions were not different from the awake values or from those measured in patients without CAD.

In another set of experiments, Reiz et al. analyzed the 12-lead ECG when lactate production was first observed in 26 patients subjected to anesthesia for major vascular surgery. Only 12 patients (45%) demonstrated diagnostic ST-segment depressions (0.1 mV) at the time of lactate production. However, all the remaining 14 patients had some kind of new ECG abnormality, most commonly an ST-segment depression which was less than 0.1 mV in one or more leads. Other abnormalities included new inverted T-waves, sudden onset of nodal or ectopic atrial rhythm and appearance of multiple premature ventricular contractions. Our approach in clinical practice is therefore to regard all new ECG abnormalities observed during anesthesia in patients with CAD as the result of myocardial ischemia until proven otherwise.

Using M-mode echocardiography, Elliot et al. [29] demonstrated periinduction LV wall dysfunction, interpreted to be ischemia in 10 of 24 patients with CAD. In comparison, the ECG was indicative of ischemia in one patient only. Strikingly similar results in comparable patients were obtained by Bellows et al. [26], who found eight of 24 patients with new periinduction CKG abnormalities, whereas the ECG indicated ischemia in only one.

Smith et al. [31], using TEE, documented new systolic wall motion abnormalities at some time during anesthesia and surgery in 24 of 50 patients with previous myocardial infarction undergoing either vascular surgery or CABG. Only six patients experienced ST-segment changes indicative of ischemia. Furthermore, all patients demonstrating an ECG abnormality also had abnormal wall motion. Häggmark et al. [7] could not find that all instances of ECG abnormality were accompanied by wall motion abnormality as detected by the CKG. It is, however, possible that wall motion abnormalities were present in areas not sampled by the CKG, or that wall motion abnormality was too slight to be detected by this technique.

The study by Häggmark et al. [7] also indicated that wall motion abnormalities are far more common than ischemic ECG changes, myocardial lactate production, or elevated PCWP with an abnormal pressure wave form (Table 4). Furthermore, it was evident that the concurrence between the various techniques was poor.

Our group has performed studies comparing the ability of the 12-lead electrocardiography, vector-cardiography, automated 2-lead electrocardiography (Siemens Sirecust 1280), transesophageal echocardiography, cardiokymography

Table 4. Incidence of myocardial ischemia in vascular surgery in relation to mode of detection. Data from Häggmark et al. [7]

Mode of detection	Incidence of ischemia [%]
Cardiokymography (wall function)	53
12-lead ECG	41
Myocardial lactate production	20
Elavated PCWP with abnormal wave form	17
All modalities	86

and hemodynamics to detect pacing-induced and afterload-change induced myocardial ischemia (as detected by metabolic indices) during anesthesia prior to coronary artery revascularization. Wall motion abnormalities were not particularly specific and only moderately sensitive for ischemia. The pulmonary capillary wedge pressure had no value as an index of ischemia. All electrocardiographic techniques were highly specific for ischemia. However, vector-cardiography was more sensitive than the scalar techniques, between which no differences could be observed.

From all these data, it appears as if electrocardiography provides the most reliable information as regards the diagnosis of myocardial ischemia. New wall motion abnormality which occurs with increased loading conditions is probably infrequently indicating ischemia. The sensitivity of scalar electrocardiography can be improved if vector-cardiography is introduced into clinical practice in the operating room. This technique may in addition give a more precise estimate of the localization and magnitude of the ischemic territory. It is desirable, however, that the influence of decision-making based on abnormal observations by this and other recent techniques upon cardiac outcome is evaluated to provide information of their real usefulness in clinical practice.

References

1. Wilkinson PL, Hamilton WK, Moyers JR, et al (1981) Halothane and morphine-nitrous oxide anesthesia in patients under-going coronary artery bypass operations – patterns of intraoperative ischemia. J Thorac Cardiovasc Surg 82:372–378
2. Lieberman RW, Orkin FK, Jobes DR, Schwartz AJ (1983) Hemodynamic predictors of myocardial ischemia during halothane anesthesia for coronary-artery revascularization. Anesthesiology 59:36–41
3. Slogoff S, Keats A (1985) Does perioperative myocardial ischemia lead to postoperative myocardial infarction? Anesthesiology 62:107–114
4. Slogoff S, Keats A (1986) Further observations on perioperative myocardial ischemia. Anesthesiology 65:539–542
5. Coriat P, Harari A, Daloz M, Viars P (1982) Clinical predictors of intraoperative myocardial ischemia in patients with coronary artery disease undergoing non-cardiac surgery. Acta Anesthesiol Scand 26:287–290
6. Roy WL, Edelist G, Gilbert B (1979) Myocardial ischemia during non-cardiac surgical procedures in patients with coronary-artery disease. Anesthesiology 51:393–397
7. Häggmark S, Hohner P, Östman M, et al (1988) Comparison of hemodynamic electrocardiographic, mechanical and metabolic indicators of intraoperative myocardial ischemia in vascular surgical patients with coronary artery disease. Anesthesiology 70:19–25
8. Knight AA, Hollenberg M, London MJ, et al (1988) Peri-operative myocardial ischemia: importance of the preoperative ischemic pattern. Anesthesiology 68:681–688
9. Fegert G, Hollenberg M, Browner W, et al (1988) Peri-operative myocardial ischemia in the noncardiac surgical patient. Anesthesiology 69:A49
10. Leung JM, O'Kelly B, Browner WS, Tubau J, Hollenberg M, Mangano D, The SPRG (1989) Prognostic importance of postbypass regional wall-motion abnormalities in patients undergoing coronary artery bypass graft surgery. Anesthesiology 71:16–25
11. Kugler G (1979) Myocardial release of lactate, inosine and hypoxanthine during atrial pacing and exercise-induced angina. Circulation 59:43–49
12. Soutter WP, Sharp F, Clark DM (1978) Bedside estimation of whole blood lactate. Br J Anaesth 50:445–450
13. Blackburn H, Katigbak R (1964) What electrocardiographic leads to take after exercise. Am Heart J 67:184–185

14. London MJ, Hollenberg M, Wong MG (1988) Intraoperative myocardial ischemia: localization of continuous 12-lead electrocardiography. Anesthesiology 69:232–241
15. Kotrly KJ, Kotter GS, Mortara D, Kampine JP (1984) Intraoperative detection of myocardial ischemia with an ST segment trend monitoring system. Anesth Analg 63:393–397
16. Ellis JE, Rolzen MF, Aronson S, et al (1988) Comparison of two automated ST-segment analysis systems, EKG (including T wave inversion analysis), and transesophageal echocardiography for the diagnosis of intraoperative myocardial ischemia. Anesthesiology 69:A5
17. Raby KE, Goldman L, Creager MA, et al (1989) Correlation between preoperative ischemia and major cardiac events after peripheral vascular surgery. N Engl J Med 321:1296–1300
18. Hollenberg M, Go MJ, Massie BM, Wisneski JA, Gertz EW (1985) Influence of R-wave amplitude on excercise-induced ST depression: need for a "gain factor" correction when interpreting stress electrocardiograms. Am J Cardiol 56:13–17
19. Frank E (1956) Accurate, clinically practical system for spatial vectorcardiography. Circulation 13:737
20. Sederholm M, Erhardt L, Sjögren A (1983) Continuous vectorcardiography in acute myocardial infarction. Natural course of ST and QRS vectors. Intern J Cardiology 4:53–63
21. Häggmark S, Johansson G, Näslund U, Reiz S (1987) Kvantifiering av infarkt och ischämistorlek med kontinuerlig datoriserad vektorcardiografi (VCG). Proceedings of the Swedish Association of Anesthetists:86/A4
22. Sederholm M, Grøttum P, Erhardt L, Kjekshus J (1983) Quantitative assessment of myocardial ischemia and necrosis by continuous vectorcardiography and measurement of creatine kinase release in patients. Circulation 68:1006–1012
23. Forrester JS, Wyatt HL, Tyberg JV, et al (1976) Functional significance of regional ischemic contraction abnormalities. Circulation 54:64–70
24. Waters HL, daLuz PL, Wyatt HL, et al (1977) Early changes in regional and global left ventricular function induced by graded reduction in regional coronary perfusion. Am J Cardiol 39:537–543
25. Lowenstein E, Foëx P, Francis CM, et al (1981) Regional ischemic ventricular dysfunction in myocardium supplied by a narrowed coronary artery with increasing halothane concentration in the dog. Anesthesiology 55:349–359
26. Bellows WH, Bode RH, Levy JH, et al (1984) Noninvasive detection of periinduction ischemic ventricular dysfunction by cardiokymography in humans: preliminary experience. Anesthesiology 60:155–158
27. Videcoq M, Arvieux CC, Ramsay JG, et al (1987) The association isoflurane-verapamil causes regional left ventricular dyssynchrony in the dog. Anesthesiology 67:635–641
28. Serruyus BN, Hooghoudt TEH, Reiber JHC, et al (1983) Influence of intracoronary nifedipine on left ventricular function, coronary vasomotility, and myocardial oxygen consumption. Br Heart J 49:427–441
29. Elliott PL, Schauble JF, Weiss J, et al (1980) Echocardiography and LV function during anesthesia. Anesthesiology 53:1980 (53) PS105.
30. Abel MD, Nishimura RA, Callahan MJ, et al (1987) Evaluation of intraoperative transesophagel two-dimensional echocardiography. Anesthesiology 66:64–68
31. Smith JS, Cahalan MK, Benefield DJ, et al (1985) Intra-operative detection of myocardial ischemia in high-risk patients: electrocardiography versus two-dimensional transesophageal echocardiography. Circulation 72:1015–1021
32. Diamond GA, Chag M, Vas R, Forrester JS (1978) Cardiokymography: quantitative analysis of regional ischemic left ventricular dysfunction. Am J Cardiol 41:1249–1257
33. Vas R, Diamond GAS, Vas R, et al (1979) Assessment of the functional significance of coronary artery disease with atrial pacing and cardiokymography. Am J Cardiol 44:1283–1289
34. Silverberg RA, Diamond GA, Vas R, et al (1980) Noninvasive diagnosis of coronary artery disease: the cardiokymographic stress test. Circulation 61:579–589
35. Vas R (1967) Electronic device for physiologic kinetic measurements and detection of extraneous bodies. IEEE Trans Biomed Eng 14:2–10
36. Vas R, Diamond GA, Wyatt HL (1977) Noninvasive analysis of regional wall motion: cardiokymography. Am J Physiol 233:H700

37. Burke JF, Morganroth J, Soffer J (1984) The cardiokymographic stress test compared to the thallium-201 perfusion exercise test in the diagnosis of coronary artery disease. Am Heart J 107:718-725
38. Weiner DA, Principal Investigators (1985) Accuracy of cardiokymography during exercise testing: results of a multicenter study. J Am Coll Cardiol 6:502-509
39. Gobel FL, Nordström LA, Nelson RR, et al (1978) The rate-pressure product as an index of myocardial oxygen consumption during exercise in patients with angina pectoris. Circulation 57:549-556
40. Moffitt EA, Sethna DH, Gray RJ, et al (1984) Rate-pressure product correlates poorly with myocardial oxygen consumption during anesthesia in coronary patients. Can Anaesth Soc J 31:5-12
41. Buffington CW, Bashein G, Sivarajan M (1987) Blood pressure and heart rate predict ischemia in collateral-dependent myocardium. Anesthesiology:A5
42. Kaplan JA, Wells PH (1981) Early diagnosis of myocardial ischemia using the pulmonary artery catheter. Anesth Analg 60:789-793
43. Reiz S, Bålfors E, Sorensen MB, et al (1983) Isoflurane – a powerful coronary vasodilator in patients with coronary artery disease. Anesthesiology 59:91-99
44. Lowenstein E, Reiz S (1987) Effects of inhalation anesthetics on systemic hemodynamics and the coronary circulation. In: Kaplan JA (ed) Cardiac anesthesia. Grune and Stratton, New York, pp 3-35

Cardiorespiratory Monitoring

Reliability of Cardiac Output Measurements by the Thermodilution Method

J. R. C. Jansen, J. J. Schreuder, and A. Versprille

Introduction

Since Fegler [1] introduced the thermodilution technique 35 years ago to measure mean cardiac output, many studies and as much discussions have been devoted to this topic. This chapter is an other extension of these discussions which serves the consideration of the reliability of the thermodilution method in patients during mechanical ventilation. In general, the method has been accepted as a clinical useful method, because it is simple, safe and swift. Commercial devices compute cardiac output instantaneously and present the value digitally together with an assessment of the quality of the thermodilution curve. By the commercial availability the thermodilution technique became extensively applied in cardiology, surgery and anesthesia. Moreover, it became an integral part of comprehensive monitoring of critically ill and severely traumatized patients.

Problems Related to the Thermodilution Technique

Although the thermodilution method has been evaluated extensively and was accepted by many investigators [2–5], we must be aware that the computation is based on the application of the Stewart-Hamilton equation. For this application a few important conditions has to be fulfilled. These conditions are: complete mixing of indicator and blood, no loss of indicator between the site of injection and that of detection, and constant blood flow.

The errors made in the estimation of cardiac output with the thermodilution method are primarily related to:

1. Violations of the above mentioned condition of constant blood flow. Variability of blood flow occurs during shivering, mechanical ventilation, variations in heart rate, cardiac arrhythmias, valvular insufficiencies, intracardiac shunts, and other causes of hemodynamic instability [2, 4].
2. Errors due to uncareful usage of the technique, as warming of injectate [4, 5], incorrect catheter positioning, or injections with an uneven rate [4, 6].
3. Changes in blood temperature in the pulmonary artery [3, 4, 7–9].
4. Cardiac output computer accuracy [10].

Taking these errors in consideration, the clinician should expect 5 to 15% data scatter, even in hemodynamically stable patients [10]. There is, however, good evidence that the mean of a large number of thermodilution measurements will lead to the estimation of an accurate mean cardiac output [8, 9, 11]. A high variance indicates the need to increase the number of measurements and to average them. How many consecutive thermodilution determinations have to be taken per estimation of mean cardiac output depends on the nature of variance (normally or not normally distributed). For a normal distribution of errors the standard deviation will decrease with the square root of the number of observations as we observed indeed in our own data [9].

The Estimation of Cardiac Output by Thermodilution During Mechanical Ventilation

Many authors have shown cyclic changes in stroke volume during mechanical ventilation [12–15], implying that the condition of constant blood flow over the period of a measurement is not fulfilled and the thermodilution method is misused on theoretically grounds. Ignorance of this misuse may lead to a considerable scatter in cardiac output values, as is demonstrated in Fig. 1. Stroke volumes of the right ventricle are modulated by the ventilation. The ventilation is illustrated by the intrapulmonary pressure (P_T). Stroke volume is smallest at peak insufflation. When the spontaneous expiration starts the stroke volume is rapidly increasing and attains an end-expiratory plateau after an overshoot. The mean value over the ventilatory cycles is constant. Injection of a bolus of cold indicator at two different moments in the respiratory cycle, 96%, and 24% from the start of an inspiration gave estimates of cardiac output of 17.4 ml/s and 28.2 ml/s respectively. Besides the differences in cardiac output also the shape of the thermodilution curve was changed, depending on the phase of the ventilatory cycle. In a period of low flow the concentration (i.e. ΔT) will be changed only slightly, whereas the increasing flow will decline the temperature-time curve more rapidly.

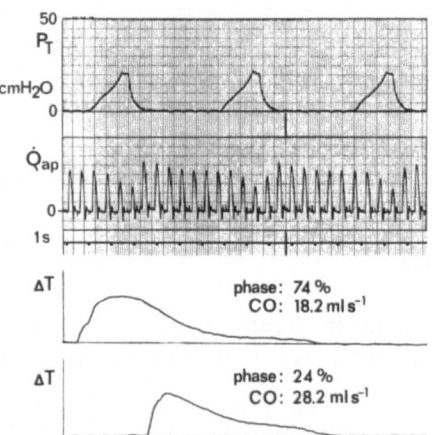

Fig. 1. Fluctuations of blood flow in the pulmonary artery ($\dot{Q}_{ap}$) in relation to the airway pressure (P_T) during artificial ventilation and 2 thermodilution curves with the corresponding estimates of cardiac output (CO) after injections at different moments in the ventilatory cycle. P_T is given in cmH$_2$O, $\dot{Q}_{ap}$ in arbitrary units

A more detailed analysis of the variation in cardiac output estimates related to the moment of injection in the ventilatory cycle is given elsewhere for animals [8, 9, 16, 17] and humans [18]. An individual example of our own observations in patients is given in Fig. 2. Twelve thermodilution measurements were performed consecutively at intervals of 1–2 min and at the phases 0, 25, 50, 75, 8, 33, 58, 83, 16, 41, 66, and 92% in the ventilatory cycle. After sorting the series of 12 measurements with respect to the moments of injection in the ventilatory cycle, a cyclic pattern of modulation of the estimates appeared with the same periodicity as the ventilation. We observed in a group of 9 patients marked differences in the amplitude and the phase of the pattern of modulation. This was also reported by Okomato et al. [18].

Improvement of Estimation of Mean Cardiac Output by the Thermodilution Method During Mechanical Ventilation

In the literature a number of suggestions have been given for improvement of the accuracy of the thermodilution method.

Injections at a Fixed Moment in the Ventilatory Cycle: This approach needs a constant phase relationship in CO variations versus the ventilatory cycle. It was demonstrated in animal and human studies that the phase relationship between the CO estimates and the ventilatory cycle is changed, when either the ventilatory pattern or the frequency or the end-expiratory pressure or the blood volume were changed [8, 9, 17, 18]. Therefore, we cannot support the recommendation of Stevens et al. to inject the cold bolus at a fixed moment in the ventilatory cycle [19].

An Increase in the Ventilatory Rate: At a higher respiratory frequency the amplitude of the real flow modulation will be smaller due to a lower tidal volume and, therefore, a smaller variation in intrathoracic pressure and venous return. Then

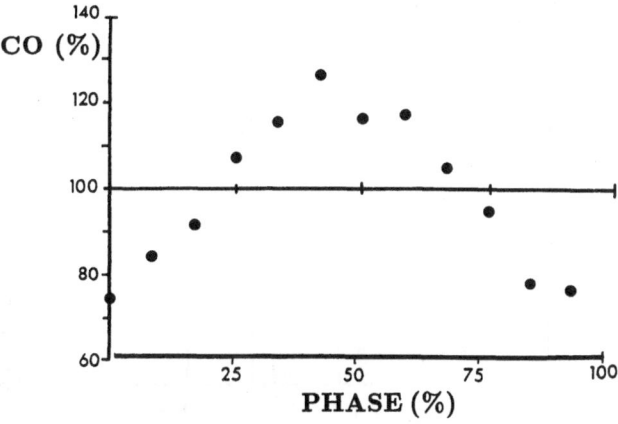

Fig. 2. An individual series of 12 cardiac output (CO) measurements in a patient, plotted against the moment of injection as a percentage phase of the ventilatory cycle. 100% is mean of each series of 12 estimates. The determinations were done with a time intervals of at least 1 minute

the estimates of mean cardiac output are less varied. Also the higher frequency in itself will diminish the range of cardiac output estimates [9, 11, 20, 21]. A change in the ventilatory settings will influence gas transport mechanisms and the hemodynamic status of a patient or animal which will affect the value of cardiac output to be determined.

Breathhold Procedures: During a prolonged expiratory pause as well as during inspiratory hold maneuvers constant hemodynamic conditions were found [22]. The cardiac output estimates during prolonged end-expiratory pauses were significantly higher than mean cardiac output during the preceding normal cycles of mechanical ventilation [23]. This overestimation was not constant in changing hemodynamic circumstances.

Averaging of Estimates: In an animal study [9] we analyzed the difference between averages of randomly performed measurements and the averages of measurements performed equally spread over the ventilatory cycle. In both situations there an improvement of accuracy was found with an increasing number of estimates to be averaged. The best result was obtained by averaging four estimates equally spread over the ventilatory cycle. The accuracy of mean cardiac output by two estimates differing half a cycle proved to be as good as the average of five randomly performed estimates.

   In a human study we performed a similar analysis (Fig. 3). The percentage of all mean values deviating more than 10% of the reference mean decreased with the number of single estimates to be averaged. This counted both for random measurements as well as measurements performed at equal intervals in the ventilatory cycle (phase selected estimates). However, the results were considerably better with phase selected estimates of cardiac output. From a data set of two series of 12 single estimates performed at equal intervals in the ventilatory cycle and obtained in 9 patients, approximately 60% of the data were within the accuracy level of 10%. Thus, with a single estimate the chance is 40% to get a value which deviates more than 10% from the reference value. All phase selected four point averages were within the accuracy level of 10%, whereas 15% of the averages from random estimates were outside this accuracy level. The results confirmed also the animal studies in another respect. The average of two measure-

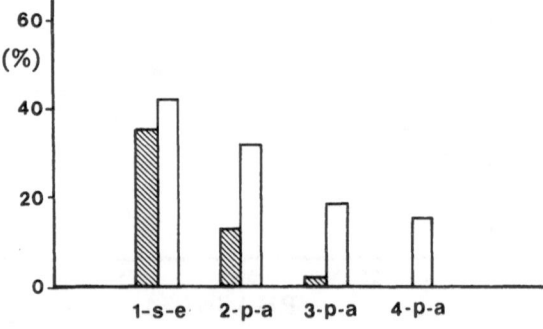

Fig. 3. Percentage of randomly and systematically determined averages open and dashed columns respectively. Vertically the percentage of the values is plotted, which deviates more than 10% of the mean. 1-s-e: single estimates; 2-p-a: two point averages; 3-p-a: three point averages; and 4-p-a: four point averages

ments differing half a ventilatory cycle was more accurate than four randomly performed measurements.

Conclusion

During mechanical ventilation mean cardiac output can be accurately estimated, even with a theoretical misuse of the Stewart-Hamilton equation. This can be done best by averaging three or four measurements equally spread over the ventilatory cycle. For this aproach manufactures of cardiac output computers have to be persuaded to adapt there apparatus, in order to extent their cardiac output computers with a phase selector.

References

1. Fegler G (1954) Measurement of cardiac output in anaesthetised animals by a thermo-dilution method. Q J Exp Physiol 39:153–164
2. Ganz W, Swan HJC (1972) Measurement of bloodflow by thermodilution. Am J Cardiol 29:241–246
3. Weisel RD, Berger RL, Hechtman HB (1975) Measurement of cardiac output by thermal dilution. N Engl J Med 292:67–72
4. Levett JM, Replogle RL (1979) Thermodilution cardiac output: a critical analysis and review of literature. J Surg Res 27:392–404
5. Runciman WB, Ilsley AH, Roberts JG (1981) An evaluation of thermodilution cardiac output measurement using the Swan-Ganz catheter. Anaesth Intens Care 9:208–220
6. Nelson LD, Houtchens BA (1982) Automatic vs. manual injections for thermodilution cardiac output determinations. Crit Care Med 10:190–192
7. Wessel HU, Paul MH, James GW Grahn AR (1971) Limitations of thermal dilution curves for cardiac output determinations. J Appl Physiol 30:643–652
8. Jansen JRC, Schreuder JJ, Bogaard JM, van Rooyen W, Versprille A (1981) The thermodilution technique for the measurement of cardiac output during artificial ventilation. J Appl Physiol 51:584–591
9. Jansen JRC, Versprille A (1986) Improvement of cardiac output estimation by the thermodilution method during mechanical ventilation. Intensive Care Med 12:71–79
10. American Edwards Laboratories COM-2. Cardiac Output Computer Operations Manual 1989
11. Bassingthwaighte JB, Knopp TJ, Anderson DU (1970) Flow estimation by indicator dilution. (Bolus injection): Reduction of errors due to time-averaged sampling during unsteady flow. Circ Res 27:277–291
12. Hoffman JIE, Guz A, Charlier AA, Wilcken DEL (1965) Stroke volume in conscious dogs: effect of respiration, posture and vascular occlusion. J Appl Physiol 20:865–877
13. Morgan BC, Martin WE, Hornbein TF, Crawford EW, Fronek A (1966) Hemodynamic effects of intermittent positive pressure ventilation with and without an end-expiratory pause. Anesthesiology 27:584–590
14. Vermeire P, Butler J (1968) Effect of respiration on pulmonary capillary blood flow in man. Circ Res 22:299
15. Versprille A (1987) Pulmonary blood flow and blood volume during positive pressure ventilation. In: Vincent JL (ed) Update in intensive care and emergency medicine. Springer, Berlin Heidelberg New York, Tokyo, pp 213–222
16. Armengol J, Man GCW, Balsys AJ (1981) Effects of the respiratory cycle on cardiac output measurements: Reproducibility of data enhanced by timing the thermodilution injections in dogs. Crit Care Med 9:852–854

17. Snyder JV, Powner DJ (1982) Effects of mechanical ventilation on the measurement of cardiac output by thermodilution. Crit Care Med 10:677–682
18. Okamoto K, Komatsu T, Kumar V, et al (1986) Effects of intermittent positive-pressure ventilation on cardiac output measurements by thermodilution. Crit Care Med 14:977–980
19. Stevens JH, Raffin TA, Mihm FG, Rosenthal MH, Stetz CW (1985) Thermodilution cardiac output measurement. Effect of the respiratory cycle on its reproducibility. JAMA 253:2240–2242
20. Scheuer-Leeser M, Morquet A, Reul H, Inrich W (1977) Some aspects to the pulsation error in blood-flow calculations by indicator dilution technique. Med Biol Eng Comput 15:118–123
21. Von Reth EA, Aerts JC, van Steenhoven AA, Versprille A (1983) Model studies on the influence of nonstationary flow on the mean flow estimate with the indicator-dilution technique. J Biomech 16:625–633
22. Versprille A, Jansen JRC (1985) Mean systemic filling pressure as a characteristic pressure for venous return. Pflügers Archiv 405:226–271
23. Jansen JRC, Bogaard JM, Versprille A (1987) Extrapolation of thermodilution curves obtained during a pause in artificial ventilation. J Appl Physiol 63:1551–1557
24. Zierler KL (1962) Circulation times and the theory of indicator-dilution methods for determining blood flow and volume. In: Handbook of physiology. Circulation. Am Physiol Soc (sect. 1) vol 1, chap 18, pp 585–615

Continuous Cardiac Output Monitoring During Cardiac Surgery

J. J. Schreuder, J. R. C. Jansen, and J. J. Settels

Introduction

For the treatment of critically ill patients in the operating room (OR) or the intensive care units (ICU) a continuous monitoring system for cardiac output is of importance since the circulatory condition of these patients can change rapidly and unexpectedly. However, the method used most often clinically, the thermodilution method allows only intermittent measurement. More seriously, each individual thermodilution estimate has substantial scatter and therefore clinically a combination of three or four subsequent estimates are taken. The reliable estimation of thermodilution cardiac output requires a stable thermal baseline and constant cardiac output, conditions that are seldomly present in particular during mechanical ventilation [1, 2].

An attractive method to monitor beat-to-beat changes in cardiac output is the pulse contour method. This method, however, only provides changes in cardiac output. To calibrate a pulse contour method to give absolute values requires comparison with an absolute method, such as a thermodilution cardiac output. In addition, pulse contour methods are unreliable under changing hemodynamic conditions unless a correction for changes in blood pressure and heart rate is carried out [3–5]. A system combining thermodilution and pulse contour cardiac output is continuous and calibrated and could prove a clinically relevant monitor.

We designed an automatic computerized system combining the two methods and used a prototype to study patients undergoing a coronary artery bypass graft (CABG) operation. During cardiac surgery great and rapid changes in hemodynamics occur caused by pharmacological action, cardioplegia, surgical intervention and total heart-lung bypass.

The Pulse Contour Method

Pulse contour methods compute an arterial flow or a volume from an arterial pressure pulse contour and are therefore based on a model relating these two quantities in arteries, either implicitly or explicitly. Sufficient information on human arterial hemodynamics is available today to provide a scientific basis for such models. The Wesseling method used in this study is explicitely based on a transmission line model of the aorta. A detailed description can be found elsewhere [3]. Basically, our computation formula can be written as:

$$CO_{pc} = HR \cdot A_{sys}/Z_0 \cdot \{correction\},$$

where CO_{pc} the pulse contour cardiac output for a beat,
A_{sys} the area under the systolic portion of the pressure wave,
Z_o the characteristic impedance of the aortic transmission line
and $\{correction\} = (a + b \cdot P_{mean} + c \cdot HR)$, with a, b and c age-dependent factors [3, 5], respectively.

The characteristic impedance calibration is not known and must be determined at least once for each patient from an absolute cardiac output estimate like thermodilution applying the formula:

$$Z_0 = CO_{pc}/CO_{td}.$$

The Thermodilution Method

Baseline temperature fluctuations in the pulmonary artery and right heart cardiac output modulation in mechanically ventilated patients require special measures to avoid potentially large errors [1, 2]. In mechanical ventilation these variations show a cyclic pattern allowing corrective action. Second, the integration of the thermodilution curve was stopped after 18 seconds since the often used exponential extrapolation may introduce large errors. In addition, since a reliable estimate of true mean cardiac output is desired a series of at least 4 precisely timed thermodilution estimates are averaged, with their injections equally spread over the ventilatory cycle [2].

Automatic Calibration

The process of calibration of pulse contour cardiac output by thermodilution was carried out automatically. The moment of injection of 5 ml of room temperature saline in the ventilatory cycle is derived from a synchronizing pulse from the ventilator. During periods of spontaneous and therefore irregular breathing the injections are timed randomly. To avoid operator variability the cold bolus is injected automatically by an electro-pneumatic injection system controlled by the computer but with a "break" switch available to the operator. Pulse contour cardiac output simultaneous with each thermodilution is averaged over 5 ventilatory cycles, starting one cycle before injection. Four or twelve measurement pairs are assumed to reflect true average cardiac output with sufficient precision and subsequently used to calibrate the pulse contour.

Calibrating measurements were always taken during hemodynamically stable periods without surgical or anesthetic intervention.

A Typical Result

Figure 1 shows an example of data obtained in the manner described. A male 50 y/o patient with normal ventricular function and stable angina pectoris, underwent an elective triple CABG operation. Lorazepam, 5 mg, was given as premedication 2 hours before induction. Peripheral venous catheters, a 20 gauge radial artery cannula and a 7F Swan-Ganz pulmonary artery catheter were placed and baseline measurements, labeled T1, were performed during a period of spontaneous breathing before induction. True average cardiac output was estimated from the mean of 12 random thermodilution estimates. Radial artery pressure was used as a substitute for the theoretically more ideal central aortic waveform.

After the initial series at T1, anesthesia was induced with an initial dose of 7.5 μg/kg sufentanyl and maintained with a continuous infusion of 3.75 μg/kg/hr of the same agent. Pancuronium bromide 0.1 mg/kg was given for muscle relax-

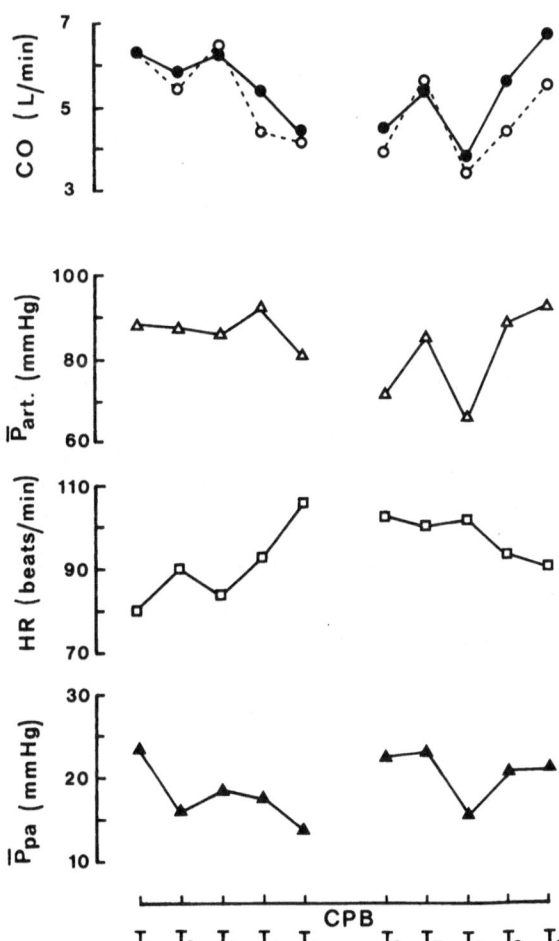

Fig. 1. Example of patient data. The figure shows cardiac output (CO, thermodilution = open circles, pulse contour = closed circles), mean arterial pressure (P_{art}), heart rate (HR), mean pulmonary pressure (P_{pa}) at the defined moments T1 to T10 as explained in the text

Table 1. Calibration measurements in a patient during cardiac surgery (see text)

Code	Moment in surgery	No.	CO_{pc} (l/min)	CO_{td} (l/min)
T2	3 min post-induction	12	5.8	5.5
T3	3 min post-sternotomy	4	6.2	6.4
T4	pre-bypass	4	5.3	4.4
T5	pre-bypass nitroprusside infusion 2 µg/kg/min	4	4.7	4.1
T6	3 min post-bypass	4	5.3	3.9
T7	8 min post-bypass	4	5.3	5.0
T8	13 min post-bypass nitroprusside as at T5	4	4.2	3.3
T9	18 min post-bypass	4	5.6	4.5
T10	end of operation	12	6.5	5.5

ation at intubation. The patient was ventilated with a Siemens/Elema Servo 900B ventilator using $FiO_2 = 0.5$ at 10 respiratory cycles per minute.

Table 1 gives the results of the calibration measurements. The measurement series at T1 was used to calibrate Z_0 which value was not changed for the other comparison pairs. In the pre-bypass period blood pressure was stable yet cardiac output decreased by 38% from thermodilution or 23% from pulse contour between T3 and T5 indicating a substantial increase in total peripheral resistance. Without the beat-to-beat availability of cardiac output, such an episode would have gone by unnoticed or would have been detected only accidentally.

References

1. Jansen JRC, Schreuder JJ, Bogaard JM, van Rooyen W, Versprille A (1981) Thermodilution technique for measurement of cardiac output during mechanical ventilation. J App Physiol 51:584–591
2. Jansen JRC, Versprille A (1986) Improvement of cardiac output estimation by the thermo-dilution method during mechanical ventilation. Intensive Care Med 12:71–79
3. Wesseling KH, de Wit B, Weber JAP, Smith NT (1983) A simple device for the continuous measurement of cardiac output. Its model basis and experimental verification. Adv Cardiovasc Phys 5 (Part II) (1983) 16–52
4. Wesseling KH, Purschke R, Smith NT, Nichols (1976) Continuous monitoring of cardiac output. Medicamundi 21/2:78–90
5. Langewouters GJ, Wesseling KH, Goedhard WJA (1984) The static elastic properties of 45 human thoracic and 20 abdominal aortas in vitro and the parameters of a new model. J Biomechanics 17:425–435

Hemodynamic Monitoring Using Aortic Doppler

M. Singer and D. Bennett

Introduction

"The fundamental problems in the circulation derive from the fact that the supply of adequate amounts of blood to the organs of the body is the main purpose of the circulation and the pressures that are necessary to achieve it are of secondary importance; but the measurement of flow is difficult while that of pressure is easy so that our knowledge of flow is usually derivatory."

Karl Ludwig (1816–1895)

With ever-increasing treatment capability there is clearly a need for accurate hemodynamic measurement to ensure both optimization of therapy and rapid detection of deterioration and adverse events. This does however need to be balanced against the safety of the technique, the risk of which increases with the degree of invasiveness and operator inexperience. A reliable, non-invasive and "user-friendly" technique would be a useful intermediate step where the pulmonary artery (PA) catheter is either unavailable or considered unwarranted.

In the United States approximately one million PA catheters are inserted annually. The technique does however carry a recognized morbidity of up to 7.2% [1] including dysrhythmias, infection, infarction and hemorrhage. A recent retrospective study has even implicated the PA catheter as a cause of increased mortality in a subset of patients with myocardial infarction [2]. Reservations still exist in the United Kingdom over its use; a recent survey revealed that they are not used by over a fifth of British Intensive Care Units (ICU) and two-thirds of Coronary Care Units [3]. Of the ICU that monitor invasively, two-thirds inserted no more than 2 catheters per month and nearly a quarter did not possess the computer necessary to measure cardiac output. Furthermore, fewer than 10% of hospitals used them perioperatively, albeit infrequently. As a consequence, usage is approximately 40-fold greater in the United States on a population-adjusted basis. Cost, complications and lack of necessary expertise were cited as major limiting factors though many British Intensivists felt that the benefit-to-risk ratio and clinical indications for insertion also restricted usage. This implied that catheters were placed (if at all) in response to an adverse event rather than in anticipation of one. As patients would need to be *in extremis* in many British ICU before insertion is considered it could be argued that the PA catheter is being used sub-optimally.

Development of non-invasive hemodynamic monitoring techniques that reduce expense, risk and the dependency on medical and nursing expertise is obviously appealing. Doppler ultrasound measurement of aortic blood flow is one such method that is currently attracting considerable attention. We have been interested for a number of years in its application to both investigation of left ventricular function and management of the critically ill. This article will introduce the theory behind aortic Doppler, summarize previous work and describe some novel approaches being launched into the marketplace. We will emphasize our belief that it should be used for trend analysis rather than for making absolute volumetric measurements, though a reasonable estimate can be made of stroke volume using Doppler alone. By avoiding the temptation of utilizing other technology to embellish the results further, and thus retaining its inherent simplicity, we feel that aortic Doppler has much to commend it as a rapid, safe and reliable means of continuous hemodynamic monitoring.

Theory

It was in 1842 that Christian Doppler described what has come to be known as the Doppler effect, namely that the shift in frequency of sound or light waves emitted by, or reflected off, a moving object is proportional to the relative velocity between object and observer. A formula was derived (Fig. 1) relating frequency shift to velocity which encompassed other parameters such as the angulation of the point of observation to the path of the moving object, and the speed of sound. If these variables were kept constant then the proportionality between changes in frequency shift and velocity would be maintained.

Doppler ultrasound is the technique whereby the Doppler effect is obtained using an acoustic carrier wave with a frequency exceeding the upper range of the human ear, i.e. greater than 20 KHz. For measurement of aortic blood flow transmitted frequencies are usually in the 2–5 MHz range, this being selected on the basis of depth of penetration required to insonate the aorta and the scale of velocities being measured. Whenever the ultrasound beam reaches a tissue interface of different acoustic impedance part of the wave is reflected back. The density difference between red blood corpuscles and plasma is thus responsible for the back-scattered Doppler shift signals used to measure blood flow. If ultrasound is reflected from a stationary tissue interface no change in frequency occurs. If the reflecting surface is however moving towards the receiver then this surface is tending to overtake waves also reflected in that direction. Hence the distance between successive waves is shorter than usual, resulting in a shorter wavelength and a higher frequency being detected by the receiver than that originally transmitted (positive shift). Similarly, if the reflecting surface is moving away from the transducer the distance between successive reflected waves becomes longer, resulting in a lower frequency (negative shift). The Doppler shift may thus be either positive or negative depending on the direction of flow of

$$v = \frac{c \ f_d}{2 \ f_T \ \cos \theta}$$

Fig. 1. Doppler equation. v = flow velocity, c = speed of sound, f_d = frequency shift (Hz), f_T = frequency of transmitted ultrasound (Hz), cos θ = cosine of angle between sound beam axis and velocity vector

blood corpuscles relative to the observer. The angular dependence of the Doppler effect, represented by cos θ in the Doppler equation, results in a smaller shift at larger angles; at 0° – when the beam is parallel to flow – the shift is maximal whereas at 90° – with the beam perpendicular to flow – no shift is detected. By the nature of the cosine curve a smaller angle of insonation will give a smaller error if the assumed angle differs from the true angle. A 15° over-estimation will result in an 18% error in flow velocity when the assumed angle is 30° and a 30% error when the assumed angle is 45°.

Doppler ultrasound may be either continuous-wave (CW) or pulse-wave (PW) by which, as the name implies, the frequency is being transmitted either continuously or in pulses. For CW Doppler a transducer comprising two piezo-electric crystals is required, one transmitting a pure tone frequency and the other receiving back-scattered shifts reflected from any flow within the entire beam volume. A single crystal is however sufficient for PW Doppler as it can receive reflected signals between the transmitted pulses. More complex electronic circuitry is required for PW to locate the depth at which flow is being monitored. Only flow occurring within an adjustable distance around that known depth – the 'range-gate' – will be monitored; this is dependent on the length of the pulse and its repetition frequency which can be varied to give depth resolution. According to Nyquist's theory the maximum frequency shift that can be measured and faithfully reconstructed is one-half of the sampling frequency of the system. If this Nyquist limit is exceeded 'aliasing' occurs whereby spurious signals are produced in the processing due to inadequate sampling. To avoid ambiguity in depth the back-scattered signal must be sampled before transmission of the next pulse. The pulse repetition frequency is inversely proportional to the maximal sampling depth because of the finite transit time of the pulsed signal. Therefore, at greater depths, the velocity level at which aliasing appears is lowered. Using higher repetition rates to an extent where several pulses in the interrogated vessel at the same time causes problems with range resolution thereby nullifying this facility of pulsed-wave Doppler. In practice, the pulse-Doppler system provides precise information at a particular depth but requires more care and time in focussing to obtain an optimal signal. Limitations in velocity measurement, which do not affect CW Doppler, may interfere with data acquisition though the risk of including other vessel flows is minimized.

The back-scattered Doppler signals can be processed to produce velocity-time waveforms which can provide useful information on the circulation being studied. The velocity-time waveforms can be displayed visually; laminar or near-laminar flows have smooth, distinct waveform envelopes whilst jagged, irregular waveform outlines are seen with turbulence. This turbulent flow may be due to flow disruption such as that occurring with either vessel or valve stenosis.

Processing of the Doppler frequency shifts can be achieved by a number of techniques. One such is spectral analysis where a real-time Fourier transform spectral analyzer will produce instantaneous estimates of the spectrum of the received signals. This spectrum can be depicted as a velocity waveform envelope containing all of the different velocities that correspond to the different Doppler frequency shifts. These are displayed in a power density distribution, using grey- or colour-scales, where the intensity of the back-scattered signal at any single frequency is proportional to the total number of cells moving at that velocity at that point in time.

Aortic blood flow can be measured by Doppler from a number of sites including suprasternal, esophageal and tracheal. Intra-cardiac and aortic root blood flow can be measured using Doppler-echocardiography; this however requires expensive equipment and specialist training not generally available to ICU staff and will therefore not be considered further in this article. The assumptions of a flat velocity profile, a laminar flow pattern, known angulation of the ultrasound beam to blood flow, and a constant aortic cross-sectional area in systole, are necessary for changes in the velocity waveform area to reflect accurately proportional changes in stroke volume. These conditions appear to be fulfilled across large variations in pressure, flow and temperature.

The suprasternal approach is where a transducer is placed on the suprasternal notch and angled towards either ascending or arch portions of the aorta. The ultrasound beam is assumed to be in line with blood flow negating any angle effect. Correct placement is achieved when maximum pitch is heard through a loudspeaker and, if a visual display of the spectral analysis is available, by seeing sharp, well-defined velocity waveforms. This approach has the advantages of ease of access and total non-invasiveness however in some 5% of patients good signals are difficult to achieve e.g. post-cardiac surgery, severe emphysema. Significant aortic valve disease will cause turbulence thereby preventing quantification of flow. Another problem has been the inability to fix the probe in position and thus achieve continuous beat-by-beat monitoring. Breathing and movement artifacts may also interfere with good signal acquisition though one benefit of having a visual display is the ability to selectively pick out the aortic flow waveforms.

The esophageal approach utilizes a probe passed approximately 35–40 cm through the mouth to obtain velocity waveforms of descending aortic blood flow. This does provide continuous beat-by-beat monitoring with high quality signals and little artifact. It is unaffected by mediastinal air and can thus be utilized both during and after cardiac surgery. Personal experience with this technique has been highly satisfactory; in well over 100 patients, both in the ICU and perioperatively, signals have always been obtained with the exception of one patient with a severe aortic coarctation. Quantification is possible even in those with aortic valve disease. No significant problems have been encountered, even in those with coagulopathies, and it has been kept in situ for up to three days. For patient comfort it has only been utilized in those being ventilated. The need for refocussing has been infrequent but easily recognized from the fisual display. Running costs are negligible as the probe can be sterilized after use. There are some drawbacks to be considered: it is invasive to some degree and does carry a potential risk of perforation or hemorrhage of the pharynx or esophagus. It should not therefore be recommended for general use in patients with known pharyngo-esophago-gastric pathology and/or significant bleeding diatheses. The probe face is angled thus the cos θ term becomes significant, and approximately 25–30% of the left ventricular output does not pass through the ultrasound beam. It must therefore be assumed that the angle of the beam to blood flow is the same as the probe face and that blood flow down the descending aorta remains in a fixed proportion of total left ventricular output over wide ranges of flow, pressure and temperature. Fourcade et al. found that a probe inserted to a depth of approximately 35 cm from the lips would be at the level of the 5th–6th thoracic vertebra at which point the esophagus runs parallel with the descending aorta [4]. The regional blood flow distribution to limbs and organs has been discussed by Wade and Bishop for normal, high and low output states [5]. Approximately three-quarters of the total cardiac output passes through the descending thoracic aorta; this changes little in high output states and decreases by only 10% in low output conditions such as heart failure. Clinical studies have also shown that, when validated against simultaneous thermodilution measurements, it follows accurately changes in output and a reasonable estimate can be made of volumetric cardiac output (q.v.). A potential source for error is during vascular surgery as aortic cross-clamping may distort both the aortic diameter proximal to it and the proportion of upper to lower body blood flow; this needs to be specifically addressed.

The tracheal approach is a recent innovation whereby a Doppler transducer is an integral part of an endotracheal tube. After oro-tracheal intubation the tube is rotated to insonate ascending aortic flow. Clinical data is somewhat sparse at the moment [6] and we have no personal experience of this technique. The tubes are obviously non-reusable thus a significant running cost is incurred. Other problems may reveal themselves with greater usage however, at present, this is a novel and potentially useful development.

A number of velocity waveform variables can be measured or derived (Fig. 2). *Stroke distance (SD)* – the systolic velocity-time integral – is the area of the waveform. This is the length a column of blood travels along the aorta with each ventricular stroke. If the assumption is made that the vessel cross-sectional area changes little during systole then the product of stroke distance and cross-sectional area is the volume of blood passing through that vessel with each ventricular stroke. In the case of the ascending aorta the stroke distance is a linear index of the total left ventricular stroke volume. *Minute distance (MD)* is the product of stroke distance and heart rate. For the ascending aorta this is a linear index of cardiac output. Changes in cardiac output will thus be reflected by proportional changes in minute distance. An *index of systemic vascular resistance*

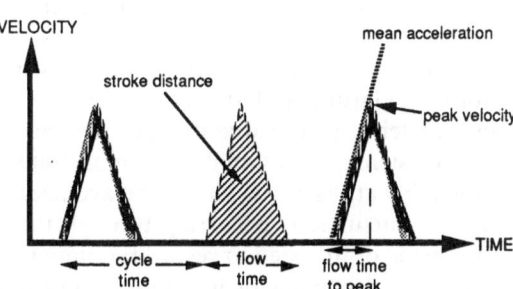

Fig. 2. Doppler velocity waveform variables

(ISVR) can be obtained non-invasively by dividing the mean arterial blood pressure by the minute distance.

Flow time (FT) is the time of systolic flow in the aorta. This corresponds to the base of the velocity waveform. *Cycle time (CT)* is the time from the beginning of one waveform to the start of the next. This corresponds to the R-R interval on an electrocardiogram. The FT_{corr} is a correction of flow time for changes in heart rate. This is achieved by dividing flow time by the square root of the cycle time – Bazett's equation. For minor changes in heart rate, flow time and the *ratio of flow time/cycle time* provide an indication of alterations in left ventricular filling. Where large changes in heart rate have occurred FT_{corr} should be used in preference (q.v.).

The *peak velocity (PV)* is the velocity at the apex of the waveform. The *maximum acceleration (MaxA)* is the greatest rate of change of velocity during systole. This occurs early in systole, within the first 30–50 ms and because of flow frequency artifact – "wall thump" – this is difficult to measure accurately using spectral analysis. The *mean acceleration (MA)* is the value of peak velocity divided by the time to peak velocity (FT_{peak}). This can be used as an alternative to *MaxA*. Both acceleration and peak velocity are indicators of left ventricular contractility and function (q.v.).

Previous Studies

In 1969 Light published the first study of aortic blood flow measurement [7]. This was achieved by placing a Doppler transducer in an intercostal space (usually the third) and aiming it at the ascending aorta. He later modified the technique – termed transcutaneous aortovelography – by placing the transducer in the suprasternal notch and aiming it postero-inferiorly and to the left to insonate the aortic arch [8]. Inter- and intraobserver variability using transcutaneous aortovelography of the aortic arch was reported to be below 6%. In 1983 Huntsman et al. [9] demonstrated close agreement between changes in Doppler stroke distance measured in the ascending aorta and simultaneous thermodilution-measured stroke volume. Many other investigators e.g. Chandraratna et al. [10] have also found close agreement between cardiac output measured by ascending aortic Doppler velocimetry - either continuous or pulsed wave – and either Fick or thermodilution. It should be pointed out that "gold standard" techniques against which Doppler-measured cardiac output is validated are themselves subject to variation, e.g. thermodilution [11]; exact agreement would not therefore be expected.

Using suprasternal pulsed-wave Doppler to insonate ascending aortic flow in normals, Gardin et al. demonstrated a mean intraobserver variability of 2.6%, a mean interobserver variability of 4.5% and a mean day-to day variability of 4.4% [12]. Kristensen and Goldberg demonstrated that a minimum of three beats, and preferably at least five, should be averaged to reduce the potential for error e.g. due to fluctuations occurring through the respiratory cycle [13]. Mention was also made of the need to record far more beats if patients with severe respiratory disease, arrhythmias or unstable hemodynamic conditions were studied. Good agreement was shown by Fisher et al. in open-chest dogs between a roller pump delivering known cardiac outputs and pulsed-wave Doppler sampling flow in a variety of ascending and descending aortic sites [14]. Labovitz et al. also studied the effects of sampling site though used patients on the ICU with thermodilution as the reference technique [15]. Once again, good correlations were shown from suprasternal ascending and descending aortic approaches, the apical left ventricular outflow tract and the parasternal long axis of the main pulmonary artery.

The first description of an esophageal Doppler probe was by Side and Gosling in 1971 [16]. They recognized its potential – *"beat-to-beat changes in the flow pattern and peak velocity and acceleration can be of considerable value to the surgeon by giving immediate warning of deteriorating cardiac efficiency"* though they did not develop it further. In 1974 Olson and Cooke reported their design of a combined esophageal Doppler and pulse-echo system whereby continuous measurement of flow could be combined with estimation of the aortic diameter [17]. Validation of flow velocity measurement was made against implanted flow probes with good agreement. They found that changes in aortic diameter were relatively small and mainly occurred in early systole thus most of the forward flow passed through an aorta of fairly constant diameter. In 1975 Daigle et al. validated descending aortic flow measurement by their prototype esophageal transducer against electromagnetic flowmetry and pulsed Doppler flow cuffs placed around the aorta of beagles at the level of the diaphragm [18]. A blunt velocity profile was demonstrated during forward flow in the descending thoracic aorta. They too observed that most of the change in aortic diameter occurred early in systole.

The esophageal system described by Lavandier et al. in 1985 had an interobserver reproducibility of below 2% [19]. There was a very high coefficient of correlation between Doppler and thermodilution-measured cardiac output though absolute values were significantly underestimated. A number of problems were identified, including the zero-crossing processing technique used and the inaccuracy of aortic diameter measurement. Mark et al. also commented on the unreliability of arotic diameter measurement [20]. They used a commercial Doppler device (Ultracom, Lawrence Medical Systems, USA) modified to accept an esophageal probe. This device relied on two additional inputs to provide a volumetric measure of total body cardiac output:

1. calibration of descending aortic blood flow to total body blood flow using a suprasternal Doppler probe to measure ascending aortic flow; and
2. measurement of ascending aortic diameter using A-mode echocardiography.

The esophageal continuous-wave Doppler probe, 6 mm in diameter and angled at 45°, was inserted and positioned approximately 35–40 cm from the incisors by maximizing both the pitch of an audible signal and the signal level seen on a digital display. Fairly good tracking of cardiac output was obtained overall however significant errors were introduced by the calibration steps of measuring aortic diameter and ascending aortic flow. Further investigations were suggested to address the need for absolute cardiac output values and that trends alone may be sufficient to aid management in many instances. The Ultracom was developed into a dedicated esophageal Doppler machine – the Accucom – which incorporated a nomogram for aortic diameter derived from patient gender, height and weight data. Again, validation studies showed reliable trend following but an inaccuracy in making absolute volumetric cardiac output measurements [21, 22].

Initial findings from our prototype esophageal probe system (Doptek, Chichester, UK) were recently reported [23]. The probe was 9 mm in diameter, its face was angled at 45° and 5MHz continuous wave Doppler ultrasound was used. Placement time took a matter of minutes and an online beat-by-beat visual display of the spectral analysis was used to achieve correct positioning. No attempt was made to measure aortic diameter or calibrate descending to ascending aortic blood flow. Changes in cardiac output compared against thermodilution showed close agreement; indeed, as Mark had found, the coefficient of variation was considerably lower for Doppler. By taking age into account (q.v.), an estimation of volumetric cardiac output could be made to within 80% accuracy. We believe this is sufficient as in most cases only an indication of low, normal or high output states is required. Thereafter it is the change in output – either spontaneous or therapeutically-induced – that is important to follow. We accept readily that flaws exist in the esophageal technique and inherent assumptions may not be totally valid. Attempts to measure or derive aortic diameter and thus make claims of accurate volumetric measurements only severe to complicate, add further error and undermine confidence in the technique.

Waveform Shape

Little attention has been paid to the shape of the waveform and changes thereof in the management of the critically ill. In conjunction with the waveform size (the stroke distance) we have found that the waveform shape and associated parameters such as peak velocity and flow time serve to provide information not only for hemodynamic management but also in diagnosis.

Mowat et al. demonstrated that aortic blood flow velocity in adults was independent of sex, body surface area and blood pressure but did decline progressively with age so that at 70 years of age the mean value of peak velocity was 55% of that at age 20 [24]. The same group showed a progressive decline in stroke distance and minute distance with age of 0.88% per annum of adult life; this could be accounted for by (1) reduction in cardiac output with age, and (2) dilatation of the aorta with age whereby an equivalent minute distance would reflect a higher cardiac output in older age groups [25]. Stroke distance could discriminate between age-matched normals, pregnancy, hypertension, atrial fibrillation and cardiac failure. Gardin et al. also confirmed the lack of relationship between gender, blood pressure, body surface area and aortic flow measurements [26]. They found that peak velocity, stroke distance and mean acceleration all decreased with increasing age whereas FT_{corr} increased and FT_{peak} did not change.

Provided age is taken into account, parameters of acceleration and velocity can be used as indicators of left ventricular function; values exceeding normal age-related ranges are seen in hyperdynamic states such as sepsis whilst lower values are seen in conditions of poor left ventricular function. A progressive increase is seen in PV and acceleration on giving increasing doses of an inotrope whilst the converse is seen with a negative inotrope or a continuing deterioration in function, e.g. cardiogenic shock.

The FT_{corr} value provides a guide to left ventricular filling; reduced values with normal or relatively normal values of acceleration and velocity indicate underfilling of the left ventricle, e.g. hypovolemia or mitral stenosis [27]. An increase in filling from an underfilled state produces an increase in FT_{corr}. Conversely, the FT_{corr} will fall with progressive reductions in preload e.g. uncorrected hemorrhage. When the ventricle is overfilled, and the compliance is thus lower, the FT_{corr} also falls. Reduction in preload, in this instance towards normal values, will now result in an increase in FT_{corr} until a situation is reached where the ventricle becomes underfilled and the FT_{corr} then starts to fall. We have recently completed a study examining changes in PA wedge pressure and FT_{corr} on

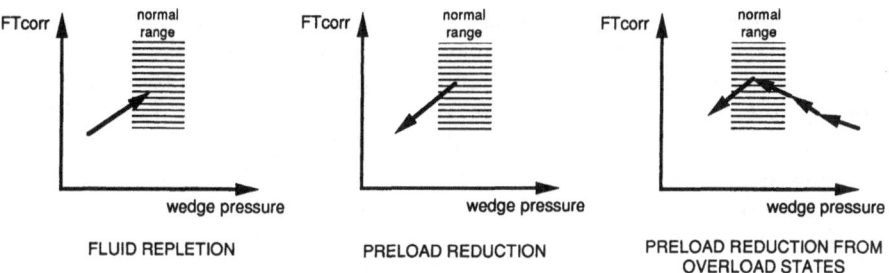

Fig. 3. Stylized changes in FT_{corr} and pulmonary artery wedge pressure on (1) fluid repletion from hypovolemia, (2) preload reduction from a 'normal' wedge pressure level and (3) progressive preload reduction from states of fluid overload

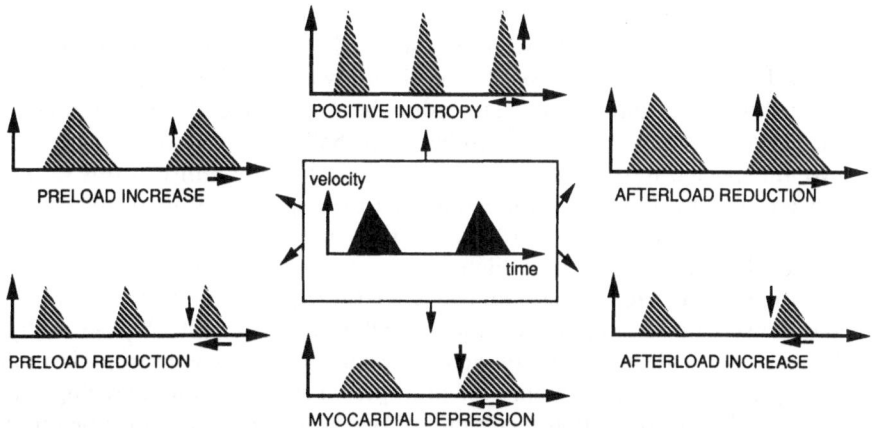

Fig. 4. Changes in peak velocity and FT_{corr} on altering left ventricular filling, inotropy and systemic vascular resistance

50 occasions in patients during volume repletion, preload reduction from normal to subnormal wedge pressure values, and preload reduction from high to normal wedge pressures. Consistent changes were seen and are depicted in Fig. 3.

A reduction in afterload will allow the ventricle to eject blood more easily; as a consequence PV and FT_{corr} will both increase. The opposite is seen with increases in afterload; this is especially marked in patients with poor ventricular function where the ventricle may have considerable difficulty in pumping against an increased resistance. A dynamic interrelationship exists between preload, afterload and inotropic state. For example, a compensatory increase in afterload occurs with both extremes of left ventricular filling, be it hypovolemia or left ventricular failure, in an attempt to maintain systemic blood pressure. Only after these compensatory reflexes are lost does the blood pressure fall, as in severe hemorrhage or cardiogenic shock. Thus the FT_{corr} falls with decreased preload/increased afterload states and increases with increasing preload/decreasing afterload. Velocity and acceleration are affected to some degree by changes in preload (the Frank-Starling effect), to a greater degree by changes in afterload and, most of all, by changes in contractility. We demonstrated these effects in patients on the ICU or undergoing cardiac surgery before and after 78 hemodynamic maneuvers which predominantly affected one variable, e.g. fluid challenge, phentolamine for afterload reduction, glyceryl trinitrate for preload reduction [23]. Consistent changes were seen and are stylized in Fig. 4. Inotropic changes mainly affected PV with relatively little change in FT_{corr}; changes in preload mainly affected FT_{corr} with lesser changes in PV whilst changes in afterload affected both in approximately equal proportions.

We have recently submitted for publication a study examining changes in Doppler parameters resulting from hemodynamic maneuvers in healthy, resting, awake and supine subjects. Their cardiovascular responses could not therefore be blunted either by anesthesia or intrinsic heart disease. The suprasternal approach was used to follow changes during administration of increasing intravenous doses of placebo, dobutamine, esmolol (a short-acting β-blocker), phentolamine (for afterload reduction), metaraminol and methoxamine (for afterload increases). Progressive fluid depletion was achieved by plasmapheresis. Consistent changes were seen and were dose-related. The findings are summarized in Fig. 5. Furthermore, a reasonable correlation was noted between the ISVR and FT_{corr} thus highlighting the relationship between preload and afterload. This correlation was not however found between ISVR and either PV or acceleration. Two unexpected findings serve to further underline the utility of this technique: we were surprised that esmolol had neither the negative chronotropic effects nor change in systemic vascular resistance that one would expect with a pure β-blocker. This infers some vasodilatory effects which may be attributable either to the drug or its carrier vehicle; indeed, we later found esmolol studies in patients that showed no change in systemic vascular resistance [28, 29]. Secondly, the changes seen with metaraminol were suggestive of positive inotropy in addition to peripheral vasoconstriction. This prompted a review of pharmacological literature which confirmed that metaraminol is a vasoconstrictor-inotrope and not a 'pure' vasoconstrictor as originally (and commonly) believed. Methoxamine, a relatively 'pure' vasoconstrictor indeed produced the expected changes.

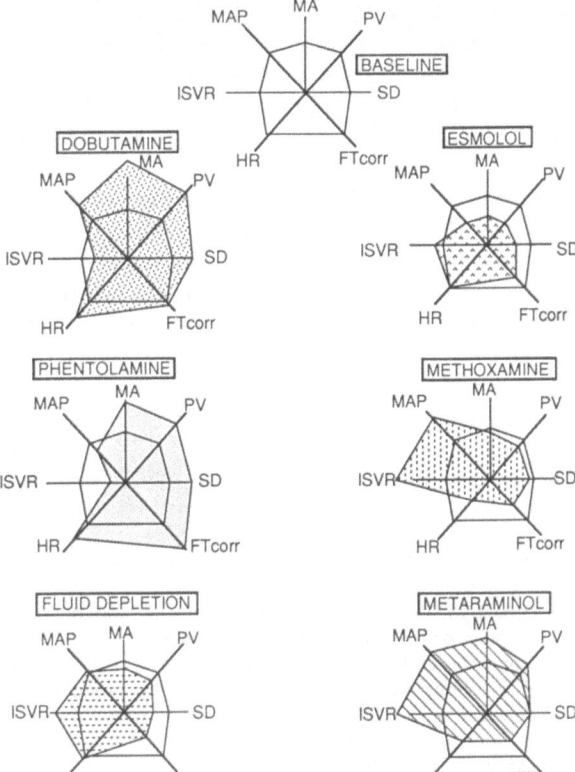

Fig. 5. Changes from resting baseline values in mean acceleration (MA), peak velocity (PV), stroke distance (SD), FT$_{corr}$ (flow time corrected for heart rate), heart rate (HR), index of systemic vascular resistance (ISVR) and mean arterial pressure (MAP) on administration of dobutamine, esmolol, phentolamine, methoxamine, metaraminol and fluid depletion

Conclusion

Doppler measurement of aortic blood flow offers a quick, safe and reliable means of hemodynamic monitoring. There is a sharp learning curve and the user can quickly identify both adequate and inadequate signals. We recommend the use of a machine with a visual waveform display to further assist in this recognition. Changes in cardiac output can be easily followed, an estimation of volumetric output made, and an indication provided of left ventricular filling, contractility and afterload. The addition of further technology e.g. to measure aortic diameter, calibrate ascending to descending flow, serves mainly to complicate and add further error. Criticism can be aimed at some Doppler enthusiasts and manufacturers for overstating claims of making accurate absolute volumetric output measurements. As a number of assumptions are made, the technique cannot provide more than an approximation of cardiac output, albeit a good one; emphasis should instead be placed on its facility to trend-follow with ease.

Its application to the management of the critically ill or hemodynamically unstable patient has still to be fully developed. For its general acceptance as a tool on the ICU it has to be simple to use and ideally provide continuous hands-off monitoring. Current technology now allows superior processing, on-line measurement and compact machinery. With relatively little expertise adequate signals of aortic flow can be obtained. The suprasternal approach provides a useful means of intermittent monitoring in either conscious or ventilated patients. When continuous monitoring is desired in ventilated patients esophageal or tracheal probes can be easily placed to provide valuable hemodynamic information.

Aortic Doppler should be viewed as complementary to the pulmonary artery catheter. There are many situations where absolute data on cardiac output, oxygen delivery and uptake, etc. ... are important to known. Likewise, many situations exist where further hemodynamic information is desirable yet the invasive technique is either unavailable or felt unwarranted.

References

1. Elliot CG, Zimmerman GA, Clemmer TP (1979) Complications of pulmonary artery catheterisation in the care of critically-ill patients. A prospective study. Chest 76:647–652
2. Gore JM, Goldberg RJ, Spodick DH, Alpert JS, Dalen JE (1987) A community-wide assessment of the use of pulmonary artery catheters in patients with acute myocardial infarction. Chest 92:721–727
3. Singer M, Bennett ED (1989) Invasive hemodynamic monitoring in the United Kingdom. Enough or too little? Chest 95:623–626
4. Fourcade C, Cathignol D, Muchada R, et al (1980) Validation de la débitmétrie aortique par capteur ultrasonore oesophagien dans la surveillance hémodynamique non sanglante. Agressologie 21:121–128
5. Wade OL, Bishop JM (1962) Cardiac output and regional blood flow. Backwell Scientific Publications, Oxford
6. Abrams JH, Weber RE, Holmen KD (1989) Continuous cardiac output determination using transtracheal Doppler; initial results in humans. Anesthesiology 71:11–15
7. Light LH (1969) Non-injurious ultrasonic technique for observing flow in the human aorta. Nature 224:1119–1121
8. Light LH (1976) Transcutaneous aortovelography. A new window on the circulation? Br Heart J 38:433–442
9. Huntsman LL, Stewart DK, Barnes SR, Franklin SB, Colocousis JS, Hessel EA (1983) Non-invasive Doppler determination of cardiac output in man. Circulation 67:593–602
10. Chandraratna PA, Nanna M, McKay C, et al (1984) Determination of cardiac output by transcutaneous continuous-wave ultrasonic Doppler computer. Am J Cardiol 53:234–237
11. Stetz CW, Miller RG, Kelly GE, Raffin TA (1982) Reliability of the thermodilution method in the determination of cardiac output in clinical practice. Am Rev Resp in Dis 126:1001–1004
12. Gardin JM, Dabestani A, Matin K, Allfie A, Russell D, Henry WL (1984) Reproducibility of Doppler aortic flow measurements: studies on intraobserver, interobserver and day-to-day variability in normal subjects. Am J Cardiol 54:1092–1098
13. Kristensen BO, Goldberg SJ (1987) Number of cardiac cycles required to accurately determine mean velocity of blood flow in the ascending aorta and pulmonary trunk. Am J Cardiol 60:746–747
14. Fisher DC, Sahn DJ, Freidman MJ, Larson D, Valdes-Cruz LM, Horowitz S (1983) The effect of variations on pulsed Doppler sampling site on calculation of cardiac output: an experimental study in open-chest dogs. Circulation 67:370–376
15. Labovitz AJ, Buckingham TA, Habermehl K, Nelson J, Kennedy HL, Williams GA (1985) The effects of sampling site on the two-dimensional echo-Doppler determination of cardiac output. Am Heart J 109:327–331
16. Side CD, Gosling RJ (1971) Non-surgical assessment of cardiac function. Nature 232:335–336

17. Olson RM, Cooke JP (1974) A nondestructive ultrasonic technique to measure diameter and blood flow in arteries. IEEE Trans Biomed Eng 168–171
18. Daigle RE, Miller CW, Histand MB, McLeod FD, Hokanson D (1975) Nontraumatic aortic blood flow sensing by use of an ultrasonic esophageal probe. J Appl Physiol 38:1153–1160
19. Lavandier B, Cathignol D, Muchada R, Bui Xuan B, Motin J (1985) Noninvasive aortic blood flow measurement using an intraesophageal probe. Ultrasound Med Biol 11:451–460
20. Mark NB, Steinbrook RA, Gugino LD, Madi R, Hartwell B, Shemin R (1986) Continuous noninvasive monitoring of cardiac output with esophageal Doppler ultrasound during cardiac surgery. Anesth Analg 65:1013–1020
21. Freund P (1987) Transesophageal Doppler scanning versus thermodilution during general anesthesia. An initial comparison of cardiac output techniques. Am J Surg 153:490–494
22. Seyde WC, Stephan H, Rieke H (1987) Non-invasive determination of cardiac output by Doppler ultrasound. Experiences and results by using the Accucom. Anaesthesist 36:504–509
23. Singer M, Clarke J, Bennett ED (1989) Continuous hemodynamic monitoring by esophageal Doppler. Crit Care Med 17:447–452
24. Mowat DHR, Haites N, Rawles JM (1983) Aortic blood velocity measurement in healthy adults using a simple ultrasound technique. Cardiovasc Res 17:75–80
25. Haites NE, McLennan FM, Mowat DHR, Rawles JM (1985) Assessment of cardiac output by the Doppler ultrasound technique alone. Br Heart J 53:123–129
26. Gardin JM, Davidson DM, Rohan MK, et al (1987) Relationship between age, body size, gender and blood pressure and Doppler flow measurements in the aorta and pulmonary artery. Am Heart J 113:101–109
27. Singer M, Bennett ED (1989) Pitfalls of pulmonary artery catheterisation highlighted by Doppler ultrasound. Crit Care Med 17:1060–1061
28. Gray RJ, Bateman TM, Czer LSC, Conklin C, Matlof JM (1985) Use of esmolol in hypertension after cardiac surgery. Am J Cardiol 56:49F–56F
29. Reves JG, Flezzani P (1985) Perioperative use of esmolol. Am J Cardiol 56:57F–62F

Real-Time Monitoring of Gas Exchange

L. D. Nelson

Introduction to Real-Time-Monitoring

The Ideal Monitor

Monitoring is the essence of critical care. It is the need for monitoring that resulted in the establishment of the initial intensive care units (ICU) in the late 1950s and early 1960s. Since the establishment of these units, physicians have sought an ideal monitoring system which would provide an early warning of untoward events in the patient's clinical course. The ideal monitoring system would be sensitive to small changes in the patient's status yet would be specific enough to suggest therapeutic alternatives which may improve the patient's course. The system would be accurate and precise yielding both correct and reproducible information. It should be easy to use, selfcalibrating, reliable, safe, noninvasive, and inexpensive.

THE IDEAL MONITORING SYSTEM DOES NOT EXIST!

Since the ideal monitoring system does not exist, we are forced with using multiple monitoring systems which increase the expense and complexity of critical care management. The purpose of this article is to review currently available real-time monitors of gas exchange and to compare and contrast the differences of the clinically available devices. Emphasis will be placed on the pitfalls and problems associated with each of the devices. A thorough understanding of problems associated with the monitoring systems should allow better utilization of these devices in the management of critically ill patients.

Goals of Real-Time-Monitoring

Since the primary function of monitoring is to provide an early warning of events which if undetected will lead to organ system dysfunction and eventually failure, the need for real-time monitors should be self-evident. Real-time monitoring allows detection of an event at a point in time in which correction of the underlying problem is most likely to have an impact on outcome. If ICU activities are to have an impact on patient outcome, prompt intervention at the earliest possible time and goal directed application of treatment is necessary. Real-time monitoring satisfies both requirements by giving information regarding changes at the earliest possible moment and allowing goal directed titration of therapy in the most time efficient manner possible.

Problems with Intermittent Measurements

Intermittent measurements made in the ICU have several disadvantages when compared with real-time monitoring. The obvious disadvantage is the time lag associated with the measurement and its relationship to a physiologic event. Unless there are appropriate real-time "triggers" which activate intermittent measurements, there will be delays in the detection of physiologic occurrences.

Blood gas sampling is classic example of intermittent measurement. When blood gases are drawn following a ventilator manipulation, an arbitrary period of time must pass in order for "steady-state" to occur. There is also an interval of time required for drawing the blood gas, sending it to the laboratory, making the measurement, and returning the data to the bedside. In the best of situations this turnover time may only be a few minutes but in a typical large ICU perhaps 10 to 15 minutes is a more realistic period of time. If 15 to 20 minutes are allowed for patient equilibration following ventilator changes and blood gases are measured following each ventilator change to assure optimal goal directed therapy, a maximum of only 2 to 4 interventions per hour can be made. With real-time monitoring since the equilibration period is defined by the patient's physiologic course rather than arbitrary times, numerous ventilatory interventions may be performed in less than one hour. This concept intuitively allows the clinician to reach a therapeutic endpoint earlier, therefore resulting in more efficient care.

Oxygenation Monitoring

Transcutaneous PO₂ Monitoring (PtcO₂)

Transcutaneous PO_2 monitoring has been used as an assessment of oxygenation in neonates and infants since the 1970s. In the late 1970s and early 1980s tremendous interest was generated in this monitoring technique in critically ill adults. It quickly became evident that transcutaneous PO_2 was determined by 3 primary factors [1]. One of the most important factors was obviously arterial oxygen tension. However, $PtcO_2$ was found to vary greatly from PaO_2 when the patients were in a low flow state [2]. The transcutaneous PO_2/PaO_2 index was used to evaluate the effect of perfusion on the transcutaneous value. While this lead to an improvement in the interpretation of $PtcO_2$ values, it detracted from the cost effectiveness of this monitoring technique. PaO_2 would have to be measured whenever there was a significant change in $PtcO_2$ in order to calculate the index and determine the effect of blood flow on the transcutaneous value [2].

It became apparent in the mid 1970s that in addition to total blood flow (i.e., cardiac index) local blood flow was also an important factor in determining $PtcO_2$. The suggestion was made to evaluate both the $PtcO_2/PaO_2$ index and the cardiac index. If there was a discrepancy between the oxygenation values, then cardiac index was measured and if found to be low, the problem was likely due to impaired cardiac output. On the other hand, if cardiac index was high, the problem was more likely to be secondary to impaired local perfusion [3].

In another study looking at the relationship between PaO_2 and $PtcO_2$ in hyperdynamic trauma patients, a positive correlation was found between the values [4]. In these selected patients with ARDS due to trauma and/or sepsis who had a high cardiac output, the transcutaneous gas analysis was found to have a high correlation with PaO_2 and could be used as an overall estimate of oxygenation. In this specific patient population the assumption must be made that there were no local cutaneous perfusion abnormalities which would have interfered with the transcutaneous measurements.

The general consensus at this time is that $PtcO_2$ measurements are a sensitive but non-specific indicator of oxygenation abnormalities. A decrease in $PtcO_2$ may be the result of a decrease in PaO_2, a decrease in cardiac index, or a decrease in local perfusion. Because of the poor specificity of transcutaneous oxygenation monitoring, it has not achieved widespread acceptance in adult critical care.

Transconjunctival PO_2 Monitoring ($PcjO_2$)

Monitoring of transconjunctival PO_2 was developed in the early 1980s as an attempt to eliminate the need of heating the skin to obtain $PtcO_2$ measurements. It was felt initially that gas exchange accross the palpebral conjunctiva would be less dependent upon blood flow and therefore a more accurate indicator of arterial oxygenation [5]. The value was demonstrated to have a good correlation with PaO_2 unless there was a fall in conjunctival temperature [6]. Initially, it was felt that $PcjO_2$ would be an indicator of cerebral oxygenation. The device was advocated during carotid artery surgery [7, 8]. Further investigation, however, found no correlation between $PcjO_2$ and cerebral blood flow during carotid artery occlusion [9].

As might be expected, $PcjO_2$ monitoring also has been found to be dependent upon total systemic and local blood flow variation. There is a relationship between $PcjO_2$ and blood volume [10, 11] and global oxygen transport [12].

One advantage of $PcjO_2$ monitoring over $PtcO_2$ monitoring seems to be a faster response time [13].

In summary, $PcjO_2$ monitoring seems to have the same limitations as $PtcO_2$ in that it is dependent upon global and local changes in blood flow. It is also a sensitive but non-specific indicator of changes in oxygen transport whether they be due to oxygen content or blood flow. $PtcO_2$ monitoring has not become widely accepted. It is used in a limited number of centers in the early acute resuscitation of patients prior to placement of more traditional monitoring techniques.

Pulse Oximetry

Without question, the most significant advance in real-time monitoring of pulmonary gas exchange occurred in the early 1980s. The refinement and clinical institution of pulse oximetry has literally changes the way critically ill patients are monitored [14]. Pulse oximetry has become a standard of care for intraoperative monitoring and is rapidly becoming standard of care for all patients receiving supplement ventilatory or oxygenation support. Some of the reasons for this great success of pulse oximetry include the ease of operation, the reliability of the measurement, and the importance of the measurement [15]. The advantages of pulse oximetry over other types of continuous oxygenation monitors have been well described [16, 17]. Several potential problems of pulse oximetry need to be discussed.

The pulse oximeter cannot measure accurately in low perfusion states. When the pulse pressure is low due to low blood flow, vasoconstriction, severe edema or venous congestion there is a reduction in the signal to noise ratio and failure to calculate oxygen saturation. These devices differ from older ear oximeters in that they do not show a diminishing arterial saturation as perfusion decreases and both tissue oxygenation and venous oxygen saturation fall. Rather than failing "soft" and giving inaccurate data, the devices "fail hard" and yield no saturation data at all. While this is an advantage in that inaccurate data are not displayed, it is a disadvantage in that no information is available in poor perfusion states.

Similar, motion artifact increases background noise and interferes with the ability of the device to differentiate between changes in light absorbence due to sensor movement or arterialized pulsatile blood flow.

Other uncommon but important sources of artifact include changes in absorbence caused by intravascular dye administration such as methylene blue, indocyan green, indigo carmine, and fluorescein [18]. Hyperbilirubinemia does not interfere with the accuracy of the measurements.

High levels of ambient light also may interfere with the pulse oximetry measurements. It is recommended that when the sensor is in a bright environment that it be covered to reduce possible artifact induced by high intensity lighting [19].

One of the most interesting problems with pulse oximetry occurs in the patients with significant levels of carboxy- and methemoglobins. Pulse oximetry, using the two wave-length method, measures *functional* oxyhemoglobin saturation rather than the *fractional* oxyhemoglobin saturation that we are used to seeing. The fractional oxyhemoglobin saturation measured by traditional laboratory cooximetry tells us the fraction of oxyhemoglobin compared to all hemoglobins measured (i.e., oxyhemoglobin, deoxyhemoglobin, carboxyhemoglobin, methemoglobin, and sulfhemoglobin). The two wave-length pulse oximeters are unable to account for the various dyshemoglobins and report a functional oxyhemoglobin saturation. The functional oxyhemoglobin saturation is equal to:

$$SfO_2 = \frac{SaO_2}{1 - (COHb + MetHb)}$$

The functional oxyhemoglobin saturation therefore always *overestimates* the fractional oxyhemoglobin saturation by an amount proportional to the total of carboxy- and methemoglobin. While at first glance these dyshemoglobins would seem to be unimportant in critically ill patients, there is actually significant relevance to the clinician. Since carboxyhemoglobin levels can reach 10% in smokers and since the half-life of carboxyhemoglobin is about 8 hours when breathing room air, significant overestimates of arterial saturation can be made in this patient population. Even greater inaccuracy can occur in patients with carbon monoxide intoxication. In both of these subsets of patients, carboxyhemoglobin levels should be markedly reduced after ventilation with increased oxygen concentrations for a period of 24 hours. However, there are other sources of carboxyhemoglobin which may affect critically ill patients.

The sources of dyshemoglobins in the ICU are often overlooked. Even though a patient has been on supplement oxygen and ventilatory support for a significant period of time, there may not be complete washout of carboxyhemoglobin from prehospitalization exposure. Of greater interest is the fact that patients who have ongoing hemolysis secondary to massive transfusions have increased levels of carboxyhemoglobin in their blood in the 2 to 3% range. This will account for a small but perhaps significant difference between functional and fractional oxyhemoglobin saturation. Methemoglobin, on the other hand, may be seen when patients receive topical anesthetics (Cetacaine) or receive high dose intravenous nitroglycerin. Either of these interventions may result in methemoglobin levels rising into the range of 10%.

Recognition that functional oxyhemoglobin saturation exceeds fractional oxyhemoglobin saturation becomes important when we look at derived oxygen transport parameters. In a recent study we were able to note marked discrepancies between arterial-venous oxygen content difference, oxygen consumption, and intrapulmonary shunt fraction when the function rather than fractional value is used [20]. Since the functional value is high on the arterial estimate when pulse oximetry is used, $C(a-v)O_2$ and $\dot{V}O_2$ will be overestimated and Qsp/Qt will be grossly underestimated.

Anemia, unless it is profound, has little affect on the accuracy of pulse oximetry [21].

The accuracy of pulse oximetry clearly deteriorates at very low arterial saturations. In a study in dogs the accuracy decreased markedly when the oxyhemoglobin saturation was less than 70 [22]. Since this situation is virtually never allowed to occur clinically for a prolonged period of time, this does not represent a limitation to the utility of continuous pulse oximetry.

Other data may be available from the pulse oximeter. Variation in the wave form obtained on some pulse oximeters may give information regarding the patient's intravascular volume status. A correlation was found in a small number of patients between pulse wave form variations and systolic blood pressure variation. While this evidence of intravascular volume depletion may be indirect, it represents an area of future investigation [23].

Mixed Venous Oximetry

Continuous mixed venous oximetry using a fiberoptic pulmonary artery catheter has opened new understanding in the real-time monitoring of oxygen supply/demand balance. Mixed venous oximetry was introduced clinically in the early

1980s. Tremendous controversy has brewed around the ability of mixed venous oxygen saturation ($S\bar{v}O_2$) measurements to correlate with cardiac output. Early studies suggested that $S\bar{v}O_2$ should correlate with cardiac output in patients who are otherwise stable. These early studies were supported by the finding of a clinical correlation under general anesthesia. Later studies in the ICU, however, failed to show a high degree of correlation between $S\bar{v}O_2$ in cardiac output [24–27].

When one examines the determinants of $S\bar{v}O_2$ by the Fick equation, it is clear that there are multiple determinants of $S\bar{v}O_2$. When arterial saturation is maintained at a high level following relationship holds:

$$S\bar{v}O_2 = 1 - \frac{\dot{V}O_2}{Hb \times SaO_2 \times 13.4 \times CO}$$

There are four determinants of $S\bar{v}O_2$: SaO_2, Hb, CO, $\dot{V}O_2$. $S\bar{v}O_2$ is determined by the balance between the consumption of oxygen (the numerator) and the delivery of oxygen (the denominator). This relationship has been defined by others as the oxygen utilization or extraction ratio. The tissues normally extract about 25% of the delivered oxygen making a normal $S\bar{v}O_2$ of about 0.75 in a patient who has a high arterial oxygen saturation. Decreases in consumption or increases in delivery which are uncompensated will lead to an increase in $S\bar{v}O_2$. On the other hand, increases in consumption or decreases in delivery which are uncompensated will lead to a decrease in $S\bar{v}O_2$ [24]. The only time in which there would be correlation between $S\bar{v}O_2$ and cardiac output would be when there is no change in SaO_2, hemoglobin, or oxygen consumption. $S\bar{v}O_2$ is not just an indicator of pulmonary gas exchange but rather an indicator of the relationship between oxygen delivery and tissue oxygen consumption. $S\bar{v}O_2$ does not tell us about tissue oxygenation per se, but rather represents the flow weighted average of the effluents of all perfused vascular beds.

A change in $S\bar{v}O_2$ alerts the clinician that the oxygen supply/demand balance has changed and further information is needed to assess the cause for this change. $S\bar{v}O_2$ measurements can help to determine the timing of other oxygen transport measurements. It will help minimize unnecessary oxygen transport measurements in the stable patient but yet will alert the clinician as to the need for further measurements in the unstable patient. Continuous $S\bar{v}O_2$ monitoring therefore may improve the efficiency of the delivery of critical care by improving the timing of our intermittent measurements [28, 29].

Dual Oximetry

Dual oximetry is the term applied to the combined monitoring of gas exchange by arterial pulse oximetry and continuous mixed venous oximetry [30]. Dual oximetry may be performed using independent monitors and observing the relationship between the arterial and venous saturation measurements. In a patient who is hypoxemic, convergence of the SaO_2 and $S\bar{v}O_2$ would indicate decreased oxygen extraction in the periphery and increased right-to-left shunting. Conversely, in a hypoxemic patient a divergence between SaO_2 and $S\bar{v}O_2$ implies increased extraction of oxygen in the periphery. Observation of these monitoring devices may guide the clinician in management of patients with unstable oxygen transport balance towards a pulmonary versus a hemodynamic cause.

Räsänen and Downs have further refined dual oximetry by combining the two monitors with a microcomputer so that the gas exchange parameters may be calculated in a real-time fashion. Right-to-left venous admixture and oxygen extraction ratio can be computed and plotted graphically by the monitoring device. This technique has been demonstrated to improve the efficiency of titrating ventilatory support [31, 32].

Ventilation Monitoring

Transcutaneous PCO$_2$ Monitoring

Transcutaneous monitoring of PCO_2 has been successful in infants and neonates. As with $PtcO_2$ monitoring, the device has been used less successfully in adults. The $PtcCO_2$ measurement yields a value which is always greater than $PaCO_2$. This is due to local production of carbon dioxide in the heated tissue below the sensor. $PtcCO_2$ measurements also tend to be flow dependent and the disparity between $PaCO_2$ and $PtcCO_2$ increases as local blood flow decreases. For these reasons, $PtcCO_2$ measurements have not become widely accepted in adult clinical care.

End Tidal CO$_2$ Measurements (PetCO$_2$)

Capnography and the measurement of end-tidal CO_2 is rapidly becoming a "standard of care" in intraoperative management of anesthetized patients [33]. Capnography allows for the evaluation of the overall balance between production of CO_2, transport of CO_2, regional changes in ventilation, changes in total alveolar ventilation, and problems with the ventilatory circuit [34, 35]. Since so may factors affect the capnogram and end-tidal CO_2, a clear understanding of the physiology of carbon dioxide excretion must be understood.

Most devices use either mass spectrometry or infrared spectrophotometry as the analysis method. They analyze CO_2 excretion throughout the ventilatory cycle and display the real-time CO_2 tension or concentration in a graphic manner. The devices use either an in line sensor attached directly to the patient's airway or a side stream device which samples gas from the patient's airway for processing in a remote sensor. Both systems have clinical advantages and disadvantages but in adult critical care yield the same information [36].

The normal capnogram is manifest by a zero inspiratory PCO_2 followed by a rapid upstroke during the beginning of exhalation. The rapid upstroke is followed by a relatively flat "alveolar plateau", the end of which is defined as the end-tidal CO_2. During spontaneous inspiration, there is a rapid fall back to a zero inspiratory CO_2. Alterations in this wave form are caused by changes in either global or regional lung ventilation. Several common patterns are seen in the capnographic wave form. A slow decrease in end-tidal CO_2 implies either decreasing CO_2 production or increasing alveolar ventilation. Conversely, a slow increase in end-tidal CO_2 implies either an increase in CO_2 production or a decrease in alveolar ventilation. Alveolar ventilation may change as a result of either a change in dead space/tidal volume ratio or a change in exhaled minute ventilation. Since end-tidal CO_2 concentration is dependent upon many variables, it is useful as a relatively sensitive but non-specific indicator of changes in CO_2 dynamics.

Recently, capnography has moved from the operating room to the ICU. Unfortunately, in the ICU many variables which are relatively well controlled during general anesthesia cannot be controlled. Marked changes in breath-to-breath tidal volume during spontaneous ventilation and marked changes in CO_2 production with changes in metabolic rates as well as changes in dead space/tidal volume ratios make the interpretation of a change in end-tidal CO_2 somewhat more difficult.

The utility of capnography in the ICU lies in its ability to display breath by breath trend information regarding CO_2 excretion. Although there are many determinants of the end-tidal CO_2 value, the trend information may be useful to detect changes in CO_2 dynamics which may adversely affect the patient's course. In large patient populations measurement of end-tidal PCO_2 tends to underestimate the $PaCO_2$ by approximately 3 to 5 torr. While this variance changes in individual patients (with changes in ventilation/perfusion ratios), there is a high degree of correlation between end-tidal CO_2 and arterial CO_2 [37]. Because of this high statistical correlation and the fact that end-tidal CO_2 nearly always underestimates $PaCO_2$, increases in end-tidal CO_2 are almost always clinically significant. Furthermore, since the precision (i.e., reproducibility) of the measurement is approximately ±6 torr, a change greater than this amount is very likely to indicate a "true" change in the patient's status [37]. For these reasons capnography is useful in the ICU as an indicator of the onset of ventilatory acidosis.

Perhaps equally important to the function of trend monitoring is the function of capnography as a tool to aid in the clinical assessment of weaning a patient from ventilatory support. To be useful in weaning patients, capnography must detect CO_2 retention in a relatively specific and sensitive manner. When patients are being weaned from ventilatory support end-tidal CO_2 monitoring is capable of detecting significant CO_2 retention. In a series of patients who demonstrated hypercarbia ($PaCO_2$ >45 torr) end-tidal CO_2 changes of >45 torr were 79% sensitive and 73% specific in detecting an arterial CO_2 of >50 torr. This makes capnography an attractive clinical adjunct in the weaning of patients from mechanical ventilation [38].

Finally, capnography may be useful in improving both safety and efficiency of weaning from mechanical ventilatory support. In a study of hemodynamically stable patients who were being weaned from ventilatory support, the combination of continuous capnography and continuous pulse oximetry detected changes in gas exchange which resulted in termination of the weaning attempt at an earlier point in time than was detected by traditional clinical evaluation and blood gas analyses. In the study 40 patients being actively weaned from ventilatory support had 13 events that necessitated increases in ventilatory support. All of the events were detected initially by pulse oximetry (in 7 events) or capnography (in 7 events). One event was detected by both pulse oximetry and capnography. The average change in arterial saturation was 5% (94.9 to 89.9) and the average change in $PetCO_2$ was 9.6 torr (37.7 to 47.3). While it is not surprising that changes were detected by the continuous noninvasive monitors, what is surprising from this study is how long a delay occurred before interventions were made on the basis of blood gas analyses. The average time from detection by the continuous monitoring technique to blood gas analysis was 73 ± 55 minutes. Additionally, the average time from blood gas analysis to a clinical response and alteration of ventilatory support was an additional 82 ± 97 minutes. Thus, the average delay in these 13 weaning failures from detection by real-time monitoring to alteration in therapy was 156 ± 106 minutes. Although no significant complications occurred as a result of these delays, obviously, delays in therapy are not clinically desirable [39].

In summary, capnography represents a relatively new advance in the real-time monitoring of gas exchange in the ICU environment. While the final answer is not in on the cost effectiveness of the monitoring technique, it clearly represents another tool to extend our clinical assessment of critically ill patients.

References

1. Shoemaker WC, Vidyasagar D (eds) (1981) Physiological and clinical significance of $PtcO_2$ and $PtcCO_2$ measurements. Crit Care Med 9:689-690
2. Tremper KK, Shoemaker WC (1981) Transcutaneous oxygen monitoring of critically ill adults, with and without low flow shock. Crit Care Med 9:706-709
3. Reed RL, Maier RV, Landicho D, et al (1985) Correlation of hemodynamic variables with transcutaneous PO_2 measurements in critically ill adult patients. J Trauma 25:1045-1051
4. Stokes CD, Blevins S, Siegel JH, et al (1987) Prediction of arterial blood gases by transcutaneous O_2 and CO_2 in critically ill hyperdynamic trauma patients. J Trauma 27:1240-1260
5. Fatt I, Deutsch TA (1983) The relation of conjunctival PO_2 to capillary bed PO_2. Crit Care Med 11:445-448
6. Isenberg SJ, Shoemaker WC (1983) The transconjunctival oxygen monitor. Am J Ophthalmol 95:803-806
7. Shoemaker WC, Lawner PM (1983) Method for continuous conjunctival oxygen monitoring during carotid artery surgery. Crit Care Med 11:946-947
8. Kram HB, Shoemaker WC, Bratanow N, et al (1986) Noninvasive conjunctival oxygen monitoring during carotid endarterectomy. Arch Surg 121:914-917
9. Gibson BE, McMichan JC, Cucchiara RF (1986) Lack of correlation between transconjunctival O_2 and cerebral blood flow during carotid artery occlusion. Anesthesiology 64:277-279
10. Smith M, Abraham E (1986) Conjunctival oxygen tension monitoring during hemorrhage. J Trauma 26:217-224
11. Abraham E, Oye RK, Smith M (1984) Detection of blood volume deficits through conjunctival oxygen tension monitoring. Crit Care Med 12:931-934
12. Shoemaker WC, Fink S, Ray CW, McCartney S (1984) Effect of hemorrhagic shock on conjunctival and transcutaneous oxygen tension in relation to hemodynamic and oxygen transport changes. Crit Care Med 12:949-952

13. Abraham E, Smith M, Silver L (1984) Conjunctival and transcutaneous oxygen monitoring during cardiac arrest and cardiopulmonary resuscitation. Crit Care Med 12:419–421
14. Neff TA (1988) Routine oximetry; A fifth vital sign? Chest 94:227
15. Taylor MB, Whitwam JG (1986) The current status of pulse oximetry. Anaesthesia 41:943–949
16. Yelderman M, New W (1983) Evaluation of pulse oximetry. Anesthesiology 59:349–352
17. New W (1985) Pulse oximetry. J Clin Mon 1:126–129
18. Scheller MS, Unger RJ, Kelner MJ (1986) Effects of intravenously administered dyes on pulse oximetry readings. Anesthesiology 65:550–552
19. Amar D, Neidzwski J, et al (1989) Fluorescent light interferes with pulse oximetry. J Clin Mon 5:135–136
20. Nelson LD (1985) Variation in derived cardio-pulmonary variables using calculated and measured venous oxygen saturation. Crit Care Med 13:321
21. Kelleher JF (1989) Pulse oximetry. J Clin Mon 5:37–62
22. Sidi A, Rush W, Gravenstein N, et al (1987) Pulse oximetry fails to accurately detect low levels of arterial hemoglobin oxygen saturation in dogs. J Clin Mon 3:257–262
23. Partridge BL (1987) Use of pulse oximetry as a noninvasive indicator of intravascular volume status. J Clin Mon 3:263–268
24. Nelson LD (1986) Continuous venous oximetry in surgical patients. Ann Surg 203:329–333
25. Magilligan DJ, Reasdall R, et al (1987) Mixed venous oxygen saturation as a predictor of cardiac output in the postoperative cardiac surgical patient. Ann Thorac Surg 44:260–262
26. Shenag SA, Casar G, Chelly JE, et al (1987) Continuous monitoring of mixed venous oxygen saturation during aortic surgery. Chest 92:796–799
27. Divertie MB, McMichan JC (1984) Continuous monitoring of mixed venous oxygen saturation. Chest 85:423–428
28. Birman H, Haq A, et al (1984) Continuous monitoring of mixed venous oxygen saturation in hemodynamically unstable patients. Chest 86:753–756
29. Orlando R (1986) Continuous mixed venous oximetry in critically ill surgical patients. 'High-Tech' cost-effectiveness. Arch Surg 121:470–471
30. Räsänen J, Downs JB, Malec DJ, et al (1987) Estimation of oxygen utilization by dual oximetry. Ann Surg 206:621–623
31. Carroll GC (1987) A continuous monitoring technique for management of acute pulmonary failure. Chest 92:467–469
32. Räsänen J, Downs JB, DeHaven B (1987) Titration of continuous positive airway pressure by real-time dual oximetry. Chest 92:853–856
33. Sedlow DB (1986) Capnometry and capnography: The anesthesia disaster early warning system. Sem Anesthesia V:194–205
34. Snyder JV, Elliot JL, Grenvik A (1982) Capnography. In: Spence AA (ed) Respiratory monitoring in intensive care. Churchill-Livingston, London, pp 100–121
35. Stock MC (1988) Noninvasive carbon dioxide monitoring. Crit Care Clin 4:511–525
36. Nelson LD, Safcsak K (1990) Side-stream vs in-line sensing for capnography in adult surgical patients. (Submitted)
37. Nelson LD, Safcsak K (1990) Accuracy and precision of pulse oximetry/capnography in assessing gas exchange. (Submitted)
38. Nelson LD, Safcsak K (1990) Specificity and sensitivity of pulse oximetry/capnography in predicting blood gas changes during weaning. (Submitted)
39. Nelson LD, Safcsak K (1990) Continuous noninvasive monitoring improves efficiency and safety during weaning of ventilatory support. (Submitted)

Continuous Assessment
of Cardiopulmonary Function

J. B. Downs

Introduction

"Assessment" of oxygenation may entail measurement and calculation of a variety of physiologic variables. However, the oxygen tension of arterial blood (PaO_2) is by far the most common measurement utilized in determining the "adequacy" of oxygenation. Because of the ease of measurement, PaO_2 often is used as a guide to oxygen therapy, ventilator adjustment, and other therapeutic interventions. Some clinicians have suggested a mathematical manipulation of PaO_2, alone or in combination with other variables, to improve diagnostic accuracy and assessment of pulmonary function. The perceived advantage of using the alveolar-arterial O_2 tension difference (AAD), the arterial/alveolar oxygen tension ratio (AAI), the PaO_2/F_IO_2 ratio (PFI), etc., rather than the PaO_2 alone, often is far greater than the actual advantage. It is apparent that the ease and efficiency of measurements and calculations have played a greater role in the determination of monitoring practices than accuracy and efficacy. Because of advances in monitoring technology during the last decade, a reassessment of monitoring techniques is indicated.

Ultimately, a primary purpose of the cardiorespiratory system is to deliver an adequate volume of oxygen to the periphery to meet metabolic demand. In the past, measurement techniques for the determination of oxygen delivery (O_2 del) and oxygen consumption ($\dot{V}O_2$) have been cumbersome, time consuming, of questionable accuracy, and difficult to apply in routine clinical situations. Thus, it is not surprising that clinicians have developed only a vague and superficial understanding of oxygen utilization (O_2 util) and its assessment. The flow directed pulmonary artery catheter has brought about significant advances in the monitoring of pulmonary and cardiovascular function. However, until recently, even this technology has allowed only intermittent monitoring of some aspects of cardiopulmonary function. Furthermore, guidelines to assist the clinician regarding the efficacy of pulmonary artery catheterization have been vague.

Although the technology for continuous measurement of oxyhemoglobin saturation has been available for more than a decade, widespread interest been generated only recently. Appropriate use of oximetry requires understanding of the dynamics of oxygen transport and the means by which alteration in cardiopulmonary function may affect arterial and venous oxyhemoglobin saturation. Recent advances in oximetry, both economic and technical, warrant a reconsideration of the appropriateness of current monitoring practices and assessment of newer, and perhaps more accurate, techniques.

For more than two decades, PaO_2 measurement has formed the basis for pulmonary function monitoring, especially in critically ill patients. For similar period of time, clinicians have debated whether arterial blood oxyhemoglobin saturation (SaO_2) or PaO_2 should be monitored. Both measurements have advantages and disadvantages in the accurate assessment of pulmonary function. Similarly, in certain clinical circumstances, oxyhemoglobin saturation will allow more accurate monitoring of pulmonary function than will oxygen tension measurement. In a different set of circumstances, the reverse will be true. Arterial hypoxemia may result when some areas of the lung have decreased ventilation ($\dot{V}_A$), with relatively higher levels of perfusion ($\dot{Q}$). In addition, as the inspired oxygen concentration (F_IO_2) is decreased, the hypoxemia producing effect of such low $\dot{V}_A/\dot{Q}$ areas will be enhanced. Only when an individual breathes pure oxygen will such areas be masked, and subsequent arterial hypoxemia be attributed only to direct, right-to-left intrapulmonary shunting of blood ($\dot{Q}_{SP}/\dot{Q}_T$). In order to assess the relative importance of areas with low $\dot{V}_A/\dot{Q}$, a two-compartment model composed of normal lung and lung with no ventilation, but persistent perfusion, was proposed. In order to calculate physiologic right-to-left intrapulmonary shunting of blood using this two-compartment model ($F_IO_2 < 1.0$), the clinician must have access to mixed venous blood from the pulmonary artery [1, 2]. Until recently, such access was relatively uncommon. This limitation led clinicians to assume a fixed value for mixed venous blood oxygen content and arterial-venous blood oxygen content difference ($C_{(a-\bar{v})}O_2$). By so doing, any variation in arterial blood oxygen content, saturation, or oxygen tension would be attributed to alteration in pulmonary function. Thus, PaO_2-based calculations of AAD, AAI, PFI, etc. were proposed to assess the efficiency of pulmonary gas exchange. Unfortunately, a fixed value for the arterial-mixed venous blood oxygen content difference may not be assumed, and any variable based on such an assumption is likely to be grossly inaccurate, especially in critically ill patients

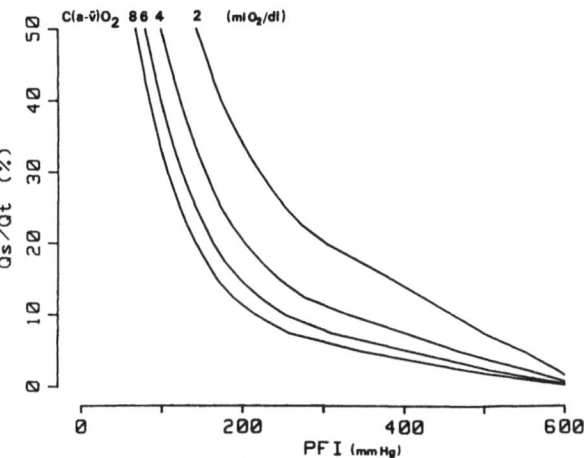

Fig. 1. Mathematical relationship between $\dot{Q}_{SP}/\dot{Q}_T$ and PFI, plotted with $C(a-\bar{v})O_2$ levels ranging from 2.0 to 8.0 ml/dl. Average normal values were set for Hgb (15.0 g/L), $PaCO_2$ (40 mmHg), and RQ (0.8). F_IO_2 was assumed to 0.5

(Fig. 1). In fact, any alteration in cardiac output, oxygen consumption, or hemoglobin concentration will have an impact on mixed venous blood oxygen content, and therefore, on arterial oxygen content, saturation, and tension.

Analysis of the oxyhemoglobin dissociation curve demonstrates the reason why PaO_2 alone will not allow accurate assessment of physiologic shunting of blood (Fig. 2). The non-linear relationship between oxygen tension and oxyhemoglobin saturation has numerous physiologic advantages in terms of oxygen uptake within the lung and oxygen delivery to the periphery. The relatively flat portion of the oxyhemoglobin dissociation curve ensures maximum O_2 loading, even when alveolar O_2 tension is somewhat reduced by $\dot{V}_A/\dot{Q}$ mismatching. At the cellular level, the vertical portion of the curve ensures a significant unloading of oxygen with little change in oxygen tension. Even though this non-linear relationship is advantageous, it causes accurate assessment of pulmonary function to be complex. Small changes in $\dot{V}_A/\dot{Q}$ mismatching may cause large changes in PaO_2 when PaO_2 is high (i.e. >115 mmHg). However, because of the vertical portion of the oxyhemoglobin dissociation curve, large increases in shunting of

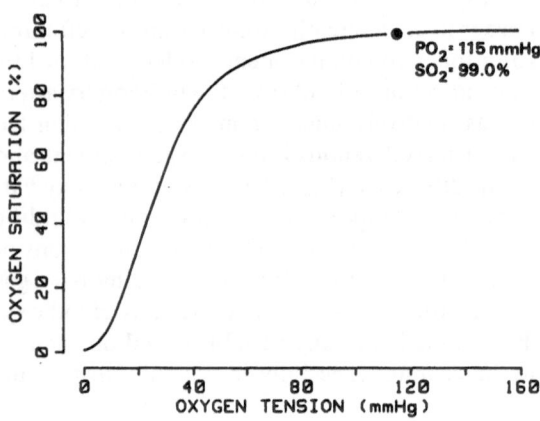

Fig. 2. The oxyhemoglobin dissociation curve plotted according to the equation published by Ruiz et al. [2]

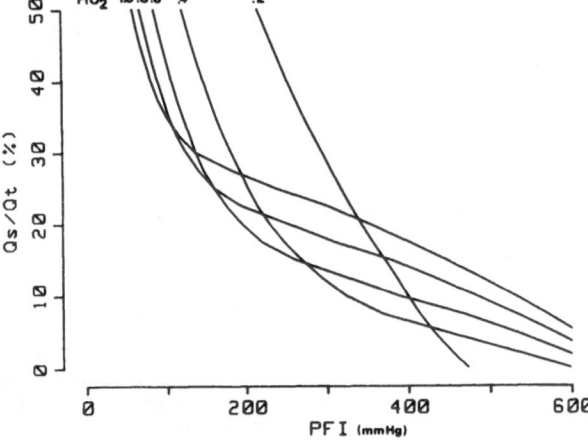

Fig. 3. Mathematical relationship between $\dot{Q}_{SP}/\dot{Q}_T$ and PFI, plotted with F_IO_2 levels ranging from 0.21 to 1.0. Average normal values were set for Hgb (15.0 g/l), $PaCO_2$ (40 mmHg), and RQ (0.8). $C(a-\bar{v})O_2$ was assumed to be 4.0 ml/dl

blood may be undetected secondary to small changes in PaO_2 associated with oxyhemoglobin desaturation. For that reason, clinicians have suggested that the F_IO_2 be elevated for PaO_2 determination, so that arterial oxyhemoglobin saturation approaches 100%. Although the F_IO_2 may be safely elevated for a short period of time on an intermittent basis, routine and continuous monitoring of pulmonary function with elevated F_IO_2 is inaccurate and impractical. When 100% oxygen is used and $C_{(a-\bar{v})}O_2$ is normal, PaO_2 based gas exchange indices reflect pulmonary gas exchange in a linear fashion only up to a $\dot{Q}_{SP}/\dot{Q}_T$ of $\approx 30\%$, and then only when $F_IO_2 = 1.0$ (Fig. 3). If $\dot{Q}_{SP}/\dot{Q}_T$ is higher, the nonlinearity of the oxyhemoglobin dissociation curve will make these indices insensitive to further impairment in gas exchange. Additional inaccuracy is introduced by the increase in $\dot{Q}_{SP}/\dot{Q}_T$ during pure oxygen breathing [3]. Because of the various sources of error, correlation coefficients between $\dot{Q}_{SP}/\dot{Q}_T$ and the oxygen tension based estimates range from 0.45 to 0.75 [4, 5]. These indices are more accurate when PaO_2 is high ($r = 0.84$–0.90; $PaO_2 > 115$ mmHg; $SaO_2 > 99.0\%$), but their accuracy is severely reduced ($r = 0.10$–0.54) when PaO_2 values fall on the descending portion of the oxyhemoglobin dissociation curve ($PaO_2 < 115$ mmHg, $SaO_2 < 99.0\%$). Recently, D. Valentine compared the AAD, PFI and AAI to calculated $\dot{Q}_{SP}/\dot{Q}_T$ in patients who received cardiopulmonary bypass. Even when F_IO_2 was elevated to 0.5, the correlation between the O_2 tension

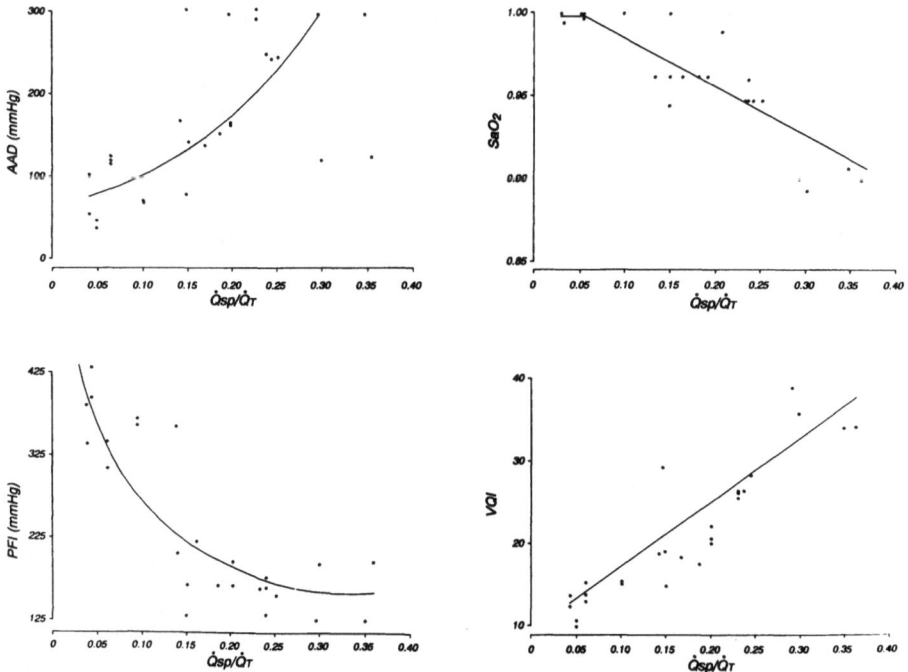

Fig. 4. Comparison of $\dot{Q}_{SP}/\dot{Q}_T$ with AAD, SaO_2, PFI and VQI (published data by Valentine, Hammond and Downs). Data derived from patients following cardiopulmonary bypass breathing 40% oxygen

based indices and $\dot{Q}_{SP}/\dot{Q}_T$ was clinically unacceptable (Fig. 4) (personal communication).

It long has been our contention that application of low F_IO_2 may have significant benefits [3, 6]. A low F_IO_2 will avoid oxygen toxicity and absorption atelectasis. In addition, the hypoxemia producing effect of areas of lung with decreases $\dot{V}_A/\dot{Q}$ will be more apparent with low F_IO_2. Most importantly, when arterial oxyhemoglobin saturation is less than 100%, accurate assessment of pulmonary function by measurement of arterial oxyhemoglobin saturation becomes possible. Because a linear relationship exists between SaO_2 and $\dot{Q}_{SP}/\dot{Q}_T$, estimation of pulmonary function is *easier* for the clinician when using SaO_2, than when using O_2 tension based indices. In contrast to intermittent sampling of blood for measurement of PaO_2, continuous measurement of arterial oxyhemoglobin saturation is clinically practical. Thus, continuous assessment of pulmonary function may occur when arterial oxyhemoglobin saturation measurement is employed. By combining measurement of arterial oxyhemoglobin saturation with mixed venous oxyhemoglobin saturation, accurate estimation of physiologic shunting of blood is possible. Right-to-left intrapulmonary shunt can be approximated by the ventilation perfusion index (VQI) derived as follows:

$$\frac{\dot{Q}_{SP}}{\dot{Q}_T} = \frac{S\dot{c}O_2 - SaO_2}{S\dot{c}O_2 - S\bar{v}O_2} \approx VQI$$

Here, SO_2 is the oxyhemoglobin saturation of arterial (a) mixed venous (v̄) and pulmonary end-capillary (ċ) blood, Thus, measurement of arterial and venous oxyhemoglobin saturation will permit continuous assessment of pulmonary function without alteration of clinically applicable F_IO_2. Calculation of VQI provides a linear estimate of $\dot{Q}_{SP}/\dot{Q}_T$ because the effect of the oxyhemoglobin dissociation curve is absent. Since changes in mixed venous oxygenation are taken into account, alterations in peripheral oxygen delivery and consumption have little effect on the estimate (Fig. 5). We found a correlation coefficient of 0.92

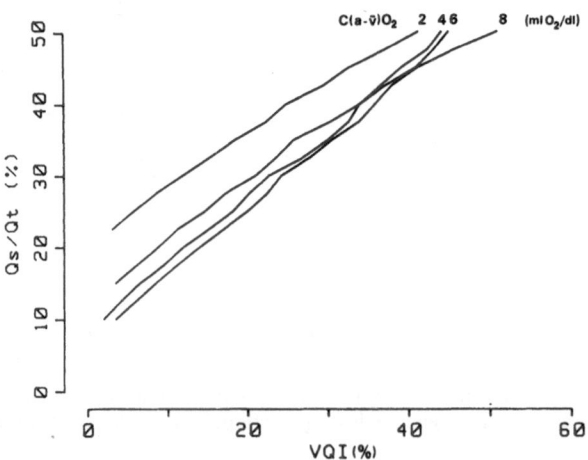

Fig. 5. Mathematical relationships between $\dot{Q}_{SP}/\dot{Q}_T$ and VQI, plotted with $C(a-\bar{v})O_2$ levels ranging from 2.0 to 8.0 ml/dl. Average normal values were set for Hgb (15.0 g/l), $PaCO_2$ (40 mmHg), and RQ (0.8). F_IO_2 was assumed to 0.5

between $\dot{Q}_{SP}/\dot{Q}_T$ and its oxyhemoglobin saturation based estimate, VQI [5]. Valentine found the same correlation (r = 0.92) when he compared the VQI to shunting by measuring with the multiple inert gas elimination technique described by Wagner, West and Saltzman (Fig. 4) (personal communication). Thus, VQI is a clinically useful and accurate calculation. The accuracy of this index is maintained as long as arterial oxyhemoglobin saturation has value other than 100%.

Alteration of respiratory therapy may occur frequently in critical care settings. Usually, major changes in therapy are assessed no more frequently than hourly. However, changes in continuous positive airway pressure (CPAP) have been shown to result in equilibration of functional residual capacity in less than one minute. Equilibration of arterial oxygen tension occurs in a similar time frame [7]. Change in F_IO_2 results in rapid alteration in PaO_2. Therefore, it is evident that major alterations in respiratory therapy should be evaluated within minutes, rather than the current practice of waiting one or two hours following change. Continuous measurement of arterial and mixed venous oxyhemoglobin saturation using combined pulse and pulmonary artery oximetry (dual oximetry) permits such assessment. In addition, clinically unsuspected changes in the patient's pulmonary function will be detected more rapidly with continuous measurement techniques than with intermittent sampling of arterial and venous blood. Alterations in therapy then will be triggered directly by the primary change in lung function rather than by secondary hemodynamic change that normally would initiate blood sampling. Data from arterial and mixed venous saturation monitors easily can be transformed to estimate gas exchange in a real-time fashion using on-line calculation of VQI. This procedure obviates the delay associated with data interpretation at the monitor-observer interface (Fig. 6).

Invasive monitoring of cardiac function has become commonplace in most critical care units. Usually, clinically appropriate assessment of cardiac function includes measurement of cardiac filling pressure and stroke volume. However, "adequacy" of cardiac performance, in terms of oxygen delivery, has only re-

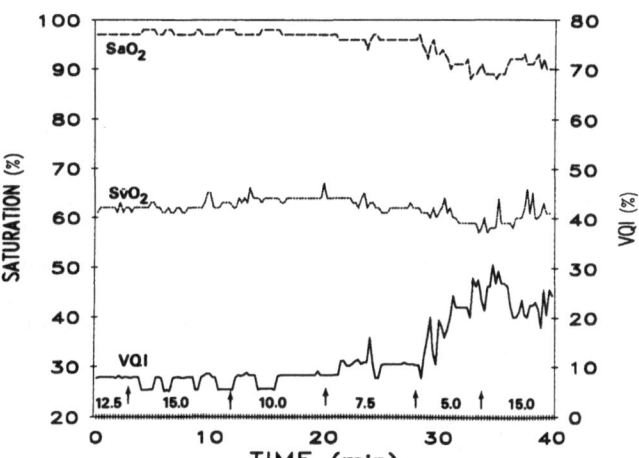

Fig. 6. Changes in SaO_2, $S\bar{v}O_2$, and VQI at varying levels of CPAP in a patient with acute pulmonary insufficiency

cently been widely appreciated. For example, a cardiac output of 10 L/min would be more than adequate in most clinical settings. However, an anemic patient with increased oxygen consumption might require an even higher cardiac output to meet peripheral oxygen demand. Ideally, the clinician should have some means of assessing oxygen delivery relative to oxygen demand. Oxygen delivery depends not only on cardiac output, but on arterial oxygen content, as well. Arterial blood oxygen content is determined by hemoglobin concentration and oxyhemoglobin saturation, and is relatively independent of the dissolved oxygen. Oxygen consumption of an organ system depends on metabolic demand. However, blood flow to the organ system, distribution of blood flow within the system, distance from the capillary to the cell, and the oxygen tension gradient between the capillary and the cell also play critical roles. The diffusion gradient may depend on the oxyhemoglobin saturation and the relative position of the oxyhemoglobin dissociation curve.

The relationship between oxygen delivery and oxygen consumption for any organ system will determine the "adequacy" of oxygenation. Although it is possible to assess oxygen utilization of some organ systems, for most such assessment is clinically difficult. It is possible to assess global oxygen utilization by measurement of systemic oxygen delivery and total body oxygen consumption.

$$O_2 \text{ utilization} = \frac{\dot{V}O_2}{O_2 \text{ del}}$$

Further expansion of this equation results in a readily applicable oxygen extraction index (O_2EI):

$$O_2 \text{ utilization} = \frac{CO \cdot Ca - \bar{v}O_2}{CO \cdot CaO_2} = \frac{Ca - \bar{v}O_2}{CaO_2} = 1 - \frac{C\bar{v}O_2}{CaO_2}$$

$$= 1 - \frac{Hgb \cdot 1.34 \cdot S\bar{v}O_2 + P\bar{v}O_2 \cdot 0.0031}{Hgb \cdot 1.34 \cdot SaO_2 + PaO_2 \cdot 0.0031} \approx 1 - \frac{S\bar{v}O_2}{SaO_2}$$

Thus, mixed venous oxygen saturation accurately represents total body oxygen utilization [8]. Several investigators have shown that mixed venous oxygen saturation more accurately predicts the ratio between oxygen consumption and oxygen delivery than does cardiac output, arterial oxygen tension, arterial oxygen delivery, oxygen consumption, or any other variable suggested for assessment of "adequacy" of oxygenation [1]. Use of $S\bar{v}O_2$ to estimate oxygen utilization assumes complete saturation of arterial blood oxyhemoglobin. When dual oximetry is used, such an assumption no longer is necessary, and the accuracy of the estimate will improve accordingly. Thus, we suggest use of the oxygen extraction index (O_2EI).

$$O_2EI = \frac{Sa\bar{v}O_2}{SaO_2}$$

There is sound physiologic basis for continuous monitoring of arterial and mixed venous oxyhemoglobin saturation. Dual oximetry will provide simultaneous, real-time estimates of two critically important body functions, pulmonary gas exchange and peripheral tissue oxygen utilization [9]. There is little doubt that application of these techniques will improve the efficacy of therapy with vasoactive and cardiotonic drugs, oxygen, mechanical ventilation, and CPAP. It is likely that time and cost savings will result and that morbidity and mortality may decrease.

References

1. Mitchell LA, Downs JB, Dannemiller FJ (1975) Extrapulmonary influences on A-aDO$_2$ following cardiopulmonary bypass. Anesthesiology 43:583–585
2. Ruiz BC, Tucker WK, Kirby RR (1975) A program for calculating intrapulmonary shunts, blood-gas, and acid-base values with a programmable calculator. Anesthesiology 42:88–90
3. Douglas ME, Downs JB, Dannemiller FJ, et al (1976) Change in pulmonary venous admixture with varying inspired oxygen. Anesth Analg 55:688–690
4. Covelli HD, Nessan VJ, Tuttle WK (1983) Oxygen derived variables in acute respiratory failure. Crit Care Med 11:646–650
5. Räsänen J, Downs JB, Malec DJ, et al (1987) Oxygen tension and oxyhemoglobin saturations in the assessment of pulmonary gas exchange. Crit Care Med 15:1058–1060
6. Register SD, Downs JB, Stock MC, et al (1987) Is 50% oxygen harmful? Crit Care Med 15:598–601
7. Rose DM, Downs JB, Heenan TJ (1981) Temporal responses of functional residual capacity and oxygen tension to changes in positive end-expiratory pressure. Crit Care Med 9:79–80
8. Nelson LD (1983) Continuous venous oximetry in surgical patients. Ann Surg 203:329–330
9. Räsänen J, Downs JB, Malec DJ, et al (1988) Real-time continuous estimation of gas exchange by dual oximetry. Intensive Care Med 14:118–121

Regulation Assessment of Cardiopulmonary Function   468

Intoxications

Intoxications

Current Topics in the Management of Poisoning

J. R. Johnston, D. L. Coppel, and J. J. Wilson

Introduction

Drug overdose remains one of the commonest causes of admission to hospital; 10% being due to self-poisoning [1]. The following reviews several topics of recent interest.

Drug Measurement in the "Stat Lab"

Measurement blood levels of poisoning are useful to:

1. Aid in the diagnosis of the unconscious patient;
2. Aid in the choice of therapy of the poisoned patient;
3. Monitor effectiveness of therapy.

Toxicological screening, if deemed necessary, is usually performed in a large clinical biochemistry laboratory. However when seriously poisoned patients are admitted to an intensive care unit (ICU) the management which can be greatly assisted by drug estimations being performed rapidly. There is now available the technology to measure drug levels in close proximity to or within the ICU environment.

 Most analyzers use reflectance spectroscopy or a photometric process for the measurement of the reaction of the sample with the test reagent. The reagent is usually a drug chemical to which the sample and or distilled water is added before it is incubated at 37°C and the measurement obtained.

Three manufacturers have suitable instruments

(a) Ames Seralyser III;
(b) Kodak Ektachem DT60 analyzer system;
(c) Merck Easy ST.

Most instruments will measure a range of electrolytes, enzymes and drugs; some may also be used for estimating prothrombin time or partial thromboplastin time. The Merck Easy ST analyzer will analyze the widest range for the common overdoses – paracetamol, salicylate and theophylline. A list is given in Table 1 of presently available drug tests.

 The Easy ST Analyzer uses a photometric process for measuring the samples reaction with the test reagent. Once the sample and reagent are mixed, incubated

Table 1. Available drug tests with cost per test, in English pounds

1) Amikacin	£3.75
2) Carbamazepine	£3.47
3) Ethosuximide	£3.75
4) Gentamicin	£3.47
5) Lidocaine	£3.75
6) N-Acetyprocainamide	£3.75
7) Paracetamol	£3.75
8) Phenobarbital	£3.47
9) Phenytoin	£3.47
10) Primidone	£3.47
11) Procainamide	£3.75
12) Quinidine	£3.75
13) Salicylate	£2.13
14) Theophylline	£3.47
15) Tobramycin	£3.75

light from a Tungsten-Halogen lamp is allowed to pass through the sample. Light exiting the sample is passed through a filter which only permits light of a specific wavelength to enter the detector which automatically calculates the difference between light entering and leaving the sample. The amount of light absorbed is proportional to the measured drug level.

These methods require serum for the analysis so it is essential to have a centrifuge available for the separation of the blood samples. For the estimation of drug levels, following overdose because they are greater than the measuring range of the instruments, it is imperative that accurate dilution are made to obtain a correct level. The purchase of automatic pipettes for this and for the accurate calibration of the instrument is required. This type of instrument is simple to use but does require a higher degree of user knowledge and is more time consuming than most analyzers usually found in satellite laboratories. It is therefore important to ensure that regular quality control and maintenance is performed on the instrument to ensure accurate results and that only trained staff are permitted to use it.

Ipecacuanha

The most common methods to prevent absorption from the gastrointestinal tract are lavage and emesis. Lavage must only be performed if a potentially harmful substance has been taken relatively recently, i.e. within 4 hours. Exceptions to

Table 2. Recommended dose of ipecacuanha

6 – 18 months	10 ml	
Older children	15 ml	one dose with water
Adult	30 ml	

this rule include substances which delay gastric emptying such as salicylates and tricyclic antidepressants.

The standard emetic is syrup of ipecacuanha [2]. This plant extract has as its active constituents the alkaloids emetine and cephaeline. Both induce vomiting by a central action, cephaeline being twice as potent as emetine and also having a direct irritant action on the gastric mucosa. This results in the initial bout of vomiting; the combined central actions causing the later vomiting. The recommended dose is given in Table 2.

Problems that may arise with the use of ipecacuanha include prolonged vomiting from using too large a dose which can mimic symptoms of poisoning and confuse the clinical picture. It may also cause diarrhea and lethargy again mimicing the signs and symptoms of poisoning. Serious side effects from forceful vomiting such as gastric rupture and barotrauma may occur. Emetine can also act as a myocardial depressant. Allied to these problems is the concern that using ipecacuanha may not be the most effective method for reducing drug absorption. Activated charcoal can reduce the absorption of paracetamol, aminophylline and tetracycline more effectively than by causing emesis [3].

Emesis however remains useful in children but must not be used if there is a risk of aspiration into the lungs or if substances such as petroleum distillates, petrol or corrosives have been taken. It must be remembered that if emesis is used that administration of agents such as methonine or activated charcoal are precluded. Clearly the use of ipecacuanha in adults must be questioned especially in the growing number of poisonings for which activated charcoal appears to be effective.

Activated Charcoal

There has recently been increased interest in activated charcoal both because of its adsorptive properties preventing drug absorption and because of its use in promoting increased drug elimination.

It is a fine black powder made by the distillation of certain organic materials (wood pulp, coconut shells or coal) which is activated by the action of steam or strong acids at high temperatures. This gives it a large surface area of 950–1200 m^2/g which along with its electrostatic properties aids binding. Its absorptive capacity is 500-1000 mg of drug per gram of charcoal. It is useful as an adsorbant to reduce drug absorption and there is some evidence that is is better than ipecacuanha [3].

Recent interest has centred on its use as an aid to drug elimination by the so called "gastro-intestinal dialysis". With repeated oral dosing the bowel, especially the small intestine, becomes the site of transfer of poison from circulation in the gut villi to the charcoal in the gut lumen. This is especially so for lipophilic compounds that are unionized in plasma, have a long elimination half-life, a small volume of distribution and are not heavily tissue bound. Those that have an enterohepatic recirculation or are actively secreted in the bowel can be particularly easy to clear using this technique.

The technique involves instilling 50–100 g activated charcoal as soon as possible after poisoning followed by instillation of 12.5 g/hour via a nasogastric tube. Precautions to protect the airway should be taken if it is at risk from aspiration. The following compounds can be eliminated using this technique – salicylates, benzodiazepines, digoxin, meprobamate, phenytoin, phenobarbitone, phenylbutazone, carbemazepine, theophylline and quinine. The cyclic antidepressants have a large volume of distribution and should theoretically not be eliminated successfully using this technique. However, patients with this type of poisoning do seem to benefit.

Apart from being unpalatable there were hazards reported with this technique. Menzies et al. [4] reported a fatal death following aspiration of gastric contents containing Medicoal (Lundbeck). This form of activated charcoal contains povidone as a nonabsorbable suspending agent; this may have worsened the pneumonitis. A further possible hazard of hypernatremia from the sodium load (Medicoal contains 18 mmol sodium/5 g sachet) has been reported [5]. Although large doses of charcoal are needed, this method of elimination is simple and cheap to perform and also relatively safe. It is practical only in those cases not associated with vomiting. It needs transport of the absorbant through the bowel and the question of the best formulation has not been answered yet. It should be noted that Medicoal may cause diarrhea while Carbomix may cause constipation.

Digoxin and Digitoxin

Digitalis and its drug compounds are widely available and serious overdose is important because it is often fatal. Following doses of 15 mg, the average mortality is approximately 18% and reaches 95% following ingestion of over 35 mg. Plasma concentrations become toxic at levels greater than 2.5 µg/l but serious problems only arise at levels above 10 µg/l. However, plasma levels may not correlate closely with severity of poisoning.

Digoxin overdose leads to an inhibition of the sodium and potassium activated ATP-ase pump which causes an increase in the plasma potassium level. This rise is correlated strongly with the clinical course. Nausea and vomiting are constant features of a toxic overdose with diarrhea occurring less frequently. Drowsiness, mental confusion and even a psychosis have been observed. Bradycardia and cardiac arrhythmias are common. There may be varying degrees of atrioventricular block. Supraventricular arrhythmias with or without heart block and less commonly ventricular ectopic beats, ventricular tachycardia and ventricular fibrillation may also occur. Treatment is supportive. Gastric lavage if indicated should be carried out with care because any increase in vagal tone may lead to cardiac arrest. Bradycardia can be treated with atropine which may need to be repeated over a period of several days. In serious poisoning transvenous cardiac pacing may be required. Hyperkalemia should be treated with intravenous glucose and insulin, although with a large overdose the potassium level may not decrease because of the severe inhibition of the Na^+/K^+ pump. In these cases treatment with Fab digoxin specific antibiody fragments (Digibind

– Wellcome Foundation Ltd) is warranted. Hypokalemia can occur in certain cases who receive chronic diuretic therapy. A cautious intravenous infusion of potassium chloride may be given until the plasma potassium level is normal. Ventricular ectopic beats should only be treated if they are compromising the cardiac output. Should these fail, amiodarone 5 mg/kg as a bolus over 5–10 minutes followed by an infusion of 900 mg over 24 hours is appropriate. Measures to increase elimination such as forced diuresis, hemodialysis or hemoperfusion are ineffective because the plasma is constantly being replenished from the extensive tissue compartment; the volume of distribution is large at 7L/kg. The results of hemoperfusion with Amberlite XAD-4 resin are more encouraging. Hemoperfusion in cases of digitoxin poisoning may be more effective because of its smaller volume of distribution (0.5 L/kg).

The treatment of choice for the elimination of digoxin is the administration of digoxin specific Fab antibody fragments [6]. IgG antibodies to digoxin are raised in sheep and then cleaved enzymatically by papain. The Fc and other Fab fragments are separated from the drug specific antibody by affinity chromatography. The Fab fragments lack complement-fixing activity and are not susceptible to immune degradation. They work because their affinity for digoxin is greater than that of digoxin for its receptor. Digoxin is therefore attracted away from the receptor on heart tissues. Fab fragments can be filtered through the glomerulus taking the drug with it. These fragments can pass from the plasma into the interstitial spaces and can easily get to the toxic sites of action. Following administration, improvements in signs and symptoms begin within 30 minutes. At this time, the plasma digoxin concentration rises (10–12 fold) the digoxin now being plasma bound. It is however, protein-bound and is pharmacologically inactive. There is also a decrease in the serum potassium.

The low molecular weight of the complex (50 000 daltons) means it is small enough to cross the glomerular basement membrane. The plasma elimination half-life after intravenous administration of Fab ranges from 16–34 hours in patients with good renal function. Experience with the use of Fab fragments in patients with severe renal impairment is limited. Such patients might exhibit a decreased elimination of the complex which eventually would be metabolized with the subsequent release of free digoxin and a recurrence of toxicity.

After the administration of Fab fragments, most of the digoxin in serum is bound and cannot displace radio-labelled digoxin in competitive binding assays. Thus it is not possible to follow serum digoxin concentrations with routine radio-immunoassays. As the Fab fragments are extremely expensive this approach must be used when specific indications are fulfilled. They are a rising and uncontrollable potassium concentration, life-threatening cardiac arrhythmias and a serum digoxin concentration of greater than 20 µ/l. Following a dose of 2 mg to test for rare allergic reactions a therapeutic dose is given diluted in 100 ml 5% dextrose over 15 minutes. The dose is calculated from the amount of digoxin ingested multiplied by 0.80 to take into account incomplete absorption and by 60 (molecular weight of drug/antibody complex = 60).

As the use of this treatment is limited the side effects are unknown. The re-exposure of animals to these fragments has led to an antibody response; in humans re-exposure could lead to severe hypersensitivity or even anaphylaxis. The immunogenic threat of Fab fragments should however be less than that from an intact immunoglobulin molecule. In patients therapeutically dependent on digoxin, the use of Digibind could precipitate a return of heart failure or arrhythmia.

Hapten specific Fab fragments could be used to treat poisoning from other drugs and toxins such as paraquat, tricylic depressants and amanita toxins.

Benzodiazepine Antagonists

Benzodiazepines probably act by facilitating the inhibitory effects of the aminobutyric acid (GABA) post synaptic receptor in the CNS producing anxiolysis, muscle relaxation and seizure control [7]. Overdose with this group of drugs produces very few serious side-effects. Symptoms include drowsiness, ataxia, dysarthria and nystagmus. They are less likely to cause respiratory depression. Their management is similar to that needed for the barbiturates and active elimination measures are not warranted.

A specific benzodiazepine antagonist, flumazenil, can reverse the effects of benzodiazepines by competitively displacing them at the benzodiazepine-GABA-chloride complex. It has a rapid onset of action of less than one minute following an intravenous injection with an effect maximal at 5 minutes. It should be administered in 0.1 mg aliquots to a total of 1.0 mg. It has a short duration of action, the elimination half-life being 54 minutes mainly due to rapid hepatic clearance. It can reverse a comatose state and return respiratory rate and blood pressure towards normal but because of its short half-life repeat administration is required [8]. An infusion of flumazenil can be useful in reversing prolonged sedation if given by infusion at a rate of 0.5–1.0 mg/hr [9].

Flumazenil should be used with caution both when used to reverse pure benzodiazepine depression and for a mixed drug overdose. Rapid reversal may cause ventricular fibrillation [10], status epilepticus or could counteract possible beneficial effects of benzodiazepines following a mixed drug overdose [11].

Carbon Monoxide

Carbon monoxide (CO) poisoning is the most common type of chemical asphyxiation, causing over 1000 deaths in England and Wales annually. It is the most common cause of death from poisoning in children [12]. It is a colourless, odourless, tasteless, non irritating gas produced by the incomplete combustion of carbonaceous materials. CO poisoning is treated in detail also in another chapter.

The causes of toxicity from CO poisoning are multifactorial. CO combines avidly with hemoglobin to form carboxyhemoglobin (COHb). The affinity of CO for Hb is 223 times as great as that of oxygen and thus oxygen is replaced by CO reducing the total oxygen carrying capacity of blood, producing an "anemia". Moreover the addition of CO to a molecule of hemoglobin shifts the HbO_2 dissociation curve to the left as the affinity of the remaining oxygen for their hemgroups is increased. This interferes with the unloading of oxygen at tissue level and results in a greater degree of tissue anoxia than would be expected from a simple loss of oxygen carrying capacity. There is also strong evidence that CO inhibits cellular respiration by combining with other hem-containing proteins such as myoglobin and the cytochrome system [13]. Combining with cytochromes only occurs under hypoxic conditions because its affinity of oxygen is 9.2 times that for CO [14]. Tissue toxicity of CO poisoning will therefore only be significant under hypoxic conditions when CO can combine with these enzymes. Once this occurs, CO may bind tightly and be resistant to reversal by conventional oxygen therapy. This tissue toxicity may be the major cause of the clinical factors of severe CO poisoning and may explain the discrepancies between clinical features and blood COHb levels.

The clinical course is directly related to the degree and duration of exposure (Table 3). The acute effects of CO poisoning are due to tissue hypoxia and as the brain and heart are the organs with the highest metabolic rate, they are the organs which demonstrate the major toxic manifestations. Individuals with pre-existing coronary and cerebral artery disease, myocardial insufficiency, pulmonary disease, or anemia are more vulnerable. The CNS, being especially vulnerable to hypoxia, tends to be the most affected and the effect ranges from lethargy to acute agitation and mental confusion to coma.

Patients in whom consciousness is maintained usually recover rapidly and completely. Those who become unconscious may continue to deteriorate clinically despite a COHb which is returning to normal. This indicates the presence of cerebral edema and is associated with papilledema, hypertension and increased reflexes. Some patients may recover completely only to develop days or weeks later a "delayed post-hypoxic encephalopathy". Myocardial ischemia is frequent and may precipitate angina and even progress to infarction. In severe poisoning the marked degree of hypoxia initially causes stimulation of the respiratory center with hyperventilation. Acute pulmonary edema may occur and respiratory center failure may follow. Visual defects including loss of vision and retinal hemorrhage may occur. Acute neuropsychiatric findings range from headache and fatigue to epilepsy and chronic cognitive and psychomotor

Table 3. Clinical effects of carbon monoxide poisoning

COHb %	Signs and symptoms
0.3 – 0.7	Normal range
< 10	No symptoms
10 – 20	Slight headache, variable vasodilatation
20 – 30	Throbbing headache, dyspnea and angina on exertion
30 – 40	Severe headache, nausea, vomiting, visual disturbance, weakness, dizziness
40 – 50	Syncope, tachycardia, tachypnea
50 – 60	Coma, convulsions, Cheynes-Stokes respiration
60 – 70	Cardiorespiratory failure, death

changes which may be permanent. Many of these abnormalities may be induced at low levels of COHb.

Various types of skin lesions can occur and vary from bullous eruptions to areas of erythema and alopecia. The pink skin color due to carboxyhemoglobin is uncommon unless poisoning is severe. Cyanosis and skin pallor are more common. It should be noted that in cyanide, atropine and phenothiazine poisoning a pink color is also seen. The distinction between the cyanide and CO poisoning is critical because appropriate treatment for one would be inappropriate for the other. Hyperpyrexia following skin sweat gland necrosis may be a feature. Myonecrosis may occur as a compartmental symptom and may even lead to rhabdomyolytic renal failure.

The most reliable method for diagnosis of CO poisoning is a direct measurement by spectrophotometry (oximetry). The correlation between COHb concentrations and clinical effects is given in Table 3. It must be borne in mind that CO is very rapidly eliminated and the blood level on arrival at hospital does not necessarily reflect the true insult if a delay occurs between exposure and COHb analysis. It should be noted that the PaO_2 is usually normal in CO poisoning as it reflects dissolved oxygen content of the blood and not hemoglobin saturation.

Treatment is initiated by terminating exposure, securing the airway and administering 100% oxygen as soon as possible using either a tightly fitting face mask or an endotracheal tube attached to a breathing circuit with a reservoir bag. The half-life of COHb in room air is 5-6 hours; with 100% oxygen and half-life decreases to 45-90 minutes; with a hyperbaric pressure of 3 Atm the half-life approximates to 23 minutes. The mechanism of action of a high inspired oxygen fraction is that the CO will be diluted and displaced by oxygen from cytochromes, myoglobin and hemoglobin by a mass action effect. Hyperbaric oxygen (HBO) also increases the amount of dissolved oxygen sufficiently to meet tissue needs even without functioning hemoglobin. Treatment with HBO will reduce the duration of coma, the incidence of the delayed encephalopathy and the long term morbidity to less than 5% [13].

The place of HBO treatment for CO poisoning still requires clarification. Arguments have been presented both for and against HBO. There is a concept that HBO may be dangerous as reactive oxygen metabolites may worsen the tissue damage on subsequent reoxygenation [15]. The delayed neurological complications of CO poisoning may be due to secondary oxidative damage which results from resuscitation of patients with HBO of high concentration of inhaled oxygen. On the other hand, advocates of HBO propose that an HBO chamber should be present in every hospital and should be used without delay following CO poisoning [16]. Furthermore evidence has been cited that HBO should be administered beyond the time that clinical recovery is evident. This could be until the EEG is shown to be normal which may be weeks after full clinical recovery.

Applying HBO to every patient with CO poisoning and continuing this treatment for weeks after recovery would require large capital purchase of HBO equipment. There is a need to confirm the usefulness of HBO in order to justify the increase of facilities. Raphael et al. [17] consider that previous trials advocating HBO were uncontrolled, retrospective or used historical controls. They compared normoxic therapy with HBO and suggested that HBO was not useful in patients who did not lose consciousness and therefore do not need it. This tends to agree with recommendations [18] that if consciousness has not been lost and there are no other symptoms other than headache or nausea or the COHb level is less than 40%, normobaric O_2 is sufficient. If however there are other symptoms or consciousness has been lost or the COHb level is greater than 40% then HBO is the treatment of choice. HBO should be applied at 2.5–3.0 Atm for periods of at least 90 min; should be repeated till there is no further improvement in the level of consciousness [19].

Further supportive treatment should be given as required espiecially if there is evidence of myocardial ischemia or cerebral edema.

References

1. Kessel N (1985) Patients who take overdoses. Br Med J 290:1297–1298
2. Vale JA, Meredith TJ, Proudfoot AT (1986) Syrup of ipecacuanha is it really useful? Br Med J 293:1321–1322
3. Neuvonen PJ, Vartiainen M, Tokola O (1983) Comparison of activated charcoal and ipecac syrup in prevention of drug absorption. Eur J Clin Pharmacol 24:557–562
4. Menzies DG, Busuttil A, Prescott LF (1988) Fatal pulmonary aspiration of oral activated charcoal. Br Med J 297:459–460
5. Gorchein A, Chong SKF, Mowat AP (1988) Hazards of oral charcoal. Lancet 1:1220
6. Wenger TL, Butler VP, Habet E, Smith TW (1985) Treatment of 63 severely digitalis-toxic patients with digoxin-specific antibody fragments. J Am Coll Cardiol 5:118A–123A
7. Whitwam JG (1987) Benzodiazepines. Anaesthesia 42:1255–1256
8. Knudsen L, Lonka L, Sorensen BH, Kirkegaard L, Jensen OV, Jensen S (1988) Benzodiazepines intoxication treated with flumazenil (Anexate, RO 15-1788). Anaesthesia 43:274–276
9. Bodenham A, Park GR (1989) Reversal of prolonged sedation using flumazenil in critically ill patients. Anaesthesia 44:603–605
10. Short TG, Maline T, Galletly DL (1988) Ventricular arrhythmia precipitated by flumazenil. Br Med J 296:1070–1071
11. Burr W, Sandham P, Judd A (1989) Death after flumazenil. Br Med J 298:1713
12. Vale JA, Meredity TJ (1985) A concise guide to the management of poisoning, 3rd edn. Churchill Livingstone, Edinburgh
13. Meredith TJ, Vale JA (1988) Carbon monoxide poisoning. Br Med J 296:77–79
14. Ball EG, Strittmatter CF, Cooper O (1951) The reaction of cytochrome oxidase with carbon monoxide. J Biological Chem 193:635–647
15. Howard RJMW, Blake DR, Pall H, Williams A, Green ID (1987) Allopurinol/N-acetylcysteine for carbon monoxide poisoning. Lancet 2:628–629
16. James PB (1988) Hyperbaric oxygen, carbon monoxide and cerebral oedema. Br Med J 296:500–501
17. Raphael JC, Elkharrat D, Jars-Guincestre MC, et al (1989) Trial normobaric and hyperbaric oxygen for acute carbon monoxide intoxication. Lancet 2:414–418
18. Broome JR, Pearson RR, Skrine H (1988) Carbon monoxide poisoning: "forgotten not gone!" Br J Hosp Med 39:298–305
19. Neubauer RA, Gottlieb SF (1989) Hyperbaric oxygen for carbon monoxide poisoning. Lancet 2:1032–1033

Carbon Monoxide Intoxication

C. A. Piantadosi

Introduction

Intoxication with carbon monoxide (CO) is a common consequence of breathing the toxic byproducts of combustion. Serious CO exposure often occurs during inhalation of smoke or automobile exhaust or as a result of industrial accidents. CO causes most of the morbidity and mortality from toxic inhalations in the United States [1] where it may be responsible for as many as 4000 deaths per year [2].

Carbon monoxide exposure results in diverse and nonspecific clinical findings which may not be diagnosed without a clear history of exposure or smoke inhalation. This is because CO generally does not produce symptoms of respiratory irritation [3]. Prompt recognition of serious CO intoxication followed by appropriate therapy will usually assure a good clinical outcome for the exposed patient. In most cases of acute intoxication, oxygen administration is the primary therapy, and in severe cases, there is a sound rationale for use of hyperbaric oxygen therapy. The purpose of this paper are to review the mechanisms and pathophysiologic features of CO intoxication and to provide the clinician with some useful guidelines for proper management of this condition.

There is some CO present normally in the body which is derived from endogenous CO production during heme catabolism [4] and pulmonary uptake of CO from exogenous sources. In normal people, the rate of endogenous CO production is low and results in an arterial carboxyhemoglobin saturation [HbCO] of about 1%. Most of the CO in the body is made during heme catabolism as a byproduct of the reaction form bilirubin from protoporphyrin [5]. In patients with accelerated red blood cell turnover, e.g. hemolysis, CO production may be enhanced eight-fold and [HbCO] may increase by a factor of three [6]. Increased production of CO may occur after induction of hepatic microsomal enzymes by certain drugs such as phenytoin and phenobarbital [7]. CO also may be produced in the body from metabolism of dihalomethanes, such as methylene chloride [8]. Exposure to methylene chloride in paint thinner has been associated with CO toxicity [9].

Exogenous uptake of CO occurs primarily from inhalation of CO-containing gases such as cigarette smoke and automobile exhaust. Heavy cigarette smokers can achieve HbCO saturations approaching 10% [10]. Nonsmokers exposed to "sidestream" cigarette smoke in poorly ventilated workplaces also absorb significant amounts of CO [11]. Exposure to CO from engine exhaust fumes on highways has been associated with HbCO levels above 5% in nonsmokers [12]. Internal combustion engines account for most of the CO generated by human activities [13] and automobile exhaust may contain up to 8% CO before it exceeds U.S. emission standards. Other common sources of CO exposure include fires, explosions and incomplete combustion of industrial hydrocarbons. CO poisoning also occurs in mines, ships and after the use of internal combustion engines in poorly ventilated spaces [14, 15]. Improperly ventilated or faulty gas furnaces and space heaters may produce large quantities of CO and are a significant factor in CO poisoning in the home [16]. Another hazardous chemical asphyxiant, hydrogen cyanide (HCN), sometimes accompanies CO poisoning in smoke inhalation and may be very difficult to recognize [17, 18]. Cyanide poisoning is common in fires, where HCN gas evolves from the combustion of plastics and other synthetic materials [19].

Mechanisms of Action of Carbon Monoxide

Carbon monoxide toxicity is a direct result of tissue hypoxia attributable primarily to the effects of CO on hemoglobin. This is known as CO hypoxia [20]. When inhaled, CO diffuses rapidyl across the alveolar capillary membrane of the lung where it binds tightly but reversibly to hemoglobin. In the pulmonary capillary, CO completes with oxygen for the ferrous iron of the iron-porphyrin complex of hemoglobin with which it equilibrates rapidly. This reaction, although slower than O_2 binding to Hb, requires only a few tenths of a second at body temperature [21]. CO uptake by pulmonary capillary blood is related to several physical and biological variables including the partial pressures of oxygen and CO in alveolar gas, alveolar ventilation, diffusion across capillary membranes, pulmonary capillary blood volume, the equilibrium constant for HbCO formation and the rates of CO production and oxidation by the body. HbCO levels after known CO exposures can be estimated from prediction equations [22].

The affinity of hemoglobin for CO is more than 200 times than for oxygen. This relationship is described by Haldane's first law:

$$[HbCO]/[HbO_2] = M(PCO/PO_2)$$

where M, the Haldane coefficient or equilibrium constant for the reaction of CO and HbO_2 varies from 210 to 230 for human hemoglobin [23]. The M value of blood is relatively constant over a range of HbCO saturations, but it may vary with temperature, pH and type of hemoglobin [20]. CO binding to hemoglobin results in two important effects that alter its ability to deliver oxygen to the body tissues. These effects are to reduce the ability of hemoglobin to transport oxygen and to increase the affinity for oxygen of the remaining heme moieties of the molecule. The latter effect shifts the oxygen dissociation curve of hemoglobin to the left which decreases oxygen unloading to the tissues.

The oxygen needs of the tissues are met normally by convective delivery of oxyhemoglobin to capillaries where oxygen diffuses into the mitochondria. The oxygen content of blood decreases from an arterial value of about 20 vol% to a mixed venous value near 15 vol% at normal cardiac output and tissue oxygen uptake. During CO hypoxia, the arterial oxygen content decreases in proportion to the HbCO saturation because HbCO does not carry oxygen. The decreasing arterial oxygen content during HbCO formation will decrease venous PO_2 if tissue oxygen requirements remain constant and blood flow does not increase [24]. Increased blood flow may minimize the fall in venous PO_2 in anemia [25], however, the CO-induced leftward shift of the oxygen dissociation curve moves the effective P_{50} of hemoglobin to a lower PO_2 for any oxygen content. Thus, HbCO decreases the driving force for diffusion of oxygen into the tissues and decreases the tissue and intracellular PO_2. HbCO is known to decrease mixed venous [26], cerebrovenous [27], and tissue PO_2 [28] in experimental animals and HbCO-related decreases in jugular venous PO_2 have been measured in man [29].

A potentially serious consequence of tissue hypoxia produced by HbCO is CO binding to intracellular proteins. Intracellular compounds that contain iron or copper will bind CO [20]. CO competes with oxygen for the active sites of hemoproteins such as myoglobin, cytochrome P450 and cytochrome c oxidase, a.k.a cytochrome a,a_3. The competition between oxygen and CO for the binding sites on these molecules is described by the Warburg partition coefficient [20], or the ratio of the partial pressures of the two gases necessary for CO to occupy half of the available binding sites. The Warburg coefficients for these compounds are inversely related to M, but are much greater than $1/M$. Thus, despite the low tissue tensions of oxygen, only about 15% of a total body store of CO is located normally in the tissues [30]. During tissue hypoxia or hypoperfusion, however, CO redistributes from the vascular space to extravascular tissues as intracellular PO_2 falls [31]. Extravascular CO binds *in vivo* to myoglobin in heart [32] and skeletal muscle [33] where it may interfere with normal mechanisms of oxygen diffusion from the capillaries to the mitochondria.

During hypoxia, CO also may bind to intracellular hemoproteins such as cytochrome c oxidase. Cytochrome oxidase is the terminal enzyme complex of the intramitochondrial electron transport system that reduces oxygen to water in the process of respiration [34]. During respiration, free energy from electron transport by mitochondria is conserved in the form of ATP, i.e. by oxidative phosphorylation. CO inhibits respiration by binding to the cytochrome a_3 component of the oxidase in the presence of two electrons [34]. A high reduction level of the enzyme has been observed in the brain, where some of the oxidase molecules are reduced at normal PO_2 [35] and reduction state varies inversely as a function of tissue PO_2 [36]. Animal studies have also indicated that low cerebral perfusion during acute CO intoxication augments pathohistological lesions in the brain [37]. Evidence for CO binding to cytochrome oxidase in the brain under similar circumstances has been obtained in laboratory animals at [HbCO] above 50% [38]. Thus, when regional brain anoxia appears during the course of CO intoxication, cytochrome oxidase rapidly becomes reduced and CO readily binds to it. This condition can be distinguished from other hypoxic or ischemic insults only after reoxygenation, when the functional capacity of the inhibited mitochondria will be restored very slowly. This concept is supported by studies of uncoupled mitochondria which indicate that very low concentrations of CO (100 ppm) will prolong the rate of reoxidation of cytochrome oxidase in the transition from anoxia to normoxia [39]. Brain mitochondria after CO poisoning also have low cytochrome oxidase and increased succinate dehydrogenase activities by histochemical methods [40]. These enzymatic changes appear to be quantitatively greater after CO than after hypoxic hypoxia. One group of investigators reported that cytochrome oxidase activity decreased in the brain only after reoxygenation, suggesting progression of injury during reperfusion [41].

Although intracellular uptake of CO is well-documented, little evidence supports the premise that it is the cause of death in lethal CO exposures. Claims that death is caused by an intracellular mechanism [42, 43] have not been confirmed [26, 44] and experiments with fluorocarbon-circulated animals indicate that animals can survive very high tissue concentrations of CO [45]. Even in these bloodless animals, however, mitochondrial redox effects in cerebral cortex can be measured by optical techniques [46]. A crisis in energy metabolism in such situations may be averted if unblocked oxidase molecules oxidize the respiratory chains of CO-blocked oxidase when oxygen is available. This does not mean, however, the intracellular effects of CO are inconsequential when cellular hypoxia is present. Whether or not the tissues escape energy failure depends on cellular oxygen availability and requirements, to some extent on intracellular CO and cytochrome oxidase concentrations, and on the duration of the exposure.

Neuropathologic Findings in CO Poisoning

Tissues that have a mandatory requirement for an uninterrupted oxygen supply such as the brain are highly sensitive to the damaging effects of CO. CO poisoning commonly produces lesions in the basal ganglia, cerebral gray matter and white matter [37, 47–50]. Three pathologically distinct categories of white matter damage have been described including 1-small multifocal necrotic lesions of the cerebral centrum and commissures, 2-extensive zones of necrosis in the hemispheric white matter, and 3-symmetric myelinopathy, characterized by patchy to extensive demyelination of the deep central white matter and periventricular zones of the hemispheres (Grinker's myelinopathy). The latter pattern of injury has been associated with delayed neurological deterioration after CO poisoning. The white matter lesions of CO poisoning, once considered pathognomonic, have been reported in other settings associated with prolonged cerebral hypoxia and oligemia [50]. The propensity to develop white matter lesions in these situations may be related to specific circulatory parameters such as elevated cerebrovenous pressure, edema and peculiarities of the arterial distribution to deep hemispheric white matter. The low concentrations of cytochrome oxidase in white matter also may predispose it to CO-induced damage [37]. A similar hypothesis has been proposed for cyanide intoxication, where two kinds of white matter damage occur commonly after acute intoxication. These include well-defined areas of necrosis and partial demyelination reminiscent of the pathological changes of CO poisoning [37].

Clinical Findings in Acute CO Poisoning

The clinical features of CO intoxication are highly variable and nonspecific. Most individuals do not develop symptoms until the [HbCO] exceeds 10%; smokers may tolerate somewhat higher [HbCO] without symptoms. The correlation between clinical presentation and measured [HbCO] is weak and the clinical findings may be more closely related to the concentration-time product of the exposure. The common symptoms are headache, nausea, dizziness, shortness of breath and lethargy [3]. Loss of consciousness also occurs and may be without warning [51]. Coma occurs often with carboxyhemoglobin saturations above 50%. Other associated symptoms include malaise, loss of memory and disorientation. When CO poisoning is unsuspected in patients who present with vague "flu-like" illness in wintertime, they may return unwittingly to a dangerous environment [51]. Patients with coronary artery disease may develop angina pectoris, arrhythmias or myocardial infarction [52], and patients with chronic obstructive pulmonary disease may have more severe shortness of breath at low HbCO saturations [53].

Physical findings in acute CO poisoning are nonspecific, but may include tachypnea, tachycardia and hypotension. Signs of smoke inhalation and burns should alert the physician to the possibility of serious CO intoxication. Ancillary physical findings may include retinal hemorrhages, retinal venous congestion and papilledema. Bullous and vesicular skin lesions and sweat gland necrosis also have been reported [54]. Cherry red capillary beds and mucous membranes, once considered classic findings in CO poisoning, are not very common [51]. Rhabdomyolysis may occur, usually in association with severe CO poisoning [55], and it may lead to renal failure [56]. Neurological findings are diverse and usually nonfocal. Common neurological abnormalities include obtundation, seizures, peripheral neuropathy, agnosia, apraxia, amnesia, Parkinsonism, cortical blindness, and incontinence [48]. Longterm neuropsychiatric disturbances may persist in many surviving victims [57], and delayed neurologic manifestations occur in about 3% of patients after a lucid interval ranging from 2 days to 6 weeks [58]. The incidence of delayed neurological sequelae correlates with the severity of the anoxic insult and the patient's age. Most patients who develop late neurological deterioration are comatose at presentation, but regain consciousness within the first 48 hours. Common manifestations of the late syndrome include intellectual and personality deterioration, incontinence, gait disturbances, frontal signs, incoordination and impaired speech.

Laboratory Diagnosis of CO Intoxication

A diagnosis of CO poisoning can be established readily by measuring the HbCO saturation in the blood. The analysis requires either a gas chromatograph or a CO-oximeter. The CO-oximeter directly measures the total hemoglobin concentration and fractional (%) values for oxyhemoglobin, deoxyhemoglobin, carboxyhemoglobin and methemoglobin [59]. The oxygen content and oxygen carrying capacity of the blood sample are calculated from the hemoglobin concentration and the fraction of oxygen-saturated hemoglobin. Standard arterial blood gas analyzers measure PO_2, PCO_2 and pH and derive the oxyhemoglobin saturation from a nomogram. These values all may be unremarkable, even during serious intoxication, since CO hypoxia usually does not produce hypoxemia. In seriously ill patients, a metabolic acidosis or a mixed respiratory alkalosis-metabolic acidosis may be present. The metabolic acidosis is accompanied by an elevated anion gap from increased lactate production by the tissues.

The severity of the CO exposure may not be reflected by the HbCO saturation when significant time has elapsed since the end of the exposure or when treatment with oxygen has been instituted before obtaining a blood sample for HbCO. This problem may arise if a CO-oximeter is not readily available, however, a heparinized blood sample drawn from the patient before beginning treatment can be stored for several hours anaerobically before analysis.

Other laboratory abnormalities accompanying CO poisoning may include elevated serum BUN, creatinine and CPK. The latter finding and myoglobinuria may indicate significant rhabdomyolysis [55, 56]. The electrocardiogram may show tachycardia, ventricular arrhythmias, nonspecific ST-T wave changes or signs of myocardial infarction [60]. The chest roentgenogram is often normal, but it may show evidence of noncardiogenic pulmonary edema [61] or aspiration. Diffuse and focal electroencephalographic (EEG) changes have been reported [62], however, EEG findings are nonspecific and suggest a diffuse metabolic encephalopathy. Computed tomography of the brain may be abnormal early in the course of the disease [63, 64]. Comatose patients may show severe diffuse brain edema, hypodensity of the central white matter and low density defects of the basal ganglia, especially the globus pallidus [63]. The severity of structural abnormalities in the brain appears to correlate with the patient's prognosis [64].

If a diagnosis of concurrent cyanide poisoning is suspected, whole blood cyanide levels should be drawn [65]. Unfortunately, cyanide levels are usually not immediately available emergently and a high clinical index of suspicion must be maintained in victims of smoke inhalation. Significant clinical signs of cyanide poisoning occur at blood concentration of 0.5–2.0 µg/ml and death usually occurs when blood levels exceed 3µg/ml. Plasma thiocyanate levels, reflecting the amount of cyanide detoxification in the body, also may help confirm the diagnosis [65]. Another useful laboratory manifestation of cyanide intoxication is an acid-base disturbance characterized by a metabolic acidosis with an elevated anion gap. The anion gap is usually explained by an elevated serum lactate concentration [66]. The patient also may have a narrow arteriovenous oxygen content difference and an O_2 saturation gap. An O_2 saturation gap, defined as the difference between calculated and measured arterial O_2 content, may occur if significant cyanhemoglobin is present [65].

Emergency Management of CO Poisoning

The patient with suspected CO poisoning should be placed immediately on 100% oxygen and an arterial blood sample drawn for measurement of HbCO saturation, blood gases and pH. Comatose patients should be intubated promptly to control the airway and assure adequate oxygenation and ventilation. In seriously ill patients, or those with underlying cardiovascular disease, the laboratory evaluation should include an EKG, chest roentgenogram, complete blood count, urinalysis and serum electrolytes, glucose, BUN, creatinine and cardiac enzymes. A drug screen should be performed when the ingestion of alcohol or other toxic substances is suspected. If cyanide intoxication is considered in the differential diagnosis of a comatose patient or victim of smoke inhalation, additional blood should be drawn for determination of cyanide and thiocyanate (SCN) levels. The patient should receive 100% oxygen to breathe, ventilation established and appropriate chemical antidotes administered quickly [65, 66].

The administration of hyperbaric oxygen (HBO) is a primary therapeutic modality in serious CO intoxication. CO poisoning is classified as a Category 1 disorder by the Undersea and Hyperbaric Medical Society to indicate that treatment with HBO is effective [67]. Cyanide intoxication is also a Category 1 disorder, however, the efficacy of HBO in cyanide poisoning is supported only by clinical anecdotes. The use of hyperbaric oxygen to treat acute CO poisoning was reported first in 1960 [68]. The rationale for its use at that time was based on studies of HbCO elimination in normal volunteers by Pace [69], although the protective effects of HBO against CO hypoxia had been known since Haldane's time. The rationale for the use of HBO in acute CO poisoning is threefold (Table 1). First, HBO greatly enhances the rate of elimination of CO from hemoglobin and tissue stores, second it allows physically dissolved oxygen to be delivered to tissues until HbCO is eliminated, and finally, it decreases cerebral edema [70].

The rate of HbCO elimination from the body is a reflection of the same variables which determine its uptake. The HbCO elimination curve tends to follow a single exponential function with a half-time of approximately 300 min in air, however, there may be significant redistribution of CO from blood to muscle for up to one hour after exposure [71]. The elimination half-time of HbCO is shortened greatly at high PO_2; it is approximately 60 min for 100% O_2 and 23 min at 3 atmospheres absolute (ATA) of O_2 with normal pulmonary gas exchange [72]. Furthermore, the amount of physically dissolved oxygen in arterial blood at 3 ATA normally will approach 6 vol%. This amount of oxygen in solution is suffi-

Table 1. Rationale for use of oxygen in CO intoxication

Principle	Mechanism
1) Enhance HbCO elimination from the body	Mass action: O_2 competes with CO for hemoglobin binding site
2) Enhance CO elimination from myoglobin and other tissue sites	Mass action: O_2 competes with CO for iron/copper binding sites in tissues
3) Maintain oxygen delivery to tissue	Oxygen, 2.1 vol% per ATA is physically dissolved in plasma
4) Reduce cerebral edema and ICP	Primarily vasoconstrictive effect of HBO

cient to meet the basal oxygen requirements of the body at a normal cardiac output without any requirement for O_2 unloading by hemoglobin.

There are no prospective, randomized clinical trials which prove greater efficacy of HBO over sea level oxygen in CO poisoning. This leaves some uncertainty about whether HBO is superior to sea levels O_2 for treatment of acute CO poisoning and if so, which patients benefit from HBO. Nonetheless, the rationale for the use of HBO in serious cases of acute CO intoxication is sound, the treatment in safe, and the clinical experience has been excellent. Three clinical criteria are used widely for treatment of CO intoxication with HBO. These are shown in Table 2 [73]. Note that a low HbCO saturation is not a reason to withhold HBO if the clinical features of the case are consistant with serious CO poisoning. Recent studies of CO poisoning have shown no difference in HbCO level between comatose patients who survived and those who died after their exposures [74]. Also, patients at any level of HbCO may have persistent, subtle neuropsychiatric abnormalities by psychometric testing [75]. Therefore, a high index of suspicion for neurological effects must be maintained at all times. Hyperbaric oxygen therapy for CO poisoning is usually given at 2.5 to 3 ATA for 90 to 120 minutes. At our facility, we use a hyperbaric protocol of 2.5 ATA for 90 minutes. A single treatment usually decreases the HbCO saturation to 5% or less and brings about complete resolution of symptoms. One or more follow up treatments may be administered to patients who do not recover completely after the first treatment.

Various other therapies have been employed or proposed in the management of CO poisoning, but these are unproven. These options include hypothermia [76] and other measures to reduce cerebral metabolic rate, as well as treatment of cerebral edema by the administration of glucocorticoids, mannitol and hyperventilation [77]. The rationale behind these strategies in CO hypoxia is analogous to the rationale for using them to treat other forms of global brain hypoxia. When a hyperbaric chamber is unavailable, exchange transfusion with whole blood or artificial blood substitutes may be considered in life-threatening CO poisoning, particularly for young children [76].

Results of Therapy for CO Poisoning

Perhaps one third of patients with serious CO toxicity die from their exposures [78]. The prognosis of a patient who survives acute CO intoxication is variable and difficult to predict because of differences in intensity and duration of exposure and individual susceptibility. About 11% of survivors suffer obvious long-term neuropsychiatric sequelae including 3% who develop delayed neurological

Table 2. Clinical criteria for treatment of CO poisoning with hyperbaric oxygen

- A HbCO saturation of 25% or greater
- Anginal pain or ischemic changes on ECG
- Any degree of neurological impairment regardless of HbCO saturation at presentation

manifestations [58]. One third of CO poisoning victims may suffer subtle, persistent deficits of memory or personality changes [57].

Hyperbaric oxygen has been proposed to decrease mortality from CO poisoning [79] as well as the incidence of both residual neurological sequelae [73, 75] and late neurological manifestations [71, 79]. Most large series of CO poisoning treated promptly with HBO report and incidence of long term residual CNS effects of 0 to 16% [74, 75, 79, 80]. The incidence of delayed neurological deterioration after prompt HBO treatment is unknown, however, some patients treated with HBO do develop delayed sequelae [79, 81]. In a retrospective study by Min of 86 patients with delayed manifestations of CO poisoning, it was noted that 32 had received HBO [81]. Information was not given about the duration of the CO exposures, the delay between CO poisoning and HBO, or the type or number of HBO treatments used. Apart from prolonged exposure and delays in treatment, other clinical factors may indicate poor prognosis in CO poisoning including altered consciousness at presentation, age over 40 [58, 81], metabolic acidosis [82, 83], EEG changes and structural abnormalities on brain CT [63, 64]. Adequacy of pulmonary gas exchange and delays of more than 2 to 6 hours between exposure and treatment also appear to affect the outcome after HBO therapy [79, 80]. Comatose patients have been shown to benefit from HBO when pulmonary gas exchange is sufficient to produce high PO_2 values in arterial blood [80]. In a recent, randomized trial involving 629 patients from Paris, Raphael et al. [84] compared the outcome of patients presenting within 12 hours of CO poisoning and without loss of consciousness who were treated with either 2 ATA of HBO or surface O_2. Patients with loss of consciousness received either one HBO period of 1 hour at 2 ATA or two HBO treatments. The data showed no differences between therapies in either arm of the study, however, the recovery rates at 1 month were only 68 and 66% in the patients who had no loss of consciousness and 54 and 52% in patients who had suffered loss of consciousness. These results are comparable to patients who have received no therapy, and questions must be raised about whether some patients were treated too late or with insufficient amounts of oxygen [85]. By comparison, the results of two other recent studies, one from Seattle using HBO therapy [74] and one from Copenhagen using sea level O_2 alone [83], suggest a difference between the two therapies. The data from these studies suggest that mortality may be lower by a factor of two in acute CO intoxication when HBO is employed in patients with loss of consciousness. There also have been cases of clinical improvement in patients treated with HBO more than 24 hours after an acute episode of intoxication [86]. The pathophysiologic basic for such delayed responses is uncertain, but it may well relate to remnant intracellular effects of CO or brain edema.

References

1. Winter PM, Miller JN (1988) Carbon monoxide poisoning. JAMA 236:1502-1504
2. Turnbull TL, Hart RG, Strange GR, et al (1988) Emergency department screening for unsuspected carbon monoxide exposure. Ann Emerg Med 17:478-483
3. Grace TW, Platt FW (1981) Subacute carbon monoxide poisoning. Another great imitator. JAMA 246:1698-1700

4. Coburn RF, Blakemore WS, Forster RE (1963) Endogenous carbon monoxide production in man. J Clin Invest 42:1172–1178
5. Yoshida T, Noguchi M, Kikuchi G (1982) The step of carbon monoxide liberation in the sequence of heme degradation catalyzed by the reconstituted microsomal heme oxygenase system. J Biol Chem 257:9345–9348
6. Lundh B, Stahl EC, Merke C (1975) Heme catabolism, carbon monoxide production and red cell survival in anemia. Acta Med Scand 197:161–171
7. Coburn RF (1970) Enhancement by phenobarbital and diphenylhydantoin of carbon manoxide production in normal man. N Engl J Med 283:512–515
8. Rodkey FL, Collison HA (1977) Biological oxidation of [^{14}C] methylene chloride to carbon monoxide and carbon dioxide in the rat. Toxicol Appl Pharm 40:39–47
9. Stewart RD, Fisher TN, Hosko MH, Peterson JE, Bartetta ED, Dodd HC (1972) Carboxyhemoglobin elevation after exposure to dichloromethane. Science 176:295–296
10. Stewart RD, Bartetta ED, Plate LR, et al (1974) Carboxyhemoglobin levels in American blood donors. JAMA 229:1187–1195
11. Collishaw NE, Kirkbridge J, Wigle DT (1984) Tobacco smoke in the workplace: an occupational health hazard. Can Med Assoc J 131:1199–1204
12. Aronow WS, Harris CN, Isbell MW, et al (1972) Effect of freeway travel on angina pectoris. Ann Intern Med 77:669–676
13. Committee on Medical and Biologic Effects of Environmental Pollutants (1977) Carbon Monoxide. National Research Council, National Academy of Sciences, Washington DC, pp 28–37
14. Whorton MD (1976) Carbon monoxide intoxication: a review of 14 patients. JACEP 5:505–509
15. Kwok PW (1983) Evaluation and control of carbon monoxide exposure in indoor skating arenas. Can J Public Health 74:261–265
16. Burney RE, Wu SC, Nemiroff MJ (1982) Mass carbon monoxide poisoning: clinical effects and results of treatment in 184 victims. Ann Emerg Med 11:394–399
17. Clark CJ, Campbell D, Reid WH (1981) Blood carboxyhemoglobin and cyanide levels in fire survivors. Lancet 1:1332–1335
18. Jones J, McMullin MJ, Dougherty J (1987) Toxic smoke inhalation: Cyanide poisoning in fire victims. Am J Emerg Med 5:318–321
19. Becker CE (1985) the role of cyanide in fires. Vet Hum Toxicol 27:487–490
20. Coburn RF, Forman HJ (1987) Carbon monoxide toxicity. In: Farhi LE, Tenney SM (eds) Handbook of physiology, section 3: The respiratory system. vol 4. Gas exchange. Am Physiol Soc, Bethesda, Maryland, pp 439–456
21. Holland RAB (1969) Rate of O_2 dissociation from O_2 Hb and relative combination rate of CO and O_2 in mammals at 37°C. Respir Physiol 7:30–42
22. Coburn RF, Forster RE, Kane PB (1965) Considerations of the physiological variables that determine blood carboxyhemoglobin concentration in man. J Clin Invest 44:1899–1910
23. Rodkey FL, O'Neal JD, Collison HA, Uddin DE (1974) Relative affinity of hemoglobin S and hemoglobin A for carbon monoxide and oxygen. Clin Chem 20:83–84
24. Forster RE (1970) Carbon monoxide and the partial pressure of oxygen in tissue. Ann NY Acad Sci 174:233–241
25. Tenney SM (1974) A theoretical analysis of the relationship between venous blood and mean tissue oxygen pressures. Resp Physiol 20:283–296
26. Gutierrez G, Rotman HR, Reid CM, Dantzker DR (1985) Comparison of canine cardiovascular responses to inhaled and intraperitoneally infused CO. J Appl Physiol 58:558–563
27. Koehler RC, Jones MD, Traystman RJ (1982) Cerebral circulatory response to carbon monoxide and hypoxic hypoxia in the lamb. Am J Physiol 243:H27–H32
28. Zorn H (1972) The partial O_2 pressure in the brain and liver at subtoxic concentrations of carbon monoxide. Staub Reinhalt Luft (Engl ed) 32:24–29
29. Paulson OB, Parving HH, Olesen J, Skinhoj E (1973) Influence of carbon monoxide and of hemodilution on cerebral blood flow and blood gases in man. J Appl Physiol 35:111–116
30. Luomanmäki K, Coburn RF (1969) Effects of metabolism in distribution of carbon monoxide on blood and body stores. Am J Physiol 217:354–363
31. Coburn RF (1979) Mechanisms of carbon monoxide toxicity. Prev Med 8:310–322

32. Coburn RF, Ploegmakers F, Gondrie P, Abboud R (1973) Myocardial myoglobin oxygen tension. Am J Physiol 224:870–876
33. Coburn RF, Wallace HW, Abboud R (1971) Redistribution of body carbon monoxide after hemorrhage. Am J Physiol 220:868–873
34. Erecinska M, Wilson DF (1981) Inhibitors of cytochrome c oxidase. In: Erecinska M, Wilson DF (eds) Inhibitors of mitochondrial function. Pergamon Press, Oxford, pp 145–164
35. Jöbsis FF, Kaiser JH, LaManna JC, Rosenthal M (1977) Reflectance spectrophotometry of cytochrome a,a_3 in vivo. J Appl Physiol 43:858–872
36. Kreisman NR, Sick TJ, LaManna JC, Rosenthal M (1981) Local tissue oxygen tension cytochrome a,a_3 redox relationship in rats cerebral cortex in vivo. Brain Res 218:161–174
37. Ginsberg MD (1979) Delayed neurological deterioration following hypoxia. In: Fahn S et al (eds) Advances in neurology, vol 26. Raven Press, New York, pp 21–43
38. Brown SD, Piantadosi CA (1988) Reversal of CO cytochrome c oxidase binding by hyperbaric oxygen in vivo. In: Rakusan K, Biro GP, Goldstick TK, Turek Z (eds) Oxygen transport to tissue XI. Plenum Press, New York, 747–754
39. Chance B, Erecinska M, Wagner M (1970) Mitochondrial responses to carbon monoxide toxicity. Ann NY Acad Sci 174:193–204
40. Somogyi E, Balogh I, Rubanyi G, Sotonyi P, Szegedi L (1981) New findings concerning the pathogenesis of acute CO poisoning. Am J Forensic Med Pathol 2:31–39
41. Savolainen H, Kurppa K, Tenhunen R, Kivisto H (1980) Biochemical effects of carbon monoxide poisoning in rat brain with special reference to blood carboxyhemoglobin and cerebral cytochrome oxidase activity. Neurosci Lett 19:319–323
42. Goldbaum LR, Ramirez RG, Absalon KB (1975) What is the mechanism of carbon monoxide toxicity? Aviat Space Environ Med 46:1289–1291
43. Goldbaum LR, Orellano T, Durgal E (1977) Studies on the relationship between carboxyhemoglobin concentration and toxicity. Aviat Space Environ Med 48:969–970
44. Halebian P, Robinson N, Barie P, Goodwin C, Shires GT (1986) Whole body oxygen utilization during acute carbon monoxide poisoning and isocapneic nitrogen hypoxia. J Trauma 26:110–117
45. Geyer RP (1976) Review of perfluorochemical-type blood substitutes. In: Proceedings of the 10th International Congress for Nutrition: Symposium on Perfluorochemical Artificial Blood. Igakushobe Osaka Jpn, pp 3–19
46. Piantadosi CA, Sylvia AL, Saltzman HA, Jöbsis-Vander Vliet FF (1985) Carbon monoxide-cytochrome interactions in the brain of the fluorocarbon perfused rat. J Appl Physiol 58:665–672
47. Lapresle J, Fardeau M (1967) The central nervous system and carbon monoxide poisoning. II. Anatomical study of brain lesions following intoxication with carbon monoxide. Prog Brain Res 24:31–74
48. Garland H, Pearce J (1967) Neurological complications with carbon monoxide poisoning. Q Jour Med 36:445–455
49. Brucher JM (1967) Neuropathological problems posed by carbon monoxide poisoning and anoxia. Prog Brain Res 24:75–100
50. Ginsberg MD, Hedley-White ET, Richardson EP Jr (1976) Hypoxic-ischemic leukoencephalopathy in man. Arch Neurol 33:5–14
51. Dolan MC (1985) Carbon monoxide poisoning. Can Med Assos J 133:392–398
52. Anderson EW, Andelman RJ, Strauch JM, et al (1973) Effect of low level carbon monoxide exposure on onset and duration of angina pectoris. Ann Intern Med 79:46–50
53. Caverley PMA, Leggett RJE, Flenley DC (1981) Carbon monoxide and exercise tolerance in chronic bronchitis and emphysema. Br Med J 283:878–880
54. Leavell OW, Farley CH, McIntyre JS (1969) Cutaneous changes in a patient with carbon monoxide poisoning. Arch Dermatol 39:429–433
55. Finley J, Van Beek A, Glover GL (1977) Myonecrosis complicating carbon monoxide poisoning. J Trauma 17:536–540
56. Bessoudo R, Gray J (1978) Carbon monoxide poisoning and non-oliguric renal failure. Can Med Assoc J 119:41–44
57. Smith JS, Brandon S (1973) Morbidity from acute carbon monoxide poisoning at 3 year followup. Br Med J 1:318–321

58. Choi IS (1983) Delayed neurologic sequelae in carbon monoxide intoxication. Arch Neurol 40:433–435
59. Brown LJ (1980) A new instrument for the simultaneous measurement of total hemoglobin, % carboxyhemoglobin, % methemoglobin and oxygen content in whole blood. IEEE Transactions Biomed Engineering 27:132–138
60. Anderson RF, Allensworth DC, DeGroot WJ (1967) Myocardial toxicity from carbon monoxide poisoning. Ann Intern Med 67:1172–1182
61. Sone S, Higushihara T, Kotake T, et al (1974) Pulmonary manifestations in acute carbon monoxide poisoning. Am J Roentgenol 120:865–871
62. Neufeld MY, Swanson JW, Klass DW (1981) Localized EEG abnormalities in acute carbon monoxide poisoning. Arch Neurol 38:524–527
63. Savada Y, Ohashi N, Maemura K, et al (1980) Computerized tomography as an indication of long term outcome after acute monoxide poisoning. Lancet 1:783–784
64. Miura T, Mitomo M, Kawai R, Harada K (1985) CT of the brain in acute carbon monoxide intoxication: characteristic features and prognosis. Am J Neuroradiol 6:739–742
65. Hall AH, Rumack BH (1986) Clinical toxicology of cyanide. Ann Emerg Med 15:1067–1074
66. Vogel SN, Sultan TR, Ten Eyck RP (1981) Cyanide poisoning. Clin Toxicol 18:367–383
67. Hyperbaric Oxygen Therapy (1986) A committee Report. Undersea and Hyperbaric Medical Society Publ. # 30, Bethesda, MD, pp 33–36
68. Smith GI, Sharp GR (1960) Treatment of carbon monoxide poisoning with oxygen under pressure. Lancet 1:905–906
69. Pace N, Strajman E, Walker EL (1950) Acceleration of carbon monoxide elimination in man by high pressure oxygen. Science 111:652–654
70. Sukoff MH, Hollin SA, Jacobson JH (1967) The protective effect of hyperbaric oxygenation in experimentally produced cerebral edema and compression. Surgery 62:40–46
71. Shephard RJ (1983) In: Charles C (ed) Carbon monoxide. The silent killer. Thomas, Springfield, Ill; pp 44–67
72. Peterson JE, Stewart RD (1970) Absorption and elimination of carbon monoxide by inactive young men. Arch Environ Health 21:165–171
73. Kindwall EP (1977) Carbon monoxide and cyanide poisoning. In: David JC, Hunt TK (eds) Hyperbaric oxygen therapy. Undersea Medical Society, Bethesda MD, pp 177–190
74. Norkool DM, Kirkpatrick JN (1985) Treatment of acute carbon monoxide poisoning with hyperbaric oxygen: a review of 115 cases. Ann Emerg Med 14:1168–1171
75. Myers RAM, Snyder SK, Emhoff TA (1985) Subacute sequelae of carbon monoxide poisoning. Ann Emerg Med 14:1163–1167
76. Boutros AR, Hoyt JL (1976) Management of carbon monoxide poisoning in the absence of hyperbaric oxygenation chamber. Crit Care Med 4:144–147
77. Safar P (1981) Resuscitation after brain ischemia. In: Grenvik A, Safar P (eds) Brain failure and resuscitation. Churchill Livingstone, New York, pp 155–184
78. Shillito FH, Drinker CK, Shanghnessy TJ (1936) The problem of nervous and mental sequelae in carbon monoxide poisoning. JAMA 106:669–674
79. Goulon M, Barois A, Rapin M, et al (1969) Carbon monoxide poisoning and acute anoxia due to breathing coal gas and hydrocarbons. Ann Med Interne 120:335–349
80. Zanetti CL (1987) A review of carbon monoxide poisoning treated at Edgewater Hospital. In: Kindwall EP (ed) Proceedings of the eighth international congress on hyperbaric medicine. Best Publishing Co, San Pedro, CA, pp 258–262
81. Min SK (1986) A brain syndrome associated with delayed neuropsychiatric sequelae following acute carbon monoxide intoxication. Acta Psychiatr Scand 73:80–86
82. Larkin JM, Brahos GJ, Moylan JA (1976) Treatment of carbon monoxide poisoning: prognostic factors. J Trauma 16:111–114
83. Krantz T, Thisted B, Strom J, Sorensen MB (1988) Acute carbon monoxide poisoning. Acta Anesthesiol Scand 32:278–282
84. Raphael JC, Elkharrat D, Jars-Guincestre MC, et al (1989) Trial of normobaric and hyperbaric oxygen for acute carbon monoxide intoxication. Lancet 1:414–419
85. Brown SD, Piantadosi CA (1989) Hyperbaric oxygen for CO poisoning. Lancet 2:1032
86. Myers RAM, Snyder SK, Linberg S, Cowley RA (1981) Value of hyperbaric oxygen in suspected carbon monoxide poisoning. JAMA 246:2478–2480

Management of the Acute Neuropsychiatric Manifestations of Cocaine Intoxication

L. Goldfrank

Introduction

Cocaine users in North America, South America and Europe number in the millions on a daily basis. The neuropsychiatric manifestations of cocaine intoxication are often an exaggeration of the sought after clinical manifestations and represent the commonest causes of visits to hospital settings. Of the thousands of patients who present to the Bellevue Emergency Department with cocaine intoxication annually approximately two-thirds have neuropsychiatric compromise. These complications included an altered mental status, seizures, agitation, suicidal ideation and cerebrovascular accidents. The prevalence of cocaine use has become so substantial that almost all patients from adolescence to adulthood presenting to the emergency department with these symptoms are considered to potentially have used cocaine and become intoxicated with the agent. During the first 11 months of 1986, 935 persons died in the city of New York with evidence of cocaine in their bodies [1]. This represented 15% of all patients brought to the Office of the Chief Medical Examiner. Neuropsychiatric abnormalities were a common cause of death: 38% died of homicide, 7% of suicide, 8% of "accidents", and 2% of cerebral hemorrhage. Of these patients 86.9% were between the ages of 11–44 years of age [1].

There does not appear to be a correlation between the route of administration, dose delivered or prior experience and the severity of complications [2]. The number of patients presenting has increased dramatically and appears to parallel the marked increase in availability of the more easily delivered cocaine alkaloid (crack), which can be smoked, yet achieves comparable rapidity of onset of action and effect to intravenous cocaine hydrochloride. In 1980, cocaine was the tenth most frequently utilized drug of abuse in the Bellevue Emergency Department following heroin and numerous sedative hypnotics. In 1989, cocaine is the most frequently used agent.

Pharmacologic Action of Cocaine with Regard to Neuropsychiatric Manifestations

Benzoylmethylecognine is an ester with the basic structure of local anesthetics. Its local anesthetic effects result from its ability in preventing the initiation and conduction of neural impulses. Cocaine stimulates the central nervous system

(CNS) initially and at low dose resulting in a stimulatory phase of alertness, euphoria and dysphoria. At a later stage and associated with higher doses increased motor activity, tremor, uncontrolled movement and seizures may result. This may progress to CNS depression including respiratory depression and death. At these higher doses marked hyperthermia may result from this increased motor activity, the associated vasoconstriction limiting heat dissipation and the central effect of cocaine on the thermoregulatory centers of the brain.

Cocaine's effect on the sympathetic nervous system results in the inhibition of the uptake of catecholamines at synaptic adrenergic terminals. This inhibition prevents the termination of adrenergic impulses and allows for the persistence of excessive sympathetic manifestations.

Experimental Basis for the Pathophysiology of the Neuropsychiatric Manifestations of Cocaine

The pharmacologic properties that lead to an increase in heat production with concomitant diminished heat dissipation have led to several consequential and at times contradictory experimental studies [3, 6].

In Catravas' dog model cocaine related increases in mean arterial pressure, heart rate, cardiac output, rectal temperature and acidemia were studied. All animals administered cocaine developed convulsions and died with a mean lethal dose of 22 ± 2 mg/kg. In the experimental design pretreatment antidotal therapy was administered. Chlorpromazine demonstrated efficacy with regard to cardiovascular complications and no animals died although all animals developed seizures. Pimozide, a D_2 antidopaminergic and adrenergic blocking agent, had no salutary effect on any parameter or lethality. Propranolol was efficacious with regard to the cardiovascular complications yet had no effect on the incidence of seizures nor the fatality rate. Pancuronium had no effect on the cardiovascular manifestations but did prevent fatalities and although there was no motor activity presumably seizures did occur. Pretreatment diazepam decreased the cardiovascular manifestations, prevented seizures and resulted in no fatalities. The use of an ambient environment of $-5\,°C$ led to a diminished cardiovascular effect of the cocaine and the absence of seizures and fatalities.

Derlet [7] also demonstrated in a rat model that diazepam was effective in preventing the tonic clonic manifestations of seizures and death inspite of a continuum of convulsant-like electrical activity. Witkin [5] further expanded research in search of a central dopamine receptor blocking agent. Dopamine antagonists with varying affinity for dopamine-1 and dopamine-2 receptor subtypes were utilized. When the established rat model was pretreated with a dopamine-2 antagonist haloperidol there was no alteration in the lethal effect of cocaine. When SCH 23390 a dopamine-1 antagonist was utilized in pretreatment the lethal dose was increased whereas as a posttreatment agent given 5 minutes after cocaine administration no benefits were appreciated. These results combined with the analysis of chlorpromazine and a D-2-dopamine antagonist pimozide [3] suggest that antidopaminergic agents currently available such as chlorpromazine and haloperidol may not necessarily be efficacious in treating cocaine toxicity but that more specific agents against D-1-dopamine receptors may be effective.

Two studies utilizing calcium channel blockers have resulted in divergent analyses. Trouve [4] utilizing nitrendipine an experimentally available calcium channel blocker as an antagonist to the cardiac toxicity of cocaine and as a potential antidote to the lethal effects demonstrated arrhythmia suppression and increased survival times. Derlet [6] in a rat model demonstrated that animals pretreated with diltiazem, nifedipine or verapamil developed seizures more rapidly than did control animals and at any specific doses the fatality rate was higher. This potentiation of seizures and death was demonstrated at 2 mg/kg nifedipine pretreatment doses with three variable cocaine doses. The Derlet study suggests that all the currently available calcium channel blockers may increase the risk and consequence of seizures associated with cocaine intoxication. The authors raise the concern of a potential hemodynamic interaction between seizures and mortality in cocaine intoxicated calcium channel blocker treated animals.

These studies suggest the importance of sedative hypnotics such as diazepam, the utility of paralyzing agents such as pancuronium and the efficacy of ambient cooling, the present risk of dopaminergic antagonists currently available, a concern over the merits and risks of currently available calcium channel blockers and the lack of efficacy of a beta blocker such as propranolol. These studies define research direction in the field of neurotransmitters, biogenic amines, sedative hypnotics, specific dopamine antagonists, calcium channel and beta blockers (or more specific beta receptor blockers) and the use of thermoregulatory control.

Neuropsychiatric Manifestations

The effects on the CNS include intense stimulation resulting euphoria, tremor, agitation, confusion and dysphoria. This initial phase is rapidly followed by depression, anxiety and paranoia. Delirium, disorientation, hallucinations (tactile and visual), psychosis as well as an aggressive behavior may ensue (Table 1). Seizures are relatively uncommon among cocaine users but have been reported using any route. These seizures may be partial or generalized and can in certain

Table 1. Psychiatric manifestations of cocaine intoxication

Decreased REM sleep
Agitation, irritability
Hallucinations: visual, auditory, tactile
Anxiety or depression
Hyperexcitability
Psychosis
Paranoia
Suicidal ideation
Violent, aggressive behavior
Confusion

instances be directly attributable to cocaine toxicity in the absence of a demonstrable critical vascular event, hypoxia or an arhythmia [8, 9].

Many of the other neurologic manifestations may be ascribed to acute vascular events associated with vasospasm or hypertension [10], include migraine headaches, transient ischemic attacks, subarachnoid hemorrhage and cerebrovascular accidents (Table 2).

The life-threatening concerns in neuropsychiatric management include controlling acute psychiatric behavior, aggressive and violent behavior, and seizures. Control of agitation, seizures and hyperthermia are necessary if rhabdomyolysis and resultant myoglobinuric acute tubular necrosis are to be prevented [11] (Fig. 1).

Controlling vasospasm or hypertension as well as evaluating the patient for a cerebrovascular catastrophe are essential.

Table 2. Neurologic manifestations of cocaine intoxication

Headache
Tremor
Restlessness
Tonic/clonic seizures (status epilepticus)
Confusion
Subarachnoid hemorrhage
Vasculitis
Intracerebral hemorrhage
Cerebral infarction
Syncope/transient loss of consciousness
Brain abscess
Movement disorders
Transient ischemic attacks
Blindness/blurred vision

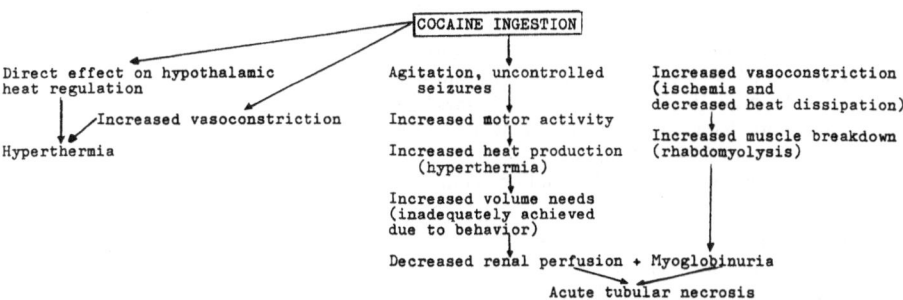

Fig. 1. Mechanistic analysis of cocaine intoxication related hyperthermia, rhabdomyolysis, and acute tubular necrosis

Management Strategies for Acute Neuropsychiatric Abnormalities

Control of acute psychiatric manifestation of cocaine intoxication should be based on supportive care that minimizes risks to patients and staff as well as reduces external stimuli. Sedation with diazepam is chosen due to its demonstrable experimental efficacy [3, 7] and the substantial experience in its use in comparable clinical states associated with agitation such as sedative hypnotic or ethanol withdrawal [12, 13] (Table 3).

Haloperidol is not suggested due to the lack of experimental support [3, 5] and comparable difficulties in sedative hypnotic withdrawal in humans [14] particularly when faced with agitation and hyperthermia. This is of consequence as loss of thermoregulatory control is a common complication in the acutely agitated psychotic patient with cocaine intoxication.

Agitation and seizures are managed in the standard manner with focus on rapid control of motor activity while protecting the patient's airway and achieving adequate ventilation and oxygenation. Restraints should be applied transiently to achieve an intravenous line. Ideally if a restraint blanket is used it should be constructed as a strong netting or a mesh to avoid increasing the patient's temperature by preventing heat dissipation. Diazepam and phenobarbital are preferable in the management of seizures in that they also achieve sedation. If they are not rapidly effective pancuronium and general anesthesia may be indicated.

Control of hyperthermia is best achieved by rapid cooling with an ice bath and a fan. Conduction and evaporation prove rapidly efficacious. Control of the associated agitation, psychosis or seizures are essential to achieve and maintain cooling while avoiding cerebral, hepatic and muscle cellular destruction. There

Table 3. Treatment of neuropsychiatric manifestations of cocaine intoxication

(A) Agitation/seizures:
  Protect airway; give 100% oxygen
  Initially physical restraints may be necessary
  Diazepam 5–10 mg IV/2 minutes repeat until sedation
  Phenobarbital 100 mg/minute to 15–20 mg/kg loading dose.
  Phenytoin 50 mg/minute to 15–20 mg/kg loading dose.
  Pancuronium 0.04–0.10 mg/kg.
  General anesthesia (pentobarbital or halothane)

(B) Hyperthermia:
  Protect airway; give 100% oxygen
  Control agitation/seizures
  Rapid cooling (ice/water bath)
  Enhance evaporation (Fan)
  Stop cooling at 38.4°C (101°F)
  Control fluids and electrolytes

(C) Psychiatric:
  Sedation: diazepam 5–10 mg IV/2 minutes
  Repeat until sedation achieved

is no evidence that other pharmacologic agents play a role in enhancing the cooling process in these patients with life threatening hyperthermia.

Conclusion

The neuropsychiatric manifestations of cocaine intoxication have become exceedingly common emergency department problems. Recent advances in the understanding of the pharmacologic interventions necessary in the management of lifethreatening cocaine emergencies have led to simple approach emphasizing sedation. Further research into the efficacy of calcium channel blockers, dopamine antagonists and safe mechanisms to control catecholamine excess will improve our therapeutic options.

References

1. Tardiff K, Gross E, Wu J, Stajic M, Millman R (1989) Analysis of cocaine-positive fatalities. J Forensic Sciences 34:53-63
2. Lowenstein DH, Massa SM, Rowbotham MC, Collins SD, McKinney HE, Simon RP (1987) Acute neurologic and psychiatric complications associated with cocaine abuse. Am J Med 83:841-846
3. Catravas JD, Waters IW (1981) Acute cocaine intoxication in the conscious dog: Studies on the mechanism of lethality. J Pharm Exp Therap 217:350-356
4. Trouve R, Nahas G (1986) Nitrendipine: An antidote to cardiac and lethal toxicity of cocaine. Proc Soc Exp Biol Med 183:392-397
5. Witkin JM, Goldberg SR, Katz JL (1989) Lethal effects of cocaine are reduced by the dopamin-1 receptor antagonist SCH 23390 but not by haloperidol. Life Sci 44:1285-1291
6. Derlet RW, Albertson TE (1989) Potentiation of cocaine toxicity with calcium channel blockers. Am J Emerg Med 7:464-468
7. Derlet RW, Albertson TE (1989) Diazepam in the prevention of seizures and death in cocaine intoxicated rats. Ann Emerg Med 18:542-546
8. Choy-Kwong M, Lipton RB (1989) Seizures in hospitalized cocaine users. Neurology 39:425-427
9. Myers JA, Earnest MP (1984) Generalized seizures and cocaine abuse. Neurology 34:675-676
10. Wojak JC, Flamm ES (1987) Intracranial hemorrhage and cocaine use. Stroke 18:712-715
11. Merigian KS, Roberts JR (1978) Cocaine intoxication: Hyperpyrexia, rhabdomyolysis and acute renal failure. Clin Tox 25:135-148
12. Sellers EM, Naranjo CA, Harrison M (1983) Diazepam loading simplified treatment of alcohol withdrawal. Clin Pharmacol Therap 34:822-826
13. Thompson WL (1978) Management of alcohol withdrawal syndromes. Arch Intern Med 138:278-283
14. Greenblatt DJ, Gross PL, Harris J (1978) Fatal hyperthermia following haloperidol therapy of sedative hypnotic withdrawal. J Clin Psychiatry 39:673-675

Acute Heroin Intoxication

G. Conti, J. L. Teboul, and A. Gasparetto

Introduction

The use of narcotics, especially morphinic, is spreading over Western Europe, and this represents a real social and economic emergency. Heroin (diacethylmorphine), a new semi-synthetic derivative of morphine, is nowadays the most widely used narcotic in Southern Europa, being responsible for the large majority (>80%) of deaths directly related to drug abuse. Heroin addicts are often referred to emergency department or intensive care units for the treatment of lifethreathening complications of drug abuse. We will briefly review the effects of acute heroin intoxication, focussing our attention to the pathophysiology of heroin induced pulmonary edema.

Heroin Overdose

Heroin overdose has been generally reported after intravenous injection (although described after subcutaneous injection, oral intake or snuffing), and is generally caused by accidental overdose or voluntary increase of the standard dose. Heroin overdose is generally characterized by coma, cyanosis, hypoventilation or apnea, and myosis that promptly regresses after IV administration of naloxone (N-allil-noroxymorphone), a pure morphine antagonist [1]. Naloxone is generally administred at a first dose of 0.4 mg IV, followed by a 3–6 hours IV continuous infusion, which is required in view of its short duration of action (25–45 min), [2].

When promptly treated and not complicated by acute pulmonary edema, aspiration pneumonia or toxic synergism with other drugs, heroin overdose is generally easy to manage and the overall mortality rate is low. However it is important to underline that the large majority of non-survivors from heroin overdose die before receiving any treatment.

Heroin overdose patients are prone to important complications listed in Table 1.

Rhabdomyolysis and Acute Renal Failure (Fig. 1)

Acute renal failure has been reported in heroin and methadone addicts as complication of rhabdomyolisis [3, 4]. It is generally induced by the muscular com-

Table 1. Complications of heroin overdose

- Heroin pulmonary edema
- Aspiration pneumonia
- Cerebral vascular accidents
- Brain edema
- Seizures
- Rhabdomyolysis
- Acute renal failure

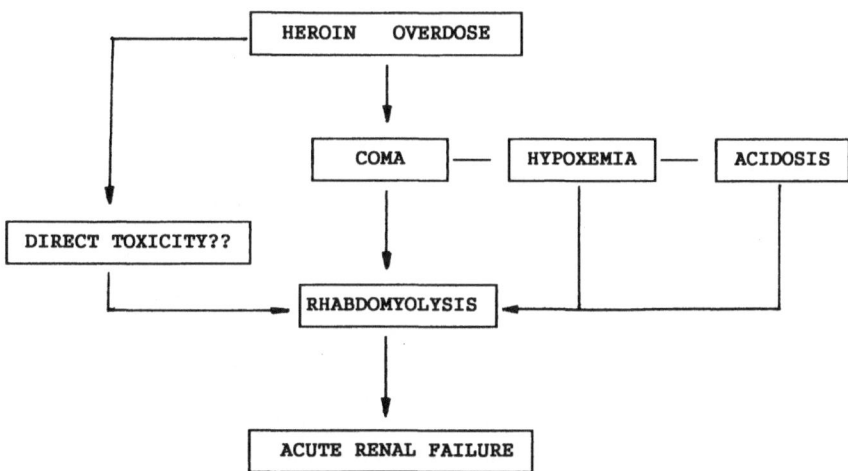

Fig. 1. Mechanisms of rhabdomyolysis in heroin overdose

pression produced by profound sedation: this compression, that is aggravated by hypoxia, acidosis and hypovolemia, induces a renal "pressure necrosis", that can be easily identified by important serum levels increase of SGOT, SGPT, CPK and LDH muscular isoenzymes. Moreover, if performed early, urine analysis shows large amount of heme and myoglobin [3]. However, a possible direct toxic effect of heroin, although difficult to prove, must be considered.

The clinical picture is similar to that of non traumatic rhabdomyolysis and the treatment is non specific. Outcome is generally good.

Heroin Induced Pulmonary Edema

Pulmonary edema following heroin overdose (HPE), is a well recognized entity and has been described more than 100 years ago by Osler. However, although there is large evidence that HPE has a non-cardiogenic origin, many pulmonary and hemodynamic aspects remain obscure. Also the real incidence among heroin overdoses is not well known. The major pathophysiologic factors that have been considered in the past are hypoxia, a particular hypersensitivity to heroin or to a contaminating excipient, and a direct toxic action of the drug.

Profound hypoxia has been reported as responsible of pulmonary edema during high altitude pulmonary edema (HAPO) [5]. Moreover HAPO develops in subjects with important individual variation in pulmonary vascular response to hypoxia [5], and can be reproduced in animals only in an experimental setting that combines profound hypoxemia and physical exercise [6].

Although hypoxia can be observed in heroin overdose patients as a consequence of marked central hypoventilation, this picture can also be observed in other intoxications characterized by respiratory depression (i.e. barbiturate overdose), in which pulmonary edema is not observed.

A hypersensitivity mechanism to heroin or excipients is also hard to prove as

(a) pulmonary edema has been described in some patients in the absence of prior exposition to opiates ([7], personal observation);
(b) pulmonary edema after opiates IV injection has been observed also after use of commercially prepared, uncontaminated solution made for medical use [3].

However, there is large evidence that heroin can produce a dramatic outpouring of large quantities of fluid from the vascular compartment into the alveoli (as shown by the constant observations of low right atrial pressure and high hematocrit value) by increasing capillary permeability. In 1972 Katz and coworkers [8], analyzed simultaneously samples of blood and pulmonary edema fluid from 5 patients mechanically ventilated for heroin pulmonary edema and 5 patients mechanically ventilated for cardiogenic pulmonary edema. While in cardiogenic edema the total proteins of the edema fluid averaged only $40 \pm 7\%$ of the blood protein concentration, in heroin induced edema the protein content of the edema fluid averaged $96 \pm 7\%$ of the blood protein content. Moreover, in the HPE patients the protein fractions were similar in edema fluid and in blood. Similar findings had been observed by Frand et al. [9], both after heroin overdose and after methadone overdose. These observations suggested a possible common pathway for the induction of pulmonary edema after morphine derivative abuse. In our experience the presence of a protein edema fluid concentration close to blood concentration is constant in HPE patients.

In the severe cases the clinical picture of HPE is similar to adult respiratory distress syndrome (ARDS): the patients are severely hypoxic, hypercapnic and their chest X-ray shows diffuse bilateral pulmonary infiltrates. Few data are available about pulmonary mechanics in the early phase of acute respiratory failure. We have recently evaluated pulmonary mechanics in a group of 6 HPE patients treated in our ICU, and observed a severe reduction in static thoracopulmonary compliance ($C_{st} < 30$ ml/cm H_2O^{-1}), and a moderate increase in airway resistance without air trapping phenomenon.

Although similar to ARDS, HPE syndrome is characterized by a rapid response to mechanical ventilation with positive end-expiratory pressure (PEEP), and by a favorable outcome. In our experience weaning from mechanical ventilation is obtained after 2–4 days and survival rate is 100%. Similar results have been reported by Frand et al. [9]. When the hemodynamic data are analyzed in the first hours after the onset of pulmonary edema, HPE patients seem relatively hypovolemic, showing low right atrial pressure values and very low pulmonary capillary occlusion pressure. These findings confirm the absence of cardiogenic mechanisms in the genesis of pulmonary edema following heroin injection. If a small amount of fluids is administered to preserve renal function, an hyperdynamic state with high values of cardiac output, low systemic vascular resistances and moderately increased heart rate can occur. However, this hyperdynamic state, always associated with low values of pulmonary capillary occlusion pressure can be observed in some patients also in the early phase.

Pulmonary function after HPE has been extensively studied by Frand et al. [9] in a group of 16 patients, 6 of which required mechanical ventilation. Interestingly, although PaO_2 levels and pulmonary volumes increased to normal values within a week in 13 of the 16 patients, CO diffusion capacity (DLCO) was still reduced after several weeks. These data are consistent with our findings: a mean three-month delay for the DLCO values to return to normality.

In conclusion, heroin-induced pulmonary edema seems to be a clinical entity produced by direct or indirect lesional permeabilization of the pulmonary microvascular tree. Although in the early phases it mimicks ARDS with respect to gas exchange alterations, pulmonary mechanics and hemodynamic pattern, HPE has generally a rapidly favorable evolution. Therefore it should probably not be considered, in its uncomplicated presentation, as a form of ARDS.

References

1. Evans LE, Swanson CF, Roscoe P, Prescott LF (1973) Treatment of drug overdosage with naloxone, a specific narcotic antagonist. Lancet 1:721–724
2. Bradberry C, Raebel M (1981) Continuous infusion of naloxone in the treatment of narcotic overdose. Drug Intell Clin Pharmacy 15:945–949
3. Fraser D (1971) Methadone overdose. JAMA 217 10:1387–1389
4. Richter RW, Challenor YB, Pearson J, et al (1970) Acute myoglobinuria associated with heroin addiction. Clin Res 18:695
5. Wiswanathan R, Ain SK, Subramanian S (1969) Pulmonary edema of high altitude: pathogenesis. Am Rev Respir Dis 100:342–349
6. Whaine TF, Severnghaus JW (1968) Experimental hypoxic pulmonary oedema in the rat. J Appl Physiol 25:729–732
7. Steinberg AD, Karliner JS (1968) The clinical spectrum of heroin pulmonary oedema. Arch Intern Med 122:122–127
8. Katz S, Aberman A, Frand UI, Stein IM, Fulop M (1972) Heroin pulmonary edema: evidence for increased pulmonary capillary permeability. Am Rev Respir Dis 106:472–474
9. Frand U, Chang HS, Henry Williams M (1972) Heroin induced pulmonary oedema. Ann Intern Med 77:29–35

Mushroom Poisoning

M. Langer, S. Vesconi, and D. Costantino

Introduction

Mushroom poisoning, a well known problem in Central Europe is now recognized as a major problem also in the United States where the gathering of wild mushroom seems to become more and more popular. Nobody can define the incidence of this medical emergency. Years ago Costantino [1] estimated only for the *Amanita* poisoning. 50–100 cases/year in Northern Italy and large patient populations are reported also from France, Germany, Hungary, Czechoslovakia and Poland. Friedman [2] reports for the USA "... more than 100 deaths each year from consumption of wild mushrooms".

Amatoxin poisoning, mainly due to ingestion of *Amanita phalloides* is by far the most frequently dangerous intoxication. The knowledge about amatoxin poisoning, which accounts for more than 90% of the fatalities, had an important evolution over the last 15 years. This intoxication is now well investigated, the toxins are identified [3], the mechanism of action is described [4, 5] many details are known about the kinetics of the toxins in experimental [6–8] and in human poisoning [9]. The capital importance of early suspicion of this uncommon diagnosis and application of aggressive treatment (before the evidence of severe liver damage) is now recognized. The use of these therapeutic principles based on fluid replacement combined with various removal approaches and drug administration allowed to lower the mortality rate to approximately 10–15% in *Amanita phalloides* poisoning [10, 11] compared to the 50% mortality reported by Friedman [2] and the 90% mortality in an earlier edition of Harrison's Textbook.

A new therapeutic option is patients with very severe amatoxin intoxication, fulminant liver failure and extremely high risk of death is now the liver transplantation. Until now only few cases are reported [12], but liver transplantation may be the only possible treatment if organ failure is otherwise irreversible.

Gastro-intestinal Symptoms After Mushroom Ingestion

Nearly all patients with mushroom poisoning suffer first from gastro-intestinal (GI) symptoms (diarrhea, vomiting, abdominal pain), but obviously not all GI symptoms after mushroom ingestion are due to intrinsic toxicity of the fungi. A differential diagnosis must include other forms of concomitant food poisoning, ethanol abuse, viral or bacterial gastro-enteritis as well as possible surgical causes of the symptoms.

The most useful criterion for the "not-mycologically trained" physician to classify the clinically relevant syndromes of fungal poisoning is the time elapsed between the mushroom ingestion and the onset of GI symptoms ("period of latency"). This allows to distinguish between short latency (less than 6 hours) and those with long latency (more than 6 hours) intoxications (Table 1). The analysis of clinical symptoms is rarely sufficient to establish a precise diagnosis, but the evidence of mushroom ingestion, the "period of latency" and the nature of the GI symptoms are sufficient for a presumptive diagnosis necessary for appropriate emergency treatment.

A definite diagnosis in this early phase is possible if a mycologist's diagnosis on mushroom residuals (preferably uncooked) is available or – in the case of

Table 1. Mushroom poisoning: "flow chart". Vomiting, diarrhea, nausea, and abdominal pain are the leading GI symptoms

Mushroom ingestion	
long latency (6–18 hours)	short latency (1/2–4 hours)
Amatoxin poisoning	**Gastrointestinal Syndrome**
mainly *Amanita phalloides*	many different species of mushrooms
Amanita virosa/verna –	*Sy: GI symptoms, rarely liver damage*
Lepiota sp (helveola, burneo-incarnata, subincarnata)	Tr: symptomatic
Galerina marginata	
Sy + Tr see text	
Gyromitra poisoning	**Muscarine-like syndrome**
Gyromitra esculenta	*Inocybe patouillardi*
Sarcxosphera coronaria	*Clitocybe sp.*
Tox: gyromitrine	Tox: muscarine
Sy: GI, CNS symptoms incl. seizures, liver/kidney failure, hemolysis	Sy: GI symptoms, sweating, salivation, myosis, bradycardia, bronchospasm
Tr: removal of toxins, pyridoxin (neurotox.)	Tr: removal of toxins, atropine
Orellanus poisoning	**Atropine-like syndrome**
Cortinarius orellanus,	*Amanita muscaria*
C. speciosissimus,	*Amanita pantherina*
C. orellanoides	Tox: different toxins
Tox: orellanine	Sy: GI symptoms, mydriasis, mental confusion, restlessness, coma, hallucinations
Sy: mild, inconstant GI symptoms (lat. 6–8 hrs)– asthenia, non specific symptoms (about 1 week)– renal failure (1–3 weeks)	Tr: removal of toxins, benzodiazepines, symptomatic
Tr: removal ??	
symptomatic treatment (hemodialysis)	
	Disulfiram-like syndrome
	Coprinus atramentarius + alcoholics
	Tox: coprine
	Sy: tachycardia, vasodilation
	Tr: symptomatic

Tox toxins, *Sy* symptoms, *Tr* treatment

amatoxin poisoning – if amatoxin determination (RIA) can immediately be performed on the urine. Besides the above mentioned criteria, also the examination of all involved commensals and the presentation of colored tables to those who collected and cooked the mushroom meal may prove helpful in a very early phase.

Mushroom Poisoning with Short Latency

A high number of wild mushrooms may be toxic or at least irritant for the human GI tract or contain neurotoxic substances. Four major clinically relevant syndromes are generally reported (Table 1) and seem useful to classify and treat the most common mushroom poisonings with a short period of latency (30 min–4 hours).

Nearly all these intoxications have a favorable prognosis and are self limiting so that the medical intervention will just shorten the course.

Gastric lavage is indicated when vomiting is absent or insufficient; cathartics and/or activated charcoal may always be useful. In isolated cases of *Clitocybe* or *Inocybe* intoxication (muscarine-like syndrome), atropine is a specific antidote, which may control potentially dangerous symptoms like bradycardia.

In amateur mycologists with very poor knowledge in wild mushrooms also the possibility of a collection and consumption of different toxic species (with short and long latency period) must sometimes be taken in account.

Mushroom Intoxications with GI Symptoms After a Long Latency Period

All dangerous mushroom poisonings show an onset of symptoms after a long latency period. This is useful to identify patients at high risk of severe organ damage but makes the removal of toxins much more difficult. From the 3 syndromes reported in Table 1 the most relevant intoxication is the Amatoxin poisoning.

Amatoxin poisoning

Chemical structure, toxin content of mushrooms: Amatoxins, a group of chemically defined octapeptides with a molecular weight of 900 daltons [3], are present in different species of wild mushroom (Table 1) and their concentration is reported as 0.2–0.4 mg/g fresh tissue of *Amanita phalloides* [13]. The concentration of toxins is however variable non only between the amatoxin containing species [13] but also from year to year, from site to site and also between the parts of the mushroom (gills > stipe > cap > bulb – spores controversial) [14].

Mode of action and tissue penetration: Amatoxins are considered the sole cause of fatalities in human poisoning [5]. They produce their severe cellular damage by binding to nuclear RNA polymerase B of eucaryotic cells, inhibiting enzymatic activity and leading to cell necrosis [4, 5]. Although amatoxins are equally toxic to all cells, in human poisoning they exhibit an apparent specific toxicity to hepatocytes, intestinal epithelium – and kidney (?) cells [5]. The mechanism of toxin uptake is not entirely clarified; the transport in liver cells apparently takes place in the same system that mediates the flux of bile salts under physiologic conditions [15].

Amatoxin concentration in biological samples – kinetics of amatoxins: Toxins can be determined in early specimens of poisoned patients [9] in concentrations of few nanograms/ml. Similar concentrations are found during experimental poisoning in blood and liver tissue of dogs [8, 7]; the toxins are eliminated through the bile and kidney and the importance of entero-hepatic circulation has been established in experimental studies [6] while the amount of toxins eliminated in the urine was determined also in clinical poisoning [9].

Figure 1 reports serum and urine detection for amatoxins in patients treated early for *Amanita phalloides* poisoning in our hospital. Not all patients had detectable (limit of the RIA determination was 0.5 ng/ml) levels in the blood, while all urine samples were positive with also very high values (> 100 ng/ml) in the first, very concentrated urine.

Figure 2 (modified from [5]) summarizes the kinetics of the toxins and emphasizes the two elimination routes which can be forced therapeutically.

Clinical presentation of patients with amatoxin poisoning: The latency period typically ranges from 6–18 hours, the GI symptoms are generally severe with marked dehydration. Emergency admission occurs, in our experience, mostly around 12 hours after ingestion. Usually all commensals have symptoms but the severity of symptoms does not reflect the prognosis.

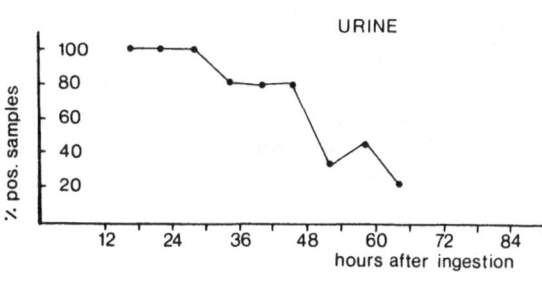

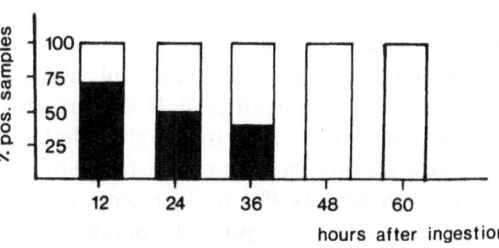

Fig. 1. Amatoxins in urine and serum: Amatoxins were demonstrable in all (7/7) initial urine samples (upper part) while the percentage of positivities in serial serum samples of 14 patients (lower part) was 75% at 12 hours and 0 at 48 hours. (From [9])

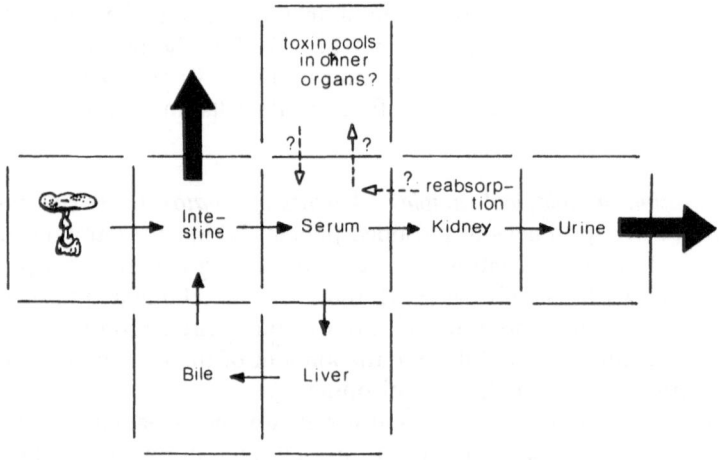

Fig. 2. Kinetics of amatoxins in human poisoning. Arrows show the two possible elimination routes, if urinary output is maintained and entero-hepatic circulation stopped. (From [5])

The diagnosis of amatoxin poisoning already at the first observation is of vital importance. It can be proven only by mycological examination (uncooked mushrooms > cooked mushrooms > rests in vomiting > spors from gastric lavage) or by the amatoxin detection in the urine.

A presumed diagnosis is therefore necessary first, and is based on:

1. evidence of wild mushroom ingestion and GI symptoms after a long latency
2. presence of similar symptoms also in other commensals.

The identification of amatoxin containing mushrooms on colored tables may corroborate the presumed diagnosis in some cases. Other laboratory tests (SGOT, SGPT, bilirubin, prothrombin time ...) at that time are normal or reflect just previous illness or severe hemoconcentration.

The loss of water and salts during this "cholera like" diarrhea, when vomiting inhibits the oral ingestion of fluids is the most striking feature and some reported early deaths as well as early renal failure are certainly related to hypovolemia, dehydration and hypokalemia rater than to the cytotoxicity of mushrooms.

The first signs of liver necrosis become evident about 36 hours after ingestion with raising transaminases and – with slight delay – prolongation of prothrombin time. The extent of liver injury has been classified according to several parameters, such as "clinical course", "maximum SGPT levels", "prothrombin complex" and "bilirubin" [10]. All patients with lethal poisoning showed maximum SGPT levels above 1000 mU/ml; high SGPT/SGOT levels however do not predict outcome. Vesconi et al. [10, 16] reported a favorable outcome also in 13 of 19 patients with a liver injury classified as "severe".

Figure 3 reports the time course of mean values of liver enzymes, bilirubin and prothrombin activity (%) in 3 patients who survived severe *Amanita phalloides* intoxication. Figure 4 reports the parallel course of two children, brother (surviv-

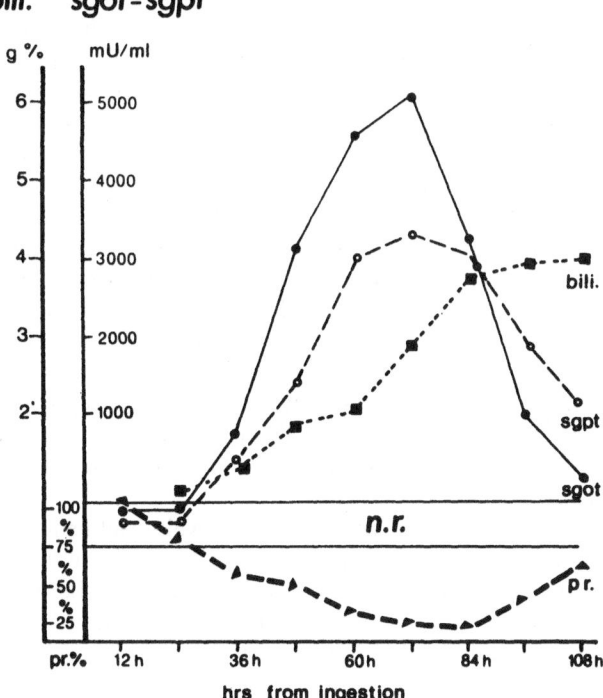

bili.   sgot-sgpt

Fig. 3. Time course of liver enzymes (SGOT, SGPT mU/ml), bilirubin (bili mg/100 ml) and prothrombin activity (pr %) in severe but not lethal *Amanita phalloides* poisoning (mean values from 3 surviving patients). At the time of hospital admission no abnormal values can be found; the raise in SGOT/SGPT is followed shortly by the prolongation of the prothrombin time. The elevation of bilirubin is a relatively late and longer persistent phenomenon. n.r. = normal range

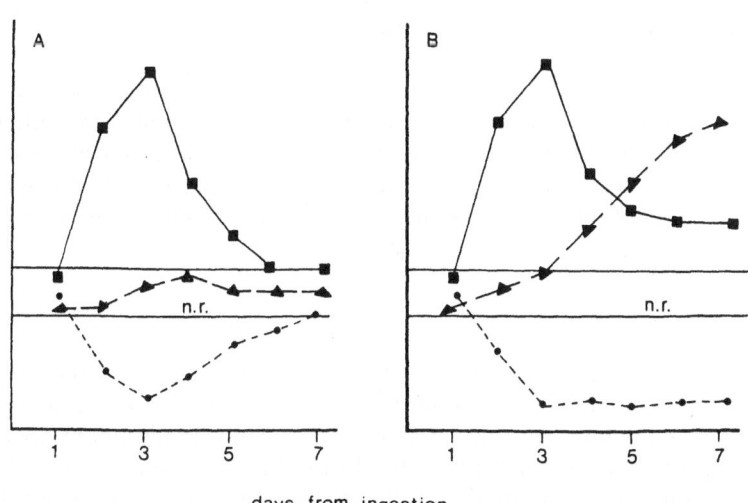

days from ingestion

Fig. 4A, B. Parallel course of two children, brother (A, surviving) and sister (B, dying) from *Amanita phalloides* poisoning. The figure reports the time course of SGPT (rectangles), alpha-amino-nitrogen (as an overall indicator of the amino acid pool; triangles) and the prothrombin activity (expressed as %; circles). n.r. = normal range

ing) and sister (dying) from amatoxin poisoning: the different evolution cannot be seen in the levels of transaminases but rather in the persistent low levels of prothrombin activity and the raising levels of alpha-amino-nitrogen.

The clinical evaluation of the patient with amatoxin poisoning and severe liver injury is the same as in other forms of fulminant hepatic failure. The most dangerous complications are bleeding, hypoglycemia, hypoxia, cerebral edema and circulatory failure.

Complete recovery is possible from a minimal, mild or severe liver damage. Also in our series patients with persistent abnormalities in liver function were observed, which were ascribed more to post-transfusional hepatitis than to toxic injury. From our past experience [10] about one-third of amatoxin poisoned patients will experience severe liver injury with a high risk of death (6 of 19 pts). In those years (1975–1979) liver transplantation was not available and all patients who progressed to severe liver failure and deep coma requiring respiratory support, died after 6–11 days. The earlier deaths were due to uncontrolled bleeding and later deaths to respiratory-, circulatory failure, infections and hepato-renal syndrome.

Today liver transplantation is a well established treatment of fulminant liver failure due to viral hepatitis as well as to toxic exposure [17]. The case reports from Fig. 4 show a clear difference between the two children at day 5: the liver of patient A is recovering (raising prothrombin activity), there is no accumulation of amino-acids (alpha-amino-nitrogen within normal range) as confirmed by a better neurological score than her brother (patient B). At day 5 patient B is clearly doing worse, despite only slightly elevated transaminases; the synthesis of clotting factors remains low and also the raising alpha-amino-nitrogen indicates that liver parenchyma is failing. Retrospectively we can state that this patient should have been included in a transplant program at day 5. In fact, in our past experience, no patient with the progression to degree 4+ of hepatic encephalopathy due to amatoxin poisoning recovered. This experience is in agreement with the review of Klein et al. [12] who found only one case report of a patient recovered from coma. In the last 10 years, however, intensive care improved and it is now possible to support patients better and for a longer time even with a failing liver. This may be a reason for the recovery of a patient at our ICU in Autumn 1989, who had no liver transplant because of lack of donors.

Case Report

A 14 year old boy showed severe GI symptoms 8 hours after ingestion of about 300 g of amatoxin containing *Lepiota burneo-incarnata* (mycologist's diagnosis). He was admitted at 12 hours to the first hospital (without any specific treatment) and transferred to a University Hospital at 36 hours because of SGOT/SGPT elevation. At 60 hours the prothrombin activity was < 10% and the patient was transferred to our unit as a possible candidate for liver transplantation. The peak SGOT/SGPT levels were reached at day 4 (4580/5350 mU/ml) with prothrombin activity mantained between 25–35% with 2000 ml FFP/day. At the same day the patient showed a 1+ grade encephalopathy. The neurological status however rapidly deteriorated and, at day 6, the patient was in hepatic coma (4 + grade encephalopathy) with high amplitude delta waves in the EEG. Respiratory support was instituted. At day 7 the coma deepened further with decorticate and decerebrate posture. Despite 4 days "urgent" italian and 1 day "superurgent" european list, no liver donor was available.

At 8–9 days the patient became more stable, neurological status was graded as 3 +, less amounts of plasma were needed to correct prothrombin time and the bilirubin level (10 mg/100 ml) was stable. At day 10 the patient localized stimuli and was for short periods responsive; he was no more considered as a candidate for liver transplantation. He was extubated at day 12 and transferred 2 days later with a fair liver function (SGOT/SGPT nearly normal, bilirubin 6.2 mg/dl, prothrombin activity 60%, alpha-fetoprotein 15x normal). Two months later the patient had no neurological sequelae and a nearly normal liver function. No liver biopsy was performed.

The evaluation of the reversibility of the liver failure seems the most difficult clinical problem in severe amatoxin poisoning. Successful transplantation in some patients on the one hand and spontaneous reversal of extremely severe liver failure on the other hand, make decisions very difficult. The possibility of liver transplantation gives the intensive support in amatoxin poisoned patients with severe encephalopathy a new end-point. The survival, with or witout graft, will certainly improve.

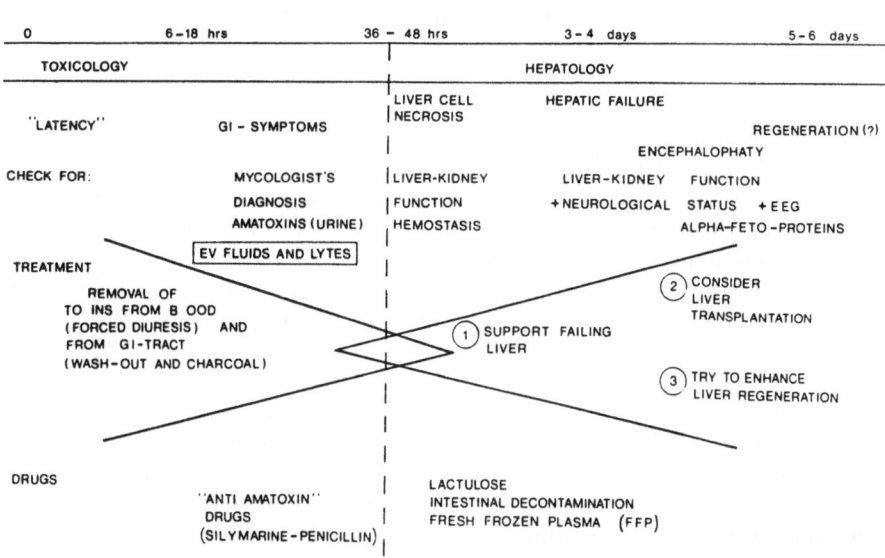

Fig. 5. Synopsis of the treatment of the amatoxin poisoning. The treatment priorities in the two principal phases are different: a toxicological approach with treatment of severe dehydration, removal of toxins and "anti amatoxin" drugs will be successful in a very early phase; later, if the toxin load was very high or the toxicological treatments failed, the liver function must be supported and the liver regeneration stimulated. Liver transplantation may be a life-saving procedure in selected patients (see text)

Treatment of amatoxin poisoning: The treatment is in two phases (Fig. 5):

- initially the goals are, as in all other intoxications, the removal of toxins, the administration of "antidotes", and the treatment of symptoms;
- in the second phase, when the parenchymal injuries become manifest and nearly no more toxins can be found in biological fluids, the patients need treatment for their liver failure.

Removal of circulating toxins: The possibility of the removal of toxins was controversial until 10 years ago and only the introduction of RIA determinations in clinical practice showed that, despite the long latency period, amotoxins are still detectable in the blood of many patients [9] and that forced diuresis is the most effective, safest and cheapest removal treatment. It can be applied without delay and simultaneously to several poisoned patients admitted together even to small hospitals, were dialysis, hemofiltration ... are not available [10, 18].

To obtain a high urinary output in a dehydrated patient, a large volume of iv fluids must be administered in the first hours and, with a small dose of furosemide (5–10 mg) as starter, a 150–400 ml/h urinary flow can be obtained already from the first hour.

Also other forms of removal are effective (hemodialysis, hemofiltration, charcoal-hemoperfusion [5]) but, in our opinion, they should be applied only if fluid and toxin elimination through the kidneys cannot be achieved.

Forced diuresis can be applied also when the diagnosis of amatoxin poisoning is still suspected but unproven. An early removal has the highest probability to eliminate considerable amounts of circulating toxins [10] and fluid administration to obtain high urine output should be started without waiting for RIA determinations or mycologist's diagnosis.

Removal of toxins from the GI tract: In the early phase the GI tract contains always residuals of mushrooms, spors and toxins eliminated with the bile. The absorption of toxins from the GI tract is only partially inhibited by patients diarrhea and vomiting and an accurate intestinal wash out and the adsorption of the toxins to activated charcoal are mandatory.

At our institution forced diuresis (with decreasing volumes after the first 12 hours) and lactulose/charcoal treatment continue until 48–60 hours from ingestion.

"Antidotes": No true antidote is available and an extremely high number of substances and drugs have been applied in patients or investigated in different experimental models [11]. Methodological difficulties make the clinical evaluation of the different protocols nearly impossible. In his review, Floersheim [11] recommends to opt for penicillin and silibenin as "the more specific antidotal therapy". Suggested doses are: penicillin G 1 000 000 U/kg/day, silymarin 20–50 mg/kg/day. The mechanism of action of those drugs is not entirely clear but both showed to exert positive effects in clinical studies, experimental animals and in vitro experiments by reducing the amatoxin uptake to hepatocytes [19].

As the removal procedures, drugs should be applied as early as possible taking into account the possible allergic reactions to penicillin.

Treatment of symptoms: The only symptom to be treated in the early phase of Amanita poisoning is the severe dehydration and the possible electrolyte imbalance. The aggressive fluid resucitation need a minimum of expertise and monitoring of the central venous pressure is suggested.

Vomiting and diarrhea cease spontaneously and any symptomatic treatment against those symptoms may be dangerous.

Prevention of secondary injuries: While the extent of the liver failure will depend only from the number of liver cells destroyed by the toxins, secondary injuries like hypoglycemia can certainly be prevented. The infusion of fresh frozen plasma should maintain the prothrombin activity above 20–25% to minimize the risk of bleeding (2000 ml/day may be required). Lactulose administration, digestive decontamination, infusion of glucose/insulin and amino acids are useful to reduce protein catabolism to limit hepatic encephalopathy.

Overhydration will enhance cerebral edema and should be avoided like hypercapnia due to hypoventilation.

Once intubated, the respiratory support should be choosen according the patients breathing pattern, mantaining – whenever possible – a spontaneous breathing activity (PS-IMV/CPAP-IMV ...). The intensive care management of an amatoxin poisoned patient with severe liver failure and coma is the same as in the fulminant liver failure due to viral infection. It is possible that regeneration will take place earlier than in viral hepatitis, the action of the toxins being limited to the initial period. Monitoring of α-fetoprotein may help to evidence if liver regeneration is going on.

Gyromitra poisoning

Gyromitra toxins were identified in the late 1960s [20] but the mechanism of action is not clear [21].

The interval between ingestion and GI symptoms is, like in amatoxin poisoning, 6–12 hours; there are no specific tests to identify the toxins in biological fluids but the fungus has a highly characteristic aspect and can be described also by non-mycologists. The GI symptoms are followed (36–48 hours from ingestion) by signs of liver cell injury but, at difference to amatoxin poisoning, also neurological symptoms become manifest (restlessness – stupor, dizziness, tremor, seizures, anisochria, diplopia, nystagmus). Hemolysis is a very typical but not constant finding. The literature reports fatal cases mainly due to liver failure.

The occurrence of Gyromitra poisoning is rather rare and, compared to amatoxin poisoning, few data are available. The chemical structure of Gyromitra toxins allows a renal excretion and forced diuresis is suggested for 24–96 hours; wash out of the GI tract and charcoal treatment should be applied as in other forms of food poisoning. The treatment of symptoms includes fluid resuscitation and the administration of pyridoxine (100–600 mg/day) for the neurological symptoms.

Orellanus poisoning

Orellanus poisoning is reported to complete this review even if initial GI symptoms are rarely observed and patients report their symptoms retrospectively when they are hospitalized because of renal failure (7–17 days from mushroom ingestion).

In 1985, Costantino [22] analyzed from the literature 44 patients regarding their renal function after Orellanus poisoning: 19 recovered without impairment, 11 were on hemodialysis, 6 had a kidney transplant and 8 had a fair but reduced renal function. Although we have no personal experience in Orellanus poisoning, we consider this possibility in all patients with GI symptoms after mushroom ingestion and without liver injury at 48 hours, requesting the mycologist's diagnosis as well as kidney function tests at 2–3 weeks.

References

1. Costantino D (1978) Mushroom poisoning in Italy. Intern J Art Organs 1:257–259
2. Friedman PA (1987) Poisoning and its management. In: Braunwald E, et al (eds) Harrison's principles of internal medicine, 11th edn. Mc Graw-Hill, New York, pp 838–850
3. Wieland T (1968) Poisonous principles of mushrooms of the genous amanita. Science 159:946–952
4. Fiume L, Wieland T (1970) Amanitins, chemistry and action. FEBS letter 8:1–5
5. Faulstich H (1979) New aspects of amanita poisoning. Klin Wochenschr 57:1143–1145
6. Fauser U, Faulstich H (1973) Beobachtungen zur Therapie der Knollenblätterpilzvergiftung. Dtsch Med Wschr 98:2259
7. Faulstich H, Fauser U (1975) Amanita poisoning in the dog. In: Keppler D (ed) Pathogenesis and mechanism of liver cell necrosis. MTP press Ltd, Lancaster, pp 69–75
8. Busi C, Fiume L, Costantino D, et al (1977) Déterminations des amanitines dans le sérum de patients intoxiqués par l'amanite phalloide. Nouv Presse Méd 6:2855–2857
9. Langer M, Vesconi S, Costantino D, Busi C (1980) Pharmacodynamics of amatoxins in human poisoning as the basis for the removal treatment. In: Faulstich H, Kommarell B, Wieland T (eds) Amanita toxins and poisoning. Witzstrock, Baden-Baden, pp 90–95
10. Vesconi S, Langer M, Iapichino G, Costantino D, Busi C, Fiume L (1985) Therapy of cytotoxic mushroom intoxication. Crit Care Med 13:402–406
11. Floersheim GL (1987) Treatment of human amatoxin mushroom poisoning. Myths and advances in therapy. Med Toxicol 2:1–9
12. Klein AS, Hart J, Brems JJ, Goldstein L, Lewin K, Busuttil RW (1989) Amanita poisoning: treatment and the role of liver transplantation. Am J Med 86:187–193
13. Seeger S, Stijve T (1980) Occurrence of toxic Amanita species. In: Faulstich H, Kommarell B, Wieland T (eds) Amanita toxins and poisoning. Witzstrock, Baden-Baden, pp 3–17
14. Bodenmueller H, Faulstich H, Wieland T (1980) Distribution of amatoxins in amanita phalloides mushrooms. In: Faulstich H, Kommarell B, Wieland T (eds) Amanita toxins and poisoning. Witzstrock, Baden-Baden, pp 18–22
15. Kroncke KD, Fricker G, Meier PJ, Gerok W, Wieland T (1986) Alpha-amanitin uptake into hepatocytes. J Biol Chem 261:12562–12567
16. Vesconi S, Langer M, Costantino D, Iapichino G, Macchi R (1980) Clinical evaluation of amatoxin removal approach in amanita phalloides poisoning. In: Faulstich H, Kommarell B, Wieland T (eds) Amanita toxins and poisoning. Witzstrock, Baden-Baden, pp 232–236
17. Starzl TE, Demetris AJ, Van Thiel D (1989) Liver transplantation. N Engl J Med 321:1014–1022
18. Langer M, Vesconi S, Iapichino G, Costantino D, Radrizzani D (1980) Die frühzeitige Elimination der Amanita Toxine in der Therapie der Knollenblätterpilzvergiftung. Klin Wochenschr 58:117–123
19. Jahn W, Faulstich H, Wieland T (1980) Pharmacokinetiks of 3H-methyl-dehydroxymethyl-alpha-amanitin in the isolated perfused rat liver, and the influence of several drugs. In: Faulstich H, Kommarell B, Wieland T (eds) Amanita toxins and poisoning. Witzstrock, Baden-Baden, pp 79–85

20. List PH, Luft P (1969) Gyromitrin, das Gift der Frühjahrslorchel. Archiv der Pharm 301:224
21. Braun R, Greef U, Netter KJ (1979) Liver injury by the false morel poison gyromitrin. Toxicology 12:155
22. Costantino D (1985) Sindrome orellanica. In: Costantino D (ed) Gli avvelenamenti da funghi a lunga incubazione. Farmitalia, pp 119-149

Poisoning by Agricultural Chemicals – Organophosphates and Paraquat

K. Koyama, M. Yamashita, and M. Takeda

Introduction

Though, there are many kinds of agricultural chemicals in the world, the most common causes of poisoning are organophosphates and paraquat. We present here some experimental and clinical results for these two chemicals in the last several years.

Organophosphates

Absorption Rate

We experienced a case of trichlorfon poisoning where the death occurred shortly after ingestion. Therefore we compared the absorption of trichlorfon to that of other organophosphates. In anesthetized dogs 200 mg/kg of one of the organophosphates was administered through the gastric tube. The blood level of organophosphates were measured. Trichlorfon and dichlorvos were absorbed more rapidly than other organophosphates (Fig. 1). This was well correlated to the water solubility of each organophosphate (Fig. 2). Rapid development of signs of poisoning from trichlorfon can be explained by these data.

DHP [1]

We studied the effect of DHP on organophosphate poisoning, because organophosphates have relatively high fat solubility and large Vd. In anesthetized dogs EDDP (20 mg/kg) was continuously i.v. infused for 120 minutes. DHP was performed during EDDP infusion. The blood level of EDDP was checked before and after DHP column. DHP was not performed for the control dogs. Only about 3.5% of total dose were removed by DHP. However the blood level of EDDP was significantly lower and AUC was slightly smaller in DHP group (Fig. 3).

The Appropriate Dose of Atropine [2]

Excessive dose of atropine causes atropine poisoning. This study was carried out to determine the appropriate dose of atropine for each case of organophosphate

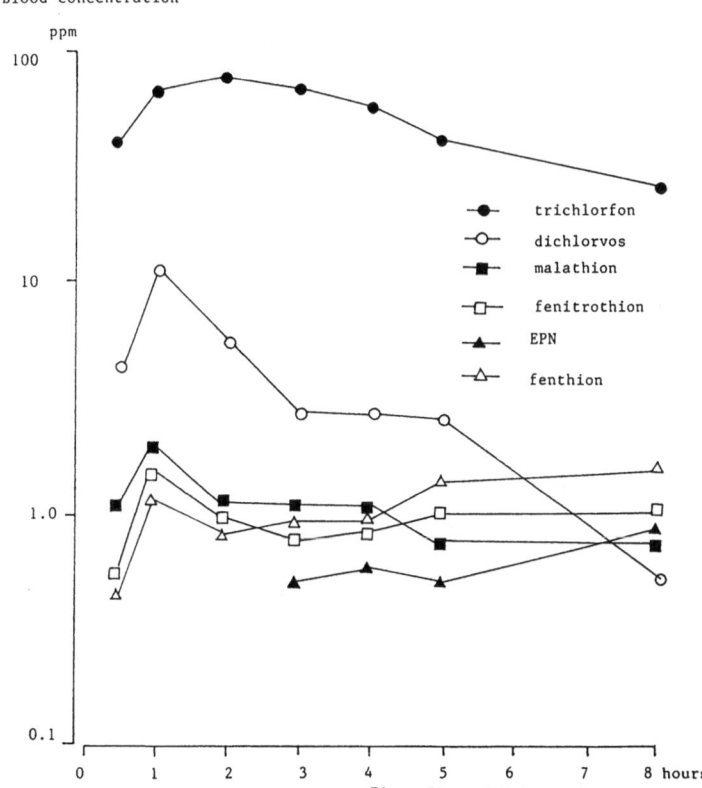

Fig. 1. Blood concentration of organophosphates after oral administration (200 mg/kg), (n = 3 for each group)

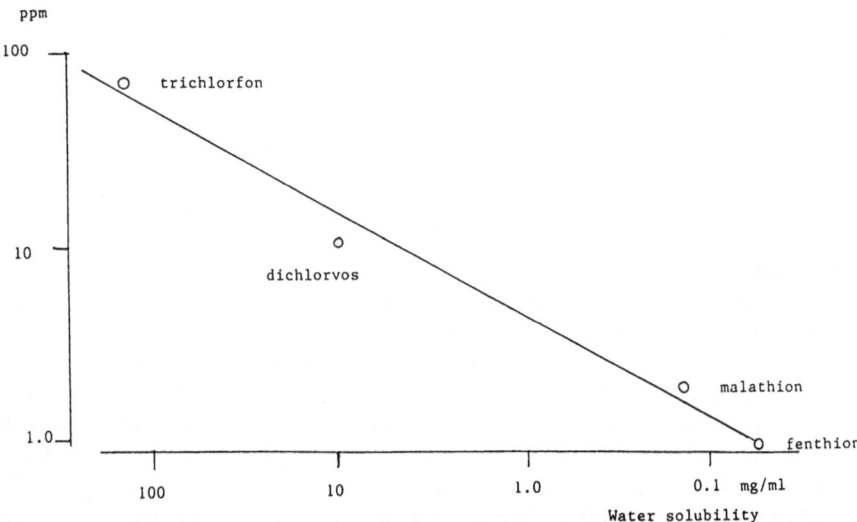

Fig. 2. Water solubility and maximum blood concentration after organophosphates administration (200 mg/kg, p.o.)

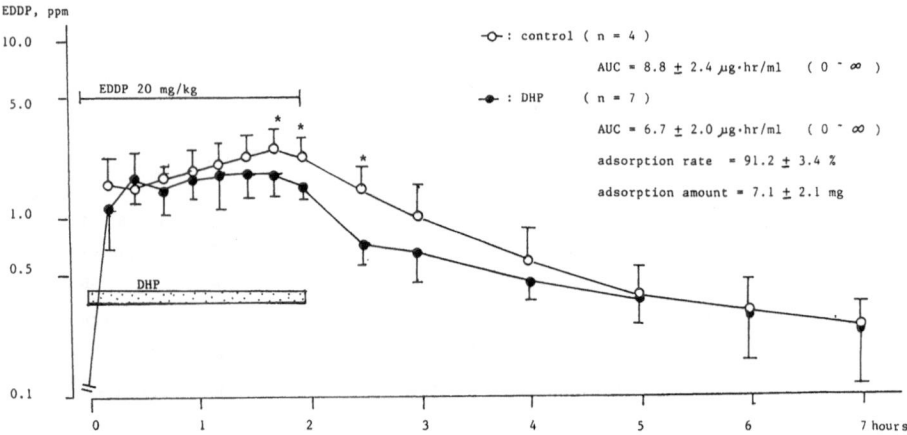

Fig. 3. The effect of DHP for blood concentration of EDDP (20 mg/kg i.v. for 120 min.). The DHP was performed during EDDP i.v. infusion; *p<0.05 vs control

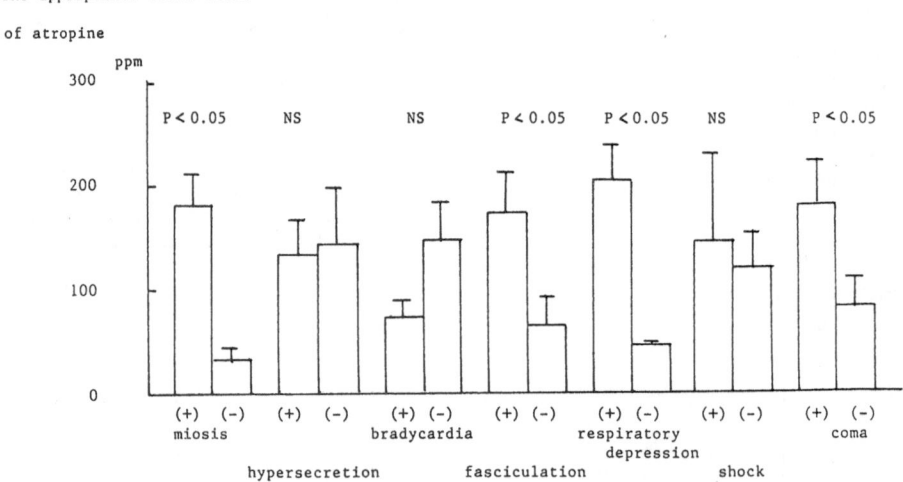

Fig. 4. The signs of admission and the appropriate blood level of atropine

poisoning. We retrospectively studied 17 cases of organophosphate poisoning in whom atropine had been infused until the signs of poisoning were disappeared. From the dose and the duration of atropine infusion, the blood atropine level (i.e. the appropriate blood level of atropine) was calculated by using the two-compartment model. Next, for every sign of organophosphate poisoning, the difference of therapeutic blood level of atropine was examined by the T-test, between the patients who had developed the signs and who had not. Then, by using the signs that showed the significant difference in the appropriate blood level of atropine, a multivariate analysis was performed to calculate therapeutic level of atropine. Myosis, fasciculation, respiratory depression, and coma showed the significant difference in the appropriate blood level of atropine (Fig.

Table 1. The appropriate blood concentration of atropine (C_A) for organophosphate poisoning; $C_A = 60.7 + X_R + X_F + X_C + X_P$ (ppm)

Respiration	Normal	$X_R = 0$
	Depressed	$X_R = 66.3$
Fasciculation	(–)	$X_F = 0$
	Local	$X_F = 115.7$
	Systemic	$X_F = 133.9$
Consciousness	Clear ¨drousy	$X_C = 0$
	Comatose	$X_C = 45$
PAM	(–)	$X_P = 0$
	Administered	$X_P = -133.2$

Multiple correlation 0.834; estimation error 64.7 (ng/ml).

4). By using these signs, the multivariate analysis was made and the formula was obtained for the appropriate blood level of atropine (Table 1). We can obtain the initial dose Xo (mg) and the infusion rate Ko (mg/kg·hr) of atropine by the following formula, derived from a two-compartment model:

$$C_A = 49.0 \text{ Ko}, \text{ Xo} = 0.4 \text{ Ko}$$

Paraquat

The effectiveness of a cation resin (Kayexalate) as an adsorbent [3, 4]. Since paraquat is completely dissociated in water, cation-exchange resins could be effective adsorbents of paraquat. Paraquat was diluted by distilled water, simulated gastric juice (J.P. first solution, pH 1.2), and simulated intestinal juice (J.P. second solution, pH 6.8). Kayexalate, Klimate, Bentonite, Adsorbin, and activated charcol were added to the paraquat solution. By determination of paraquat concentration in the solution, adsorption capacity of each adsorbent was calculated. In an animal study, wister rats were administered 0.5, 1 and 2 g/kg of Kayexalate, Adsorbine immediately after oral administration of 200 mg/kg paraquat, and the survival curve for seven days was obtained. Kayexalate adsorbed 5–6 times as much paraquat as Adsorbin did (Table 2). Survival curve of animal study (Fig. 5) indicates that Kayexalate is more effective than Adsorbine on animal survival.

Table 2. Langmuir constants of adsorption (mg/g) of paraquat by various adsorbents from aqueous solution, first solution and second solution at 37°C

	H_2O	First solution (pH 1.2)	Second solution (pH 6.8)
Kayexalate	526	357	419
Kalimate	400	305	409
Activated charcoal	54	20	70
Bentonite	60	44	61
Adsorbin	88	68	81

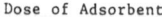

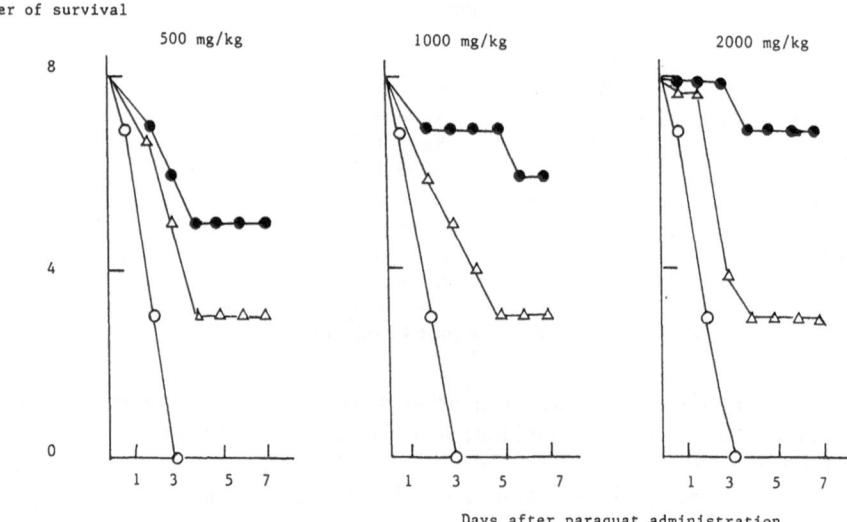

Fig. 5. Alleviation of paraquat toxicity by adsorbents in rats. o—o, paraquat; ●—●, paraquat + kayexalate; △—△, paraquat + adsorbin. Paraquat and adsorbents were given orally

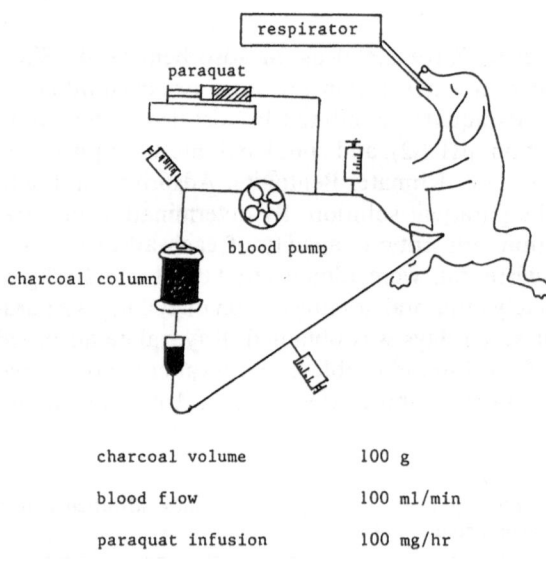

charcoal volume	100 g
blood flow	100 ml/min
paraquat infusion	100 mg/hr

Fig. 6. The sites of paraquat infusion, DHP column, and blood sampling

DHP

Because paraquat has large Vd, DHP should be performed for a long period. We studied adsorption mode of one column for 20 hours. The changes of platelet count in the systemic blood was also observed. In anesthetized dogs (n = 12), DHP was performed for 20 hours. The site of paraquat infusion and blood sampling is shown in Fig. 6. Almost all of the paraquat was adsorbed by the column for 10 hours, but paraquat could pass the column 15 hours after DHP started (Fig. 7). The systemic platelet count was decreased by 40%, 1 hour after DHP started, but did not change thereafter. If we changed the column every three

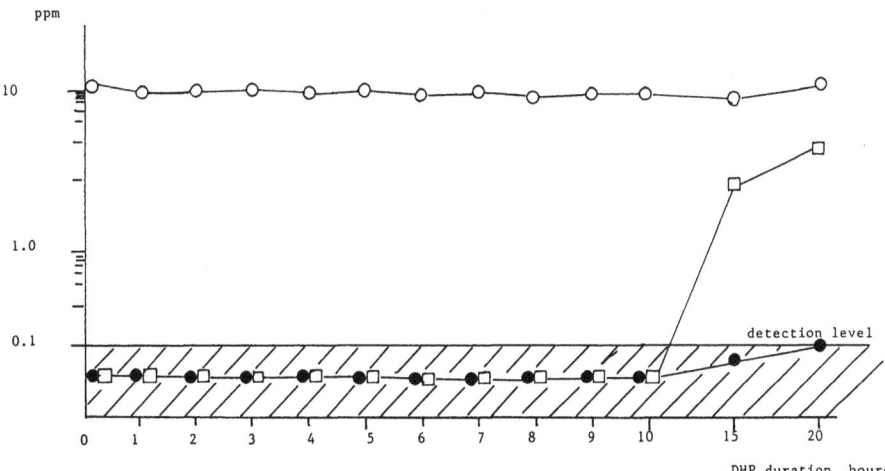

Fig. 7. Blood paraquat concentration during DHP of single column. Paraquat was continuously infused before column, and blood was sampled in each 3 sites. o—o After paraquat infusion; •—• before paraquat infusion; □—□ after column

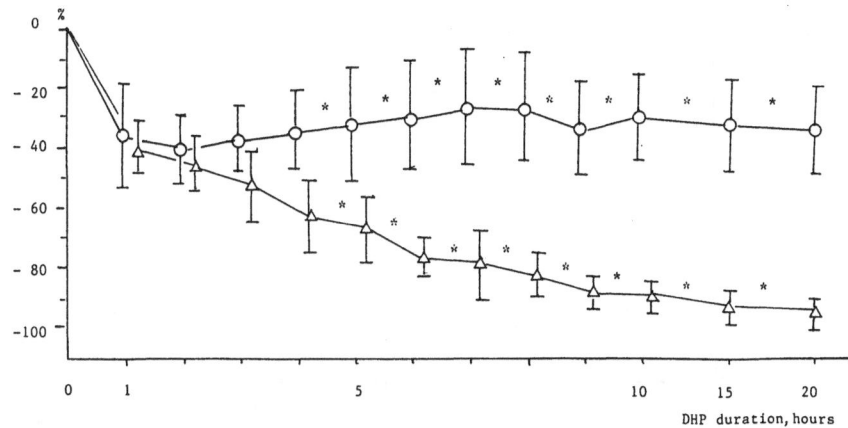

Fig. 8. Changes of platelet count during DHP. o—o One column for 20 h; ∆—∆ change column every 3 h; * $p < 0.05$

hours, the platelet count continued to decrease as long as DHP performed. Therefore, one DHP column should be used for about 10 hours in this model (Fig. 8).

Free Radical Scavengers [5]

Because the lipid peroxidation is supposed to be the cause of organ failure in paraquat poisoning, the effect of many kinds of free radical scavengers, radical catabolizing enzymes, or its activators on paraquat poisoning were studied in vivo. We studied the effects of chlorpromazine (CPZ) on paraquat poisoning for

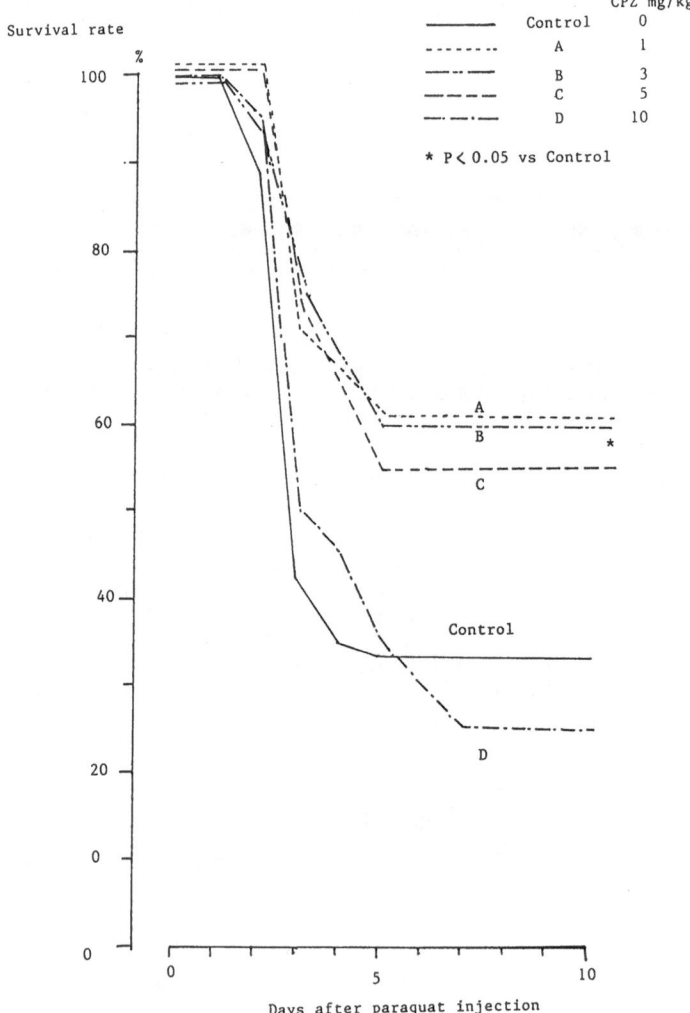

Fig. 9. Dose of CPZ and survival rate of paraquat poisoned rats

the following reasons. First, CPZ inhibits uptake and enhances efflux of paraquat in rat lung slices [6]. Second, CPZ is a free radical scavenger [7]. Third, CPZ accumulates in high concentration in the lung [8]. Fourth, CPZ has high lipid solubility and can easily penetrate into the biological membrane [9].

Sprague-Dawley rats were injected CPZ (1–10 mg/kg, s.c.) and paraquat (30 mg/kg, i.p.). Survival rate, observed for 10 days, was significantly higher in rats receiving 1–5 mg CPZ than in controls (Fig. 9). However, further studies should be performed to reveal the mechanism of CPZ effect on paraquat poisoning.

References

1. Takeda M, Yamashita M (1988) Hemoperfusion for organophosphate poisoning. Jap J Toxicol 1:55–60
2. Yamashita M (1988) Pharmacokinetics of organophosphate and its antidotes. Jap J Toxicol 1:49–54
3. Takagi S, Yamashita M, Suga H, Naito H (1983) The effectiveness of cation exchange resin as an adsorbent of paraquat both in vitro and in vivo. Vet Hum Toxicol 25 (Suppl 1):34–35
4. Yamashita M, Naito H, Takagi S (1987) The effectiveness of a cation resin (Kayexalate) as an adsorbent of paraquat: experimental and clinical studies. Hum Toxicol 6:89–90
5. Koyama K, Yamashita M, Tai T, Tajima K, Mizutani T, Naito H (1987) The effect of chlorpromazine on paraquat poisoning in rats. Vet Hum Toxicol 29:177–121
6. Siddik ZH (1979) The effect of chlorpromazine on uptake and efflux of paraquat in rat lung slices. Toxicol Appl Pharmacol 50:443–450
7. Cohen HJ (1980) Chlorpromazine inhibition of granulocyte superoxide production. Blood 56:23–29
8. Syrota A (1981) Pulmonary extraction of C-11 chlorpromazine, measured by residue detection in man. J Nucl Med 22:145–148
9. Luxnat M (1984) Membrane solubility of chlorpromazine. Biochem J 224:1023–1026

Emergency and Trauma

The Shock Index Revisited

R. A. Little, D. Gorman, and M. Allgöwer

Introduction

Trauma has been described as the last major plague of the young [1]. This is undoubtedly the case as injury is responsible for more deaths in those less than 44 years of age than, for example, heart disease and malignancies combined. Such a problem should ensure that the treatment of the injured, which has a history as long as that of surgery itself, would now be of the highest quality. That this is not the case was clearly demonstrated by Trunkey et al. in the U.S.A. They showed that as many as 73% of deaths following injury were preventable [2]. A very similar picture was revealed more recently in the U.K. [3]. This retrospective analysis of 1000 trauma deaths indicated that 63–71% of non-head and 29–37% of head injuries were preventable. An important factor in many of these deaths was a failure to recognize the presence and/or extent of blood loss. The inexperience of those first treating such patients may be part of the problem but limitations on the usefulness of the clinical signs of blood loss, an increase in heart rate and hypotension, may also be important.

In the First World War it was noted that traumatic shock was not always accompanied by a tachycardia [4], and Robertson and Bock [5] concluded that "blood pressure is of assistance in judging blood volume only when it is below a certain point, for there may be a considerable reduction of blood volume without any appreciable drop in the pressure." A study of air-raid casualties during the Second World War was also most informative [6]. All cases studied were shocked and they were categorised as hypertensive (9%), normotensive (28%) or hypotensive (63%) on initial observation. The authors stressed that the normotensive group had suffered severe injury and hemorrhage with a mortality rate of 25%. The hypotensive group (systolic blood pressure < 100 mmHg) were further divided into slow pulse rate (< 70 beats/min − 14%) normal pulse rate (43%) or rapid pulse rate (> 100 beats/min − 43%). Overall only 27% of these patients observed within the first few hours after injury had hypotension and tachycardia.

In a summary of a large amount of war-time data, Grant and Reeve [7] related systolic blood pressure to blood volume. In 68 of 70 cases with a systolic blood pressure above 100 mmHg blood volume was at least 70% of "normal", while in 22 out of 28 cases with a systolic pressure below 100 mmHg blood volume was below 70% of "normal". They concluded that systolic blood pressure was the next most useful sign after wound size "assessed as hands full of tissue damage" of blood loss. Pulse rate was not found to be of individual value confirming the findings of Keith [8] and Emerson and Ebert [9] that there was no consistent correlation between pulse rate and the degree of oligemia. When it is further considered that Grant and Reeve [7] noted that the situation was even worse once transfusion had begun it is perhaps surprising that so much weight is attached to pulse rate in the assessment of the injured patient [10].

Shock Index (SI)

The obvious shortcomings of blood pressure and pulse rate for assessing the degrees of hypovolemia led to the development of the SI [11]. This index is derived by dividing the pulse rate by the systolic blood pressure. It was hoped that by combining the changes in both pulse rate and blood pressure that the SI would be a more sensitive indicator of blood loss and a low flow state than either variable used alone. Indeed the SI was found, in a group of 175 patients with either gastro-intestinal bleeding, bleeding from open wounds or intra-abdominal/thoracic bleeding following blunt trauma, to be directly related to the magnitude of blood loss (Fig. 1). The admission values for SI were directly related to mortality, for example in a group of 80 patients with a ruptured spleen and a SI greater than 1.2 there was a 40% mortality whereas in those with a SI below 1.2 the mortality rate was 20%. Unfortunately despite this early promise the SI does not seem to have been used very widely and so it was decided to reinvestigate its usefulness as a guide to the severity of shock in a number of experimental models.

Hemorrhage in the Unanesthetized Rat

The heart rate response to hemorrhage (2.2% blood volume/min) in the unanesthetized rat is biphasic. There is an initial tachycardia up to a loss of 10-15%

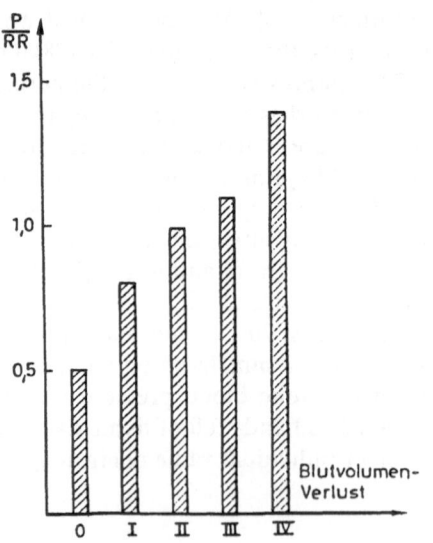

Fig. 1. The original figure showing the relationship between shock index and blood volume loss in man. (From [11] with permission)

Table 1. Shock index in the unanesthetized rat (mean ± SEM)

	Blood loss (% estimated blood volume)			
	0	11	25	33
Control	4.37 ± 0.14	5.09 ± 0.20[a]	5.75 ± 0.54[b]	–
+ 30 min BHL1 (9)	3.84 ± 0.11	4.83 ± 0.12[a]	5.48 ± 0.31[a]	8.44 ± 0.84[a]
+ 3½ hr BHL1 (6)	3.90 ± 0.09	5.00 ± 0.21[a]	6.22 ± 0.47[a]	7.09 ± 0.93[b]

[a] $P < 0.05$ (Wilcoxon matched pair signed rank test).
[b] = non significant, hemorrhage-induced bradycardia.

blood volume, followed by a marked bradycardia as the blood loss increases reaching a maximum at a loss of approximately 25% blood volume [12–14]. Blood pressure is well maintained during the tachycardia but falls as the brady-cardia develops. With greater blood losses there is a profound fall in blood pressure and asystolic cardiac arrest. The changes in heart rate are due, almost entirely, to changes in efferent cardiac vagal activity. Although the pattern of heart rate and blood pressure changes are complex there is a progressive increase in SI as the magnitude of blood loss increases (Table 1 – in these studies mean rather than systolic arterial blood pressure was used to calculate SI).

Hemorrhage and Concomitant Tissue Ischemia in the Unanesthetized Rat

The presence of concomitant tissue injury modifies the cardiovascular response to hemorrhage [14, 15]. The effect is mediated by nociceptive impulses arising in the injured tissues ascending to the spinal cord in non-myelinated fibers. They are transmitted to the brain in long-fiber tracts projecting to the periaqueductal gray matter and thereby modifying, by some means, the activity of vagal cardio-motor neurones [16].

If the hemorrhage was started when tissue ischemia, produced by bilateral hind-limb tourniquets, had been present for 30 minutes it was noted that a larger blood loss (16%) than in controls was required to produce an equivalent increase in heart rate. The main change, however, was that continued hemorrhage in the injured animals failed to induce a significant bradycardia. Also hemorrhage now produced a smaller fall in arterial blood pressure than in uninjured controls. Despite these marked alterations in the cardiovascular response to hemorrhage the SI showed a similar pattern to that seen with "simple" hemorrhage (Table 1). The index at a given blood loss is not significantly different from that seen in control animals (without hind-limb ischemia), however the relationship has been extended and can be seen to hold for blood losses as great as 33% blood volume.

The hypovolemia induced bradycardia returned if the tourniquets were left in place for 3.5 hours but a greater blood loss (27.5%) was required for its onset compared with uninjured animals (20%). Although the influence of tissue injury was changed and the pattern of heart rate and blood pressure responses to hemorrhage was further modified the relationship between SI and blood loss was maintained (Table 1).

Hemorrhage in the Anesthetized Pig

This study has been done in young large white pigs anesthetized with nitrous oxide-oxygen (FiO$_2$ = 0.5) and 1.5% isoflurane following induction with ketamine. The cardiac output was measured with a thermodilution pulmonary artery catheter. Hemorrhage at a rate of 1% estimated blood volume per minute up to a total loss of 40% blood volume reduced blood pressure and increased heart rate with a resultant progressive increase in SI (Table 2). Reinfusion of the shed blood (2 ml/min/kg) 30 minutes after the end of hemorrhage restored the SI to pre-hemorrhage levels but, in the absence of further therapy, cardiovascular status then deteriorated such that 30 minutes after reinfusion SI had again increased (Table 2).

Hemorrhage with Concomitant Nociceptive Afferent Fiber Stimulation in the Anesthetized Pig

The hemorrhage protocol described above was repeated in a further series of pigs but this time the hemorrhage was done against background of somatic afferent nerve stimulation. Both brachial nerves were dissected in the axillae and stimulated electrically in such a way as to activate afferent C-(nociceptive) fibers. The stimulation was started 1 hour before hemorrhage and was maintained thoughout the rest of the experiment. It was hoped that such stimulation would mimic the barrage of afferent neural impulses associated with tissue injury and

Table 2. Shock index in the anesthetized pig (mean ± SEM)

	Blood loss (% estimated blood volume)				Reinfusion	
	0	20		40	+5 min	+30 min
Control (7)	1.57 ± 0.19	2.16 ± 0.26[a]		2.91 ± 0.29[a]	1.76 ± 0.16[b]	2.19 ± 0.26[a]
	0	0 + STIM	20	33–37		
+ STIM (5)	1.47 ± 0.11	1.62 ± 0.07[b]	2.43 ± 0.17[a]	2.80 ± 0.11[a]	1.75 ± 0.17[a]	2.19 ± 0.19[a]

STIM: Somatic afferent nerve stimulation.

[a] P < 0.05 (Wilcoxon matched pair signed rank test, vs controls).

[b] Non significantly different from 0.

ischemia. Nerve stimulation did not alter the pre-hemorrhage SI or its increase following a 20% hemorrhage (Table 2). However such stimulation did modify the response to hemorrhage in that it was now not possible to achieve a 40% blood loss without the animals dying acutely. The maximum blood loss tolerated to allow a 30 minute period before reinfusion and survival for at least 2 hours after reinfusion was reduced to 33–37% (median 35%). Once again reinfusion of the shed blood restored the SI to normal but this effect was transient (Table 2).

All of the experiments described above suggest that SI is reflecting the cardiovascular response to hemorrhage with or without the influence of concomitant tissue injury. What aspect of cardiovascular activity is the SI reflecting? By applying Ohm's law (pressure = cardiac output · total peripheral resistance) SI becomes 1/(stroke volume · total peripheral resistance) which approximates to an inverse function of cardiac work. This is confirmed by analysis of the relationship between SI and left ventricular stroke work (LVSW). SI is negatively related to LVSW ($r = -0.8162$, $n = 49$). The correlation is markedly improved by taking the inverse of SI ($r = 0.9204$) (Fig. 2a). This putative relationship between SI and cardiac function is supported by the finding of a negative relationship, in the same experiments, between SI and cardiac output ($r = -0.6854$), in other words the higher the SI the lower the measured cardiac output (Fig. 2b).

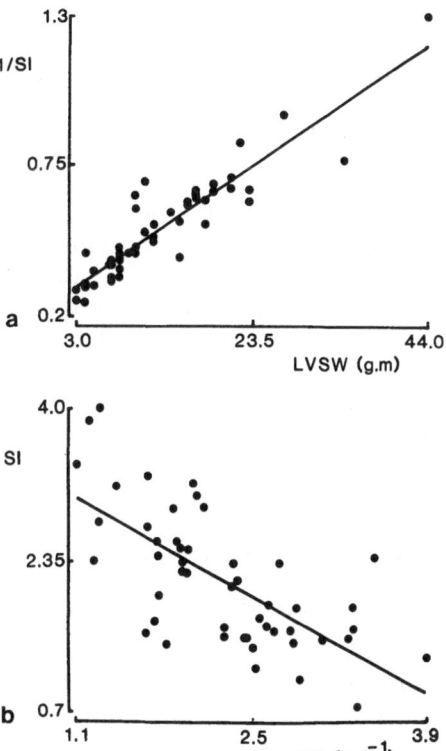

Fig. 2a, b. Relationships between a the inverse of shock index (1/SI) and left ventricular stroke work (LVSW) ($r = 0.9204$; $n = 49$) and b shock index (SI) and cardiac output (CO) ($r = -0.6854$; $n = 49$) in the anesthetized pig during "simple" hemorrhage (see text) and reinfusion of the shed blood

Thus it seems from these experimental studies that SI provides a simple non-invasive method for assessing left ventricular function in shock states. A re-investigation of its clinical usefulness would seem to be warranted.

Shock Index Following Accidental Injury in Man – Preliminary Results

The North Western Injury Research Centre is the U. K. co-ordinating center for the MTOS developed by Champion and his colleagues in Washington, USA [17]. This study utilizes the measurement of the severity of injury by the Abbreviated Injury Scale [18] and the assessment of the systemic response to that injury by the Revised Trauma Score (RTS) [10, 19] for calculating the probability of survival. The RTS is the sum of weighted values assigned to the Glasgow Coma Scale, systolic blood pressure and respiratory rate. Our early experience, with data from approximately 500 patients has suggested that if the elapsed time from accident to arrival at hospital and calculation of RTS is short (e. g. 30 min or less) compensation of the physiological changes elicited by injury is still effective. Thus blood pressure is well maintained, indeed some patients may be hypertensive, and hence the RTS is not reflecting the true severity of injury and a falsely high probability of survival may be derived. Perhaps, as indicated above, SI may be a more sensitive indicator of the physiological disturbance associated with injury.

A SI was calculated for a group of 193 patients all primary referrals to one center (Hope Hospital, Salford, UK) and who were admitted to that center for at least 72 hours or died within that period. All patients had received a blunt injury and the index was calculated before fluid therapy was started, within 30 minutes following injury. The distribution of severity of injury and mortality is shown in Table 3. There was no clear relationship between severity of injury and SI, however there seemed to be a trend towards higher values in the more severely injured (Table 4). In the minor injury group the distribution of SI is asymmetrical although the mode is close to the control value of 0.5 described by Allgöwer and Burri [11]. As the severity increases the distribution is skewed increasingly towards high values with a corresponding increase in the mode value.

A surprising feature was the number of patients with a SI below the normal value of 0.5. In a previous study [11], only one such value was noted however, in a very recent analysis of data from 288 patients, aged 15–54, they were recorded in 3 of the minor, 22 of the moderate and 8 of the severe injury groups. None of the low values could be considered agonal. A low value was associated with both

Table 3. Severity of injury and mortality in 193 patients assigned to study

Severity of injury (ISS)	(n)	Deaths	Mortality (%)
Minor (1–8)	55	0	0
Moderate (9–14)	98	10	10
Severe (> 14)	40	12	30
very severe (> 24)	18	11	61

Table 4. Relationship between Shock Index (SI) and severity of injury in 193 patients. (From [11])

SI	Blood volume loss (%)	No of patients with a given SI within each injury severity band (deaths)		
		1–8	9–14	>14
>1.79				1 (1)
1.7–				2
1.6–			1	
1.5–				
1.4–				
1.3–	40–50			
1.2–			2	
1.1–	30–40		1	2 (1)
1.0–		1		1
0.9–	20–30	4	2 (1)	1
0.8–		3	7	5 (2)
0.7–	10–20	8	10 (1)	6 (1)
0.6–		15	29 (2)	8 (3)
0.5–	0	19	23 (3)	5
0.4–		3	16 (3)	6 (2)
0.3–		2	7	1 (1)
<0.3				2 (1)
		1–8	9–14	>14
			Severity of injury (ISS)	

a bradycardia (range 44–72, median 62 beats/min) and an increase in systolic blood pressure (range 130–220, median 150 mmHg). The small number of patients precludes further meaningful analysis although a number of points which merit further study emerged. Firstly the lowest values (SI <0.45, n = 18) were all associated with blunt and not penetrating injuries. No deaths were noted when the initial value was between 0.43 and 0.60 (close to the normal range), however with values <0.43 the mortality rate rose to 45%. Eight of the 18 patients with SI values of 0.44 or less had a significant closed head injury (AIS for the head ≤3) and this might reflect a Cushing reflex (high systolic blood pressure and bradycardia) elicited by a raised intracranial pressure [20].

It seems, therefore, that the SI is reflecting the systemic response to injury and is in some complex way related to survival/mortality. The question arises as to whether it is a more sensitive indicator of the extent of the response than RTS. The present study does not provide the answer but suggests that this may be the case. For example 160 of the first 193 patients in whom it was possible to calcu-

Table 5. The distribution of shock index (SI) values within a group of 160 trauma victims with a revised trauma score of 7.84

	SI									
	0.3 –	0.4 –	0.5 –	0.6 –	0.7 –	0.8 –	0.9 –	1.0 –	1.1 –	1.2 – 1.3
No of patients	8	23	44	47	17	11	5	1	3	1

late, from the notes provided, both a RTS and a SI had an RTS value of 7.84. In spite of this apparent physiological normality the SI showed a much wider distribution with many clearly abnormal values (Table 5).

Conclusion

A number of experimental studies and a preliminary clinical survey support the suggestion by Allgöwer and Burri in 1967 that the SI is a more sensitive indicator of the response to fluid loss from the circulation than either pulse rate or blood pressure used alone. We suggest that its clinical usefulness should be more systematically studied after traumatic injury and in other shock (e. g. septic and cardiogenic) states where cardiac function may be compromised.

Acknowledgements: We are grateful to the Medical Research Council (UK), North Western Regional Health Authority and Delta Biotechnology Limited for their support and E. Kirkman, M. Rady, I. D. Anderson, M. Woodford, and M. Misra for prividing data used in this paper.

References

1. Committee on Trauma Research (1985) National Research Council and the Institute of Medicine "Injury in America". National Academy Press, Washington DC
2. West J. Trunkey DD, Lim RC (1979) Systems of trauma care. Arch Surg 114:455–460
3. Anderson ID, Woodford M, DeDombal FT, Irving M (1988) Retrospective study of 1000 deaths from injury in England and Wales. Br Med J 296:1305–1308
4. Cowell EM (1919) The initiation of wound shock. Special report series. Medical Research Committee 25:99–108
5. Robertson OH, Bock AV (1919) Memorandum on blood volume after haemorrhage. Special report series. Medical Research Committee 25:213–244
6. Grant RT, Reeve EB (1941) Clinical observations on air-raid casualties. Br Med J 2:293–297
7. Grant RJ, Reeve EB (1951) Observations on the general effects of injury in man with special reference to wound shock. Special report series. Medical Research Committee:277
8. Keith NM (1919) Blood volume changes in wound shock and primary haemorrhage. Special report series. Medical Research Committee 27:3–16
9. Emerson CP, Ebert RV (1945) A study of shock in battle casualties. Ann Surg 122:745–772
10. Champion HR, Sacco WJ, Carnazzo AJ, et al (1981) Trauma score. Crit Care Med 9:672–676
11. Allgöwer M, Burri C (1967) Schockindex. Deutsche Med Wochensch 43:1–10
12. Little RA (1986) Homeostatic reflexes after injury. In: Vincent JL (ed) Update in intensive care and emergency medicine, vol 1. Springer, Berlin Heidelberg New York Tokyo, pp 377–383
13. Little RA (1989) Heart rate changes after haemorrhage and injury – a reappraisal. J Trauma 29:903–906
14. Little RA, Marshall HW, Kirkman E (1990) Attenuation of the acute cardiovascular responses to haemorrhage by tissue injury in the conscious rat. Q J Exp Physiol (in press)
15. Redfern WJ, Little RA, Stoner HB, Marshall HW (1984) Effect of limb ischaemia on blood pressure and the blood pressure-heart rate reflex in the rat. Q J Exp Physiol 69:763–779
16. Jones RO, Kirkman E, Little RA (1990) The involvement of the midbrain periaqueductal grey in the cardiovascular response to injury in the conscious and anaesthetized rat. Q J Exp Physiol (in press)

17. Boyd CR, Tolson MA, Copes WS (1987) Evaluating trauma care: the TRISS method. J Trauma 27:370–378
18. Baker SP, O'Neill B, Haddon W, et al (1974) The injury severity score: a method for describing patients with multiple injuries and evaluating emergency care. J Trauma 14:187–196
19. Champion HR, Sacco WJ, Copes WS, Gann DS, Gennarelli TA, Flanagan ME (1989) A revision of trauma score. J Trauma 29:623–629
20. Cushing H (1901) Concerning a definite regulatory mechanism of the vasomotor center which controls blood pressure during cerebral compression. Johns Hopkins Hosp Bull 12:290–292

Prevention of Post-traumatic Complications

K. Hillman

Introduction

Trauma is the greatest cause of mortality in the under 40 year old age group in the Western world. Just as important as the high mortality, is the huge burden on the State, as well as friends and relatives of the maimed survivors, many of whom need constant care for the rest of their lives. Trauma is increasingly becoming a multi-disciplinary specialty. The initial management is usually undertaken by the emergency room physician, as well as a surgeon and anesthetist or intensivist. Other specialists such as orthopedic surgeons and neurosurgeons are often consulted after the initial resuscitation.

The patient's course is largely dictated by the events of the first hour – the so-called "Golden Hour". While the intensivist is waiting in his department, the effectiveness of the initial resuscitation is determining whether the patient will remain overnight in the Intensive Care Unit (ICU), to be discharged to the general ward the following morning, or will suffer a stormy and prolonged course, often involving multi-organ failure. It is important the intensivist understands that the outcome of his trauma patient is determined by factors largely outside the skills of his own ICU.

"The Golden Hour"

The concept of the "Golden Hour" in trauma has been emphasized for many years. It has been instinctively felt that a successful outcome is largely determined by the effectiveness of the system to restore homeostasis within the first hour. The principle of establishing an effective Airway, Breathing and Circulation is well known to all of us. However, the pathophysiology of the "Golden Hour" is only recently being determined and it is largely determined by the Circulation. To be more specific, the circulation of the gastrointestinal tract (GIT).

Hypovolemia is common after severe trauma. The body adapts well to this insult. Blood flow is reduced to all but the vital organs and the blood pressure is maintained. Non-vital organs such as the muscles and skin, have an abundance of alpha receptors in their circulation. The sympathetic nervous system (SNS) and endogenously released catecholamines sacrifice blood supply to the so-called non-vital organs. While this is a life-saving response, we are now learning that it can also be a life-threatening response. The weak-point in this response is the GIT.

The GIT is a dirty organ. It is full of micro-organisms. As one goes further down the GIT from the stomach to the large intestine, the number of micro-organisms increases. This potential threat to a normal organism is controlled by a complicated and sophisticated series of defenses, especially in the GIT mucosa. The few micro-organisms that manage to cross into the circulation from the GIT are filtered by an intact immune system, based on the reticulo-endothelial system. However, when blood flow is decreased to the GIT, the mucosal barrier is compromised and micro-organisms readily cross, or translocate, and enter the systemic circulation. The reticulo-endothelial system is also compromised by ischemia.

Bacteremia, septicemia and multi-organ failure (MOF) will occur if perfusion to the GIT is not rapidly re-established. It is not surprising then, that the GIT is being increasingly recognized as the motor of MOF.

Even after a short period of ischemia during cardiopulmonary resuscitation (CPR), bacteremia is common [1]. In both animal models of hemorrhagic shock [2-4] and hypotensive patients after trauma [2, 5], bacteremia and endotoxemia is common. It is also proposed that the same mechanism may be responsible for septicemia and MOF in seriously ill patients in intensive care [6].

Overgrowth by intestinal microbes, especially in an alkaline environment is common in intensive care [7]. These micro-organisms translocate across the GIT mucosal barrier in the presence of ischemia and become the source of continuing bacteremia and MOF. It is assumed that the SNS plays the major role in GIT vasoconstriction during shock states. However, it is more likely that a disproportionate sensitivity to the renin angiotensin axis is a more important factor [8]. Whatever the reason there is little doubt that ischemia of the GIT is deterimental to the organism.

Recognizing that the reservoir of micro-organisms in the GIT may play an important role in MOF in patients with trauma has led to recent interest in the use of oral anti-microbials. The rationale is that appropriate non-absorbable antimicrobials will decrease the number or organisms that are available to translocate into the circulation. The incidence of septicemia and nosocomial pneumonia can be reduced with this technique – so-called selective decontamination of the digestive tract (SDD) [9]. Further prospective, controlled trials are needed to confirm this, as the technique is expensive, time-consuming and may eventually predispose to the emergence of resistant organisms. A more logical solution for multi-trauma patients may be to increase the integrity of the mucosal barrier to prevent translocation rather than to kill the micro-organisms within the lumen of the GIT.

This is the basis of the importance of the "Golden Hour". It is no longer good enough to maintain the function of the so-called vital organs – the brain, heart and kidneys. We must consider the GIT in these circumstances as a vital organ. With more aggressive and compulsive fluid transfusion, intestinal ischemia is reduced [10] and it may be that techniques such as the use of oral antibiotics will become less necessary.

The Pre-intensive Care Management

Our resuscitative attempts must be aimed at rapidly restoring the circulation to normal. New systems, if they do not already exist, must be developed to achieve this. Otherwise our efforts in the ICU may be prolonged, expensive and eventually in vain. The battle is won and lost before the patient reaches the ICU. This involves the skills of many people before the patient actually reaches the ICU.

The first response must be by ambulance personnel, trained in techniques such as cannulation and rapid infusion of fluid. A hospital trauma team must be called with the rapidity of a cardiac arrest team. The team must not only be capable of sustaining life but of resuscitating the GIT mucosa. In practical terms the skin and the GIT mucosa have a similar perfusion in shock states. While the skin is in anyway shut down, it can be assumed that GIT mucosa is compromised. Fluid must be aggressively transfused until the skin of the most distal digit is warm and well perfused. Recently a simple technique for monitoring intramucosal pH has been shown to correlate well with GIT mucosal perfusion [11]. It is almost impossible to over-transfuse an actively bleeding patient with multi-trauma, whereas it is very common to under-transfuse them. Maintaining an adequate blood pressure is not good enough. Blood pressure is maintained at the expense of perfusion to the so-called non-vital organs such as the GIT. By aiming for a normal blood pressure, urine output, pulse rate, filling pressures and skin perfusion we should also guarantee adequate GIT perfusion. The markers of underperfusion of the GIT are not immediately recognized. They occur several days later in the ICU as jaundice, renal failure, sepsis and MOF.

The importance of giving the right fluid in the right circumstance is also important. The major problem in multi-trauma is hypovolemia and the most efficient way to restore intravascular volume is with either blood or colloid [12]. The probability of compatibility with a rapid saline cross-matching technique taking less than 10 minutes is 99.4% and with full compatibility testing, 99.95%. In other words there should be minimal delay in safely delivering a blood transfusion. Blood should be given early and rapidly in actively bleeding patients.

Dextrose solutions should not be used for hypovolemia because the water is mainly distributed to the intracellular space. Similarly because crystalloid solutions are mainly distributed to the interstitial space, they are not efficient for the correction of hypovolemia. Moreover, salt and water retention is an early and efficient response to multi-trauma. To give extra salt and water in the form of crystalloid solutions in these circumstances encourages pulmonary and peripheral edema [13]. This in turn causes hypoxia and decreased oxygen consumption. Salt and water loss is not a problem in the acute management of trauma, it is hypovolemia from blood loss. The most efficient method for correcting hypovolemia in these circumstances is with either blood or colloid.

There is little place for monitoring preload during acute correction of hypovolemia [13]. There may be more of a place for central venous pressure (CVP) measurements and pulmonary artery wedge pressure (PAWP) in the fine tuning of fluid replacement once the patient is stable. Initially simple measurements such as blood pressure, pulse rate, peripheral perfusion and urine output are the best guides to accurate fluid replacement.

The patient often needs further investigation (e.g. CT scan, angiography) or surgery. It is crucial that a system is developed for continued resuscitation and that it is as efficient during transport and at the sites of further investigation and treatment as it was initially in the emergency room. It is common for the patient to need continued fluid transfusion to maintain perfect perfusion.

The investigative suite or operating room becomes an extension of the emergency room. This is becoming more important as early fixation of orthopedic fractures is increasingly used [14]. While early fixation has many advantages, especially in the long term management of patients, the initial surgery can be prolonged and associated with large blood loss. Resources and expertise must be devoted to the trauma patient during this crucial period. Nursing and medical assistance may be needed to assist the anesthetist to resuscitate, stabilize, transfuse and monitor the patient. Concurrent pathology needs to be considered and constant clinical reassessment needs to be undertaken. For example, an urgent laparotomy may have been necessary before a CT scan could be performed to exclude intracranial hematoma. Thoracic injuries, such as a pneumothorax, aortic dissection or pulmonary hemorrhage may become obvious during surgery. Assessment is difficult while the patient is under anesthesia and definitive investigation would have to be delayed until urgent surgery is completed. Awareness of the possible complications is essential.

Other Factors in the Early Management of Trauma

Our attention has recently been focussed on other developments in the early management of trauma, apart from the importance of re-establishing an ideal circulation. One of these factors is the re-assessment of high intra-abdominal tamponade as a protective mechanism in order to decrease intra-abdominal bleeding. The severity of the tamponade is usually assessed by abdominal girth measurements. Both of these assumptions need to be elaborated on. Firstly, girth measurements are of no value in assessing abdominal bleeding [15]; and secondly, while raised intra-abdominal pressure may tamponade bleeding, it also seriously affects intra-abdominal organ function as well as adversely affecting cardiorespiratory function [16–18].

Intra-abdominal pressure can be accurately and simply estimated by measuring intravesicle pressure [19, 20]. This is readily achieved by placing a needle or cannula into the urinary catheter or by using a specially designed T-piece attachment [20]. The urinary catheter is clamped distal to this insertion and 50 ml of sterile isotonic saline run into the bladder. The fluid in the bladder is then connected via a continuous column of fluid to a CVP manometer. Readings are taken from the pubic symphysis. Less than 20 cmH$_2$O is acceptable; 20–25 cmH$_2$O causes a reduction in organ flow, particularly to the kidneys and at more than 25 cmH$_2$O, oliguria occurs, eventually resulting in anuria. It may not always be possible to prevent abdominal tamponade as it is sometimes necessary in order to prevent bleeding. However, intravesical pressure should always be measured and options such as embolization of venous bleeding or laparotomy should be seriously considered in order to prevent otherwise certain renal failure and other intra-abdominal organ damage.

With the high incidence of chronic ill health, especially due to smoking related diseases in the community, an attempt should be made to get a relevant past history and drug history. Ischemic heart disease and chronic lung disease are very common and important in terms of eventual outcome to the patient. Drugs such as β-blockers, calcium channel blockers are important considerations in intra-operative management. Aspirin is becoming very common as a prophylactic drug in ischemic heart disease in over 40-year old males and may be responsible for prolonged and abnormal bleeding after multi-trauma.

It would be irresponsible to discuss any specific problem in medicine without seeing it in its overall context. The best way to treat multi-trauma is to prevent it. There is no doubt that in the past, resources have been wrongly placed. The medical profession assumed others would sort these priorities out. However, by our very involvement in spending large amounts of the finite health budget on acute management and long term support of these patients, we have left little for other options. It is crucial that our profession lobby at all levels to collect data on the effectiveness of preventative measures and then to put these measures into effect.

Similarly, we need a system which will effectively manage patients with multi-trauma before and after our own involvement – the so-called "networking" of a problem. We need to be involved with primary retrieval and management, together with our Ambulance Service. We need to have the most capable and experienced doctors involved in the initial resuscitation in accident and emergency and not, as in the past, the most junior and least experienced. Our Emergency Departments will largely determine the clinical course of patients. All larger hospitals have organisational and teaching responsibilities to other hospitals and services involved in the trauma system. Trauma teams and multi-disciplinary committees are essential. Data collection and quality assurance are also essential in order to test our own performance and rigorously compare them with others.

References

1. Gaussorgues P, Gueugniaud P-Y, Vedrinine J-M, Salord F, Mercatello A, Robert D (1988) Bacteremia following cardiac arrest and cardiopulmonary resuscitation. Intensive Care Med 14:575–577
2. Rush BF Jr, Sori AJ, Murphy TF, Smith S, Flanagan JJ, Machiedo GW (1988) Endotoxemia and bacteremia during hemorrhagic shock. Ann Surg 207:549–554
3. Wilder Baker J, Deitch EA, Berg RD, Specian RD (1988) Hemorrhagic shock induces bacterial translocation from the gut. J Trauma 28:896–906
4. Berg RD, Garlington AW (1979) Translocation of certain indigenous bacteria from the gastrointestinal tract to the mesenteric lymph nodes and other organs in a gnotobiotic mouse model. Infect Immun 23:403–411
5. Border JR, Hassett J, LaDuca J, et al (1987) The gut origin septic states in blunt multiple trauma (ISS = 40) in the ICU. Ann Surg 206:427–448
6. Marshal JC, Christou NV, Horn R, Meakins JL (1988) The microbiology of multiple organ failure. Arch Surg 123:309–315

7. Hillman KM, Riordan T, O'Farrell SM, et al (1982) Colonization of the gastric contents in critically ill patients. Crit Care Med 10:444–447
8. Bailey RW, Hamilton SR, Morris JB, Bulkley GB, Smith GW (1986) Pathogenesis of non-occlusive ischemic colitis. Ann Surg 203:590–599
9. Stoutenbeek CP, van Saene HKF, Miranda DR, Zandstra DF (1984) The effect of selective decontamination of the digestive tract on colonization and infection in multiple trauma patients. Intensive Care Med 10:185–193
10. Jamieson WG, Pliagus G, Marchuk S, et al (1988) Effect of antibiotic and fluid resuscitation upon survival time in experimental intestinal ischemia. Surg Gynecol Obstet 167:103–108
11. Fiddian-Green RG (1988) Splanchnic ischaemia and multiple organ failure in the critically ill. Ann R Coll Surg Engl 70:128–134
12. Hillman KM (1989) Fluid therapy. In: Atkinson RS, Adams AP (eds) Recent advances in anaesthesia and analgesia. Churchill Livingstone, London, pp 105–123
13. Hauser CJ, Shoemaker WC, Turpin I, Goldberg SJ (1980) Oxygen transport responses to colloids and crystalloids in critically ill surgical patients. Surg Gynecol Obstet 150:811
14. Seibel R, LaDuca J, Hassett JM, et al (1985) Blunt multiple trauma (ISS) femur traction and pulmonary failure septic state. Ann Surg 202:283–295
15. Finlayson DF, Muirhead AG (1983) Is measurement of girth of value in assessing intraperitoneal bleeding after trauma? Br Med J 287:728
16. Richards WO, Scovill W, Shin B, Reed W (1983) Acute renal failure associated with increased intra-abdominal pressure. Ann Surg 197:183–187
17. Cullen DJ, Coyle JP, Teplick R, Long MC (1989) Cardiovascular pulmonary, and renal effects of massively increased intra-abdominal pressure in critically ill patients. Crit Care Med 17:118–125
18. Robotham JL, Wise RA, Bromberger-Barnea B (1985) Effects of changes in abdominal pressure on left ventricular performance and regional blood flow. Crit Care Med 13:803–808
19. Iberti TJ, Lieber CE, Benjamin E (1989) Determination of intra-abdominal pressure using a transurethral bladder catheter: clinical validation of the technique. Anesthesiology 70:47–50
20. Jacques T, Lee R (1988) Improvement of renal function after relief of raised intra-abdominal pressure due to traumatic retropoeritoneal haematoma. Anaesth Intensive Care 16:478–494

Pathophysiological Mechanisms in Severe Head Trauma

S. Cotev, Y. Shapira, and E. Shohami

Introduction

Severe head injury (SHI) in man, defined in terms of an admission Glasgow Coma Scale score ≤ 8 is still associated with an overall mortality rate exceeding 50% and poor functional outcome despite extensive clinical and experimental research efforts, as well as the development of sophisticated diagnostic and therapeutic modalities in its management.

Outcome after SHI seems to depend on the extent of neuronal damage in two phases along the time-axis. In the first phase, occurring immediately at or very soon after the impact, a variable degree of irreversible structural injury occurs. It involves vascular dysruption with the development of hematomatous mass lesions, early neuronal ischemic death, and often intracranial hypertension. Diffuse axonal injury may also occur in this phase, particularly in acceleration/deceleration injuries. The second phase of injury is less well defined. It develops gradually following the impact, and in theory, at least, is partially if not completely preventable and reversible. A cascade of events which are still poorly defined, is presumably triggered by the impact and set into motion, leading to expanding secondary neuronal injury. Recent investigative efforts, therefore, are primarily directed to explore the nature of this cascade of events in an effort to intervene and interrupt its development, and thus minimize secondary neuronal death to improve outcome after SHI.

The basic premise of most investigators is that ischemic alterations are of paramount importance in the extension of neuronal death during the second phase of SHI [1]. Graham et al. [2] have shown that pathological evidence of foci of cerebral ischemia can be found in over 90% of brains of victims after SHI.

Even though cerebral hyperemia may characterize the early phase of SHI [3], regional or even global ischemia due to unfavorable oxygen balance between demand and supply, are likely to develop in the second phase of SHI. This is due to reduced cerebral blood flow (CBF) secondary to regional vascular compression from mass lesions and edema, or global intracranial hypertension. Additionally, endogenous mediators may be involved in the biochemical cascade that is triggered by SHI. The eicosanoids have been suggested as possible mediators in the cascade leading to secondary ischemia [4]. They possess vasoregulatory and "inflammatory" (including vascular permeability) properties, as well as being able to modulate neurotransmission [5]. With this background in mind we have recently described a rat model of SHI [6] that we feel simulates blunt SHI in man, and in which we have studied steps in the cascade leading to secondary CNS dysfunction after SHI.

The Experimental Model

Blunt SHI is induced by allowing a weight-drop device to freely fall over the convex surface of the exposed skull of lightly-anesthetized Sabra strain of rats, 250–350 g body weight, 2–3 mm to the left of the midline. The energy impacted on the skull is reproducable and easily controlled by varying the height from which the device is allowed to fall. In the following experiments the height was chosen such that results in a 30–40% immediate mortality to simulate clinical circumstances. Figure 1 demonstrates the macroscopic nature of the injury, immediately after the impact. In ten rats we measured intraarterial pressure and observed a maximal rise in mean pressure of about 20 mmHg 10 min after the impact which gradually dissipated in the following hour.

We followed surviving rats for as long as ten days after the injury. Increased H_2O content in the left hemisphere was determined by both the dry/wet weight and the specific gravity (SG) method, using linear gradient columns [7]. Edema of the injured hemisphere starts 15 min and peaks 18–24 h after trauma (Fig. 2). The maximal increase in H_2O content is calculated at 5–6%. Edema subsequently subsides, and is no longer apparent ten days after injury. In this model, the extent of left hemisphere edema positively correlates with a specifically de-

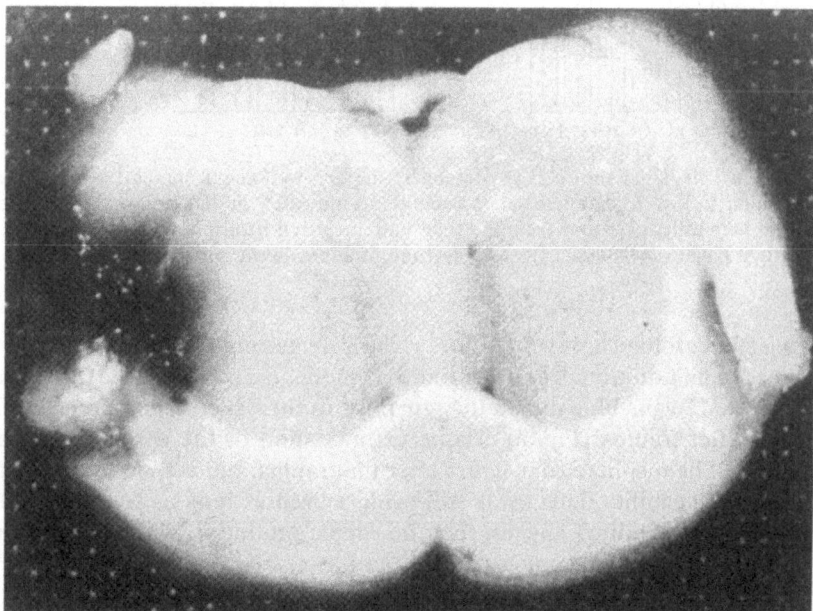

Fig. 1. Coronal section of cerebral hemispheres of a traumatized rat sacrificed immediately after the impact. Note hematomatous swelling of the left hemisphere

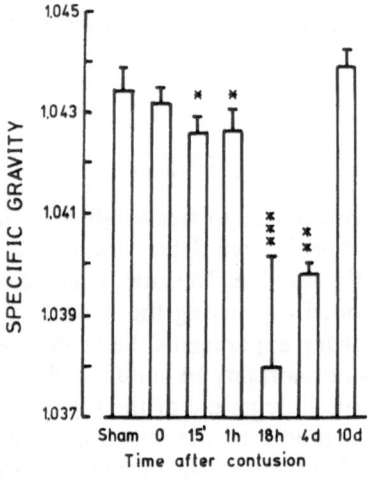

Fig. 2. Tissue specific gravity of the left (injured) hemisphere in 7 groups of rats. Sham = non-traumatized rats. O = control rats. 15′, 1h, 18h, 4d and 10d = traumatized rats decapitated at the assigned times. * p < 0.001 as compared to 0 group rats (Mann-Whitney U test)

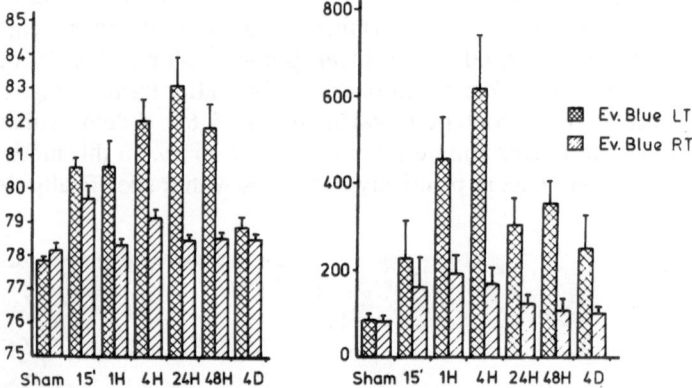

Fig. 3. Left panel shows H$_2$O content by the dry/wet weight method. (Group designation is similar to Fig. 2.) The left bar in each group indicates the left (injured) hemisphere, and the right-equivalent sections from the right untraumatized hemispheres.

Right panel shows tissue Evans blue concentrations in the same groups of rats

vised neurological severity score (NSS), suggesting clinical relevance of the edema. In an additional study of our SHI model (to be published) we intravenously injected Evans blue dye to the rats prior to their sacrifice at predetermined periods after trauma (Fig. 3). Tissue extravasation of the dye was maximal in the injured hemisphere four hours after the trauma, but a residual blood-brain-barrier permeability defect was still evident even as long as four days after the insult. These findings suggest that the edema produced by the trauma was at least in part of the vasogenic type.

The Eicosanoid Synthesis Profile

Previous investigators had demonstrated in several animal models significant increases in cerebral eisosanoid synthesis after variable experimental insults, including trauma and ischemia [4]. Small cortical tissue slices were similarly obtained in our rat model of SHI immediately after sacrifice at various time periods after trauma.

The rate of synthesis and release of PGE_2, 6-keto-PGF_1 (the stable metabolite of prostacyclin), TXB_2 (the stable metabolite of thromboxane) and of 5-, 12- and 15-HETE was measured in these tissue sections by radio-immunoassay [8, 9].

PGE_2 synthesis was markedly elevated 18 hours after trauma in both the injured (left) and the right hemispheres, although the degree of rise in synthesis was larger in the former (Fig. 4). This peak rise was closely related to that of edema formation along the time axis, although significant edema was already apparent before PGE_2 levels began to rise. Statistical correlation could not be established between the elevations in PGE_2 and H_2O content.

The rise in 6-keto-$PGF_{1\alpha}$ and TXB_2 synthesis was less dramatic (i.e., only 2-fold, as compared to sham operated, untraumatized rats). Their peak preceded the rise of PGE_2, and was almost equal in the injured and uninjured hemispheres. 12- and 15-HETE levels were not elevated by trauma. The synthesis of 5-HETE, however, was significantly increased in the injured hemisphere as early as 15 min after trauma, but was no longer apparent four hours later, when edema was still increasing [9].

Augmented synthesis of arachidonic acid metabolites in the injured brain is customarily attributed to ischemic disturbances that promote massive intracellular flux of free calcium ions from extracellular fluid, as well as from intracellular binding sites, such as mitochondria and endoplasmic reticulum [10].

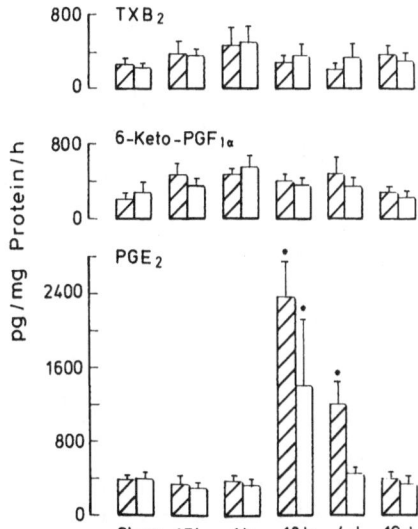

Fig. 4. Release rate of TXB_2, 6-keto-$PGF_{1\alpha}$ and PGE_2 from sections of tissue removed (<1 min) after sacrifice of rats. (Group designations are as in Fig. 2.) The left and right bars in each group indicate the left (injured) and right hemispheres, respectively; * $p < 0.05$

Indeed, in the SHI rat model, total cerebral tissue Ca^{++} content, measured by atomic absorption spectroscopy, was increased 3–4 folds (as compared to sham-operated non-traumatized rats) at 24–48 h after trauma [11]. This increase occurred in both the injured (left) and uninjured hemispheres, although it was most marked in the grey matter of the left hemisphere (over 60 µmol/g, dry weight) when it significantly correlated with increased H_2O content (Fig. 5).

Our methodology did not permit to pin-point the rise in total tissue calcium concentration to the intracellular compartment, but this is highly plausible as it complements existing data in other models of cerebral injury.

Massive intracellular flux of Ca^{++} results in ATP depletion and may well be the final common pathway in causing neuronal death from a variety of injurious insults [10]. It also activates cellular membrane phospholipases (especially PLA_2), resulting in hydrolysis of membrane phospholipids and release of free fatty acids, including arachidonic acid, and subsequently the eicosanoids. In tissue slices from the SHI model, PLA_2 activity was indeed determined to be 170% and 300% of normal at 4 hours and 24 hours after trauma, respectively [12].

The demonstration of increased tissue concentrations of Ca^{++}, raised PLA_2 activity and augmented synthesis of arachidonic acid metabolites, triggered by blunt cerebral trauma, and closely associated with vasogenic edema formation, suggested but could not prove their possible etiological role in the cascade of events that lead to neurological dysfunction in our experimental model, and possibly also, by inference, in the second phase of clinical head injury.

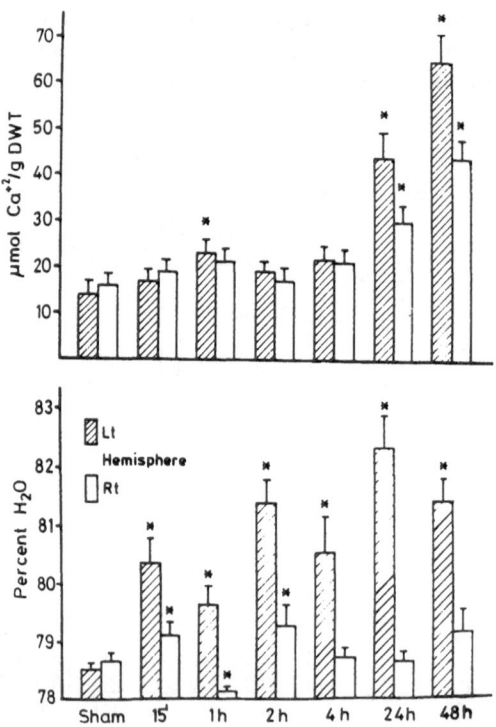

Fig. 5. Bottom panel indicates H_2O content of tissue sections in groups of rats (as in Fig. 3). The upper panel indicates tissue Ca^{++} concentrations in adjacent sections of the same rats. The left and right bars in each group indicate left and right hemispheres, respectively; * $p < 0.05$

Thus, the following studies were undertaken with the aim to elucidate the pathophysiological relevance of the eicosanoids in the genesis of delayed neuronal injury.

Experiments to Inhibit Arachidonic Acid Metabolism

Some of the preceding data suggests that a cascade of biochemical events is triggered by blunt cerebral trauma in rats, and that the breakdown of membrane phospholipids to release arachidonic acid, and subsequently the eicosanoids, might play a central role in the pathogenesis of vasogenic edema and delayed neuronal dysfunction.

If this assumption that credits the eicosanoids as mediators of neuronal injury is correct, then a whole spectrum of therapeutic modalities, based on blocking the eicosanoid cascade, may be open, to improve outcome after SHI. The other possibility that can not be ruled out is that raised eicosanoid levels in this context of head trauma are merely markers rather than mediators of cerebral ischemia and injury; under these circumstances blockers or inhibitors of the cascade are unlikely to have a salutary effect.

Dexamethasone: The almost universal practice of using the drug in the management of SHI only a few years ago is now fading in the face of both clinical and experimental evidence of its uselessness. Steroids are known to induce lipomodulin, which inhibits in turn the action of phospholipases. As such, these compounds could be expected to slow down arachidonic acid release and eicosanoid synthesis. In our model, however, free dexamethasone given at, and 8 hours after trauma, was ineffective in significantly preventing edema formation or improving neurological score, even though it decreased PGE_2 and TXB_2 synthesis [13].

Indomethacin: Similarly, this drug, a nonsteroidal cycloxygenase inhibitor, had no effect on raised H_2O content in the injured hemisphere when given even in massive doses either as pre- or post-treatment to SHI [13]. This finding contrasts that of Yen and Lee [14] who recorded decreased brain edema, induced by a freezing lesion in rats with indomethacin, but only when the drug was given as pretreatment 48 hours prior to injury.

OKY-046: This agent is a specific thromboxane synthetase inhibitor. In the rat model it decreased both the basal and the elevated levels of TXB_2 after trauma, but totally failed to prevent edema accumulation and to improve neurological status of the rats after trauma [15]. Failure to halt edema formation and neurological deterioration in these last experiments, despite obvious effects of the agents to inhibit PG synthesis (as they are expected to do), suggested to us at least two possibilities: PG's may be markers of ischemic processes in trauma, but not causative mediators of the cascade, or, alternatively, that inhibition of the cycloxygenase pathway by these drugs merely caused the arachidonic acid metabolism to be shifted towards the lipoxygenase pathway, the products of which might be the true mediators of ischemic injury. The results of the following experiment (unpublished) suggest that the latter possibility may be operational. Nordihydroguaiaretic acid (NDGA) is a 5-lipoxygenase inhibitor. When it was given to our SHI rats (in doses of 3 mg/kg, intraperitoneally, twice daily, from 48 hours pre-trauma until 12 hours after trauma) it prevented both edema formation and neurological deterioration 24 hours after trauma in a statistically significant fashion (Table 1).

Comment

Measures to improve mortality and morbidity after severe traumatic injury to the brain must be directed along several venues. First of these is obviously prevention of injury, although modern society is exposed as helpless in this task. Spotty success in diminishing the impact of injury, once it had occurred, seems to be related to the advancement forwards, to the site of injury and to the transport to the neurosurgical facility of appropriate care of the victims by trained medical and paramedical personnel, providing early management of the airway, adequate oxygenation, hyperventilation to control intracranial pressure and volume resuscitation from hypovolemia [16]. It may be suggested that provision of these measures during "the golden hour" after SHI limits the extension of cerebral ischemia/hypoxia and thus improves outcome [1]. Once in the appropriate medical facility (i.e. containing experienced neurosurgical and neuroanesthetic teams and computerized tomographic equipment), emphasis is directed towards reduction of intracranial pressure by either surgical interventions to extirpate intracranial hematomas, and/or medical therapeutic modalities. These measures, too, aim to decrease ischemia secondary to regional or global vascular compression and vasospasm.

Our work, and that of many others, focuses on the biochemical cascade of events that is triggered by ischemic conditions leading to secondary neuronal death. Mediators of this cascade are probably many, but we chose to work in the laboratory on the chain of events that apparently involves the intracellular flux of free Ca^{++} ions, activation of membrane phospholipases, liberation of free

Table 1. The effect of nordihydroguaiaretic acid (NDGA) administration on tissue specific gravity and neurological severity score 24 hours after blunt head trauma

	Specific gravity		Neurological severity score (points)	
	Right-hemisphere (uninjured)	Left-hemisphere (injured)	1 hour (max 24)	24 hours (max 20)
Control	1.0397 ± 0.0012	1.0366 ± 0.0018^a	15	8.6 ± 0.8^b
NDGA	1.0433 ± 0.0004	1.0407 ± 0.0010	14.1	5.0 ± 0.9

[a] $p < 0.05$ As compared to right hemisphere in the same group and to left hemisphere in the NDGA-treated group.

[b] $p < 0.01$ As compared to NDGA-treated group at 24 hours.

fatty acids (mainly arachidonic acid) and the subsequent metabolic release of eicosanoids. The latter are known to have vasoregulatory effects as well as damaging properties that result in vascular permeability and edema [5]. Also, during prostaglandin synthesis, free O_2 radicals are known to be released, which have cytotoxic effects. It is hoped that the understanding of these biochemical events will lead to the addition of new, clinically applicable, therapeutic agents that may block or diminish the extent of this injurious biochemical evolution.

The rat model of SHI seems to be appropriate for this purpose as it closely simulates the pathology and events that occur after head trauma in man, including the development of secondary regional vasogenic edema [6]. Increased eicosanoid synthesis indeed occurs in this rat model [8, 9]. Attemps to attenuate or diminish the extent of edema formation by blocking the cyclooxygenase pathway of prostaglandin synthesis, however, have not proven successful [13]. Lipoxygenase pathway inhibition, in very preliminary studies, seems to reduce edema formation as well as improve neurological status of the rats after SHI, providing early evidence that its metabolites are mediators of secondary neuronal dysfunction after SHI. It remains to be seen if this and future experiments will eventually provide clinicians caring for patients with SHI with a new type of armamentarium that will lower the devastating impact that is still inherent to this injury.

References

1. Miller JD (1985) Head injury and brain ischaemia – implications for therapy. Br J Anaesth 57:120–129
2. Graham DI, Adams JH, Doyle D (1978) Ischemic brain damage in fatal non-missile head injuries. J Neurol Sci 39:213–234
3. Nilsson B, Nordstrom CH (1977) Experimental head injury in the rat: Part III. Cerebral blood flow and oxygen consumption after concussive impact acceleration. J Neurosurg 47:262–273
4. Gaudet JR, Alam I, Levine L (1980) Accumulation of cyclooxygenase products of arachidonic acid metabolism in gerbil brain during reperfusion after bilateral common carotid occlusion. J Neurochem 35:653–658
5. Wolfe LS (1982) Eicosanoids: prostaglandins, thromboxanes, leukotrienes and other derivatives of carbon 20 unsaturated fatty acids. J Neurochem 38:1–14
6. Shapira Y, Shohami E, Sidi A, Soffer D, Freeman S, Cotev S (1988) Experimental closed head injury in rats: Mechanical, pathophysiologic, and neurologic properties. Crit Care Med 16:258–265
7. Marmarou A, Tanaka K, Shulman K (1982) An improved gravimetric measure of cerebral edema. J Neurosurg 56:246–253
8. Shohami E, Shapira Y, Sidi A, Cotev S (1987) Head injury induces increased prostaglandin synthesis in rat brain. J Cereb Blood Flow Metab 7:58–63
9. Shohami E, Shapira Y, Yadid G, Cotev S, Feuerstein G (1989) Increased 5-HETE production in the brain following head injury. Ann NY Acad Sci 559:485–487
10. Raichle ME (1983) The pathophysiology of brain ischemia. Ann Neurol 13:2–10
11. Shapira Y, Yadid G, Cotev S, Shohami E (1989) Accumulation of calcium in the brain following head trauma. Neurol Res 11 (in press)
12. Shohami E, Shapira Y, Yadid G, Reisfeld N, Yedgar S (1989) Brain phospholipase A2 is activated after experimental closed head injury in the rat. J Neurochem 53:1541–1546
13. Shapira Y, Davidson E, Weidenfeld Y, Cotev S, Shohami E (1988) Dexamethazone and indomethacin do not affect brain edema following head injury in rats. J Cereb Blood Flow Metab 8:395–402

14. Yen MH, Lee SH (1987) Effects of cyclooxygenase and lipoxygenase inhibitors on cerebral edema induced by freezing lesions in rats. Europ J Pharmacol 144:369-373
15. Shapira Y, Yadid G, Cotev S, Shohami E (1989) OKY-046 inhibits thromboxane synthesis with no effect on brain edema and neurological status in head traumatized rats. Prostagland Leukotrien Essen Fatty Acids 36:49-55
16. Klauber MR, Marshall LF, Toole BM, et al (1985) Cause of decline in head injury mortality rate in San Diego County, California. J Neurosurg 62:528-531

Primary Treatment in Severe Head Injury

C. Simon and D. Scheidegger

Introduction

Brain injury remains the primary cause of death in the majority of all severe head accidents [1]. One-fourth of the more than 400 000 patients hospitalized yearly in the United States after head injury suffer from severe brain injury and are admitted to intensive care with a Glasgow Coma Scale (GCS) of 8 or less. As mortality in this group is very high [2], head injury remains a major medical and socio-economic problem.

Pathophysiology

Four mechanisms cause brain damage after head injury:

1. Primary brain injury results from a direct biomechanical impact on the brain with its negative consequences on neurons and blood vessels;
2. Bleeding in the parenchyma of the brain;
3. Edema that develops around a contusion or a hematoma;
4. Ischemia caused by brain swelling or a shifting of the brain.

Primary brain injury is frequently followed by complications, including hypoxemia, hypotension, hypercarbia, and acidosis which contribute to further brain damage [3]. In contrast to primary brain injury, these secondary systemic insults, which lead to delayed recovery and a high mortality rate, are avoidable. A primary aim is to correct respiratory insufficiency and hypotension at the accident site; this will reduce adverse outcome after severe head injury [4].

Securing Respiration and Circulation

Various causes of arterial hypoxemia and hypercapnia often occur after severe head injury, including airway obstruction, aspiration, neurogenic lung edema, atelectasis and additional injury of thorax and/or lung.

Severe arterial hypoxemia induces cerebral vasodilation. CO_2 retention leads to the cessation of autoregulation (the capacity of the normal brain to maintain a constant level of perfusion despite a large variation of the perfusion pressure [MAP between 50 and 150 mmHg]) as well as the dilation of blood vessels [5]. In the normal brain, blood supply varies by about 2 ml/100 g of brain tissue for a change of 1 mmHg CO_2. For a CO_2 pressure range of 20–80 mmHg the calculated change in intracranial blood volume is about 33 ml. Normally this variability does not cause a significant rise in intracranial pressure (ICP), as there is resistance to variation in intracranial pressure/volume changes, expressed by the term "compliance". Cerebrospinal fluid (CSF), for example, can escape from the intracranial space to the spinal channel. Under pathological conditions such as caused by edema or an intracranial hematoma, a small increase in volume may prevent these normal autoregulating processes. In this manner the venous low pressure and capillary system compresses leading to ischemia which, by producing an edema, provokes a further rise in ICP. Therefore, each patient must receive sufficient ventilation. When the cough and swallowing reflex is absent or reduced, the patient must be intubated.

Although intubation in the daily operating room procedure is generally quite routine, intubation in brain-injured patients is often difficult with disastrous consequences. Intubation should only be performed by experienced personnel who should ensure that the stimulation caused by intubation does not lead to a rise in ICP. This can be avoided by supplying oxygen, relaxation, and hyperventilation prior to intubation. ICP can be lowered by intravenous administration of barbiturates, if the hemodynamic condition permits it, or if the circulation is unstable, by administration of 1.5 mg/kg lidocaine one minute before intubation [6]. Lidocaine lowers the ICP in a similar way as thiopental by reducing cerebral blood flow. Systemic pressure remains stable, in contrast to the reaction to barbiturates. While turning and intubating a patient, special attention must be given to the movement of the head, as fractures or luxations of the cervical spine are often associated with head injury.

In addition to ventilation, the maintenance of proper circulation is an essential component of primary care after head injury. To prevent the development of ischemia, cerebral perfusion pressure (mean arterial pressure minus ICP) must remain between 60 and 100 mmHg.

Following brain injury autoregulation is lost in the damaged areas. This loss produces a cerebral blood flow which is dependent on pressure.

Hypotension after head injury is generally a sign of extracranial trauma, such as heavy bleeding from a scalp wound, large hematomas in the area of a fracture, or intrathoracical or intraabdominal bleeding. Hypotension is only caused by a cerebral pathology in a terminal state with brain-stem trauma. It follows that hypovolemia is considered the most frequent origin of hypotension and must be corrected. Infusions like Ringer's lactate or plasma expander should be immediately administered through large peripheral catheters. Infusion therapy should not be reduced because of concern of brain edema. Moreover, glucose solutions existing as free water must not be administered. Results of studies from England and the United States demonstrated a two-fold increase in mortality in brain-injured patients who arrived at the emergency ward in a hypotensive condition [7].

However, it can be questioned whether hypertension should be corrected in patients arriving at the emergency ward in a hypertensive state, which occurs in about 25% of all severely head-injured patients. Hypertension may be caused by a release of catecholamines. These initiate, through an arachidonic acid cascade, an increased production of prostaglandins (prostacyclin and thromboxane A_2), causing cerebral vasodilation and damage in the endothelium, which results in brain edema and in an increase of ICP.

On the other hand, some brain-injured patients are hypertensive prior to trauma while others develop hypertension because of an ischemia in the brain stem or as a protective reaction of the circulation caused by an elevated ICP. In these patients a reduction in blood pressure would lead to cerebral ischemia. In the ideal case, then, ICP should be measured in order to guarantee an appropriate perfusion pressure. As this is impossible during the first acute phase, an elevated ICP should be assumed and appropriate clinical measures taken to reduce it.

Abnormal ECG suggestive of ischemia or arrhythmia of various kinds which may occur after brain injury are generally caused by an increased activity of the autonomous nervous system. After successful treatment of hypoxemia, they should be corrected with adrenergic blockers.

Prevention of Cerebral Ischemia

Once proper ventilation and circulation are ensured, it is important to prevent or to control cerebral ischemia by the following means:

1. Intracranial hematomas must be evacuated before the development of irreversible damage;
2. Cerebral edema and elevated ICP must be avoided.

In the case of an acute subdural hematoma, the time factor and the age of the patient have a direct influence on prognosis [8]. If the interval between accident and evacuation of the hematoma exceeds four hours, mortality increases from 30% to above 90%.

Brain edema and elevated ICP, which are present in about half of all severely brain-injured patients, lead to irreversible cerebral ischemia and consequently must be corrected as soon as possible [9]. A reliable assessment of an increased ICP is possible only if direct and continuous monitoring is performed. This should be done in all cases where GCS is less than 8. Clearly, arterial blood pressure must be continuously monitored to obtain the cerebral perfusion pressure. Cerebral perfusion pressure must not be reduced by the therapy used to lower ICP. The aim is to maintain an ICP below 20 mmHg and a perfusion pressure above 60 mmHg.

Therapy of Intracranial Hypertension

Extracranial factors which can cause an increase in ICP must be excluded or eliminated. In addition to factors previously discussed can be added: extreme positions of the body or the head, such as lateral rotation or flexion of the neck, pyrexia, electrolyte abnormalities, such as a reduced sodium level, and the influence of various drugs including volatile anesthetics or vasodilators.

ICP can be reduced by several procedures. Controlled hyperventilation is a fast and efficient method. The aim is to achieve a $PaCO_2$ between 3.4 and 4 kPa. Hyperventilation can reduce an elevated cerebral blood flow in a head-injured patient over a span of several days. Normalization of pH in the CSF takes 6 to 8 hours in a normal brain, but is markedly slowed down after injury.

It is often impossible to hyperventilate a patient without using sedation. In the case of additional trauma, analgesia and even muscle relaxants can be used. Clearly, the required medications must not increase brain damage. Benzodiazepines, e.g. midazolam, reduce oxygen metabolism in the brain and cerebral perfusion by 35%. Increasing doses have no further cerebral effect [10]. The effect of midazolam can be stopped by flumazenil, a benzodiazepine antagonist. Midazolam has a similar effect on intracranial pressure as that of thiopental.

Similar to barbiturates, etomidate induces a decrease in cerebral oxygen metabolism, blood perfusion, and ICP. Depending on the dose, etomidate can cause the latter to drop only until the zero line in EEG is reached [11]. However, the suppressive side effect of etomidate on the cortex of adrenal glands limits its use in trauma patients.

In the view of neuroanesthetists propofol also has problems associated with its use. This drug often causes a lowering of cerebral perfusion pressure below the critical value of 60 mmHg, parallel to a reduction of ICP [12].

Opiates may safely be administered to the brain-injured patient, together with the technique of hyperventilation, as opiates do not alter the CO_2 reactivity in blood vessels.

Muscle relaxants do not cross the blood-brain barrier. With the exception of vecuronium, they influence brain dynamics by a direct effect on systemic circulation or by metabolites. d-Tubocurarine increases ICP by causing a release of histamine. Pancuronium may have the same effect by increasing systemic pressure in the absence of autoregulation. The atracurium metabolite, laudanosine, if used at a high dose, provokes central convulsions. Succinylcholine increases cerebral blood perfusion and ICP primarily through afferent activities of muscle spindles and secondarily by a succinylcholine induced rise of the $PaCO_2$. This effect could be mitigated but not eliminated by using precurarization [13]. Insofar as the brain is concerned, since vecuronium is the most inert muscle relaxant, it is the preferred relaxant for patients having a reduced cerebral compliance.

Weaning from hyperventilation must be executed carefully and by small degrees, as a small rise in CO_2 may provoke a drastic increase of ICP if the cerebral compliance remains reduced.

In the past, corticosteroids were administered to brain-injured patients, because they decrease perilocal edema in patients with brain tumors. Recently, it has been found that steroids have no beneficial effects on brain-injured patients and such treatment has been discontinued [14].

Hyperosmotic solutions, e.g. 20% mannitol, can be used to decrease intracranial pressure. In this case, the solution is given at 0.25 to 1.0 g/kg within 10 to 20 minutes. This decrease can be achieved by three possible mechanisms:

1. dehydration of the brain;
2. a vasoconstriction caused by a change in viscosity as long as autoregulation is functioning properly [15]; and
3. by a reduction of CSF.

The degree of dehydration and alteration of electrolyte levels must not be extreme. The use of osmodiuretics may be dangerous during the acute phase after head injury, since generally brain swelling does not occur immediately and preventing shock is more important than trying to dehydrate the brain. In addition, intracranial bleeding may increase because of a reduction of brain volume caused by an osmodiuretic therapy. Osmodiuretics are not recommended for posttraumatic cerebral hyperemia, which is often observed in children. Hyperemia can be intensified by an osmotically induced increase of plasma volume. The use of osmodiuretics is indicated in instances of acutely increased ICP, cerebellar or midbrain impaction, peaks of ICP, and as a preparation for an operation. Diuretics, e.g. furosemide, dosed 1 mg/kg, also lower ICP. In addition, they reduce production of cerebrospinal fluid.

In the event that these measures do not sufficiently lower ICP, a barbiturate coma must be considered. Barbiturates reduce cerebral oxygen metabolism and increase cerebrovascular resistance, thereby reducing perfusion and ICP. Cerebral oxygen metabolism is reduced by more than 50%, leading to a suppression in the EEG. This effect is used to reduce epileptic attacks which are resistant to other treatment or within the scope of transitory incomplete ischemia (reverse steal). The protective effect occurs only in the presence of incomplete ischemia and only as long as there is some brain function. When global ischemia occurs, as after cardiac arrest, a barbiturate coma had no favorable effects in either animal experiments or in man.

In prospective studies, no evidence was found for a reduction in ICP and mortality by prophylactically applying barbiturate therapy in severely braininjured patients [16, 17]. In one of these studies pentobarbital was compared with mannitol [16], whereas in the other pentobarbital was prophylactically randomized and administered to patients with a low GCS, independent of their ICP [17]. In contrast to a prophylactic administration of barbiturates, it was reported in a third study that only 12% of the patients required barbiturates after randomization, because ICP remained elevated despite intense conventional therapy [18]. In this case, one out of three patients who received barbiturates had reduced ICP compared with one out of six who received only conventional therapy. It was concluded that barbiturates may have a beneficial effect, when other intensive measures prove unsuccessful in lowering ICP.

Barbiturate therapy has a cardiodepressive effect. Moreover, since the restriction of fluid intake and the use of diuretics result in volume depletion, it is most important to assure adequate filling of volume, especially during hyperventilation, to avoid hypotension. Frequently, despite fluid replacement, vasoactive drugs must also be administered. Dopamine, epinephrine, and norepinephrine do not have any direct cerebrovascular effect, if autoregulation is functioning normally. If the blood-brain barrier is defective, catecholamines will increase cerebral oxygen metabolism and perfusion; these effects are counteracted by barbiturates.

The requirement for pharmacological protection of the brain remains. Although some drugs such as nimodipine, offer favorable indications, beneficial effects on long-term outcome remain unproven. To date, only hypothermia has provided some protection for the brain in cases of complete ischemia. Artificially induced hypothermia is not generally recommended for clinical use due to the variability of injuries.

In conclusion, at the present time, the main problem in acute care of brain-injured patients is the prevention of secondary brain damage.

References

1. Five D, Jagger J (1984) The contribution of brain injury to the overall injury severity of brain-injured patients. J Neurosurg 56:697–699
2. Langfitt TW, Gennarelli TA (1982) Can the outcome from head injury be improved? J Neurosurg 56:19–25
3. Miller JD, Butterworth JF, Gudemann SK, et al (1981) Further experience in the management of severe head injury. J Neurosurg 54:289–299
4. Klauber MR, Marshall LF, Toole BM, Knowlton SL, Bowers SA (1985) Cause of decline in head-injury mortality rate in San Diego County, California. J Neurosurg 62:528–531
5. Lassen NA (1974) Control of cerebral circulation in health and disease. Circ Res 34:749–759
6. Bedford RF, Persing JA, Pobereskin L, Butler A (1980) Lidocaine or thiopental for rapid control of intracranial hypertension? Anesth Analg 59:435–437
7. Miller JD (1985) Head injury and brain ischaemia – implications for therapy. Br J Anaesth 57:120–130
8. Seelig JM, Becker DP, Miller JD, Greenberg RP, Ward JD, Choi SC (1981) Traumatic acute subdural hematoma: major mortality reduction in comatose patients treated within four hours. N Engl J Med 304:1511–1518
9. Miller JD, Becker DP, Ward JD, et al (1977) Significance of intracranial hypertension in severe head injury. J Neurosurg 47:503–516
10. Fleischer JE, Milde JH, Moyer TP, Michenfelder JD (1988) Cerebral effects of high-dose midazolam and subsequent reversal with Ro 15-1788 in dogs. Anesthesiology 68:234–242
11. Milde LN, Milde JH, Michenfelder JD (1985) Cerebral functional, metabolic, and hemodynamic effects of etomidate in dogs. Anesthesiology 63:371–377
12. Herregods L, Verbeke J, Rolly G, Colardyn F (1988) Effect of propofol on elevated intracranial pressure. Preliminary results. Anaesthesia 43 Suppl:107–109
13. Lanier WL, Laizzo PA, Milde JH (1989) Cerebral function and muscle afferent activity following intravenous succinylcholine in dogs anesthetized with halothane: the effects of pretreatment with a defasciculating dose of pancuronium. Anesthesiology 71:87–95
14. Dearden NM, Gibson JS, McDowall G, Gibson MR, Cameron MM (1986) Effect of high-dose dexamethasone on outcome from severe head injury. J Neurosurg 64:81–88
15. Muizelaar JP, Lutz HA, Becker DP (1984) Effect of mannitol on ICP and CBF and correlation with pressure autoregulation in severely head-injured patients. J Neurosurg 61:700–706
16. Schwartz ML, Tator CH, Rowed DW, et al (1984) The University of Toronto head injury treatment study: a prospective, randomized comparison of pentobarbital and mannitol. Can J Neurol Sci 11:434–440
17. Ward JD, Becker DP, Miller JD, et al (1985) Failure of prophylactic barbiturate coma in the treatment of severe head injury. J Neurosurg 62:383–388
18. Eisenberg HM, Frankowski RF, Content CF, Marshall LF, Walker MD and the comprehensive central nervous system trauma centers (1988) High-dose barbiturate control of elevated intracranial pressure in patients with severe head injury. J Neurosurg 69:15–23

The Role of Alcohol in Trauma

D. W. Yates

Alcohol Use and Abuse

Doctors are increasingly aware of the medical consequences of alcohol abuse and the general public professes to be concerned about its effect on family life, public safety and crome. However, affluence appears to generate an increased demand for drink, consumption is increasing world wide and its acute and chronic effects are seen to permeate all levels of society. Although there is some evidence that doctors have moderated their drinking habits in recent years – the profession's death rate due to cirrhosis has fallen substantially – and that the incidence of drunken driving is decreasing in some Western countries, the general trend remains upward on a global scale with specific increases in alcohol use amongst young people in developing countries.

During the 1970s the total world alcoholic beverages trade increased by more than 15% each year. Alcohol consumption has risen over the past 3 decades in all countries for which W. H. O. has reliable statistics – with the exception of France, which showed a slight decline whilst remaining at the top of the list. Industrialisation and greater mobility bring with them increased risk of accidental injury. It is clear that alcohol related trauma will become much more important in most countries outside North America and Europe in the coming decade and will remain a significant and preventable cause of morbidity in the West.

The medical response to this challenge must recognise the complex relationship between alcohol and injury. This review provides a summary of the extensive and sometimes contradictory literature on the subject and attempts to distinguish the various ways that alcohol can influence the incidence and management of and the responses to trauma.

The Incidence of Intoxication in Trauma Victims

Honkanen and Visuri [1] reported from Finland that alcohol use was associated with 19% of industrial accidents, 38% of traffic accidents, 36% of home accidents and 69% of assaults. In contrast Lings and Jensen [2] concluded that less than 3% of Danish occupational accidents could be linked to alcohol abuse. This is in agreement with the work of Yates et al. [3] who found that only 7 out of 275 patients referred to a UK Emergency Department from their place of work had a blood alcohol concentration (BAC) greater than 80 mg%. However they found that 60% of assaulted patients were intoxicated, the majority having sustained head injuries. The Annual Report of the Royal Life Saving Society for 1984 records that 19% of all known drownings were associated with alcohol use – the largest contributory factor. There is little information about the frequency with which alcohol is associated with domestic injury, but Yates [3] reported a 19% incidence.

More is known about motor vehicle accidents. In 1974 one third of drivers killed in road accidents in the UK had blood alcohol levels above 80 mg%. Between 10 pm and 4 am this rose to 51% during the week and 71% at the weekend [4]. Recent surveys from the US and UK suggest that the incidence of drunken driving is beginning to fall, particularly amongst the young. For example in a random survey in the US, the incidence of drivers with a BAC greater than 100 mg on weekend nights fell by 37% between 1973 and 1986 [5]. Nevertheless 25% of the teenage drivers killed in the UK in 1985 still had a BAC greater than 80 mg% and it should be remembered that for every trauma death there are two survivors with major permanent disabilities. Most are young and head injured.

Whilst this association between alcohol and head injury in vehicle occupants has received much attention, Galbreith et al. [6] have noted the much commoner link between alcohol and other forms of brain trauma. They reported a mean BAC of only 54 mg% in road accident patients, compared with levels of 137 mg% and 92 mg% in victims of assault and in pedestrians respectively.

A Causal Link

These epidemological surveys provide some measure of the incidence of alcohol use in various populations and point to an association between abuse and injury. However a causal link cannot be proven unless case controlled studies are undertaken and the whole spectrum of incidents is investigated. This is an obvious weakness in some reports – for example those exclusively concerned with patients admitted to hospital which do not take into account patients pronounced dead at the scene. Such methodological problems are often difficult to resolve in alcohol research – due to the complexity of matching control patients (and the ethical issues that this often raises) and the collection of information from unrelated sources. Much of the conflicting laboratory and clinical work in this area is a result of the use of inappropriate sampling techniques or unrepresentative animal models. Waller has written extensively on the methodical problems encountered in studying the relationship between alcohol and trauma [7].

The classical case controlled study designed to resolve this problem was reported by Borkenstein et al. in 1974 [8]. By comparing large matched groups of drivers (who had and had not had accidents and who had and had not been driving) they calculated the probability of an accident for each of the subgroups in relation to their measured blood alcohol concentrations. The curve of accident probability against BAC was age dependent and influenced to some extent by drinking experience. A young experienced driver had a six fold increase in accident risk at BAC of 80 mg/dl and the average driver a 10 fold increase at 150 mg/dl.

Waller et al. have recently reviewed over 1000 patients admitted to a Level 1 Trauma Center in North America and showed that alcohol impairment was strongly associated with greater injury in those patients seen but not admitted to hospital [7]. Severity of impact and age were taken into account, leaving a clear difference which could only be attributed to the presence or absence of alcohol.

The influence of alcohol on causation varies with the type of accident, being more important in falls from a height and in pedestrian and single vehicle accidents than in sports injuries and multiple vehicle incidents. Additionally protective devices are less likely to be worn by the intoxicated. Luna et al. found that only 11% of intoxicated motor cyclists wore their safety helmets compared with 38% of sober riders in a US survey [9]. Similar variations in the use of seat belts has been noted and yet Waller showed that belt use was of greater benefit to the intoxicated driver than to the sober driver in her study population [7].

The injuries sustained by the alcohol impaired road user are thus greater as a direct consequence of failure to use protective devices – for example Luna et al. [9] reported a mean Injury Severity Score (ISS) of 24.3 in their intoxicated group compared to an ISS of 15.1 in the sober group. However they further analysed their results to compare a subset of patients who had sustained similar head injuries (with a similar mean ISS). The mortality rate for the intoxicated group was 80% compared with 43% for the sober group. The ISS is a variable interval scale and the use of mean ISS values has been criticised. There are also problems with comparison of multiple injuries in different body regions, particularly when this involves the brain. Nevertheless such a large discrepancy does suggest that alcohol may influence outcome after trauma even when the circumstances of the incident and the injuries sustained are identical.

The results of many clinical and laboratory studies are however, inconclusive. Huth et al. [10] did not find any deleterious effect of alcohol in patients receiving Level I Trauma Center care. Some laboratory studies have also failed to show any effect [11] whilst others support a positive correlation [12]. Ward et al. [13] suggested that their intoxicated patients might have fared better than their equally severely injured sober controls. Zink et al. [14] used an unanesthetised swine hemorrhagic shock model in an attempt to more closely approximate the clinical situation and found that blood pressure was lower and hematocrit higher in the intoxicated animals. However, there was no sognificant difference in survival rates.

The chronic abuse of alcohol was not taken into account in these laboratory and clinical studies yet it may influence outcome. It could, for example, increase tolerance to the drug and even reduce the severity of consequential injury. More probably, the presence of chronic disease would increase the likelihood of injury and impair the recovery process. Waller [7] found that chronic alcohol abuse was associated with a higher ISS and Trauma Score and in increased probability of admission. She postulated that the inconsistent relationship between increasing injury severity and increasing BAC may be explained by the extent and duration of alcohol use and also the "biological vulnerability to injury". Hervé et al. [15] have emphasised the importance of chronic alcohol abuse in France. Fifty-nine per cent of their patients with raised glutamyltransferase (GT) and increased mean corpuscular volume (MCV) died, compared to a general mortality of 34%.

In summary, very carefully controlled clinical studies show that alcohol adversely affects outcome after injury, even when its effects on incidence and the accident environment have been taken into account. The most comprehensive survey, by Waller et al. [16] studied over one million US traffic accidents and found a two-fold increase attributable to alcohol (after controlling for speed, vehicle deformation, seat belt use and age). Rapid volume replacement, masking any peripheral vasodilation, could explain why Huth [10] was unable to show any adverse systemic effect of alcohol ingestion. In contrast Luna [9] has postulated a direct action on the CNS, which could potentiate the deleterious effect of a head injury on the central co-ordination of the cardiovascular responses to multiple trauma.

Problems with Diagnosis

Clinical detection of inebriation is unreliable [17] and causes major difficulties in the initial assessment of patients who have sustained apparently mild head injury [18]. However, patients rarely refuse to blow into a pocket alcometer. This measures mid stream exhaled air alcohol concentration, which correlates closely with blood alcohol concentration [19]. The determination of BAC for clinical purposes has no legal value if, as is usually the case, it has not been carried out in accordance with legal procedures. The patient can, therefore, be reassured on this point.

Whilst knowledge of the presenting BAC is valuable in long-term management (hematological complications, drug interactions, potential for withdrawal problems and need for support), and for research purposes, it is potentially dangerous information in the Emergency Department. Clearly a positive result should not influence the management of a patient with any altered level of consciousness. Neither should a negative result be taken as evidence of a sober lifestyle (vide infra). The intoxicated patient may have a reduced score on the Glasgow Coma Scale, and this in turn will alter his or her Trauma Score. It is difficult to separate out the influence of alcohol from other causes of deterioration in these parameters, adding to the problem of assessing the extent of physiological derangement after alcohol related trauma.

The blunting of sensation and the potential for aggressive behaviour further complicate the diagnostic process. Peripheral nerve injuries are often overlooked. Patient compliance is reduced, often resulting in motion artefact on radiographs and electrocardiographs. The risk of contamination of staff by the patient's blood, either by direct contact or by aerosol, is always greater in such circumstances, hence the use of gloves should be mandatory. There is increasing evidence that eye protection is important. Goggles should be available.

The Influence of Acute Intoxication on Trauma Management

Intoxicated patients are more likely to have full stomachs, more likely to have brain injuries and, therefore, more likely to vomit soon after injury. Many will have inhaled vomit before arrival at hospital. Pre-hospital and emergency department care must be concerned initially with the maintenance of a clear airway.

The acute ingestion of alcohol in previously normal subjects induces a diuresis. Hypotension has been observed, even after a relatively minor injury when associated with significant alcohol impairment [20]. This is probably due to a peripheral pooling secondary to loss of vasomotor tone, but another factor may be depression of the myocardium which is known to occur in normal subjects with quite low doses of ethanol [21].

Patients who have a history of chronic alcohol abuse tend to be overhydrated due to salt and water retention, and if they are cirrhotic may be hypokalemic with a metabolic alkalosis [22]. Cardiac function may be impaired without overt evidence of cardiac disease [23]. These distinct effects of acute and chronic alcohol abuse may explain some of the apparent inconsistencies highlighted in the epidemological studies mentioned previously.

The liver is a major heat source and patients with chronic liver disease tend to become hypothermic. This also occurs during acute intoxication, probably secondary to peripheral vasodilation. Fluid shifts from the circulation into the extracellular space as the core temperature falls. This has implications for retransfusion when the patient is being rewarmed simultaneously.

Lee et al. [24] have reported a doubling of anesthetic related mortality when the BAC exceeds 250 mg%. The pharmacological management of the trauma patient is compromised by liver damage increasing resistance to some anesthetic drugs and reducing tolerance to analgesics and psychotropic agents. Again the relationship is often influenced by the duration of exposure. For example, in acute intoxication the half-life of pentobarbital is prolonged, but after chronic ingestion it is significantly shortened.

Thrombocytopenia and impaired platelet function in the chronic alcoholic impair hemostasis but sudden alcohol withdrawal may result in a rebound thrombocytosis increasing the risk of venous thrombosis and pulmonary embolism [25]. Depression of neutrophil production, migration and killing ability leads to impairment of reticulo-endothelial clearance and a deficiency of host defenses [26].

These wide-ranging effects of acute and chronic alcohol use will have a significant impact on the initial management of the multiply injured patient. Subsequent care may be complicated by the development of withdrawal symptoms – fits are quite common – and the rarer presentation of delerium tremens.

Management of the Alcohol Problem

It has been estimated that alcoholics are twice as likely to die from trauma as from any of the more generally recognized complications of the disease [27]. The patient's involvement in an accident may be the first pointer to alcohol abuse and the admitting team have a responsibility to attend to this aspect of the patient's management once the care of the injuries has been organised and accomplished. Early treatment of patients with alcohol related problems is more likely to be successful if it is begun before advanced physical, psychiatric or social problems have developed. However, the detection of problem drinkers in the Emergency Department is not easy. In one series 64% of patients who admitted to drinking more that 10 units of alcohol on at least 5 occasions each week has a zero BAC [17]. The combination of a brief questionnaire and the measurement of GT and MCV is much more sensitive.

A recent US Survey revealed that only 32% of Level I Trauma Centers employed an alcohol councillor [28]. Yet alcohol has a greater influence on the frequency of trauma related deaths than it does on the mortality associated with any other disease process. The integration of alcohol treatment programes with trauma services is long overdue.

Intoxication Without Alcohol Ingestion

It is now well recognized that alcohol can be produced in the intestine of sober patients when a high carbohydrate diet is associated with a slow transit time and the proliferation of Candida Albicans. This syndrome was first described in Japan where it is known as Meitei-sho [29]. Although very rare in Western countries, it should be considered if the intoxicated injured patient subsequently denies alcohol consumption. Of more relevance to the pathologist is the finding that alcohol can be produced post mortem by gram negative rods from glucose and plasma at 4°C [30].

Conditions Simulating Drunkenness

The resuscitation team should be aware that intoxication can be mimicked by a wide spectrum of medical conditions. Whilst this knowledge must not influence the initial management and particularly the search for and treatment of intracranial pathology, it may help to explain apparently bizarre behaviour which is inconsistent with the evident injuries and the BAC. Abuse of other drugs is the commonest problem. This may be difficult to diagnose if alcohol has been taken concurrently and screening assays are unavailable. Hypoglycemia may present with aggressive unco-ordinated behaviour and the patient may have a grand mal fit. Alcoholic encephalopathy, cerebellar ataxia, stroke and disseminated sclerosis are other possibilities.

Future Strategies

The importance of alcohol in the causation of accidents has been emphasized and its effect on outcome discussed. Those responsible for the management of the injured should become more involved in the public debate about alcohol misuse and use their specialist knowledge to influence political opinion. Research has been shown to be inadequate and often poorly designed. In the UK £ 0.62 m was committed to alcohol research in 1986. The estimated cost of alcohol abuse was £ 1909,48 m. In the US it has been estimated that the economic cost of alcohol abuse in 1978 was almost as high as that due to cardiovascular disease and over twice that due to cancer. Work is required to more clearly define how alcohol influences outcome after injury, to identify target population for prevention campaigns, and to monitor trends.

Many countries have raised the minimum legal drinking age form 18 to 21 (Australia and most US States), and some have introduced random breath tests for car drivers. In the UK only 13% of drivers who are involved in accidents have their BAC measured. Random breath testing in New South Wales was associated with a 37% fall in vehicle occupant fatalities. There is increasing support for these measures in many developed countries and for the introduction of stricter enforcement of sensible drinking policies at work, in sport, and in public places. The co-operation of doctors in these developments at an international level will help to ensure that the upward trend of alcohol related accidents worldwide is gradually reversed.

References

1. Honkanen R, Visuri T (1976) Blood alcohol levels in a series of injured patients with special reference to accident and type of injury. Ann Chirurg Gynae 65:287–294
2. Lings S, Jensen J (1984) Occupational accidents and alcohol. Int Arch Occ Envir Hlth 53:321–329
3. Yates DW, Hadfield JM, Peters K (1987) Alcohol consumption of patients attending two accident and emergency departments in Northwest England. J Roy Soc Med 80:486–489
4. Royal College of Psychiatrists (1986) Alcohol – our favourite drug. Tavistock, London p 82
5. Insurance Institute for Highway Safety (1987) Drinking and driving drops sharply across nation. IIHS Arlington VA, USA 22:4 Jan 24
6. Galbraith S, Murray WR, Patel AR, Knill-Jones R (1976) The relationship between alcohol and head injury and its effect on the conscious level. Br J Surg 63:128–130
7. Waller PF, Hanson AR, Stewart JR (1989) The potentiating effects of alcohol on injury: a clinical study. In: Proceedings of 33rd Annual Conference, AAAM Des Plaines IL, USA Assoc Adv Automotive Med 1–16
8. Borkenstein RF, Crowther RF, Shumate RP, Ziel WB, Zyman R (1974) Report on the grand rapids survey. Indiana University: Department of Police Administration
9. Luna GK, Maier RV, Sowder L, Copass MK, Oreskovich MR (1984) The influence of ethanol intoxication on outcome of injured motor cyclists. J Trauma 24:695–699
10. Huth JF, Maier RV, Simonowitz DA (1983) Effect of acute ethanolism on the hospital course and outcome of injured automobile drivers. J Trauma 23:494–498
11. Hadfield JM, Stoner HB (1983) Interaction between ethanol and the response to injury. J Trauma 23:518–522
12. Gettler DT, Allbritten FF Jr (1963) Effect of alcohol intoxication on the respiratory exchange and mortality rate associated with acute hemorrhage in anesthetised dogs. Ann Surg 158:151–158
13. Ward RE, Flynn TC, Miller PW, Blaisdell WF (1982) Effects of ethanol ingestion on the severity and outcome of trauma. Am J Surg 144:153–157

14. Zink BJ, Syverud SA, Dronen SC, Barsan WG, Van Ligten P, Timerding BL (1988) The effect of ethanol on survival time in hemorrhagic shock in an unanesthetised swine model. Ann Emerg Med 17:15–19
15. Hervé C, Gaillard M, Roujas F, Huguenard P (1986) Alcoholism in polytrauma. J Trauma 26:1123–1126
16. Waller PR, Stewart JR, Hansen AR (1986) The potentiating effects of alcohol on driber injury. JAMA 256:1461–1466
17. Yates DW, Hadfield JM, Peters K (1987) The detection of problem drinkers in the accident and emergency department. Br J Addict 82:163–167
18. Rutherford WH (1977) Diagnosis of alcohol ingestion in mild head injuries. Lancet 1:1021–1023
19. Jones AW, Coldberg L (1978) Evaluation of breath alcohol instruments. In vitro experiments with alcometer pocket model. Forensic Sci Int 12:1–9
20. Swan K, Vidaver R, Lavigne JE, Brown CS (1977) Acute alcoholism, minor trauma and "shock". J Trauma 17:215–218
21. Ahmed SS, Levinson GE, Regan TJ (1973) Depression of myocardial contractility with low doses of ethanol in man. Circulation 48:378–385
22. Sereny G, Rapaport A, Husdan H (1966) The effect of alcohol withdrawal on electrolyte and acid base balance. Metabolism 15:896–904
23. Spodick DH, Pigott VM, Chirife R (1972) Preclinical cardiac malfunction in chronic alcoholism. N Eng J Med 287:677–680
24. Lee JF, Gliesecke AH, Jenkins MT (1967) Anesthetic management of trauma. Influence of alcohol ingestion. Southern Med J 60:1240–1243
25. Haselager EM, Vreeken J (1977) Rebound thombocytosis after alcohol abuse: a possible factor in the pathogenesis of thromboembolic disease. Lancet 1:774–775
26. Smith FE, Palmer DL (1976) Alcoholism, infection and altered host defences: A review of clinical and experimental observations. J Chronic Dis 29:35–49
27. Reyna TM, Hollis HW Jr, Hulsebus RC (1985) Alcohol related trauma: the surgeons responsibility. Ann Surg 201:194–197
28. Soderstrom CA (1987) Trauma, trauma centers and alcohol perspectives. J Assoc Adv Automotive Med 9:12–15
29. Kaji H, Asanuma Y, Yanara O, et al (1984) Intragastrointestinal alcohol fermentation syndrome: report of two cases and review of the literature. J Forensic Sci Soc 24:461–471
30. Vuori E, Renkonen OV, Lindbohm R (1983) Validity of post mortem blood alcohol values. Lancet 1:761–762

Emergency Management of Acute Lower Limb Ischemia

H. Haljamäe and L. Jivegård

Introduction

Acute nontraumatic lower limb ischemia is associated with very high mortality rates, often exceeding 25% [1-3]. Systemic atherosclerotic cardiovascular disease is present in most of these patients and the clinical risk index is therefore usually high due to old age, congestive heart failure, prior myocardial infarction, prior stroke, arrhythmia and abnormal electrocardiogram [4-6]. Acute arterial ischemia results in a high degree of energy metabolic impairment in the muscle [7] and the ischemic leg constitutes a source of complement activation increasing plasma anaphylatoxin concentrations [8], which in turn may further impair cardiac function [9]. Mortality in connection with acute limb ischemia seems related to the severity of the metabolic consequences of the ischemia, i.e. to the amount of tissue involved and the severity and duration of the circulatory disturbance.

Although a straightforward surgical approach to the vascular obstruction with removal of the embolic or thrombotic material by the use of a Fogarty catheter may seem the most relevant approach to a non-specialist in vascular surgery, alternative approaches based on a proper clinical assessment of the patient, may sometimes be more advantageous [1-3, 10]. Despite the long experience accumulated since the year 1911 when the first successful surgical treatment of a femoral artery embolus was carried out the emergency management of acute lower limb ischemia is still controversial.

Clinical Picture

From a surgical viewpoint, there are two major causes of acute non-traumatic lower limb ischemia, arterial embolism and thrombosis. Embolism may occur in patients with or without peripheral atherosclerotic occlusive disease, while acute arterial thrombosis almost exclusively occurs in patients with significant occlusive disease. Most patients with acute limb ischemia present with a history of a sudden onset of numbness, weakness and pain in the limb. Clinically, the limb is often waxy pale or shows mottled cyanosis, and in addition distal coolness and absence of pulses are found. Due to initial arterial spasm [1, 11], the symptoms are commonly maximal within 30 minutes from the onset. The initial spasm is in our experience usually diminished within 2-3 hours. If collateral circulation exists and is sufficient to avoid the immediate risk of limb loss, there is no further thrombotization in the arterial tree (unpublished observations). Development of collateral circulation and relief of initial arterial spasm is experienced by the patient as diminishing sensory and motor dysfunction and relief of the ischemic pain. This type of clinical course occurs in 60–70% of patients with acute limb ischemia, and emergency embolectomy usually is not necessary in these patients [3]. In the remaining 30–40% of the cases, collateral blood flow is insufficient due to poor cardiac output, preexisting occlusive disease and rheological factors. The clinical picture then obviates the need for emergency revascularization as pain is increasing and further impairment or loss of motor and sensibility functions are observed indicating that secondary thrombotization may occur in the arterial tree distal to the occluding clot [1].

The nerves of the limb are sensitive to ischemia, and the sensation to light touch and the neuro-muscular transmission are affected early, if the ischemia is critical. Nervous function and the degree of ischemic pain can therefore be used as valuable markers of the severity of the limb ischemia. If a patient has only moderate pain and impairement of sensory and motor functions in the foot of the ischemic leg there is no immediate risk of limb loss [3]. Energy demands in skeletal muscle during rest are small, and the skeletal muscle has a rather large store of potential energy present. Yet, irreversible damage to skeletal muscle occurs after some 3 to 5 hours of total or near total ischemia [12]. In acute limb ischemia of embolic or thrombotic origin the ischemia is seldom total.

Vital Organ Dysfunction

The mortality rate in patients with acute lower limb ischemia is due to impairment of vital organ function. The major causes of death are cardiopulmonary failure, accounting for 50–65% of the deaths, thromboembolic complications, accounting for 15–20% of the deaths, and myonephropathic-metabolic complications responsible for death of 5–10% of the patients [1–3]. There is a significant relationship between gangrene of the limb and fatal outcome [14], suggesting a relationship between the severity of the limb ischemia and the function of vital organs.

Cardiac Dysfunction

Most arterial emboli originate from the heart, the main causes being atrial fibrillation or acute myocardial infarction due to atherosclerotic heart disease [2, 15, 16]. Recent studies have shown that cardiac output and myocardial contractility often are low in patients with acute lower limb ischemia, whereas systemic vascular resistance is high [17]. The already low cardiac output is further decreased following embolectomy and reperfusion, thus reducing the already critically reduced blood flow to vital organs such as the heart, brain and kidneys. There is a significant relationship between the cardiac output and the severity of the limb ischemia on admission suggesting either that factors depressing myocardial function are released from the ischemic limb or that the limb ischemia is worsened by poor cardiac pump function, or both. Ongoing experimental studies at our department in a pig model for aortic saddle embolism have demonstrated that lower limb ischemia and reperfusion per se decrease myocardial contractility and cardiac output, suggesting that acute severe limb ischemia is associated with a cardiodepressive effect.

Thromboxane A_2 (TxA$_2$) has been suggested to be one mediator of such cardiodepressive effects [18], and we have in ongoing studies found a significant relationship between in vivo TxA$_2$ biosynthesis, measured as urine levels of a stable TxA$_2$-metabolite, and cardiac output, but not to the severity of the limb ischemia in patients with acute embolic lower limb ischemia. Limb ischemia also activates the complement cascade [8], and complement activation may negatively affect cardiac function [9]. The nutritive blood flow within the heart and other vital organs may be further impaired due to reduced red blood cell deformability as indicated by ongoing studies. The impairment in red blood cell deformability is strongly related to the severity of the limb ischemia and it is abolished by successful revascularization [19].

The available information thus suggests that cardiac function is often critically reduced in patients with acute limb ischemia and cardiac dysfunction is a major cause of death in these patients implying that monitoring and support of the failing heart is important and must have supreme priority. Cardiac function can rapidly and without risks non-invasively be monitored by computerized thoracic electrical bioimpedance technique [17]. Since the information given by such cardiac monitoring with reasonable accuracy predicts the risk of cardiac death, also the choice of surgical treatment for the limb may partly be based on the cardiac performance data [17].

Thromboembolic Complications

Ischemia and gangrene in vital organs such as the brain or organs of the gastrointestinal tract is not infrequently seen in patients with limb ischemia and may be caused by thromboembolism. Also pulmonary embolism due to secondary venous thrombotization is reported to be common following arterial embolectomy and reperfusion [1]. Thromboembolic complications may theoretically be counteracted by heparin infusion. However, there are as yet no prospective randomized studies demonstrating the efficacy of heparin in preventing thromboembolic complications in such patients [20], although several retrospective studies suggest a beneficial effect by heparin [13, 21]. Preliminary data from a large ongoing prospective multicenter study comparing the results in patients undergoing arterial embolectomy with and without anticoagulant medication suggest that the rates of good results are similar in the two groups. Although theoretically heparin may reduce thromboembolic complications and reduce the risk of rethrombosis or recurrent embolization to the limb, heparin increases the risk of severe bleeding complications. It is conceivable, however, that, heparin may have a beneficial effect in selected patients.

In order to prevent systemic cascade system activation by tissue components from the ischemic leg it has been suggested that phlebotomy of the femoral vein should be performed during embolectomy prior to restitution of the arterial blood flow. The efficacy of such a procedure in preventing postoperative complications is unproven, however. Hemorrheological treatment with low molecular weight dextran is considered an additional beneficial factor in the management of the ischemic limb and for prevention of postoperative thrombosis following difficult lower extremity bypass [22, 23].

Myonephropathic-Metabolic Syndrome

The myonephropathic-metabolic syndrome has been described in detail by Haimovici [24]. The initiating event is ischemic rhabdomyolysis and myoglobin release. During the ischemic phase, the clinical manifestations are rigidity of the muscles of the ischemic limb, and usually oliguria, acidosis, myoglobinemia and hyperkalemia are present. Some of the metabolic changes are easily correctible, whereas the hyperkalemia and myoglobinemia due to manifest massive muscle necrosis following reperfusion may reach deleterious levels leading to death of the patient. The syndrome is reported to occur in 7.5-10% of cases of acute limb ischemia. The mortality rate in this syndrome is reported to 30-80% [24]. The patient with massive muscle rigidity is best treated by emergency amputation. In the absence of massive muscle rigidity, optimal treatment consists of emergency revascularization in those patients who have immediately threatened viability of the limb. Whenever the syndrome is suspected alkalinization and enforced diuresis should promptly be instituted thereby diminishing the precipitation of myoglobin in the renal tubules. In the presence of edema and stiffness of the muscle compartments, emergency fasciotomy should be employed. In advanced cases, hemodialysis should be performed as an emergency procedure to avoid the lethal effect of severe hyperkalemia. Electrolyte balance should be reestablished.

Surgical Management

Methods for Revascularization of the Acutely Ischemic Limb

It is obvious from previously published studies of the spontaneous course of embolic limb ischemia that a fraction of the patients will have restituted arterial blood flow without any therapeutic measures having been instituted [11]. Whether this is due to fragmentation or lysis of the embolus, or to major collateral blood flow is unknown. It is clear, however, that most patients with acute limb ischemia will need some kind of revascularization procedure. In cases of arterial embolism and no or minor atherosclerotic occlusive disease, some reconstructive procedure must at times be added to the embolectomy; procedures such as a patch graft, thrombendarterectomy or even a bypass procedure. Reconstructive procedures are nearly always needed in cases of acute arterial thrombosis in order to eliminate the stenoses which elicited the acute thrombosis.

Some patients may not tolerate even the minor operative procedure of thromboembolectomy, and vascular reconstruction is thus neither a possible alternative. Furthermore, use of the Fogarty catheter is known to be associated with early and late arterial damage [25] suggesting that alternative treatment, if effective may be indicated.

Lysis of the occluding clot may be achieved by infusion of streptokinase, urokinase or tissue plasminogen activator either alone [26] or as an adjunct to operative thromboembolectomy [27, 28]. Transluminal angioplasty with or without laser recanalization may then be added to improve long-term patency. Thromboembolectomy may also be performed by angioscopic techniques, which possibly could decrease the operative trauma in critically ill patients [29].

Although significant experiences have accumulated in some centers in recent years with the mentioned techniques, these therapeutic principles are not yet widely accepted as safe and effective procedures.

Widely Accepted Principles for Surgical Management

The goals of treatment are salvage of the limb and survival of the patient. Occasionally, the first goal must be sacrificed to achieve the other. In the patient without significant heart failure with embolic arterial occlusion of short duration and without signs of muscle necrosis and who has no evidence of peripheral atherosclerotic occlusive disease, early embolectomy by use of the Fogarty catheter offers rewarding results [14]. In definite cases of *acute arterial thrombosis* due to atherosclerotic occlusive disease, it is reasonably well established that treatment is best brought about by initial heparin infusion, and early arteriography followed by a vascular reconstruction [2, 3, 14]. A commonly used management policy is to differentiate on admission between arterial embolism and thrombosis as the cause of the acute ischemia, and to employ emergency operation in all cases believed to have *embolic occlusion*. Unfortunately, the differentiation between arterial embolism and thrombosis is often difficult. The only sign of discriminating value between arterial thrombosis and embolism seems to be cardiac arrhythmias [30]. The differential diagnosis between arterial embolism and thrombosis is even more difficult in the group of patients (about 20–30% in our experience) who have a history of peripheral vascular disease and who present with atrial fibrillation on admission.

Overall, an admission diagnosis of embolism is incorrect in 10–20%, the correct diagnosis in these cases instead being acute arterial thrombosis or cardiac failure [30, 31]. Such patients do not benefit from emergency embolectomy. In the patients with a correct admission diagnosis of arterial embolism, we have in a study in which emergency arteriography was routinely performed observed that more than half have moderate or severe peripheral atherosclerotic occlusive disease [31]. Early embolectomy is associated with significantly higher mortality and amputation rates in patients with embolization to atherosclerotic arteries [31]. This may in part be due to the increasing operative hazards, and difficulties in reestablishing adequate blood flow by thromboembolectomy alone in patients with significant local atherosclerosis. Vascular reconstruction may be needed in such patients, and this is best performed during daytime by a specialist vascular surgeon. We therefore believe that initial conservative treatment may be beneficial also in a substantial fraction of patients with embolic occlusion, provided that the ischemia does not immediately threaten limb viability.

Selective Initial Conservative Treatment

Due to the difficulties described above, we have employed a selective conservative approach in patients with acute limb ischemia during the last 7-year period [3]. Initial treatment is chosen solely on the basis of an examination of the severity of the acute ischemia, regardless of the presumed etiology of the acute occlusion. Patients with immediately threatened viability of the limb, as evidenced by severe pain and loss of motor and sensibility functions, are taken to the operating room and undergo emergency thromboembolectomy unless there is regidity of the skeletal muscle. If, on the other hand, the patient has preserved or only moderate impairment of sensory and motor functions on admission, conservative treatment is initially employed. The patient is then given heparin infusion (350 units/kg per day intravenously) and is subjected to arteriography. The state of the heart and of the ischemic limb must be continuously carefully assessed, and cardiac function is supported whenever considered necessary. If the state of the limb deteriorates or fails to improve during heparin infusion, operation is performed. This is performed during the first week from admission, and is necessary in approximately 60% of these cases in our experience. During the operation, every step judged necessary to achieve adequate revascularization is undertaken, and in our experience some 40% will need reconstructive procedures, whereas 60% undergo thromboembolectomy alone [31]. We have found that a major advantage with the present management policy is that most patients in this way can be operated upon electively, during daytime, by a specialist vascular surgeon [10].

Until 1981 we routinely employed emergency operation in nearly all patients with acute limb ischemia [3]. At present this is only performed in approximately 30% of the cases. Overall the rate of gangrene in our total series of patients with acute limb ischemia (all cases, i.e. both cases of arterial thrombosis and embolism) has been reduced by about 50%. Limb salvage rate in embolic cases is near 100%, whereas there still remains a significant failure rate in patients with arterial thrombosis due to atherosclerotic occlusive disease. Overall, there has also been a reduction in the mortality rate, and the rate of good results has improved significantly.

Conclusions

The patient with acute lower limb ischemia is a high surgical risk. The emergency treatment should be based on a careful clinical assessment of the severity of the local ischemia and of vital organ function. Patients with immediately threatened viability of the limb should be acutely operated upon, whereas the remaining majority with less severe ischemia initially are managed by heparin infusion and an early arteriography. If the arteriogram does not show significant occlusive disease and the patient fails to improve during heparin infusion a simple embolectomy can safely be performed during the first days after admission unless the patient has very poor cardiac output. In the latter group of patients every effort must be made to improve cardiac function preoperatively. In cases with arteriographic findings of moderate or severe occlusive disease an elective operation, which often will include vascular reconstruction, is performed during the first days.

References

1. Blaisdell FW, Steele M, Allen RE (1978) Management of acute lower extremity arterial ischemia due to embolism and thrombosis. Surgery 84:822-834
2. Lusby RJ, Wylie EJ (1983) Acute lower limb ischemia: pathogenesis and management. World J Surg 7:340-346
3. Jivegård LE, Arfvidsson B, Holm J, Scherstén T (1987) Selective conservative and routine early operative treatment in acute limb ischemia. Br J Surg 74:798-801
4. Cooperman M, Pflug B, Martin Jr EW, Evans WE (1978) Cardiovascular risk factors in patients with peripheral vascular disease. Surgery 84:505-509
5. Hertzer NR (1981) Fatal myocardial infarction following lower extremity revascularization. Two hundred seventy-three patients followed six to eleven postoperative years. Ann Surg 193:492-498
6. Fowkes FGR (1988) Epidemiology of atherosclerotic arterial disease in the lower limbs. Eur J Vasc Surg 2:283-291
7. Aldman Å, Larsson J, Elfström J (1987) Muscle energy stores in relation to clinical findings and outcome in acute arterial ischemia of the lower leg. Eur J Vasc Surg 1:415-420
8. Bengtson A, Holmberg P, Heideman M (1987) The ischemic leg as a source of complement activation. Br J Surg 4:697-700
9. Hachfeld del Balzo U, Levi R, Polley MJ (1985) Cardiac dysfunction caused by purified human C3a anaphylatoxin. Proc Natl Acad Sci USA 82:886-890
10. Nachbur B (1988) Treatment of acute ischaemia: Every general surgeon's business? Eur J Vasc Surg 2:281-282
11. Haimovici H (1950) Peripheral arterial embolism. A study of 330 unselected cases of embolism of the extremities. Angiology 1:20-45
12. Walker PM (1986) Symposium on acute arterial insufficiency. 1. Pathophysiology of acute arterial occlusion. Can J Surg 29:340-342
13. Takolander R, Lannerstad O, Bergqvist D (1987) Peripheral arterial embolectomy, risks and results. Acta Chir Scand 154:567-572
14. Jivegård L, Holm J, Scherstén T (1986) The outcome in arterial thrombosis misdiagnosed as arterial embolism. Acta Chir Scand 152:251-256
15. Abbott WM, Maloney RD, McCabe CC, Wirthlins LS (1982) Arterial embolism. A 44 year perspective. Am J Surg 143:460-464
16. Elliot JP, Hageman JH, Szilagyi E, Ramakrishnan V, Bravo JJ, Smith RF (1980) Arterial embolization: problems of source, multiplicity, recurrence, and delayed treatment. Surgery 88:833-845
17. Jivegård L, Arfvidsson B, Frid I, Haljamäe H, Holm J (1990) Cardiac output in patients with acute lower limb ischemia of presumed embolic origin. A predictor of severity and outcome? Eur J Vasc Surg (in press)
18. Matiesson M, Dunham BM, Huval MV, et al (1983) Ischemia of the limb stimulates thromboxane production and myocardial depression. Surg Gynecol Obstet 157:500-504
19. Jivegård L, Belboul A, Bergman P, Al-Khaja N, Holm J, Roberts D (1990) Red cell deformability in patients with acute embolic lower limb ischemia. Eur J Vasc Surg (in press)

550   H. Haljamäe and L. Jivegård

20. Jivegård L, Holm J, Scherstén T (1986) Arterial thromboembolectomy, should anticoagulants be administered? Acta Chir Scand 152:493–497
21. Hammarsten J, Holm J, Scherstén T (1978) Positive and negative effects of anticoagulant treatment during and after embolectomy. J Cardiovasc Surg 19:373–379
22. Dormandy JA (1983) Significance of hemorrheology in the management of the ischemic limb. World J Surg 7:319–325
23. Rutherford RB, Jones DN, Bergentz S-E, et al (1984) The efficacy of dextran 40 in preventing early postoperative thrombosis following difficult lower extremity bypass. J Vasc Surg 1:765–773
24. Haimovici H (1979) Muscular, renal, and metabolic complications of acute arterial occlusions: myonephropathic-metabolic syndrome. Surgery 85:461–468
25. Dobrin DP (1989) Mechanisms and prevention of arterial injuries caused by balloon embolectomy. Surgery 106:457–466
26. Earnshaw JJ, Westby JC, Gregson RHS, Makin SS, Hopkinson BR (1989) Local thrombolytic therapy of acute peripheral arterial ischemia with tissue plasminogen activator: a dose-ranging study. Br J Surg 75:1196–1200
27. Norem RF, Short DH, Kerstein MD (1988) Role of intraoperative fibrinolytic therapy in acute arterial occlusion. Surg Gynecol Obstet 167:87–91
28. Parent FN, Bernhard VM, Pabst TS, McIntyre KE, Hunter GC, Malone JM (1989) Fibrinolytic treatment of residual thrombus after catheter embolectomy for severe lower limb ischemia. J Vasc Surg 9:153–160
29. White GH, White RA; Kopchok GE, Wilson SE (1988) Angioscopic thromboembolectomy: Preliminary observations with a recent technique. Vasc Surg 7:318–325
30. Cambria RP, Abbott WM (1984) Acute arterial thrombosis of the lower extremity. Its natural history contrasted with arterial embolism. Arch Surg 119:784–787
31. Jivegård L, Arfvidsson B, Holm J (1989) Femoral embolectomy for embolic lower limb ischemia. The influence of coexisting atherosclerotic occlusive disease. Vasc Surg (in press)

Emergency Medicine in France: Examples of Organization and Services Provided

F. Carpentier, M. Guignier, and J. Mingat

Introduction

A veritable "problem child" in French hospital system, and for many years "underpriviliged" in comparison with other disciplines, emergency medecine in France is undergoing major reorganization. Continuous 24 hour operation in Regional and University Hospital emergency departments (ED) has become a health care priority. Indeed, nearly 6 million patients are admitted each year in medical and surgical emergency rooms in the country, and 50% of all hospitalizations are the result of initial evaluation and treatment in the ED which serves as liaison between primary care physicians and hospital medicine. Both suitable standards of procedure and the nature of patient problems motivating emergency care "consumption" need to be specified in order to:

1. define the essential roles of the ED and the qualifications of medical and paramedical staff;
2. determine the architectural requirements for providing optimal and pleasant reception, and for responding to all types of medical and surgical emergencies;
3. evaluate the need for technical facilities (lab, radiology) in the vicinity of the ED.

Emergency Care: Patient Profile

Knowledge of emergency patient socio-demographic parameters is important to establish reception procedures and prepare the organizational framework (medical and administrative staff, structural set-up, etc.). Armed at determining these parameters, a prospective multi-center inquiry was carried out over a one month period (November 1987) in 17 French hospital centers (10 university hospitals and 7 regional hospitals). A total of 11 items were studied including age, sex, marital status, profession, nationality, ethnic origin and conditions of admission and discharge [Carpentier F., 1989, personal communication]

Population

During this month, 21 122 patients were admitted (704 patients/day) with numbers varying according to hospital (121 to 3431 patients/month). Patient age is

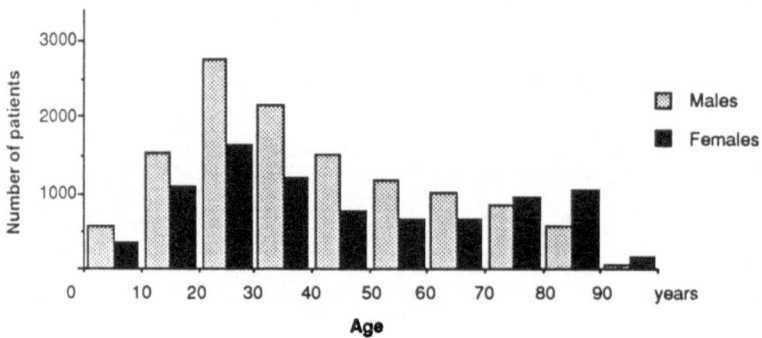

Fig. 1. Age and sex distribution of patients admitted to emergency departments

42 ± 23 years (range 0–99 years), but more than 25% of patients are over age 60 (Fig. 1). The sex ratio is 1.42. 82% of patients are French and 89% originate from the region served by the hospital. The majority of hospitals have an essentially urban patient recruitment. 35% of patients are salaried workers and 25% are retired.

Mode of Arrival

51% of patients arrive by their own means (Fig. 2), while 7% are transported by hospital ambulance (in France: Service d'Aide Médicale Urgente ou SAMU) and 24% by private ambulance.

The distribution of ED admissions according to day of the week is relatively homogeneous with, however, 2 peaks: Monday and Saturday (Fig. 3A). 73% of patients are admitted between 10 A.M. and 10 P.M. (Fig. 3B), the hour of arrival depending on patient age: 23% of patients admitted between 6 A.M. and 10 A.M. are in the 20–29 year age group while 29% of patients arriving between 2 P.M. and 6 P.M. are over age 60 years. The day of admission also varies with age: on Sunday, 44% of patients are under age 30, versus 36% on Monday, for example.

Mean Length of Stay

The mean length of stay (MLS) is 6 ± 17 hours. This important variability is due to 2 types of emergency service in France:

1. ED (n = 10) with short MLS (1h 25 min) admitting both trauma cases requiring punctual care and medical cases needing brief hospitalization;
2. ED (n = 7) with long MLS (11 h 20 min) and without independant hospitalization units where patients arriving and patients undergoing evaluation are managed in the same area.

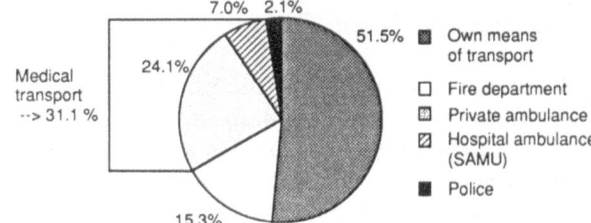

Fig. 2. Frequency distribution of mode of arrival

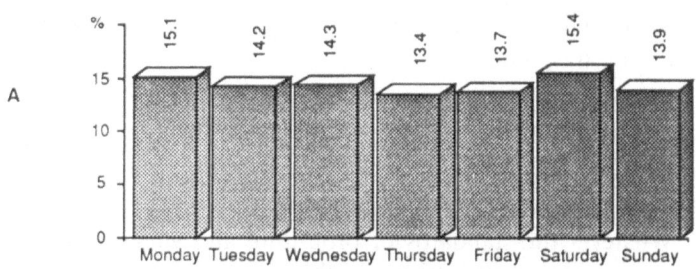

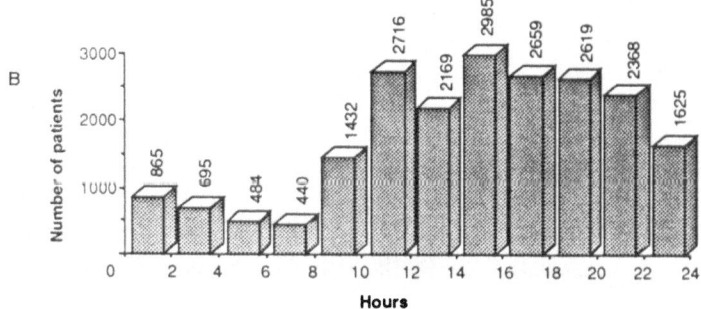

Fig. 3 A, B. Distributions of admissions: **A** according to the day of the week, **B** according to the hour of the day

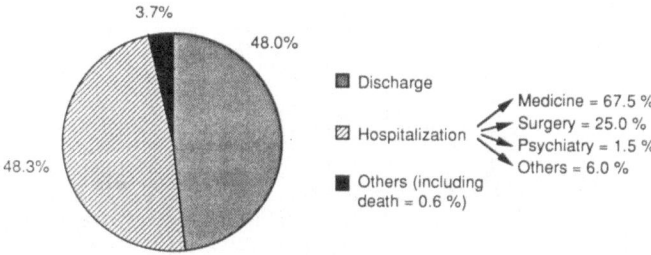

Fig. 4. Frequency distribution of patient discharge from ED

Conditions of Patient Discharge

48% of patients admitted to the ED return home (Fig. 4) and 48% are hospitalized, the majority of whom in medicine (70%). The percentage of patients hospitalized varies from one hospital to another (17% to 73%) depending on the number of trauma cases and whether or not pediatric emergencies are handled in the same facility. Conditions of discharge are modified by age: the number of hospitalizations increases with age (Fig. 5A). Orientation in medicine or surgery also varies with patient age (Fig. 5B). Young patients are more often hospitalized in surgery because of the increased incidence of trauma in this age group. Professional status also influences discharge mode: 76% of students and 68% of salaried workers are discharged, while 64% of retirees and 65% of agricultural workers are hospitalized.

Conclusions

Whatever the standards of procedure and whatever the patient recruitment, it appears that characteristics of the population seeking emergency care are identi-

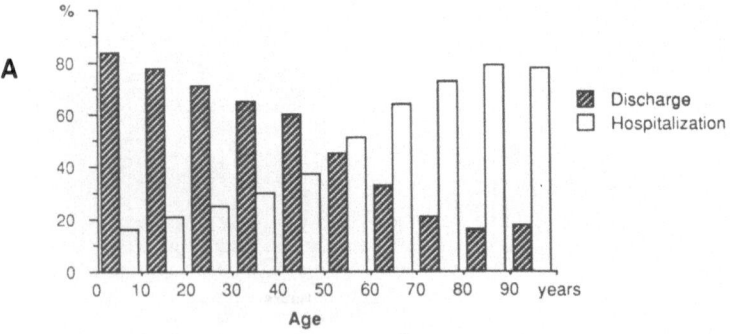

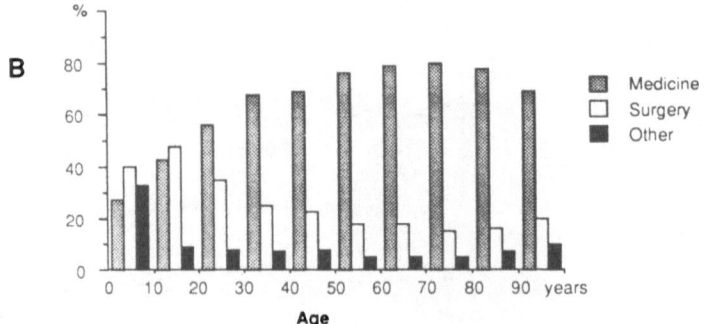

Fig. 5. A Outcome of patients according to age. **B** Department of admission according to age

cal from one hospital center to another: relatively young patients [1, 2] arrive at the ED by their own means of transport which demonstrates that the ED can be used, in good or bad earnest, as a "walk-in" consultation service [3, 4]. Half of all patients admitted to the ED are discharged, while the percentage of those hospitalized increases with age.

The Emergency Department at Grenoble: Pathology Profile

The ED for adult patients at the Grenoble University Hospital Center is separated into 2 wards:

1. the surgical emergency ward receives only trauma cases involving 22000 patients/yr (hospitalization = 25%)
2. the medical emergency ward, which is the subject of this study, is subdivided into 3 functionally and geographically distinct units:
   - the medical ED, open 24 hours a day, receives 11000 patients/year whatever the nature and urgency of the problem. It is staffed by 2 full-time physicians assisted by interns, who make 3 complete rounds each day.
   - the ICU (4 beds) receives 1300 patients/year who are in vital distress and require close cardiovascular and/or neurological surveillance with intensive therapeutic measures. It is staffed by the same physicians and interns responsible for the medical ED.
   - the walk-in clinic admits 5500 patients/year and is open 6 days a week (8 A.M. to 7 P.M. Monday through Friday and 8 A.M. to noon on Saturday). Consultations are provided without appointment by private general practitioners with house-staff privileges.

From a prospective study during 24 days evenly distributed over a 4 month period involving 1066 patients in these 3 medical emergency services, we were able to determine the different pathologies as well as the outcome of the patients after admission to the ED [5].

The Medical ED

638 patients (26.5 patients/day), with a mean age of 52 yrs and a sex ratio of 1.18 were admitted during the period studied. 72% of all patients and 93% of patients over 65 years of age are referred by a private physician. A small number of patients (38%) arrive by their own mean in this unit in contrast with other reports in the literature [3]. 67% are hospitalized after a MLS of 12 hours.

We established 12 diagnostic categories keeping in mind that the same patient can present one or more affections. Three diagnostic stages are compared in this study (Table 1) in order to determine the role and effectiveness of the ED: reason for admission, ED discharge diagnosis and final diagnosis after hospitalization.

The reason for admission is influenced by whether or not the patient is referred by a physician (Fig. 6 A1 and A2). 64% of referred patients present neurolo-

Table 1. Distribution of different pathologies for 638 patients admitted to the medical emergency department (ED)

	Reason for admission %	ED discharge diagnosis %	Final diagnosis % (for 427 patients)
Neurology	19.1	19.5	18.0
Gastro-enterology	18.2	18.5	20.6
Systemic symptoms	15.9	12.5	6.3
Cardiology	14.6	19.4	23.4
Intoxications	14.6	19.4	15.2
Psychiatry	13.6	16.4	12.2
Pulmonary	8.5	11.6	12.9
Nephrology	7.1	9.9	12.1
Endocrinology	3.3	3.6	5.1
Infectious diseases	1.3	3.9	5.8
Malignant diseases	1.1	2.5	4.2
Others	11.3	16.5	18.4

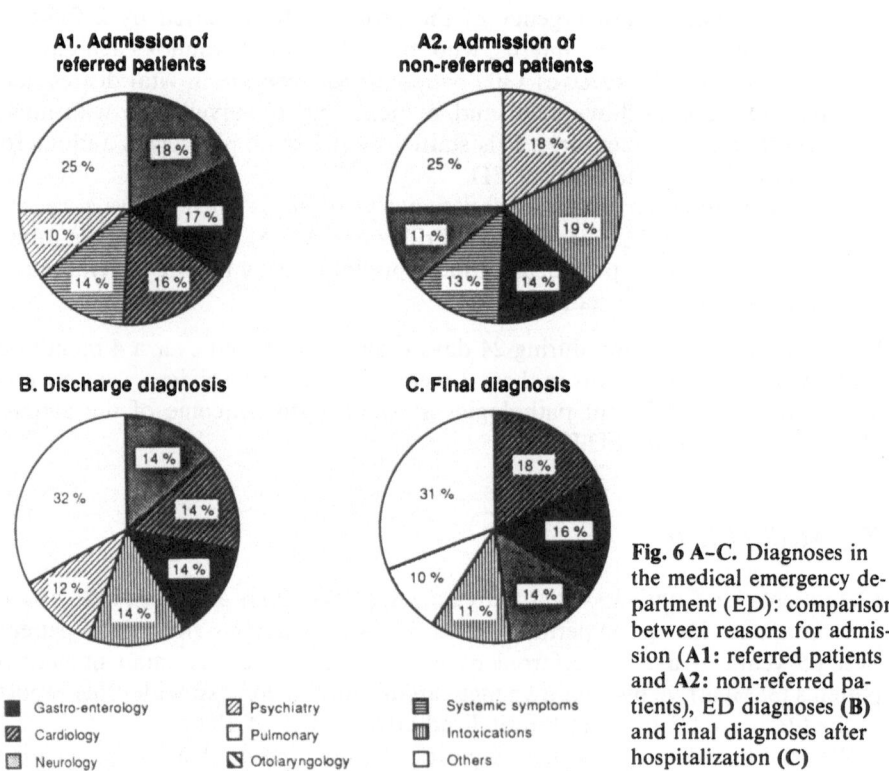

Fig. 6 A–C. Diagnoses in the medical emergency department (ED): comparison between reasons for admission (**A1**: referred patients and **A2**: non-referred patients), ED diagnoses (**B**) and final diagnoses after hospitalization (**C**)

gical, cardiovascular or digestive problems. 37% of non-referred patients present an intoxication or a psychiatric problem. Referred patients are more often hospitalized (77%) than non-referred patients (41%). ED discharge diagnoses (Fig. 6B) involve 4 major pathologies: neurological, cardiovascular, gastroenterological and intoxications. Among final diagnoses after hospitalization (Fig. 6C), cardiovascular diseases are the most common.

An evaluation of ED efficacy is also based on the number of correct diagnoses made. 71% of final diagnoses are already made in the ED before transfer to another hospital unit with the aid of a careful physicial exam, several basic lab tests and radiologic explorations, and sometimes (25%) a specialist opinion. In addition:

1. when patients are referred by private physicians, the correct diagnosis is already established in only 42% of cases.
2. 29% of final diagnoses made after transfer to an hospital bed are made only after the performance of complementary analyses impossible to carry out in an emergency context and usually unmodified (1%) within the first 24 hours of hospitalization.

The Walk-in Clinic

342 patients (19 patients/day), with a mean age of 42 yrs and a sex ratio of 1.19, were received in this department. 58% of these patients arrive on their own and 92% by their own means of transport. 31% of these patients are hospitalized after a brief MLS of 2 h 45 min.

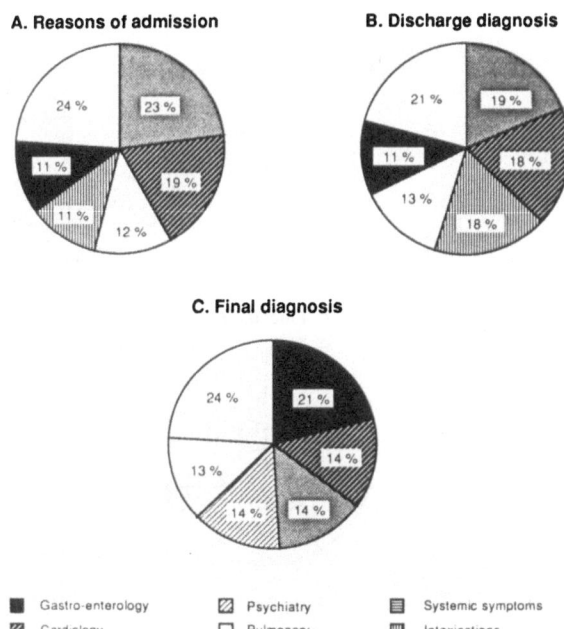

Fig. 7 A–C. Diagnoses in the walk-in clinic: comparison between reasons for admission **(A)**, discharge diagnoses **(B)** and final diagnoses after hospitalization **(C)**

The pathologies encountered in this unit are mostly minor (94%) and do not modify the vital or functional prognosis. Reasons for hospitalization (Fig. 7A) include systemic (malaise, pain, etc.), neurological, digestive or psychiatric symptoms. The discharge diagnosis (Fig. 7B) after physical examination and an eventual specialist opinion (16% of patients) is predominantly based on psychiatric and gastro-enterological problems. Few patients are hospitalized and their final principal diagnoses (Fig. 7C) involve digestive, cardiac and psychiatric pathology.

Diagnostic performance in the walk-in clinic is lower because of the shorter MLS and the smaller number of complementary exams ordered in this unit.

The Intensive Care Unit (ICU)

86 patients (3.6 patients/day) are admitted in this unit either directly or following initial evaluation in the medical ED. Mean patient age is high (65 years), and the sex ratio is 1.23. All patients are referred by a physician while 66% are transferred by hospital ambulance and 29% by private ambulance. 88% of these patients present severe disease engaging the immediate vital prognosis and correlated with a high mortality rate (12%) and high hospitalization rate (74%). Neurological disease (essentially strokes) and acute cardiac affections (myocardial infarction or acute pulmonary edema for example) constitute the majority of admission motives (Fig. 8A). Diagnoses at discharge from ICU (Fig. 8B) after an average stay of 21 h 15 min are based on neurological or cardio-vascular disease or an intoxication.

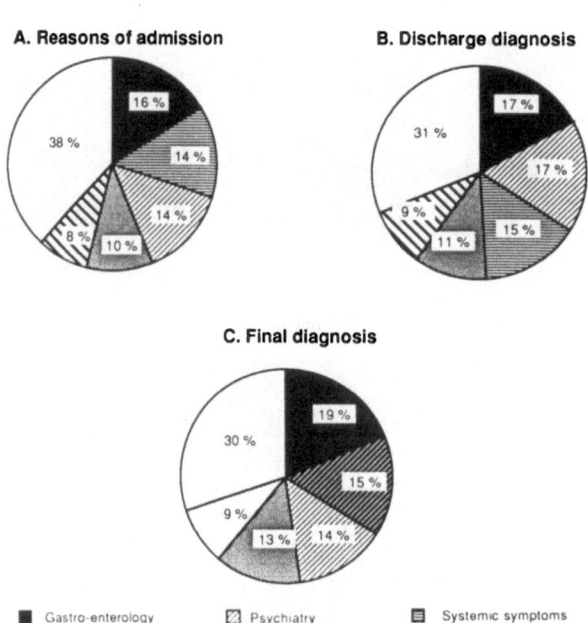

Fig. 8 A–C. Comparison of intensive care unit diagnoses: comparison between reasons for admission **(A)**, discharge diagnoses **(B)** and final diagnoses after hospitalization **(C)**

The final diagnosis of hospitalized patients most often involves cardiovascular problems (Fig. 8C) while the majority of deaths occurring in the ICU are due to neurological causes. A comparaison of ICU diagnoses and final diagnoses after hospitalization reveals a global performance of 77%.

Synthesis

From these two examples of organization, it clearly appears that knowledge of both admission profiles and different pathologies encountered is the first step to understand emergency care standards of procedures in France. From this, one may foresee the ideal organization of such services. ED managers now want to prove their ability to serve patients and their families, to provide accurate diagnoses with a high degree of confidence and to initiate appropriate therapeutic measures [6].

The Personnel

The mission of an Emergency Room is to accept patients 24 hours a day, whatever their pathologies and degree of urgency [7, 8]. This main objective can only be met under the following conditions:

1. The ED head physician must be a senior staff member assigned on a full-time basis [6]. ED services should no longer be put under the responsibility of physicians whose only motivation is to become "department head", nor be left to young and inexperienced interns [9]. Unlike in the United States [10], emergency medicine in France is not a recognized speciality. The ED are most often staffed by internists, anesthetists, cardiologists, surgeons, etc.
2. A frequency of psychiatric cases (12% in our study) suggests an efficient participation of psychiatrists either through a system of staff priviliges or by scheduled assignment.
3. The paramedical staff must be polyvalent (nurses, secretaries, administrative personnel, ...). It must be large enough to avoid endless waiting periods and provide a service of quality. Some countries, such as Switzerland and Belgium [11] have set up specific training for the nursing staff.
4. The presence of social workers appears necessary, for instance to place elderly persons or to orient the homeless toward appropriate centers.

The Facilities

The current renovation of ED facilities in most French hospitals [12] should make us ready to face the problems we routinely encountered (including the massive influx of patients). An Emergency Room must no longer resemble a "railway station". It seems necessary for each center to have:

- rooms or individual compartments for private clinical exams;
- consultation rooms for walk-in patients who should in no case remain in the Emergency Room;
- an ICU with two to four beds, depending on the size of the Hospital Center, with advanced monitoring and resuscitation equipment;
- one or two isolation rooms for agitated patients;
- rooms for orthopedic casting and minor surgery if the service provides traumatology;
- an area for short-term hospitalization in order to keep patients awaiting paraclinical exams or hospital rooms in comfortable conditions.

Obviously an ED must also have the technical support it needs around-the-clock i.e. an analytical lab, radiography room, ultra-sound room and permanent access to a CT scan [13].

Computer Data Processing

Because of the very large number of patient admissions each year in an ED, the quantity of data managed (patient files, medical files, exam reports, billing, etc.) is beyond the capacity of traditional methods. The creation of computer files [14] must be a priority so as to facilitate the tasks of each participant and speed up the procurement of clinical care [15, 16]. This project must be integrated into the present system of emergency care organization without changing its standards of procedure, and must at the same time take into account the need for easy accessibility by a large variety of personnel often untrained (nurses, secretaries, receptionists, physicians and medical students).

Conclusions

French hospital ED must strive to advance in the field of emergency medicine as a discipline in its own right and to obtain recognition of their services which, no longer limited to a sorting process, involve diagnostic evaluation and therapeutic initiatives. The objectives of an ED include limiting the number of unnecessary hospitalizations, orienting the patient towards an appropriate specialized hospital department and responding effectively in critical situations [17]. ED should therefore be staffed by competent "senior" physicians. Once these standards of procedure are obtained, the ED will undoubtedly become an ideal place for the education of future primary care practitioners, a remarkable source of epidemiological data, and an important center for clinical and therapeutic research.

References

1. Askenasi R, Rasquin C, Van Reeth O, et al (1984) What is emergency? Analysis of a population presenting to an emergency room. Acta Anaesth Belg 35:53–63
2. Franaszeck JB, Guterman JJ, Murdy D, et al (1985) The 1980 patient urgency study: further analysis of the data. Ann Emerg Med 14:1191–1198

3. Buesching DP, Jablonowski A, Vesta A, et al (1985) Inappropriate emergency department visits. Ann Emerg Med 14:672–676
4. Askenasi R, Gillet JB, Lheureux P (1987) Profil des admissions dans un service d'urgences. Réan Soins Intens Méd Urg 3:201–205
5. Miquel C, Veyrat P (1986) Approche sociologique, analyse de la mortalité et de l'efficacité dans la prise en charge des patients aux urgences médicales du centre hospitalier universitaire de Grenoble. Medicine Thesis, University of Grenoble
6. Mills JD (1986) Organization and staffing. In: Schwartz Gr, Safar P, Stone JH, et al (eds) Principles and practice of emergency medicine, 2nd edn. Saunders, Philadelphia, pp 622–625
7. Cayten CG, Murphy JG (1986) Evaluation. In: Schwartz Gr, Safar P, Stone JH, et al (eds) Principles and practice of emergency medicine, 2nd edn. Saunders, Philadelphia, pp 633–640
8. Gifford MJ, Franaszeck JB, Gibson G (1980) Emergency physicians' and patients' assessments: urgency need for medical care. Ann Emerg Med 9:502–507
9. Bleichner G, Manet P, Desdoudard P (1988) Rapport sur le fonctionnement des services d'accueil et d'urgences des hôpitaux généraux. In: Conférence nationale des présidents de CME des hôpitaux généraux
10. Riggs LM (1981) A vigorous new speciality. N Engl J Med 304:480–483
11. Askenasi R (1983) Plaidoyer pour une nouvelle spécialité. Acta Clin Belg 38:265–270
12. Denance AM, Fraisse F (1989) Réaménagement d'un service d'urgences. Réflexion sur une structure. Agressologie 30:201–205
13. Cazejust D (1989) L'organisation des urgences dans le futur hôspital du XVème arrondissement de Paris. In: Réanimation et médecine d'urgence. Expansion Scientifique Française, Paris, pp 54–60
14. Dupraz F, Perez P (1989) Contributions à l'informatisation du dossier médico-administratif des patients admis au service des urgences médicales du centre hospitalier universitaire de Grenoble. Medicine Thesis, University of Grenoble
15. Cantril SV (1987) Use of computers in emergency department practise. Emerg Med North Am 5:155–165
16. Wears RL (1989) Use of computers in emergency medicine. Am J Emerg Med 7:120–126
17. Gibson G, Mac Kenzie EJ (1986) Epidemiologic factors in emergency care. In: Schwartz Gr, Safar P, Stone JH, et al (eds) Principles and practice of emergency medicine, 2nd edn. Saunders, Philadelphia, pp 689–691

Cardiopulmonary Resuscitation

Current Standards and Future Directions of Basic and Advanced Cardiopulmonary Resuscitation

P. E. Pepe

Introduction

Sudden cardiac arrest is not only extremely common, but it is also a dramatic entity in the realm of medical care. Most people who die in our communities do so as a result of out-of-hospital "sudden death", generally as the result of underlying coronary artery disease. It is estimated that sudden death is the first symptom of significant coronary artery disease in as many as 25% with this underlying problem. In addition, many other deaths occur both in and out of the hospital because of a cardiac or respiratory arrest that has resulted from a multitude of etiologies, including chronic heart disease, chronig lung disease, seizure, asthma, toxic overdose, drowning, electrocution, and so on.

Cardiopulmonary arrest is also the final mode of exodus for many patients with terminal diseases. And it is clear that when a terminal disease has devastated a patient to the point of circulatory demise, resuscitation attempts are often unwarranted (or simply unsuccessful) when attempted. Because of this, many physicians have very little enthusiasm for attempting CPR in general or are quick to call an end to the CPR attempt and "pronounce the patient" as dead. On the other hand, though most cardiac arrest clinically appear the same, all cardiac arrests should not be lumped together as carrying a bleak prognosis. In fact, in today's "Western society", more people die from coronary artery disease-related sudden death than from any other single disease process, and yet, ironically, a large percentage of these deaths can still be prevented given the rapid provision of certain basic and advanced life support (BLS and ALS) techniques. Although it is the number one killer in the American population (nearly 350,000 deaths/yr in the United States alone) and while serious underlying ischemic heart disease is the major pathophysiologic factor, it is now known that, under certain circumantances, nearly half of these patients are salvageable and that many have an underlying problem that is amenable to subsequent therapy (i.e., isolated ischemic coronary artery disease).

In other words, sudden death in the community is also the number one cause of death that is potentially treatable. As a result, proper management of sudden death syndrome becomes the most tangible form of lifesaving therapy that the medical profession can offer. Therefore, practitioners who maintain a general across-the-board lack of enthusiasm about resuscitation attempts are often those who lack a clear understanding of the delineation of the various pathophysiologies of cardiac arrest. If cardiac arrest is seen as a single or generic disease process, it would be easy to develop misconceptions. But if the various pathways leading to this common-appearing clinical condition are better understood, appropriate enthusiasm for resuscitation can be better-directed.

Because the overwhelming majority of resuscitations are now initiated in the prehospital setting by physician-directed professional emergency medical services (EMS) systems, this discussion will tend to focus in great part on this unique and evolving venue of medical practice. Ironically, resuscitation success rates can be much higher in the out-of-hospital setting because the patient population is generally "less sick" to begin with. We have now learned that perhaps only half of the patients successfully resuscitated after out-of-hospital sudden death associated with ventricular fibrillation (VF) or ventricular tachycardia (VT) have sustained any evidence of permanent heart damage (i.e., no evidence of infarction by ECG or enzymes). As Dr. Claude Beck (who performed the first successful human defibrillation in 1947) pointed out, oftentimes "The heart's too good to die". Anyone who has worked in a busy emergency department or a coronary care unit certainly has not only witnessed a sudden cardiac arrest in monitored patients with cardiac ischemia, but also witnessed the relative ease with which most monitored patients who arrest with VF or VT are resuscitated – if they are treated immediately. Indeed, studies have even demonstrated a very high salvage rate for those patients who have their VF/VT associated cardiac arrest in the out-of hospital setting in the presence if a paramedic who can immediately provide defibrillation and other ALS interventions (Fig. 1). Approximately two-thirds (or more) of these patients can be resuscitated and successfully discharged from the hospital neurologically intact (and quite functional). Therefore, while VF, a sudden, unexpected chaotic twitching of the heart muscle

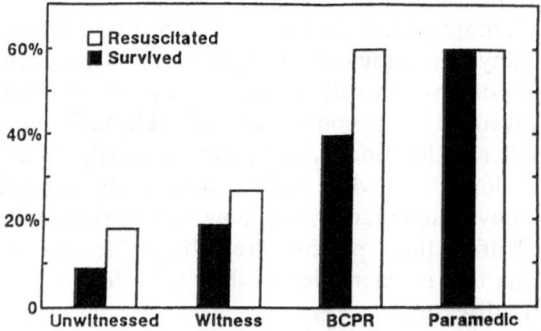

Fig. 1. The effect of witnessing persons on the outcome of sudden death associated with out-of-hospital ventricular fibrillation/tachycardia. If no one hears or sees the collapse (Unwitnessed), chances for long-term survival (successful hospital discharge) are only one in ten. Even without performing CPR, a bystander witnessing the event (Witness) more than doubles the chances of long-term survival (successful hospital discharge). If that witness performs "bystander CPR" (BCPR), the survival rate is again doubled (to about 40%). Meanwhile, if an advanced life support (ALS) provider (Paramedic) witnesses the event (monitored arrest), the great majority (nearly two-thirds) survive. The chances of resuscitation of the cardiovascular system (resuscitation of spontaneous circulation) is also nearly the same with BCPR as that achieved by ALS providers, indicating a key physiologic contribution of BCPR. From [18]

which results in immediate loss of all cardiac output, is obviously lethal, it is also quite treatable. Furthermore, studies have also shown that essentially all patients resuscitated (pulses restored) after arresting in front of a paramedic with VF/VT can eventually be successfully discharged from the hospital, alive and intact. Interestingly, the few who do not survive, are simply not even resuscitated. On closer analysis, *those not surviving generally had hypotension* when they presented to paramedics while most of the *survivors had good vital signs before* they suddenly arrested. This implies that in the smaller group not surviving, the VF/VT was probably "secondary" to evolving cardiogenic shock and severe myocardial dysfunction, whereas the VF was more of an ischemic primary "electrical" problem in the much larger group of survivors.

It is possible that when VF/VT occurs after paramedics arrive (being called for some other symptomatology), the pathophysiology may be slightly different than when it occurs as the initial (or a very early) symptom. However, even assuming that ALS-witnessed (monitored) VF/VT has a different pathophysiology, the rate of successful resuscitation (restoration of spontaneous circulation) can still be strikingly high even when "unmonitored" sudden death occurs (before paramedics are called). Studies have shown that paramedic resuscitation rates for unmonitored VF can be >60%, particularly when a bystander performs basic cardiopulmonary resuscitation (CPR). Again, this rate of resuscitation is nearly equivalent to that achieved during paramedic monitored arrests (Fig. 1). Although ultimate long-term survival rates may be somewhat less with bystander-initiated CPR (BCPR), more than likely this only reflects a delay or an inadequacy of BCPR in being able to protect the brain against irreversible ischemic damage for extended periods of time, such as those instances when ALS care is delayed of when a single rescuer must leave temporarily to call for help. This successful resuscitation rate still serves to reflect Beck's adage ("The heart's too good to die.") in cases of VF or VT. Most studies indicate that when BCPR is performed, it is usually initiated within the first four minutes. As a result, on the average, 40% of the patients who received BCPR from someone who witnessed the VF/VT-associated arrest are successfully discharged from the hospital (Fig. 1). This clearly represents a remarkable rate of reversibility for such an unpredicted clinical entity that occurs out in the community, far from a coronary care unit, and one that is "99.9%" fatal left untreated. These same approximate results for BCPR-associated VF/VT cases have now been confirmed in multiple EMS systems (e.g., Seattle, Sydney, Milwaukee, Pittsburgh, Houston).

Before going on, it should be reiterated that these favorable statistics reflect the save rates following out-of-hospital cardiac arrest that is associated with *VF or VT as a presenting ECG rhythm*. The long-term survival rates for those initially found in cardiac arrest presenting with asystole (or even with organized complexes) are much less favorable. Nevertheless, VF/VT rhythms are found in nearly half of the cases of primary cardiac arrests in the out-of-hospital setting. Some EMS systems with a very rapid response of so-called "first responder" crews with monitoring equipment show even higher rates of VF/VT on presentation (over 50%). In fact, as discussed below, the presenting ECG rhythm is not only indicative of pathophysiology and outcome, but it can also be indicative of both the response time for initiating aid as well as an individual's relative tolerance to circulatory arrest.

Interestingly, the average age of VF victims is about 60 years. It is most really a disease of "the elderly". As sudden death is generally reported as the first symptom in 25% of those with coronary artery disease, it is not totally surprising to see VF in 40 year old men, as some U.S. studies find that 20% of males with coronary artery disease will experience their first symptom by the age of 50. Therefore, sudden death from VF is clearly a major, if not *the* major health issue of out time, not only because of the sheer numbers (over a ¼ million Americans annually) but also because of what we now know about its reversibility.

Initial Presentation and Pathophysiology

Asystole (cardiac standstill) generally indicates that the patient has no electrical activity, probably as the result of high-energy phosphate depletion in the heart's tissues, such as that occuring after prolonged periods of VF. Cardiac arrest is often seen as a rather static process. However, major physiologic processes are on-going, particularly in the case of VF. In VF, the immediate loss of organized heart beat due to the suddeen, charotic, short-circulating of the heart's electrical system leads to immediate loos of coronary artery perfusion. Therefore, the sources of the necessary metabolic nutrients to produce the high-energy phosphates (e.g., adenosine triphosphates) necessary to fuel the heart's various functions including pacemaker activity, conduction of electrical impulses, and myocardial contractility are suddenly shut off. Depending on the individual, the degree of previous underlying cardiac disease and external factors such as the timing (or absence) of BCPR, the VF activity consums all remaining energy sources. As minutes pass, the VF is less vigorous and its ECG appearance becomes less "coarse". Eventually, the VF becomes more and more "fine" until the complete depletion of energy supplies leaves the heart at a standstill (Fig. 2). In some cases, after the VF completely dissipates, an agonal electrical impulse may even be observed, but usually asystole (evidenced by confirmed flat line on ECG) is

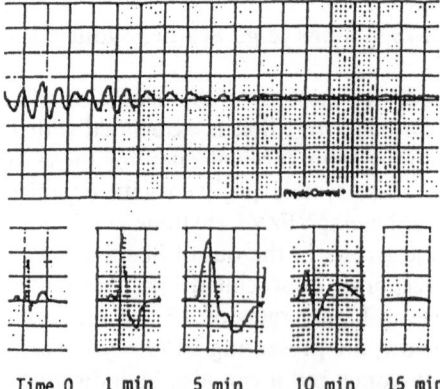

Fig. 2. A sample time-course of the ventricular fibrillation waveform (on the upper panel) demonstrating a deterioration of coarse to fine fibrillation. The lower panel shows samples of the conversion rhythms one might expect as time elapses

Time 0   1 min   5 min   10 min   15 min

the end-point. In other words, asystole or agonal rhythms reflect long downtimes and depletion of the energy sources necessary to resume spontaneous circulation. With certain exceptions, this presentation generally predicts a very poor prognosis, at least within our current understanding and techniques for managing cardiac arrest. Even in the best of EMS systems, the long-term survival prognosis for unmonitored cardiac arrests presenting with asystole in ECG is rarely greater than 3% to 4% in cases of primarily cardiac-related arrests. This is why most "last-ditch" attempts to resuscitate with artificial pacemakers are futile, despite "capture". In fact, the save rate generally is near zero in most places. Even when the arrest is monitored, the changes of survival for those immediately losing their ECG complexes rarely exceed 15%. Those who do survive usually are patients who had an easily-reversible underlying cause of arrest such as transient hypoxemia of transient loss of blood pressure. In general, however, asystole portrays extended downtime and a relatively poor prognosis in unmonitored arrests.

In contrast, if the presenting ECG rhythm still is VF, this suggests a potential for reversibility. VF usually occurs as a sudden primary short-circuiting of the heart's electrical system. This generally is the result of acute ischemia associated with coronary artery disease. On occasion, it may result because of some other factor (Table 1) such as serum chemical imbalances or drug toxicity (such as hypokalemia/hypomagnesemia and/or digitalis-related arrhythmias). Because the short-circuiting can occur suddenly (before other symptoms of ischemia become manifested), VF (or VT-associated arrest) has been often nicknamed "Sudden Death Syndrome." Frequently, without much warning, the alert, conscious victim suddenly collapses (occasionally with a brief hypoxic seizure) because of the sudden loss of organized, effective heart beat.

VF may initially begin as sustained VT, which may often persist for as much as a minute. However, VT may immediately deteriorate into VF or it may go on

Table 1. External factors, biochemical imbalances and drug toxicities associated with sudden ventricular dysrhythmias

---

Digitalis (esp. with hypokalemia, hypomagnesemia)
Quinidine (and other drugs predisposing to long Q–T interval)
Tricyclic anti-depressants
Adrenergic Drugs (e. g., isoproterenol, levarterenol, dopamine dobutamine, epinephrine, etc.)

Cocaine +
Amphetamines

Hypercalcemia[b]
Hypokalemia[a]
Hypomagnesemia[a]

Unsynchronized cardioversion attempt[a]
Synchronized cardioversion[a, b]

Electrocution (including accidental countershock contact)
Factors exacerbating coronary atery ischemia (e. g., hypoxemia[b], CO poisoning[b], hypoperfusion due to hypovolemia[b], poor ejection fraction or rapid, tachycardia)

---

[a] Especially with Digoxin.
[b] Less usual.

for extended periods (with or without associated palpable pulse) before deterioration into VF. *Sustained* VT (more than several minutes duration) may spontaneously convert back to a normal rhythm, but this is uncommon without therapy (e. g., lidocaine, electrical cardioversion or countershock). It may never even lead to cardiac arrest. However, in VF or in VT, once there is a true loss of the pulse, this obviously indicates the onslaught of a completely lethal process as permanent, irreversible brain damage can begin to occur within minutes.

But as shown earlier, despite the sudden, insidious appearance and the immediate fatal course, VF is generally easy to reverse and the earlier the interventions, the better the result. This is most obvious in a monitored VF situation in which an alert person suddenly fibrillates and foes into circulatory arrest. Because the majority of functioning heart tissues, be they pacemakers, nervous conduction tissue, or even the contractile tissue of the myocardium, have not yet been subject to prolonged hypoxia, they should still be capable of functioning fairly well (were it not for the chaotic electrical disturbance). Therefore, if an appropriate electrical depolarization (standard countershock) is immediately delivered and the fibrillation cleared, the heart should usually be able to return to near-normal function within seconds (as indicated by return of a "sinus" rhythm, narrow QRS complexes on EKG and the return of an adequate spontaneous blood pressure). If, however, defibrillation is delayed by one or two minutes, even with basic CPR (which usually offers suboptimal perfusion), the heart may be somewhat compromised by the period of inadequate perfusion (Fig. 2). As a result, the post-defibrillation pacemaker firing, nervous conduction, and myocardial contraction may be sluggish due to diminishing energy sources (as evidence by a decreased rate, widened QRS complex, or diminished or absent pulse/BP). If the residual cardiac activity is adequate enough to begin a heartbeat and reperfuse the coronary arteris, the necessary continued spontaneous improvement (and subsequent return) of cardiac function should occur, particularly with supportive therapy (oxygen, CPR). However, if the defibrillation is delayed even more (e. g., 5 to 10 min), the residual post-defibrillatory response may reflect a severely compromised state manifested by spontaneous return of only a wide, bizarre, slow ventricular complex on the ECG that is not accompanied either by any detectable atrial depolarization or by an adequate contractile state (pulselessness). This is not surprising if one considers, the concept of adenosine triphosphate (ATP) depletion and the resulting "O_2 debt" that quickly develops over minutes in the fibrillating heart. Not only is the usual steady-state high demand for circulatory O_2 supply not matched by basic CPR techniques, but there is now this additional "energy debt" to overcome. In such a situation, advanced therapeutic adjuncts will be needed in order to augment perfusion of the coronary arteries (such as peripheral vasoconstriction with epinephrine administration to enhance the effect of basic CPR). Even so, the patient may now be well beyond either cerebral or cardiac resuscitation.

Certainly, those patients who receive defibrillation but have no residual rhythm despite several minutes of good oxygenation (e. g., endotracheal intubation with adequate tidal volumes and oxygen flows), basic CPR, and epinephrine administration have been without adequate coronary artery circulation for a significant period of time. By the same token, some patients respond well to initial therapy, but eventually their condition deteriorates, presumably because of a significant major coronary artery occlusion that originally precipitated the event or perhaps because of an irreversible abberation in the peripheral circulatory system after having gone too long without perfusion. On the other hand, some patients who have a poor initial response may also do well after persistent efforts. But, overall, the response to initial therapy is one of the more reliable indications of downtime (and prognosis) in the patient with VF. Although an initial presenting rhythm of coarse VF is more likely to be converted to a rhythm that restores spontaneous circulation than is fine VF, this observation may be less reliable than the actual observed response to initial therapeutic interventions. Studies are currently underway that will correlate VF-waveform amplitude and downtime. It is possible therefore that, in the future, outcome may be better predicted even earlier in the evaluation process.

Meanwhile, those cardiac arrests not associated with VF or VT have a different outlook. The presence of ECG complexes in a patient who is found apneic and pulseless may be better in terms of survival prognosis than asystole, but the prognosis still is much poorer than that of VF or VT-associated arrest. The presentation of either an idioventricular rhythm (IVR) associated with no pulse (commonly nicknamed pulseless idioventricular rhythm or PIVR) or even a more organized ECG complex that should be (but is not) associated with an adequate heartbeat (commonly called electromechanical dissociation or EMD) usually herald a different pathophysiology (or several different pathophysiologies) than that occurring in VF.

Intuitively, EMD conveys the situation in which the cardiac electrical system has not lost its perfusion for very long and the heart theoretically should beat (but it does not). Theoretically, it either means that there is a readily-reversible underlying problem such as transient hypoxemia, or it means significant myocardial damage and a severe cardiogenic shock state in which the ventricle may be barely twitching in response to relatively intact electrical depolarization.

In contrast, PIVR may reflect a late phase along a spectrum of cardiovascular deterioration resulting from inadequate coronary artery perfusion due to one of multiple potential etiologies. For example, some patients, such as those with hemorrhage and severe hypoxia, will experience global loss of perfusion to the coronary arteries and the result is the "dwindling heart" syndrome. Because of the more global compromise to cardiac oxygenation under these circumstances, the three major functional tissues of the heart, namely pacemaker, conduction, and contractile myocardial tissue, all become steadily impaired, resulting in slowing rates, widening QRS complexes, and the loss of BP and pulses. Rarely does a moribund hypovolemic patient arrest with VF. These manifestations are those of global cardiac ischemia and they should be progressive. The progressive diminution of heart rate and contractility leads to a further compromise in coronary artery perfusion, resulting in a vicious cycle. Eventually there will be an absence of ECG-detected impulses altogether (asystole or agonal impulses at best). Therefore, PIVR represents a temporal snapshot of a deteriorating heart. In essence, it is also a manifestation of evolving high-energy phosphate depletion which may or may not be reversible deplending on the underlying mechanism and ease of reversibility. Even in arrests witnessed by ALS providers, the survival probability rarely exceeds 15% to 20% with this presentation, particularly when dealing with primary cardiac etiologies (i.e., those cases in which primary respiratory, toxicologic, and injury mechanisms have been ruled out).

While asystole is often the end stage of prolonged VF which has progressively deteriorated from a very active "coarse VF" to a less and less active "fine VF" (and eventually asystole), it may also represent the end-point of the "dwindling heart syndrome" as well. Again, no matter what, asystole *generally* means that the downtime for coronary artery perfusion has been long enough to predict a very grim prognosis. But because it represents a physiological endpoint, the frequency of asystole patients presenting in and the associated grim prognosis, can be altered by external factors. As stated before, from an epidemiologic point of view, VF/VT is by far the single, largest potentially-reversible clinical entity causing death in North American society. Of the hundreds of thousands of primary cardiac arrests that occur annually in the United States, it is estimated that as many as 75% or more of out-of-hospital primary cardiac arrests *initially* begin as a VF/VT-induced event. However, depending on the therapeutic response time to these events, the patient may or may not present in VF. If too much time has elapsed, the ALS-responder may only find asystole in the monitor at the time of arrival. Therefore, in most EMS systems, many patients have already progressed to states of asystole and VF/VT is the presenting ECG tracing in only 30% to 50% of out-of-hospital cardiac arrest cases. Again, these figures may be higher or lower depending on the EMS system's overall average response times, the use of first-responders with automatic defibrillation capabilities, and the rate of BCPR performance in that community. For example, in Houston, prior to 1983, BCPR was seen in less than 1% of cases and there was no rapid emergency telephone access system (i.e., 9-1-1 system). At that time the frequency of VF on initial EKG presentation was 25%. Despite slightly longer response times for paramedics, the frequency had steadily risen to over 40% in 1988 following the introduction of a 9-1-1 system, implementation of a neighborhood fire department first responder program and the appearance of BCPR in 15–20% of cases over the five year interim period. The rate is in excess of 50% in places like Milwaukee and King County, Washington where extremely rapid first response programs and/or high BCPR rates are found. Therefore, the overall number of potentially salvageable cases of cardiac arrest is dynamic related to several logistic and system-related factors.

Relative Contributions of Therapeutic Modalities

Based on the above discussion, access to the EMS system via a specialized telephone number (9-1-1, 9-9-9 or some equivalent) is key. One essential aspect of the training of the lay public in basic CPR techniques is simply the fact that we also instruct them in the "when and how" of accessing the EMS system quickly. The other obvious aspect of public CPR training is that the earlier BLS is performed, the better the results. For example, there is a commonly-held tenet that starting basic CPR within four minutes and initiating ALS within the next four minutes will result in a 40% ling-term survival rate for victims of out-of-hospital

VF, and that if either of these two time limits are exceeded, the chances of survival fall dramatically. More recently, it has also been recognized that if the BCPR is actually begun within seconds (and continued), this may be more apt to "buy the patient more time" (e. g., survival despite the passage of more than 10 to 15 minutes before ALS arrives). On the other hand, if BCPR is not initiated until three minutes after collapse, this may also buy some time, but in such an instance, the basic CPR may be of value for only a couple more minutes. Studies also show that very early BCPR is more apt to be associated with an initial rhythm of coarse VF and a more organized conversion rhythm (e. g., sinus tachycardia) after initial countershocks. The patient is also apt to be still trying to make respiratory efforts or even have some observable motor function when ALS arrives. Therefore, early BCPR may have a more pronounced physiologic effect if it is provided almost immediately (i. e., the earlier the better). It should be emphasized, that this observation should not prevent the bystander rescuer from first calling for professional help. Preferably, if there are two bystanders, one should call for help while the other immediately begins BLS.

Studies of out-of-hospital VF which can show successful outcomes (overall average long-term survival rates > 20%), are usually conducted in EMS systems in which there is a minimum of two ALS providers (paramedics) accompanied by several BLS providers (e. g., neighborhood firetruck personnel) who assist with the basic CPR, ventilation, and drug set-ups, and who are dispatched *simultaneously* and often arrive within minutes as the neighborhood "first-responder" (FR) to provide BCPR. In addition, community CPR training is usually a major feature. For example, in the City of Seattle where there has been a 27% save rate for VF, BCPR has been reported in nearly 40% of cases. In addition to rapid defibrillation, the paramedics in these systems provide endotracheal intubation (ETI) on a regular basis in addition to all the other typical intravenous (IV) drugs used for cardiac emergencies. Currently, the addition of semi-automatic

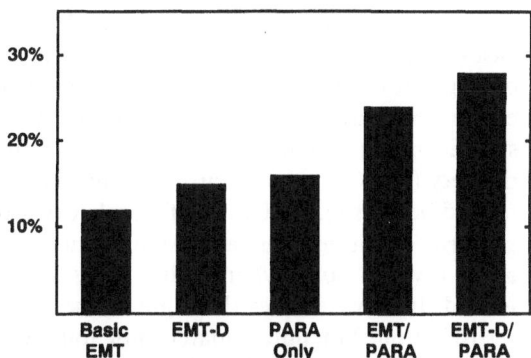

Fig. 3. A comparison of average survival (successful hospital discharge) rates following out-of-hospital sudden death associated with ventricular fibrillation among various types of emergency medical service (EMS) system configurations including those with: *1)* basic emergency medical technicians (Basic EMT) only; *2)* EMTs that can defibrillate (EMT-D); *3)* Paramedics (PARA) only; *4)* "tiered" EMT/PARA services; and *5)* tiered systems in which EMTs also defibrillate (EMT-D/PARA). (From [12])

defibrillators on neighborhood FR firetrucks in some communities has increased the changes of survival even further (Fig. 3), not only by earlier delivery of defibrillatory countershocks, but also by increasing the number of cases presenting in VF/VT (because of earlier arrival). So while VF survival rates may approach (or even surpass) 30% in many communities with FR semi-automatic defibrillation, the absolute number of patients saved also increases even further because more patients actually present in VF. Often, patients receiving FR defibrillation will already have pulses long before the other ALS modalities and care are available. While a large percentage of patients defibrillated from VF will refibrillate (on the average this is about 60% of defibrillated patients), there is still a very significant percentage who remain converted. It has now been shown in systems where BLS providers also have a defibrillator that lives can be without the immediate provision of other ALS modalities such as endotracheal intubation (ETI) and IV lidocaine (Fig. 3). Therefore, while paramedic services are still important, the earliest possible initiation of BCPR and defibrillation, accompanied minimally by basic ventilatory adjuncts (oral airway, bag-valve mask, and oxygen) are clearly the most key lifesaving factors in cardiac arrest management. The question remains whether or not those other ALS procedures improve outcome as well. Most of us have very strong biases that both ETI and antiarrhythmic drug administration are also key adjuncts, but the scientific data confirming these biases are lacking. There does exist some significant inferential evidence to support the value of ETI (and the same applies to lidocaine administration), namely that higher survival rates are found in systems using them versus those without these modalities. Nevertheless, any documented effects of ETI and lidocaine administration are still far overshadowed by the necessary contributions of early BCPR and early defibrillation. Similarly, while *experimental* data support the concept of improved outcomes following epinephrine administration, the absolute clinical value of epinephrine (and other such drugs) has not yet been clearly delineated in a rigorous scientific fashion.

Interestingly, recent experimental evidence suggests that our current methodologies of drug administration may actually be ineffectual in a large percentage of cases. For example, the current recommended dose of epinephrine in adultes during cardiac arrest is 0.5 to 1.0 mg (about 0.01 mg/kg) every 5 minutes. However, recent studies in canines and swine have now demonstrated that there is no significant improvement in aortic diastolic pressure (AODP), myocardial oxygen delivery (MDO_2), or myocardial blood flow (MBF) at this dosage following extended periods (e. g., 10 min) of circulatory arrest. Human studies have now been performed that demonstrate a significant increase in AODP following prolonged arrest (over ½ hour) when higher doses of epinephrine (5 to 10 mg) are administered. In those studies the higher doses were also associated with unexpected resuscitation, but unfortunately not long-term survival. Clinical experience in our own EMS system has demonstrated several cases in which not only was resuscitation, but also long-term survivorship, achieved in patients given similar doses (e. g., 10 mg) of IV epinephrine after the patients had remained in a refractory VF for >20 min using standard approaches. However, the success rate of such single large doses was not frequent and was more likely to be successful in cases in which BCPR was performed.

Upon closer analysis, the dose of epinephrine required for therapeutic efficacy is probably dependent of multiple factors, and is particularly time-related. In terms of serum catecholamine levels, 1 mg of IV epinephrine may be considered almost a "physiologic dose" soon after the time of cardiac arrest. Progressively higher doses may be indicated as time passes in order to reverse progressive circulatory collapse. Recent experimental studies have brought us a better understanding of both the pathophysiology of the cardiac arrest state as well as our current strategies for reversing that process. During normal sinus rhythm (NSR) and with normal systemic blood pressure (BP), the heart is perfused during diastole by the "backwash" from the aorta into the coronary arteries. Therefore, the typical perfusion pressure that permits MBF is about 80 to 100 mm Hg. Following cardiac arrest, the AODP rapidly falls, and despite immediate basic CPR, may be no more than half of that provided during normal perfusion. Furthermore, as time passes, this BLS-generated AODP continues to fall and, as a result, MBF (as well as cerebral blood flow) may rapidly become negligible despite the basic CPR. Depending on several factors, the rate of AODP fall may vary, but within minutes can be as low as 10–15 mm Hg.

As indicated by experimental studies of epinephrine administration, the reason for this fall in AODP (and therefore MBF) appears to be a progressive fall in systemic vascular resistance. It is postulated that this occurs within just a few minutes as the result of systemic vascular collapse due to hypoxia, acidosis, and ischemia, as well as a possible tachyphylactic (uncoupling) phenomenon, occuring at vascular α-receptors, receptors which have already been stimulated by high endogenous catecholamine release (300 times normal) immediately after arrest. This progressive relaxation of peripheral vascular resistance and fall in central aortic pressure (to about 10 to 15 mm Hg) probably diminishes coronary artery and central blood flow by $\geq 90\%$, often within 10 minutes of cardiopulmonary arrest. It is speculated however, that if basic CPR is initiated *immediately* (within 15–30 seconds), the rate of deterioration may be delayed. Such patients are more apt to be found in coarse VF, still trying to breathe and even moving on occasion. They will also usually convert into a sinus rhythm after defibrillation, even after 10 minutes or more of CPR. It is thought therefore that the immediate basic CPR allows enough perfusion to ameliorate the rate of vascular collapse. Still, in most cases, the basic CPR is not done immediately and, as a result, hemodynamic deterioration has already unravelled. In turn, the basic CPR quickly becomes ineffective, accelerating the deterioration.

After 10–15 minutes of VF, it would not be surprising that most high-energy phosphates in the heart are totally depleted and, as a result, a severe oxygen debt is created. Therefore, the demand for MBF and MDO_2 rises. Yet, at this point, in view of the minimal AODP, MBF generated by basic CPR is almost negligible. As a result, not only is the steady-state demand for O_2 supply far from being met, but the depleting energy reserves must be restored as well. So even after defibrillation, there is nothing left to fuel the heart's functioning tissues, including the pacemakers, conduction system and the myocardium whose contraction is the only hope of survival. Therefore, even with artificial pacing, the chance for resuscitation has fallen dramatically.

Given that MBF generally becomes inadequate during prolonged basic CPR and that this is due to peripheral vascular collapse, it appears that peripheral vascular constriction would be the absolute key to restoring O_2 perfusion to the heart so that the necessary energy supplies can be regenerated. Current data suggest, ar this point, that a standard dose of epinephrine (about 0.01 to 0.02 mg/kg) appears to add very little to endogenous serum catecholamine levels. On the other hand, Brown, et al, have now shown significant elevations in AODP (up to 50 mm Hg) when 0.20 mg/kg of IV epinephrine was used versus standard therapy (0.2 mg/kg) in pigs subjected to 10 minutes of VF. In the same model, less impressive results were obtained with methoxamine and phenylephrine, while slightly better results were obtained with norepinephrine (although more post-resuscitation arrhythmias were observed with this latter drug). These observations may imply the development of a possible down-regulation of α_1-receptors or a continued (but still somewhat resistant) clinical effect at the α_2-receptor sites. It may also be that the α_2-receptor sites are anatomically closer to the blood vessel lumen and therefore are easier to stimulate with circulating catecholamines than the less-accessible α_1-receptor sites where methoxamine and phenylephrine primarily work. Therefore α_2 stimulating vasoconstrictors may be the most appropriate drugs to use. Various new vasoconstrictors are presently being evaluated experimentally, but in the meantime, epinephrine (and norepinephrine) appear to be the current drugs of choice during prolonged CPR conditions.

There is experimental evidence to suggest that the clear resuscitative effect of epinephrine is, for the most part, extra-cardiac, at least initially. In other words, epinephrine's effect during CPR is not as a direct cardiac stimulant. For example, it does no "coarsen-up" VF (as one often hears), rather, it acts as an indirect stimulant by causing the peripheral vasoconstriction that helps to raise central AODP and therefore better restores MBF during CPR. Therefore, epinephrine primarily achieves its resuscitative effect by enhancing reperfusion of the heart. It is not clear, however, that once reasonable perfusion has been restored, whether or not epinephrine then also provides a direct stimulant effect (i.e., beta-agonist properties that stimulate the "three C's" of chronicity, conductivity, and contractility). Most likely it does cause direct cardiac stimulation, even in low doses, once a pulse returns. Regardless, current experimental data support the concept that prior to restoration of spontaneous circulation, very little of the drug gets directly into the coronaries following several minutes of CPR because of the negligible MBF.

But despite the experimental data, the proposed doses of epinephrine required to affect resuscitations in humans are still speculative, and more importantly, dosage requirements are probably determined by multiple factors. Furthermore, sound scientific investigations must be conducted to examine not only the proper dosing required for efficacy, but also to clearly rule out undesirable complications (i.e., successful long-term resuscitations accompanied by irreparable brain damage, or a large number of patients who infarct more myocardium than those resuscitated while receiving lesser doses of epinephrine).

As alluded to above, clinical variables that might affect epinephrine dosing probably include the time of the administration as well as the timing of BCPR. It is less likely that those with a monitored arrest who are treated immediately will need any epinephrine (let alone the higher doses discussed above). Also, as discussed earlier, the timing of BCPR may have a profound physiologic effect if administered within seconds. Therefore, the time of BCPR may alter the rate at which vascular receptors lose their tone as well as their sensitivity to administered epinephrine. Finally, both relative weight (lean body versus actual) and individual variation may also play significant roles in determining the relative need and dosing of epinephrine.

In view of the previous discussion, the efficacy and proper dosing of other ALS drugs such as atropine and lidocaine *during CPR conditions* may also need to be re-examined. For example, the common understanding that 2 mg of atropine is the "total vagolytic dose" may be true in a human adult with normal circulation. On the other hand, this dose may not be as effective in the setting of profound vascular collapse and minimum circulatory blood flow.

Still, despite all the experimental data, most current drug therapy may be simply "icing on the cake" with respect to the contributions of *very* early BCPR and early defibrillation. Perhaps in the future, drugs that restore energy supplies, or mechanical devices that immediately restore more-than-adequate MBF will be found to be more efficacious. Until then, the present initial approach of VF will be to provide the earliest possible difibrillation, airway protection and adequate lung inflation usually with an endotracheal tube oxygen, basic CPR techniques and, if needed, enhancement of the basic CPR effect by epinephrine (and other α_2 vasopressors) followed by appropriate administration of stabilizing antiarrhythmic agents. Given this background, the following sectins will review the latest rationales and accepted clinical approaches to cardiac arrest management.

Management of Cardiac Arrest

The main purpose for reviewing the latest experimental evidence regarding resuscitative modalities primarily has been to help create a better understanding of rationales for our contemporary resuscitation strategies. In fact, those actually conducting the latest research will be the first to state that proposed approaches such as larger dose of epinephrine are still somewhat premature for widespread recommendations as clinical standards. Clinical guidelines recommended for advanced cardiac life support (ACLS) should be based preferably on scientific, peer-reviewed, published studies. Therefore, the remainder of this chapter will discuss guidelines for BLS and ACLS as most recently recommended by the American Heart Association Committee on Emergency Cardiac Care. While these contemporary guidelines may change in the near future, the critical care practitioner must still be expert in these recognized standards, regardless of any promising experimental reports. But at the same time, the discussion will still provide personal suggestions and recommendations for care of the patient found in cardiopulmonary arrest. Such suggestions will represent an assimilation of both our latest understanding of the pathophysiology as well as a practical clinical approach to this dramatic and common medical entity. No doubt, by the time these words reach the reader, further advances will have been made that may even alter these most current suggestions.

Basic Life Support

Current standards for BLS involve the restoration and continued provision of adequate lung inflation in the patient who has had cardiopulmonary arrest. Such patients have rapid lung deflation (especially following chest compressions), and adequate red blood cell oxygenation may not occur as a result of dependent airway closure. Therefore, two large breaths are given after every 15 typical chest compressions. If the compressions are delivered at 80 to 100/min, it is easier for the average rescuer to better deliver a proper up-down stroke ratio to effect the best possible cardiac output. Therefore, the 15 compressions being given to depress the sternum by 1.5 to 2 inches in the average adult will take about 9 to 11 sec, followed by the two large breaths. For children 1 to 8 years of age, the recommended compression depth is about 1 to 1.5 inches, while it is ½ to 1 inch in those <1 year of age. Also, the recommended compression rate is 100/min and one rescue breath for every five compressions in children. Once a patient has received endotracheal intubation, however, asynchronous compressions and breathing are not only acceptable, they are recommended in view of our current understanding of how intra-thoracic pressures inter-relate to basic CPR effectiveness.

Advanced Life Support

BLS may occasionally restore circulation in those who may simply need a "jump-start," such as the occasional elderly patient with "presbycardia" who has transient bradycardia, ot the occasional near-drowning victim who is stimulated by the basic CPR techniques. However, ALS will usually be mandatory to effect successful resuscitatioion in the majority of cardiac arrest victims. At the very least, ALS monitoring should be instituted as soon as it is feasible.

Practical Approach to Cardiac Arrest Management

Perhaps one of the most critical aspects of resuscitation of the cardiac arrest patient is maintaining a organized, prioritized approach that will effectively accomplish the appropriate interventions as rapidly as possible.

While the pathophysiologies and outcomes of various cardiac arrests may be different, the approach to management still can be simplified. In essence, the approach to all cases is to *rapidly* restore brisk coronary artery perfusion with oxygenated blood. Therefore, in all cases, the primary mechanisms used to achieve this goal are to:

1. adequately inflate the lungs bilaterally (tidal volume of 15 ml/kg) with 100% O_2 (which should always allow for nearly full O_2 saturation of red cells);

2. circulate the oxygenated red cells with basic CPR (chest compressions); and
3. enhance the basic CPR with potent vasopressors (epinephrine, norepine-phrine) as needed (pulselessness, persistent hypotension).

Obviously, in the electrical short-circuiting syndromes (i.e. VF/VT), one must first clear out a pathway for organized electrical impulse and then help to maintain electrical stability with anti-arrhythmics (e.g. lidocaine). But these are the simple "bookend" additions to the basic strategies of proper lung inflation, chest compressions and enhancement of the basic CPR effect with vasopressors. Additional drugs like atropine and sodium bicarbonate are considerations, but their use must be considered supplemental to the basic strategies to restore strong perfusion of the coronaries. To be more specific, when one defibrillates a victim of unmonitored VF and finds the post-conversion ECG rhythm to be one with wide QRS complexes and a rate of 40/minute, a common reaction is to administer atropine because of the bradycardia. While it may actually be helpful in some patients, it must be remembered that, in the pulseless state, the bradycardia is most likely to be secondary to an O_2-starved conduction system that needs to be dramatically reperfused. Particularly, it must be remembered that sucessful drug actions during CPR conditions will usually be by *indirect* stimulation of the heart such as restoration of adequate AODP. Therefore, atropine would be an afterthought to the priorities of basic CPR, ETI, O_2 and epinephrine. Nevertheless, it is still not un unreasonable supplement under such circumstances.

Table 2. General approach to non-traumatic cardiac arrest management

---

Clear out VFIB/VTACH, while considering spinal injury and follow "ABC's" below:

A *Adequate Lung Inflation* Bilaterally with O_2 (check ET tube centimeter mark, stomach sounds, bite block)

B *BP* or CPR adequate? (check CPR depth, and rate 80–100/min.)

C *Catheter(s)* Drips and patency? (use large bore if possible)

D *Drugs* = "LEAP ABC" Consider each one and go back again.
  L *Lidocaine* - Always in VF/VT (except with wide, slow QRS not driven by P wave). Remember to load (3 mg/kg).
  E *Epinephrine* - Pulseless despite good O_2 and CPR *or* pulseless and definite long downtime.
  A *Atropine* - 1) Hypotensive *and* 2) rate 60 or less (or AV block).
  P *Pressors* - (e. g., levarternol or dopamine) - pulses present but hypotensive (or epi wearing off). Set up ahead of time in anticipation or need.
  A *Altered Mental Status* Considerations (e. g., glucose, naloxone)
  B *Bicarbonate* - no significant response to initial therapy
  C *Chemical Imbalances* (Mg^{++}, Ca^{++}, K^+, etc.)

E *ECG* Functions ("GAMES") and Pacemaker Trial
  Gain
  Attached
  Mode
  ECG Vector
  Strip

F *Further History and Physical* (e. g., medications, recent symptoms/injury, ChemStrip Auto-PEEP, etc.)

Repeat above steps over and over

In view of this simplified concept, a singular mnemonic approach can be memorized that will assist the practitioner in the sudden turmoil of a cardiac arrest (Table 2). This approach represents a check list that can be applied almost universally to nontraumatic cardiac arrest management in which other factors such as hypovolemia, tension pneumothorax, pericardial tamponade and other reversible processes have at least been considered and tentatively ruled out. The following sections will elaborate on each of the various parts of this useful approach.

Clearing Ventricular Fibrillation

As stated before, if the strategy for cardiac arrest management could be summarized into a single phrase, it would be that the sooner a strong spontaneous circulation is restored, the better the outcome. So in the case of the most treatable form of primary cardiac arrest, namely that occurring as the result of VF, spontaneous circulation will almost uniformly not occur until the VF is therapeutically removed. Therefore, the priority in VF or VT-associated circulatory arrest is to *clear out the ventricular arrhythmia* with defibrillatory countershocks in order to allow a clear path for spontaneous, organized, cardiac electrical impulse. While it can be argued that defibrillation may not occur until a better environment is first created, such as facilitating blood oxygenation by ETI or by reversing acidosis with sodium bicarbonate, it is actually more likely that very early defibrillation will not only allow the heart to spontaneously beat again and thus restore spontaneous circulation, but it may also result in spontaneous respiration and rapid wakening. In turn, this might even obviate the need for these other ALS procedures. Therefore, in VF/VT-associated arrest, the patient should receive successive countershocks until the VF/VT clears, at least for the first several shocks.

A certain percentage of VF patients can be successfully defibrillated even with only 100 Joules (or less) of defibrillatory energy. However, well over 90% of patients can be successfully cleared of VF using three shocks (or less) at 200 Joules. Therefore, this seems to be the most efficient lower energy level. There is some evidence that suggests that cardiac arrest "stuns" the myocardium and that the conduction system is more apt to be stunned by the higher energies, at least transiently. Nevertheless, a small percentage of patients may have a larger than usual mass of fibrillating myocardium. Therefore, it is felt by some that these patients should receive higher energies if the first shock or two fail to convert the VF, using the rationale that the sooner the defibrillation occurs the better. Thus, the current ACLS algorithm calls for 200 Joules for the first shock, 200 (or 300) for the second, and "up to 360 Joules" for the third if necessary. As a result, this wording leaves leverage for clinical judgment, let alone different points of view.

These energy levels are relatively standard for adults, as most adults have about the same heart size (regardless of body weight), as opposed to a child whose heart size and mass of fibrillating myocardium are obviously much smaller. As a result, it is recommended that children receive the starting "dose" of 2

Joule/kg as a rough guideline. Currently, however, the correct level of defibrillation energy has not yet been clearly established for the pediatric population.

Adequate Lung Inflation Bilaterally with Oxygen

Because of the experimental data supporting the effectiveness of epinephrine in augmenting the effects of basic CPR, IV epinephrine is often considered to be next on the recommended list of actions if the patient remains pulseless (with or without VF). While most agree that airway control is a priority, the latest American Heart Association ACLS algorithm appears to rank epinephrine above ETI because of the experimental evidence supporting its efficacy. Nevertheless, in most settings, at least two ALS providers are available and ETI can be performed simultaneously.

The importance of ETI is recognized not only in terms of airway protection from aspiration of gastric contents, but also because it is the definitive way to restore the adequate lung inflation required to reserve the critical hypoxemia that usually occurs when gas exchange units collapse after cardiopulmonary arrest. Because lung compliance falls dramatically during apnea and chest compressions, it may be difficult to re-inflate the lung with a bag-valve mask system alone. The use of ETI will guarantee the 10 to 15 ml/kg that will probably be needed to reverse the intrapulmonary shunt resulting from CPR-associated collapse of gas-exchange units. If the patient receives ETI, properly-placed and accompanied by the delivery of 10 to 15 ml/kg tidal volumes and 100% oxygen, PaO_2 levels leading to significant red blood cell (hemoglobin) desaturation will rarely be seen regardless of the etiology and severity of any accompanying lung disease.

Blood Pressure

The "B" in this mnemonic approach is not the well-known "breathing" of basic life support but rather "blood pressure" (BP). If the "A" of adequate lung inflation bilaterally with O_2 guarantees red cell saturation in virtually all cases, the next end-point is to briskly perfuse the coronaries with those oxygenated cells by restoring a *strong* AODP. In fact, if the BP is less than 110–120 mm Hg systolic, the coronary artery perfusion pressure (AOCP) may not be so adequate, especially when the end-diastolic pressure typically is not even clinically detectable. While chest compressions may not be so essential in a patient primarily presenting with hypotension, in the post-CPR situation when the myocardium has been underperfused for a while, it is not unreasonable in some cases to sustain chest compressions in order to augment spontaneous circulation. Despite the fact that pulses have returned, it the BP remains less than 90–100 mmHg (e.g. absence of radial pulse or *strong* femoral pulses), this still may not be enough to adequately restore the O_2 debt to be "stunned myocardium", let alone supply the steady state circulation required to support coronary perfusion.

Catheters

While endotracheal administration of drugs (such as epinephrine) can be an alternative approach in adults in whom IV access is not available, this method is probably a poor route in the absence of adequate circulation. This is particularly true in the case of lidocaine and atropine which are not even absorbed very well in the patient with normal circulation. Therefore, one should "go where the money is" and quickly establish an IV catheter placement (or several) with as large a bore cannula as is feasible (e.g., 14 or 16 G). This is obviously best accomplished either at the antecubital, forearm or external jugular sites. As drugs are administered during CPR conditions, they should be subsequently flushed in vigorously. For example, in an antecubital site, the IV solution (e.g., D5W) can be squeezed in under pressure with the arm elevated well above heart level. In this situation a 20–30 second flush is probably adequate especially if positive pressure breathing and chest compressions are transiently withheld during the last 5 or 10 seconds of the flush in order to overcome any obstruction of flow from associated increases in intrathoracic pressures. In the case of external jugular or direct central venous access, a shorter flush (with immediate CPR and ventilation interruption) is obviously acceptable.

Multiple cannulations are preferred, at least eventually, as long as the initial therapeutic interventions are not delayed. This is encouraged so that there are multiple sites for various interventions (lidocaine drip, norepinephrine drip, etc.) and in anticipation of IV site inflation or accidental dislodging. So the "C" is for Catheter(s).

Drugs

The "D" is for drugs. It should be remembered that even those who regain their pulse after a period of cardiac arrest are at great risk for refibrillation or further deterioration if the perfusion of the coronaries is not adequate enough to restore sorely needed nutrients for functional cardiac requirements. Therefore, in hypotensive post-resuscitative patients, the aggressive use of pressor agents is generally recommended to transiently augment AODP enough to establish a stabilized and adequate spontaneous circulation (e.g., systolic BP > 100 or 110 mm Hg). This may take several minutes or even hours of continued pressor support before this stabilization will occur.

In cases of ventricular dysrhythmias, lidocaine administration is strongly recommended, particularly when pressors are being used. A minimum dose of 1 mg/kg is usually ordered initially. However, the patient then receives further loading doses of up to 3 mg/kg to achieve a reasonably "suppressive" level. In our own system, we aggressively pugh 100 mg IV in most adults, followed by another dose within minutes if VF persists, and often 50–100 mg more within another few minutes if it still remains. Once an adequate spontaneous circulation is achieved, a maintenance drip of 2 mg/min (initially) is also provided and is often increased to 3 or 4 mg/min if ventricular ectopy persists. Bretylium is now considered a second-line drug in VF because of its potential hypotensive effects and, with our current approach, is rarely needed.

Sodium bicarbonate administration is generally not recommended early in the arrest. Many practitioners now believe that the correction of blood pH is largely "cosmetic" and dies not alter outcome. Others even believe it harmful. While a lower blood pH usually correlates with a bad outcome, this may simply mean that the degree of metabolic acidosis is just a marker for the patient's tolerance of the cardiac arrest state. For example, sprinters and seizure patients often lower their blood pH substantially without adverse effect. Thus, this agent is usually not given until after the fist round of therapy has failed. This usually occurs about 10 minutes into the arrest, thus the current ACLS recommendations. Therefore, the restoration of spontaneous circulation generally suggests that sodium bicarbonate should be deferred. Nevertheless, there now exists some reassessment of this concept and clinical trials are even being considered to examine which subset of patients are benefited (or even harmed) by supplemental bicarbonate.

ECG Functions

The "E" is for ECG functions. It is important to properly interpret the ECG. Asystole is not a "flatline" on ECG. It is a *clinical state* evidenced by pulseless, apnea and no detectable electrical activity in the heart. Therefore one must be assured of the detection apparatus. Proper adjustment of the ECG monitor gain position should be performed to establish standard amplitude calibration. If gain adjustment is desired, notation of the increased or decreased gain should accompany the ECG interpretations. Standard coarse VF may resemble torsades de pointes (atypical polymorphic VT) if the gain is too high or a NSR may be mistaken for asystole if the gain is too low, particularly in some patients such as those with chronic obstructive pulmonary disease (COPD) who have electrical "insulation". This misinterpretation might be more apt to occur if the patient has an axis deviation and an incorrect vector (e.g., Lead I) is examined.

Obviously, detachment of an ECG lead is a key problem in patients receiving continuous chest compressions and multiple body jolts (during countershocks), not to mention the relatively chaotic emergency situation that predisposes to accidental detachment and no notice of such.

One of the mistakes occasionally made by prehospital care providers is failure to recognize that they did not switch from the "quick-look" paddle mode to the "lead" mode once they have placed the standard ECG leads. Thus absent electrical activity on the monitor can be very misleading. Clearly, the best safeguard is to always check for pulses and/or apical heart beat (no matter what shows up on the monitor). In addition, constant reassessment is deserved and in cases of flatline or possible atypical VF waveforms, one should consider looking at both modes and various ECG vectors before drawing final conclusions.

Further History and Physical Examination

The "F" is for "further history and physical examination". Although there is no time to get much of a history when one must act quickly, still one should try to establish whatever background information might be useful in guiding further therapy as soon as it is feasible. A history of hypoglycemic medications might make one consider glucose administration, for example. Although there is some current thinking that hyperglycemia may be harmful or exacerbate the neurological insult following cardiac arrest, hypoglycemia should not go untreated. We now routinely measure blood glucose by Chemstrip which is generally very sensitive in ruling out hypoglycemia. A history or discovery of tricyclic antipressant use might steer one away from the use of anti-arrhythmics that might widen the Q-T interval while a history or furosemide and digoxin in coarse VF or recurrent VT might make one consider hypomagnesemia and/or hypokalemia and prompt one to treat accordingly. Medications such as beta-blockers (e.g. propanolol) or vasodilators (nitroglycerin, hydralazine or other afterload reducers) may explain refractory bradycardia or hypotension. Make sure nitroglycerin pads on the chest wall are removed and wiped clean during resuscitations.

A patient with a prolonged expiratory phase (e.g., COPD or asthma patient) may appear to be in EMD when pulses have simply been diminished by an "Auto-PEEP effect". In such cases there is a severely diminished venous return due to persistently high intrathoracic pressures. This occurs because of overzealous ventilation in patients who unable to rapidly expel an entire tidal volume prior to delivery of the next positive pressure breath, resulting in inadvertent positive end-expiratory pressure (PEEP). Under such circumstances, a transient (10 second) cessation of breathing that allows complete expulsion of gas may then allow return of palpable pulses. Treatment directed at bronchospasm, slowing of respiratory rates and even fluid challenges may be of value here.

In all cases, reversible causes of shock (e.g., tension pneumothorax, cardiac tamponade and hypovolemia) should be considered.

Conclusion

The future directions of cardiac arrest management standards have been speculated in earlier parts of this discussion. Regardless of whether or not these hypotheses are eventually validated, the key to successful cadiac arrest management is the fastest possible restoration of adequate spontaneous circulation. Over the past two decades, we have clearly learned that the earlier the intervention, the better the results. At the present time, the earliest possible BCPR, along with the earliest possible defibrillation (and probably the aggressive use of epinephrine and ETI) are the keys to achieving better survival rates. Lidocaine probably also plays a significant role in preventing the recurrence of VF, particularly once adequate perfusion is restored. In the future, other modalities, such as emergency cardiopulmonary bypass (ECPB) may even replace our present methodologies. For example, it may be found that immediate restoration of an adequate circulation with a modified, rapid ECPB procedure may become a priority over other interventions. However, whatever the future holds, cardiac arrest management will remain one of the most important skills that the critical care practitioner must master.

Acknowledgements: The author thanks his mentors Drs. Michael Copass and Leonard Hudson as well as the City of Houston Fire Department dispatchers, first-responders, paramedics and EMS command staff for their leadership and example, their enthusiasm and compassion and for having made modern miracles possible. Also Denise Mann and Nina Meher-Homji for their patience, fortitude and skill in preparing this manuscript.

References

1. Alvarez H III, Miller RH, Cobb LA (1975) Medic I: The Seattle advanced paramedic training program. In: Proceedings of the National Conference on Standards for Cardiopulmonary Resuscitation (CPR) and Emergency Cardiac Care (ECC). Dallas, American Heart Association, pp 43–37
2. Bergner L, Bergner M, Hallstrom AP, et al (1983) Service factors and health status of survivors of out-of-hospital cardiac arrest. Am J Emerg Med 3:259–263
3. Bonnin MJ, Pepe PE, Clark PS (1989) Survival prognosis for the elderly after out-of-hospital arrest. Ann Emerg Med 18:469–472
4. Brown CG, Taylor HA, Luu T, et al (1988) Effect of standard doses of epinephrine on myocardial oxygen delivery and utilization during cardiopulmonary resuscitation. Crit Care Med 16:536–539
5. Brown CG, Werman HA, Davis EA, et al (1987) The effects of graded doses of epinephrine on regional myocardial blood flow during cardiopulmonary resuscitation in swine. Circulation 75:491–498
6. Callaham MA (1986) Advances in the management of cardiac arrest – Medical Staff Conference. West J Med 145:670–676
7. Cobb LA, Alvarez H, Copass MK (1976) A rapid response system for out-of-hospital cardiac emergencies. Med Clin North Am 60:283–290
8. Cobb LA (1982) Prehospital cardiac care. Does it make a difference? Am Heart J 103:316–318
9. Crampton RS, Aldrich RF, Gascho JA, et al (1975) Reduction of prehospital, ambulance and community coronary death rates by the community-wide emergency cardiac care system. Am J Med 58:151–154
10. Eisenberg MS, Bergner L, Hallstrom A (1979) Paramedic programs and out-of-hospital cardiac arrest: I. Factors associated with successful resuscitation. Am J Public Health 69:30–35
11. Eisenberg MS, Bergner L, Hallstrom A (1979) Cardiac resuscitation in the community – Importance of rapid provision and implications for program planning. JAMA 241:1905–1908
12. Eisenberg MS, Horwood BT, Cummins RO, Hearne TR (1990) A tale of 28 cities: Cardiac arrest and Resuscitation. Ann Emerg Med 19 (in press)
13. Emergency Cardiac Care Committee, American Heart Association (1986) Standards and guidelines for cardiopulmonary resuscitation and emergency cardiac care. JAMA 255:2841–2857
14. Griffith BP (1988) Some futuristic possibilities for resuscitation. Crit Care Med 16:1007–1010
15. Koscove EM, Paradis NA (1988) Successful resuscitation from cardiac arrest using high-dose epinephrine therapy. JAMA 259:3031–3035
16. Pepe PE, Copass MK, Joyce TH (1985) Prehospital endotracheal intubation – Rationale for training emergency medical personnel. Ann Emerg Med 14:1085–1092
17. Pepe PE (1988) Whom to resuscitate In: Civetta JM (ed) Intensive and critical care medicine. Lippincott, pp 93–102
18. Pepe PE, Bonnin MJ, Clark PS (1989) Clinical predictors of survival in paramedic – witnessed cardiac arrest. Prehospital and Disaster Medicine 4:71
19. Pepe PE, Bonnin MJ, Almaguer DR, et al (1989) The effect of tiered system implementation on sudden death survival rates. Prehospital and Disaster Medicine 4:71

Acidosis in CPR: Pathophysiology and Treatment*

M. von Planta

Introduction

During cardiac arrest and cardio-pulmonary resuscitation (CPR) only limited blood flow and consequently organ perfusion can be maintained by chest compression. Cardiac output during CPR averages only 25 to 35% of normal and thus severely reduces oxygen delivery to the tissues. The metabolism therefore turns to its energetic emergency pathway resulting in the production of anaerobic metabolites. The buildup of lactic acid is slow, while the CO_2 concentration rapidly increases during CPR. After onset of cardiac arrest intramyocardial CO_2 progressively increases to levels exceeding 400 mmHg. These increases in CO_2 can only be reversed by improving coronary blood flow and its associated oxygen delivery.

The critical reduction in systemic and pulmonary blood flow curtails alveolar CO_2 clearance which in association with continuous CO_2 production in the organs explains the accumulation of CO_2 in the pre-pulmonary venous vascular bed and in the tissues. Indeed, experimental and clinical studies demonstrated decreases of the expired PCO_2 ($P_{ET}CO_2$) in association with hypercarbic acidosis in venous blood and hypocarbic alkalosis in arterial blood. In the cardiac venous blood i.e. the venous effluent of the left ventricle, marked increases in the $[H^+]$ and PCO_2 together with lactic acid accounted for drastic decreases in intramyocardial $[H^+]$ during experimental CPR.

For the treatment of this "triple acid-base defect" alkalinizing agents are conventionally used. However, the administration of CO_2 generating or CO_2 consuming alkalinizing agents neither increased the resuscitability rate nor did it improve the long term outcome after CPR. Therefore, the current controversy regarding the rationale and therapeutic effectiveness of buffer agents as part of the pharmacotherapy of CPR is reviewed in the light of recent research developments in the acid-base management of cardiac arrest.

Acid-Base Changes During CPR

During conventional closed chest CPR, there is a critical reduction in cardiac output and consequently in systemic and coronary blood flow [1]. Therefore,

* With support of the Swiss National Science Foundation.

oxygen transport is drastically reduced and anaerobic energy production is responsible for increases in CO_2 and lactic acid with development of acidemia during the low flow state of CPR. The highly diffusible CO_2 rapidly crosses from the cells into the capillaries and increases the venous CO_2 concentration with resultant hypercarbic venous acidosis. These excesses in CO_2 may be removed from the small amount of blood circulating through the alveolar-capillary exchange bed of the lungs. Consequently, arterial blood is less acidotic than venous blood. This phenomenon of hypercarbic venous acidosis coincident with hypocarbic arterial alkalosis was termed the arterio-venous paradox [2, 3]. Since the advent of modern CPR, correction of the acidosis was recommended as Jude stated already in 1961: *"continued cardiac arrest, even though the circulation is artificially maintained, will result in metabolic acidosis. Sodium bicarbonate is beneficial in maintaining blood pH close to the normal value"* [4].

However, it was later recognized that the initial phase of CPR was characterized more often by arterial alkalemia than by acidemia [2, 3]. The alkalemia was attributed to marked increases in the ventilation/perfusion ratio during vigorous mechanical ventilation. Accordingly, minor metabolic acidosis was well compensated by concurrent respiratory alkalosis since severe arterial acidosis is usually due to inadequate ventilation. Consequently, the recent Standards and Guidelines for Cardiopulmonary Resuscitation and Emergency Cardiac Care state: *"adequate alveolar ventilation is the mainstay of the control of acid-base balance in the cardiac arrest circumstance"* [5].

Marked increases in venous CO_2 are associated with decreases in the arterial CO_2 and time coincident decreases in the $P_{ET}CO_2$ [6, 7]. Prospective investigations of the aorto-venous gradients of pH, CO_2 and HCO_3^- in experimental animals and in patients demonstrated increases in the gradients for pH and CO_2 but not for HCO_3^- [3, 8]. Even greater gradients were observed when blood was sampled selectively in the venous effluent of a single organ such as the heart [9].

Myocardial Acid-Base Changes: During ischemia coronary blood flow is reduced and anaerobic myocardial metabolism results in the production of $[H^+]$, CO_2 and lactate (Fig. 1). Recent studies demonstrated severe hypercarbic acidosis in the great cardiac vein with increases in CO_2 to levels exceeding 150 mmHg during experimental CPR. Since simultaneously sampled aortic CO_2 was less than 50 mmHg, the excess of cardiac vein CO_2 is best explained by myocardial CO_2 production [9]. The accumulation of CO_2 within the myocardium reflects the balance between local production of CO_2, endogenous myocardial buffering of CO_2 and its clearance by blood flow. Therefore, intramyocardial CO_2 increases when coronary blood flow is impaired [10, 11]. These increases in intramyocardial CO_2 are strikingly correlated with the coronary perfusion pressure during CPR [12].

CO_2 is the predominant determinant of muscle pH. Extracellular HCO_3^- has only a minor effect on intracellular pH. Partial "respiratory compensation" of extracellular metabolic acidosis readily prevents intracellular acidosis; however, increases in extracellular HCO_3^- fail to correct intracellular acidosis [13]. The buffering capacity of myocardial muscle is higher than that of skeletal muscle,

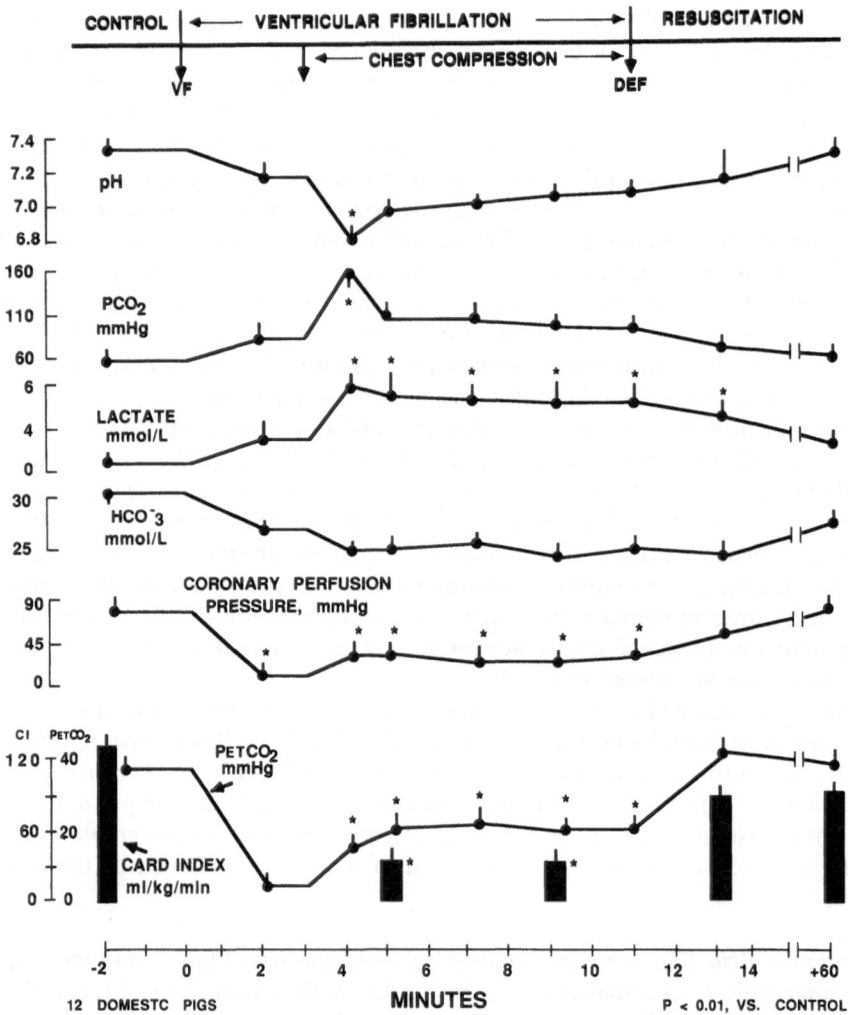

Fig. 1. Great cardiac vein pH, PCO_2, lactate and HCO_3^- together with coronary perfusion pressure, $P_{ET}CO_2$ and cardiac index prior to ventricular fibrillation (VF), during chest compression and after defibrillation (DEF) with successful resuscitation. Cardiac vein acidemia during CPR is reversed within 60 min after return of spontaneous circulation. $P_{ET}CO_2$ parallels the decrease in coronary perfusion pressure and cardiac index during CPR in 12 domestic pigs

nervous tissue or blood and bicarbonate buffering of the anaerobically generated lactate may explain increases in intramyocardial CO_2 [14].

Adverse effects of hypercapnia involve primarily the cardiovascular and central nervous systems, including increased adrenergic activity. Increases in myocardial CO_2 are associated with reduced myocardial contractility [11]. Progressive hypercarbic acidosis favors the competition of [H^+] ions with calcium ions for binding to troponin and cross bridging between actin and myosin is therefore inhibited. The dysfunction of the sarcoplasmic reticulum with decreases in both calcium uptake and ATPase activity may be responsible for the ultimate break-down in the myocardial excitation-contraction coupling system. Indeed, recent data from Koretsune et al. demonstrated fourfold increases in free intracellular calcium during ventricular fibrillation which would further account for decreases in myocardial contractility and prolonged postresuscitation contractile dysfunction, known as stunned myocardium [15].

Buffer Therapy During CPR

During CPR a triple acid-base defect consists of venous hypercarbic acidosis, of arterial hypocarbic alkalosis and of metabolic (lactic) acidosis. Thus, the choice of an optimal buffer agent for CPR is a difficult and controversial task since organic and anorganic options are open to the clinician's judgment (Fig. 2).

THAM [(CH$_2$OH)$_3$ C—NH$_2$]: The organic proton acceptor, THAM (Tris-Hydroxymethyl-Amino-Methane) decreases the CO_2 concentration of blood and tissues and reverses acidosis according to its buffer reaction:

$$(CH_2OH)_3C—NH_2 + HA \leftrightarrow (CH_2OH)_3C—NH_3^+ + A^-$$

THAM rapidly crosses cell membranes and acts as an intracellular buffer whereas NaHCO$_3$ acts predominantly as an extracellular buffer [16]. It exerts positive inotropic effects and increases myocardial contractility.

However, unexpected decreases in resuscitability and survival after CPR with THAM were observed. Of the animals which received THAM only 40% were successfully resuscitated; whereas, in the NaHCO$_3$ group 70% and in the saline placebo group 80% were resuscitated. Accordingly, neither THAM or NaHCO$_3$ improved outcome when compared to saline placebo. THAM induced arterial vasodilation and reduced systemic resistance with consequent decreases in mean

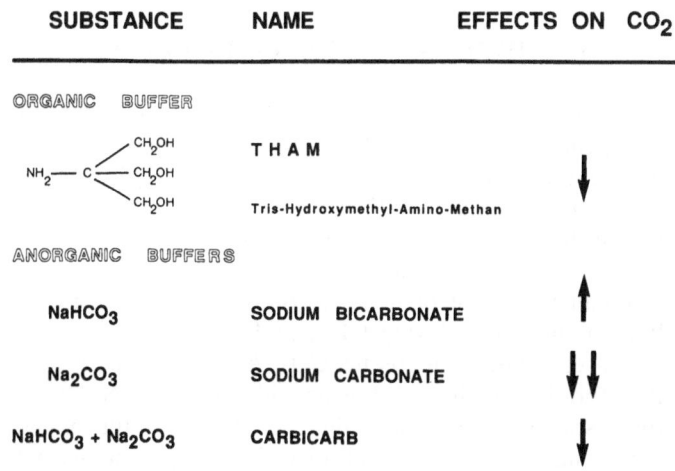

Fig. 2. Effects of buffer agents on CO_2

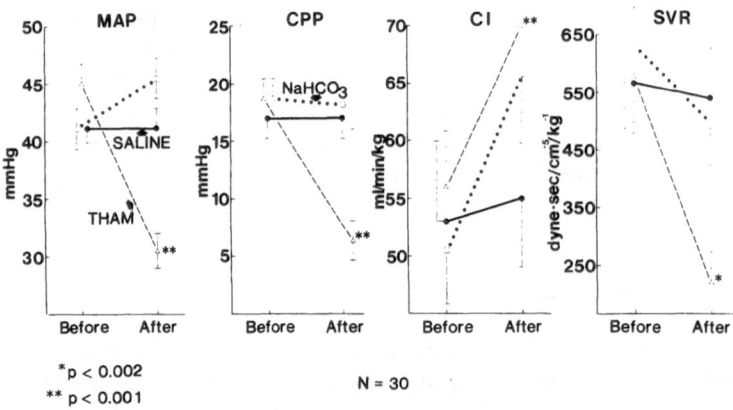

*p < 0.002

** p < 0.001

N = 30

Fig. 3. Mean aortic pressure (MAP), coronary perfusion pressure (CPP), cardiac index (CI) and systemic vascular resistance (SVR) before and after administration of THAM, NaHCO₃ and saline placebo during external chest compression (10 pigs in each treatment group)

aortic and coronary perfusion pressures to levels which were previously shown to preclude survival (Fig. 3).

However, the carbon dioxide tension after THAM infusion was significantly reduced in expiratory, aortic, mixed venous and coronary venous blood. This indeed contrasted with NaHCO₃ in which significant increases of the PCO₂ were observed. Accordingly, THAM was an efficient buffer agent which consumed CO_2 but exerted arterial vasodilator effects which of themselves adversely affected outcome [17].

Sodium Bicarbonate (NaHCO₃): NaHCO₃ dissociates to sodium and bicarbonate which, in the presence of hydrogen ions, is converted to carbonic acid and thence to carbon dioxide which is subsequently excreted by the lungs. Under conditions of normal perfusion and ventilation bicarbonate forms the easily excretable CO_2 which permits its function as an efficient buffer:

$$H^+ + HCO_3^- \leftrightarrow H_2CO_3 \leftrightarrow H_2O + CO_2$$

In hemodynamically stable conditions with adequate alveolar ventilation, the CO_2 generated by NaHCO₃ can be eliminated by the lungs, and NaHCO₃ therefore may effectively neutralize excesses of $[H^+]$. As the pK of the bicarbonate system is 6.1, bicarbonate would be expected to function poorly as a buffer within the clinically relevant pH range of 6.9 to 7.9. However, Kruse et al. demonstrated in 20 patients during CPR, that the pK of blood carbonic acid is not different from that of healthy controls [18]. Since the removal of CO_2 by the lungs is impaired during CPR, NaHCO₃ cannot act as efficient buffer and it increases venous and tissue CO_2. A decrease in myocardial contractility can therefore be anticipated. Further side effects of NaHCO₃ include among others increases in plasma osmolality, left shifts of the oxyhemoglobin dissociation curve and hypernatremia, all of which are potentially deleterious.

Thus, restraint in the use of $NaHCO_3$ was advised. In the 1985 Standardization Conference on CPR the consensus was to abandon the initial use of $NaHCO_3$ and constrain its use to after 10 minutes of conventional CPR [5].

Sodium Carbonate (Na_2CO_3): Na_2CO_3 acts as $[H^+]$ acceptor and reverses acidosis by binding $[H^+]$ ions. In the extracellular fluid space, the following reaction is anticipated in the presence of CO_2 and H_2O:

$$HCO_3^- + H^+$$
$$Na_2CO_3 + CO_2 + H_2O \leftrightarrow 2HCO_3^- + 2Na^+$$

Thereby not only HCO_3^- is generated but CO_2 is bound. However, very little has been published regarding the effects of sodium carbonate on acid base disturbances during CPR. The very alkaline Na_2CO_3 (pH of 11) prevented a decline in arterial blood pH and increased plasma sodium, HCO_3^-, and osmolality in an apnea model in dogs and it increased coronary blood flow and myocardial contractile force whereas $NaHCO_3$ decreased both.

Carbicarb ($Na_2CO_3 + NaHCO_3$): The disadvantages of the high pH of Na_2CO_3 alone were overcome with the introduction of a mixture composed of equimolar amounts of $NaHCO_3$ and Na_2CO_3 which subsequently was termed Carbicarb [19]. In dogs with hypoxic lactic acidosis, the combined buffers normalized arterial blood pH without increasing arterial CO_2. The limited data currently available therefore confirm that Na_2CO_3 reduces CO_2 and that $NaHCO_3$ increases CO_2 in blood.

However, Gazmuri recently demonstrated in a porcine model of CPR that neither mean arterial pressures nor cardiac index were adversely affected after the administration of Carbicarb [20]. However, significant decreases in the coronary perfusion pressure were observed which were attributed to a vasodilator effect of the hyperosmolal buffer mixture in association with an increase in the right atrial pressure. Furthermore, Carbicarb failed to reduce intramyocardial acidosis, myocardial CO_2 production or to increase the resuscitability rate.

Conclusions

Venous and tissue CO_2 rapidly rises after onset of cardiac arrest and increases in myocardial CO_2 are associated with decreases in myocardial contractility. Venous blood gas data – in contrast to arterial – reflect with greater accuracy the actual acid-base state of the tissues during CPR. Neither CO_2 generating or CO_2 consuming buffer agents improve survival after cardiac arrest. $NaHCO_3$ may be contraindicated, in part due to CO_2 production, while THAM reduces coronary perfusion pressures under levels consistent with survival. Carbicarb failed to decrease coronary vein CO_2 or to mitigate intramyocardial acidosis or to improve resuscitability.

In the absence of preexisting acidosis, adequate ventilation in association with efficient cardiac compression may eliminate the CO_2 generated during cardiac arrest. Metabolic acidosis may be counterbalanced by concurrent respiratory alkalosis in the first phase of CPR.

References

1. Ditchey RV, Winkler JV, Rhodes CA (1982) Relative lack of coronary blood flow during closed-chest resuscitation in dogs. Circulation 66:297–302
2. Grundler WG, Weil MH, Rackow EC (1986) Arteriovenous carbon dioxide and pH gradients during cardiac arrest. Circulation 74:1071–1074
3. Weil MH, Rackow EC, Trevino R, Grundler W, Falk J, Griffel M (1986) Difference in acid base state between venous and arterial blood during cardiopulmonary resuscitation. N Engl J Med 315:153–157
4. Jude JR, Kouwenhoven WB, Knickerbocker GG (1961) Cardiac arrest: Report of application of external cardiac massage on 118 patients. JAMA 178:1063–1070
5. Standards and guidelines for cardiopulmonary resuscitation and emergency cardiac care (1986) JAMA 255:2905–2984
6. von Planta I, Weil MH, von Planta M, et al (1988) Cardiopulmonary resuscitation in the rat. J Appl Physiol 65:2641–2647
7. Falk JL, Rackow EC, Weil MH (1988) End-tidal carbon dioxide during cardiopulmonary resuscitation. N Engl J Med 318:607–611
8. Adrogué HJ, Rashad MN, Gorin AB, Yacoub J, Madias NE (1989) Assessing acid-base status in circulatory failure. N Engl J Med 320:1312–1316
9. von Planta M, Weil MH, Gazmuri RJ, Bisera J, Rackow EC (1989) Myocardial acidosis associated with CO_2 production during cardiac arrest and resuscitation. Circulation 80:684–692
10. Brantigan JW, Perna AM, Gardner TJ, Gott VL (1972) Intramyocardial gas tensions in the canine heart during anoxic cardiac arrest. Surg Gyn Obstet 134:67–72
11. MacGregor DC, Wilson GJ, Holness DE, et al (1974) Intramyocardial carbon dioxide tension: A guide to the safe period of anoxic arrest of the heart. J Thor Cardiovasc Surg 68:101–107
12. Kette F, Weil MH, Gazmuri RJ, Bisera J, Rackow EC (1989) Increases in myocardial PCO_2 during CPR correlate inversely with coronary perfusion pressures (CPP) and resuscitability (Abstract). Circulation 80 (in press)
13. Adler S, Roy A, Relman AS (1965) Intracellular acid-base regulation. II. The interaction between CO_2 tension and extracellular bicarbonate in the determination of muscle cell pH. J Clin Invest 44:21–30
14. Bettice JA, Wang BC, Brown EB jr (1976) Intracellular buffering of heart and skeletal muscles during the onset of hypercapnia. Resp Physiol 28:89–98
15. Koretsune Y, Marban G (1989) Cell calcium in the pathophysiology of ventricular fibrillation and in the pathogenesis of postarrhythmic contractile function. Circulation 80:369–379
16. Nahas GG (1959) Use of an organic carbon dioxide buffer in vivo. Science 129:782–783
17. von Planta M, Gudipati CV, Weil MH, Kraus LJ, Rackow EC (1988) Effects of tromethamine and sodium bicarbonate buffers during cardiac resuscitation. J Clin Pharmacol 28:594–599
18. Kruse JA, Hukku P, Carlson RW (1988) Constancy of blood carbonic acid pK in patients during cardiopulmonary resuscitation. Chest 93:1221–1224
19. Bersin RM, Arieff AL (1988) Improved hemodynamic function during hypoxia with carbicarb, a new agent for the management of acidosis. Circulation 77:227–233
20. Gazmuri RJ, von Planta M, Weil MH, Rackow EC (1990) Cardiac effects of CO_2 consuming and CO_2 generating buffers during cardiopulmonary resuscitation. J Am Coll Cardiol (in press)

Modern Drug Therapy During Cardiopulmonary Resuscitation

H. W. Gervais and W. F. Dick

Introduction

Based on the recommendations of the American Heart Association (AHA), four classes of drugs are considered of major importance during cardiopulmonary resuscitation (CPR), and a fifth class of experimental drugs, although currently still under investigation holds the possibility of gaining significance for the future:

1. Oxygen;
2. Drugs to improve cardiac output and blood pressure (vasopressor agents);
3. Drugs to improve cardiac rhythm and heart rate (antiarrhythmic agents, atropine, isoproterenol);
4. Drugs to improve acid-base disturbances (buffer solutions);
5. Experimental drugs under investigation.

Oxygen

The AHA recommends the administration of oxygen during CPR as early as possible at the highest concentration available, because hypoxemia and inadequate oxygen delivery to all tissues can be expected to occur rapidly after cardiopulmonary arrest [1]. The most important determinants of oxygen supply are pulmonary gas exchange and organ perfusion by the heart.

Inadequate tissue oxygenation may be due to various factors, i.e. inadequate oxygenation of the blood, a decrease in hemoglobin concentration, a reduction in the percentage of hemoglobin saturated with oxygen in arterial blood, impaired affinity of hemoglobin for oxygen, and finally a dimished or – as under conditions of cardiac arrest – totally absent oxygen transport due to inadequate cardiac output. The distribution of perfusion is an additional factor of major importance to the oxygen supply-demand balance [2]. There are no restrictions with regard to a critical upper limit of oxygen concentration during CPR. An inspired concentration of 100% oxygen appears to be generally safe for at least 6 hours without the development of undesirable side effects. Though tissue oxygenation is not solely determined by blood oxygenation, an adequate PaO_2 level should be maintained. "Adequate PaO_2 values could be considered those high enough to maintain oxygen uptake without the need for compensatory changes, a reduction in tissue energy levels or anaerobic metabolism" [3].

Vasopressor Agents

The cornerstone of pharmacological therapy during CPR is the choice of the correct pressor agent. Two classes of vasoactive drugs have been shown to be effective during CPR: "pure" α-adrenergic receptor agonists such as phenylephrine, methoxamine, and norepinephrine or mixed α-β receptor agonists such as epinephrine.

The efficacy of epinephrine during CPR has been confirmed by numerous studies. Epinephrine improves myocardial and cerebral blood flow by selectively redirecting the artificial cardiac output to brain and heart and thus affecting a raise in coronary and cerebral perfusion pressures. Peripheral vasoconstriction of other, noncerebral, noncoronary vascular beds leading to improved systolic and diastolic aortic pressures without adverse alterations of right atrial or intracranial pressure is believed to be the underlying mechanism of this process [4].

Alpha-agonists have also been shown to increase arterial pressure although their effects on cerebral and myocardial blood flow, oxygen consumption, and recovery of brain electrical function after CPR have only recently been clarified [5, 6].

Moreover, each class of drugs has distinct advantages or disadvantages over the other. Epinephrine given during ventricular fibrillation for example can increase the frequency in amplitude of fibrillatory contractions. This in turn could raise myocardial oxygen demand, thus disturbing the balance between myocardial oxygen supply and demand while impairing subendocardial blood flow [7]. The mechanism responsible for impairing subendocardial flow appears to be coronary vascular compression at increased muscular wall tension [8]. In contrast to the potentially harmful effects of epinephrine on subendocardial blood flow, methoxamine, a pure α-agonist, improved subendocardial flow during open-chest CPR [9]. Comparing epinephrine and norepinephrine, Lindner and coworkers recently observed a smaller increase in myocardial oxygen demand and an improved myocardial oxygen extraction ratio with norepinephrine, resulting in effective defibrillation and restoration of spontaneous circulation [10]. Although it is widely accepted that ventricular fibrillation of increased frequency and amplitude can be terminated more easily by defibrillation and that the required energy for countershock is reduced by epinephrine, Yakaitis et al. were unable to demonstrate any beneficial effect of epinephrine on defibrillation or on a reduction of energy requirements [11].

With regard to the effects of adrenergic agents on the central nervous system, the situation is still more complex: when epinephrine gains access to cerebral β-receptors, it can cause an increase in cerebral oxygen demand. Should this occur while blood flow to the brain is restricted, an adverse effect on recovery of brain function during and after resuscitation might result. However, stimulation of cerebral β-receptors can also cause cerebral vasodilation, thereby improving cerebral blood flow. Pure α-adrenergic vasoconstriction by drugs like phenylephrine unopposed by β-receptors mediated vasodilation may on the other hand result in lower cerebral blood flow compared to epinephrine. Two recent investigations studied the effects of equipotent pressor doses of phenylephrine (bolus injection of 1 mg followed by a continuous infusion of 20 µg/kg/min) and epinephrine (bolus injection of 1 mg followed by a continuous infusion of 4 µg/kg/min) on cerebral blood flow, metabolism, and brain electrical function, as assessed by somatosensory evoked potentials and brainstem auditory evoked responses during and after CPR in a closed-chest dog model. They were unable to observe any differences between epinephrine and phenylephrine, independently of whether CPR was started immediately after initiating cardiac arrest or whether there was an 8 minute delay in the onset of CPR after cardiac arrest [5, 6]. These findings confirm results by other authors who were unable to demonstrate differences between epinephrine (bolus injection of 1 mg) and phenylephrine (bolus injection of 10 mg) on neurologic outcome and 24-hour survival when CPR was commenced 3 minutes after cardiac arrest, and vasopressor infusion was started 12 minutes after arrest [12]. It has to be kept in mind that most comparison studies of epinephrine and other pressor agents do not report whether equipotent pressor doses were used. However, equipotent pressor doses are an unconditional prerequisite in determining differences between the drugs during and after CPR.

A critical issue in dealing with epinephrine mediated effects on the brain is the functional integrity of the blood-brain barrier. Although preliminary results of the studies cited above do not confirm the evidence of a blood-brain barrier impairment, the possibility cannot be excluded that in the presence of more prolonged ischemic periods prior to the onset of CPR, a disruption of the blood-brain barrier allowing access of large amounts of adrenergic agonists to the brain can result. Even after very short ischemic periods due to maximal dilatation of cerebral vessels, the blood-brain barrier will be more prone to disruption by rapid pressure fluctuations.

The blood-brain barrier issue is also of key interest in the immediate postresuscitation period due to a generalized hyperemic pattern frequently observed at that time. Some studies reported blood-brain barrier disruption after resuscitation by fluorescence microscopy using Evans Blue as a blood-brain barrier tracer. They could not confirm a statistical relationship between the magnitude of postresuscitation blood pressure increase and the severity of Evans Blue extravasation, although the rapidity of blood pressure increase after restoration of ventricular function appears to be a contributing factor of major importance. Furthermore, blood-brain barrier dysfunction is more likely to occur during extreme hypoxia and hypercapnia of sufficient duration [13]. Further investigations of these important factors are still needed.

With regard to current recommendations on the use of epinephrine by the AHA [1]: 0.5–1.0 mg IV every 5 minutes during CPR, two major differences to the studies mentioned above become apparent: first, those studies focus on animal models whose limits are well known and not on human subjects; second, the investigators used continuous infusions of high-dose pressor agents rather than low-dose bolus injections as recommended in humans. The currently recommended AHA dosage regimen provides only between 8.5 µg/kg to 15 µg/kg of epinephrine every five minutes. This dose is significantly lower than that needed to successfully resuscitate most animal species. A recent study determining the effect of epinephrine, 15 μg/kg, 45 μg/kg, or 75 μg/kg during late closed-chest CPR in human beings (epinephrine was given only after almost 60 minutes of CPR without pressor agents) observed a direct relationship between the dose of epinephrine and the level of systolic and diastolic blood pressure which could be achieved during CPR [14].

In view of the above results and of results reported in case reports, it becomes apparent that a reevaluation of the AHA recommendations is required with the suggestion of a considerable increase in the dosage recommendation on epinephrine, it has to be kept in mind that the currently recommended epinephrine dosage surprisingly does not vary with the weight of the patient. With regard to pure α-adrenergic agents, the evidence in support of the superiority of one of those agents over epinephrine is inconclusive. Any change of the recommendations in favor of an α-adrenergic agent would therefore be without any sound scientific foundation at the present time.

Drugs to Improve Cardiac Rhythm and Heart Rate
(antiarrhythmic agents, atropine, isoproterenol)

The drug of choice for use during ventricular fibrillation or pulseless ventricular tachycardia resistent to defibrillation is lidocaine. In accordance with the AHA, after a bolus injection of 1 mg/kg, repeated additional doses of 0.5 mg/kg should be given every 8 to 10 minutes up to a total dose of 3 mg/kg, thus permitting rapid achievement and maintenance of therapeutic blood levels. However, bolus injections are recommended for use in the setting of CPR only. Once spontaneous circulation has been restored, a continuous infusion of 2 to 4 mg/min is preferable in order to prevent the reocurrence of ventricular ectopy. The dose has to be reduced in patients with decreased cardiac output, in patients older than 70 years and those with hepatic dysfunction, since its principal clearance mechanism is hepatic elimination [1].

Lidocaine belongs to group 1b of the membrane stabilizing antidysrhythmic drugs, decreasing phase 4 depolarization. Its primary effects are inhibition of retrograde conduction, and inhibition of reentry mechanisms. Advantages of lidocaine compared with other antiarrhythmic agents such as quinidine or procainamide include a more rapid onset and prompt disappearance of effects after discontinuation of therapy.

Bretylium tosylate is the drug of second choice to be used in case lidocaine proves to be ineffective. Bretylium, a quarternary ammonium compound, acts by prolonging the ventricular action potential and the refractory period. Bretylium 5 mg/kg IV as is recommended in refractory ventricular fibrillation, to be followed by another defibrillation attempt. In case of persistent ventricular fibrillation, further bolus injections of up to 10 mg/kg can be given at 15- to 30-minute intervals up to a cumulative maximal dose of 30 mg/kg. The main effect of bretylium given during ventricular fibrillation is its ability to facilitate defibrillation. Bretylium is also recommended for use during persistent or recurring ventricular tachycardia. Under these conditions bretylium should be given as a loading dose of 5 to 10 mg/kg, followed by continuous infusion of 1 to 2 mg/min [1].

Procainamide hydrochloride is recommended in case of ventricular tachycardia unresponsive to lidocaine treatment or when lidocaine is contraindicated. Its principal electrophysiological actions are very close to those of lidocaine. Procainamide should be given in incremental doses of 50 mg each, slowly administered IV, and repeated every 5 minutes, until either arrhythmia is suppressed, hypotension occurs, the QRS complex is widened by 50% of its original width, or a total cumulative dose of 1 g has been given. Because of immediately developing hypotension after too rapid injection of procainamide, continuous monitoring of blood pressure and ECG has to be warranted [1]. Other antiarrhythmogenic agents are of only minor importance in the setting of cardiopulmonary resuscitation.

Atropine sulfate is recommended for use in asystolic cardiac arrests or in bradycardia with hemodynamic compromise. It should however be emphasized, that atropine is not the drug of first choice in the treatment of asystole. Before administering atropine, basic measures of cardiac life support, i.e. ventilation and thoracic compression have to be established, and epinephrine is most importantly given to improve cerebral and myocardial perfusion. Atropine completely abolishes vagal influence on the heart at the level of the sino-atrial nodal pacemaker. It enhances the rate of discharge of the sinus node and decreases atrio-ventricular conduction time. It has been shown that atropine is most effective in cases of asystole caused by toxic effects of choline esters, anti cholinesterase agents, or by other parasympathomimetic drugs. In addition to this, atropine is a suitable agent for treatment of cardiac arrest resulting from electrical stimulation of the vagus. The recommended dose of atropine for the treatment of asystole is 1 mg IV, repeated after 5 minutes. Unless asystole is caused by intoxication with choline esters or anticholinesterase agents, a total dose of 2 mg is sufficient to result in complete vagal blockade. In cases of bradycardia with hemodynamic compromise, atropine should be given at a dose of 0.5 mg IV, repeated every 5 minutes up to a total dose of 2.0 mg [1]. In patients where bradycardia is a consequence of myocardial infarction or myocardial ischemia, care should be taken to avoid excessive increases in heart rate which may increase the area of infarction or the amount of ischemia.

Isoproterenol during CPR is indicated only in the treatment of hemodynamically compromising extreme bradycardia in patients with a pulse does not respond to treatment with atropine. This treatment regimen is only temporary until a pacemaker is inserted. The recommended dose is 2 to 10 µg/min as a continuous infusion. It is the most potent synthetic catecholamine acting almost exclusively at β-1 and β-2 receptors. In clinical doses, isoproterenol is totally devoid of α agonistic properties. Isoproterenol lowers peripheral vascular resistance, which leads to a fall in diastolic blood pressure. This is compensated by an increased cardiac output due to its positive inotropic and chronotropic actions. As a final result, systolic blood pressure is usually maintained or raised, even in the presence of reduced mean arterial pressure. Since isoproterenol increases myocardial oxygen demand, patients with impaired ventricular function are prone to exacerbation of ischemia and rhythm disturbances [1]. A recent study in dogs with chronic left ventricular failure found harmful effects of isoproterenol on systolic and diastolic function, and a significant impairment of the endocardial to epicardial blood flow ratio during drug treatment, indicating subendocardial hypoperfusion [15].

Drugs to Improve Acid-Base Disturbances (Buffer Solutions)

There has been a dramatic change concerning the use of buffer substances during CPR. The AHA currently explicitly discourages the routine administration of sodium bicarbonate during CPR [1]. If used at all, bicarbonate can be administered only after at least 10 minutes of ongoing advanced cardiac life support at the discretion of the physician in charge of the resuscitative efforts. If bicarbonate is given, 1 mEq/kg should be administered as an initial dose. No more than half this dose can be given 10 minutes thereafter [1]. This recommendation is based on a lack of experimental evidence for improved resuscitability after infusion of sodium bicabonate. By contrast, there are many studies showing that adequate ventilation is the mainstay in maintaining acid-base homeostasis during CPR. During cardiac and respiratory arrest, a respiratory acidosis with the subsequent accumulation of CO_2 which is freely diffusible across cellular and organ membranes is likely to develop very rapidly. CO_2 removal can be accomplished most effectively by vigorous hyperventilation. However, data guiding the amount of hyperventilation to be be aimed at are not available. At the present time, it is not known whether CO_2-reactivity of the cerebral vessels is preserved under CPR or whether cerebral vessels are unable to constrict or to dilate, paralleling changes in PCO_2. The duration of the preceeding ischemic period before the onset of CPR could furthermore influence cerebrovascular reactivity.

In addition to "adequate" hyperventilation, resuscitative efforts should aim to generate sufficient myocardial perfusion pressures. In presence of effective CPR leading to adequate coronary perfusion pressures, Michael et al. were able to resuscitate animals without sodium bicarbonate or other buffers even after one hour of ventricular fibrillation and CPR – despite arterial pH values of less than 7.0 [4]. Many clinical and experimental studies have documented an arteriovenous gradient for pH and PCO_2 during CPR. Two factors are contributing to this phenomenon: first, the presence of metabolic acidosis due to the accumulation of lactic acid and other metabolites of anaerobic metabolism. Second, a respiratory acidosis affecting the venous system. The disparity between the amount of alveolar ventilation and the lack of adequate pulmonary blood flow may account for the phenomenon of venous acidosis in the presence of arterial alkalosis [16, 17].

Most of the data currently available in the literature caution against the use of sodium bicarbonate during resuscitation [18–20]. However, a recent study by Hennes et al. evaluating the effects of three buffer substances (sodium bicarbonate, Tribonat [a buffer mixture of tris, acetate, sodium bicarbonate, and disodium phosphate], and tromethamine [tris] observed no adverse effects of sodium bicarbonate with respect to defibrillation and outcome [21]. Their results showed Tribonat not to be superior to bicarbonate, while tris led to a marked arterial and central venous alkalosis which adversely affected defibrillation and survival rate. A possible explanation of their results could be the slow infusion rate of bicarbonate: bicarbonate was administered at a dosage of 1 mmol/kg over 10 minutes. Prolonged infusion of small doses of bicarbonate might therefore be preferable to administering rapid infusion or bolus injections.

While sodium bicarbonate has a number of disadvantages, the major drawback is its CO_2 generating mechanism of action. CO_2 will accumulate in the venous system due to insufficient blood flow towards the pulmonary vascular bed where it could be eliminated by ventilation. In other words, the volume of distribution into which sodium bicarbonate is infused during CPR cannot be compared to the volume of distribution under spontaneous circulation. As mentioned previously, CO_2 is furthermore freely diffusible across cell and organ membranes, thus increasing the degree of intracellular acidosis. This may have an adverse effect on the heart and the brain in particular. A recent investigation by von Planta and coworkers found a disproportionate myocardial production of CO_2 during CPR, which was accompanied by an only modest decrease in myocardial bicarbonate concentration [22]. Accordingly, myocardial CO_2 production during ischemia seems to be the predominant mechanism accounting for myocardial acidosis during CPR [22].

It is well known that intracellular acidosis exerts negative inotropic actions. Hence, administration of bicarbonate would further exacerbate the already existing myocardial acidosis and decrease ventricular performance. Myocardial acidosis not only causes strong negative inotropic actions, but ultimately leads to a total impairment of cardiac function: the so-called "stone heart".

By virtue of its free diffusibility bicarbonate generated carbon dioxide will enter the cerebral spinal fluid (CSF) containing compartment much faster than bicarbonate ions, thus at least initially further exacerbating the CSF acidosis and impairing cerebral blood flow and brain electrical function [23, 24]. It is well documented by clinical studies that cerebrospinal fluid acidosis is far more deleterious to brain function than acidosis in the blood [23].

A study in dogs by Berenyi et al. found a marked decrease in CSF pH and an increase in CSF PCO_2 during 20 minutes of CPR after 4 minutes of cardiac arrest, when sodium bicarbonate was administered. In contrast, no significant change in CSF pH or PCO_2 was found in those animals receiving only CPR without bicarbonate administration [25]. Apart from other shortcomings and potentially harmful effects, tromethamine (tris), a non-CO_2-generating buffer, is also unable to prevent brain acidosis, even in the presence of adequate CO_2 elimination by cardiopulmonary bypass during CPR [26]. A more promising agent to maintain cerebral intracellular pH seems to be carbicarb (a combination of 0.33 M Na_2CO_3 and 0.33 M $NaHCO_3$). This recently formulated buffer does not elevate PCO_2 and led to both systemic and cerebral intecellular alkalinization when given during systemic metabolic or respiratory acidosis as confirmed by magnetic resonance spectroscopy [24].

Another concern with respect to the use of sodium bicarbonate is the danger of sodium overload and rapidly increasing serum osmolality. Both bear the risk of irreversible cerebral damage. Mattar and coworkers found bicarbonate mediated increases in osmolality in patients undergoing CPR with an average serum osmolality of 377 mOsm/L and an average serum sodium concentration of 170 mEq/L after bicarbonate administration. All of their patients died [27]. These results confirm the results obtained from many other clinical and experimental studies indicating that a plasma osmolality in excess of 350 mOsm/l is potentially fatal while blood osmolality close to normal values is optimal for recovery [28]. Although in depth investigations are not available at present, hyperosmolality might be one of the factors leading to a breakdown of the blood-brain barrier. It should be kept in mind that in addition to a sodium bicarbonate mediated increase in serum osmolality, hyperglycemia due to endogenous release and/or exogenous administration of catecholamines will always occur during CPR, thus further contributing to increased osmolality.

Sodium bicarbonate produces arterial alkalosis, causing a shift in the oxygen dissociation curve to the left. This will exacerbate oxygen transport to the cells. On the other hand, metabolic acidosis up to pH values of 7.20 is known to improve tissue oxygen oxygenation by shifting the oxygen dissociation curve to the right. However, in the presence of acidosis the dose of epinephrine has to be increased in order to exert sufficient pressor effects.

It is of practical importance to also remember that bicarbonate is going to inactivate simultaneously administered catecholamines such as epinephrine.

Experimental Drugs

Calcium and Calcium Channel Blocking Agents

During CPR and reperfusion, an intracellular calcium overload takes place, in particular impairing oxidative phosphorylation of the mitochondria. This mechanism is of key importance in the smooth-muscle cells of cerebral vessels due to the fact that vascular spasm predominantly contributes to the so-called cerebral no-reflow phenomenon. This term describes the state of postischemic hypoperfusion in the cerebral microvasculature which takes place after initial hyperperfusion. Presently, there is some experimental evidence that calcium antagonists like nimodipine can promote cerebral blood flow and neurologic recovery after global ischemia. The data on lidoflazine hydrochloride and other calcium channel blocking agents are not consistent. Before general recommendations for use of calcium antagonists during CPR can be given, further data are needed (for overview see [29].

Calcium should only be administered during CPR in the presence of documented hyperkalemia, hypocalcemia, or intoxication with calcium channel blocking agents [1].

Free Oxygen Radical Scavengers and Related Agents

The pathophysiological function of free oxygen radicals during ischemia and reperfusion is an area of ongoing intense research. Since reoxygenation after ischemia has been shown to contribute to the so-called reperfusion injury via promotion of the formation of free radicals such as superoxide and hydroxyl radicals and consecutive peroxidation of cell membrane lipids, the beneficial role of oxygen during the initial phase of CPR (= reperfusion) has been challenged. However, further studies are needed before any recommendations with respect to drugs like free radical scavengers or iron chelating agents can be given.

Barbiturates

After initial enthusiasm about the use of barbiturates in the treatment of patients with cardiac arrest, which was mainly based on single case reports and theoretical considerations, they were never included into the routine drug therapy during CPR. Although barbiturates are known to reduce cerebral metabolism, edema formation, intracranial pressure, seizure activity, and structural damage by focal or global ischemia, a large study of 262 comatose survivors of cardiac arrest showed no benefits of barbiturate therapy on postischemic cerebral function of survial [30]. The use of barbiturates during CPR can therefore not be advocated.

Drug therapy during CPR has to be directed toward restoration of the patient's pre-arrest state. Main focuses or organ preservation are brain and heart. This implies that a multioriented balanced combination of agents acting at different levels of body functions has to be instituted in order to successfully resuscitate a victim of cardiac arrest.

References

1. (1986) Standards and guidelines for cardiopulmonary resuscitation (CPR) and emergency cardiac care (ECC). JAMA 255:2905-2989
2. Snyder JW (1987) Oxygen transport: the model and the reality. In: Snyder JV, Pinsky MR (eds) Oxygen transport in the critically ill. Year Book Medical Publishers, New York, pp 3-15
3. Bryan-Brown C (1987) Oxygen transport variables and the management of the critically ill: Rationalization in pursuit of uncertainty? In: Bryan-Brown C, Ayres SM (eds) Oxygen transport and utilization. Society of Critical Care Medicine, Fullerton, pp 1-11
4. Michael JR, Guerci AD, Koehler RC, et al (1984) Mechanisms by which epinephrine augments cerebral and myocardial perfusion during cardiopulmonary resuscitation in dogs. Circulation 69:822-835
5. Schleien CL, Koehler RC, Gervais H, et al (1989) Organ blood flow and somatosensory evoked potentials during and after cardiopulmonary resuscitation with epinephrine or phenylephrine. Circulation 79:1332-1342
6. Gervais H, Schleien CL, Koehler RC, et al (1988) Effect of adrenergic drugs on cerebral blood flow, metabolism and evoked potentials after delayed onset of CPR in dogs. Anesthesiology 69:A 843
7. Ditchey RV, Lindenfeld JA (1988) Failure of epinephrine to improve the balance between myocardial oxygen supply and demand during closed-chest resuscitation in dogs. Circulation 78:382-389
8. Downey J (1976) Compression of the coronary arteries by the fibrillating canine heart. Circ Res 39:53-57

9. Livesay JJ, Follette DM, Fey KH, et al (1978) Optimizing myocardial oxygen supply/demand balance with alpha-adrenergic drugs during cardiopulmonary resuscitation. J Thorac Cardiovasc Surg 76:244-251

10. Lindner KH, Ahnefeld FW, Schürmann W, Pfenninger E, Bowdler (1988) A comparison of epinephrine and norepinephrine on myocardial oxygen delivery and consumption during cardiopulmonary resuscitation. Anesthesiology 69:A 96

11. Yakaitis RW, Otto CW, Blitt CD (1979) Relative importance of alpha and beta adrenergic receptors during resuscitation. Crit Care Med 7:293-296

12. Brillmann J, Sanders A, Otto CW (1987) Comparison of epinephrine and phenylephrine for resuscitation and neurologic outcome of cardiac arrest in dogs. Ann Emerg Med 16:11-17

13. Arai T, Watanabe T, Nagaro T, Matsuo S (1981) Blood-brain barrier impairment after cardiac resuscitation. Crit Care Med 9:444-448

14. Gonzalez ER, Ornato JP, Garnett AR (1989) Dose-dependent vasopressor response to epinephrine during CPR in human beings. Ann Emerg Med 18:920-926

15. Huttinger L, Shannon RP, Kohin S, et al (1989) Isoproterenol-induced alterations in myocardial blood flow, systolic and diastolic function in conscious dogs with heart failure. Circulation 80:658-668

16. Weil MH, Rackow EC, Trevino R, Grundler W, Falk JL, Griffel MI (1986) Differences in acid-base state between venous and arterial blood during cardiopulmonary resuscitation. N Engl J Med 315:153-156

17. Grundler W, Weil MH, Rackow EC (1986) Arteriovenous carbon dioxide and pH gradients during cardiac arrest. Circulation 74:1071-1074

18. Bishop RL, Weisfeldt ML (1976) Sodium bicarbonate administration during cardiac arrest. Effect on arterial pH, PCO_2, and osmolality. JAMA 235:506-509

19. Graf H, Leach W, Arieff AJ (1985) Evidence for a detrimental effect of bicarbonate therapy in hypoxic lactic acidosis. Science 227:754-756

20. Guerci AD, Chandra N, Johnson E, et al (1986) Failure of sodium bicarbonate to improve resuscitation from ventricular fibrillation in dogs. Circulation 74:IV75-79

21. Hennes HJ, Eberle B, Jantzen JP, Dick WF (1990) Effects of three buffer solutions on acidosis and survival in a porcine model of CPR (Abstr). Anesth Analg (in press)

22. von Planta M, Weil MH, Gazmuri RJ, Bisera J, Rackow EC (1989) Myocardial acidosis associated with CO_2 production during cardiac arrest and resuscitation. Circulation 80:684-692

23. Posner JB, Plum F (1967) Spinal-fluid pH and neurologic symptoms in systemic acidosis. N Engl J Med 277:605-613

24. Shapiro JI, Whalen M, Kucera R, Kindig N, Filley G, Chan L (1989) Brain pH responses to sodium bicarbonate and carbicarb during systemic acidosis. Am J Physiol 256:H1316-H1321

25. Berenyi KJ, Wolk M, Killip T (1975) Cerebrospinal fluid acidosis complicating therapy of experimental cardiopulmonary arrest. Circulation 52:319-324

26. Rosenberg JM, Martin GB, Paradis NA, et al (1989) The effect of CO_2 and non-CO_2-generating buffers on cerebral acidosis after cardiac arrest: a P^{131} NMR study. Ann Emerg Med 18:341-347

27. Mattar JA, Weil MH, Shubin H, Stein L (1974) Cardiac arrest in the critically ill. II. Hyperosmolal states following cardiac arrest. Am J Med 56:162-158

28. Hossmann KA (1988) Resuscitation potentials after prolonged cerebral ischemia in cats. Crit Care Med 16:964-971

29. Kirsch JR, Dean JM, Rogers MC (1986) Current concepts in brain resuscitation. Arch Int Med 146:1413-1419

30. Brain resuscitation clinical trial I study group (1986) Randomized clinical study of thiopental loading in comatose survivors of cardiac arrest. N Engl J Med 314:397-403

Cardiac Arrest and the Brain

N. S. Abramson

Introduction

Sudden cardiac arrest claims approximately 400,000 lives each year in the United States alone. It is the leading cause of death in men between 20 and 55 years of age. Despite advances in pre-hospital resuscitation, rapid transport and inhospital management, cardiopulmonary arrest is still highly lethal. Various reported series indicate that restoration of spontaneous circulation and admission to hospital occurs in 40–60% of out-of-hospital cardiac arrests. Of those patients who have been resuscitated and admitted to the hospital, approximately 60% die, most within two weeks. In 10–40% of long-term survivors, varying degrees of permanent brain damage occurs [1–4]. The economic cost of brain-damaged survivors is estimated to be billions of dollars.

Although the brain as a functioning organ is exquisitely sensitive to ischemia, individual cerebral neurons may tolerate normothermic ischemia of up to 30–60 minutes duration [5, 6]. Clinically, the rapid loss of consciousness which occurs with cardiac arrest (ϱ 15 sec) and the failure of brain stem function, (i.e. apnea and fixed pupils by 60 seconds) parallels the rapid depletion of brain oxygen by ϱ 15 seconds and glucose and ATP stores by 4–5 minutes. After normothermic cardiac arrest (no flow) $\geq$ 5 min, secondary post-reperfusion derangements occur, i.e. the post-resuscitation syndrome (PRS) or postischemic-anoxic encephalopathy (PIE) [7–10]. We hypothesize the two principle components of this to be:

1. cerebral "no reflow"[9, 11] followed by transient global hyperemia and then by protracted (multifocal and global) hypoperfusion; and
2. reoxygenation injury initiated by chemical cascades leading to cell necrosis [12, 13].

Current approaches to brain resuscitation, i.e. attempts to mitigate the devastating effects of ischemia on the brain, focus on methods to improve reperfusion, decrease metabolism and block the generation of cytotoxic substances during cardiac arrest and early after resuscitation. Therapeutic efforts started before the insult may be termed, "brain protection", those started during the cardiac arrest, "brain preservation" and those started with or shortly after reperfusion "brain resuscitation". Since brain protection is rarely possible in the treatment of cardiac arrest, we will focus on brain preservation and resuscitation.

Brain Preservation

As Crile pointed out in 1906 "success in resuscitation is inversely proportional to the lapse of time after the onset of arrest" [14]. Toward this end, widely publicized efforts have been implemented to develop rapid response pre-hospital emergency medical systems and to educate the public about coronary artery disease and bystander CPR. Data from our brain resuscitation clinical trials confirm the work of others showing that the arrest time (time from cardiac arrest until resuscitative measures are started) and CPR time (duration of artificial circulation prior to restoration of spontaneous circulation) are the most important factors determining survival and neurologic recovery. Additionally, our data demonstrate the interaction between these two components of the brain ischemic insult. Figure 1 shows moving averages of percentage of patients with good neurologic recovery (capable of independent life) as function of brain insult times. CPR effectiveness was found to be time limited and related to prior arrest time in a dichotomous fashion. If prior arrest time was ≤ 6 minutes, CPR appeared to be initially more effective and this effectiveness was more lasting. However, even if CPR time exceeded 30 minutes, good recovery still occurred occasionally, especially if the preceeding arrest time was short. These clinical findings are consistent with the results of animal experiments which measured cerebral blood flow during CPR. Thus, standard CPR provides a window of opportunity for the restoration of spontaneous circulation or for implementation of more effective means of artifical circulation.

In addition to developing ways to minimize the duration of brain ischemia, current efforts are also focused on developing more effective techniques of artificial circulation. Although some experimental CPR techniques have demonstrated increased pressures, flows or improved physiologic or metabolic parameters in laboratory experiments, no clinical studies have demonstrated improved outcome in either animals or man. Thus, new techniques of CPR have not yet been accepted in clinical practice.

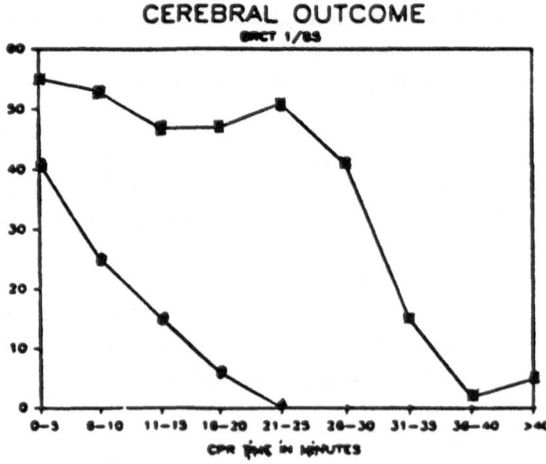

Fig. 1. The effect of the duration of CPR on the percentage of survivors achieving a cerebral performance category (CPC) level of 1 or 2. Data are presented as moving averages and grouped according to ATs above (●) or below (■) 6 min. (From [1], with permission)

Epinephrine

Another method to improve the effectiveness of CPR currently being investigated is modification of the usual vasopressor drug protocols. Epinephrine, still the key drug for cardiac resuscitation [14], increases arterial pressures during cardiac massage [15]. Its α-receptor agonist (vasoconstrictor) effect increases coronary perfusion, thereby increasing the chance for successful defibrillation and restoration of spontaneous circulation [16, 17]. Its effect on defibrillation threshold is not clear, but increased perfusion pressures make ventricular fibrillation (VF) more vigorous and thus probably more reversible [15, 16]. Whether epinephrine reduces subendocardial blood flow during CPR is not clear [17, 18]. During external CPR without epinephrine, cerebral blood flow (CBF) is unpredictable [19], often below 20% normal (the hypothesized viability threshold) [20]. The longer the period of no flow (cardiac arrest) preceeding CPR, the less likely external CPR without epinephrine is capable of producing viable levels of CBF. Epinephrine improves CBF probably because of its systemic vasoconstrictive effect; and coronary blood flow probably because of its combined α- and β-agonist effects. Its combined α-plus β effects transiently increase pressure and flow after restoration of heart beat which may improve cerebral reperfusion [5].

American CPR standards currently recommend epinephrine doses equivalent to 0.01–0.02 mg/kg. These have resulted in low reperfusion pressures and many CPR failures. Recently, Brown et al. in a swine model of cardiac arrest found that external CPR with epinephrine 0.2 mg/kg produced better regional CBF [21] and myocardial blood flow [22] compared with epinephrine 0.02 mg/kg, phenylephrine 0.1 mg/kg, and methoxamine 10 mg/kg. Comparable flows were generated by phenylephrine 10 mg/kg. Mean arterial pressure produced during and after restoration of heart beat by a given epinephrine dose differs between animals with normal hearts and people with sick hearts. However, CBF and metabolism during CPR seem to be influenced by perfusion pressure, irrespective of the use of epinephrine or phenylephrine.

The risks of using increased epinephrine dosage include increased cardiac arrhythmias, increased post-ischemic ventricular dysfunction, catecholamine-induced contraction band necrosis and post-ischemic hypertension, although this appears to be beneficial for the diseased myocardium as well as for the brain [23]. Recent evidence suggests that epinephrine favorably affects oxygen supply: demand ratios in the heart and doses not compromise subendocardial: subepicardial flow ratios. Overall, the preponderance of current evidence suggests a beneficial effect of higher dose epinephrine administration on the heart, in terms of CPR generated coronary perfusion, rate of successful defibrillation and preferential vasoconstriction favoring vital organ perfusion.

There is continuing controversy concerning the direct effects of epinephrine on the brain. If epinephrine crosses the blood brain barrier during cardiac arrest, its β-adrenergic effects might increase oxygen demand, by direct stimulatory effect on neurons, in excess of the increase in cerebral blood flow. Recent evidence suggests that this does not occur. Relevant clinical trials have been few and anecdotal. Controlled clinical studies are needed.

Hypothermia: Another Technique of Brain Preservation

Cerebral protection by pre-cooling has been suggested before [24]. Hossman showed that mild pre-cooling improves recovery of EEG and evoked potentials in cats [6]. Mild pre-cooling reduces lactate production during ischemia [24] and improves brain ischemic histologic damage.

Moderate hypothermia (28–32°C) induced before circulatory arrest for heart surgery protects the brain [25]. Deep hypothermia (<25°C) provides greater protection, but causes circulatory arrest and therefore can be used only with cardiopulmonary bypass. With hypothermia of 30°C, recovery of normal brain function has been achieved in man after complete global brain ischemia or cardiac arrest of 15–30 minutes. However maintaining moderate hypothermia over days poses significant management problems and complications.

Cooling of the homeothermic organism without anesthesia elicits a sympathetic discharge (hypertension, tachycardia, shivering, vasospasm, transiently increased O_2 consumption). This response can be suppressed by anesthesia and paralysis; it is absent in postischemic coma. Without shivering, cooling causes a 7–10% reduction in cerebral O_2 and glucose consumption per °C decrease of temperature [26]; slower depletion of brain ATP during ischemia [27]; reduced metabolic needs for functional and structural integrity; and increased blood viscosity, because of increased plasma viscosity, hematocrit [23], fibrinogen, and red cell aggregation.

Moderate hypothermia seems to be beneficial in focal ischemia and brain contusion even if induced after the insult [26]. Its use after cardiac arrest has been documented only by clinical anecdotes; and by uncontrolled studies in dogs, with inconclusive results. We recently obtained the first outcome data with mild hypothermia (T 34–36°) induced *before* [33] or *after* prolonged VF cardiac arrest in dogs. Mild hypothermia induced *before* cardiac arrest had a protective effect. Previous CPR studies showed similar protective effects. Mild hypothermia induced *after* the onset of cardiac arrest of 12.5 minutes (preservation and resuscitation), with clinically feasible head cooling during VF and total-body cooling by CPB continued to 1 hour postarrest, as well as hypertension and hemodilution, resulted in good (although not all dogs were entirely normal) in ten dogs compared with 9 of 10 normothermic, normotensive dogs who had poor recovery. Histopathologic scores were also better in the hypothermic group and CBF was improved.

The potential beneficial effects of post-arrest hypothermia at the molecular and cellular level, might be offset by its deleterious effect on the microcirculation. However, hematologic effects, such as elevation of hematocrit secondary to plasma loss and increased viscosity, only become significant at temperatures <27°C. Significant cardiac dysfunction is not expected from mild hypothermia, but hypothermia is known to decrease insulin secretion and may exacerbate hyperglycemia. Hypothermia is currently used in the treatment of a variety of clinical problems, e.g. cardiac surgery, adult respiratory distress syndrome. Extension of this therapeutic modality, in well controlled trials, to the treatment of post-ischemic encephalopathy now seems reasonable.

Brain Resuscitation

Post-ischemic Reperfusion

After normotensive reperfusion following cardiac arrest, diffuse hyperemia of all brain regions, including the cortex brainstem and basal ganglia is found for the first 30 minutes (Peter Safar – personal communication, 1989). Following this, diffuse hypoperfusion of varying levels develops. While this might reflect matching of blood flow to low post-ischemic oxygen demands, this hypoperfusion is suspected to hamper post-ischemic neuronal recovery. However, controversy exists about the details of post-arrest flow patterns and factors influencing them [11] Changes in cerebral blood flow should be interpreted with caution as they may not correlated with foci of injury. Furthermore, the degree of post-ischemic hypoperfusion does not necessarily correlate with outcome.

Following restoration of spontaneous circulation, the multifocal no reflow demonstrated by Ames [11] can be mitigated by moderately high reperfusion pressures [28]. In Hossman's cat model, recovery of post-ischemic evoked potentials and EEG activity correlated with higher reperfusion pressures (MAP > 140 mmHg vs. 90–140 mmHg) [6].

In our recent studies, using a reproducible dog model of VF cardiac arrest of 12.5 min, epinephrine/norepinephrine generated hypertensive reperfusion (MAP 140–110 mmHg over 4 hours), improved neurologic recovery. In studies of multifocal (local) CBF measurements, using stable xenon-enhanced CT scanning [29], we found many low flow (CBF < 20 ml/100 g per min) and trickle flow (< 10 ml) regions with normotensive reperfusion. Hypertension post-arrest (MAP > 140–110 mmHg) normalized lCBF, but low flow recurred when MAP returned to 100 mmHg. In our Brain Resuscitation Clinical Trial II, MAP < 70 mmHg early after restoration of spontaneous circulation correlated with worse cerebral outcome. As discussed before, epinephrine administration in doses modified from those now recommended may improve CPR generated perfusion as well as minimize post-ischemic hypoperfusion, resulting in improved neurologic outcome.

Neuron-Benefitting Pharmacologic Agents

Once post-ischemic hypoperfusion has been overcome, neuron benefitting pharmacologic agents may be successfully delivered to the microcirculation resulting in salvage of still viable cells. Based on our current understanding of the complex pathophysiology of post-ischemic brain damage, many such therapies have been investigated. Early studies suggested benefit of barbiturate loading [30]. However, thiopental loading in patients (BRCT I) did not show a statistically significant improvement in neurologic recovery [2].

Promising results were found in animal studies of calcium entry blockers [31, 32]. However, a clinical trial of lidoflazine administration after cardiac arrest (BRCT II) also did not demonstrate improvement in neurologic recovery. Results of additional European clinical studies on calcium entry blocker administration after cardiac arrest are expected in the near future. Anti-reoxygenation injury "cocktails" have not yet been shown to improve outcome; nor has an excitatory neurotransmitter receptor blocker. We attribute all these negative results to the multifactorial nature of the post-resuscitation syndrome for which multifaceted combination therapies may be needed [7]. Although there is an evergrowing list of potentially promising therapeutic interventions to prevent post-ischemic brain damage, no specific brain resuscitative interventions have yet been proven beneficial (Table 1).

Emergency Cardiopulmonary Bypass

After no flow of >5 min, standard CPR does not reliably produce cerebral and coronary perfusion sufficient to maintain cell viability. Nor does it provide prolonged control over blood pressure, flow, composition, or temperature. Emergency closed-chest cardiopulmonary bypass (CPB) has been suggested as a resuscitative intervention for selected cases [33]. In six separate studies, 179 dogs that received CPB after prolonged cardiac arrest (no-flow) or CPR (low-flow) had restoration of stable spontaneous circulation [33]. The use of CPB, compared with standard CPR, enhanced survival and neurologic recovery. With CPB and standard intensive care, normothermic cardiac arrest of up to 15 minutes could be reversed to survival without brain damage. VF of up to 20 minutes reversed with brain damaged survival; and VF of up to 30 minutes reversed only transiently [33]. The findings of others, in general, agree with these results [34, 35].

The use of CPB alone may be beneficial by restoring adequate perfusion, while unloading the heart, which might support recovery of the myocardium. CPB may also allow the use of other brain damage ameliorating therapies that would otherwise be too dangerous in this situation, e.g., hypothermia or drugs with cardiovascular depressant side effects (e.g. calcium entry blockers). The risks of CPB include arterial injury or embolization which could cause claudica-

Table 1. Potential brain resuscitation therapies

Pharmacologic	Procedures
Steroids	Hemodilution
Indomethacin	Hypertension
Heparin	Cardiopulmonary Bypass
Lidocaine	Dialysis
Phenytoin	Plasmapheresis
Diazepam	
Etomidate	
Prostacyclin	
Naloxone	
ATP-MgCl$_2$	

tion or loss of limb; pseudoaneurysm formation; venous injury which could cause deep venous thrombosis with the risk of pulmonary embolism; and infection. The CPB circuit itself carries the risk of air embolism, which could cause a stroke. The necessary anticoagulation could cause bleeding. Platelet, electrolyte abnormalities, and hemolysis may occur as a result of blood trauma by the circuit. Potential uses of CPB include cases of VF, asphyxia, trauma, pulmonary emboli, temperature emergencies, drug overdoses, and electrolyte abnormalities. Feasibility trials are now needed to work out the logistical problems of emergency implementation of this intervention and other possibilities for emergency CPB should be investigated.

Outcome Prediction

Survival after cardiac arrest has been widely investigated [36-39]. Considerably less information is available on post-ischemic neurologic function and even less on predictive factors which accurately predict neurologic outcome. In one series of patients remaining in deep coma for at least 6 hours after resuscitation, 22% ultimately regained consciousness, but only 12% achieved a reasonable degree of independence [3]. In our first Brain Resuscitation Clinical Trial (BRCT I), a study of cardiac arrest survivors who remained comatose at least until randomized (i.e. within two hours of resuscitation), 43% regained consciousness and 34% achieved independent existence [2]. The difference in outcome between these two series reflects the importance of carefully defining the study population. Individuals who are either arousable or fully alert within 12 hours of resuscitation usually do well neurologically [40]. Patients who are still decorticate, decerebrate, or flaccid and unresponsive to stimulation 24 hours after arrest have a 7% chance of awakening. No patients with these findings on the third or fourth day after cardiac arrest survived [40]. In BRCT I, we found that patients with absent motor response to pain after three days of coma never awakened. Absent pupillary or corneal reflexes for more than 3 days after arrest is also virtually incompatible with survival or neurologic recovery [3, 4].

Conclusion

In the United States alone, one treatable case of sudden death occurs every five minutes. It is estimated that 30,000-50,000 lives could be saved annually with improved cardiac resuscitation and brain resuscitation techniques. Today there is over 50% chance of not surviving to leave the hospital even if CPR is started within four minutes of collapse, and over 80% chance of not surviving to hospital discharge if standard CPR is started later than four minutes. With the use of current standard CPR and post-resuscitation techniques, 20-40% of survivors have permanent brain damage [36]. In light of this poor prognosis, new more effective therapies must be developed.

References

1. Abramson NS, Safar P, Detre KM, et al (1985) Neurologic recovery after cardiac arrest: effect of duration of ischemia. Crit Care Med 13:930-931
2. Abramson NS, Safar P, Detre K, et al (1986) Brain resuscitation clinical trial (BRCT) I study group: Randomized clinical study of *thiopental loading* in comatose cardiac arrest survivors. N Engl J Med 314:397-403
3. Levey DE, Bates D, Caronna JJ, Singer BH, et al (1985) Predicting outcome from hypoxic-ischemic coma. J Am Med Assoc 253:1420-1424
4. Longstreth WT, Diehr P, Inui TS (1983) Prediction of awakening after out-of-hospital cardiac arrest. N Engl J Med 308:1378-1381
5. Hossman KA (1982) Review: Treatment of experimental cerebral ischemia. J Cereb Blood Flow Metab 2:275-279
6. Hossman KA (1988) Resuscitation potentials after prolonged global ischemia in cats. Crit Care Med 16:964-971
7. Safar P (1988) Resuscitation from clinical death: Pathophysiologic limits and therapeutic potentials. Crit Care Med 16:923-941
8. Safar P (1986) Cerebral resuscitation after cardiac arrest. A review. Circulation 74 (suppl IV):138-153
9. Negovsky VA, Gurvitch AM, Zolotokrylina ES (1983) Postresuscitation disease. Elsevier, Amsterdam
10. Siesjo BK (1988) Mechanisms of ischemic brain damage. Crit Care Med 16:954-963
11. Ames A, Wright RL, Kowada M, et al (1968) The no-reflow phenomenon. Am J Pathol 52:437-453
12. Ernster L (1988) Biochemistry of reoxygenation injury. Crit Care Med 16:947-953
13. McCord JM (1985) Oxygen-derived free radicals in postischemic tissue injury. N Engl J Med 312:159-163
14. Crile GW, Colley DH (1906) An experimental research into the resuscitation of dogs killed by anesthetics and asphyxia. J Exp Med 8:713-717
15. Wiggers CJ (1940) The physiological bases for cardiac resuscitation from ventricular fibrillation. Method for serial defibrillation. Am Heart J 20:413-416
16. Otto CW, Yakaitis RW, Ewy GA (1985) Effect of epinephrine on defibrillation in ischemic ventricular fibrillation. J Emerg Med 3:285-291
17. Livesay JJ, Follette DM, Fey KH, et al (1978) Optimizing myocardial supply/demand balance with adrenergic drugs cardiopulmonary resuscitation. J Thorac Cardiovasc Surg 76:244-251
18. Ditchey RV, Lindenfeld J (1988) Failure of epinephrine to improve the balance between myocardial oxygen supply and demand during closed-chest resuscitation in dogs. Circulation 78:382-389
19. Michael JR, Guerci AD, Koehler RC, et al (1984) Mechanisms by which epinephrine augments cerebral and myocardial perfusion during cardiopulmonary resuscitation in dogs. Circulation 69:822-835
20. Symon L (1985) Flow thresholds in brain ischemia and the effects of drugs. Br J Anaesth 57:34-37
21. Brown CG, Werman HA, Davis EA, et al (1986) Comparative effect of graded doses of epinephrine on regional brain blood flow during CPR in a swine model. Ann Emerg Med 15:1138-1144
22. Brown CG, Werman HA, Davis EA, et al (1987) The effects of graded doses of epinephrine on regional myocardial blood flow during cardiopulmonary resuscitation in swine. Circulation 27:491-497
23. Buffington CW (1985) Hemodynamic determinants of ischemic myocardial dysfunction in the presence of coronary stenosis in dogs. Anesthesiology 53:651-662
24. Berntman L, Welsh FA, Harp JR (1981) Cerebral protective effect of low-grade hypothermia. Anesthesiology 55:495-499
25. Vandam LD, Burnap TK (1959) Hypothermia. N Engl J Med 261:546-553, 595-603
26. Rosomoff HL (1959) Protective effects of hypothermia against pathological processes of the nervous system. Ann NY Acad Sci 80:475-479

27. Michenfelder JD, Van Dyke RA, Theye RA (1970) The effects of anesthetic agents and techniques on canine cerebral ATP and lactate levels. Anesthesiology 33:315-318
28. Fischer EG, Ames A (1972) Studies on mechanisms of impairment of cerebral circulation following ischemia: effect of hemodilution and perfusion pressure. Stroke 3:538-542
29. Gur D, Good WF, Wolfson SK Jr, et al (1982) In vivo mapping of local cerebral blood flow by xenon-enhanced computed tomography. Science 215:1267-1268
30. Bleyaert AL, Nemoto EM, Safar P, et al (1978) Thiopental amelioration of brain damage after global ischemia in monkeys. Anesthesiology 49:390-398
31. Vaagenes P, Cantadore R, Safar P, et al (1984) Amelioration of brain damage by lidoflazine after prolonged ventricular fibrillation cardiac arrest in dogs. Crit Care Med 12:846-855
32. Steen PA, Gisvold SE, Milde JH, et al (1985) Nimodipine improves outcome when given after complete cerebral ischemia in primates. Anesthesiology 62:406-414
33. Safar P, Abramson NS, Cantadore R, Tisherman S, et al (1988) Emergency cardiopulmonary bypass for prolonged cardiac arrest (CA) in dogs. Am J Emerg Med (in press)
34. Mattox KL, Beall AC (1976) Resuscitation of the moribund patient using portable cardiopulmonary bypass. Ann Thorac Surg 22:436-442
35. Phillips SJ, Ballentine B, Slonine D, et al (1983) Percutaneous initiation of cardiopulmonary bypass. Ann Thorac Surg 36:223-255
36. Detre KM (1988) Epidemiologic evaluation of reports on survival after CPR. ACTA Anes Belg (Suppl 2) 39:109-113
37. Bergner L, Bergner M, Hallstrom AP, et al (1983) Service factors and health status of survivors of out-of-hospital cardiac arrests. Am J Emerg Med 3:259-263
38. Hallstrom AP, Cobb LA, Swain M, Mensinger K (1985) Predictors of hospital mortality after out-of-hospital cardiopulmonary resuscitation. Crit Care Med 13:927-929
39. Weaver WD, Cobb LA, Hallstrom AP, et al (1986) Considerations for improving survival from out-of-hospital cardiac arrest. Ann Emerg Med 15:1181-1186
40. Snyder BD, Tabbaa MA (1987) Assessment and treatment of neurological dysfunction after cardiac arrest. Stroke 22:1-6

Cerebral Resuscitation in Children

J. M. Dean

Introduction

Management of children and infants with severe intracranial pathology is often a discouraging prospect, and clinicians naturally are eager to discover the breakthrough as they search for ways to ameliorate the outcome of these unfortunate patients. Over the past decade and a half, the subject of cerebral resuscitation has sprung from these roots, and numerous therapies, both heroic and ordinary, have been proposed to help preserve neuronal function following various illnesses or injuries. At the outset of this discussion, brain resuscitation can be divided into two categories: non-controversial and controversial. Most of this discussion will concern the latter, but a few words are in order about the non-controversies in this area.

While one may have a spirited argument about the benefits of barbiturate coma or even intracranial pressure (ICP) monitoring, no one today seriously questions the need for an airway and adequate ventilation in brain injured patients. Ten years ago, elective intubation of head trauma patients was not universal and could even engender disagreement. Today, airway control and ventilation are standard foundations of neurointensive care. Today no one will seriously question the need for an adequate blood pressure, normal temperature, absence of seizures, and expeditious surgical intervention when indicated. The *state of the art* for brain resuscitation in children centers around good basic measures of intensive care [1]; little substantive progress has really been made with the more esoteric subjects often incorporated into the term "cerebral resuscitation" [2, 3]. Throughout this discussion, keep in mind that certain facets of neurointensive care are assumed to already be present. The child's airway must be patent and protected; gas exchange must occur, and blood flow must carry oxygen to the surviving brain. If these goals cannot be reached, then further aspects of cerebral resuscitation should not be entertained.

The most common scenario in which this issue arises concerns placing an ICP monitor into a brain injured patient with ventricular arrhythmias and hypotension. The need for an ICP monitor in such a patient is dubious unless hemodynamic stability can be achieved and the arrhythmias controlled. Only in the context of good basic intensive care should there be a discussion about cerebral resuscitation.

Types of Cerebral Injury

Cerebral resuscitation is a topic which engenders enthusiasm or disdain, has issues of clear agreement but remains controversial, and is confused by problems in terminology. For purposes of this discussion, cerebral injuries are considered to be of three types. *Global ischemic injury* is ischemia which affects the entire brain in a relatively uniform initial manner. While subsequent secondary injury may be focal in nature, the initial insult is global. Examples would include drowning, asphyxia, hanging, cardiac arrest, and perhaps even the low flow state which occurs during cardiopulmonary resuscitation. *Focal ischemic injury* is ischemia which involves a specific vascular bed or perhaps several specific vascular beds. Subsequent secondary injury may be more global in scope and may extend beyond the vascular supply area of the original insult, but the initial insult is focal. Both global and focal ischemia may be further divided into complete and incomplete. Complete ischemia (e.g. ventricular fibrillation) means there is total cessation of blood flow; during incomplete ischemia (e.g. cardiopulmonary resuscitation) an inadequate amount of blood flow is present. The third type of cerebral injury is *direct traumatic injury*, such as might be seen with a bullet wound, a knife slice, etc. In this type of injury, certain neurons are transected, crushed, or otherwise killed by a direct external force.

Injury may then be generally broken into *primary* and *secondary* phases. Primary injury refers to the initial insult, such as the direct death of neurons from 8 minutes of anoxia or ischemia, or the death of a neuron from being burned by a bullet. Subsequently, edema and further ischemic injury occur, which may extend the injury to otherwise viable parts of the brain. Reperfusion with oxygenated blood may cause sudden release of reactive free radicals, which may in turn cause lipid peroxidation and membrane dysfunction. This process probably also includes excitatory neurotransmitter mechanisms, alterations in the eicosanoids, etc. The summation of these processes which follow the initial injury is termed secondary injury. With advances in our understanding of cell death and reperfusion injury, we may need to redefine the boundaries between primary and secondary injury. Brain resuscitation is oriented solely to secondary injury, as primary injury is pragmatically definable as the injury that occurs before a physician has a chance to intervene.

Experimental Models

The literature about cerebral resuscitation is vast, and it is important to understand the different types of models that are employed in laboratory investigations. It is helpful to consider each of the three types of brain injury separately.

Models of global ischemia include aortic occlusion, cardiac arrest, and increasing ICP enough to eliminate or reduce cerebral blood flow. Aortic occlusion involves a thoracotomy and isolating the root of the aorta beyond the coronary arteries, and simply clamping the vessel. The heart continues to be perfused, though with increasingly cyanotic blood, and after a period of time, the occlusion is relieved and the brain is reperfused. The entire body is also ischemic in this type of preparation, and whatever factors and magic humours are produced by gut ischemia and so forth will hamper the purity of this type of experiment. The major advantage of the method is that you can control the ischemic period well, and usually you can restore perfusion easily. A more clinically appealing method of ischemia is ventricular fibrillation, but this turns out to be difficult to precisely control. Resuscitation may take one to ten minutes, and you have to exclude animals based on previously agreed criteria. The whole body is ischemic in this situation, just as after aortic cross clamping, so that the only advantage of this technique over aortic occlusion is the lack of thoracotomy and the "clinical relevance". Increasing the ICP with an epidural ballon or by infusion mock CSF into the ventricles until cerebral perfusion is eliminated can result in "pure cerebral ischemia", and the body can go on without much distress. A variant of this is the famous neck tourniquet, except that the ICP method results in bloodless ischemia. This may make the results totally irrelevant if, for instance, factors produced in the blood are important in reperfusion or ischemic injury.

Models of focal ischemia include permanent and transient occlusion of the middle cerebral artery (MCA), usually via a transorbital approach, carotic occlusion in gerbils, and combinations of vessel occlusions with hypotension. It is important to distinguish permanent MCA clipping from transient, and the relevance of either model to human stroke is difficult to establish. Permanent occlusion may be more close to the human scenario, but if a patient has developed ischemia over a period of years, collateral flow may exist which will not be present in the acute animal model. Transient MCA clipping may help us understand TIAs but once again, humans have an underlying disease process that is not modelled in the animal systems. Gerbil models rely on incomplete circles of Willis, but unfortunately gerbils vary among themselves. Thus, confirmation of ischemia is needed when this model is employed. The use of rodents may itself be difficult to interpret in light of human events, since it takes a connaisseur to detect subtle neurological changes in these animals.

Finally, direct trauma is modeled by thermal injuries, impact injuries, etc. These are most often employed to cause various degrees of edema; the clinical relevance of thermal injury is difficult and the public emotional aspects of impact head injuries are making these experiments less common.

It is important to understand the precise model that is being employed when reading a paper about some magical drug that "cures ischemia". As an example, a study several years ago demonstrated that a calcium channel blocker ameliorated post ischemic hypoperfusion when compared with controls [4]. However, this model involved cardiac bypass. The ischemia was caused by turning off the bypass machine, and reperfusion occurred when the machine was turned on again. The investigators were able to set the reperfusion pressure at whatever level they wished, and it remained there, absolutely stable and completely adequate. Unfortunately, blood pressure stability is not a constant feature of animal models involving ventricular fibrillation for ten minutes, or aortic occlusion for 12 minutes, and brain injured human children are often hypotensive and unstable. A conclusion that this calcium channel blocker should be employed in patients would be unjustified – the results were obtained in a specific animal model under specific conditions.

Regulation of cerebral blood flow may differ both between ages and between species. While there are some papers on asphyxia in immature dogs [5, 6] and swine [7–9], most papers concerning ischemic or traumatic injury are based on mature animal studies. Extrapolation of the results to human infants and children is hazardous.

Intracranial Hemodynamics

The intracranial vault is a closed space, and its contents determine the pressure relationships within the head. The normal contents of the intracranial vault are brain, CSF, and blood. Brain consists of cells and interstitium, and the total volume of brain can be manipulated to an extent by osmotic means. Blood volume is proportional to cerebral blood flow, and is controlled by perfusion pressure and vascular resistance. Cerebral blood flow is exquisitely sensitive to changes in carbon dioxide and oxygen tension, as well as changes in perfusion pressure beyond the autoregulatory range [10]. CSF normally represents about 10% of the intracranial volume, and is produced in adults at a rate of about 0.35 ml/min, or about 20 ml/hour. There is pressure dependent resorption at the subarachnoid villi.

Abnormal conditions affect these contents. Perhaps most obvious is the presence of a brain tumor – this is a new content for the intracranial vault. But the normal constituents of the cranium are potentially changed as well. The brain may become edematous, and cerebral volume therefore increases. CSF production may remain constant as blood clots and obstructs the subarachnoid villous reabsorption, resulting in hydrocephalus. Hypoventilation may occur and cerebral blood flow and volume increase. Each of these events will increase ICP, potentially affecting cerebral perfusion pressure.

Cerebral perfusion pressure is usually calculated as

$$CPP = MAP-ICP,$$

where MAP refers to mean arterial pressure. But this simple equation hides several concepts and at least one controversy. The inflow pressure to the head is the carotid artery pressure, and the outflow pressure is the jugular venous pressure, not the ICP. There is a vascular waterfall, or a Starling resistor, and therefore the greater downstream pressure, either jugular or intracranial, becomes the effective downstream pressure. Thus, one should more correctly state that CPP = MAP – [Maximum of ICP, JVP]. Indeed, this relationship has been experimentally demonstrated [11]. The MAP is usually measured somewhere other than the carotid artery, so the next assumption is that blood pressure is constant in different arterial beds. This brings us to the controversy about where to reference transducers when one is monitoring ICP and MAP. In order to validly subtract these two values and calculate CPP, the transducers must be referenced to the same level. The traditional approach of referencing the MAP at the right atrium and the ICP at the external auditory meatus introduces fundamental errors into calculations of perfusion pressure. As an example, raising the head of the bed will reduce ICP when referenced at the head, while the arterial pressure will not change. This will improve the cerebral perfusion pressure that is calculated. However, raising the head of the bed also reduced carotid arterial pressure, often by the same amount that the ICP appeared to drop. The author does not have the ultimate answer about whether to level the ICP monitor at the head or the heart, but if cerebral perfusion pressure calculations are anticipated, the arterial and ICP transducers must be leveled at the same level.

The possibility that jugular pressure may exceed ICP should also be borne in mind. When a patient returns from the operating room where he has been on cardiac bypass with a mean perfusion pressure of 50 mm Hg, and the thoracic resident has inadvertently been leaning on the right atrium with his retractor, raising CVP to 30, then the cerebral perfusion pressure may have been reduced to 20 mm Hg. It ought be no surprise when such a patient develops cerebral herniation while on a nitroprusside drip that evening.

Intracranial Pressure Monitors

ICP monitoring has been practiced off and on for two decades. There are at least four major types of monitoring devices. Intraventricular drains have the advantage of permitting CSF drainage, but the disadvantage of traversing much brain matter and potentially introducing organisms into the ventricle. Epidural monitors can be implanted in the epidural space, but suffer disadvantages of drifting zero baseline and difficulty with calibration. Subarachnoid bolts have been used because they are relatively non-invasive, but suffer from inadequate signal fidelity and frequent dysfunction. In order to perform well, it is important to actually resect a portion of dura to insure a continuous fluid column in the monitoring system – this is rarely done, but instead multiple needle punctures are made in the dura. Finally, transducer tipped catheters have been used over the last several years. These catheters transmit exquisite signals with excellent fidelity. The devices also suffer from the problem of drifting zero baseline, but this problem is insignificant over a few days.

It remains controversial whether ICP ought to be monitored at all, particularly with asphyxial injuries such as near drowning [12–14]. However, this author believes that knowledge of the ICP is often valuable and need not force irresponsible medical decisions. With the exception of asphyxia, our institution monitors ICP in cerebral injuries if the children have Glasgow coma scores less than 8.

Intracranial Hypertension Therapy

Intracranial hypertension is treated by addressing each of the contents on the intracranial vault with a specific reduction therapy. The contents consist of brain matter itself, blood, CSF, and other miscellaneous contents such as tumors, hematomas, etc. The brain substance can be reduced in bulk by the scalpel [15], ore more commonly with osmotherapy such as mannitol. Cerebral blood volume can be reduced by decreasing cerebral blood flow, using hyperventilation therapy. Maintenance of oxygen delivery also helps reduce cerebral vasodilation, and in this context a normal hematocrit is useful. CSF can be drained if a ventricular catheter is in place, and production can be reduced with diazoxide. Finally, miscellaneous intracranial contens such as tumors can be resected.

The use of barbiturates to reduce ICP still causes a brawl in many educated circles, and there remains little proof that this type of management is efficacious. However, these drugs are quite efficacious in reducing ICP, and the controversy revolves around whether ICP reduction itself is helpful. That question remains as valid today as ten years ago, and ICP monitoring and therapy have yet to be proven effective in improving the outcome of patients who have suffered brain injuries. There are essentially no data available in pure pediatric populations, but a recent study of human adult head injury victims suggests that barbiturate therapy may indeed provide benefit in selected instances [16]. This use of barbiturates (reduction of ICP) is to be distinguished from barbiturate coma therapy, described in the next section.

Barbiturate Coma Therapy

Barbiturates might be considered as a prototype of brain resuscitation research, perhaps contributing to the controversy evoked by the term. While barbiturate coma has little place in current management of patients, the history of these agents is interesting and instructive.

The earliest demonstration of amerlioration of neuronal injury occurred in the 1960s, when anesthetics were noted to increase the survival time of mice subjected to hypoxia. Subsequent studies have demonstrated clearly that barbiturate anesthetics are associated with less severe brain injuries when compared with inhalational anesthetics. While these results were originally interpreted to mean that barbiturates ameliorate injury, a more current interpretation is that inhalational anesthetics are harmful to the injured brain because of cerebral vasodilation.

In focal ischemia, there have been numerous studies that demonstrate slight to major amelioration of ischemic damage when animals or patients are treated with barbiturates. The more important clinical application has been to employ barbiturates before elective cerebral ischemia, such as during carotid endarterectomy. However, more aggressive use of barbiturates or barbiturate coma in stroke patients has not been widely adopted, because the laboratory evidence is not strong and the risks are great.

In global ischemia, barbiturates have been employed in numerous models. The most famous results came from studies performed by the Pittsburgh group in primates, using a neck tourniquet model of ischemia. In these studies, high dose thiopental reduced injury in baboons subjected to 17 minutes of ischemia [17]. Subsequent results by other investigators and by the same group have failed to confirm the early interpretation that thiopental in fact ameliorated injury [18]. These experiments are difficult to perform, the investigators became more proficient with the preparations, etc. Subsequent trials conducted in humans have confirmed the absence of a major clinical effect of barbiturate coma on outcome after global ischemia [19].

The global ischemia experiments are instructive for our review because they demonstrate the initial points of this discussion: cerebral resuscitation rests on good neurointensive care. The original protocol included aggressive mainte-nance of many physiological parameters, and animals which could not be kept on the protocol were not included in the original results. When errors of proto-col occured, the outcomes were dismal [20]. The human situation is, of course, more likely to be similar to the latter group, since human patients are generally unstable and difficult to maintain after serious intracranial injuries.

Calcium Channel Blockers

Calcium channel blockers were employed in numerous studies during the past 8 years, based on considerably more theoretical knowledge than were the pre-viously described barbiturate experiments. Data from various sources demon-strated a crucial role of calcium in mitigating cell death, and it became an ob-vious interest to somehow block calcium from playing such a role.

When most of these studies were conducted, calcium channels were consid-ered to be receptor operated, potential sensitive, or intracellular. Receptor oper-ated channels (ROC) are typified by those excited by serotonin. The role of se-rotonin and calcium channels in cerebral vasospasm following subarachnoid he-morrhage was worked out in the laboratory by George Allen, leading to clinical use of calcium channel blockers in patients following subarachnoid hemorrhage. Potential sensitive channels and intracellular calcium fluxes have not been speci-fically nailed down in the etiology of cell death, but the notion that mito-chondrial accumulation of calcium and cristal breakage might be blocked with different drugs has motivated many studies.

There are numerous classes of calcium channel blockers, but it should be pointed out that many of the studies have been based on the availability of a drug, either in intravenous or oral form, or simply availability on the shelf of the particular investigator. Drugs which have been investigated include flunarazine, lidoflazine, verapamil, nimodipine, nifedipine, nocardipine, diltiazem, etc. Re-sults of these studies have been variable. Lidoflazine has no effect on cerebral blood flow [21, 22], but may ameliorate damage after ventricular fibrillation and ischemia [23]. Nimodipine favorable affects both cerebral blood flow and out-come, while nicardipine improves flow and has no effect on outcome. Verapamil may be widely available, for which reason it was studied, but it has no effect on either cerebral blood flow or outcome after ischemia.

Over the last several years, much new information has been obtained concern-ing calcium channels in neurons, and research has suggested a role of excitatory neurotransmission in delayed cell death following cerebral ischemia. It is quite possible that calcium channel blockade needs to be revisited from this newer vantage point.

Glutamate and aspartate are released during ischemia, though the precise mechanism is not clear. These excitatory neurotransmitters are partially released via stimulation of N type presynaptic calcium channels, and transmission is at least partly mediated via postsynaptic receptor stimulation by these amino acids. There are at least three major groups of postsynaptic receptors, including the N-methyl-d-aspartate receptor (NMDA), kainic acid receptors (KA), and quisqualic acid sites. There are at least two other types of presynaptic calcium channels, as well as postsynaptic calcium channels. It is interesting that most of the previously tested calcium channel blockers were identified because of peripheral cardiovascular effects, and exhibit little potency at the N type presynaptic calcium channel. Thus, when specific blockers are available for N channel blockade, it will be worthwhile to consider their effect following cerebral injuries. NMDA receptor blockade has been investigated in ischemia, and some of the results have been very exciting.

Another way to block excitatory neurotransmission is to flood the synapse with magnesium. Several studies have suggested that magnesium might be useful following ischemic injury, but no systematic work has been done in this regard. There would be obvious side effects to such therapy in children, but it is clear that improved understanding of the role of synaptic transmission following ischemia will probably reveal novel therapies in the future.

References

1. Dean JM, Rogers MC, Traystman RJ (1987) Pathophysiology and management of the intracranial vault. In: Rogers MC (ed) Textbook of pediatric intensive care. Williams & Wilkins, Baltimore, pp 527–555
2. Kirsch JR, Dean JM, Rogers MC (1986) Current concepts in brain resuscitation. Arch Intern Med 146:1413–1419
3. Dean JM, Kirsch JR, Ackerman A, Rogers MC (1987) Theories of brain resuscitation. In: Rogers MC (ed) Textbook of pediatric intensive care. Williams & Wilkins, Baltimore, pp 557–595
4. White BC, Gadzinski DS, Hoehner PJ, et al (1982) Effect of flunarizine on canine cerebral cortical blood flow and vascular resistance post cardiac arrest. Ann Emerg Med 11:119–126
5. Ment LR, Stewart WB, Petroff OAC, Duncan CC (1989) Thromboxane synthesis inhibitor in a beagle pup model of perinatal asphyxia. Stroke 20:809–814
6. Ment LR, Stewart WB, Gore JC, Duncan CC (1988) Beagle puppy model of perinatal asphyxia: alterations in cerebral blood flow and metabolism. Pediatr Neurol 4:98–104
7. Armstead WM, Mirro R, Busija DW, Leffler CW (1988) Postischemic generation of superoxide anion by newborn pig brain. Am J Physiol (Heart Circ Physiol) 24:H401–H403
8. Laptook AR, Stonestreet BS, Oh W (1982) The effects of different rates of plasmanate infusions upon brain blood flow after asphyxia and hypotension in newborn piglets. J Pediatr 100:791–796
9. Goperlund JM, Wagerle LC, Delivoria-Papadopoulos M (1989) Regional cerebral blood flow response during and after acute asphyxia in newborn piglets. J Appl Physiol 66:2827–2832
10. Traystman RJ (1981) Control of cerebral blood flow. In: Vanhoutte PM, Leusen I (eds) Vasodilation. Raven Press, New York
11. Wagner EM, Traystman RJ (1986) Hydrostatic determinants of cerebral perfusion. Crit Care Med 14:484–490
12. Dean JM, McComb JG (1981) Intracranial pressure monitoring in severe pediatric near drowning. Neurosurgery 9(6):627–630

13. Allman FD, Nelson WB, Pacentine GA, McComb G (1986) Outcome following cardiopulmonary resuscitation in severe pediatric near-drowning. Am J Dis Child 140:571-575
14. Nussbaum E, Galant SP (1983) Intracranial pressure monitoring as a guide to prognosis in the nearly drowned, severely comatose child. J Pediatr 102:215-218
15. Cushing H (1902) Some experimental and clinical observations concerning states of increased intracranial tension: The Mutter Lecture for 1901. Am J Med Sci 124:375
16. Eisenberg HM, Frankowski RF, Contant CF, Marshall LF, Walker MD (1988) High dose barbiturate control of elevated intracranial pressure in patients with severe head injury. J Neurosurg 69:15-23
17. Bleyaert AL, Nemoto EM, Safar P, et al (1978) Thiopental amelioration of brain damage after global ischemia in monkeys. Anesthesiology 49:390-398
18. Gisvold SE, Safar P, Hendrickx HHL, Rao G, Moossy J, Alexander H (1984) Thiopental treatment after global brain ischemia in pigtailed monkeys. Anesthesiology 60:88-96
19. Abramson NS, Safar P, Detre K, et al (1983) Results of a randomized clinical trial of brain resuscitation with thiopental. Anesthesiology 59(Suppl):A101
20. Bleyaert A, Safar P, Nemoto E, Moossy J, Sassano J (1980) Effect of postcirculatory arrrest life support on neurological recovery in monkeys. Crit Care Med 8:153-156
21. Dean JM, Hoehner PJ, Rogers MC, Traystman RJ (1984) Effect of lidoflazine on cerebral blood flow following twelve minutes of total cerebral ischemia. Stroke 15:531-535
22. Dean JM, Hoehner PJ, Rogers MC, Traystman RJ (1985) Use of calcium blockers after cardiac arrest. Proceedings of the 5th International Congress in Intensive Care
23. Vaagenes P, Cantadore R, Safar P, et al (1984) Amelioration of brain damage by lidoflazine after prolonged ventricular fibrillation cardiac arrest in dogs. Crit Care Med 12:846-855

Out-of-Hospital Cerebral Resuscitation

R. O. Roine

Introduction

The aim of resuscitation is invariably the preservation of brain function. Cerebral resuscitation was first introduced by Safar in the 1970s and soon became an intrisic part of resuscitation from cardiac arrest. This has led to the new concept of cardiopulmonary-cerebral resuscitation (CPCR) instead of CPR [1]. Measures starting after the restoration of spontaneous circulation are sometimes called post-resuscitative brain-oriented therapy. The term cerebral protection is usually reserved for treatment initiated before an ischemic insult, for example during open-heart surgery or after subarachnoid hemorrhage. The rationale of cerebral resuscitation, which actually means all measures limiting the brain injury after ischemia, anoxia or trauma, is found in experimental neurology. The rapidly increasing data base of pathophysiologic mechanisms in cerebral anoxia has opened completely new vistas in this field, although most of the decisive experimental findings have not yet been clinically tested. This short review is an attempt to summarize some of the general principles of brain resuscitation which could be applied to the treatment of out-of-hospital cardiac arrest. Therapeutic approaches that are clinically available will be emphasized more than experimental and speculative drug treatments.

Pathophysiology of Cerebral Ischemia

In experimental models, neurons can recover their high energy metabolism, enzymatic functions and action potential generation even after up to 60 minutes of complete ischemia [2]. Global ischemic anoxia of the brain is typically followed by initial hyperemia and by delayed hypoperfusion which reflects a mismatch between metabolic rate and blood flow in the brain [3]. Finally, the ischemic-anoxic brain injury has been shown to develop progressively during several hours of reperfusion while the accumulation of intracellular calcium continues [4, 5]. Calcium dependance of toxic and hypoxic cellular injury was first demonstrated in the hepatocyte [6].

Global ischemia induces depletion of high-energy phosphates and ATP in minutes, which seems to trigger the ischemic cascade [7]. This is followed by potassium efflux, depolarization of the cell membrane and massive calcium influx resulting in intracellular calcium overload. The intracellular calcium accumulation is believed to cause impaired blood flow and neuronal death by following mechanisms [3, 8]:

1. Activation of phospholipases and proteases, destruction of cellular membranes, free fatty acid liberation and free radical formation,
2. Activation of the cyclo-oxygenase and lipo-oxygenase pathways leading to formation of thromboxane A_2 and leukotrienes, smooth muscle spasm and increased vascular wall permeability,
3. Intracellular uncoupling of the oxidative phosphorylation in mitochondria,
4. Release of excitatory neurotransmitters (e. g. glutamate and aspartate) at synaptic terminals.

The excitotoxic hypothesis of neuronal ischemic damage is connected to the calcium hypothesis in several ways: it has been shown both that glutamate receptor activation can lead to intracellular calcium accumulation and that calcium overload in turn can lead to liberation of glutamate [9, 10]. Although difficult to prove, it is widely believed also that the reperfusion injury might be caused by oxygen-derived free radicals, which has led to experimental use of free radical scavengers in cerebral protection [11].

Considerable progress has also been made in the field of brain acidosis [12], which is a key element in the pathophysiology of neuronal ischemic injury. Brain tissue acidosis is accentuated by hypercapnia and hyperglycemia and the decline of pH correlates with the extent of cellular necrosis [13]. Neuronal injury can also be caused directly by the hydrogen ion, which seems to be one of the mediators of cellular death [14].

Post-resuscitation Syndrome

'Post-resuscitation disease' is a still incompletely understood multiple organ failure that often results during reperfusion after prolonged cardiac arrest [15]. In the brain, it is characterized by multifocal hypoperfusion (possibly caused by microcirculatory changes related to oedema, vasospasm or vasoparalysis and change of rheological properties of the blood), continuing cerebral acidosis, hypermetabolism often accompanied by seizure activity and maturation of the ischemic neuronal damage during several days, which has been demonstrated both in animals and in man [16, 17]. Depending on the circumstances during the first minutes, hours and days after resuscitation, this condition can lead either to recovery or to severe brain injury, persistent vegetative state and brain death.

Cerebral Resuscitation

The main alternative approaches to prevent or treat the post-resuscitation syndrome of the brain after cardiac arrest can be categorized as follows:

1. General measures aiming at normalization of blood pressure, blood gases and blood chemistry.

2. Normalization of cerebral blood flow (CBF).
3. Limitation of metabolic rate in the brain.
4. Prevention or treatment of increased intracranial pressure (ICP).
5. Specific cytoprotective approaches.

General Measures

The most important methods of cerebral resuscitation are relatively simple measures aiming at restoration of systemic homeostasis as soon as possible, e.g. normalization of blood pressure, blood gases and blood chemistry. Generally, the use of more specific methods should be considered only after these basic requirements have been fulfilled. Because the delay of basic and especially advanced life support is of utmost importance to the brain, all measures shortening these critical delays also serve the purpose of cerebral resuscitation. Basically, these critical delays can be reduced by minimizing the alarm center delay, using a two-tiered response system, early defibrillation and education of professionals and laymen.

Ventilation and Blood Pressure

The ventilation is particularly important in neurological emergencies. Although the cerebral circulation frequently loses its ability to adjust to blood pressure changes after ischemia, vasodilatory response to increased $PaCO_2$ as well as to hypoxia can still be present and lead to increased ICP. The role of hyperventilation is controversial. The usefulness of hyperventilation has never been demonstrated after global ischemia, on the contrary, the effect of prolonged hyperventilation on ICP and CBF is unfavorable in animals [18]. Hyperventilation at normothermia results in decline of CBF and no change in $CMRO_2$ in cats, whereas hyperventilation at 32° C produces a more significant fall in both suggesting that this combination may be advantageous [19]. Nevertheless, slight hyperventilation is usually recommended to guarantee that carbon dioxide does not rise above normal values at any time [1, 20]. Hyperventilation is also effective in normalizing the pH in cerebrospinal fluid and probably also in the acidotic brain because of the free diffusion capacity of CO_2. Sodium bicarbonate does not have such beneficial effect in cerebral acidosis but may produce paradoxical acidosis due to production of carbon dioxide and may worsen CBF. 100% oxygen is recommended to be used during advanced cardiac life support [20]. However, prolonged use of excess oxygen is not beneficial. Hyperbaric oxygen has been shown to increase experimental ischemic cellular injury, presumably by activating peroxidative reactions and by causing cerebrovascular spasm [21]. 100% oxygen is thus not useful and may be harmful for the brain after restitution of normal partial pressure of oxygen in the blood. One should not forget however, that hypoxia is more harmful than hyperoxia and PaO_2 of at least 100 mmHg should be maintained to assure adequate oxygenation. Based on current knowledge, it is probably safe to recommend brief initial hyperventilation with 100% oxygen and normo- or slight hyperventilation with normoxia if spontaneous hyperpnea or straining are present. Too early extubation should be avoided. Aspiration pneumonia should be prevented, specifically looked for and treated when necessary. For the same reason, the gastric contents should be emptied and the nasogastric tube should be kept in place long enough to prevent aspiration commonly even in intubated patients.

Cerebral Blood Flow, Autoregulation and Blood Pressure

During external cardiac compressions, CBF is insufficient to maintain viability of the brain for more than a limited time. CBF is probably not more than 20% of normal (about 10 ml/100g/min) in most cases of closed-chest CPR, whereas open-chest cardiac compression can produce nearly normal CBF. It is also inversely related to the time delay before CPR is started. The ischemic threshold for intracellular K^+ release which corresponds to irreversible cellular injury is 6 to 8 ml/100g/min in the baboon and the threshold for somatosensory cortical evoked potentials about 15 ml/100g/min [22]. Keeping CBF in the range between these thresholds, it is theoretically possible to maintain the brain nonfunctional but viable in a state of so called 'ischemic penumbra' for a time period depending on the flow. Experimentally, 8 ml/100g/min sustains the potential for recovery for 30 minutes in the awake monkey – which corresponds roughly the clinical upper limit of duration of external cardiac compression [23, 24]. Correspondingly, flows exceeding 18 ml/100g/min were able to prevent brain necrosis almost indefinitely. This means that any innovation providing only a minor increase in the CBF during CPR would probably have an effect on the neurological outcome and overall outcome of out-of-hospital resuscitation. For example in dogs, the simultaneous compression-ventilation technique provides CBF values more than 10 times higher than the non-simultaneous technique up to $32 \pm 7\%$ of prearrest CBF [25].

When CBF is restored after a period of global cerebral ischemia exceeding some 5 minutes, the initial phase of hyperemia is often replaced by a more prolonged hypoperfusion which can be either diffuse or more localized [26]. In experimental settings, CBF can be restored and maintained much better by CPR instituted immediately after arrest than after several minutes [1]. Clinically, it is possible that in patients with long delays of advanced life support different pathophysiological mechanisms are operative as compared to patients with shorter delays. Consequently, the neurological state of the patient would be more decisive for the prognosis in the former patient group. Thus, this group might benefit most of efforts focused on cerebral preservation after cardiac arrest.

The first blood pressure values after restoration of spontaneous circulation often seem to be higher than the following ones. This could perhaps represent the transient effect of epinephrine. Slight hypertension is usually considered beneficial because it might improve the cerebral reperfusion initially [1].

Unfortunately, increase of CBF is no guarantee of good neurological outcome. On the contrary, there is evidence that increased CBF about 24 hours postarrest correlates with permanent coma and death [27]. This probably reflects the total loss of cerebrovascular autoregulation leading to cerebral perfusion that passively follows the changes in blood pressure. It is also unlikely that drugs that mainly increasing CBF would be beneficial after global ischemia. Normally, CBF remains almost constant between mean arterial pressures of about 50 and 160 mmHg. After all kinds of cerebral ischemia, as well as after head trauma, cerebral autoregulation is at least initially lost. Because of impaired cerebral autoregulation in extended hypoxemia, hypercarbia or both, careful control of blood pressure is mandatory. Even mild hypotension as well as severe hypertension must be avoided because they can be directly reflected in the cerebral blood flow. In cases of suspected increase of ICP, low blood pressure is naturally even more detrimental. According to some studies, elevated ICP is rare during the first days after cardiac arrest [28, 29] but, according to others, it is elevated above 20 mmHg already within a few hours after cardiac arrest in almost 30% of patients, who do not recover [30]. Routine ICP monitoring is not recommended after cardiac arrest, but in selected cases the detection and treatment of increased ICP may be worthwhile. Development of increased ICP, perhaps several days after arrest, predicts poor outcome and often precedes anoxic brain death, which is relatively uncommon in contrast to the higher frequency of vegetative state after cardiac arrest. As CBF correlates with the cerebral perfusion pressure (MAP – ICP), all activity increasing ICP – such as straining and coughing, even during tracheal suction – should also be restricted. The head should also be slightly elevated (approximately 30° C) intracranial venous stasis with resultant increase in ICP [20].

Cerebral Hypermetabolism, Temperature and Seizures

A severe mismatch between increased metabolic rate and reduced CBF flow sometimes ensues during a so called delayed post-ischemic hypoperfusion. Both hyperthermia and seizure activity increase the oxygen requirements of the brain [31, 32]. Electroencephalographic seizure activity has been observed in up to 30% of cases after cardiac arrest during acute stage [33].

From the theoretical point of view, it would be tempting to limit the metabolic rate in the brain. This can be accomplished either by hypothermia or by using central nervous system depressant drugs. Hypothermia, pentobarbital and lidocaine all inhibit cerebral oxygen and glucose consumption in the dog [34]. The result of a large multicenter trial of thiopental after cardiac arrest was clearly negative and thiopental cannot be recommended in routine use after cardiac arrest [35]. On the other hand, in one trial thiopental slightly reduced the neuropsychological complications of open-heart surgery [36]. The possibility of hemodynamic instability and the potential of increasing myocardial infarct size in the dog should strictly limit the use of thiopental to clear-cut indications after cardiac arrest [37]. Nevertheless, thiopental often seems to be effective in reducing postarrest seizure activity in the brain, which often occurs without any visible seizure manifestations in comatose patients. There are no clinical studies demonstrating the effectiveness of any drugs in limiting this activity or the clinical usefulness of anticonvulsant treatment in general in the post-resuscitative care.

Based on purely experimental data, it can probably be recommended that post-arrest seizure activity in the EEG-monitor as well visible seizures should be treated using thiopental, especially if benzodiazepines and phenytoin are ineffective. Phenytoin, which also has unspecific calcium antagonistic properties, might be the drug of choice for the treatment (and perhaps prevention) of post-arrest seizure activity, supported perhaps by the fact that it has been demonstrated to limit anoxic injury in animals and even seemed to improve neurological outcome in a small uncontrolled clinical study [38, 39]. Although central nervous system depressants are not routinely recommended, they are still often indicated for sedation, even out-of-hospital. Barbiturates should probably not be used outside the hospital. Diazepam is usually effective against excessive straining and also extensor posturing that commonly occur even in recovering patients during the acute stage. The rationale of such treatment is to prevent increased demands on the cardiovascular system and particularly to prevent increases of intracranial pressure which might lead to deterioration of the already compromised intracranial circulation. Hypothermia is known to be very effective in cerebral protection both clinically and experimentally, but the use of therapeutic hypothermia is not practical after cardiac arrest [40]. According to experimental results, even a slight drop (from 36°C to 34°C) in brain temperature can markedly reduce the extent of ischemic neuronal injury [41]. Prolonged hypothermia has also been reported to be harmful in regional ischemia and it bears an additional risk of cardiovascular problems and infection [42]. On the other hand, rapid warming of the moderately hypothermic patient is probably not indicated after cardiac arrest. The development of hyperthermia must be prevented, and it can usually be controlled by physical means.

Hyperglycemia

The harmful effect of high blood glucose concentration for the ischemic brain deserves to be mentioned. Very substantial amount of data has accumulated of the detrimental effect of hyperglycemia both in complete ischemia produced by cardiac arrest and especially in incomplete ischemia produced by CPR [43-45]. It has also been shown that increased blood glucose level on admission to hospital predicts poor outcome after out-of-hospital cardiac arrest [46]. The typical rise of blood glucose after cardiac arrest is often considered as a secondary stress reaction. For the brain suffering from incomplete ischemia, the elevated level of blood glucose per se is more critical than the cause of hyperglycemia. This should have at least two consequences: (1) unnecessary glucose administration should be avoided after cardiac arrest, (2) elevated blood glucose levels should be treated promptly. 5% glucose without electrolyte additions is still widely used but theoretically a bad choice after cardiac arrest; not only because it contains glucose but also because it is hypotonic and may worsen cerebral edema. In Helsinki, glucose is currently administered only to cardiac arrest patients with verified hypoglycemia.

Pharmacological Agents

Of the drugs routinely used in the treatment of out-of-hospital cardiac arrest, only epinephrine has been shown to be beneficial for cerebral circulation, although perhaps in higher doses than those used clinically [47]. There is also some evidence of the cerebroprotective action of lidocaine which may be linked with its suppressive effect on synaptic transmission and inhibition of metabolism [34, 48]. The use of sodium bicarbonate has been limited because of its several potential harmful effects, including cerebral ones, and lack of proved efficacy [20]. As corticosteroids are not effective in reducing cytotoxic edema and are ineffective or harmful in global as well as focal ischemia by enhancing hyperglycemia and infarction according to several studies, they are definitely not indicated in the routine treatment of ischemia and their use in cardiac arrest should also be discontinued [49]. According to large controlled clinical studies, they are generally not indicated in cerebral trauma either [50].

Although an enormous amount of different compounds have been studied experimentally in models of global and focal ischemia and also demonstrated to have varying cerebroprotective effects, the use of other drugs in the treatment of global cerebral ischemia remains still experimental.

These drugs include:

1. various metabolic depressants, such as barbiturates, etomidate, phenytoin, lidocaine and diazepam,
2. vasoactive agents such as prostacyclin, indomethacin, thromboxane A_2 synthetase inhibitors, eicosapentaenoic acid,
3. anticoagulants,
4. solvents such as Fluosol DA,
5. osmotic diuretics,
6. opiate antagonists such as naloxone,
7. calcium entry blockers and
8. glutamate (NMDA-receptor) antagonists.

Of these new experimental drugs, calcium entry blockers are the ones most thoroughly investigated and, based on animal and preliminary data, also the most promising ones. Nimodipine is a dihydropyridine derivative calcium entry blocking drug with predilection for cerebral circulation. It has been documented to ameliorate the delayed postischemic hypoperfusion of the brain, with prevention of neurologic deficits and death [51, 52]. Nimodipine has some selectivity for cerebral vessels and it has high affinity for specific receptors in brain tissue, which are identical with calcium channels and have also been identified in human cerebral cortex [53–55]. Nimodipine inhibits noradrenaline release from cerebral arteries in humans and dopamine release in the rat [56, 57] and has an anticonvulsant effect against seizures produced by ischemia and reperfusion or certain convulsive agents [58]. More importantly, nimodipine improved but lidoflazine did not improve neurological outcome in a primate global ischemia model relevant from the clinical point of view, since the treatment was started 5 minutes after 17 minutes of complete cerebral ischemia [59, 60]. In the cardiovascular side, nimodipine has been demonstrated to dilate coronary arteries, increase cardiac output, elevate PaO_2 and diminish pulmonary vascular resistance without an effect on intrapulmonary shunting [61–63]. Nimodipine does not increase ICP after ischemia. On the contrary, it decreases ICP after MCA occlusion in baboons at all pressure and PCO_2 levels and has no adverse effect on ICP after human cardiac arrest either [30, 64]. Nimodipine is effective in reducing ischemic damage after subarachnoid hemorrhage [65, 66]. Substantial experimental evidence suggests that it may also be beneficial after human cardiac arrest.

In 1989, two large placebo controlled studies of calcium antagonists in cardiac arrest have been completed. The first one was an international multicenter trial of 505 patients, which demonstrated no difference between lidoflazine and placebo in the outcome of comatose survivors of various in-hospital and out-of-hospital cardiac arrests [67]. The other one was a randomized, placebo controlled single center study of 155 patients with out-of-hospital ventricular fibrillation resuscitated by one mobile intensive care unit in Helsinki. In this study, nimodipine or placebo was started as a bolus dose of 10 µg/kg followed by a 24 hours infusion of 0.5µg/kg/min approximately only 23 minutes after estimated cardiac arrest time. A standardized, protocol defined cerebral resuscitation therapy was used in both studies. The results of the latter study will be published soon. This study has led to a large scale European multicenter trial of nimodipine in out-of-hospital ventricular fibrillation starting in the beginning of 1990.

The next group of compounds expected to follow calcium antagonists into clinical trials will probably be the NMDA-receptor antagonists, and of these perhaps MK-801, which has been studied more carefully than other members of this group. However, insufficient clinical data and potential side effects do not make NMDA-receptor antagonists feasible for controlled trials yet.

In the future, the combination of different approaches will probably be the most logical attempt to improve neurological outcome in out-of-hospital cerebral resuscitation, since it is unlikely that any single agent could solve all the problems in the extremely complex process of cellular injury during global cerebral ischemia and reperfusion.

References

1. Safar P, Bircher NG (1988) Cardiopulmonary cerebral resuscitation, 3rd edn. Saunders Company Ltd, London
2. Hossmann K-A, Kleihues P (1973) Reversibility of ischemic brain damage. Arch Neurol 29:375–384
3. Siesjö BK (1981) Cell damage in the brain: a speculative hypothesis. J Cereb Blood Flow Metabol 1:155–186
4. Pulsinelli WA, Brierley JB, Plum F (1984) Temporal profile of neuronal damage in a model of transient forebrain ischemia. Ann Neurol 11:491–498
5. Deshpande JK, Siesjö BK, Wieloch T (1987) Calcium accumulation and neuronal damage in the rat hippocampus following cerebral ischemia. J Cereb Blood Flow Metabol 7:89–95
6. Schanne FAX, Kane AB, Young EE, Farber JL (1979) Calcium dependence of toxic cell death: a final common pathway. Science 206:700–703
7. Hass WK (1983) The cerebral ischemic cascade. Neurol Clin 1:345
8. Raichle ME (1983) The pathophysiology of brain ischemia. Ann Neurol 13:2–10

9. Benveniste H, Jørgensen MB, Diemer NH, Hansen AJ (1988) Calcium accumulation by glutamate receptor activations is involved in hippocampal cell damage after ischemia. Acta Neurol Scand 78:529–536
10. Rothman SM, Olney JW (1986) Glutamate and the pathophysiology of hypoxic-ischemic brain damage. Ann Neurol 19:105–111
11. McCord JM (1985) Oxygen-derived free radicals in post-ischemic tissue injury. N Engl J Med 312:159–163
12. Rehncrona S (1985) Brain acidosis. Ann Emerg Med 14:770–776
13. Rehncrona S, Rosen I, Siesjö BK (1981) Brain lactic acidosis and ischemic cell damage: 1. Biochemistry and neurophysiology. J Cereb Blood Flow Metab 1:297–311
14. Kraig RP, Petito CK, Plum F, Pulsinelli WA (1987) Hydrogen ions kill brain at concentrations reached in ischemia. J Cereb Blood Flow Metab 7:379–386
15. Negovsky VA, Gurvitch AM, Zolotokrylina ES (1983) Postresuscitation disease. Elsevier, Amsterdam
16. Petito CK, Pulsinelli WA (1984) Delayed neuronal recovery and neuronal death in rat hippocampus following severe cerebral ischemia: Possible relationship to abnormalities in neuronal processes. J Cereb Blood Flow Metabol 4:194–205
17. Petito CK, Feldmann E, Pulsinelli WA, Plum F (1987) Delayed hippocampal damage in humans following cardiorespiratory arrest. Neurology 37:1281–1286
18. Albrecht RF, Miletich DJ, Ruttle M (1987) Cerebral effects of extended hyperventilation in unanesthetized goats. Stroke 18:649–655
19. Frewen TC, Sumabat WO, Han VK, Campbell K, Tiffin N (1989) Effects of hyperventilation, hypothermia, and altered blood viscosity on cerebral blood flow, cross-brain oxygen extraction, and cerebral metabolic rate for oxygen in cats. Crit Care Med 17:912–916
20. American Heart Association (1986). Standards and guidelines for cardiopulmonary resuscitation (CPR) and emergency cardiac care (ICC). JAMA 255:2905–3044
21. Mickel HS, Vaishnav YN, Kempski O, Von Lubitz D, Weiss JF, Feuerstein G (1987) Breathing 100% oxygen after global brain ischemia in mongolian gerbils results in increased lipid peroxidation and increased mortality. Stroke 18:426–430
22. Astrup J, Symon L, Branston NM, Lassen NA (1977) Cortical evoked potential and extracellular K^+ and H^+ at critical levels of brain ischemia. Stroke 8:51–57
23. Jones TH, Morawetz RB, Crowell RM et al (1981) Treshold of focal cerebral ischemia in awake monkeys. J Neurosurg 54:773–782
24. Heiss W-D, Rosner G (1983) Functional recovery of cortical neurons as related to degree and duration of ischemia. Ann Neurol 14:294–301
25. Koehler RC, Chandra N, Guerci AD et al (1983) Augmentation of cerebral perfusion by simultaneous chest compression and lung inflation with abdominal binding after cardiac arrest in dogs. Circulation 67:266–275
26. Ames A III, Wrigth RL, Kowada M, Thurston JM, Majno G (1968) Cerebral ischemia. II. The no-reflow phenomenon. Am J Pathol 52:437–453
27. Cohan SL, Mun SK, Petite J, Correia J, Da Silva AT, Waldhorn RE (1989) Cerebral blood flow in humans following resuscitation from cardiac arrest. Stroke 20:761–765
28. Sakabe T, Tateishi A, Miyauchi Y, et al (1987) Intracranial pressure following cardiopulmonary resuscitation. Intensive Care Med 13:256–259
29. Schmidt A, Binner L, Mayer U, Stauch M (1988) The role of intracranial pressure (ICP) monitoring after cardiopulmonary resuscitation (CPR). Abstract. Crit Care Med 16:389
30. Gueugniaud P-Y, Vaudelin T, Gaussorgues P, Petit P (1989) Out-of-hospital cardiac arrest: The teaching of experience at the SAMU of Lyon. Resuscitation 17:S79–S98
31. Carlsson C, Hagerdal M, Siesjö BK (1976) The effect of hyperthermia upon oxygen consumption and upon organic phosphates, glycolytic metabolites, citric acid cycle intermediates and associated amino acids in rat cerebral cortex. J Neurochem 26:1001–1006
32. Meldrum BS, Nilsson B (1976) Cerebral blood flow and metabolic rate early and late in prolonged epileptic seizures induced in rats by bicuculline. Brain 99:523–542
33. Prior PF (1975) The EEG in acute cerebral anoxia. Excerpta Medica, Amsterdam
34. Astrup J, Sørensen PM, Sørensen HR (1981) Inhibition of cerebral oxygen and glucose consumption in the dog by hypothermia, pentobarbital and lidocaine. Anesthesiology 55:263–268

35. Brain Resuscitation Clinical Trial I Study Group (1986) Randomized clinical study of thiopental loading incomatose survivors of cardiac arrest. N Engl J Med 314:397–403
36. Nussmeier NA, Arlund C, Slogoff S (1986) Neuropsychiatric complications after cardiopulmonary bypass: cerebral protection by a barbiturate. Anesthesiology 64:165–170
37. Jugdutt BI, Rogers MC, Hutchins GM, Becker LC (1986) Increased myocardial infarct size by thiopental after coronary occlusion in the fog. Am Heart J 112:485–494
38. Cullen JP, Aldrete JA, Jankovsky L, et al (1979) Protective action of phenytoin in cerebral ischemia. Anesth Analg (Cleve) 58:165–169
39. Aldrete JA, Romo-Salas F, Mazzia VDB, Tan SL (1981) Phenytoin for brain resuscitation after cardiac arrest. An uncontrolled clinical trial. Crit Care Med 9:474–477
40. Dempsey RJ, Combs DJ, Maley ME, Cowen DE, Roy MW, Donaldson DL (1987) Moderate hypothermia reduces post-ischemic edema development and leukotriene production. Neurosurgery 21:177–181
41. Busto R, Dietrich WD, Globus MYT, Valdes I, Scheinberg P, Ginsberg M (1987) Small differences in intraischemic brain temperature critically determine the extent of ischemic neuronal injury. J Cereb Blood Flow Metabol 7:729–738
42. Steen PA, Soule EH, Michenfelder JD (1979) Detrimental effect of prolonged hypothermia in cats and monkeys with and without regional cerebralischemia. Stroke 10:522–529
43. Pulsinelli WA, Waldmann S, Rawlinson D, Plum F (1982) Moderate hyperglycemia augments ischemic brain damage: a neuropathologic study in the rat. Neurology 32:1239–1246
44. Plum F (1983) What causes infarction in ischemic brain? The Robert Warttenberg lecture. Neurology 33:222–233
45. Siemkowicz E (1985) The effect of glucose upon restitution after transient cerebral ischemia: a summary. Acta Neurol Scand 71:417–427
46. Longstreth WT, Diehr P, Cobb LA, et al (1986) Neurologic outcome and blood glucose levels during out-of-hospital cardiopulmonary resuscitation. Neurology 36:1186–1191
47. Koehler RC, Michael JR, Guerci AD, et al (1985) Beneficial effect of epinephrine infusion on cerebral and myocardial blood flows during CPR. Ann Emerg Med 14:744–749
48. Dutka AJ, Clark J, Evans D, Hallenbeck JM (1987) Lidocaine improves recovery following transient multifocal cerebral ischemia induced by air embolism. Neurology 37:S250
49. Norris JW (1976) Steroid therapy in acute cerebral infarction. Arch Neurol 33:69–71
50. Cooper PR, Moody S, Clark WK, et al (1979) Dexamethasone and severe head injury. A prospective double-blind study. J Neurosurg 51:307–316
51. Kazda S, Hoffmeister F, Garthoff B, Towart R (1979) Prevention of the postischaemic impaired reperfusion of the brain by nimodipine. Acta Neurol Scand 60 (Suppl 72):302–303
52. Steen PA, Newberg LA, Milde JH, Michenfelder JD (1984) Cerebral blood flow and neurologic outcome when nimodipine is given after complete cerebral ischemia in the dog. J Cereb Blood Flow Metabol 4:82–87
53. Bellemann P, Schade A, Towart R (1983) Dihydropyridine receptor in rat brain labeled with [3H]nimodipine. Proc Natl Acad Sci USA 80:2356–2360
54. Middlemiss DN, Spedding M (1985) A functional correlate for the dihydropyridine binding site in rat brain. Nature 314:94–96
55. Peroutka SJ, Allen GS (1983) Calcium channel antagonist binding sites labeled by [3H]nimodipine in human brain. J Neurosurg 59:933–937
56. Porter ID, Gardiner IM, de Belleroche J (1985) Nimodipine has an inhibitory action on neurotransmitter release from human cerebral arteries. J Cereb Blood Flow Metabol 5:338–342
57. Woodward JJ, Leslie SW (1986) Bay K 8644 stimulation of calcium entry and endogenous dopamine release in rat striatal synaptosomes antagonized by nimodipine. Brain Res 370:397–400
58. Meyer FB, Anderson RE, Sundt TM Jr, Sharbrough FW (1986) Selective central nervous system calcium channel blockers – a new class of anticonvulsant agents. Mayo Clin Proc 61:239–247
59. Steen PA, Gisvold SE, Milde JH, et al (1985) Nimodipine improves outcome when given after complete cerebral ischemia in primates. Anesthesiology 62:406–414

60. Fleischer JE, Lanier WL, Milde JH, Michenfelder JD (1987) Lidoflazine does not improve neurologic outcome when administered after complete cerebral ischemia in primates. J Cereb Blood Flow Metabol 7:366-371

61. Haws CW, Heistad DD (1983) Cardiovascular effects of nimodipine: I. Effects on distribution of blood flow. II. Inhibition of cerebral vasoconstrictor responses. J Cereb Blood Flow Metabol 3:S524-S525

62. Satoh K, Kawada M, Wada Y, Taira N (1984) Cardiovascular actions of the dihydropyridine calcium antagonist nimodipine in the dog. Arzneim Forsch 34:563-568

63. Boldt J, Von Bormann D, Kling D, Ratthey K, Hempelmann G (1987) Influence of nimodipine and nifedipine on intrapulmonary shunting - a comparison to other vasoactive drugs. Intensive Care Med 13:52-56

64. Hadley MN, Spetzler RF, Fifield MS, Bichard WD, Hodak JA (1987) The effect of nimodipine on intracranial pressure. Volume-pressure studies in a primate model. J Neurosurg 66:387-393

65. Öhman J, Heiskanen O (1988) Effect of nimodipine on the outcome of patients after aneurysmal subarachnoid hemorrhage and surgery. J Neurosurg 69:683-686

66. Pickard JD, Murray GD, Illingworth R, et al (1989) Effect of oral nimodipine on cerebral infarction and outcome after subarachnoid hemorrhage: British aneurysm nimodipine trial. Br Med J 298:636-642

67. Abramson NS and the Brain Resuscitation Clinical Trial (BRCT) II Study Group (1989) Effect of calcium entry blocker (lidoflazine) administration on comatose survivors of clinical cardiac arrest. Abstract. Crit Care Med 17:S132

When to Stop CPR?

M. Gauthier and J. Lacroix

Introduction

Basic life support techniques (BLS) and more advanced therapies for emergency treatment and stabilization of patients in the postarrest phase (ACLS) are well known to emergency physicians and intensivists. The medicolegal considerations of resuscitation, namely the obligation to provide, and the indications for withholding or withdrawing cardiopulmonary resuscitation (CPR) [1] are less familiar to most health care providers.

Discussion of the termination of CPR, which is the purpose of this article, is important for several reasons. The results obtained in terms of survival and neurologic morbidity using the techniques of BLS and ACLS are far from ideal and they are, in general, inversely proportional to the duration of the maneuvers. Therapy may become futile, if prolonged beyond a point where there is no hope for long-term survival and acceptable neurologic recovery. If survival rates were better, if neurologic sequelae were almost never encountered, or if the success obtained with CPR was the same no matter its duration, nobody would argue that CPR is sometimes prolonged improperly. Inappropriately excessive maneuvers have human and financial consequences that are not negligible. Transient survival of a patient in coma who will die days, weeks or months after his "successful" resuscitation is an extremely distressing experience for the victim's family and, to a lesser degree, for the hospital team responsible for his care. The decision to limit aggressive support is often taken in these circumstances; in most cases, this is an emotionally draining process for both the family and the physicians. The care of such patients in intensive care units, on hospital wards, or in a nursing home setting is extremely costly, increasing the financial burden for the families and draining medical resources which could be used more productively [2].

In the following discussion, the results obtained today with conventional CPR will be summarized. Already published guidelines on withdrawing of CPR will be mentioned, and the usefulness of some clinical variables as predictors of outcome will be discussed. Lastly, practical recommendations about CPR will be proposed.

Outcome Following CPR

Outcome following CPR is usually measured by two different parameters: 1) the percentage of resuscitations initially successful, that is, return to an effective spontaneous cardiac function and pulse for at least 30–60 minutes after cardiac standstill or ventricular fibrillation (VF), and 2) the percentage of patients surviving who are discharged from the hospital. Successful CPR percentage is based on the number of CPR cases, and not the number of patients. The percentage who returned home is based on the number of patients, and not the number of cases. Most authors consider the rate of survival to discharge as the most significant measure of outcome.

Survival up to discharge following out-of-hospital CPR in adults varies between 8 and 28% (Table 1). Variability of results among series may be explained in part by the definition of "arrest" used by different authors. The category of excellent results can be inflated with patients who have experienced a respiratory arrest without true cardiac arrest, a vasovagal syncope, or with patients who respond to a single chest thump. Some series involve only arrests associated with VF [3] or heart disease [4, 5], where resuscitation is more successful. Data depicted in Table 1 seem to indicate a positive influence of early CPR involving bystanders on the survival rates. However, in a 10-year review of 1905 prehospital witnessed cardiac arrests, Stueven et al. failed to demonstrate increased save rates in bystander CPR patients [6]. No prospective randomized evaluations of the independent effect of early CPR have been conducted so far.

Table 2 summarizes rates of survival reported over the last fifteen years following in-hospital CPR in adults. Although 22 to 57% of CPR were considered as initially successful, only 6 to 24% of the victims survived up to discharge from hospital. There has been no tendency for outcome to be more successful in the more recent studies [7]. The lack of improved survival may be due in part to a more aggressive attitude with more resuscitation attempts in a larger number of

Table 1. Survival following out-of-hospital cardiopulmonary resuscitation in adults

Study	Year	Location	No. of pts	Survival up to discharge from hospital		
				With bystander CPR	Without bystander CPR	Total group
Lund and Skulberg [24]	1976	Oslo	631	36%	8%	11%
Thompson et al. [3]	1979	Seattle	316	43%	21%	28%
Rockswold et al. [18]	1979	Minneapolis	514	NA[a]	NA	16%
Tweed et al. [25]	1980	Winnipeg	226	25%	5%	11%
Gudjonsson et al. [26]	1982	Reykjavik	122	42%	6%	17%
Vertesi et al. [27]	1983	Vancouver	315	21%	6%	8%
Guzy et al. [28]	1983	Los Angeles	243	22%	5%	11%
Roth et al. [5]	1984	Pittsburgh	187	17%	5%	10%
Cummins et al. [4]	1985	Seattle	2043	27%	13%	18%

[a] NA, data not available.

Table 2. Survival following in-hospital cardiopulmonary resuscitation in adults

Study	Year	Location	No. of CPR	Initially successful CPR	Survival up to discharge
Messert and Quaglieri [20][a]	1976	Wisconsin	218	22%	14%
Peatfield et al. [29]	1977	England	1063	33%	9%
Wernberg and Thomassen [30]	1979	Denmark	1172	NA[b]	6%
Tweed et al. [25]	1980	Winnipeg	2091	41%	13%
De Bard [10]	1981	Ohio	1073	57%	24%
Bedell et al. [21][a]	1983	Boston	294	44%	14%
Woog and Torzillo [11][a]	1987	Australia	174	44%	16%
Rozenbaum and Shenkman [7][a]	1988	Israël	71	41%	18%

[a] Prospective study.
[b] NA, data not available.

patients [7]. It may also indicate that newer techniques and more sophisticated equipment have not had a major impact on outcome [7].

Pediatric CPR is substantially different compared to adult CPR, due to anatomical, physiologic, and pathologic differences. Outcome after out-of-hospital CPR is significantly worse in children than in adults, with 3–8% of victims surviving to leave hospital (Table 3). Factors which may explain this difference in outcome include the fact that most pediatric arrests are secondary to hypoxia, that the majority of out-of-hospital arrests in children are unwitnessed, and that the terminal arrhythmia is different. There is a much higher incidence of asystole in children, rendering restoration of a cardiac rhythm much more difficult than in most adult arrests.

Contrary to adults, children have been reported to be more likely to survive an in-hospital than an out-of-hospital arrest [8], with 9 to 55% surviving to discharge after in-hospital CPR (Table 4). Here again, the extreme variability in survival rates between different series may be due to differences in inclusion criteria. In one study, for example [9], cardiopulmonary arrest was defined as a call for the ACLS team and only 60% of the patients described required external cardiac compression. With the available data, it is surely impossible to conclude at this

Table 3. Survival following out-of-hospital cardiopulmonary resuscitation in children

Study	Year	Location	No. of pts	Survival up to discharge		
				Witnessed	Cardiac Arrest Unwitnessed	Total group
Eisenberg et al. [12]	1983	Seattle	119	15%	3%	7%
Torphy et al. [13]	1984	Wisconsin	92	NA[a]	NA	3%
Losek et al. [19]	1987	Wisconsin	114	NA	NA	8%

[a] NA, data not available.

Table 4. Survival following in-hospital cardiopulmonary resuscitation in children

Study	Year	Location	Patients		
			Total no.	Initially resuscitated	Survived up to discharge
Lewis et al. [22][a]	1983	Wisconsin	58	NA[b]	15%
Ludwig et al. [9]	1983	Philadelphia	130	82%	55%
Wark and Overton [14][a]	1984	Australia	49	66%	42%
Gillis et al. [15]	1986	Toronto	33	55%	9%
Nichols et al. [8][a]	1986	Philadelphia	34	NA[b]	44%
Davies et al. [23][a]	1987	Atlanta	67	75%	37%
Zaritsky et al. [16][a]	1987	Washington D.C.	53	34%	9%

[a] Prospective study.
[b] NA, data not available.

point in time that success rate of inside hospital CPR is better in children than it is in adults.

Survival rate is the major variable used to evaluate the effectiveness of CPR, but neurologic outcome must also be considered. Surprisingly enough, neurologic sequelae among survivors are not mentioned in many publications on CPR outcome in adults [3–5, 10, 11], and in the majority of articles on the subject in children [8, 12–16]. Very few data are available concerning neurologic morbidity after out-of-hospital cardiac arrests. Longstreth et al. studied 459 adults initially resuscitated [17]. Sixty-one per cent (279/459) regained consciousness, 67% (188/279) without and 33% (91/279) with persistent neurologic deficits. Rockwold et al. [18] reviewed 514 adults. Eighty three (16%) were discharged alive from hospital. Forty-nine of these long-term survivors were ambulatory with normal neurologic function when discharged; most of the remaining 34 patients had some degree of neurologic impairment. Eight per cent of a group of 114 children with out-of-hospital arrest survived to be discharged from the hospital, 67% of them (3/9) with neurologic sequelae [19].

Neurologic outcome following in-hospital CPR is more documented. In a series of 218 CPR efforts in 183 adults, the rate of chronic vegetative state was 10.4% among the initial survivors [20]. Ninety-two per cent (12/13) of the adult survivors described by Rozenbaum et al. [7] were fully functional. Bedell et al. evaluated mental status, depression, and functional capacity among 41 adults discharged from hospital [21]. Gross impairment of mental status occurred for the first time in only one patient. All patients reported some decrease in functional capacity, often attributed to fear; thirty per cent (10/33) were newly homebound. Eight children discharged after an in-hospital cardiac arrest were evaluated by Lewis et al. [22]. Twenty-two per cent (2/9) of the survivors had severe neurologic sequelae. In 25 similar patients, reported by Davies et al. [23], only 8% (2/25) had evidence of hypoxic/ischemic damage at the time of discharge.

Outcome after CPR varies according to the location of the arrest (inside vs outside hospital), and the presence or absence of witnesses. Results are different in children compared to adults. Regardless of the age of the patient or the circumstances of the arrest, the probability for any individual victim to be initially resuscitated is 50% at best. In addition, only 3 to 5 patients out of ten who are initially resuscitated will survive to be discharged from the hospital. CPR as it is practiced today may be lifesaving, but only for a minority of patients. The great majority of the victims either die on site of the arrest or before being discharged from hospital.

This reality plus the scarcity of data concerning neurologic sequelae among survivors should prompt the clinician to critically assess the indications for termination of CPR.

Historical Perspective on Recommendations

Based on a study of 198 consecutive patients treated for cardiac arrest in the emergency department at Stanford University Medical Center, and on a survey of the literature, Eliastam et al. in 1977 proposed specific recommendations concerning termination of CPR [2]. These criteria were listed as follows:

1. apnea and pulselessness known to have exceeded 10 minutes;
2. no response after more than 30 minutes of ACLS, including that administered in the pre-hospital setting;
3. no ventricular electrocardiographic activity (asystole) for over 10 minutes during ACLS; and
4. pre-existing terminal illness.

These authors were among the first to suggest guidelines concerning termination of CPR. Their recommendations were clear and based on a good knowledge of the predictors of outcome (see below). However, their set of criteria was rather rigid and did not take into account exceptional circumstances, such as hypothermia, which could affect the outcome of CPR, and the decision to stop resuscitation.

In 1985, the fourth national conference on CPR and emergency cardiac care was sponsored by the American Heart Association (AHA), and major recommendations concerning medicolegal considerations were published following discussions at this meeting [1]. Indications for physicians as well as for nonphysicians to withdraw BLS were described. Concerning termination of CPR, the national conference stipulated that the major criteria to be used by clinicians should be a "finding of cardiovascular unresponsiveness", indicating that the heart has died. "The judgment that a cardiac arrest victim is unresuscitable and that CPR should be terminated must mean that BLS and ACLS were employed in a manner and for a time adequate to test the responsiveness of the victim's cardiovascular system. The use of this end point eliminates not only speculation as to recoverability of the brain but also arbitrary end points based on the duration of the resuscitative effort, the age of the patient, or the presence or absence of certain neurological signs" [1]. In the opinion of the national conference's panel, "if cardiovascular function is reestablished by CPR, neurologic status must be determined and suspension of life support may then need to be considered".

There are several problems with these recommendations. The time adequate to test the responsiveness of the victim's cardiovascular system was not defined by the panel of experts; the relative importance of duration of CPR, the age of the patient, and the presence or absence of certain neurologic signs as predictors of outcome were not considered (see below). Most importantly, cardiovascular responsiveness is definitely not synonymous with hope for survival as proved by the discrepancy already noted between the rates of initial CPR success and the rates of discharge from hospital (Tables 2 and 4). To consider cardiovascular unresponsiveness as the endpoint to terminate CPR surely eliminates more arbitrary endpoints but may also lead directly to futile therapy.

Predictors of Outcome

Many efforts have been made to define accurate predictors of outcome after CPR. Variables which have been determined to be predictive of outcome are listed in Table 5. Other factors such as age of the adult [7, 21, 29, 31] or pediatric victim [8], and the location of the arrest in the hospital [7, 10, 21], do not influence outcome.

Duration of CPR

Duration of CPR is usually defined as the interval of time between initiation of resuscitation effort and return to an effective spontaneous circulation. Anecdotal cases of patients surviving without sequelae after very prolonged CPR have been reported; the majority of them were near-drowning victims with severe associated hypothermia. Despite these rare anecdotal cases, most authors agree that duration of CPR is of critical importance as determinant of outcome in adults [7, 11, 20, 21, 32, 33] as well as in children [8, 15, 16, 23]. Rates of survival are significantly worse when CPR time is over 15 minutes (Table 6). The adult and pediatric literature of the last fifteen years seems also to indicate that a CPR time of more than 30 minutes in normothermic conditions is almost incompatible with survival (Table 6).

Table 5. Factors predictive of outcome after a cardiac arrest

Duration of resuscitation
Number of drugs administered during CPR
Unsuccessful prehospital ACLS
Down time
Duration of out-of-hospital CPR
Underlying diseases
Electrocardiographic rhythm at the time of initial resuscitation

Table 6. Rates of survival following cardiopulmonary resuscitation in relation to duration of CPR

Study	Survival (%) up to discharge from hospital	
	CPR ≤ 15 min	CPR > 15 min
Adults		
Bedell et al. [21]	56% (27/48)[a]	5% (12/241)
Rozenbaum and Shenkman [7]	35% (9/27)	9% (4/44)
Children		
Gillis et al. [15]	22% (2/9)	0% (0/21)
Nichols et al. [8]	60% (12/20)	16% (4/25)
Zaritsky et al. [16]	NA[b]	0%
	CPR ≤ 30 min	CPR > 30 min
Adults		
Bedell et al. [21]	NA[b]	0% (0/179)
Woog and Torzillo [11]	20% (27/133)	0% (0/35)
Children		
Davies et al. [23]	46% (25/54)	0% (0/13)

[a] Number of patients figure in parentheses.
[b] NA, data not available.

Number of Drugs Administered During CPR

Nichols et al. [8] established a relation between survival and the number of drugs required during CPR in children. Among a group of 21 patients who received more than two doses of epinephrine and bicarbonate, none survived. Gillis et al. [15] reported the same 0% discharge rate in 18 children who received two doses or more of epinephrine. Zaritsky et al. [16] reported no survivors in 31 cardiac arrest victims receiving more than two doses of epinephrine. Failure to establish spontaneous circulation during the time required to administer 2 doses of epinephrine appears to be a very powerful predictor of eventual hospital mortality in children [16]. In certain circumstances, epinephrine and bicarbonate may be detrimental. The β-adrenergic effect of epinephrine may increase myocardial oxygen demand in the fibrillating heart and cerebral metabolic rate if the blood-brain barrier is disrupted [8]. Nonetheless, the relation that exists between the number of drugs and survival is most probably due to the fact that the longer the duration of resuscitation, the more numerous are the drugs used. Although it has not been documented yet in adults, this relation seems to be another proof of the crucial importance of the duration of CPR as a prognostic marker.

Failure to Respond to Prehospital ACLS

Failure to respond to prehospital ACLS is also very highly predictive of death prior to hospital discharge. Kellermann et al. combined their data with the results of seven other authors; they found only ten out of more than 1440 patients (0.69%) to have survived to hospital discharge after arriving in cardiac arrest following prehospital ACLS [34]. Regardless of the factors associated with failure to respond in any given case, non-response to prehospital ACLS must thus be considered as a significant marker of bad prognosis.

Down Time

Down time is defined as the interval of time between the arrest itself and the onset of CPR maneuvers. Survival rates are inversely proportional to down time [32, 33]. Nonetheless, the use of this variable as a predictor of outcome has several problems. Down time is often difficult to document accurately [33]. Moreover, the concept that a normothermic cardiac arrest longer than 4 to 5 minutes cannot be reversed with normal brain function has become debatable. Animals have survived with good brain function after normothermic cardiac arrest of up to 15 minutes [35]. Occasionally, patients have been resuscitated to recovery after normothermic estimated cardiac arrest times of 10 to 15 minutes [35]. "Critical down time" must be better defined, although one should consider that a cardiac arrest of more than 15 minutes without CPR is probably hopeless.

Duration of Out-of-Hospital CPR

Smith et al. reviewed the data on prehospital CPR published from 1970 through 1983 and concluded that prolonged prehospital CPR (more than 30 minutes) is a predictor of poor outcome [36]. The global survival rate of patients with prolonged prehospital CPR was 5.5% (96/1733 patients) [36]. Most people (93/96) resuscitated in the emergency department had relatively short periods of prehospital CPR (less than 30 minutes). Only three patients survived after more than 30 minutes of prehospital CPR, with two of the three survivors either hypothermic or a victim of a cold-water-near-drowning [36].

Underlying Diseases

Survival rates after in-hospital CPR in adults are negatively influenced by the presence of some underlying disease. Pneumonia [7, 21], sepsis [7, 21], hypotension [21], renal failure [7, 21], and cancer [7, 21] are all associated with a very high mortality rate. In children, the response to CPR is also related to the cause of arrest. Although respiratory diseases account for the majority of cardiac arrests in the pediatric population, they have the most favourable prognosis; trauma and sepsis carry a grave prognosis.

Table 7. Survival following CPR in adults according to initial rhythm

Study	Year	Location of arrest[a]	Survival up to discharge	
			VF/VT[b]	BA[c]
Castagna et al. [37]	1974	I	NA[d]	0% (0/60)[e]
Myerbyurg et al. [38]	1980	O	27% (67/244)	0% (0/108)
Bedell et al. [21]	1983	I	27% (26/97)	8% (15/192)
Roth et al. [5]	1984	O	15% (15/98)	3% (3/89)
Woog and Torzillo [11]	1987	I	27% (15/56)	8% (7/89)
Rozenbaum and Shenkman [7]	1988	I	30% (7/23)	9% (3/35)

[a] I, in-hospital; O, out-of-hospital.
[b] VF/VT, ventricular fibrillation/ventricular tachycardia.
[c] BA, bradysystolic arrest (asystole, heart block, electromechanical dissociation, pulseless idioventricular rhythm).
[d] NA, data not available.
[e] Number of patients figure in parentheses.

Initial Rhythm

The initial cardiac rhythm is another predictive variable in determining successful prehospital as well as in-hospital CPR. Adults with ventricular fibrillation or ventricular tachycardia have significantly better survival rates than do patients in asystole, blocks electromechanical dissociation, or idioventricular rhythm (Table 7). This observation also applies to children [19].

Conclusions

More clinical research is needed to evaluate outcome and define accurate predictors of survival after CPR. In the mean time, clinicians must use current data as best as they can to decide when to stop CPR. The decision to terminate CPR must be made by the physician bearing primary responsability for the patient's management during the arrest [31].

CPR should be withhold in patients who are obviously dead. Decapitation, rigor mortis, and evidence of tissue decomposition are usually reliable criteria of death [1]. CPR should not be initiated in case of competent refusal of such treatment by the patient or if do-not-resuscitate orders have been written prior to arrest [1]. When it is realized that CPR was inappropriately initiated, it should be stopped. In addition, we suggest to stop CPR when the probability for survival is almost zero or is exceedingly low. This happens in the following circumstances:

1. after 25–30 minutes or more of CPR without resumption of spontaneous cardiac activity;
2. non-response to prehospital ACLS;

3. brady/asystolic arrest that persits despite attempted myocardial pacing or pharmacologic therapy [31];
4. non-response to more than two doses of epinephrine in a child.

The continuation of maneuvers even in these circumstances may be justified by special considerations, which increase the probability for the resuscitation to be successful, such as hypothermia (below 30–32°C), drug overdose, and uncorrected electrolyte disturbance [31].

We realize that this attitude differs somewhat from published recommendations of the AHA [1]. However, we are convinced that physicians must weigh the anticipated result of further treatment when deciding whether to persist with resuscitative efforts. As Montgomery already mentioned, "the purpose of CPR is the prevention of sudden, unexpected death, not the prolongation of meaningless life. The decision to perform CPR – when, when not to, or how much – remains a difficult one for practitioners ... and involves sensitive and informed decision making at many levels" [39].

References

1. 1985 National Conference on Cardiopulmonary Resuscitation and Emergency Cardiac Care (1986) Standards and Guidelines for Cardiopulmonary Resuscitation and Emergency Cardiac Care. Part VIII: Medicolegal considerations and recommendations. JAMA 255:2979–2984
2. Eliastam M, Duralde T, Martinez F, Schwartz D (1977) Cardiac arrest in the emergency medical service system: guidelines for resuscitation. JACEP 6:525–529
3. Thompson RG, Hallstrom AP, Cobb LA (1979) Bystander-initiated cardiopulmonary resuscitation in the management of ventricular fibrillation. Ann Intern Med 90:737–740
4. Cummins RO, Eisenberg MS, Hallstrom AP, Litwin PE (1985) Survival of out-of-hospital cardiac arrest with early initiation of cardiopulmonary resuscitation. Am J Emerg Med 3:114–118
5. Roth R, Stewart RD, Rogers K, Cannon GM (1984) Out-of-hospital cardiac arrest: factors associated with survival. Ann Emerg Med 13:237–243
6. Stueven H, Troiano P, Thompson B, et al (1986) Bystander/first responder CPR: ten years experience in a paramedic system. Ann Emerg Med 15:707–710
7. Rozenbaum EA, Shenkmann L (1988) Predicting outcome of in-hospital cardiopulmonary resuscitation. Crit Care Med 16:583–586
8. Nichols DG, Kettrick RG, Swedlow DB, Lee S, Passman R, Ludwig S (1986) Factors influencing outcome of cardiopulmonary resuscitation in children. Pediatr Emerg Care 2:1–5
9. Ludwig S, Kettrick RG, Parker M (1983) Pediatric cardiopulmonary resuscitation. A review of 130 cases. Clin Pediatr 23:71–75
10. DeBard ML (1981) Cardiopulmonary resuscitation: analysis of six years' experience and review of the literature. Ann Emerg Med 10:408–416
11. Woog RH, Torzillo PJ (1987) In-hospital cardiopulmonary resuscitation: prospective survey of management and outcome. Anaesth Intens Care 15:193–198
12. Eisenberg M, Bergner L, Hallstrom A (1983) Epidemiology of cardiac arrest and resuscitation in children. Ann Emerg Med 12:672–674
13. Torphy DE, Minter MG, Thompson BM (1984) Cardiorespiratory arrest and resuscitation in children. Am J Dis Child 138:1099–1102
14. Wark H, Overton JH (1984) A pediatric "cardiac arrest" survey. Br J Anaesth 56:1271–1274
15. Gillis J, Dickson D, Rieder M, Steward D, Edmonds J (1986) Results of inpatient pediatric resuscitation. Crit Care Med 14:469–471

16. Zaritsky A, Nadkarni V, Getson P, Kuehl K (1987) CPR in children. Ann Emerg Med 16:1107–1111
17. Longstreth WT, Inui TS, Cobb LA, Copass MK (1983) Neurologic recovery after out-of-hospital cardiac arrest. Ann Intern Med 98 (Part 1) 588–592
18. Rockswold G, Sharma B, Ruiz E, Asinger R, Hodges M, Brieter M (1979) Follow-up of 514 consecutive patients with cardiopulmonary arrest outside the hospital. JACEP 8:216–220
19. Losek JD, Hennes H, Glaeser P, Hendley G, Nelson DB (1987) Prehospital care of the pulseless, nonbreathing pediatric patient. Am J Emerg Med 5:370–374
20. Messert B, Quaglieri CE (1976) Cardiopulmonary resuscitation. Perspectives and problems. Lancet 2:410–411
21. Bedell SE, Delbanco TL, Cook EF, Epstein FH (1983) Survival after cardiopulmonary resuscitation in the hospital. N Engl J Med 309:569–576
22. Lewis JK, Minter MG, Eshelman SJ, Witte MK (1983) Outcome of pediatric resuscitation. Ann Emerg Med 12:297–299
23. Davies CR, Carrigan T, Wright JA, Ahmann PA, Watson C (1987) Neurologic outcome following pediatric resuscitation. J Neurosci Nurs 19:205–210
24. Lund I, Skulberg A (1976) Cardiopulmonary resuscitation by lay people. Lancet 2:702–704
25. Tweed WA, Bristow G, Donen N (1980) Resuscitation from cardiac arrest: assessment of a system providing only basic life support outside of hospital. Can Med Assoc J 122:297–300
26. Gudjonsson H, Baldvinsson E, Oddsson G, et al (1982) Results of attempted cardiopulmonary resuscitation of patients dying suddenly outside the hospital in Reykjavik and the surrounding area, 1976–1979. Acta Med Scand 212:247–251
27. Vertesi L, Wilson L, Glick N (1983) Cardiac arrest: comparison of paramedic and conventional ambulance services. Can Med Assoc J 128:809–813
28. Guzy PM, Pearce ML, Greenfield S (1983) The survival benefit of bystander cardiopulmonary resuscitation in a paramedic served metropolitan area. Am J Public Health 73:766–769
29. Peatfield RC, Sillet RW, Taylor D, McNicol MW (1977) Survival after cardiac arrests in hospital. Lancet 1:1223–1225
30. Wernberg M, Thomassen A (1979) Prognosis after cardiac arrest occurring outside intensive care and coronary units. Acta Anesthesiol Scand 23:69–77
31. Bickell WH, Rice MM, Dellinger RP (1988) Termination of resuscitation. In: Civetta JM, Taylor RW, Kirby RR (eds) Critical care. Lippincott Co, Philadelphia, pp 121–124
32. Brain Resuscitation clinical trial I Study group (1985) Neurologic recovery after cardiac arrest: Effect of duration of ischemia. Crit Care Med 13:930–931
33. Chipman C, Adelman R, Sexton G (1981) Criteria for cessation of CPR in the emergency room. Ann Emerg Med 10:11–17
34. Kellermann AL, Staves DR, Hackmann BB (1988) In-hospital resuscitation following unsuccessful prehospital advanced cardiac life support: "Heroic efforts" or an exercise in futility? Ann Emerg Med 17:589–594
35. Safar P (1989) Cardiopulmonary cerebral resuscitation. In: Shoemaker WC, Ayres S, Grenvik A, Holbrook PR, Thompson WL (eds) Textbook of critical care, 2nd edn. WB Saunders CO, Philadelphia, pp 5–40
36. Smith JP, Bodai B (1985) Guidelines for discontinuing prehospital CPR in the emergency department – A review. Ann Emerg Med 14:1093–1098
37. Castagna J, Weil MH, Shubin H (1974) Factors determining survival in patients with cardiac arrest. Chest 65:527–529
38. Myerburg RJ, Conde CA, Sung RJ, et al (1980) Clinical, electrophysiologic and hemodynamic profile of patients resuscitated from prehospital cardiac arrest. Am J Med 68:568–576
39. Montgomery WH (1986) The 1985 conference on standards and guidelines for cardiopulmonary resuscitation and emergency care. JAMA 255:2990–2991

Teaching CPR for Citizen:
Lessons from a Belgian Experience

L. L. Bossaert, R. A. F. Van Hoeyweghen, and the Scientific Committee of the CPR Campaign "3 Minutes for a Life"

Introduction

In cardiac arrest early initiation of bystander-CPR, before arrival of the Emergency Medical System (EMS) and initiation of Advanced Life Support (ALS), is widely accepted as a determinant of survival. Since the citizen is the most likely potential witness of a cardiac arrest event, this knowledge was a major incentive to train citizens in basic CPR all over the world in small and large scaled courses.

In 1981, a Gallup survey indicated that more than 20% of American citizens had attended a CPR course by that time. In Belgium we have learned from a nationwide telephone inquiry that in 1987 about 13% of adult Belgian citizens had previously attended a CPR course including training on a manikin. Important socio-demographic differences were observed in terms of CPR training level and overall attitude towards CPR and emergency cardiac care. Recently it was suggested that in some systems and structural environments bystander-CPR has probably a less important contribution providing an EMS system where very early ALS and defibrillation are available.

To evaluate the usefulness of teaching CPR to the Belgian citizens we investigated the incidence of bystander-CPR in case of cardiac arrest (CA) and its impact on survival in the Belgian context. In 1983–1987, the Cerebral Resuscitation Study Group of the Belgian Society for Intensive Care analysed 3053 cases of out-of-hospital CA, treated in 7 Belgian EMS systems [3, 8]. In this study on epidemiology and outcome of cardiac arrest in Belgium, it was observed that the majority of the studied cardiac arrests happened at home (69%), in male patients aged > 50 years (76%), and usually during office hours (71%). From this observation, the profile of the individual most likely to be the first witness of a cardiac arrest could be deduced.

In the study population of 3053 out-of-hospital cardiac arrest events, bystander CPR was performed in 33% of recorded cases (n = 998). Cardiac arrest events where bystander-CPR was performed (n = 998) were compared to cardiac arrest events without bystander-CPR (n = 2055) in terms of outcome, time intervals, characteristics of the cardiac arrest-patient and of the bystander. Bystanders providing CPR were laymen in 41% and health care workers in 59%. The use of bystander-CPR was significantly related to patient-related conditions (e.g. age and underlying disease of the CA victim, site where the CA happened, whether the CA event was witnessed or not).

Table 1. Impact on short and long time survival of bystander-CPR in 2274 cases of out-of-hospital cardiac arrest of cardiac origin

	Short term	Long term
Bystander CPR	183[a]	89[b]
(n = 775; 34%)	23.6%	11.5%
No bystander CPR	296	91
(n = 1499; 66%)	19.7%	6.1%

[a] $p < 0.05$; [b] $p < 0.001$.

Comparing early and late outcome in 2274 cases of out-of-hospital CA of cardiac origin, survival was significantly higher if bystander-CPR (B-CPR) was performed (Table 1).

Late survival declined with increasing time to ALS. In CA events where the time to ALS exceeded 8 minutes but was less than 18 minutes, the beneficial effect of bystander-CPR on survival was most significant.

From these and other observations it was concluded that in the Belgian context, where a wide range of time to BLS (9.5 ± 15.2 min; mean $\pm$ SD) and to ALS (18.8 ± 11.7 min; mean $\pm$ SD) is observed, citizen CPR is of high value. Subsequently it was recommended that citizen CPR teaching programs should be stimulated and addressed to both target groups: the potential bystander for immediate help in case of CA and the general public (e. g. school population) for long-term improvement of attitude.

Implementation of the Citizen-CPR Campaign

In 1986–1988 a nationwide citizen CPR campaign was organised in Belgium by the Belgian Heart Association, the Belgian Red Cross and the Belgian Society for Intensive Care. The slogan was "3 minutes for a life". The objective of this citizen CPR teaching program was to instruct in 2 years time at least 100 000 adult citizens in the techniques of basic CPR of the adult cardiac arrest victim, in a strictly standardised single 3-hour course according to the 1986 standards and guidelines for Cardio-Pulmonary Resuscitation and Emergency Cardiac Care of the American Heart Association (AHA).

It was advised by the scientific steering committee to audit the CPR campaign in a detailed evaluation program. The objectives of this evaluation project were:

- to study the socio-demographic characteristics of CPR-courses, instructors and trainees;
- to analyse the immediate teaching results and how they were influenced;
- to analyse the degree of retention of the acquired knowledge and skills.

Teaching Methods

The educational package was realised according to the 1986 standards and guidelines for CPR and ECC of the AHA.

Uniformity of teaching methods was obtained by a strictly standardized teaching protocol, to be used by every instructor, and consisting of a set of teaching manual, flip charts, poster, training manikin and evaluation forms. Teaching methods were described previously [4].

Evaluation forms were generated for each individual trainee (n = 102692), instructor (n = 1292) and course (n = 9930), describing knowledge and attitude of the trainee towards CPR prior to the course, socio-demographic characteristics of courses, instructors and trainees, teaching results expressed as cognitive score and practical skills at the end of the course.

Testing Methods

Theoretical knowledge was scored by 14 multiple choice questions, retrieved from the AHA test data base, and selected in such a way that all major aspects of adult basic life support were covered.

Practical skills were evaluated using a scoring system where all items, that were not or incorrectly performed by the trainee during the final practical test, had to be scored by the instructor. For analysis, this practical test was reduced to a 32-point score, allocating different weights to different errors.

A randomly selected study sample of 17491 trainees was used for analysis.

The subjective method used for testing practical skills was validated by comparing the obtained scores to the more objective test results of a simultaneously recorded stripchart on a Recording Resusci-Anne (n = 138 test individuals) or the display of a Skillmeter Resusci-Anne (n = 114 test individuals). Sensitivity, specificity and positive predictive values were calculated. Positive predictive value of testing practical performance using the subjective scoring method was 78-95% compared to recording manikin and 79-100% compared to Skillmeter-

Table 2. Validation of methods used for testing practical skills. Comparison of subjective method to recording Manikin in 138 test subjects. A test with ≥ 10% incorrectly performed items is considered as a "fail" score

		Sensitivity	Specificity	Positive predictive value
External chest compression	depth	44	79	89
	place	90	38	93
	rate	40	78	78
Ventilation	volume	42	72	83
	rate	37	82	84
Timing		43	75	95

Table 3. Validation of methods used for testing practical skills. Comparison of subjective method to Skillmeter score in 114 test subjects. A test with $\geq 10\%$ incorrectly performed items is considered as a "fail" score

		Sensitivity	Specificity	Positive predictive value
External chest compression	number	93	25	94
	depth	19	95	88
	place	65	89	95
	frequency	88	43	87
	overall correct	19	100	100
Ventilation	number	69	50	97
	volume	25	87	79
	overall correct	34	93	89

scores (Tables 2 and 3). This finding indicated that in mass citizen-CPR instructions a subjective scoring system can be used effectively to detect major errors.

Progression of the Campaign

Prior to the start of the campaign "3 minutes for a life", and in perspective of uniformity of teaching and testing, all participating instructors were trained for their job in a one-day instruction. Two types of instructors were recruited: "monitors" being experienced first aid instructors (mainly Red Cross instructors), and "animators", being volunteering doctors, nurses and teachers. After 2 years, 9930 courses were given by 1292 instructors, and 102 692 citizens were trained.

Looking at the penetration of the campaign in the different districts and provinces of the country, expressed as numbers of trainees related to the population density, we observed an equal distribution of the number of trainees over the country, showing no differences between the Flemish and French communities (Fig. 1). However some interesting differences in the type of instructors and courses were found comparing both communities, reflecting structural and organizational differences: class sizes were significantly larger in the Flemish community; significantly less doctors and nurses participated in the French community (Fig. 2).

Profile of the CPR-Course, CPR-Instructor, CPR-Trainee

Analyzing a randomly selected representative study sample of 17 491 trainees it was possible to describe the kind of target group reached by the citizen-CPR campaign, the motivation of the trainees, the characteristics of courses and instructors, and the influence of these variables on the acquired psychomotor skills.

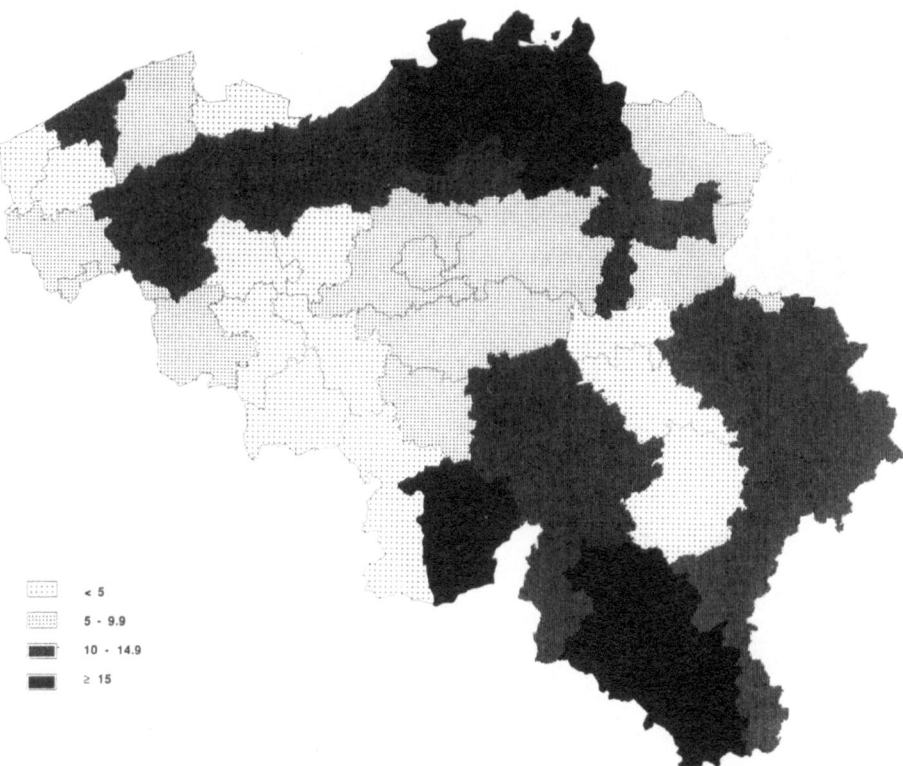

Fig. 1. Belgium and its districts. Distribution of CPR-trainees per 1000 inhabitants during the citizen-CPR campaign "3 minutes for a life"

This description was a valuable source of information for reorientation of promotional efforts throughout the course of the actual campaign, and for the design of subsequent teaching programs.

Motivation (Fig. 3)

The motivation to attend a CPR-course was highly related to socio-demographic characteristics of the trainee. General education (38.2%) and moral obligation (41.8%) were the most frequent incentives. Having a family member with a heart disease (mean 2.9%) and previously witnessing a cardiac arrest (mean 2.3%) was a motivation to attend a CPR course which was highly influenced by age and social status of the trainee: in trainees aged > 60 years these figures were respectively 11.3 and 4.5%, indicating a more rational motivation in elderly course attendants. Moreover, attitude towards emergency cardiac care (e.g. reaction in case of witnessing a cardiac arrest: active personal help or find somebody else to help) was significantly influenced by age, sex, social and demographic status of the trainee.

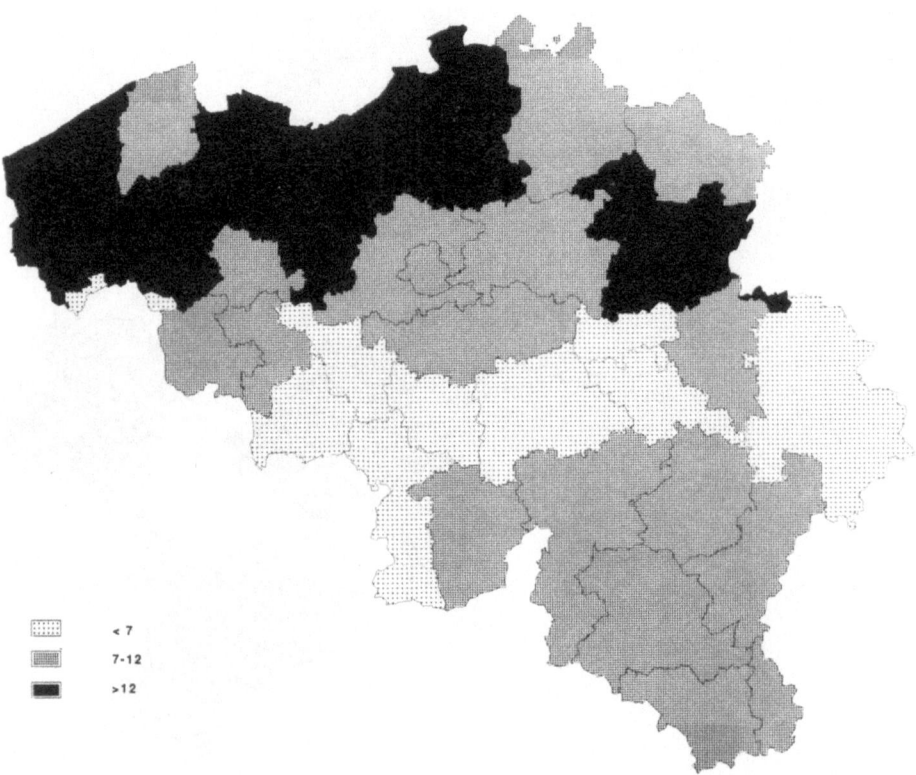

Fig. 2. Belgium and its districts. Distribution of CPR-class sizes during the citizen-CPR campaign "3 minutes for a life"

Profile of the CPR-Trainee

The individual attending a CPR course was usually young (71% ≤ 40 years), and had a high previous knowledge of "first aid" (38%). Most were students (32%) or employees (31%). Study level was high: 65% attended at least upper high school. Trainees belonging to working class (13%), housewives (10%) and retired people (4%) were underrepresented.

Regional and socio-demographic differences were observed in terms of characteristics of the courses and the instructors, but characteristics of the trainees were similar in the different regions of the country. In the Flemish speaking community (Northern part of Belgium), mean class size was 12.7 trainees/course, 32% of courses were organized in schools; 54% of courses was given by less experienced animators; 34% of instructors were doctors or nurses and 72% of instructors was <40 years of age. In the French speaking community (Southern part of the country), mean class size was 6.7 trainees/course, courses were given in schools in 19%, by more experienced monitors in 63%, being older (47% ≥ 40 years) and less doctors and nurses (21%).

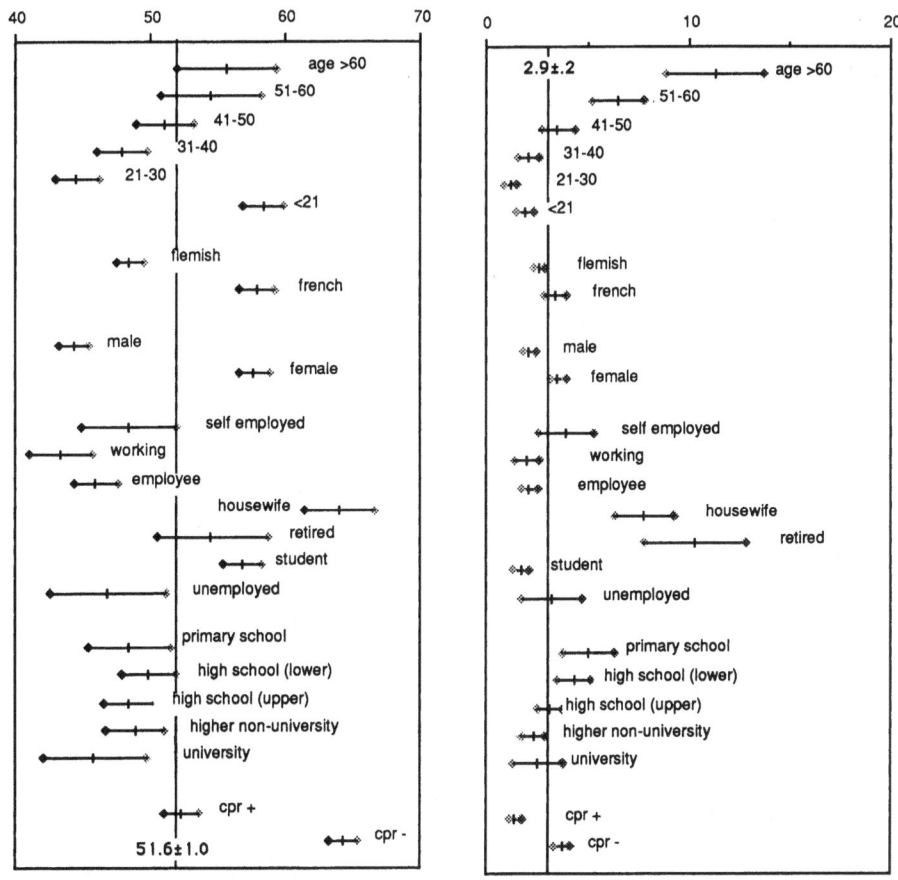

Fig. 3. Motivation and attitude of the CPR-trainee according to socio-demographic characteristics: age, language, sex, profession, study level, previous CPR-teaching (yes = +, no = −). Values are expressed as mean values ±95% confidence limits. A difference is considered as significant if 95% confidence limits do not include the overall mean value

Teaching Results (Table 4)

According to the "adaptive learning principle" (i.e. "mastery learning"), the teaching objective was to reach a good level of theoretical knowledge and practical skills (i.e. a score of ≥80% in both tests) in most (≥80%) of the trainees. Therefore, evaluating the test results, the limits for a "pass" or "fail" score were set at 80%.

Theoretical test results were mainly influenced by characteristics of the trainee. Statistical analysis (contingency table, analysis of variance) indicated that theoretical test results were higher in class size of 6–15 trainees, in trainees who previously attended a CPR course, with a study level of at least high school, aged 21–60 years, employees. Age <21 and >60 years, lower study level, ab-

Table 4. Influence of different variables on teaching results in a study sample of 17 491 trainees. Characteristics of CPR-courses, instructors and trainees are indicated as % of the total number. Theoretical (T) and practical (P) teaching results are indicated as % of trainees reaching a "pass" score (T ≥ 80% and P ≥ 80%). The significance level is indicated per category of variables

		[%]	T ≥ 80%	P ≥ 80%
1. CPR-Course				
Class size	1–5	7	77[c]	74[c]
	6–10	39	73	72
	11–15	41	74	75
	> 15	13	67	77
Applicant	association	31	71[c]	71[c]
	work	21	72	77
	school	27	73	77
	open	21	76	75
Time	morning	26	74[c]	77[b]
	afternoon	36	71	74
	evening	38	74	74
2. CPR-Instructor				
Age	> 60	4	75[b]	67[c]
	51–60	12	74	78
	41–50	17	73	73
	31–40	30	72	73
	21–30	36	74	76
	< 21	1	65	72
Sex	male	52	71[c]	72[c]
	female	48	75	77
Profession	doctor	5	71[c]	87[c]
	nurse	32	76	77
	teacher	20	73	76
	other	42	71	69
Function	monitor	57	71[c]	73[c]
	animator	43	75	76
CPR-teaching experience	≤ 5 course	29	74[c]	74[ns]
	6–15	28	73	75
	16–25	14	72	74
	> 25 courses	29	72	75
3. CPR-Trainee				
Age	> 60	5	57[c]	60[c]
	51–60	9	65	65.5
	41–50	5	73	74
	31–40	19	76	76
	21–30	25	81	77
	< 21	26	72	77
Sex	male	47	72[b]	76[c]
	female	53	74	73
Profession	self-employed	6	74[c]	72[c]
	working	13	68	72
	employee	31	79	78
	housewife	10	69	68
	retired	4	56	64
	student	32	73	76
	unemployed	4	75	69

Table 4 (continued)

		[%]	$T \geq 80\%$	$P \geq 80\%$
Study level	primary	10	55[c]	65[c]
	high school (lower)	25	66	72
	high school (upper)	37	77	76
	higher non university	21	83	78
	university	7	83	78
Previous CPR	yes	38	77[c]	76[c]
	no	62	71	73
Language	Flemish	66	73[ns]	76[c]
	French	34	73	70

[ns] Not significant; [a] $p < 0.05$; [b] $p < 0.001$; [c] $p < 0.0001$.

sence of previous CPR-training, excessive class sizes of > 15 trainees were more frequently associated with a "fail" score ($p < 0.001$).

Practical test results were more influenced by characteristics of the instructor: a "pass" score was more easily obtained by doctors and nurses ($p < 0.001$). A "fail" score was more frequently associated with instructors aged < 21 or > 60 years. Interestingly, monitors ($= 57\%$) reached the teaching objectives ("pass" score) in 71% of their trainees for the theoretical test and in 73% for the practical test; for trainees instructed by animators ($= 43\%$), these figures were 75% and 76%, respectively. Similar results were obtained subdividing instructors according to their teaching experience (≤ 5, 6–15, 16–25, > 25 CPR courses) and profession (doctor, nurse, teacher, other). These results indicate that in mass CPR training less experienced but well-motivated animators can obtain equally good teaching results than experienced monitors, providing a well-standardized educational program.

Retention of CPR-Psycho-Motor Skills

The retention of the acquired CPR practical skills and theoretical knowledge after a standardized single 3-hour course was also evaluated. At 3 time intervals after the initial course a selected sample of CPR trainees was retested: after 6 months ($n = 124$), 12 months ($n = 81$), 24 months ($n = 98$), and after a refresher course ($n = 303$). The test population consisted of students, police officers and employees.

Table 5. Retention of acquired psycho-motor skills 6, 12 and 24 months after the initial CPR-course. Results are expressed as % of trainees reaching a "pass" score (test result $\geq 80\%$)

Interval (months)	0	6	12	24	Refresher
Number	144	124	81	98	303
Knowledge (% $\geq 80\%$)	90	89	82	76	–
Skills (% $\geq 80\%$)	94	81	68	54	91

The method for evaluating retention of practical skills and theoretical knowledge was identical during the initial test and during the retention tests. Theoretical knowledge remained excellent after 6 and 12 months. Practical skills however declined rapidly: after 12 months only 68% of trainees could obtain a "pass" score, and after 24 months this figure dropped to an unacceptable level of 54%. However, after a short refresher course the initial levels of knowledge and skills were restored (Table 5).

Some Conclusions and Lessons

The quantitative objectives of the Belgian citizen-CPR campaign have been reached: in 2 years time 102 692 trainees were instructed by 1292 instructors in 9930 courses.

Some significant regional differences in the type of CPR-courses and instructors is observed, indicating some structural and organizational differences in the Flemish and French community. However, no regional differences in the type of CPR-trainees were observed.

In this untargeted large scaled citizen CPR campaign mostly "easy target groups" were reached (young, student, employee, well-educated). To reach the primary "difficult target groups" (housewife and elderly family members of cardiac patients, retired, working class), representing the large majority of the population, but above all the potential bystander of a cardiac arrest event, specific social marketing techniques and specific teaching methods are required.

To reach this large number of trainees, less experienced "animators" were needed. Teaching objectives (an immediate "pass" score in $\geq 80\%$ of trainees) were reached as well by experienced first aid instructors as by less experienced but highly motivated animators, providing a strictly standardised educational lay-out. Theoretical teaching results are mainly influenced by socio-demographic characteristics of the trainee; practical test results are primarily influenced by characteristics of the instructor.

There is a linear decline of practical CPR-skills, most markedly after 12 and 24 months. However after a short refresher course the initial levels of knowledge and skills were restored. Therefore, to maintain good knowledge and skills a short refresher CPR course is advised between 12 and 24 months after the initial CPR course.

Acknowledgement: This evaluation programme was realised with the major help of M. Hap (Centre Universitaire de Charleroi), H. Meulemans and E. Van Hove (Department Social Sciences, University Antwerp) and of the members of the steering committee of the campaign, and was supported by research grants of the Laerdal Foundation for Acute Medicine, the Fondation Bekales, the ICI and BYK companies.

References

1. American Heart Association (1986) Standards and guidelines for cardiopulmonary resuscitation and emergency cardiac care. JAMA 255:2841–3044
2. American Heart Association (1989) Basic life support instructors manual. Dallas, USA
3. Bossaert L, Van Hoeyweghen R, The Cerebral Resuscitation Study Group (1989) Bystander CPR in out-of-hospital cardiac arrest. Resuscitation 17:S55–S69
4. Bossaert L (1988) Teaching citizen-CPR: a Belgian experience. In: Vincent JL (ed) Update in intensive care and emergency medicine, vol. 5. Springer, Berlin Heidelberg New York Tokyo, pp 455–461
5. Cummins R, Eisenberg M, Hallstrom A, Litwin P (1985) Survival of out-of-hospital cardiac arrest with early initiation of CPR. Am J Emerg Med 3:114–119
6. Cummins R, Eisenberg M (1985) Prehospital cardiopulmonary resuscitation: is it effective? JAMA 253:2408–2412
7. Mandel L, Cobb L (1982) Initial and long-term competency of citizens trained in CPR. Emerg Hlth Serv Quart 1(3):49–63
8. Mullie A, Lewi P, Van Hoeyweghen R, The Cerebral Resuscitation Study Group (1989) Pre-arrest conditions and final outcome of CPR. Resuscitation 17:S11–S21
9. Stueven H, Troiano P, Thompson J, et al (1986) Bystander/first responder CPR: Ten years experience in a paramedic system. Ann Emerg Med 15:707–710
10. Stueven H (1989) Prehospital CPR: a review in perspective. Resuscitation 17:S71–S77

References

Cerebral Crisis

Cerebral Cortex

Pathophysiological Mechanisms and Therapeutic Aspects in Stroke and Ischemic Brain Injury

S. E. Gisvold

Introduction

The brain represents 2% of the body weight, but is responsible for 20% of total body oxygen consumption in the resting situation. With no stores of oxygen and a low capillary density, the brain is critically dependent on a continuous and adequate supply. Things happen rapidly if the supply is suddenly shut off: the patients will be unconscious in less than 10 s and the EEG will be isoelectric in 10–20 s. After about 5 min, stores of high energy phosphates are gone. Thus, it is not surprising that the brain is vulnerable to oxygen deprivation, with some areas being more susceptible than others, areas of so-called selective vulnerability.

Ischemia of the central nervous system is a commonly occurring clinical problem which we are faced with daily in our clinical work (Table 1). It is more than cardiac arrest and stroke. It is frequently said that brain ischemia is something you face *after* it has happened, and that therapeutic possibilities therefore are limited. This is not correct. We often know about it, or should at least suspect it before it happens. This is certainly the case for cardiac surgery, carotid artery surgery, cerebral aneurysm surgery, during the evolution of a stroke, in the post-injury phase of head injuries, and during extensive aortic surgery. The fact that many of these situations with incomplete CNS ischemia may be anticipated, should call for a more active therapeutic attitude in everyday clinical life. We could start protective/therapeutic measures prophylactically in many of these situations if it became common practice to think about it.

Table 1. Ischemia of the central nervous system.
Clinical situations where the oxygen supply may be reduced

- Stroke and transient ischemic attacks
- Subarachnoid hemorrhage: Before, during and after surgery
- Carotid artery surgery
- Prolonged cardiopulmonary bypass during heart surgery
- Head injuries
- Cardiac arrest: During arrest and recirculation
- Aortic surgery: Spinal cord ischemia
- Severe hypoxia/hypoxemia
- Severe hypoperfusion/shock states

Therapies which are being attempted in CNS ischemia are based on increased understanding of the pathophysiology. There are some excellent review articles on this topic [1–3]. The objective of the present article is to give a brief overview on the most important pathophysiologic changes during and after ischemia. The increased understanding has opened interesting therapeutic avenues and I am going to try to link the different pathophysiologic changes with possible therapies. The point I am trying to make is that future therapy in brain ischemia will consist of a combination of therapies aimed at different aspects of the pathophysiologic disturbance (Table 2). It is highly unlikely that one single agent or treatment modality will stand out as a kind of "penicillin" for the brain.

Oxygen Supply/Demand Mismatch

In situations of brain ischemia, we have by definition a mismatch between oxygen supply and demand, globally or in parts of the brain. The brain has an ability to increase oxygen extraction from the blood as the cerebral blood flow (CBF) decreases, thus postponing the potential disaster. However, at CBF levels below 20 ml/100 g/min dramatic EEG changes take place, signalling that the brain is suffering. When CBF reaches a level around 10 ml/100 g/min, there are signs of massive membrane failure indicating imminent breakdown of cellular integrity [4].

Although there is much controversy regarding therapy in brain ischemia, all investigators agree on the basic principle of trying to improve the O_2-supply/O_2-demand ratio [5].

In this context, hypothermia and barbiturates have been highlighted by investigators for many years as methods for decreasing cerebral oxygen demand and restoring a better supply/demand ratio. Hypothermia decreases cerebral metabolism by 5–7% degree Celsius [6], while barbiturates may lower $CMRO_2$ by up

Table 2. Pathophysiology of cerebral ischemia and potential corresponding therapies

Pathophysiology	Potential corresponding therapy
Oxygen supply/demand mismatch	Hypothermia, barbiturates
Membrane failure, Ca^{++} overload	Ca^{++} antagonists Membrane stabilizers
Impaired microcirculation	Hemodilution, BP elevation Ca^{++} antagonists
Excess neurotransmitter release	Glutamate receptor antagonists, α_e-adrenergic antagonist
Tissue acidosis	Avoid hyperglycemia
Free oxygen radicals	Scavengers
Brain edema	Osmotic dehydration
Spreading depression	Glutamate receptor antagonists Membrane stabilizers Ca^{++} antagonists

to 50% [7]. However, there may be different mechanisms at work. Barbiturates probably lowers only that part of the metabolism which is linked to active function as reflected by the EEG, while hypothermia seem to lower all aspects of cellular metabolism including the part linked to maintaining cellular integrity [8]. This may in part explain why barbiturates so far has failed to show a protective effective in complete anoxia [9], while there may be beneficial effects in incomplete/focal ischemia as indicated by the study of Nussmeier et al. in patients on cardiopulmonary bypass [10].

Hypothermia has an undisputed protective effect during cerebral hypoxia. Yet, its application in everyday clinical work is laboursome, and not often used, except during heart surgery. However, there are indications that even very moderate hypothermia may be protective in situations with incomplete cerebral ischemia [11].

Membrane Failure and Disturbed Ionic Homeostasis

During ischemia, oxygen, glucose, and high energy phosphates are rapidly depleted, and ionic homeostasis is disturbed [1, 2]. Maintenance of normal ionic equilibrium is an energy demanding process, and with energy failure, ionic gradients can no longer be maintained: Na^+ moves into the cell, K^+ moves out, and when the extracellular K^+ has reached a certain level, a sharp increase is seen in intracellular Ca^{++}. This is mainly caused by Ca^{++} inflow from the extracellular space through voltage sensitive channels which open in response to depolarization. However, some of the intracellular increase also comes from intracellular storage sites (e.g. endoplasmatic reticulum).

As is well known, Ca^{++} is incriminated as one of the key factors in promoting ischemic cell death [3]. The increase in intracellular Ca^{++} also seems to affect the microcirculation, partly by causing vasospasm and by decreasing red cell deformability. The net effect is an impaired microcirculation and reduced tissue oxygen supply. This might add to the deleterious cellular effect of Ca-entry triggered by ischemia.

Many therapeutic trials with Ca-antagonists have been done. Among the different Ca-antagonists, the dihydro-pyridins appear to be well tested and offers some promise [12, 13]. Clinical studies have also been done in subarachnoid hemorrhage and stroke with apparently promising results [14, 15]. It is still uncertain, however, whether the beneficial effects of Ca-antagonists are due to improved blood flow, or strictly a cellular effect independent of flow improvements [12].

Neurotransmitters

Neurotransmitters have received growing attention as important factors in the development of neuronal demage in ischemia and hypoglycemia. Among these, the amino acid neurotransmitter *glutamate* has received considerable attention lately. Excessive release (and possibly reduced uptake) of glutamate takes place during ischemia and may exert an excitatory or toxic effect, promoting cell death. Glutamate and aspartate are particularly abundant as neurotransmitters in areas of the brain which are selectively vulnerable to ischemia, such as the CA1 layer in the hippocampus.

Activation of the N-methyl D-aspartate (NMDA) postsynaptic receptor by glutamate is especially implicated in ischemic cell damage. Interestingly, activation of this receptor also promotes calcium entry into the cell [3]. Thus the calcium ion again seems to have a key position, although its entry is by another type of channels, a receptor operated channel in contrast to the voltage sensitive channels which I mentioned above.

It has also been found that the excess release of glutamate transmitter is a threshold phenomenon, linked to CBF. In a recent study of graded cerebral ischemia by Shimada et al., glutamate was found to increase when CBF fell below 20 ml/min [18]. This is the same CBF level were the EEG normally starts to deteriorate. Thus, it seems likely that this mechanism may be at work in moderate incomplete ischemia, such as experienced in the penumbra zone of a cerebral infarct.

A number of therapeutic trials have been done with glutamate receptor antagonists, the most well known being MK801, which is a non-competative NMDA-receptor antagonist. Based on animal studies, the picture appears promising regarding incomplete or focal cerebral ischemia [19]. There also seems to be an additive effect if one combines an NMDA receptor antagonist with a calcium antagonist which blocks the voltage sensitive calcium channels, two different ways of blocking calcium entry into the cell. However, when it comes to complete brain anoxia or very severe incomplete ischemia, results so far seem largely negative [20].

Neurotransmitters in the ascending noradrenergic system originating in the locus coeruleus may also be important. In a recent investigation, Gustavson et al. found an α_2-receptor antagonist to protect against ischemic damage in a rat model of temporary incomplete ischemia [21].

Spreading Depression

Another interesting phenomenon is the so-called spreading depression (SD), which may be triggered by ischemia or trauma [3]. It is a kind of propagated membrane disturbance/depolarization which may spread over the cortical surface by a kind of domino mechanism. This may be caused by activation of an unspecific conductance mechanism with extracellular K^+ and glutamate as possible mediators. Although this mechanism is probably a transient one, it may be involved in post-traumatic and post-ischemic worsening of injury if a sufficient area is energy compromised and SD is triggered repeatedly.

Hyperglycemia/Acidosis

Acidosis develops during ischemia. With more sugar available, the acidosis gets worse [1-3]. At a certain level of brain tissue lactic acidosis there is a sharp increase in neuronal death. Hyperglycemia has been shown to substantially worsen neurologic function after ischemia in a variety of different insults [22]. It is interesting that this effect seems to be important even with very moderately elevated blood glucose levels [23]. This may explain why in some experiments a trockle of blood flow seems to worsen neurologic deficit compared to a situation of no flow at all.

Although it seems clear that a low pH triggers increased cell death, it is not clear by what mechanism this effect is executed. It has been speculated that acidosis promotes formation of free oxygen radicals, thereby accelerating lipid peroxidation and cell destruction. A recent study by Rehncrona et al. seems to support this idea [24]. Interestingly, they find that acidosis due to lactic acid accumulation is significantly worse than acidosis induced by CO_2. Possibly, the effect of lactic acid is caused by dissocation of catalytic iron from proteins of the transferrin type. Recently, studies have been done with a rapidly acting intracellular buffer, which improves intracellular pH more rapidly than sodium bicarbonate. However, in spite of this, there is no difference in the recovery of neurologic function [25]. However, the deleterious effects of hyperglycemia in brain ischemia is well documented, and many neurosurgical centers today avoid the use of sugar solutions in situations where the whole brain or parts of the brain may be subjected to ischemia as for example during aneurysm surgery, carotid artery surgery, and other situations with a compromised brain.

Hypoperfusion/No-reflow

During focal or incomplete cerebral ischemia, there is often an area of dense/complete ischemia surrounded by a so-called penumbra, with some but reduced blood flow [4]. After complete anoxia where circulation is restored, we often have multifocal areas in the brain with very limited or no-reflow, like multiple focal ischemic areas, in spite of a normal systemic circulation. There may be many reasons for this phenomenon, such as obstruction of parent vessels, clotting, red cell sludging, vasospasm, and pericapillary edema. It is likely that an impaired microcirculation may worsen the initial injury in focal and global ischemia [26].

Rheologic and pharmacologic measures have been tried in order to improve cerebral circulation [26]. A number of studies indicate that a high hematocrit predisposes for stroke and may worsen the outcome [27]. Data from the Framingham study have had a strong influence in promoting this view. Hemodilution is in many places a routine part of the therapy in ischemic stroke, and there are indications that this may reduce infarct size. From patients with subarachnoid hemorrhage and vasospasm, there is some support for the use of hypervolemia and blood pressure elevations in order to improve microcirculation and clinical outcome.

Pharmacologically, the Ca-antagonists of the dihydropyridine type have been shown to improve cerebral blood flow in focal as well as global ischemia [12, 13]. However, it is still debated whether the beneficial effects of nimodipine are related to flow improvement at all.

Oxygen Radicals

There is a growing body of evidence that the oxygen radicals are somehow involved in the pathophysiology of CNS injury post-ischemia. These radicals are formed when at least some oxygen is present, such as during focal/incomplete ischemia or during recirculation after complete anoxia [1–3]. Free oxygen radicals have an unpaired electrone in an outer orbital, they are normally produced in small amounts by univalent reduction of O_2 to water. During ischemia, radicals are produced in large amounts as a bi-product in the prostaglandin biosynthesis and during breakdown of ATP. They are highly reactive substances and may cause tissue destruction, mainly by lipid peroxydation and by disturbing Ca homeostasis. The body has a normal defense system against free oxygen radicals, so-called scavengers such as superoxide dismutase (SOD) and catalase. Experimental studies with myocardial ischemia indicate that therapy with scavengers may limit the damage. In brain ischemia, results have so far been largely negative [28]. However, a new type of scavengers have recently been developed, the 21-aminosteroids. These substances are derived from glucocorticoids, but are almost devoid of glucocorticoid action. However, they have an ability to limit lipid peroxidation induced by free radicals. Therapeutic trials have been done in experimental focal ischemia [29] as well as global ischemia [30] with very promising results. The same authors also indicate that post-ischemic hypoperfusion and edema may be beneficially influenced by these drugs. To my knowledge, human trials have so far not been done.

Ischemic Brain Edema

The development of edema is common after tissue trauma or ischemia. However, there are different types of edema, and the magnitude and importance of the edema also varies, depending on the depth and duration of ischemia and the quality of reperfusion [31].

The two main types of edema are: cytotoxic and vasogenic. In addition, brain swelling can be due to vascular congestion, i.e. increased blood volume in the brain. This is often and wrongly talked about as brain edema. The two most common causes of brain swelling are hypoxemia and hypercapnia, which may cause maximal dilatation of cerebral vessels and increased brain volume.

Cytotoxic edema is an early event in severe cellular hypoxia, caused by sodium and water influx secondary to energy failure and impaired membrane function. The cytotoxic edema is also called "dry" edema, since in its pure form it represents a shift of fluid from the extracellular to the intracellular space, a dehydrated interstitium, and unchanged total brain water and brain bulk.

However, if the ischemia insult is severe enough to disrupt the blood brain barrier (BBB), extravasation of fluid may occur, leading to vasogenic edema and then usually an increase in total brain water and brain volume. However, the blood brain barrier is relatively resistant and it is generally thought that ischemia must be severe and long-lasting to disrupt the BBB. In a recent study from the cerebral edema research group in London, rats were subjected to 15 and 30 min of temporary global ischemia. The authors found a transiently increased permeability of the BBB to small molecules, but no sign of protein extravasation. At 24 hours post-ischemia, the situation was normalized [32].

The blood pressure during recirculation and the degree of metabolic recovery may also influence the development of edema and the integrity of the BBB. Besides, edema development may not reach its maximum until 2–4 days after an ischemic episode, and it is often very unpredictable.

Cerebral edema may be worth attacking from a therapeutic point of view, partly because cellular function is impaired by intracellular edema, and partly because intracranial pressure (ICP) may be raised due to the increased brain volume. However, there is no universal agreement as to the place for specific anti-edema therapy in ischemic brain insults. It is often felt that if edema is severe enough to cause dangerous increase in ICP, it probably reflects very severe and widespread damage which is unlikely to be influenced beneficially by anti-edema therapy.

Conclusion

Our knowledge concerning the pathophysiology of brain ischemia has increased tremendously. This article merely touches the surface and presents some of the important aspects of this complex picture. Therapeutically new potential avenues are opened up. Although the general principal of improving the ratio of oxygen supply to demand still applies, new data on the role of calcium, neurotransmitters, oxygen radical scavengers, and avoidance of hyperglycemia are exciting and promising. Although therapeutic possibilities in brain ischemia are still limited, there is room for optimism. It is increasingly clear that future therapy in brain ischemia will be a multifaceted one, a combination of single drugs and treatment modalities "tailored" by the increased pathophysiologic understanding (Table 2).

References

1. Siesjö BK (1981) Cell damage in the brain: A speculative synthesis. J Cereb Blood Flow Metabol 1:155–185
2. Raichle ME (1983) The pathophysiology of brain ischemia. Ann Neurol 13:2–10
3. Siesjö BK, Bengtsson F (1989) Calcium fluxes, calcium antagonists, and calcium related pathology in brain ischemia. Hypoglycemia, and spreading depression: A unifying hypothesis. J Cereb Blood Flow Metabol 9:127–140
4. Symon L (1985) Flow thresholds in brain ischemia and the effect of drugs. Br J Anaesth 57:34–43
5. Gisvold SE, Steen PA (1985) Drug therapy in brain ischemia. Br J Anaesth 57:96–109
6. Rosomoff HL (1956) The effects of hypothermia on the physiology of the nervous system. Surgery Aug:328–337

7. Michenfelder JD, Theye RA (1973) Cerebral protection by thiopental during hypoxia. Anesthesiology 39:510-517
8. Astrup J (1982) Energy requiring cell functions in the ischemic brain. J Neurosurg 56:482-497
9. Brain resuscitation clinical trial I study group (1986) Randomized clinical study of thiopental loading in comatose survivors of cardac arrest. N Engl J Med 314:397-403
10. Nussmeier NA, Ralund C, Slogoff S (1986) Neuropsychiatric complications after cardiopulmonary bypass. Cerebral protection by a barbiturate. Anesthesiology 64:165-170
11. Berntmann L, Welsh SA, Harp JR (1981) Cerebral protective effects of lowgrade hypothermia. Anesthesiology 55:495-499
12. Meyer FB, Anderson RE, Yaksh TL, Sundt TA (1986) Effect of nimodipine on intracellular brain pH, cortical blood flow, and EEG in experimental focal cerebral ischemia. J Neurosurg 64:617-626
13. Steen PA, Gisvold SE, Milde JH, et al (1985) Nimodipine improves outcome when given after complete cerebral ischemia in primates. Anesthesiology 62:406-414
14. Öhman J, Heiskanen O (1988) Effect of nimodipine on the outcome after aneurysmal subarachnoid hemorrhage and surgery. J Neurosurg 69:683-686
15. Gelmers HJ, Gorter K, de Weert CJ, Wiezer HJA (1988) A controlled trial in acute ischemic stroke. N Engl J Med 318:203-207
16. Wieloch T (1985) Neurochemical correlates to selective neuronal vulnerability. Prog Brain Res 63:69-85
17. Meldrum B (1985) Possible therapeutic application of antagonists of excitatory amino acid neurotransmitters. Clin Sci 68:113-122
18. Shimada N, Graf R, Rosner G, Wakayama A, George CP, Heiss W-D (1989) Ischemic flow thresholds for extracellular glutamate increase in cat cortex. J Cereb Blood Flow Metabol 9:603-606
19. Ozyurt E, Graham DI, Woodruff GN, McCulloch J (1988) Protective effect of the glutamate antagonist MK 801 in focal cerebral ischemia in the cat. J Cereb Blood Flow Metabol 8:138-143
20. Lanier WL, Perkins WJ, Karlsson BR, et al (1989) Effect of the excitatory amino acid antagonist NK 801 on cerebral injury following complete ischemia in primates. J Cereb Blood Flow Metabol 9 (suppl 1):S 744
21. Gustafson I, Miyauchi Y, Wieloch T (1989) Post-ischemic administration of idazoxan, an α-2 adrenergic receptor antagonist, decrease neuronal damage in the rat brain. J Cereb Blood Flow Metabol 9:171-174
22. Myers RE (1979) Lactic acid accumulation as cause of brain edema and cerebral necrosis resulting from oxygen deprivation. In: Korobkin R, Guilleminault G (eds) Advances in perinatal neurology. New York Spectrum Publishers, pp 85-114
23. Lanier W, Stangeland KJ, Scheitauer BW, Milde JH, Michenfelder JD (1987) The effects of dextrose infusion and head position on neurologic outcome after complete cerebral ischemia in primates. Anesthesiology 66:39-48
24. Rehncrona S, Nielsen Hauge S, Siesjö BK (1989) Enhancement of iron catalyzed free radical formation by acidosis in brain homogenates: Difference in effect by lactic acid and CO_2. J Cereb Blood Flow Metabol 9:65-70
25. Rosenberg JM, Martin GB, Paradis A, et al (1989) Effect of CO_2 and non CO_2 generating buffers on return of brain function and phosphate metabolism after global ischemia. J Cereb Blood Flow Metabol 9 (suppl 1):S 649
26. Fischer EG, Ames A III (1972) Studies on mechanism of impairment of cerebral circulation following ischemia: Effect of hemodilution and perfusion pressure. Stroke 3:538-542
27. Harrison MJG, Kendall BE, Pollock S, Marshall J (1981) Effect of haematocrit on carotic stenosis and cerebral infarction. Lancet 2:114-115
28. Forsmann M, Fleischer JE, Milde JH, Steen PA, Michenfelder JD (1988) Superoxide dismutase and catalase failed to improve neurologic outcome after complete cerebral ischemia in the dog. Acta Anaesth Scand 32:152-155
29. Natale JE, Schott RJ, Hall ED, Braughler JM, D'Alcey LG (1988) The 21-aminosteroid U74006F reduces systemic lipid peroxidation, improves neurologic function and reduces mortality after cardiopulmonary arrest in dogs. Stroke 19:1371-1378

30. Hall ED, Pazara KE, Braughler JN (1988) The 21-aminosteroid lipid peroxidation inhibitor U74006F protects against cerebral ischemia in gerbils. Stroke 19:997–1002
31. Klatzo I (1985) Brain oedema following brain ischemia and the influence of therapy. Br J Anaesth 57:18–22
32. Dobbin J, Crockard A, Ross-Russell R (1989) Transient blood brain barrier permeability following profound temporary global ischemia: An experimental study using ^{14}C-AIB. J Cereb Blood Flow Metabol 9:71–78

Treatment of Experimental Central Nervous System Trauma and Ischemia: Use of a Novel 21-Aminosteroid

E. D. Means, J. M. Braughler, and E. D. Hall

Introduction

There is an urgent need for new therapeutic modalities in the treatment of central nervous system (CNS) trauma and ischemia. Physicians often look upon the treatment of CNS trauma and ischemia with reservation because effective therapy in these areas has not significantly advanced over recent years. Moreover, treatment is often delayed in these entities as a consequence of inadequate and inefficient emergency medical care. The therapeutic window is frequently closed as a result. Therapeutic nihilism however is unwarranted. A better understanding of the pathophysiology of these conditions has led to a more directed research which doubtless will lead to new and effective therapies. Moreover, recognition of the emergency nature of these conditions has resulted in the formation in many metropolitan areas, of elaborate and effective emergency medical systems. This has allowed many patients to reach medical facilities in time for effective treatment.

A complex series of pathophysiological events follow an initial traumatic or ischemic insult to the CNS [1, 2]. These "secondary" factors include such events as:

1. ion shifts into and out of cells;
2. activation of destructive enzymes;
3. accumulation of harmful neurotransmitters and amino acids; and
4. the excess formation of toxic free radicals.

Free radical induced lipid peroxidation is potentially one of the most critical factors leading to secondary CNS injury following trauma or ischemia. The focus of this article is to describe a series of experimental studies in CNS trauma and ischemia with a new and novel compound, U-74,006F – a 21-aminosteroid which is a potent inhibitor of free radical induced lipid peroxidation.

The 21-aminosteroids were the result of an effort to develop non-glucocorticoids that mimicked the protective effects of high doses of synthetic glucocorticoids (e.g. methylprednisolone) in the injured CNS. It was hypothesized that the beneficial effect of methylprednisolone in the CNS was a nonglucocorticoid action, most likely the ability of the compound to inhibit lipid peroxidation both in vivo and in vitro [3–5]. An effort ensued to synthesize compounds that were potent inhibitors of lipid peroxidation that lacked glucocorticoid activity. Since 1985, several hundred of these compounds have been synthesized, one of which,

U-74,006F, was selected for clinical development. A series of preclinical studies with this compound in the areas of CNS trauma and ischemia will be described below.

The Basic Mechanism of Action of U-74,006F

The role of oxygen radicals and lipid peroxidation in ischemic injury to the central nervous system (CNS) has been recently reviewed [6, 7]. While direct and unequivocal evidence for the participation of free radical-mediated events as a primary cause of neuronal death associated with cerebral ischemia awaits to be established, numerous studies support the occurrence of such reactions in the ischemic central nervous system. Perhaps some of the most convincing evidence for the involvement of oxygen radicals and lipid peroxidation comes from studies demonstrating the efficacy of antioxidants and inhibitors of lipid peroxidation, like U-74,006F, in experimental models of cerebral ischemia and stroke.

A considerable amount of mechanistic information concerning the inhibition of lipid peroxidation and the generation of oxygen radicals has been reviewed extensively [6, 8–10] and will only be briefly considered here for the sake of providing a foundation for discussing the pharmacology of U-74,006F.

Oxygen free radicals may arise from a number of sources within injured or ischemic tissue [8–10]. Because of an unpaired electron in their outer atomic orbital, free radicals are generally highly reactive and depending upon the radical in question, can attack any of a number of important cellular constituents including proteins, nucleic acids, and lipids. Unsaturated fatty acids comprising much of the phospholipid environment of cell and organelle membranes are particularly susceptible to free attack. This may particularly be a problem in tissues rich in unsaturated fatty acids such as the CNS.

A lipid radical chain reaction within a membrane environment may be initiated when a free radical (R•) abstracts a hydrogen from an unsaturated fatty acid (LH) forming a lipid radical (L• reactions 1–3). The lipid radical readily combines with oxygen dissolved within the membrane to form a lipid peroxyl radical (LOO•) (reaction 2). Once a peroxyl radical is formed, it may attack a second unsaturated fatty acid resulting in the formation of a lipid hydroperoxide (LOOH) and a second lipid radical (L•) (reaction 3). In this way, a lipid radical chain reaction may damage many unsaturated fatty acids within the membrane (e.g. reactions 2 and 3) before the chain terminates.

$$R\bullet + LH \text{----------} RH + L\bullet \tag{1}$$

$$L\bullet + O_2 \text{------------} LOO\bullet \tag{2}$$

$$LOO\bullet + LH \text{------} LOOH + L\bullet \tag{3}$$

The radical chain reaction may be terminated by so-called chain breaking antioxidants such as Vitamin E. Vitamin E stops the lipid chain reaction by combining with LOO•, thus sparing unsaturated fatty acids in the membrane [6, 11,

12]. As the primary natural lipid-soluble antioxidant, Vitamin E is the most important antioxidant in cell membrane and plasma [11–13].

The involvement of iron in oxygen radical formation and lipid peroxidation has been extensively studied and has been reviewed [14]. Iron may not only facilitate the initiation of lipid radical chain reactions through the generation of oxygen radicals [6, 8, 14] but may catalyze lipid radical chain branching reactions through the iron-mediated decomposition of lipid hydroperoxides (LOOH) to either peroxyl (LOO•) and alkoxyl (LO•) radicals (reactions 4 and 5). Just as for LOO•, LO• may also initiate lipid chain reactions by attacking unsaturated fatty acids as in reaction 6. In that regard, LO• is naturally more reactive than LOO•. Recent studies have shown that the major driving force for lipid peroxidation is probably these iron-catalyzed decomposition reactions [15].

$$LOOH + FeII \text{-------} LO\bullet + FeIII \qquad (4)$$

$$LOOH + FeIII \text{------} LOO\bullet + FeII \qquad (5)$$

$$LO\bullet + LH \text{------------} LOH + L\bullet \qquad (6)$$

The 21-aminosteroids have been shown to be potent inhibitors or iron-catalyzed lipid peroxidation in vitro [16]. In rat brain homogenates or purified brain synaptosomes micromolar concentrations of U-74,006F have been shown to inhibit lipid peroxidation in the presence of iron. While the mechanism by which U-74,006F inhibits lipid peroxidation is not completely clear, it does appear to involve the inhibition of lipid chain reactions through scavenging of both LO• and LOO• [17]. Using in vitro systems involving pure LOO• or LO• inhibition constants for U-74,006F have been determined as 1.4×10^3 and 3.3×10^{-6} M-1 s-1, respectively, suggesting that reactivity toward LOO• is considerably greater than for LO•. The ability of U-74,006F to scavenge LOO• or LO• is considerably less than Vitamin E; nevertheless, U-74,006F is nearly as effective as Vitamin E at inhibiting lipid peroxidation in intact membranes [16]. In fact, U-74,006F can actually spare Vitamin E from utilization during lipid peroxidation [17] suggesting that mechanisms in addition to scavenging LOO• or LO• may be involved in its action.

In addition to its ability to scavenge radicals and inhibit lipid peroxidation U-74,006F has other stabilizing effects on cell membranes. The release of free arachidonic acid from injured cell membranes is blocked by U-74,006F [18]. In other unpublished studies using cultured bovine brain microvessel endothelial cells, the 21-aminosteroids have been shown to localize within the hydrophobic core of cell membranes and cause an increase in lipid ordering (e.g. decrease fluidity) of the phospholipid bilayer (Audus and Braughler, unpublished observations).

In summary, U-74,006F has been shown to inhibit lipid peroxidation and to scavenge radicals. This activity is believed to be responsible for its activity in vivo in experimental models of cerebral ischemia. Evidence for an antioxidant effect of U-74,006F has been obtained from studies demonstrating its ability to preserve tissue and plasma Vitamin E in experimental animals following experimental stroke or global ischemia associated following cardiac arrest [19, 20].

Actions in Models of Central Nervous System Trauma

Treatment of Experimental Head Injury with U-74,006F

U-74,006F has been tested in three different experimental head injury models consistently showing a beneficial effect. In an initial study, acute/intravenous administration of the compound to male CF-1 mice was shown to facilitate the early neurological recovery and one week survival after severe concussive head injury [21]. One hour post-traumatic recovery (grip test score) was significantly benefitted over a broad range of doses (0.003–30.0 mg/kg) as a single i.v. bolus within 5 minutes after injury. A 1 mg/kg dose given within 5 minutes and again at 1.5 hours after severe injury increased 1 week survival by nearly three fold, 27,3% in vehicle treated mice versus 78,6% in the U-74,006F treated. U-74,006F was also effective in improving recovery after more moderate injury.

In a cat severe concussive head injury model, U-74,006F given in a 1 mg/kg i.v. dose at 30 minutes post-injury and again at 2,5 hours has been shown to significantly reduce 4 hour cerebral cortical and white matter lactic acid accumulation [22]. In view of the likelihood that the brain tissue lactic acidosis is the result post-traumatic ischemia, its attenuation to near normal levels by U-74,006F suggests a beneficial effect of the compound on cerebral blood flow. While direct blood flow studies have not been carried out in experimental head injury, U-74,006F has been shown to attenuate post-traumatic spinal cord ischemia after either contusion [23] or compression [24] injury.

U-74,006F has further been demonstrated to facilitate 72 hour neurological recovery in rats subjected to moderate fluid percussion head injury plus a secondary 45 minute period of hypoxia (L. H. Pitts, personal communication).

Treatment of Experimental Spinal Cord Injury with U-74,006F

U-74,006F has been shown to promote recovery from compression injury of the spinal cord in cats [25] and prevent the phenomenon of post-traumatic hypoperfusion of the contused spinal cord also in cats [26]. Anderson and colleagues in a randomized blinded placebo controlled study evaluated the dose-response characteristics and capability of U-74,006F to promote functional recovery in cats subjected to compression trauma of the lumbar spinal cord [25]. U-74,006F was administered i.v. in doses ranging from 0.048 to 160.0 mg/kg. The animals were evaluated weekly for neurological recovery and animals receiving accumulated doses of U-74,006F ranging from 1.6 to 160.0 mg/kg/48 hours exhibited nearly 75% of normal neurological function by four [4] weeks after injury. These findings show that over a 100-fold dose range, U-74,006F has a remarkable capacity to promote functional recovery in spinal cord injured cats. Hall studied the effect of U-74,006F on the phenomenon of post-trauma hypoperfusion in the cat spinal cord 30 minutes after contusion injury of the lumbar area [26]. Blood flow in the spinal cord white matter was measured with the hydrogen clearance technique, and blood flow in the vehicle treated group was reduced by 63.5% compared to pre-injury controls. U-74,006F in contrast, almost completely prevented the development of post-traumatic hypoperfusion at a single dose of 10 mg/kg. In more recent unpublished studies, U-74,006F in doses as low as 1 mg/kg, was found to antagonize the development of post-traumatic ischemia in the spinal cord in a compression injury model (Hall, unpublished observation).

Treatment of Experimental Subarachnoid Hemorrhage with U-74,006F

Delayed cerebral vasospasm following subarachnoid hemorrhage (SAH) is a leading cause of death and long-term disability [27]. There is an urgent need for effective treatment of vasospasm following SAH. Studies have been conducted in cats [28], rabbits [29], and monkeys [30] using U-74,006F for the treatment of cerebral vasospasm. Initial studies using a single intravenous bolus of U-74,006F following the introduction of autologous blood into the subarachnoid space of cats, prevented post-SAH induced cerebral hypoperfusion as measured in the caudate nucleus [28]. Vollmer et al. conducted a study to determine if U-74,006F would prevent the development of delayed cerebral vasospasm after experimental SAH in a rabbit model [29]. Autologous blood was introduced into the subarachnoid space of rabbits and U-74,006F (1 mg/kg) or placebo was injected once every 12 hours for a total of 6 doses, starting 12 hours prior to the SAH. The animals were sacrificed 24 hours after SAH and the luminal diameter of the basilar artery was measured. U-74,006F treated animals showed only a 15% reduction in luminal diameter while a 44% reduction occurred in the luminal diameter of placebo animals. Steinke et al. evaluated U-74,006F in the prophylaxis of chronic cerebral vasospasm in a randomized, blinded, placebo-controlled trial in monkeys [30]. Experimental SAH was produced by introducing autologous clot next to the middle cerebral artery following craniectomy. U-74,006F or placebo were administered from day 1 to 6, i.v. every 8 hours. Angiography was performed at baseline and at 7 days. CT or MRI were done if there was evidence of delayed ischemic deficit. There was a significant difference in the degree of angiographic vasospasm in the internal carotid and middle cerebral arteries between the placebo and U-74,006F treated animals due to a greater degree of vasospasm in the control group.

Treatment of Experimental Cerebral Ischemia with U-74,006F

Initial focal ischemia studies with U-74,006F in gerbils demonstrated that treatment (10 mg/kg i.p.) 10 min before and immediately after a 3-h period of unilateral carotid occlusion improved 28 and 48-h survival. A histological examination of the brain at 24 hrs post-ischemia in another group of vehicle treated animals revealed marked neuronal loss in the hippocampus and lateral cerebral cortex. In contrast, the neuronal densities in the ischemic hemisphere of U-74,006F treated gerbils were significantly preserved in both brain regions [20]. More recent physiological studies in the same model have shown that U-74,006F acts to reduce the post-ischemic depletion of brain Vitamin-E at 2 and 24 hrs. after reperfusion together with a facilitated recovery of extracellular calcium

(E. D. Hall and J. M. Braughler unpublished data). The protection of brain Vitamin-E supports the view that the U-74,006F cereprotective effect is due to inhibition of post-ischemic lipid peroxidation. The enhanced recovery of calcium (i.e. reversal of intracellular accumulation) may be due to the consequent protection of membrane calcium extrusion mechanisms.

U-74,006F has also been shown to reduce post-ischemic brain damage in the cat following a 1-h temporary occlusion of the middle cerebral artery [31]. Beginning 15 min after occlusion release, U-74,006F was administered as a multiple bolus regimen that was continued for 12 hours. At one week, using classical histological and quantitative 2-deoxy-glucose autoradiographic techniques, the area of cerebral infarction was significantly reduced compared to that in vehicle treated cats.

The effects of U-74,006F on brain ionic shifts and edema have been examined in a permanent middle cerebral artery occlusion model in rats [32]. In those studies, U-74,006F given as a 3 mg/kg intravenous bolus dose 10 min and 3 h after occlusion significantly reduced 24 hour post-ischemic brain Na^+ accumulation, K^+ loss and edema around the infarct site. In other studies, U-74,006F pretreatment has been found to block the formation of vasogenic edema in the brain of rats induced by intracerebral injection of arachidonic acid [33].

U-74,006F has also been demonstrated to improve post-ischemic cerebral blood flow (CBF). In cats, following a 5 min period of near total global cerebral ischemia, CBF was found to decline progressively during the 3-h post-ischemic period in vehicle-treated animals [34]. In comparison, CBF remained significantly greater in animals receiving a single 1 mg/kg intravenous bolus of U-74,006F at 15 min post-ischemia. In addition, U-74,006F treatment significantly enhanced the recovery of somatosensory evoked potentials, reduced postischemic arterial acidosis, and improved post-ischemic blood pressure. The improved support of CBF is probably due to both a better maintenance of cerebral perfusion pressure (i.e. arterial blood pressure) and a direct protection of the cerebral microvasculature.

Conclusion

In summary, U-74,006F has proven to be an effective therapy in the treatment of experimental head trauma, spinal cord trauma, SAH, global cerebral ischemia and stroke. Clinical trials are planned in the near future with this compound in traumatic head injury, SAH and stroke.

References

1. Means ED, Anderson DK (1987) The pathophysiology of acute spinal cord injury. In: Davidoff RA (ed) The spinal cord handbook, vol 5. Decker, pp 16–61
2. Siesjo BK (1988) Mechanisms of ischemic brain damage. Crit Care Med 16:954–963
3. Hall ED, Braughler JM (1981) Acute effects of intravenous glucocorticoid pretreatment on the *in vitro* peroxidation of cat spinal cord tissue. Exp Neurol 73:321–324

4. Kurihara M (1985) Role of monamines in experimental spinal cord injury: relationship between $Na^+ + K^+$ ATPase and lipid peroxidation. J Neurosurg 62:743–749

5. Anderson DK, Means ED (1983) Lipid peroxidation in spinal cord: $FeCl_2$ induction and protection with antioxidants. Neurochem Path 1:249–264

6. Braughler JM, Hall ED (1989) Central nervous system trauma and stroke: I. Biochemical considerations for oxygen radical formation and lipid peroxidation. J Free Rad Biol Med 6:289–301

7. Hall ED, Braughler JM (1988) Central nervous system trauma and stroke: II. Physiological and pharmacological evidence for the involvement of oxygen radicals and lipid peroxidation. J Free Rad Biol Med 6:303–313

8. Halliwell B, Gutteridge JMC (1985) Free radicals in biology and medicine. Claredon Press, Oxford

9. Halliwell (1987) Oxidants and human disease: some new concepts FASEB J 1:358–364

10. Southern PA, Powis G (1988) Free radicals in medicine II. Involvement in human disease. Mayo Clin Proc 63:390–408

11. Machlin LJ, Bendich A (1987) Free radical tissue damage: protective role of antioxidant nutrients. FASEB J 1:441–445

12. McCay PB, Vitamin E (1985) Interactions with free radicals and ascorbate. Ann Rev Nut 5:323–340

13. Ingold KU, Webb AC, Witter D, Burton GW, Metcalf TA, Muller DPR (1987) Vitamin E remains the major lipid-soluble, chain-breaking antioxidant in human plasma even in individuals suffering severe Vitamin E deficiency. Arch Biochem Biophys 259:224–225

14. Aust SD, Morehouse LA, Thomas CE (1985) Role of metals in oxygen radical reactions. J Free Rad Biol Med 1:3–25

15. Braughler JM, Pregenzer JF, Chase RL (1987) Oxidation of ferrous iron during peroxidation of various lipid substrates. Biochem Biophys Acta 921:457–464

16. Braughler JM, Pregenzer JF, Chase RL, Duncan LA, Jacobsen EJ, McCall JM (1987) Novel 21-aminosteroids as potent inhibitors of iron-dependent lipid peroxidation. J Biol Chem 262:10438–10440

17. Braughler JM, Pregenzer JF (1989) The 21-aminosteroid inhibitors of lipid peroxidation: reactions with lipid peroxyl and phenoxy radicals. J Free Rad Biol Med 7:125–130

18. Braughler JM, Chase RL, Neff GL, et al (1988) A new 21-aminosteroid antioxidant lacking glucocorticoid activity stimulated ACTH secretion and blocks arachidonic acid release from mouse pituitary tumor (AtT-20) cells. J Pharmacol Exp Ther 244:423–427

19. Natale JE, Schott RJ, Hall ED, Braughler JM, D'Alecy LG (1988) The 21-aminosteroid U-74,006F reduces systemic lipid peroxidation, improves neurological function, and reduces mortality after cardiopulmonary arrest in dogs. Stroke 19:1371–1378

20. Hall ED, Berry KP, Braughler JM (1988) The 21-aminosteroid lipid peroxidation inhibitor U-74,006F protects against cerebral ischemia in gerbils. Stroke 19:997–1002

21. Hall ED, Yonkers PA, McCall JM, Braughler JM (1988) Effects of the 21-aminosteroid U-74,006F on experimental head injury in mice. J Neurosurg 68:456–461

22. Dimlich RVW, Tornheim PA, Kindel RM, Hall ED, Braughler JM, McCall JM (1989) The effects of a 21-aminosteroid on cerebral metabolites and edema after severe experimental head injury. Adv Neurol (in press)

23. Hall ED (1988) Effect of the 21-aminosteroid U-74,006F on post-traumatic spinal cord ischemia. J Neurosurg 68:462–465

24. Hall ED, Yonkers PA, Braughler JM (1988) Attenuation of post-traumatic ischemia by the lipid peroxidation inhibitor U-74,006F: comparison in a contusion vs compression model. Neurosc Abst 14:1154

25. Anderson DK, Braughler JM, Hall ED, Waters TR, McCall JM, Means ED (1988) Dose-response effects of U-74,006F on neurological recovery in an experimental model of spinal cord injury. J Neurosurg 69:562–567

26. Hall ED (1988) Effects of the 21-aminosteroid U-74,006F on post-traumatic spinal cord ischemia in cats. J Neurosurg 68:462–465

27. Heros RC, Zervas NT, Varsos V (1983) Cerebral vasospasm after subarachnoid hemorrhage: an update. Ann Neurol 14:599–608

28. Hall ED, Travis MA (1988) Effects of the non-glucocorticoid 21-aminosteroid U-74,006F on progressive brain hypoperfusion following experimental subarachnoid hemorrhage. Exp Neurol 102:244–248

29. Vollmer DG, Kassell NE, Hongo K, Ogawa H, Tsukahara T (1989) Effect of the non-glucocorticoid 21-aminosteroid U-74,006F in the treatment of experimental cerebral vasospasm. Surg Neurol 31:190–194

30. Steinke DE, Weir BKA, Findlay JM, Tanabe T, Grace M, Krushelnychy BD (1989) A trial of the 21-aminosteroid U-74,006F in a primate model of chronic cerebral vasospasm. Neurosurgery 24:179–186

31. Silvia RC, Piercey MF, Hoffmann WE, Chase RL, Braughler JM, Tang AH (1987) U-74,006F, an inhibitor of lipid peroxidation protects against lesion development following experimental stroke in the cat: Histological and metabolic analysis. Neurosci Abst 13:1499

32. Young W, Wojak JC, DeCrescito V (1988) Aminosteroid lipid peroxidation inhibitor reduces ionic shifts and edema in the rat middle cerebral artery occlusion model of regional ischemia. Stroke 19:1013–1019

33. Hall ED, Travis MA (1988) Inhibition of arachidonic acid-induced vasogenic brain edema by the non-glucocorticoid 21-aminosteroid U-74,006F. Brain Res 451:350–352

34. Hall ED, Yonkers PA (1988) Attenuation of post-ischemic cerebral hypoperfusion by the 21-aminosteroid U-74,006F. Stroke 19:340–344

Current Management of Aneurysmal Subarachnoid Hemorrhage

D. Chyatte and T. M. George

Introduction

The outlook following aneurysmal subarachnoid hemorrhage (SAH) remains dismal despite modern therapy [1-3]. Although the incidence of thromboembolic stroke has been decreasing over the last three decades, the incidence of SAH has remained constant and it is estimated that 26000 people in the U.S. are affected each year. Aneurysmal SAH is a devastating disease with nearly half of all patients dying as a result of the initial hemorrhage (Fig. 1). Of those surviving initial hemorrhage, delayed cerebral ischemia and aneurysmal rebleeding can be linked to most management failures.

Effective management of patients after aneurysmal SAH requires early transfer to well-equipped neurosurgical facilities. Unfortunately, many patients present to primary care centers where transfer is delayed as a consequence of the difficulty in making the initial diagnosis. Although there is a near pathognomonic cluster of signs and symptoms produced by aneurysmal SAH, the diagnosis has been confused with migraine headaches or sinusitis, particularly in young

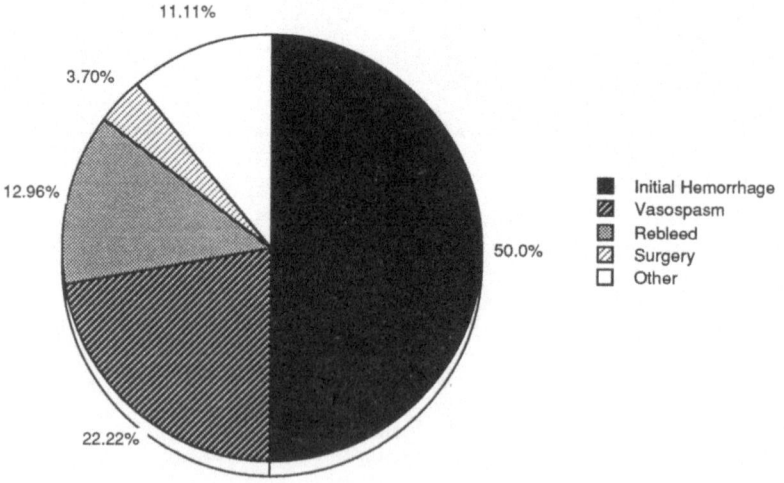

11.11%

3.70%

12.96%

50.0%

22.22%

Initial Hemorrhage
Vasospasm
Rebleed
Surgery
Other

Fig. 1. Causes of death after subarachnoid hemorrhage in all patients (n = 57)

patients with minor bleeds. Only education and a high index of clinical suspicion will avoid these errors in diagnosis and management delay.

Clinical Presentation

The *abrupt* onset of a *severe* headache is the "hallmark" of SAH. Most patients report that this headache is the worst ever experienced in their lives. Many patients will describe this by using phrases such as "a bomb went off in my head" or "it felt as if I was hit in the head with a board!". Alterations in sensorium or frank loss of consciousness often coincide with the ictus and may be accompanied by focal neurologic deficits and vomiting. Although seizures also occur, they are considerably less common. Postictally, many patients are left anxious and complain of a persistent headache, photophobia, and stiff neck. Even though the cause or causes of aneurysm formation and rupture remain controversial, hypertension, age, cigarette smoking, and use of oral contraceptives appear to be risk factors [4, 5]. Many patients report a stressful event which they believe precipitated their ictus. Seasonal variations and, in particular, rapid temperature changes appears to be associated with aneurysm rupture; however, this phenomena is less well documented [5].The most important premonitory clue is the "sentinel headache" which occurs in one fourth of patients and predates the ictus by approximately 2 weeks.

Categorization of patients into "grades" based on neurological function and meningeal signs has allowed surgeons and neurologists to predict management results and plan optimal treatment strategies soon after subarachnoid hemorrhage has occurred [6]. Patients with severe meningeal signs and profound neurological abnormalities do less well than "better" grade patients (Table 1 and Fig. 2).

Diagnosis

Computerized tomography (CT) is the diagnostic procedure of choice when SAH is suspected. Lumbar puncture is still useful in some situations and remains a sensitive test for detecting blood in the cerebrospinal fluid (CSF) [7]. CT is positive in 90–95% of patients with a subarachnoid hemorrhage if the study is obtained within 5 days of the bleed. When the CT scan is performed seven days or more after the bleed, subarachnoid blood may appear isodense with brain

---

Table 1. Modification of botterell grading system. Grades 1 and 2 are considered to be "good" grades. Grades 3 and 4 are considered to be "poor" grades

---

Grade 1: With or without mild headache, alert oriented, with no motor or sensory deficits

Grade 2: Severe headache and major meningeal signs, mild alteration in sensorium or minor focal deficit

Grade 3: Major alteration in sensorium or major focal deficit

Grade 4: Semi-comatose with or without major lateralizing findings

---

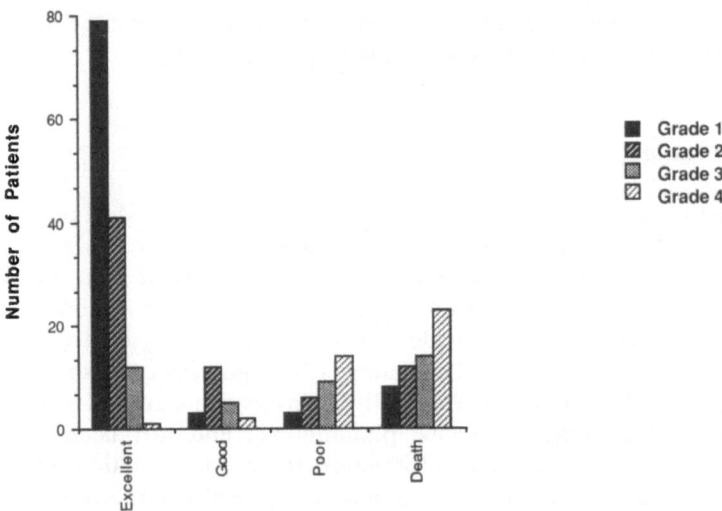

Fig. 2. Overall management results by admitting grade. Each grade is based on modified butterell grading system (n = 244)

parenchyma. As a consequence, the CT may appear normal unless there is a substantial blood clot associated with mass effect. The pattern of subarachnoid blood on CT scan may suggest the likely location of the ruptured aneurysm. This may be particularly important if more than one aneurysm is seen on angiography and may direct surgical treatment toward the symptomatic aneurysm (Fig. 3). Less commonly, the pattern of blood seen on the CT does not correlate to the aneurysm found on angiography. In these situations, the possibility of missing the symptomatic aneurysm should be considered. At times, contrast-enhanced computed tomography is useful in outlining the wall and lumen of the aneurysm, revealing its true size and degree of thrombosis. This is particularly valuable when the presence of a giant partially thrombosed aneurysm is suspected. The lesion size seen on angiography can be quite misleading in these situations.

Lumbar puncture should be performed in all patients with the appropriate clinical picture and a negative CT scan. Avoiding a traumatic tap simplifies the interpretation of the spinal fluid findings. The finding of xanthochromic, or bloody fluid that does not clear in sequential tubes indicates that a subarachnoid hemorrhage has occurred. Prior to sending the CSF for all routine studies, the first and last tubes should be spun-down and examined for xanthochromia. Xanthochromia is the result of the breakdown of hemoglobin to bilirubin and occurs if blood has been present in the CSF for a minimum of 6 hours [7]. Analysis of the CSF glucose and protein levels, cultures, and cell counts may point to other causes of hemorrhagic spinal fluid such as herpes encephalitis. Lumbar puncture is contraindicated in the setting of a coagulopathy or when a significant risk of herniation exists due to the presence of an intracranial mass lesion or obstructive hydrocephalus.

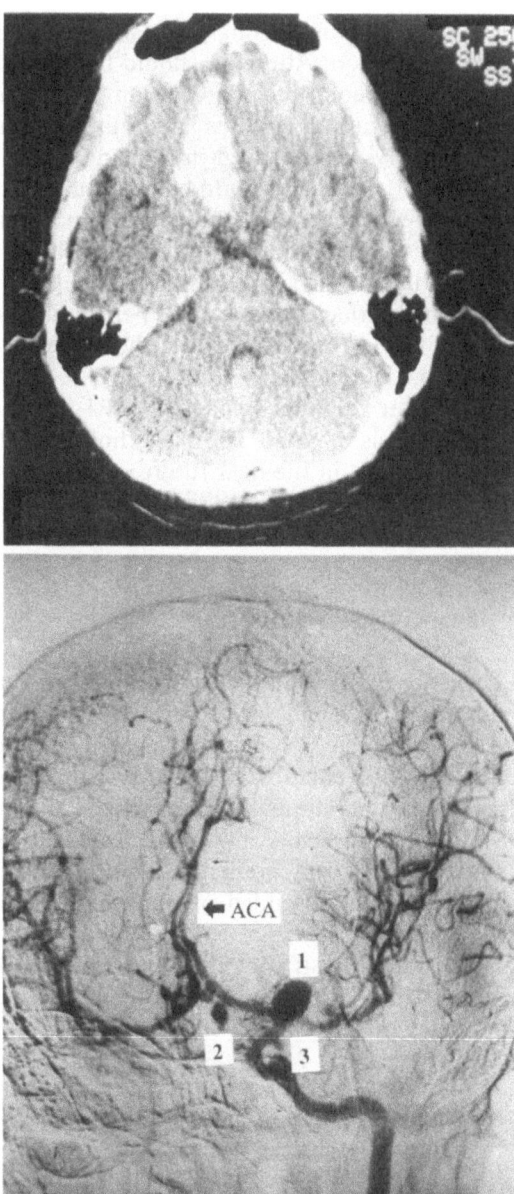

Fig. 3. Non-contrast CT revealing acute hemorrhage extending into right frontal lobe **(top)**. Anteroposterior subtraction angiogram revealing multiple intracranial aneurysms along with medial displacement of anterior cerebral arteries. *1* Internal carotid artery bifurcation aneurysm; *2* Anterior communicating artery aneurysm; *3* Posterior communicating artery aneurysm **(bottom)**.
* For details, see text. $^+$ ACA = Anterior cerebral artery

Angiography is the single best way to determine the source of the hemorrhage, and its location. Attention should be paid to the degree of vasospasm and the extent of cerebral cross-circulation when interpreting the angiogram. Complete angiography (both carotids and both vertebrals) should be performed since multiple aneurysms can occur in as many as 20% of patients [8]. If the angiogram is negative, the patient should be medically stabilized and then repeat angiography considered if the initial study was of poor-quality, had evidence of vasospasm or there was a high index of clinical suspicion. The incidence of negative panangiography in SAH is significant (13–22%) [9]. It has been suggested that these patients hemorrhaged from small perforating vessels located in the basal cisterns. Regardless of the true source of hemorrhage in these patients, their risk of rehemorrhage is quite small [10].

Magnetic resonance imaging (MRI), currently plays little role in establishing the diagnosis of SAH. The MRI, however, shows intracranial vessels extremely well and may, in the near future, replace angiography in identifying the source of the hemorrhage and its location [11].

Management

There are certain guidelines for care of patients who have sustained aneurysmal subarachnoid hemorrhage. All patients require meticulous and frequent assessment of their neurological status along with constant monitoring of blood pressure and fluid balance. In addition, painstaking attention should be paid to oxygenation, ventilation and maintenance of electrolyte balance. Central venous or Swan-Ganz catheters may provide useful information particularly in patients who have delayed cerebral ischemia or severe hemodynamic and fluid disturbances. In the obtunded or inadequately ventilated patient, urgent intubation should be considered.

The nursing staff should be instructed to place patients on "aneurysm precautions" which are a group of guidelines aimed at reducing the patient's stress, pain and anxiety, thereby lowering the risk of rebleeding (Table 2). Treatment of

Table 2. Aneurysm precautions. (For details see text)

1. All visitors must report to nursing station prior to seeing patient
2. Only 2 visitors, maintaining a quiet environment
3. Darken room
4. Food restriction cc
5. Head of bed .... °
6. No smoking
7. No rectal procedures
8. No television
9. No telephone
10. Patient needs feeding and bathing assistance
11. Food restriction, no caffeine
12. Head rotation restriction .... °

pain requires paracetamol or codeine for analgesia. Often small doses of decadron may relieve discomfort associated with meningeal irritation. Stool softeners reduce straining and counteract the inhibition of gastrointestinal function secondary ot narcotic use. The use of rectal temperature measurements and placement of a Foley urine drainage catheter should be done only when indicated. The patient's room should be dimly lit and quiet, particularly when photophobia is severe. Television viewing, frequent telephone conversations, and multiple visitors should be avoided. Soft music, restricted telephone use, and limited visitation should be implemented. Anxiety may be reduced by using drugs such as phenobarbitol, which also has excellent anticonvulsant properties.

One the patient is stabilized, efforts are directed at management of rebleeding, delayed cerebral ischemia, increased intracranial pressure and seizures.

Rebleeding

Acute neurologic deterioration due to rebleeding occurs in 15-20% of patients [12-14]. Sudden impairment of consciousness or change in vegetative functions usually occurs. Prompt investigation by repeat CT scanning often reveals evidence of a new hemorrhage, even if rebleeding occurs soon after the first bleed. Modern data suggests that the peak risk period for a re-hemorrhage is within the first 24 to 48 hours following the initial hemorrhage [1, 12-14]. The mortality associated with rebleeding is dismal (21%) [1].

Rebleeding may be prevented by:

1. obliteration of the aneurysm;
2. prevention of early clot lysis sealing the aneurysmal wrent; and
3. lowering the systemic blood pressure.

Obliteration of the Aneurysm

Craniotomy for clipping of the aneurysm remains the standard method for prevention of rerupture. With the use of the operating microscope, microsurgical techniques, and modern neuroanesthesia, skilled neurosurgeons have made the risks of aneurysm surgery minimal in most instances. The timing of aneurysm surgery, however, remains controversial [6, 15, 16].

Recently, early surgery has regained popularity [6, 15]. The expected benefits of early surgery are prevention of rebleeding and the ability to manage delayed cerebral ischemia more aggressively. The principle drawback of early surgery, poor surgical exposure due to a red, swollen, angry brain, has been overcome by modern brain relaxation techniques making early surgery technically feasible in most instances. Unfortunately, overall management results with early surgery have been less than expected. Most management morbidity is a direct result of the severity of the inital hemorrhage rather than being a consequence of delayed cerebral ischemia or rebleeding.

It is our policy to operate early on "good" grade patients. These patients have escaped the devestating direct effects of the initial hemorrhage and management results can be optimized by preventing rebleeding and effectively managing delayed cerebral ischemia. Patients who are in poor neurological condition as a direct result of the initial hemorrhage are unlikely to recover regardless of the treatment strategy chosen.

Newer endovascular techniques have made it possible to obliterate some aneurysms utilizing a detachable balloon [17]. With the present state of experience, detachable balloon therapy appears to be warranted for aneurysms deemed inoperable or of high surgical risk as a result of either poor medical condition or risky location and size. These endovascular techniques avoid a surgical incision, brain retraction, and use of a general anesthetic. As experience is gained and management results improve, it may be possible to treat many aneurysms safely that are presently approached by an open surgical procedure.

Antifibrinolytic Therapy

In situations where delayed surgery is planned, rebleeding may be reduced by the use of the antifibrinolytic agents. The antifibrinolytic agents, epsilon aminocaproic acid (Amicar) and transexamic acid, inhibit the conversion of plasmin to plasminogen; thereby, retarding lysis of the clot that seals the wrent in the aneurysm wall [18]. The beneficial effects of these drugs are often offset by an increased incidence of complications such as delayed cerebral ischemia, hydrocephalus, deep venous thrombosis and pulmonary embolism [19, 20]. As a result, it has been difficult to demonstrate a net improvement in the overall management results with their use.

Control of Systemic Hypertension

Control of systemic hypertension is important in reducing the risk of rebleeding. Systemic hypertension, seen commonly in patients after SAH, may be the result of pain, anxiety, fever, hypoxia, or reflect a relex response to cerebral ischemia or increased intracranial pressure. Experimentally, SAH results in increased levels of circulating catecholamines that leads to a hyperdynamic state and high blood pressure [21]. If significant hypertension persists after analgesics and sedatives, antihypertensive therapy should be considered. Antihypertensives should be used prudently as their injudicious use may lower cerebral perfusion pressure and precipitate or worsen delayed cerebral ischemia.

If antihypertensive therapy is used, it should be titrated against neurologic deterioration as a consequence of worsening cerebral ischemia. Initially, enteral therapy using calcium channel blockers such as nifedipine or beta-blockers can be used. We prefer to use nifedipine since β-blockers can decrease cerebral blood flow by lowering cardiac output and by directly causing cerebral vasoconstriction. The calcium-channel blockers produce an increase in cerebral blood flow but, theoretically, can increase the incidence of rebleeding. Labetalol, a relatively selective beta-1 antagonist, does not have the effects on cerebral blood flow seen with other beta-blockers, and is useful enterally or intravenously. Sodium nitroprusside is used for control of severe hypertension, which persists despite these measures. If it is continued for several days, thiocyanate levels should be measured. Toxic effects and tachyphylaxis are rare. Diuretics should be avoided since they only contribute to intravascular volume depletion and hyponatremia. Experimental evidence reveals that many patients have a negative sodium balance secondary to release of circulating natriuretic factors [22]. Therefore, effective fluid management requires volume replacement therapy in these hypovolemic hyponatremic patients and avoidance of diuresis [23].

Delayed Cerebral Ischemia

Delayed cerebral ischemia (DCI) is the most common cause of neurologic deterioration in patients who survive the initial ictus. Clinical symptoms typically appear 7 to 14 days after the inital SAH. The risk of developing DCI increases in proportion to the amount of subarachnoid blood [24, 25].

Symptomatic ischemia occurs when the large conducting arteries at the base of the brain narrow ("vasospasm") and the resistance vessels along with collateral flow are unable to compensate for these hemodynamic changes. Once regional cerebral blood flow falls below ischemic thresholds, neurological dysfunction occurs.

The cause of "vasospasm" remains uncertain. Vasospasm appears to be due to structural changes (i.e., "vasculopathy") in the vessel wall and not an active contraction of smooth muscle cells. The pathogenesis of this vasculopathy may be inflammatory, resulting from the liberation of vasotoxic substances as the blood in the subarachnoid space degrades leading to an inflammatory response. Other explanations are also possible [26].

The diagnosis of delayed cerebral ischemia secondary to vasospasm is made on clinical grounds and confirmed by non-invasive diagnostic tools. Cerebral blood flow measurements can reveal reductions in regional blood flow as a consequence of vasospasm, but cannot measure lumenal narrowing directly [27]. Transcranial Doppler ultrasonography can be used to monitor increases in flow velocity which correlate closely with vessel lumenal narrowing [28, 29]. Measures of flow velocity appears to be quite useful and can easily be performed at the bedside of an ill patient. Often accelerated flow velocity herald "vasospasm" before symptoms become clinically apparent. Treatment, therefore, can be instituted promptly.

Angiography should not be used to detect the presence of vasospasm. This invasive technique may actually worsen ischemic insults. However, preliminary experience with endovascular balloon angioplasty suggests that angiographic vasospasm can be treated by dialating the vessel directly using the balloon technique [17]. So far, no cases of neurologic deterioration secondary to ischemia or angiographic vasospasm has been documented after angioplasty. It is possible that the use of angiography will increase as a therapeutic rather than diagnostic tool. The safety and efficacy of balloon angioplasty for vasospasm has not yet been established and its use should be considered experimental.

Prevention

Currently, only clinical trials using the calcium channel blocking agents, nimodipine and nicardipine, have been shown to effectively prevent permanent ischemic deficits [30–32]. The exact mechanism of action of this class of drugs is unknown. It has been confirmed that calcium channel blockers do not reverse angiographically documented vasospasm. Whether these agents act by dilating parenchymal arterioles, promoting collateral circulation, improving red blood cell deformability, or improving neuronal and glial cell calcium homeostasis remains unclear.

Because "vasospasm" may be an inflammatory vasculopathy, high-dose steroids have been used in preliminary human trials to prevent delayed cerebral ischemia. Pilot studies suggest a substantial improvement in management outcome with these anti-inflammatory drugs, however, their safety and efficacy has not been established on larger patient samples [33].

Aggressive surgical removal of the subarachnoid blood clot, accompanied by the use of cisternal drainage has been used to lower the incidence of DCI [24, 25, 34]. However, this technique remains unproven and complications associated with its applications have tempered widespread use.

Treatment

When "vasospasm" becomes established, the brain loses its ability to autoregulate blood flow and resistence arterioles become maximally dilated. Induced volume expansion increases cerebral blood flow in this setting and is the initial therapy for post-hemorrhagic delayed cerebral ischemia [35, 36]. Colloids in the form of 5% albumin or blood products are excellent volume expanders. Their use must be guided by measurements of central venous pressure or pulmonary capillary wedge pressure and cardiac output to avoid intravascular volume overload and congestive failure.

If volume expansion fails to reverse ischemic defects, induced hypertension may improve cerebral perfusion and as a consequence, neurological symptoms [37]. Institution of induced hypertension may be risky in patients with unclipped aneurysms. Dopamine and dobutamine are excellent pressors with the latter being a better agent in patients with cardiomyopathy. Isoproterenol is effective in increasing the cardiac output, and subsequently, cerebral blood flow, but must be used concomitantly with lidocaine to prevent arrhythmias.

It is important to remember that cerebral blood flow is also dependent on intracranial pressure (ICP). Normalization of an elevated ICP may improve cerebral blood flow [37].

Intracranial Pressure

Elevated ICP is usually the consequence of hydrocephalus [37, 38]. Less commonly, cerebral edema secondary to ischemia is the cause. An altered sensorium represents the most common symptom and can be confused clinically with cerebral ischemia. In general, we treat increased ICP only when it is associated with depressed neurologic function. Lowering ICP in patients with unclipped aneurysms has the theoretical risk of promoting rebleeding.

Hydrocephalus occurs in approximately 20% of patients after SAH [37, 38]. Usually the ventricular system communicates with the subarachnoid space, but reabsorbtion of spinal fluid is depressed. When necessary, serial lumbar punctures or external ventricular drainage are used to control hydrocephalus. In dwelling lumbar spinal drains are avoided due to high incidence of infection. Permanent ventricular shunts are used if long-term hydrocephalus is expected.

Seizures

Seizures occur in approximately 3–5% of patients after aneurysmal SAH. Phenobarbitol is usually begun preoperatively because of its sedative and anticonvulsant properties. When there is significant depression in level of consciousness or the patient is over-sedated by phenobarbitol, diphenylhydantoin is preferred. Unless the patient develops a seizure disorder, all anticonvulsants can be discontinued after convalescence is completed.

References

1. Nishioka H, Turner JC, Gref CJ, Kassell NF, Sohs AL, Goettler LC (1984) Cooperative study of intracranial aneurysm and subarachnoid hemorrhage: a long-term prognostic study. Arch Neurol 41:1142–1146
2. Ropper AH, Zervas NT (1984) Outcome 1 year after SAH from cerebral aneurysm. J Neurosurg 60:909–915
3. Saveland H, Sonesson B, Lunggren B, et al (1986) Outcome evaluation following subarachnoid hemorrhage. J Neurosurg 64:191–196
4. Bell B, Symon L (1979) Smoking and subarachnoid hemorrhage. Br Med J 1:577–578
5. Keller A (1970) Hypertension, age and residence in the survival with subarachnoid hemorrhage. Am J Epidemiol 91
6. Chyatte D, Fode NC, Sundt TM (1988) Early versus late intracranial aneurysm surgery in subarachnoid hemorrhage. J Neurosurg 69:326–331
7. Marton KI, Geer AD (1986) The spinal tap: a new look at an old test. Ann Intern Med 104:840–848
8. Ostergaard JR, Hog E (1987) Incidence of multiple intracranial aneurysms. J Neurosurg 63:49–55
9. Alexander MSM, Dias PS, Uttley D (1986) Spontaneous subarachnoid hemorrhage and negative cerebral panangiography. J Neurosurg 64:537–542
10. Nishioka H, Turner JC, Graf CJ, Kassell NF, Sahs AL, Goettler LC (1984) Cooperative study of intracranial aneurysm and subarachnoid hemorrhage: A long-term prognostic study III. Arch Neurol 41:1147–1151

11. Jenkins A, Hadley DM, Teesdale GM, Condon B, MacPherson P, Patterson (1988) Magnetic resonance imaging of acute subarachnoid hemorrhage. J Neurosurg 68:731–736
12. Vermeulen M, Van Gigen J, Hydra A, Van Crevel H (1984) Causes of acute deterioration in patients with a ruptured intracranial aneurysm. J Neurosurg 60:935–939
13. Rosenborn J, Eskesen V, Schmidt K, Ronde F (1987) The risk of rebleeding from ruptured intracranial aneurysms. J Neurosurg 67:329–332
14. Hydra A, Vermeulen M, Van Gijn J, Van Creuel H (1987) Rerupture of intracranial aneurysms: a clinico-anatomic study. J Neurosurg 67:29–33
15. Ljunggren B, Saveland H, Brandt L, Zygmunt S (1985) Early operation and overall outcome in aneurysmal subarachnoid hemorrhage. J Neurosurg 62:547–551
16. Disney L, Weir B, Petruk K (1987) Effect on management mortality of a deliberate policy of early operation on supratentorial aneurysms. Neurosurgery 20:695–701
17. Hieshima GB, Higashide RT, Wapenski J, Holbach VV, Cohan L, Benston JR (1986) Balloon embolization of a large distal basilar artery aneurysm. J Neurosurg 65:413–416
18. Gibbs JR, O'Gorman P (1967) Fibrinolysis in subarachnoid hemorrhage. Postgrad Med 42:779–784
19. Adams HP, Nibbelink DW, Torner JC, et al (1980) Antifibrinolytic therapy in patients with aneurysmal subarachnoid hemorrhage: A report of the cooperative aneurysm study. Arch Neurol 38:25–29
20. Chandra B (1978) Treatment of subarachnoid hemorrhage from ruptured intracranial aneurysms with transexamic acid: A double blind clinical trial. Ann Neurol 3:502–504
21. McCormack BM, Swift DM, Hagemann MT, Solomon RA (1988) Increased norepinephrine synthesis in the cerebral hemispheres of rats following subarachnoid hemorrhage. Brain Res 382:395–398
22. Wigdick EFM, Vermeulen M, Van Brummelen P, Den Bor NC, Van Gryn J (1987) Digoxin-like immunoreactive substance in patients with aneurysmal subarachnoid hemorrhage. Br Med J 294:729–732
23. Wydicks ERM, Vermeulen M, Haaf JA, Hydra A, Bakker WH, Van Gyn J (1985) Volume depletion and natriuresis in patients with a ruptured intracranial aneurysm. Ann Neurol 18:211–216
24. Honda Y, Weir BKA, Nosko M, Mosewich R, Tsji T, Orace M (1987) The effect of timing of clet removal on chronic vasospasm in a primate model. J Neurosurg 67:558–564
25. Findlay JM, Weir BK, Steinkke D, Tanabe T, Gordon P, Grace M (1988) Effect of intrathecal thrombolytic therapy on subarachnoid clot and chronic vasospasm in a primate model of SAH. J Neurosurg 69:723–735
26. Chyatte D, Sundt TM (1984) Response of chronic experimental cerebral vasospasm to methylprednisolone and dexamethosone. J Neurosurg 60:923–926
27. Rawluk D, Smith FW, Deans HE, Gemmell HG, MacDonald AF (1988) Technetium 99m HMPAO scanning in patients with subarachnoid hemorrhage: a preliminary study. Br J Radiol 61:26–29
28. Harders AG, Gilsbach JM (1987) Time course of blood velocity changes related to vasospasm in the circle of Willis measured by transcranial Doppler ultrasound. J Neurosurg 66:718–728
29. Seiler RW, Grolimund P, Anslid R, Huber P, Nornes H (1986) Cerebral vasospasm evaluated by transcranial ultrasound correlated with clinical grade and CT-visualized subarachnoid hemorrhage. J Neurosurg 64:594–600
30. Flamm ES, Adams HP, Beck DW, et al (1988) Dose-escalation study of intravenous nicardipine in patients with aneurysmal subarachnoid hemorrhage. J Neurosurg, pp 393–400
31. Ohman J, Heiskanen O (1988) Effect of nimodipine on the outcome of patients after aneurysmal subarachnoid hemorrhage and surgery. J Neurosurg 69:683–686
32. Petruk, West M, Mohr G, et al (1988) Nimodipine treatment in poor-grade aneurysm patients. J Neurosurg 68:505–517
33. Chyatte D, Fode NC, Nichols DA, Sundt TM (1987) Preliminary report: effect of high dose methylprednisolone on delayed cerebral ischemia in patients at high risk for vasospasm after aneurysmal subarachnoid hemorrhage. Neurosurg 21:157–160
34. Mizukami M, Kawase T, Usami T, et al (1982) Prevention of vasospasm by early operation with removal of subarachnoid blood

35. Kassell NF, Peerless SJ, Duruard QJ, Beck DW, Drake CG, Adams HP (1982) Treatment of ischemic deficits from vasospasm with intravascular volume expansion and induced arterial hypertension. Neurosurg 11:337-343
36. Finn SS, Stephensen SA, Miller CA, Drobrich L, Hunt WE (1986) Observations on the perioperative management of aneurysmal subarachnoid hemorrhage. J Neurosurg 65:48-62
37. Yasargil MG, Yonekawa Y, Zumstein B, Stahl HJ (1973) Hydrocephalus following spontaneous subarachnoid hemorrhage: Clinical features and treatment. J Neurosurg 39:474-479
38. Black PM (1986) Hydrocephalus and vasospasm after subarachnoid hemorrhage from ruptured intracranial aneurysms. Neurosurgery 18:12-16

Gastro-Intestinal Crisis

Prevention of Stress Associated Gastric Mucosal Erosions

W. L. Thompson and M. Cloud

Introduction

Erosive lesions of the upper gut that occur in association with stress and complicate critical care include:

Curling ulcers (1842) classically are deep gastric or duodenal ulcers or both that bleed extensively and may perforate. Today this term is also used to describe multiple superficial erosions in the stomach that are common in patients with burn of one-third or more of the body surface.

Cushing ulcers in association with primary CNS trauma and surgery are often deep ulcers of the esophagus, stomach, or duodenum associated with hypersecretion of gastric acid, pepsin, and gastrin. This is one of the few stress associated gut erosions that seems clearly related to excess gastric acid secretion.

Drug-induced lesions are associated with ingestion of ethanol and administration of aspirin, other inhibitors of prostaglandin synthetase, and glucocorticoids.

Exacerbation of *chronic acid-peptic* disease may occur in the critical care setting with shallow or deep ulceration, and scarring, in the non-acid-producing areas of the stomach (antrum) and duodenum (bulb).

Stress associated gut mucosal erosions (SAGME) are usually asymptomatic superficial multiple lesions in acid-producing mucosa (gastric body and fundus) in patients with no recent gut pathology who are subjected to physical stress such as trauma, surgery, sepsis, and failure of lungs, liver, or kidneys. These lesions may be present on admission to critical care units and can form in hours after stress.

Pathophysiology

Hans Selye recognized the importance of the gut as a target organ in stress by defining the stress triad as:

- GI erosions and ulcers;

- adrenal enlargement;
- thymus, spleen, and lymphoid atrophy.

The mechanism by which stress leads to gut mucosal damage is complex and involves deflections from their balance points of numerous neuroendocrine, circulatory, exocrine, and motility functions.

Brain events associated with stress include pain, anxiety, and depression which in consciousness are *perceived* in the new outer cerebral cortex but are *felt* in the older limbic system. These probably act via the hypothalamus to increase activity of the sympathetic and vagus nerves and increase secretion of glucocorticoids, vasopressin, histamine, and other hormones and neurotransmitters.

Excess protons and pepsin in the gut lumen seem to permit but may not cause SAGME. The parietal cell K^+/H^+-ATPase can maintain an intraluminal free proton concentration of 100 000 µmol/L (pH 1). SAGME is uncommon at concentrations less than 320 µmol/L (pH 3.5), a 300-fold reduction. Pepsin is no longer active at free proton concentrations less than 32 µmol/L (pH 4.5). Some authorities believe that coagulation abnormalities may favor rebleeding at even lower free proton concentrations, thereby providing some rationale for neutralizing the lumen (0.1 µmol/L free protons; pH 7). Actually almost half of seriously-ill patients are unable to maintain intraluminal free proton concentrations greater than 10 µmol/L [1].

Bile reflux into the stomach may be increased by adynamic ileus and may compromise normal mucosal protective factors.

Mucosal permeability to free protons is increased and the transmucosal electrical potential difference is reduced by mucosal application of bile salts, alcohol, urea, or aspirin and in some animal models of stress.

Mucosal ischemia is a major factor in SAGME [2]. Ischemia, especially with starvation, causes a defect in mucosal ATP concentrations and also increases back diffusion of free protons into the mucosa and impairs mucosal defenses [3]. Ischemia also leads to generation of free radicals that may cause mucosal damage.

Intramucosal alkalinization during proton secretion, which is manifest systemically as the alkaline tide, may afford mucosal protection.

The mucus proton barrier secreted by healthy mucosal cells is a matrix of glycoproteins that resists proton diffusion. Thin layers can maintain 100 000-fold gradients in proton concentration. Fasting and glucocorticoids decrease hexosamine concentrations, and bile salts reduce the proton gradient.

Prostaglandins (PGE_2 and PGI_2) are protective factors that are present in high concentrations in gastric mucosa. They decrease secretion of free protons, enhance mucosal blood flow, stimulate secretion of mucus and bicarbonate, increase mucosal cyclic-AMP activity, and stabilize proton permeability of mucosal cells [3].

Epithelial renewal of limited superficial erosions may be accomplished quickly with sliding of epithelial cells over the basal lamina; this is inhibited by luminal acid and tissue acidosis [4]. Deeper injuries require cell replication which may be impeded by malnutrition.

Assessment of Damage

Mucosal damage can be assessed directly by endoscopy, but the clinical significance may be best measured by bleeding. Brown et al. [5] recently studied bleeding in 1328 *consecutive* medical and surgical critical care patients (excluding burned patients), 39.6% of whom had significant bleeding from some site at or after admission. After admission 138 patients bled significantly from 218 sites; 37% bled from more than one site. The upper GI tract was the site of bleeding in 48 patients (3.6% of 1328) with an average bleeding duration of 6 days. Twelve patients required a total of 19 units of blood replacement. Of interest in this study, reflective of general critical care patients, are the 940 patients who were not bleeding on admission. Of these, upper GI bleeding occurred in 0.6% of 479 who had no special prophylaxis for bleeding, 7.6% of 238 who received antacids, 6.2% of 81 given H_2 antagonists, and 15.5% of those who received both antacids and H_2 antagonists. Apparently the physicians were able to identify patients at greater risk and tailor their therapy accordingly. Perhaps the focus of efforts to prevent SAGME should focus on identification of patients at risk and appropriate tailoring of their prophylactic regimens.

Prevention of Stress Associated Gastric Mucosal Erosions

Antacids prevent SAGME in most studies [6]. Continuous infusions are more effective than hourly injections in maintaining consistently high intraluminal pH values. Doses of standard-strength antacids may vary from 20 to 160 ml/h. In studies of antacids, intragastric shielded mucosal surface electrodes record lower pH values than pH paper measurements on withdrawn luminal fluids [7].

In one of the initial controlled studies in critically-ill patients, Hastings et al. [8] observed GI bleeding in 4% of 51 patients given hourly antacids to maintain luminal fluid pH > 3.5 as compared with 24% of 49 control patients (p < .005). Zinner et al. [9] compared groups of 100 patients given antacid, 80 ml q2h to maintain luminal fluid pH > 4, or no therapy. Upper GI bleeding was observed in 5% and 20% of these patients (p < .002).

Antacids may be said to have a *cytoprotective* effect against NSAID damage, though the definition of cytoprotection is becoming clouded. A recent study examined the effect of aluminum hydroxide gel, 8 g tid, or placebo on transmucosal gastric potential difference two hours after aspirin, 1 g. Transmucosal potential was halved promptly after aspirin, but changes were reduced to about one-third of control with antacid pretreatment [10].

An optimal study of antacids, as a control for newer therapies, might be continuous monitoring of mucosal pH values with shielded intragastric electrodes. Antacids could be infused into the stomach continuously or intermittently to control pH values at desired levels. In routine SAGME prophylaxis, aluminum and magnesium antacids, adjusted according to colonic output, may be given continuously with intermittent measurement of the pH of aspirated luminal fluids.

Histamine H$_2$ Receptor Antagonists now marketed include cimetidine, famotidine, nizatidine, and ranitidine. Those in clinical trials include: BMY25271, BMY25368-01, BMY326539, ebrotidine, FRG8701, FRG8813, mifentidine, roxatidine, SKF94428, sufotidine, and zaltidine.

Numerous studies have compared H$_2$ antagonists with placebo, antacid, and each other in prevention of SAGME. Results are variable. In one large metanalysis of 16 prospective controlled studies in 2133 patients [11], the incidence of overt bleeding was 15% in 720 patients treated with placebo, 3.3% in 458 given antacids, and 2.7% in 402 given an H$_2$ antagonist.

Comparative studies of H$_2$ antagonists on overt GI bleeding are complicated by variable administration patterns. All marketed H$_2$ antagonists have brief half-times of elimination. Nizatidine elimination in healthy volunteers has half-times of 1 to 2 h. Cimetidine and ranitidine have half-times of 1.6 to 2.1 h and famotidine 2.5 to 3.5 h [12]. Bolus intravenous administration at intervals of 6 to 12 hours would not be expected to effect continuous suppression of proton secretion in all patients. For example, in one careful comparison of ranitidine, 50 or 75 mg iv q6h, with hourly boluses of antacid, about one-sixth of patients in both groups did not have consistent increments in gastric aspirate pH values to 4 or more [13].

Infusions of H$_2$ antagonists are more effective. Cimetidine, up to 50 mg/h, was more effective in maintaining gastric intraluminal pH >4 than equivalent doses given as bolus injections q6h [14]. Cimetidine, 83 mg/h, in critically ill patients resulted in 75% of gastric intraluminal pH values being >4 [15]. If continuous infusions are to be used, an initial "loading" dose is appropriate [16].

Anacidity from H$_2$ antagonists compromises the antimicrobial activity of gastric acid. This was shown first in 1982 by Kahn et al. [17] and duMoulin et al. [18]. Enteric pathogens spread rapidly from the stomach to trachea. Patients with greater consistency of alkalinization may be at greater risk of pneumonitis with these organisms [19]. This risk of SAGME prophylaxis was recently reviewed [20].

If desired, closed loop delivery systems could administer H$_2$ antagonists intravenously to maintain gastric intraluminal pH values at desired levels with occasional infusion interruptions to permit transient acidity to sterilize the stomach. Alternatively, prophylactic therapy with poorly-absorbed antimicrobial drugs may minimize risk of nosocomial pneumonia.

Proton Pump Inhibitors include omeprazole, AG1749, BY1023/SKF96022, NC1300, SKF95601, and WY26769. These inhibit the parietal cell H$^+$/K$^+$-ATPase to produce a long-lasting suppression of gastric acidity. Their activity in preventing SAGME is not yet defined.

Sucralfate is a non-absorbable aluminum salt of sucrose octasulfate with cytoprotective effects that may be mediated in part by enhanced gastric prostaglandin synthesis [21]. In critically-ill patients, sucralfate therapy is associated with lesser suppression of gastric intraluminal acid and a lower incidence of nosocomial pneumonia than therapy with antacids and H_2 antagonists [22]. Nosocomial pneumonia was observed [23] three times more often in patients on mechanical ventilation treated with antacids (11/34) than in those receiving sucralfate (3/29). In one study of 59 mechanically-ventilated patients given hourly antacid, cimetidine q6h iv, or sucralfate 1 g q6h, five patients had overt upper GI bleeding; one was in the cimetidine group and four in the antacid group [24].

Prostaglandins protect gastric mucosa against injury caused by acid, bile acids, ethanol, and boiling water. With severe insults, superficial layers may be lost, but are repaired rapidly [25]. Current prostaglandin analogues include enprostil, misoprostol, ornoprostil, rosaprostol, trimoprostil, and, in trial, arbaprostil dimoxaprost, enisoprost, mexiprostil, nileprost, nocloprost, rioprostil, and tiprostanide. Despite evidence of the role of prostaglandins in pathogenesis of some kinds of SAGME, their cytoprotective actions in experimental models, and their clinical utility in preventing NSAID and aspirin gut damage, there are only a few small studies in use of these agents to prevent SAGME and the results have not been impressive [26, 27].

Cytoprotective drugs of indefinite pharmacology include solfacone and plaunatol that are popular in Japan for treatment of gastritis and ulcers. Their efficacy in preventing SAGME is unknown. A possibly related drug, DQ2511, is described as a dopamine derivative.

Epidermal growth factors include MG111, prepared from human urine, and Chiron's rDNA EGF. These products are being tested in patients with ulcers; their effects in preventing SAGME are not reported.

Antimuscarinic agents include pirenzepine, darenzepine, nuvenzepine, telenzepine, timepidium, and tiquizium bromide. These are said to be more potent and selective than atropine-like drugs. Tiquizium bromide is also said to have other cytoprotective effects [28]. In 400 postoperative patients in critical care given pirenzepine or ranitidine, gastric pH was kept >4 to a greater extent by ranitidine, pneumonia among patients with mechanical ventilation was more common in those receiving ranitidine, and overt bleeding was observed in six patients receiving ranitidine and three receiving pirenzepine [29].

Somatostatin inhibits gastric acid secretion and decreases mucosal blood flow. Although it has shown some protective effect in animal models, there are no convincing controlled clinical trials in prevention of SAGME.

Tranexamic Acid is antifibrinolytic and has been tested in treatment of patients with upper GI bleeding, but efficacy has not been established in controlled trials of prevention of SAGME.

Other drugs being studied for prevention of SAGME include glucagon and allopurinol [26, 27]. Glucagon decreases gastric acid production and alters gut tone; allopurinol may prevent formation of oxygen-derived free radicals.

As the complex physiology of gastric acid secretion unfolds [30] and as we begin to understand mucosal protective factors, there will be many more therapeutic opportunities to minimize dysfunction of the energy acquisition organs in syndromes of multisystem failure.

Conclusion

Major interventions to prevent SAGME today are antacids, H_2 antagonists, or both. The preferred mode of therapy is by continuous administration that can be accomplished easily with mechanical infusion devices. H_2 antagonist prophylaxis should begin with an appropriate initial "loading" dose.

Effects on proton secretion are best monitored by recording gastric mucosal pH with shielded luminal electrodes; alternatively gastric aspirates may be monitored to maintain aspirate pH values > 4.

Constant gastric anacidity in seriously-ill patients predisposes to tracheopulmonary colonization and infection with enteric bacteria; careful monitoring, intermittent gastric "acidification", or prophylactic use of poorly-absorbable antimicrobials may be considered.

The dozens of newer agents with differing pharmacology will promote a confusing array of claims. One benefit is that demonstrating their relative efficacy, used alone and in combinations, should guarantee that every critical care physician can be ensured of numerous controlled clinical trials of SAGME among which to choose and every patient can have more attention paid to gastric pH and bleeding than ever before. That alone may be the greatest clinical benefit.

References

1. Stannard VA, Hutchinson A, Morris DL, Byrne A (1988) Gastric exocrine "failure" in critically ill patients: incidence and associated features. Br Med J 296:155–156
2. Yabana T, Yachi A (1988) Stress-induced vascular damage and ulcer. Dig Dis Sci 33:751–761
3. Miller TA (1987) Mechanisms of stress-related mucosal damage. Am J Med 83(6A):8–14
4. Silen W (1987) The clinical problem of stress ulcers. Clin Invest Med 10:270–274
5. Brown RB, Klar J, Teres D, Lemeshow S, Sands M (1988) Prospective study of clinical bleeding in intensive care unit patients. Crit Care Med 16:1171–76
6. Lanza FL, Sibley CM (1987) Role of antacids in the management of disorders of the upper gastrointestinal tract. Review of clinical experience 1975–1985. Am J Gastroent 82:1223–1241
7. Meiners D, Clift S, Kaminski D (1982) Evaluation of various techniques to monitor intragastric pH. Arch Surg 117:288–291

8. Hastings PR, Skillman JJ, Bushnell LS, Silen W (1978) Antacid titration in the prevention of acute gastrointestinal bleeding. A controlled, randomized trial in 100 critically ill patients. N Engl J Med 298:1041–1045
9. Zinner MJ, Zuidema GD, Smith PL, Mignosa M (1981) The prevention of upper gastrointestinal tract bleeding in patients in an intensive care unit. Surg Gynecol Obstet 153:214–220
10. Bergmann J-F, Caulin C, Simoneau G, Dorf G, Segrestaa J-M (1988) Persistent gastric-protective effect of antacid evaluated by measurement of transmucosal gastric potential difference. Clin Pharmacol Ther 44:546–549
11. Shuman RB, Schuster DP, Zuckerman GR (1987) Prophylactic therapy for stress ulcer bleeding: a reappraisal. Ann Intern Med 106:562–567
12. Ostro MJ (1987) Pharmacodynamics and pharmacokinetics of parenteral histamine (H_2)-receptor antagonists. Am J Med 83(6A):15–22
13. Noseworthy TW, Shustack A, Johnston RG, Anderson BJ, Konopad E, Grace M (1987) A randomized clinical trial comparing ranitidine and antacids in critically ill patients. Crit Care Med 15:817–819
14. Ostro MJ, Russell JA, Soldin SJ, Mahon WA, Jeejeebhoy KN (1985) Control of gastric pH with cimetidine: boluses versus primed infusions. Gastroent 89:532–537
15. Tome G, Fiasse R, Reynaert M, Mahieu P, Hanssens F (1988) Effect of a 2 g cimetidine infusion on twenty-four-hour intragastric pH in critically ill patients. Intensive Care Med 14:379–383
16. Morris DL, Markham SJ, Beechey A, et al (1988) Ranitidine-bolus or infusion prophylaxis for stress ulcer. Crit Care Med 16:229–232
17. Kahn RJ, Serruys-Schoutens E, Brimioulle S, Vincent J-L (1982) Influence of antacid treatment on tracheal flora in mechanically ventilated patients. Crit Care Med 10:229
18. du Moulin GC, Hedley-Whyte J, Paterson DG, Lisbon A (1982) Aspiration of gastric bacteria in antacid-treated patients: a frequent cause of postoperative colonisation of the airway. Lancet 1:242–245
19. Daschner F (1987) Stress ulcer prophylaxis and the risk of nosocomial pneumonia in artificially ventilated patients. Eur J Clin Microbiol 6:129–131
20. MacLean LD (1988) Prophylactic treatment of stress ulcers: first do no harm. Can J Surg 31:76–77
21. Tarnawski A, Hollander D, Gergely H (1987) The mechanism of protective, therapeutic and prophylactic actions of sucralfate. Scand J Gastroent 22(140):7–13
22. Driks MR, Craven DE, Celli BR, et al (1987) Nosocomial pneumonia in intubated patients given sucralfate as compared with antacids or histamine type 2 blockers. The role of gastric colonization. N Engl J Med 317:1376–1382
23. Tryba M (1987) Risk of acute stress bleeding and nosocomial pneumonia in ventilated intensive care unit patients: sucralfate versus antacids. Am J Med 83 (suppl 3B):117–124
24. Cannon LA, Heiselman D, Gardner W, Jones J (1987) Prophylaxis of upper gastrointestinal tract bleeding in mechanically ventilated patients. A randomized study comparing the efficacy of sucralfate, cimetidine, and antacids. Arch Intern Med 147:2101–2106
25. Sontag SJ (1986) Prostaglandins in peptic ulcer disease. An overview of current status and future directions. Drugs 32:445–457
26. Knodell RG, Garjian PL, Schreiber JB (1987) Newer agents available for treatment of stress-related upper gastrointestinal tract mucosal damage. Am J Med 83(6A):36–40
27. Knodell RG, Rosenthal LE (1987) Stress-related mucosal damage: critical evaluation of potential new therapeutic agents. Pharmacotherap 7:104S–109S
28. Morikawa K, Aratani T, Mizutani F, Kato H, Ito Y (1987) Cytoprotective activity of tiquizium bromide (HSR-902) and its mechanism. Folia Pharmacol Japon 90:285–293
29. Tryba M, Zevounou F, Wruck G (1988) Stressblutungen und postoperative Pneumonien bei Intensivpatienten unter Ranitidin oder Pirenzepin. Deutsch Med Wschr 113:930–936
30. Wolfe MM, Soll AH (1988) The physiology of gastric acid secretion. N Engl J Med 319:1707–1715

Management of Severe Acute Pancreatitis

T. Dugernier and M. S. Reynaert

Introduction

Acute pancreatitis is a confounding illness that implies particular skill in its diagnosis, early prognosis and treatment. In no other abdominal emergencies is the outcome of the patient so impredictable at the time of admission. Fortunately, 90% of the attacks are morphologically characterized by edematous interstitial inflammation of the pancreas that resolves spontaneously following a period of bowel rest and simple supportive therapy. Complications arise rarely and the overall mortality rate does not exceed 3% [1]. However a small subset of patients will progress into a devastating illness. Severe acute pancreatitis (SAP) is defined as fatal attack [2] or as any episode which fails to settle on conservative treatment because of serious complications [3].

Pathogenesis of Acute Pancreatitis: Therapeutic Implications

The primary factor ascribed to the development of acute necrotizing pancreatitis is autodigestion of the gland and the surrounding tissues by locally generated active proteolytic and lipolytic enzymes. The combination of a direct initiating factor: the flood of activated enzymes into the glandular epithelial cells and interstitium of the gland, and secondary effects such as massive invasion of the pancreas by polymorphonuclear leukocytes, local protease-antiprotease imbalance and subsequent activation of the different cascade systems of proteases result in direct injury to tissues, accumulation of platelets and fibrin and alteration in vascular permeability. Edema, hemorrhage and ischemia of affected regions of the pancreas ensue and result eventually in focal necrosis [4].

Autodigestion of pancreatic and peripancreatic tissues by prematurely activated enzymes implies a breakdown of the natural safeguards defending the pancreas against its own enzymes. These protective mechanisms include intracellularly the presence of enzymes such as sequestered inactive zymogens and the cellular one-way permeability. Protection is maintained in the tissue by the mucous film on the surface of the duct epithelium, by the presence of pancreatic proteinase inhibitors and by the immediate discharge of pancreatic juice into the duodenum.

Although several etiologic factors (heredity, alcohol abuse, biliary stones, surgery, trauma, drugs, viruses and neoplasm) are identified in approximatively

75% of the cases, it remains poorly understood how these various factors overcome existing safeguards to initiate pancreatitis. Nonetheless early recognition of the precipitating insult may be of paramount importance as in gallstone pancreatitis it exerts a direct influence on the initial therapeutic approach.

The pathogenesis of acute gallstone pancreatitis relies on the concept of a migrating gallstone temporarily impacting at the ampulla before passing into the intestine [5, 6]. Small stones or microlithiasis, multiplicity of gallbladderstones, adequate size of the biliary tree, the length of the common channel and the presence of pancreatic duct reflux on operative cholangiograms are factors that influence stone passage. This suggests that patients with gallstone pancreatitis have a biliary tree which facilitates migration of calculi and subsequent reflux into the pancreatic duct [7]. Since bile reflux enables permeation of activated proteases into the interstitium through the pancreatic duct [8], early relief of papillary obstruction by endoscopic or surgical papillotomy is expected to reduce the severity of pancreatitis by altering the progression towards pancreatic necrosis.

The pathophysiologic mechanisms underlying other forms of acute pancreatitis remain obscure. This lack of understanding precludes the development of effective therapeutic strategies to prevent the disease and to counteract the inflammatory process and thereby the progression towards regional necrosis.

Natural History of Severe Acute Pancreatitis

Severe pancreatitis is associated with extensive and prolonged pancreatic and retroperitoneal inflammation with patchy or generalized areas of tissue necrosis and hemorrhage in and around the pancreas [9, 10]. Schematically the course of SAP can be divided in 2 successive phases. The massive inflammatory reaction that takes place in the pancreatic region (with regional necrosis and sometimes hemorrhage) characterizes the *early toxemic phase*. At this stage lifethreatening complications arise from damage to distant organs and resultant multiple organ failure (MOF). The key role in this process has been attributed to active pancreatic enzymes (trypsin, phospholipase A_2, ...) released by the pancreas and spilled into the circulation [11, 12]. The main route of auto-intoxication of the organism by these products is direct transfer into pancreatic and retroperitoneal lymphatics which enter the thoracic duct [13]. Saturation of protease inhibitors [α_{-2} macroglobulin and α_{-1} proteinase inhibitor] results in local and systemic free proteolytic activity and the subsequent activation of the kallikrein-kinin, complement, coagulation and fibrinolytic systems [14]. Recent evidence supports the hypothesis that excessive stimulation of leukocytes (neutrophils, macrophages) by pancreatic injury plays a pivotal role in the pathogenesis of MOF [15]. These cells when activated at the site of pancreatic injury are able to generate and release a large variety of toxic substances including proteases, phopholipases, lysosomal hydrolases, reactive oxygen metabolites and many others (PAF, TNF, leukotrienes) that all result in additional damage to the pancreas and distant organs.

The regional inflammatory process abates by the 2d or 3d week after onset of symptoms. This sets the stage for the *necrotic phase* of SAP. At that time up to

70% of the patients go on to spontaneous and uneventful resolution of pancreatic and peripancreatic necrotic areas [9]. Ten to 20% develop acute pseudocysts. As necrosis creates a culture medium for bacterial invasion from the digestive tract, abdominal infection and systemic septic complications evolve in 20 to 40% [9, 16, 17]. Pancreatic infection originates from the digestive tract either by translocation, infected bile or hematogeneous/lymphatic spread. The risk of infection is closely related to the severity of the acute episode and the extent of regional necrosis [16]. It should be emphasized that bacterial contamination of those devitalized areas could be documented by operative findings or needle aspiration in 30–50% of the patients within 14 days after onset of symptoms [16, 17]. Even though infected pancreatic necrosis and pancreatic abscess are part of the same continuum, their nature, timing and prognosis differ. Pancreatic abscess tends to be well encapsulated collection of pus as it manifests in the late stage of SAP when the necrotizing process due to pancreatic enzymes has ended and the necrosis is fully liquified [18]. Infected pancreatic necrosis presents earlier and is associated with a higher mortality since the early mixing of bacteria with the ongoing enzymatic and necrotizing process generates a highly toxemic course [19]. Anyhow with the progress in the intensive care of early MOF pancreatic infection and secondary septic complications appear to be the dominant cause of death in SAP.

A better understanding of the pathophysiology of SAP with its complications, natural course and prognosis led recently to the development of new strategies and to a precipitous fall in the number of deaths below 25%.

Whatever the phase of the disease, two extremes of therapeutic policy exist. The first is the surgical removal of necrotic material to reduce MOF and to prevent further bacterial contamination of devitalized tissues [20, 21]. The second is an intensive conservative approach delaying surgery until infection is proven or complications such as massive hemorrhage or symptomatic pseudocyst develop.

Early Prognostic Evaluation

Early and accurate assessment of severity as well as monitoring of the course of the attacks is necessary in severe forms

1. to monitor the patient closely through admission to an intensive therapy area;
2. to anticipate early complications;
3. to consider agressive treatment directed to necrosis and its local and systemic consequences;
4. to evaluate the response to therapy; and
5. to select high risk patients for therapeutic trials and comparison between different centers.

1. *Multiple clinical and laboratory prognostic factors:* three major grading systems of multiple clinical and laboratory criteria have been tested recently in order

to identify high risk patients with acute pancreatitis [22–24]. So far the Acute Physiology and Chronic Health Enquiry (APACHE II) score seems the best scoring system for early detection of severity and prediction of pancreatic collection [24]. Unlike the Imrie and Ransom systems, APACHE II score can be obtained easily at the time of admission and may be recalculated at any time, allowing monitoring of pancreatic necrosis and accurate prediction of late septic complications.

2. *Single prognostic factors:* several biochemical markers and imaging procedures have recently emerged to help to early identify pancreatic necrosis, monitor its progression and assess the response to therapy. Peritoneal lavage [25], arterial hypoxemia [26] and α_2-macroglobulin determination [27] are either insensitive or poor predictors of late complications. So far the dosage of the C-reactive protein provides the best discriminent factor between mild and complicated attacks [28]. This quick and simple assay seems a reliable indicator of pancreatic necrosis and its sequential monitoring enables the anticipation of septic complications. Contrast enhanced computed tomography (CT) with prolonged bolus scanning techniques (dynamic pancreatography) is the best imaging tool for the early detection of necrosis and its extent [29]. Serial CT examinations are most valuable for the early identification of local complications (abscess, pseudocyst, hemorrhage).

Caution should be exercised as these prognostic data should be interpreted on an individual basis and in conjunction with clinical findings. Nonetheless a combination of single biochemical indicators, imaging techniques and a set of clinical criteria, if adjusted to local population and facilities, should allow the identification of most patients with SAP within a few hours of admission.

Conservative Treatment

So far there is no specific treatment which lessens the inflammatory process in SAP and prevents the progression towards pancreatic necrosis. Attempts to neutralize proteases by antienzyme therapy, to rest the pancreas (glucagon, calcitonin, somatostatin), or to inhibit phospholipase A_2 have failed to substantially reduce morbidity and mortality in SAP.

The primary objectives of medical therapy are first to prevent and/or to treat the MOF of the toxemic phase and second to detect the bacterial invasion of regional necrosis.

Baseline management: besides the prompt admission to an intensive therapy area for careful monitoring and support of vital functions the basic medical therapy of SAP is largely empirical. It includes withholding of oral H_2-antagonists feeding, nasogastric suction for paralytic ileus, prevention of stress ulceration with H_2-antagonists, antacids or sucralfate, careful volume replacement, correction of hydroelectrolytic and acid-base disorders and early parenteral nutrition [30]. Non-morphinic analgesic drugs and sedatives are often needed because of pain and mental confusion. Prophylactic antibiotic therapy should be considered in this subset of patients owing to the incidence of early bacterial contamination [16].

Considering the pathophysiologic mechanisms underlying the development of regional necrosis and distant organ damage that characterize the early phase of SAP, 3 additional therapeutic modalities are of interest.

Peritoneal lavage: the role of peritoneal lavage in the treatment of SAP remains controversial. Although a striking attenuation of the early cardiorespiratory disturbances has been demonstrated with peritoneal lavage [31, 32], this treatment did not reduce the overall mortality since the progression of tissue injury, necrosis and infection were not influenced [1]. The greatest benefit from lavage was reported in patients with alcohol-related pancreatitis [32, 33]. Since lavage acts by limiting the systemic absorption of vasoactive substances released in the peritoneal cavity, its early institution is mandatory. However it seems unlikely that enough lavage fluid gets access to the lesser sac where the concentration of toxic agents must be greatest. The addition of a low molecular weight protease inhibitor to the lavage fluid may extent the benefit by inhibition of proteolytic processes in and around the pancreas [34]. Despite these potential shortcomings, peritoneal lavage should be considered as part of the initial therapeutic approach to SAP, particularly of alcohol origin, when typical "prune juice" ascitic fluid is present in the peritoneal cavity [35].

Thoracic duct drainage: Owing to the crucial role of lymphatic pathways in the transfer of toxic substances released by the pancreas we assessed the value of drainage of the thoracic duct lymph in the prevention and treatment of lifethreatening remote complications of SAP [36]. Thoracic duct drainage was surgically carried out with a 7 F Swan-Ganz catheter in 12 patients who were admitted early in the course of fulminant necrotizing acute pancreatitis. Entry criteria included persistent circulatory failure and severe respiratory dysfunction despite and intensive conservative therapeutic regimen and peritoneal lavage. Adult respiratory distress syndrome (ARDS) was present in one half of the patients and

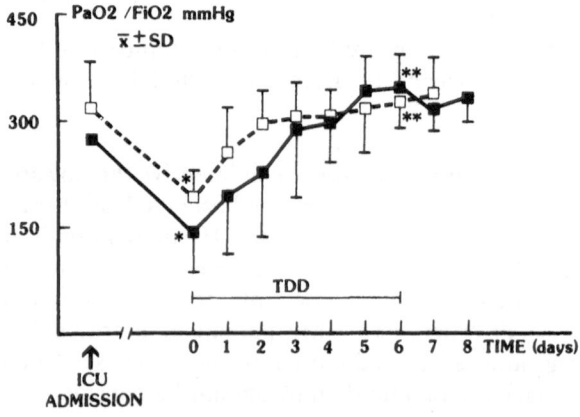

Fig. 1. Changes in PaO_2/FiO_2 as a function of time before, during and after thoracic duct drainage (TDD). Day O represents onset of TDD. Closed squares and continuous line: patients with ARDS (n = 6). Open squares and discontinuous line: patients at risk of developing ARDS (n = 6). * $p < 0.05$ compared with baseline; ** $p < 0.05$ compared with onset of TDD. (From [36] with permission)

severe hypoxemia without widespread pulmonary infiltrates was seen in the other half. As a result of drainage cardiorespiratory dysfunctions were rapidly corrected (Fig. 1) and all patients survived the early-shock phase. Like peritoneal lavage, thoracic duct drainage did not reduce the incidence of late complications (infection, pseudocyst). During the necrotic phase one patient died of MOF originating from infected pancreatic necrosis. The 11 patients left were discharged from hospital.

Substantial amounts of enzymatically active trypsin and leukocyte myeloperoxidase were isolated in the thoracic lymph, supporting the pathogenetic concepts underlying distant organ damage that occur early in the course of SAP [11, 12, 15].

Endoscopic papillotomy: Endoscopic retrograde cholangiopancreatography and emergent papillotomy if impacted ampullary stones are present seem the best therapeutic approach for severe acute gallstone pancreatitis. Early endoscopic dislodgment of impacted stones is undertaken with intent to lessen the inflammatory process and to hamper the progression towards pancreatic necrosis, which is still unproven. However in a recent study this procedure achieved within 72 hours of admission for SAP significantly reduced the morbidity of the attack without exacerbation of the disease process, hemorrhage and pseudocyst formation [37]. Cholecystectomy may be delayed safely during the same hospital admission until pancreatitis subsides since early biliary surgery carries a high mortality in these severely ill patients [23].

Conservative approach to regional necrosis and pancreatic infection: Both peritoneal lavage and thoracic duct drainage enable removal of potential mediators of MOF. These therapeutic options together with intensive supportive care and endoscopic papillotomy in case of gallstone pancreatitis keep the patients with SAP alive through the toxemic phase. However, they leave them with extensive areas of regional necrosis which are at risk of bacterial contamination.

Spontaneous and complete resolution of these necrotic areas have been demonstrated in 50-70% of the patients [9] so that conservative medical management including nasogastric suction, total parenteral nutrition and antibiotics remain sensible [38, 39]. Surgery (and its 20% attendant risk of postoperative complications: hemorrhage, fistula, infection ...) is delayed until complicated pseudocyst or infection is proven.

Sterile and infected collections cannot usually be differentiated on clinical and laboratory grounds since fever and white cells count are notoriously misleading in those patients with large necrotic areas. Serial CT examinations are the best tool for early diagnosis of infection either by demonstration of extraintestinal gas within the pancreatic mass [9, 16] or more reliably by repeated needle aspiration sampling of inflammatory collections [17]. If applied systematically and serially to patients with pancreatic necrosis, this diagnostic work-up may help to define the appropriate time for surgical debridement without jeopardizing those patients with pancreatic infection. Although surgery remains the treatment of choice for complicated pseudocyst and infected pancreatic necrosis, CT guided percutaneous drainage has a role as a temporary measure to buy time in severely ill patients before surgical debridement and drainage [40]. The small caliber of the drains and the thick necrotic material often preclude complete evacuation of the collections and lead to recurrences [9, 40].

Surgical Treatment

Besides rare instances of diagnostic uncertainty, surgical procedures in SAP are usually restricted to the treatment of complications of the disease. They have no curative role except for cholecystectomy and common duct exploration for prevention of recurrences in gallstone pancreatitis.

During the *toxemic phase* early subtotal or total pancreatectomy failed to abate the systemic effects of inflammation and necrosis. The incidence of septic complications was not reduced and the overall mortality rate exceeded 30% [41]. Postoperative diabetes developed in the majority of survivors. These unfavourable results are best explained by the poor delineation of the necrotic process in the first week of the disease [10].

Massive arterial hemorrhage almost exclusively results from regional necrosis and infection. Bleeding is usually fatal under conservative treatment. Angiographic occlusive techniques enable preoperative identification of the bleeding vessel. Arteriographic embolization should be combined with subsequent surgical ligation, drainage and thorough debridement in order to control sepsis and prevent recurrences of bleeding [42].

Persistance of overwhelming MOF and infection of regional necrosis are the most frequent indications for surgery in the early phase of SAP. Necrosectomy and drainage with [10] or without [20] local lavage of the lesser sac resulted in removal of infected necrotic tissues and elimination of activated enzymes. This surgical approach to the toxemic phase of SAP reduced the mortality rate of these patients to 10–20%. However most of these patients were operated upon because of persistant MOF and not because of generalized sepsis. Considering the 20–30% reoperation rate for postoperative complications it remains unproven that surgical drainage of sterile necrosis limits the remote complications of SAP and prevents abdominal sepsis.

Surgical indications during the *necrotic phase* of SAP include symptomatic pseudocyst and pancreatic abscess. Acute pseudocyst should be drained internally as soon as hemorrhage, infection or organ compression occur. External drainage should be considered only in patients with thin-walled and immature pseudocysts as this procedure is often complicated by fistula and abscess.

Undrained pancreatic abscess are always lethal. Several surgical approaches, either transperitoneally [18, 21, 43, 44], via the flank or the retroperitoneum [45] have been used to gain access to infected collections. Several methods of drainage with or without lavage have been reported with a survival rate of these patients between 75 to 95% [18, 21, 43–45]. Nevertheless early, aggressive and thorough debridement of necrotic areas with wide opening of infected spaces are essential. In this setting a preoperative CT scan is helpful in localizing all the areas of necrosis. Multiple reoperations are often needed because of fistula, hemorrhage and ongoing sepsis.

Conclusion

So far there is no single therapeutic agent or procedure that lessens the inflammatory reaction in acute pancratitis, hampers the progression towards regional necrosis and thereby reduces the severity of distant organ damage and the incidence of pancreatic infection. Both the medical and surgical approaches to SAP are intended to face the specific complications of the 2 distinct phases of the attack. It is only be the timely application of the several modes of therapy during the course of the disease that patients with SAP might be granted a better outcome.

References

1. Mayer DA, Mc Mahon MJ, Corfield AP, et al (1985) Controlled clinical trial of peritoneal lavage for the treatment of severe acute pancreatitis. N Engl J Med 312:399–404
2. Corfield AP, Cooper JM, Williamson RCN, et al (1985) Prediction of severity in acute pancreatitis: prospective comparison of three prognostic indices. Lancet 2:403–407
3. Mc Mahon MJ, Playforth MJ, Pickford IR (1980) A comparative study of methods for the prediction of severity of attacks of acute pancreatitis. Br J Surg 67:22–25
4. Bockman DE, Büchler M, Beger HJ (1987) Ultrastructure of human acute pancreatitis. In: Beger HG, Büchler M (eds) Acute pancreatitis. Springer, Berlin Heidelberg New York Tokyo, pp 12–22
5. Acosta JN, Pellegrini CA, Skinner DB (1980) Etiology and pathogenesis of acute biliary pancreatitis. Surgery 88:118–122
6. Kelly TR (1980) Gallstone pancreatitis: the timing of surgery. Surgery 88:345–350
7. Armstrong CP, Taylor TV, Jeacock J, Lucas S (1985) The biliary tract in patients with acute gallstone pancreatitis. Br J Surgery 72:551–555
8. Reber HA, Farmer RC, Maslin SC (1982) Effects of bile on the permeability of the pancreatic duct to macromolecules. Gastroenterology 82:1156–1160
9. Sostre CF, Flournoy JG, Bova JG, Goldstein HM, Schenker S (1985) Pancreatic phlegmon. Clinical features and cause. Dig Dis Sci 30:918–927
10. Kivilaasko E, Fraki O, Nikki P (1981) Resection of the pancreas for acute fulminant pancreatitis. Surg Gynecol Obstet 152:493–498
11. Balldin G (1987) Release of vasocative substances in ascites and blood in acute pancreatitis. In: Beger HG, Büchler M (eds) Acute pancreatitis. Springer, Berlin Heidelberg New York Tokyo, pp 63–70
12. Warshaw AL, Lesser PB, Rie M, Cullen DJ (1975) The pathogenesis of pulmonary edema in acute pancreatitis. Ann Surg 182:505–510
13. Mayer AD, Hodgson M, Mc Mahon MJ (1985) Enzyme transfer from pancreas to plasma during acute pancreatitis. The contribution of ascitic fluid and lymphatic drainage of the pancreas. Gut 26:876–881
14. Balldin G, Ohlsson K (1979) Demonstration of pancreatic protease-antiprotease complexes in the peritoneal fluid of patient with acute pancreatitis. Surgery 85:451–456
15. Rinderknecht H (1988) Fatal pancreatitis, a consequence of excessive leukocyte stimulation? Int J Pancreatol 3:105–112
16. Beger HG, Bittner R, Block S, Büchler M (1986) Bacterial contamination of pancreatic necrosis: a prospective clinical study. Gastroenterology 91:433–438
17. Gerzof SG, Banks PA, Spechler SJ, et al (1984) Role of guided percutaneous aspiration in early diagnosis of pancreatic sepsis. Dig Dis Sci 29:950–976
18. Warshaw AL, Jin G (1985) Improved survival in 45 patients with pancreatic abscess. Ann Surg 207:408–417
19. Beger HG, Krautzberger W, Bittner R, Block S, Büchler M (1985) Results of surgical treatment of necrotizing pancreatitis. World J Surg 9:972–979

20. Rattner DW, Warshaw AL (1988) Surgical intervention in acute pancreatitis. Crit Care Med 16:89-95
21. Levy E, Hannoun L, Parc R, Honiger J, Huguet C, Loygue J (1984) Le drainage actif prolongé des pancréatites aigues nécrotico-hémorragiques. Ann Chir 38:351-356
22. Ranson JHC (1979) The timing of biliary surgery in acute pancreatitis. Ann Surg 189:654-663
23. Osborne DH, Imrie CW, Carter DC (1981) Biliary surgery in the same admission for gallstone-associated acute pancreatitis. Br J Surg 68:758-761
24. Larvin M, Mc Mahon MJ (1989) APACHE-II score for assessment and monitoring of acute pancreatitis. Lancet 2:201-205
25. Mayer DA, Mc Mahon MJ (1985) The diagnostic and prognostic value of peritoneal lavage in patients with acute pancreatitis. Surg Gynecol Obstet 160:507-512
26. Cooper MJ, Williamson RCN, Pollock AV (1982) The role of peritoneal lavage in the prediction and treatment of severe acute pancreatitis. Ann R Coll Surg Engl 64:422-425
27. Lasson A, Ohlsson K (1984) Acute pancreatitis. The correlation between clinical course, protease inhibitors, and complement and kinin activation. Scand J Gastroenterol 19:707-710
28. Wilson C, Heads A, Shenkin A, Imrie CW (1989) C-reactive protein, antiproteases and complement factors as objective markers of severity in acute pancreatitis. Br J Surg 76:177-181
29. Maier W (1987) Early objective diagnosis and staging of acute pancreatitis by contrast-enhanced computed tomography. In: Beyer HG, Bückler M (eds) Acute pancreatitis. Springer, Berlin Heidelberg New York Tokyo, pp 132-140
30. Creutzfeldt W, Lankisch PG (1981) Intensive medical treatment of severe acute pancreatitis. World J Surg 5:341-350
31. Ranson JHC, Spencer FC (1978) The role of peritoneal lavage in severe acute pancreatitis. Ann Surg 187:565-575
32. Stone HH, Fabian TC (1980) Peritoneal dialysis in the treatment of acute alcoholic pancreatitis. Surg Gynecol Obstet 150:878-882
33. Alle JL, Reynaert MS, Azagra JS, Massaut J, Dive A, De Maeght S (1988) Expérience belge de la dialyse péritonéale percutanée dans le traitement de la pancréative aigue nécrotico-hémorragique alcoolique. Acta Gastroent Belg 51:23-31
34. Niederau C, Crass RA, Silver G, Ferrell LD, Grendell JH (1988) Therapeutic regimens in acute experimental hemorrhagic pancreatitis. Effects of hydratation, oxygenation, peritoneal lavage, and a potent protease inhibitor. Gastroenterology 95:1648-1657
35. McMahon MJ, Lankisch PG (1987) Peritoneal lavage and dialysis for the treatment of acute pancreatitis. In: Beger HG, Büchler M (eds) Acute pancreatitis. Springer, Berlin Heidelberg New York Tokyo, pp 278-284
36. Dugernier TH, Reynaert MS, Deby-Dupont G, et al (1989) Prospective evaluation of thoracic-duct drainage in the treatment of respiratory failure complicating severe acute pancreatitis. Intensive Care med 15:372-378
37. Neoptolemos JP, Carr-Locke DL, London NJ, Bailey IA, James D, Fossard DP (1988) Controlled trial of urgent endoscopic retrograde cholangiopancreatography and endoscopic sphincterotomy versus conservative treatment for acute pancreatitis due to gallstones. Lancet 2:979-983
38. Reynaert MS, Bshouty ZH, Otte JB, Kestens PJ, Trémouroux J (1985) Percutaneous peritoneal dialysis as an early treatment of acute necrotic hemorrhagic pancreatitis. Intensive Care Med 11:123-128
39. Reber HA (1986) Surgical intervention in necrotizing pancreatitis. Gastroenterology 91:479-482
40. Van Vyve E, Reynaert M, Dardenne A, Pringot J, Kestens PJ (1988) Pancréatite aigue nécrosante: place du drainage percutané dans le traitement des masses nécrotiques stériles et infectées. Med Chir Dig 17:18-19
41. Aldridge MC, Urnstein M, Glazer G, Dudley HAF (1985) Pancreatic resection for severe acute pancreatitis. Br J Surg 72:796-800

42. Waltman AC, Luers PR, Athanasoulis CA, Warshaw AL (1986) Massive arterial hemorrhage in patients with pancreatitis. Complementary roles of surgery and transcatheter occlusive techniques. Arch Surg 121:439–443
43. Bradley EL, Fulenwider JT (1984) Open treatment of pancreatic abscess. Surg Gynecol Obstet 159:509–513
44. Büchler M, Block S, Krautzberger W, et al (1984) Necrotizing pancreatitis: peritoneal lavage (PL) or local lavage (LL) of the lesser sac? Dig Dis Sci 29:944–976
45. Van Vyve E, Reynaert MS, Passelecq E et al (1988) Pancréatite aigue nécrosante. Traitement des masses nécrotiques stériles et infectées. Acta Gastroent Belg 51:44–50

Perioperative Management of the Liver Transplant Patient*

P. A. Sheiner, P. D. Greig, and G. A. Levy

Introduction

Orthotopic liver transplantation (OLT) has become the accepted and preferred treatment for end stage irreversible liver disease [1]. In recent years, improvement in survival of liver transplant patients has approached 80%. This improvement in survival has been not only due to improvements in immunosuppression, but also due to our increasing understanding of the management of the transplant patient in the perioperative period.

Peri-operative Assessment

A patient is only considered a suitable candidate for liver transplantation when the diagnosis of end-stage irreversible liver disease is made. In children, the indications for OLT are primarily, biliary atresia and liver disease secondary to metabolic causes. In adults however, the liver disease is usually acquired or may be a result of a chronic primary liver disease [2, 3] (Table 1).

Pre-operative Work-up

The principles behind the liver transplant workup are to firmly establish the etiology of the liver disease and to assess liver reserve (Table 2). In addition to tests which firmly establish the diagnosis and severity of liver disease, patients must be assessed with regards to their ability to withstand extensive surgery. Medical conditions which are contraindications to liver transplantation are severe cardiopulmonary disease, extrahepatic malignancy, sepsis occuring outside of the hepatobiliary tree and the acquired immune deficiency syndrome (AIDS).

Management: Once accepted into the program, liver transplant candidates are followed at regular intervals. Transplant candidates may present preoperatively with complications that require urgent attention.

One of the major complications is gastrointestinal bleeding. Common causes of hemorrhage are duodenal ulcer, gastritis, or variceal hemorrhage. These pa-

* This work was supported by Grants from the Medical Research Council of Canada (MA 6787) and Upjohn Canada Inc.

Table 1. Indications for liver transplantation at the University of Toronto (n = 105)

	Number	[%]
Adult	76	72
Cirrhosis	41	40
Cryptogenic	18	17
Primary Biliary	12	12
Hepatitis B	5	5
Alcoholic	4	4
Other	2	2
Tumor	5	5
Hepatoma	3	2
Cholangiocarcinoma	2	2
Other	6	6
Sclerosing Cholangitis	4	4
Alpha$_1$ Antitrypsin	2	2
Fulminant hepatitis	15	15
Non A, Non B	11	11
Hepatitis B	2	2
Wilson's	1	1
Toxic	1	1
Budd-Chiari	2	2
Retransplantation	7	7
Pediatric	29	28
Biliary atresia	11	11
Metabolic disorders	4	4
Tyrosinemia	3	3
Glycogen Storage Disease	1	1
Cirrhosis	2	2
Fulminant hepatitis	6	6
Non A, Non B	4	4
Wilson's	1	1
Toxic	1	1
Retransplantation	6	6

% represent percent of total transplants.

tients must be evaluated and resuscitated aggressively. The etiology of the bleeding is usually established by endoscopy. The goal of investigations and therapy is to stabilize patients prior to surgery. For those few patients with variceal hemorrhage who do not respond to nonoperative measures, emergency liver transplantation may be necessary although the results are not as favourable.

Spontaneous bacterial peritonitis (SBP) is a serious complication seen in patients with ascites. Patients with a diagnosis of SBP are admitted to hospital and placed on appropriate antibiotics. Although the presence of SBP is not a contraindication to liver transplant (patients are given a full course of antibiotics in the postoperative period) it is preferable to transplant the patient after the infection has been fully treated.

Table 2. Liver transplant work-up

Bloodwork	
Hematology	CBC, group and reserve; PT; PTT
Renal	Electrolytes, blood glucose, BUN, creatinine, magnesium, phosphate, calcium
Liver	AST, ALT, ALP, bilirubin, proteins (A/G), amylase

Other

Serum Fe/TIBC; ferritin; transferrin; sickle cell (only if pt black); serum copper; ceruloplasmin; immunoelectrophoresis; alpha$_1$ antitrypsin; alpha feto-protein; antimitochondrial antibody; rheumatoid factor; anti nuclear factor; anti-smooth muscle.

Serology

HBsAg; anti-HBsAg; HBeAg; anti-HBeAg; anti-HBcAg; anti-HAV: IgM IgG; EBV titres; CMV titres; varicella titres.
If patient has Hepatitis B+ send 1 red top HBV-DNA.
HIV (with consent).

Tissue Typing

HLA tissue typing

24 hour Urine Collection

creatinin clearance, Ca, Mg, PO$_4$ (3 days)

Radiologic

Chest X Ray (PA and lateral)
Abdominal ultrasound with Doppler hepatic vessels
Abdominal angiogram (if non-visualization of hepatic and portal veins and hepatic artery on ultrasound)
Gastroscopy
Pulmonary function test
ECG
2-D Echocardiogram
Transjugular liver biopsy with hepatic vein pressures

Consults

Anesthesia	Pharmacist
Dentistry	Dietician
Hematology	Social work
Psychiatry	

M.A.L.G skin test (consent required)

The patient with fulminant hepatic failure (FHF) provides a challenge for the transplant team. Acute fulminant hepatic failure is defined as development of severe liver disease in less than 8 weeks after the onset of the illness. When liver failure occurs 8–28 weeks after the onset of symptoms, it is classified as subacute liver failure [4]. The predominant causes have been non-A, non-B hepatitis, hepatitis B and toxic hepatitis. Overall mortality rates have been reported in the range of 50–60%. Mortality rates of patients in stage III or IV hepatic encephalopathy (HE) are as high as 80–90%. Preliminary results from uncontrolled trials have suggested a role for prostaglandins in the treatment of FHF [5]. Although there are presently clinical trials in the use of prostaglandins for the treatment of FHF, liver transplantation is now the accepted form of treatment for patients with FHF.

Success of emergency transplantation for patients with FHF ranges from 55 to 75%, although once the patient reaches stage IV hepatic encephalopathy the results are markedly diminished [6, 7].

The most common cause of death from FHF is brain stem herniation from cerebral edema from an altered permeability in the blood/brain barrier. This results in brain swelling and raised intracranial pressure. These patients must be managed in the ICU preoperatively. Swan-Ganz catheters should be placed to maintain an adequate intravascular volume. The monitoring of the intracranial pressure (ICP) has been found to be useful in management of the patient. At our institution, all patients undergoing emergency liver transplantation for FHF have ICP bolts placed preoperatively. This aids in the management of the patient both intraoperatively and postoperatively. Hyperventilation and loop diuretics are used to maintain an ICP of less than 20.

Post-operative Management

Issues that must be adressed in the post-operative period include management of fluid and electrolysis, respiratory function, monitoring of neurologic status as well as graft function. All patients are managed in an intensive care setting by individuals who have demonstrated expertise in the care of ICU patients (Table 3).

Management of Respiratory Function

All patients are taken to the intensive care unit and intubated until the anesthetic agents have been metabolized. In most cases, these patients may be quickly weaned and extubated. The usual respiratory parameters (negative inspiratory force, tidal volume) are obtained to determine the patients ability to be extubated. Most patients with a functioning liver are extubated within 24 hours although delayed graft function, the presence of pleural effusions, or pulmonary infiltrates may delay extubation.

Hemodynamics

Postoperative liver transplant patients are often volume depleted. This is usually secondary to a) operating room losses and b) vasodilation. Volume replacement with red blood cells, plasma, cryoprecipitate and platelets are often required in the early postoperative period. This is usually given in addition to a maintenance of crystalloid solutions. Pulmonary capillary wedge pressure, blood pressure and urine output are used to determine the adequacy of fluid replacement.

Coagulation

Hepatic insufficiency is associated with abnormalities in coagulation. These are routinely assessed by measurements of prothrombin time (PT) and partial

Table 3. Immediate postoperative orders

Vital signs q1H
Ventilation: FiO$_2$ _____ Vt _____ Rate _____ PEEP
Warming blanket to increase rectal temperature to 37°C
Chest X Ray (portable) and ECG STAT and daily at 0630
NPO
N/G to straight drainage. Irrigate with 10-15 ml N/S q4H and PRN
Replace losses with N/S + 20 mEq KCI/IQ/shift
IV's: (a) S/G catheter – proximal port _____
               (b) Cordis _____
               (c) Peripheral _____
               (d) Second central IV _____
               (e) _____
               (f) _____
Drains: (a) T-tube to straight drainage (bile bag)
               (b) 3 Jackson Pratt drains – check and reset suction q1H and PRN
               (c) Foley to straight drainage
CBC, blood sugar, lytes, BUN, creat, bili, AST, ALP, PT, PTT and ABG's STAT and q4H (24H)
– then reassess
Absolute lymphocyte count STAT and once daily
DAILY (0630) Bloods: CBC, blood sugar, lytes, BUN, creat, bili, prop, alb, glob, Ca, Mg, PO$_4$,
amyl, AST, ALP, PT, PTT, ABG's
Cultures: urine, sputum, oropharynx, bile and all drainage for C & S and yeast on:
PO DAY 2 _____   PO DAY 4 _____   PO DAY 6 _____   PO DAY 8 _____   then q Monday
Urine for CMV q Tuesday
Weigh daily and record on flow sheet
Medications: (a) Gammimmune N (Cutter) 5 g in 250 ml N/S at 30 ml/hr for 1 hr.
                 If tolerated give remainder over 2 hrs. Daily (3 doses)
             (b) Heparin _____ units + Persantine _____ mg
                 in _____ ml D5W at _____ ml/hr
             (c) MgSO$_4$
             (d) Antibiotic
             (e) Zantac 50 mg IV q8H
             (f) Vitamin K1 (Aquamephyton) 10 mg IV daily
             (g) Folate 10 mg IV daily
             (h) Riopan 30 ml via N/G q1H PRN for pH <4.0
Immunosuppression:
(a) Minnesota Anti-Lymphoblast Globulin (horse or _____) _____ mg in ml N/S + _____ units
    heparin at _____ ml/hr (dose 10-20 mg/kg/day via central line).
    Reassess daily
(b) SoluMedrol: 80 mg IV on PO DAY at 1000 _____
                60 mg on PO DAY 2 at 1000 _____
                40 mg on PO DAY 3 at 1000 then reassess _____
No sedation, no analgesia until patient awake – then:
                              Morphine _____ mg IV q1H PRN
                              Valium _____ mg IV qIH PRN

---

thromboplastin time (PTT). Recently, the measurement of coagulation factors V and VII have been shown to be predictive of early graft function [8]. Following successful liver transplantation, factor V and VII actively should return to normal levels promptly and failure of these activities to normalize is an ominous sign of graft failure.

Renal Function

Renal insufficiency (occasionally requiring dialysis) is frequently reported postoperatively in the liver transplant patients [2, 9]. This may be due to a combination of factors such as pre-existing renal insufficiency (hepato-renal syndrome), intraoperative blood loss, hypotension leading to acute tubular necrosis, poor liver function and sepsis.

In the early postoperative period, the goal is to maintain a urine output of 0.5 ml/kg/hr. Volume and the addition of low dose dopamine (3–5 μg/kg/min) are used to maintain renal perfusion. Poor urine output in the face of adequate filling pressures may necessitate the need for diuretics (usually loop diuretics).

Neurologic Function

Patients with FHF usually have ICP monitors placed preoperatively and ICP is monitored continuously in the postoperative period. The aim is to maintain adequate blood pressure and urine output while maintaining and ICP of less than 20 mmHg. Neurological status is ascertained by frequent neurological checks (pupil reaction responsiveness) and narcotics are kept to a minimum. Because of risk of infection, the ICP bolt is removed as soon as the patient's neurological status appears to be stable.

Confusion and seizures can be seen even in patients with chronic liver disease in the postoperative period. The incidence of reported seizures has been reported to be high as 22% [2]. There is usually no focal deficit noted, but high cyclosporine levels along with low serum magnesium levels have been implicated as contributing factors [2, 10]. In our centre, all patients are placed on continuous infusions of magnesium sulfate for the first 72–96 hours postoperatively.

Nutrition

Most patients undergoing liver transplantation present with poor nutritional status secondary to long standing liver failure. In addition, they are subjected to the usual catabolic stresses that are seen in patients who undergo major surgery. In those patients who recover quickly, oral alimentation is usually started by postoperative day 3. Hyperalimentation (TPN) is usually started in patients in whom complications such as graft dysfunction, infections or respiratory insufficiency occur as soon as the patient is hemodynamically stable. TPN is then continued until the patient has demonstrated the ability to maintain an adequate oral intake.

Medications

Prophylactic Antibiotics: Prophylactic antibiotics are given preoperatively and continued for 24 hours postoperatively. The use of broad spectrum antibiotics has resulted in a decrease in perioperative bacterial infections but an increase in the incidence of antibiotic induced enterocolitis.

Prophylaxis for Cytomegalovirus Infection: There have been a number of studies to suggest that CMV immune globulin is able to reduce the incidence of CMV infection in the transplant patient [11]. At our institution we routinely give patients high titered CMV immune globulin for the first three postoperative days and our overall incidence of CMV is only 16%.

Anticoagulation: In order to minimize the risk of deep vein thrombosis, patients are placed on heparin and persantine and patients are mobilized early and are usually fully ambulatory but the fourth postoperative day.

Antacids: In order to prevent stress ulceration, all patients are placed on H_2 antagonists as well as liquid antacids or sucralfate in order to keep the gastric pH above 4.

Immunosuppression

Before the introduction of cyclosporin A (CsA), immunosuppression of the transplant patient consisted of Imuran and high dose corticosteroids. Using this regimen, one year and five year survival rates were only 32.9% and 20%, respectively [12]. With the intriduction of CsA in 1980, one and five year actuarial survival rates rose to 70% and 63%, respectively [12]. However, CsA usage has resulted in an increased incidence of nephrotoxicity and Epstein-Barr related lymphomas. This has been significantly reduced by lowering the dosage of CsA although nephrotoxicity still remains a significant problem. Sequential immunotherapy has now become routine in most centers. Induction immunosuppression with an antilymphocyte globulin preparation (monoclonal or polyclonal) has become an accepted routine in order to minimize the neurotoxic and nephrotoxic side effects of CsA which were seen in the early postoperative period. Once renal and neurologic function are stable, CsA is intruduced in either intravenous or oral form and continued for life.

Steroids

All patients receive 100 mg of Solumedrol preoperatively. Subsequently, this is reduced rapidly until a dose of 0.3 mg/kg/day is reached. Side effects of prednisone include an increased susceptibility to infections, hyperglycemia and impaired wound healing.

Polyclonal Antilymphoblast Globulin

This is a biological product derived by sensitizing an animal (horse or goat) with T-lymphoblasts and extracting the sera which contains high titers of immunoglobulin IgG to human T lymphoblasts. Polyclonal antilymphoblast products (ALG) are potent immunosuppressive agents that are effective both in induction immunotherapy and in the treatment of episodes of acute rejection [13]. Induction therapy with ALG has been reported to reduce the incidence of significant postoperative rejection, however, it is associated with an increased incidence of CMV infection. ALG is adjusted daily to maintain an absolute lymphocyte count of 100 to 200 cells/mm^3. Cyclosporin is usually added by postoperative day 4 or 5 and ALG is continued until adequate CsA levels are reached. Side effects of ALG include fever, thrombocytopenia, leukopenia, anaphylaxis, joint pain, serum sickness and increased susceptibility to infection (candida or viral).

Monoclonal Antilymphocyte Products (OKT3)

Several monoclonal antibodies which recognize human lymphocytes have now been developed and are used routinely in the setting of liver transplantation [14]. OKT3 is a murine, monoclonal antibody to the T3 antigen of human T cells. It has been used both as a primary immunosuppressive agent as well as in the treatment of severe rejection. OKT3 being a mouse immunoglobulin is extremely antigenic and usually its use results in antibody formation. To prevent formation of antibodies, azathioprine is used concommitantly. Serious lift-threatening side effects have been observed with its use. High fever, tremors, diarrhea, vomiting and nausea, chest pain, rigors and wheezing have all been seen. Life-threatening pulmonary edema has been seen in 10% of cases, usually when given to patients who are volume overloaded. Prior to giving the initial does of OKT3, patients are usually given a bolus dose of Solumedrol to prevent allergic reactions. These patients are monitored closely for the first 48 hours and antihistamines and acetominophen may be required to prevent side effects.

Cyclosporine

CsA is an antibiotic isolated from the fungus Tolypocladium gans. It is the central immunosuppressive agent used today. It binds to a specific receptor (cyclophilin) and interferes with activation of T cells.

The drug is given preferably by the oral route as rapid intravenous infusion may cause anaphylaxis and is associated with increased nephro and neurotoxicity. This is largely due to the carrier solvent (cremaphor). The dosage of CsA is adjusted to maintain a trough cyclosporin whole blood level of 300–500 mg/L (monoclonal RIA assay). CsA is lipid soluble and absorption is dependent upon the availability of bile and bile acids. Therefore, until adequate bile flow is restored, adequate cyclosporin levels are difficult to obtain with oral preparations. If therapeutic cyclosporin levels cannot be achieved with oral CsA, IV CsA is begun at 1–15 mg/kg/day by continuous infusion. CsA must be placed in glass containers and infused through nitroglycerin-coated intravenous tubing.

BUN and creatinine are drawn daily as cyclosporine is highly nephrotoxic. Other side effects include hypertension, tremors, confusion, agitation, anorexia, increased risk of malignancy (especially Epstein-Barr related lymphomas which usually respond to lowering or removing immunosuppression), hypertrichosis, headaches, hearing loss, gum hyperplasia, gynecomastia and a decrease in serum magnesium levels (Table 4). Cyclosporin is metabolized by the cytochrome P-450 oxidase system and the contribution of cyclosporin metabolites both to immuno-suppression and toxicity is unknown. Any drug which enhances P450 activity will decrease CsA levels, whereas P450 inhibitors result in enhanced parent CsA, levels. Thus caution must be exercised in giving any drugs to patients who are taking CsA (Table 5) [15].

New Immunosuppressive Agents

FK506, a product of Streptomyces Tsukubaensis, has been shown to have potent immunosuppressive activity in heart, kidney and liver transplants in rats, dogs and primates. A number of studies have shown this agent to be associated with unacceptable toxicity including widespread arteritis. A recent study however has suggested that FK506 may be a useful immunosuppressive agent and may even reverse rejection which is unresponsive to cyclosporin A. Based upon these results future controlled studies are warranted [16].

Table 4. Side effects of cyclosporin A

Major	[%]		Minor	[%]
Renal dysfunction	51.7		Hypertrichosis	32.9
Hypertension	38.6		Tremor	20.7
Lymphoma	0.2		Paresthesiae	5.2
Malignant tumour	0.6		Headaches	0.8
Infection			Gum hyperplasia	14.8
bacterial	18.3			
viral	12.6			
fungal	3.2			

Table 5. Drug interactions with cyclosprin A

Decreased excretion	Increased metabolism	Increased nephrotoxicity
Erythromycin	Phenytoin	Amphotericin B
Ketoconazole	Rifampicin	Aminoglycosides
Corticosteroids	Isoniazid	Melphalan
Cimetidine	Sulphonamides/	Trimethoprim
Verapamil	trimethoprim,	Co-trimoxazole
	sulphadimidine	Non-steroidal anti-inflammatory agents

Postoperative Complications

Results of liver transplantation have improved in the past 5 to 10 years. Despite the significant improvements noted in survival, liver transplantation still carries with it a high morbidity and mortality. Most of the deaths occur from complications in the initial postoperative period.

Postoperative Hemorrhage

The incidence of postoperative hemorrhage ranges from 3-18% and is associated with a high mortality [2, 9]. This is in agreement with out own adult experience (17%). The incidence of postoperative hemorrhage appears to correlate with previous upper abdominal surgery, acute or chronic active hepatitis, and the degree of coagulopathy seen in the patient preoperatively. Patients are monitored in the ICU with frequent determinations of hematocrit. A rapidly dropping hematocrit, hemodynamic instability of abdominal distension are suggestive of ongoing intra-abdominal bleeding and may necessitate an explorative laparotomy.

Hepatic Artery Thrombosis

Hepatic artery thrombosis is a devastating complication seen in 5-10% of adults and up to 38% of children who undergo orthotopic liver transplantation [2, 3, 12]. Risk factors thought to be associated with hepatic artery thrombosis include the size of vessel, type of vascular anastomosis (end to end versus the use of conduits) and non-technical factors including the presence of rejection, infection, hemoconcentration or dehydration [17, 18]. Acute hepatic artery thrombosis is characterized by a dramatic increase of liver enzymes and associated by progressive coagulopathy. If unrecognized, it may progress to fulminant hepatic necrosis.

Clinical presentations to hepatic artery thrombosis include biliary strictures (secondary to ischemia in the donor anastomosis) and intrahepatic abscesses (usually a late manifestation). Relapsing bacteremia may also be a clinical presentation of hepatic artery thrombosis. Diagnosis is made by a doppler ultrasound combined with real time ultrasonography. If the hepatic artery flow cannot be identified by sonography an arteriogram should be obtained.

Hepatic artery thrombosis may occasionally be left untreated, however, the patient will usually require retransplantation either semi-electively or on an emergency basis. There may be a role for thrombectomy and revision of the hepatic artery if diagnosed early.

Portal Vein Thrombosis

This is an uncommon complication and clinical presentation depends on the timing of the thrombosis. Early postoperative portal vein thrombosis resembles hepatic artery thrombosis. It is characterized by rising liver enzymes (AST) and the patient may progress to FHF. However, when thrombosis occurs 4–5 weeks post-transplant, patients may have a non-specific rise in liver function tests, or may present with evidence of portal hypertension such as upper GI bleeding, ascites or ileus.

Diagnosis is made again by ultrasonography. Angiography or transhepatic portal venography may be required if sonography fails to provide and accurate diagnosis. Treatment consists of emergency surgery (thrombectomy) or retransplantation.

Biliary Tract Complications

Biliary tract complications following orthotopic liver transplantation are reported to be in the range of 15–25% [19]. Factors felt to contribute to this high complication rate includes inadequate blood supply or ischemic damage to the bile ducts. Other factors such as local infection, graft rejection, changes in bile secretion, drug toxicity and operative technique have also been implicated [20].

Bile leakage may occur from the first day postoperatively up to 3 weeks post-transplant. Localized leaks may present with minimal symptomatology and may only be discovered on routine cholangiogram or by ultrasound. However, they may also present as an intra-abdominal abscess or as frank bile peritonitis. This is manifested by fever, abdominal pain and the sustained rise in bilirubin with or without elevation of alkaline phosphatase. Diagnosis of a bile leak may be made by cholangiogram or by HIDA scan in patients with choledochoenterostomies.

Treatment depends upon the timing and presentation of the leak. Early leakage with intra-abdominal peritonitis require reexploration with repair and drainage. Contained leaks in the stable patients have been managed by percutaneous drainage and conservative therapy.

Primary Non-function

Postoperative liver function can be measured by transaminases and bile production and the return of coagulation factors V and VII to normal. There appears to be a correlation between the correction of these coagulation factors and liver function [21]. Primary graft non-function (PNF) is defined as initial poor hepatic function following orthotopic liver transplant. Evidence of deterioration includes minimal bile output, uncorrectable coagulopathy, continual elevation of transaminases, acidosis and hypoglycemia. Liver biopsy shows severe ischemic necrosis especially in zone 3. The incidence of PNF is reported to be in the range of 2–23% and carries with it a significant mortality. Although there is no known, effective treatment (other than retransplantation) for PNF, preliminary studies have suggested that the use of prostaglandin E_2 (PGE_2) may be beneficial in this setting [22].

Allograft Rejection

Allograft rejection in the early postoperative period occurs in 60–100% of transplant patients [8, 15]. Rejection is suspected in patients with rising liver enzymes which may be accompanied by fever and malaise and right uper quadrant discomfort. The diagnosis is confirmed by a percutaneous liver biopsy. The histologic findings are that of periportal inflammation with mononuclear cells and eosinophils. Bile duct inflammation and endothelialitis are also pathognomonic of acute rejection.

Episodes of acute rejection usually respond to bolus doses of corticosteroids. Those who fail to respond to steroids are then given a ten to fourteen day course of ALG (monoclonal or polyclonal). Failure to respond to immunosuppressive therapy may result in loss of the graft and necessitate retransplantation.

Infections

The major cause of death following liver transplantation is infection. Immunosuppressed patients are at risk for bacterial, viral and fungal infections (Table 6). Bacterial infections are usually seen in the early postoperative period. Wound infections and intra-abdominal abscesses account for the majority of bacterial infections seen in transplant patients.

Viral infections are seen frequently in immunosuppressed patients and if not recognized may prove to be fatal. CMV is present in over half the population

Table 6. Infections in the liver transplant patient in the post-transplant period

First Month

Infection present in recipient prior to transplant (e.g., hepatitis, S. stercoralis, tuberculosis, smoldering bacterial infection)

Infection transmitted with the allograft (e.g. hepatitis, HIV, acute bacterial and candidal infections)

Infection related to technical complications of the transplant procedure (e.g., pneumonia, wound infection, liver abscess, biliary sepsis)

One to Six Months

Lingering effects of infection acquired earlier

Viral infections (e.g., Cytomegalovirus, Epstein-Barr virus, hepatitis)

Opportunistic infection (e.g. Pneumocystis, Listeria, Nocardia)

Greater than Six Months

Patients with chronic cytomegalovirus, Epstein-Barr virus, or hepatitis virus infection are at risk for progressive chorioretinitis, B-cell lymphoproliferative disease, hepatocellular carcinoma or cirrhosis

Patients with good graft function and minimal immunosuppression have a minimal risk of opportunistic infections but remain at risk for community-acquired infections (e.g., influenza, pneumococcal pneumonia)

Patients with chronic rejection and a history of excessive acute and chronic immunosuppression are at high risk for opportunistic infections (e.g., Cryptococcus, Listeria, Pneumocystis)

and in non-immunosuppressed individuals is virtually non pathogenic. However, CMV infection in the transplant patient which may account for 30% of the infections seen, has been a major source of morbidity and mortality and has recently been implicated in the vanishing bile duct syndrome, characteristic of chronic rejection [23]. CMV infection is characterized by high spiking fevers usually associated with anorexia, malaise and arthralgias. Laboratory tests that suggest CMV infection may include a marked leukopenia and elevated liver function tests suggestive of an acute hepatitis (AST). In one third of the patients with fever due to CMV, pulmonary manifestations develop. A liver biopsy is mandatory in patients to make the diagnosis. Pathological evidence of CMV infection includes polyclusters of neutrophils, and CMV inclusion bodies. CMV infection is treated first by reducing or stopping the immunosuppression, however recent studies have shown that the use of the antiviral agent gancyclovir (DHPG) is associated with increased survival [24].

Other viral infections seen in the liver transplant patient include herpes simplex virus usually due to a reactivation of a dormant virus. It usually responds to treatment with acyclovir. Fungal infections (candida) have been noted in up to 20% patients and carry with it a 20–100% mortality rate [10].

Pancreatitis

Postoperative pancreatitis carries with it a grave prognosis. If pancreatitis is recognized in the preoperative assessment it is now considered a relative contraindication to transplantation.

Conclusion

Liver transplantation is the most effective treatment for end stage irreversible liver disease. Careful management of the patient in the perioperative period has resulted in a marked improvement in survival. Future advances in the production of even more selective immunosuppressive and antiviral agents should result in even better long term results.

References

1. Maddrey WC, Van Thiel DH (1988) Liver transplantation: an overview. Hepatology 4:948–959
2. Busuttil RW, Colonna JO, Hiatt JR, et al (1987) The first 100 liver transplants at UCLA. Ann Surg 206:387–402
3. Krom RAF, Wiesner RH, Rettke SR, et al (1989) The first 100 liver transplantations at the Mayo clinic. Symposium on liver transplantation – part I. Mayo Clin Proc 64:84–94
4. Tygstrup N, Panek L (1981) Fulminant hepatic failure. Clin Gastroenterol 10:191–208
5. Sinclair SB, Greig PD, Blendis LM, et al (1989) Biochemical and clinical response of fulminant viral hepatitis to administration of prostaglandin E. J Clin Invest 84:1063–1069
6. Bismuth HD, Samuel J, Gugenheim D, et al (1987) Emergency liver transplantation for fulminant hepatitis. Ann Intern Med 107:337–341

7. Gallinger S, Greig PD, Levy G, et al (1989) Liver transplantation for acute and subacute fulminant hepatic failure. Trans Proc 21 (1):2435–2438
8. Forster J, Greig PD, Glynn MFX, et al (1989) Coagulation factors as indicators of early graft function following liver transplantation. Trans Proc 21:2308–2310
9. Kirby RM, McMaster P, Clements D, et al (1987) Orthotopic liver transplantation: postoperative complications and their management. Br J Surg 74:3–11
10. Busuttil RW, Brems JJ, Hiatt JR (1988) Pediatric transplantation. In: Maddrey WC (ed) Transplantation of the liver. Current topics in gastroenterology. Elsevier, New York, pp 309–330
11. Winston D, How W, Lin C, et al (1987) Intravenous immune globulin for prevention of cytomegalovirus infection and interstitial pneumonia after bone marrow transplantation. Ann Intern Med 106:12–18
12. Gordon RD, Shaw BW, Iwatsuki S, Esquivel CO, Starzl TE (1986) Indications for liver transplantation in the cyclosporine era. Surg Cli North Am 66:541–554
13. Greig PD, Levy G, Superian RA, et al (1989) Antilymphoblast globulin (ALG) as initial prophylaxis against rejection following liver transplantation. Trans Proc 21:2244–2246
14. Colonna JO, Goldstein LI, Brems JJ, et al (1987) A prospective study on the use of monoclonal anti-T_3 cell antibody (OKT_3) to treat steroid resistant liver transplant rejection. Arch Surg 122:1120–1123
15. Neuberger J, Williams R (1987) Long-term use of cyclosporin in liver grafting. In: Calne R (ed) Liver transplantation. Grune and Stratton, Harcourt Brace Jovanovich, London UK, pp 319–327
16. Starzl TE, Fung J, Venkataramman R, Todo S, Demetris AJ, Jain A (1989) FK506 for liver, kidney and pancreas transplantation. Lancet 1:1000–1004
17. Mazzaferro V, Esquivel CO, Makowka L, et al (1989) Trans Proc 21:2466–2467
18. Hesselink EJ, Klompmaker IJ, Grond J, Gouw ASH, van Schilfgaarde R, Sloof MJH (1989) Hepatic artery thrombosis (HAT) after orthotopic transplantation (OLT) – The influence of technical factors and rejection episodes. Trans Proc 21:2468
19. Hiatt JR, Quinones-Baldrich WJ, Ramming KP, Brems J, Busuttil RW (1987) Operations upon the biliary tract during transplantation of the liver. Surg Gynecol Obstet 165:89–93
20. Ringe B, Oldhafer K, Bunzendahl H, Bechstein WO, Kotzerke J, Pichlymayr R (1989) Analysis of biliary complications following orthotopic liver transplantation. Trans Proc 21:2472–2475
21. Forster J, Greig PD, Glynn MFX, Poon A, Levy GA (1989) Predictors of graft function following liver transplantation. Trans Proc 2:3356–3357
22. Greig PD, Woolf GM, Abecassis M, et al (1989) Treatment of primary liver graft nonfunction with prostaglandin E_1 results in increased graft and patient survival. Trans Proc 21:2385–2388
23. Arnold JC, Portmann BC, O'Grady JG, Naoumov NV, Alexander GJM, Williams R (1989) Persistence of cytomegalovirus (CMV) genome in the liver during development of the vanishing bile duct syndrome. Hepatology 37
24. Paya CV, Hermans PE, Smith TF, et al (1988) Efficacy of ganciclovir in liver and kidney transplant recipients with severe cytomegalovirus infection. Transplantation 46:229–234

Sedation of the Critically Ill

Long-term Sedation in the Critically Ill

R. Ritz, M. Spoendlin, and W. Haefeli

Introduction

Patients in the intensive care unit often need to be sedated for several reasons: to apply artificial ventilation, to treat convulsions or to control agitation or anxiety [1-4]. The goal of sedation is the reduction of perception and pain. In the most frequent application of sedative drugs, namely in patients on a respirator, the attitudes have changed over the last 15 years. Initially, complete sedation, mostly combined with relaxation, was thought necessary to apply completely controlled ventilation; analgesics were usually added. More recently, after a short period of controlled ventilation cooperation of the patient has been preferred; consequently, sedation changed from complete to partial sedation, combined with analgesia but without relaxation in most cases [5]. Instead of long-acting drugs, such as diazepam [6-8] sedatives with a shorter half-life are now preferred. Besides new therapeutic regimens, the interest of intensivists for monitoring and individualization of sedation has also increased.

Desired Level and Monitoring of Sedation

Generally accepted *requirements* of a sedation regimen are: the relief of anxiety and pain, and sometimes the reduction of the patient's respiratory drive. The drug administration should be simple and safe. The *extent* of sedation, and thereby the choice of the drug, including dosage and type of administration, depend on the *strategy* of sedation planned in an individual patient.

The possible extent of sedation was investigated in 34 ICUs in Great Britain in 1981 [1], at a time when heavy sedation was still commonly desired (Table 1). In a recent own inquiry in 63 Swiss ICUs, called "Swiss Sedation 88" [7], the aimed depth of sedation was characterized by 43 ICUs (68%) as *"sedate to the point of no distress"*, 13 units (21%) preferred "deep sedation, the patient reacting only on stimuli", and 7 units had no general strategy of sedation.

This change from complete to partial sedation over the last years parallels changes in the ventilation techniques, namely from complete controlled to only supportive ventilation, implying some spontanous breathing effort by the patient. In addition, heavy sedation is not a benign treatment; the disadvantages include respiratory muscle fatigue and all the complications threatening a comatous patient such as deep venous thrombosis, general muscle wasting, risk of

Table 1. Sedation techniques in ventilated patients; investigation in 34 ICUs. (The results are taken from [1])

Extent of sedation	Most frequently used (number of ICUs)[a]
– Analgesic drugs only for painful procedures	9
– Patient completely detached from environment (woken only on occasions)	23
– Sedated to the point of no distress	9

[a] Several answers possible.

compression injuries to peripheral nerves and infection. Prolonged coma can be due to sedative overdose followed by weaning problems.

The parameters of *monitoring* the degree of sedation are rather poor and, so far, not well investigated. *Clinically,* repeated examinations of the quantitative and qualitative state of consciousness are, at the moment, most frequently performed, using the Glasgow coma scale [9], supplemented by questions concerning the orientation of the patient. In the intubated patient where verbal response is impossible some modified scoring systems are in use [3]. *Physical examination* to determine the extent of sedation include the observation of the patient's pupils, corneal reflex, painful stimuli etc. During patient's care in ICU the nursing staff will judge the depth of sedation also by the patient's *hemodynamic responses* to invasive procedures, e.g. endotracheal suctioning. Correlations between the plasma levels of a sedative agent and the extent of sedation are better known so that *drug monitoring* becomes important [10]. Intermittent or continuous EEG recording is probably the best parameter to evaluate the sedation level [11]; recently, we confirmed the good correlation between the clinical estimation of sedation following the Glasgow coma scale and the EEG findings (Fig. 1). Digital plethysmography testing the automatic response to pain is not routinely used yet to estimate the degree of sedation in intensive care. Measure-

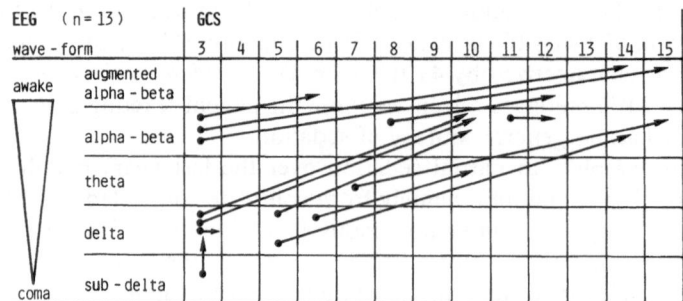

Fig. 1. Correlation between clinical evaluation of consciousness following the Glasgow coma scale (GCS) ranging from 3 (deep coma) to 15 points (fully awake), and the EEG pattern in 13 intoxicated patients

ments of the variability of the pulse rate, probably combined with other parameters, might also help to monitor sedation.

Choice of Sedative Agents and Regimens

Ten years ago ventilated patients were "totally sedated" and relaxed, usually with pancuronium, so that a fixed regimen of sedation and analgesia was generally used [12, 13]. Today, the indications for relaxation became rare and "partial sedation" combined with analgesia is performed according to the patient's need, usually judged by the nursing staff. For sedation and analgesia the following agents are in general use.

First, the *benzodiazepines* have replaced the barbiturates for long-term sedation, except possibly in patients with raised intracranial pressure. The benzodiazepines are preferred for their anxiolytic, sedative, muscle relaxant and anticonvulsant effects.

According to the inquiry performed by Merriman et al. in 1981 [1] among 34 ICUs the benzodiazepine diazepam was regularly used in 31 units to sedate ventilated patients, followed by lorazepam. In 1983, however, we described some cases of prolonged coma due to sedation with diazepam in therapeutic high

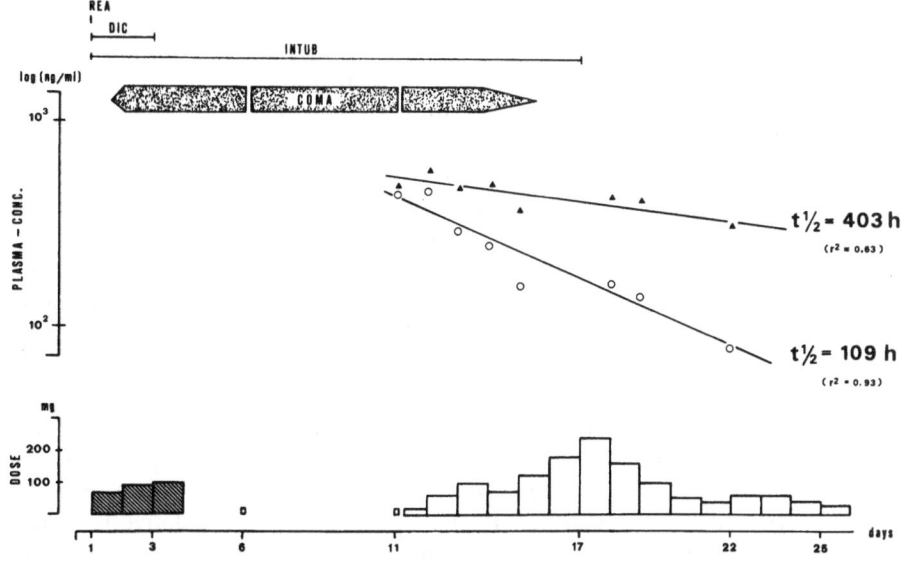

Fig. 2. Clinical course of a patient (female, 70 years old) during and following artificial ventilation and sedation with diazepam (see text). Doses of diazepam (hatched bars) and the benzodiazepine antagonist Ro 15-1788 (open bars), by i.v. injection at the 6th and 11th day, and perorally starting on the 12th day after admission. Plasma concentrations and half-lives t½ of diazepam (open circles) and desmethyldiazepam (closed triangles). *REA*, cardiopulmonary resuscitation; *DIC*, disseminated intravascular coagulopathy; *INTUB*, duration of intubation/artificial ventilation

doses [8, 14]. In addition to the advantages of a rapid passage through the blood-brain barrier, a broad therapeutic range and uncommon side effects, the benzo-diazepines also have some disadvantageous pharmacokinetic properties. The plasma half-lives of the almost 40 different types of benzodiazepines available in Europe range from 3 hours to more than 24 hours. When benzodiazepines are used repeatedly, especially in elderly patients with retarded elimination and/or reduced liver function, accumulation may lead to prolonged coma following withdrawal of the drug (Fig. 2). Among the newer benzodiazepines with shorter half-lives, midazolam is therefore preferred. In our own inquiry, "Swiss Sedation 88" [7], 94% of the 63 ICUs investigated used benzodiazepines to sedate ventilated patients, and midazolam was the most commonly used. Verwaest et al. [15] compared the effects of midazolam with those of diazepam during postoperative sedation. Quality of sedation and cardiovascular stability was better with mida-zolam. There was no evidence of accumulation and prolonged recovery. These positive effects of midazolam were confirmed by others [3, 16]. In our experience on six ventilated patients, including pharmacokinetic studies, midazolam permit-ted optimal sedation without cardiovascular or other side effects, and without weaning problems. The pharmacokinetic properties of midazolam, however, in-cluded a wide and unpredictable range of half-lives in the individual patients. Therefore, the dosage regimen can not follow an fixed schedule. Similar varia-tions in pharmacokinetics were described with halflives of midazolam between 0.7 and 15 hours by Behne et al. and Oldenhof et al. [17, 18]. However, a good correlation between midazolam plasma levels and degree of sedation was ob-served in a study by Person et al. [19]. After a loading dose, midazolam should be administered by continuous infusion and not by intermittent injections only [20]. It is usually combined with an analgesic drug. If the degree of sedation is inad-equate the serum level of midazolam should first be increased by 1 to 3 small i.v. bolus injections, since the stepwise increase of a continous infusion may lead to cumulation of the drug.

Besides benzodiazepines, drugs like alfathesin, etomidate, phenoperidine, ket-amine and propofol have been or are still in use to sedate ventilated patients in ICUs. *Alfathesin*, in which the active drugs were alphaxalone and alphadolone, almost represented the ideal sedative agent in intensive care [21], but its solvent was associated with a high proportion of anaphylactoid reactions [22] so that the drug has been withdrawn. *Etomidate* too, showed satisfactory properties when used to sedate ventilated patients and included the advantages of minimal car-diovascular and respiratory depression [23]. However, in 1983 Ledingham and Watt reported an increased mortality in their ICU patients, apparently asso-ciated with the use of etomidate [24] and possibly due to inhibition of endoge-nous corticosteroid production. The use of etomidate as a sedative is therefore no longer recommended. The enthusiasm for the use of *phenoperidine,* a popular sedative agent in the ICUs of Great Britain [1], was tempered by recent reports of cardiovascular collapse following its administration [25]. In patients who were not adequately sedated by a continuous infusion of midazolam, Park et al. showed that *ketamine* infusion resulted in better sedation, an increased in arter-ial pressure and a diminution of bronchospasm [26]. The most promising drug of the newer agents for long-term sedation in ventilated patients is probably *propo-*

fol. Its application by continuous infusion provides satisfactory and controllable sedation with rapid recovery after cessation [27]; The cardiovascular depressant properties of the drug are still under investigation.

Among the opioids *alfentanil* was compared to pethidine by Yate et al. [28], showing similar quality of sedation and similar recovery in both patient groups.

The main advantages of an older analgesic drug like *morphine* administered either by continuous infusion or by intermittent injections, are the low cost and the long experience with its use. Disadvantages might be accumulation during prolonged infusion and the dependence on renal function [29, 30]. Ledingham et al. [31] compared morphine with midazolam in 60 patients requiring mechanical ventilation; they found that morphine more often met the desired sedation criteria.

Conclusions and Outlook

Sedatives are among the most commonly used and abused drugs in intensive care. As Merriman stated, "While acknowledging the stresses to which medical and nursing staff are subjected, it sometimes appears that sedation is used more for staff convenience than patient benefit" [1]. Inquiries about ICUs practices showed that a great number of patients are sedated [6]. Patients on the ventilator usually receive a combination of sedatives, analgesics and, to a lesser degree, muscle relaxants. The number and variety of drugs used suggest that there is no single agent or combination of agents providing ideal sedation for ventilated patients at the moment [4]. Surprisingly little work has been done to evaluate the drugs used for prolonged sedation and analgesia in the ICU. The ideal agent for prolonged sedation should include advantageous pharmacokinetic properties, i.e. a broad therapeutic range and a short half-life, a rapid passage through the blood-brain barrier and a metabolism by pathway independent of renal and hepatic function. Ideally it should have no effect on the respiratory and cardiovascular systems and no interactions with other drugs. This drug does not exist. Optimal sedation can probably only be reached using several sedative and analgesic agents in combination. Today a short-acting opioid such as alfentanil or a short-acting benzodiazepine such as midazolam seem to be the drugs of choice. In case of cumulation midazolam has the additional advantage of the existence of the benzodiazepine antagonist *flumazenil*. The titration of these two drugs might lead to an optimal and balanced sedation in ventilated intensive care patients in the future [32].

References

1. Merriman HM (1981) The techniques used to sedate ventilated patients. Intensive Care Med 7:217–224
2. Hofer P, Schwander J, Ritz R (1985) Tetanus. In: Dtsch E, Kleinberger G, Lenz K, Ritz R, Schuster HP (eds) Die Hämodynamik kritisch kranker Patienten. Aktuelle Intensivmedizin. Schattauer, Stuttgart, pp 417–424

3. Hoffmann P, Imhoff M (1988) Analgesie und Sedierung beatmeter Patienten in der Intensivmedizin. Zent B1 Chir 500–513

4. Dobb GJ, Murphy DF (1985) Sedation and analgesia during intensive care. Clin Anaesth 3:1055–1085

5. Hannich H-J, Schere R, Wendt M (1983) Der Stellenwert von Sedierung und Mobilisation im Therapiekonzept beatmeter Patienten. Anaesth Intensivther Notfallmed 18:177–180

6. Buchanan N, Cane RD (1978) Drug utilisation in a general intensive care unit. Intensive Care Med 4:75–77

7. Ritz R, Spoendling M (1990) Swiss sedation 88 (in preparation)

8. Rapold HJ, Follath F, Scollo-Lavizzari G, Kehl O, Ritz R (1984) Verlängertes Koma durch Sedation mit Diazepam bei beatmeten Patienten. D M W 109:340–344

9. Teasdale G, Jennett B (1974) Assessment of coma and impaired consciousness. A practical scale. Lancet 2:81–83

10. Follath F (1988) Problems of drug elimination in intensive care patients. Resuscitation 16:63–66

11. Lehmkuhl P, Lips U, Pichlmayr I (1985) EEG-Parameter in der Überwachung beatmeter Intensivpatienten unter verschiedenen Sedierungsstrategien. Anaesth Intensivther Notfallmed 20:6–11

12. Parker MM, Schubert W, Shelhamer JH, Parrillo JE (1984) Perceptions of a critically ill patient experiencing therapeutic paralysis in ICU. Crit Care Med 12:69–71

13. Green D (1980) Paralysis or sedation for controlled ventilation. Lancet 1:715

14. Rapold HJ, Follath F, Scollo-Lavizzari G, Ritz R (1983) Diazepam: hazardous sedation of ventilated patients. Intensive Care Med 9:218

15. Verwaest Ch, Demeyers R, Ferdinande P, Schetz M, van Damme K, Lauwers P (1987) The use of midazolam and diazepam for sedation following aorto-coronary bypass surgery. Acta Anaesthesiol Belg (Suppl 1) 38:9–16

16. Ex P (1987) Use of midazolam infusion as sedative in a multidisciplinary intensive care unit. Acta Anaesthesiol Belg (Suppl 1) 38:5–8

17. Behne M, Zobel R, Asskali F, Förster H, Kessler P, Seiz W (1987) Die Pharmakokinetik des Midazolam während verschiedener Anaesthesie-Bedingungen. Anaesthesist 36:634–639

18. Oldenhof H, de Jong M, Steenhoek A, Janknegt R (1988) Clinical pharmacokinetics of midazolam in intensive care patients, a wide interpatient variability? Clin Pharmacol Ther 43:263–269

19. Persson P, Nilsson A, Hartvig P (1988) Relation of sedation and amnesia to plasma concentrations of midazolam in surgical patients. Clin Pharmacol Ther 43:324–331

20. Mathews HML, Carson IW, Collier PS, et al (1987) Midazolam sedation following open heart surgery. Br J Anaesth 59:557–560

21. Stewart GO, Dobb GJ, Craib IA (1983) Clinical trial of continuous infusion of alphaxalone/alphadolone in intensive care patients. Anaesth Intens Care 11:107–112

22. Fisher MM, Baldo BA (1984) Anaphylactoid reactions during anesthesia. Clin Anaesth 2:677–692

23. Newby DM, Edbrooke DL, Mather SJ, Bird TM, Hebron BS (1983) Etomidate as a sedative agent in intensive care: observations on its cardiovascular effects. Acta Anaesth Scand 27:218–221

24. Ledingham IM, Watt I (1983) Influence of sedation on mortality in critically ill multiple trauma patients. Lancet 1:1270

25. Green DW (1981) Severe cardiovascular collapse following phenoperidine. Anaesthesia 36:617–619

26. Park GR, Manara AR, Mendel L, Bateman PE (1987) Ketamine infusion. Anaesthesia 42:980–983

27. Newman LH, McDonald JC, Wallac GM, McA Ledingham I (1987) Propofol infusion for sedation in intensive care. Anaesthesia 42:929–937

28. Yate PM, Thomas D, Short SM, Sebel PS, Morton J (1986) Comparison of infusions of alfentanil or pethidine for sedation of ventilated patients on the ICU. Br J Anaesth 58:1091–1099

29. Ball M, Mc Quay HJ, Moore RA (1985) Renal failure and the use of morphine in intensive care. Lancet 2:784–786

30. Bion JF, Logan BK, Newman PM, et al (1986) Sedation in intensive care: morphine and renal function. Intensive Care Med 12:359–365
31. Ledingham I, Bion JF, Newman PM, Mc Donald JC, Wallace PGM (1988) Mortality and morbidity amongst sedated intensive care patients. Resuscitation 16 (Suppl):69–77
32. Ritz R, Elsasser S, Schwander J (1988) Controlled sedation in ventilated intensive care patients. Resuscitation 16 (Suppl):83–89

Pharmacokinetic and Pharmacodynamic Modeling of Sedation in the ICU: Future Perspectives

A. F. Ghouri, A. K. Mills, and P. F. White

Background

In the intensive care unit (ICU) environment sedation is often an integral component of critical care therapy. Patients who are being mechanically ventilated frequently require sedation because the endotracheal tube is extremely irritating and the ICU is an anxiety-provoking environment. In addition to alleviating anxiety, sedation may prevent sleep deprivation [1], a common problem for mechanically ventilated patients. Sleep deprivation may lead to disorientation and agitation (so-called "ICU psychosis"), as well as results in a decreased ventilatory response to hypoxia and hypercapnia [2], both of which may interfere with weaning from ventilatory support [3]. Furthermore, there is anecdotal evidence to suggest that restoration of a normal sleep-wake cycle can improve patient outcome in the ICU, and reduce the need for additional medications [4]. Thus, a sedation technique which would allow patients to rest comfortably (or sleep) may be of benefit in weaning patients from mechanical ventilation. Finally, effective sedation can decrease stress hormone levels in healthy patients and might produce similar effects in ICU patients. Since stress hormones can significantly increase both metabolic rate and protein catabolism, sedation may have the added benefit of decreasing ventilatory requirements.

In a survey of modes of sedation in 34 ICUs, Merriman [5] described a wide variety of drugs and techniques. In managing the agitated, ventilator-dependent patient, benzodiazepines, opioids, butyrophenones, and muscle relaxants are frequently used in the intensive care setting. If agitation is uncontrolled, it might prove hazardous to the critically-ill. Problems related to agitation include cardiopulmonary instability, injuries to patients and hospital personnel, inability to cooperate with nursing care, failure to maintain optimal positioning in bed, and disruption of life-sustaining tubes and catheters. Thus, the ability to provide safe, controllable, and reversible sedation can be extremely important in the care of the critically ill patient.

Providing adequate sedation, analgesia, and hemodynamic stability without prolonging the ICU stay presents a major challenge. Determining the optimal dose of sedative or analgesic medication is difficult because the presence of an endotracheal tube and the use of neuromuscular blocking agents complicate efforts to communicate with the patient. The physiological response to pain includes an increase in sympathetic activity (with tachycardia, hypertension, and increased systemic vascular resistance) which can increase myocardial oxygen demand, and lead to ischemia. Although management of these physiological responses is especially important in critically ill patients, there is no consensus regarding the best sedation technique [6].

The multitude of drugs used to control agitation attests to the lack of an ideal drug or combination of drugs for this purpose. The most widely used compounds are the benzodiazepines of which diazepam is the prototypical agent. However, diazepam is not ideally suited for use in this situation because it is a venoirritant [7] with a long elimination half-life (30–90 hours) [8]. Desmethyldiazepam, its principal metabolite, has an even longer elimination half-life, and is pharmacologically active [9]. Morphine sulfate, the prototypic opiate analgesic, produces dose-related respiratory depression, hemodynamic instability, chest wall rigidity, inhibition of gastrointestinal motility, as well as the development of tolerance and physical dependence which can result in a withdrawal syndrome. Haloperidol, a commonly used antipsychotic tranquilizer with sedative and antiemetic properties, produces dysphoria and hypotension. The sedative-hypnotic etomidate can provide effective sedation in both mechanically ventilated [10] and spontaneously breathing [11] patients. However, critically-ill patients receiving etomidate for prolonged sedation have an increased incidence of sepsis (compared with patients receiving benzodiazepines and opiates) [12] as a result of its ability to inhibit adrenal steroidogenesis [13].

Midazolam is a water-soluble imidazobenzodiazepine with a rapid onset of action and short elimination half-life compared with diazepam or lorazepam (another commonly used benzodiazepine) [14]. As a sedative, midazolam is two-to-four times more potent than diazepam, and its water solubility results in a lower incidence of venous complications [15]. Its fused imidizole ring undergoes rapid hepatic metabolism, resulting in a shorter elimination half-life (2–4 h) than the other commonly used parenteral benzodiazepines [16–18]. When administered intravenously, midazolam has a more rapid onset of action than other benzodiazepines due to its greater lipophilicity [19]. Furthermore, a recent study has demonstrated that midazolam infusions provide effective sedation while decreasing opioid analgesic requirements [20].

In summary, it is evident that the wide variety of agents as well as techniques for providing sedation in the ICU is a reflection of our limited understanding of sedation in general.

Continuous Infusion for Sedation

During the last decade, there has been increased interest in the use of intravenous anesthetic techniques. The introduction of rapid and short-acting IV anesthetic and analgesic drugs has led to the realization that these agents can be made more controllable, and therefore more like the volatile anesthetics, if they are administered by continuous variable rate infusion rather than by intermittent bolus injections [21]. As a result, there have been major developments in the use of infusion techniques, both for anesthesia and for sedation in the intensive care setting [22]. Potential benefits of using a continuous infusion (versus intermittent injections) of sedative agents in the ICU include the ability to:

- More precisely control the level of sedation, increasing or decreasing the rate of drug administration depending on the clinical situation, as well as potentially reducing the need for polypharmacy to provide adequate sedation;
- Minimize undesirable cardiovascular and respiratory depression, as well as side effects and drug toxicity by avoiding the "peaks and valleys" in blood and brain concentrations which occur with intermittent bolus administration; and
- Decrease the total amount of sedative and analgesic medication required to achieve the desired clinical state.

Indeed, a more in depth understanding of infusion techniques and the availability of inexpensive microcomputers offers the possibility of improved delivery of sedative agents in the future. However, in order to more effectively design IV drug dosing regiments a greater understanding of drug pharmacokinetics and pharmacodynamics is required. The following discussion will attempt to illustrate some of the current perspectives on the pharmacokinetic and dynamic modeling of sedation.

Theoretical Basis of Pharmacokinetic and Pharmacodynamic Modeling

Future progress in pharmacology and therapeutics will depend on furthering our understanding of drug dose-effect relationships in humans. It is clinically important to understand the relationship between drug dose and blood concentrations (kinetics), as well as the relationship between drug level and biological effect (dynamics). Improved analytical techniques for determining drug concentrations *in vivo* have been catalysts to the development of pharmacokinetic models for describing the relationship between the administered dose and blood levels of drugs. Pharmacodynamic modeling, on the other hand, has received considerably less attention. As one might imagine, a unified description of the relationship between dose and effect (a so-called *pharmacokinetic-pharmacodynamic model*), could serve as a basis for optimizing drug administration in critical environments such as the ICU.

Conventional pharmacokinetic models are mathematical descriptions of how drug concentrations change in various tissues as a function of dose and time. Pharmacodynamic models, however, typically do not include time as a variable. Rather, they seek to describe the observed effect as a function of a given concentration of drug in the plasma. However, pharmacokinetic (PK) and pharmacodynamic (PD) models can be integrated using plasma concentration, a common factor in both models. The resultant combination can then convey a more generalized relationship between dose and effect [23]:

$$\text{Dose} \rightarrow \text{PK Model} \rightarrow C_p \rightarrow \text{PD Model} \rightarrow \text{Effect}$$

Plasma concentration, C_p, is usually the common link in this description because it is easier to measure than drug concentrations in other body fluids and tissues (eg. concentrations of drug in CSF, aqueous humor of the eye). In practice, however, the drug level at the site at which the effect occurs is *not* simultaneously in equilibrium with the plasma, hence more sophisticated models have been developed which reflect the action of the drug at a hypothetical *effect* site. Such models, which can link dose and effect, are known as a *pharmacokinetic-pharmacodynamic* (PK/PD) models [23]:

$$\text{Dose} \rightarrow \text{PK Model} \rightarrow C_p \rightarrow \text{PK/PD Model} \rightarrow C_e \rightarrow \text{PD Model} \rightarrow \text{Effect}$$

where C_p represents the plasma concentration and C_e is the concentration of the drug at a hypothetical "effect" site.

The majority of biological systems which are acted upon by pharmacological agents exhibit a characteristic hyperbolic (or approximately hyperbolic) relationship between drug concentration and physiological effect. For this reason, the E_{max} *pharmacodynamic* model has been used extensively to depict this behavior because it accurately describes drug effects over wide concentration ranges. Although there are more sophisticated pharmacodynamic models in use, for illustrative purposes the E_{max} model is simple to understand, and has frequently been used with success. Basically, the E_{max} pharmacodynamic model seeks to model the system using a generalized equation of the following type:

$$E = E_0 + \frac{[E_{max} \cdot C_p(t)^S]}{[EC_{50}{}^S + C_p(t)^S]}$$

where E is the measured effect, $C_p(t)$ is the plasma concentration of the drug at time t, E_{max} is the maximum possible effect attributable to the drug, E_O is the baseline effect in the absence of any drug, S is a sigmoidicity factor influencing the slope of the E_{max} versus $C_p(t)$ relationship (and in certain instances reflects the number of receptor binding sites), and EC_{50} is the concentration of drug producing 50% of the E_{max} effect. An important attribute of the E_{max} model is that it imposes no constraints on how the effect (E) component is defined. For example, the E_{max} model has been used frequently to describe Michaelis-Menten enzymatic behavior, where the effect is defined to be the velocity of a chemical reaction.

The E_{max} model illustrates a common biological phenomena in which disproportionately higher drug concentrations are required to increase the drug's effect when one is near the maximum effect. Mathematically, this property is easily visualized, since as $C_p(t)$ approaches infinity, E approaches $E_0 + E_{max}$, a constant. Furthermore, when $C_p(t)$ is zero, the model predicts only the baseline effect, E_0. The ability of the E_{max} model to successfully describe "limiting" pharmacological effects at both extremes is a desirable property that is not shared by most other pharmacodynamic models [24], and is one reason why the E_{max} model is widely employed.

However, the E_{max} model also has some major shortcomings. For example, its use requires simultaneous measurement of plasma concentration and effect, which can be extremely difficult, especially since C_p can change rapidly. Furthermore, in clinical practice the expected direct relationship between the *serum* drug concentration and the magnititude of effects is often not observed due to equilibration delays (referred to as hysteresis). Investigators have sought solutions to such problems by combining pharmacodynamic models (such as the E_{max} model) with pharmacokinetic models, and hence developing pharmacokinetic-pharmacodynamic models which can address these limitations.

In principle, the use of a sufficiently detailed *pharmacokinetic* model may permit better prediction of the acutal concentration at the time of the effect, obviating the need for simultaneous measurements of both concentration and effect. The time course of drug concentrations in plasma, urine, and other sampled sites (eg. CSF) is usually modeled by compartmental analysis. It has been shown that a pharmacokinetic model can account for the hysteresis observed with E_{max} models by introducing what is called an "effect compartment". Equilibration between the plasma (central) compartment and the hypothetical "effect" compartment can often be accurately described mathematically using systems of ordinary first-order differential equations (with appropriate boundary conditions) of the form:

$$d\,Ce/dt = \sum_{i=1}^{n} C_i k_i$$

where C_e is the drug concentration in the effect compartment, C_i is the drug concentration in the ith compartment, k_i is the rate constant characteristic of movement from the ith compartment, t is time, and n is the number of compartments within the model. Models of this type typically lead to solutions of the form:

$$C_e(t) = S \sum_{i=1}^{n} Q_i \exp(x_i t)$$

where $C_e(t)$ is the concentration of the drug in the effect compartment at time t, S is an empiric constant, and Q_i and x_i are hybrid constants of a sum of n exponentials that are determined by $k_1, k_2, k_3, \ldots k_n$.

Incorporation of the expression for $C_e(t)$ based on the *pharmacokinetic* model into the E_{max} *pharmacodynamic* model has been one of the approaches used to combine the two systems. Substitution of $C_e(t)$ into the expression for $C_p(t)$ in the E_{max} model gives:

$$E = E_0 + \frac{[E_{max} \cdot C_e(t)^S]}{[EC_{50}{}^S C_e(t)^S]}$$

where the observed effect (E) is now a function of drug concentration in the hypothetical "effect" compartment, $C_e(t)$. Integration of $C_e(t)$ (a pharmacokinetically-derived function of time) in this manner can serve to explain complex phenomena such as latency and hysteresis.

The E_{max} model, as depicted above, has been used successfully for modeling centrally active drugs. For example, Koopmans et al. used it to quantify the effect of midazolam on suppression of electroencephalographic (EEG) alpha activity and the latency of visual evoked response (VER) in volunteers [25]. Furthermore, Kroboth et al. have recently shown that a modified version of the E_{max} model could be used to describe the development of benzodiazepine tolerance [26]. In their study, the effect of the benzodiazepine was determined by measuring psychomotor performance using digit symbol substitution test (DSST) scores and changes in EEG spectral edge (SE).

EEG-SE is defined to be the frequency below which 95% of the power of the EEG waveform lies, and is calculated by integrating the area under the frequency versus power histogram, and finding the frequency below which 95% of the area is found. It has become a commonly measured variable in the field of anesthesiology as it provides a single number which can be used as a quantitative index of cortical EEG activity, thereby simplifying much more complex analyses which would be required to describe individual changes in alpha, beta, theta, and delta EEG waveforms. (Not surprisingly, use of SE has drawbacks which inevitably result from compressing the EEG into a single number, resulting in the loss of other potentially useful information that is contained in the waveform itself).

In their preliminary study of benzodiazepine tolerance, Kroboth et al. demonstrated that tolerance to alprazolam could be predicted by allowing EC_{50} (the concentration of the drug required to achieve 50% of the maximal response) to be itself a pharmacokinetic parameter that is modified by a function of time [26]. Succinctly, these investigators demonstrated that:

$$E = E_0 + \frac{[E_{max} \cdot C_e(t)^S]}{[(1 - \exp(-k_{tol}t))^S EC_{50}{}^S + C_e(t)^S]}$$

where k_{tol} is a tolerance rate constant that describes the change in EC_{50} as a function of time. In studying the effects of thiopental as measured by changes in spectral edge, Hudson et al. used the E_{max} model to demonstrate that there are no changes observed in IC_{50} (analogous to EC_{50} in situations where inhibition of an effect is being modeled). Based on the assumption that IC_{50} represents sensitivity to the central effects of thiopental, the authors have suggested that "acute" tolerance to barbituates does *not* occur, as IC_{50} remains constant in time. However, a major shortcoming in the studies by Koopmans et al., Kroboth et al., and Hudson et al. is that they all utilized a small group of subjects ($n \leq 10$), perhaps limiting their ability to make additional statistically significant clinical inferences [25-27].

The particular mathematical details of the above equations are not important for our discussion; however, they do serve to illustrate one of the popular approaches toward unifying what is known about what the body does to a drug (pharmacokinetics) with what the drug does to the body (pharmacodynamics). Indeed, combined pharmacokinetic-pharmacodynamic models are particularily useful, since not only can they enhance our understanding of the pharmacodynamics of a drug, but they can offer insight into the underlying physiological process.

Future Directions

The detailed *pharmacokinetics* of most sedative and anesthetic drugs have been well-characterized using widely available analytical techniques (eg. *in vivo* drug assays, receptor binding studies, etc). Microcomputer-controlled infusion methods, which can accurately titrate drugs to any desired level, are also becoming readily available [28–31]. Bolus-elimination-transfer (BET) infusion devices, for instance, have recently been introduced to overcome the major problems with commonly used bolus infusion systems. Traditionally, infusions are performed by administering a loading dose (bolus) to achieve a high plasma concentration, followed by a maintenance dose that compensates for the clearance of the drug, thereby maintaining therapeutic drug levels in the blood and tissues. However, administration of the bolus usually leads to an initial overshoot, which can have undesirable effects. Bolus-elimination-transfer (BET) is a microprocessor-controlled process whereby an exponentially declining infusion rate is given during the initial bolusing (loading) period, precisely accounting for the transfer of the drug from the central compartment to various peripheral ones. Consequently, it is possible to establish a constant drug level predictably and rapidly, without the initial overshoot. Indeed, devices will soon become available whereby the anesthesiologist simply has to enter a targeted drug level, and the computer performs the pharmacokinetic calculations necessary to control the infusion pump on a second-by-second basis.

On the other hand, *pharmacodynamics* is poorly understood because it is exceedingly difficult to define the effect end-point in an objective manner. In the ICU, for example, the desired therapeutic effect is to achieve an optimal level of sedation. The measurement of this effect, however, is a formidable problem, since an objective definition of sedation does not exist. For this reason, the development of useful pharmacokinetic-pharmacodynamic models to improve the delivery of sedatives in the ICU requires further advances in the field of dynamic modeling.

Currently, many investigators use modified Ramsay and Glasgow coma scales for assessing levels of sedation, which are quite limited and often highly subjective. Recently, there has been much interest in using the EEG as a tool which would allow one to use well-defined criteria for providing sedation. Use of EEG and VER is promising since these signals are generated by the CNS, and may allow one to measure sedation noninvasively and continuously in the ICU without irritating or fatiguing critically-ill patients.

Indeed several recent studies (including those mentioned earlier) have demonstrated that the use of EEG to establish objective criteria for sedation may be possible. Various other forms of mathematical analysis have been applied to the EEG in attempt to define recognizable patterns which change in a consistent manner during different physiological states. For example, the alterations seen in the awake adult have been compared to those seen during the various stages of sleep. A popular form of mathematical analysis of EEG is the Fourier transform of the second order correlation function, better known as the power spectrum (from which EEG-SE is determined). This analytical technique treats the EEG waveform as the algebraic summation of sinusoidal functions, and is the basis of the majority of studies reported in the medical literature.

Unfortunately, power spectral analysis suppresses phase relations, and is limited by the fact that it treats the waveform as a linear function, which is inherently an incorrect oversimplification. The limited utility of EEG spectral analysis is reflected in recent studies which have demonstrated a lack of correlation between electroencephalographic and hemodynamic changes during general anesthesia [32, 33]. What is necessary, therefore, is a more sophisticated analysis of EEG waveforms, as the phase changes which occur with regard to the synchronization of the various nuclei generating the EEG are essentially transparent to the technique of spectral analysis. Until such methods are developed, objective pharmacodynamic modeling of CNS sedation may not be realistically feasible using the EEG. Nevertheless, the notion that we will one day be able to construct closed-loop, automated systems whereby sedatives are administered in the ICU using EEG parameters as titratable endpoints, is attractive. Moreover, a better understanding of pharmacodynamics will allow us to integrate newer monitoring techniques to provide a more complete assessment of sedative effects in critically ill patients.

References

1. Aurell J, Elmqvist D (1985) Sleep in the surgical intensive care unit: continuous polygraphic recording of sleep in nine patients receiving postoperative care. Br Med J 290:1029–1032
2. Ochiai R, Motoyama EK, Winter PM, Walczak SA (1986) Sleep deprivation attenuates ventilatory response to hypoxia. Anesthesiology 65:A491
3. Ochiai R, Motoyama EK, Winter PM, Walczak SA (1987) Sleep deprivation attenuates hypercapnic ventilator response in man. Anesthesiology 67:A331
4. Shapiro MD, Westphal LM, White PF, Sladen RN, Rosenthal MH (1986) Midazolam infusion for sedation in the intensive care unit: effect on adrenal function. Anesthesiology 64:394–398
5. Merriman HM (1981) The techniques used to sedate ventilated patients. Intensive Care Med 7:217–224
6. Dobb GJ, Murphy DF (1985) Sedation and analgesia during intensive care. Clinics in Anesthesia 3:1055–1085
7. Korttila K, Aromaa U (1980) Venous complications after intravenous injection of diazepam, flunitrazepam, thiopentanon, and etomidate. Acta Anaesthesiol Scand 24:227–230
8. Greenblatt DJ, Allen MD, Marmatz HS, Shader RI (1980) Diazepam disposition determinants. Clin Pharmacol Ther 27:301–312
9. Greenblatt DJ (1987) Simulataneous gas chromatographic analysis for diazepam and its major metabolite, desmethyldiazepam, with use of double internal standardization. Clin Chem 24:1838–1841
10. Edbrooke DL, Newby DM, Mather SJ, Sixon AM, Hebron BS (1982) Safer sedation for ventilated patients – a new application for etomidate. Anaesthesia 37:765–771
11. Bird TM, Edbrooke DL, Newby DM, Hebron BS (1984) Intravenous sedation for the intubated and spontaneously breathing patient in the intensive care unit. Acta Anaesthesiol Scan 28:640–643
12. Ledingham IM, Watt I (1983) Influence of sedation of mortality in critically ill, multiple trauma patients. Lancet 1:1270
13. Wagner RL, White PF, Kan PB, Rosenthal MH, Feldman D (1984) Inhibition of adrenal steroidogenesis by the anesthetic etomidate. N Engl J Med 310:1415–1421

14. Greenblatt DJ, Locniskar A, Ochus HR, Lauven PM (1981) Automated gas chromatography for studies of midazolam pharmacokinetics. Anesthesiology 55:176–179
15. White PF, Vasconez LO et al. (1988) Comparison of midazolam and diazepam for sedation during plastic surgery. J Plastic Recon Surg vol 81, 5:703–709
16. Smith MT, Eadie MJ, Brophy TO (1981) The pharmacokinetics of midazolam in man. Eur J Clin Pharmacol 10:271–278
17. Allonen H, Ziegler G, Klotz U (1981) Midazolam kinetics. Clin Pharmacol Ther 30:653–661
18. Heizmann P, Eckert M, Ziegler WH (1983) Pharmacokinetics and bioavailability of midazolam in man. Br J Clin Pharmacol 16:43s–49s
19. Greenblatt DJ, Arendt RM, Abernathy OR, Giles GH, Sellers EM, Shader RI (1983) In vitro quantitation of benzodiazepine lipophilicity: relation to in vivo distribution. Br J Anaesth 55:985–989
20. Westphal LM, Cheng E, White PF, Sladen RN, Rosenthal MH (1987) Use of midazolam infusion for sedation following cardiac surgery. Anesthesiology 66:223–226
21. White PF (1983) Use of continuous infusion versus intermittent bolus administration of fentanyl or ketamine during outpatient anesthesia. Anesthesiology 59:294–300
22. White PF (1989) Clinical uses of intravenous anesthesic and analgesic infusions. Anaesth Analg 68:161–171
23. Holford NH, Sheiner LB (1981) Understanding the dose-effect relationship: clinical application of pharmacokinetic-pharmacodynamic models. Clin Pharm 6:429–453
24. Holford NH, Sheiner LBL (1982) Kinetics of the pharmacological response. Pharm Ther 23:2–24
25. Koopmans R, Dingemanse J, Danhof M, Horsten GPM, van Boxtel CJ (1988) Pharmacokinetic and pharmacodynamic modeling of midazolam effects on the human central nervous system. Clin Pharmacol Ther 44:14–22
26. Kroboth PD, Smith RB, Erb RJ (1983) Tolerance to alprazolam after intravenous bolus and continuous infusion: psychomotor and EEG effects. Clin Pharmacol Ther 43:270–277
27. Hudson RJ, Stanski DR, Saidman LJ, Meathe E (1983) A model for studying depth of anesthesia and acute tolerance to thiopental. Anesthesiology 59:301–308
28. Schwilden H (1981) A general method for calculating the dosage scheme in linear pharmacokinetics. Eur J Clin Pharmacol 20:379–386
29. Schwilden H, Schuttler J, Stoeckel H (1983) Pharmacokinetics as applied to total intravenous anesthesia. Anaesthesia 38:51–56
30. Alvis JM, Reves JG, Govier AV, et al (1985) Computer-assisted continous infusions of fentanyl during cardiac anesthesia – comparison with a manual method. Anesthesiology 63:41–49
31. Glass P, Jacobs J, Alvis M, Bai S, Reves JG (1987) Computer-assisted continous infusion of alfentanil during noncardiac anesthesia – a comparison with a manual method. Anesthesiology 65:A546
32. Mills AK, Ghouri AF, Monk TG, White PF (1990) Lack of correlation between electroencephalographic and hemodynamic changes during general anesthesia. Anesth Analg (in press)
33. White PF, Boyle WA (1989) Relationship between hemodynamic and electroencephalographic changes during general anesthesia. Anesth Analg 68:177–181

The Use of Benzodiazepines in Surgical Patients

L. Barvais and P. Sylin

Introduction

The benzodiazepines produce dose-dependent central nervous system (CNS) depression analogous to that produced by other sedative-hypnotic drugs. The action of the benzodiazepines on the CNS include anxiolytic, sedative, hypnotic, anticonvulsivant, amnesic and muscle relaxant effects. Their mechanism of action may be related to facilitation of inhibitory action of GABA and glycine within the CNS.

In surgical patients, benzodiazepines are generally used as premedicants, as induction agents to produce rapid loss of consciousness, as anesthetic maintenance agents or as sedative agents during local or regional anesthesia. However, benzodiazepines do not replace barbiturates as induction agents because they are not as rapid acting nor as predictable in their hypnotic effect.

Midazolam is an imidazobenzodiazepine with unique properties. Midazolam is water soluble in its acid formulation but is highly lipid soluble in vivo. When compared with other benzodiazepines, midazolam does not produce venous irritation, has a relatively rapid onset of action and a high metabolic clearance. So among all the available parenteral benzodiazepines, midazolam is preferable.

The purpose of this paper is not to describe the pharmacokinetics of midazolam, its indication and its effect on the anesthetic requirement. Such a review article has already been published [1]. Our purpose is to study the various influences on the midazolam pharmacokinetic parameters and to concentrate upon the pharmacokinetic-pharmacodynamic relationship of midazolam in order to improve the use of this agent in surgical patients.

Midazolam Pharmacokinetic Parameters

Table 1 compares the physicochemical properties of midazolam, flunitrazepam and diazepam. Table 2 summarises the pharmacokinetic parameters of these benzodiazepines. A lot of factors influence the pharmacokinetics of the benzodiazepines. We will review the factors which influence the pharmacokinetics of midazolam.

Table 1. Physicochemical properties of diazepam, flunitrazepam and midazolam

	Diazepam	Flunitrazepam	Midazolam
Liposolubility	+ + +	+ +	+
Hydrosolubility	–	–	+
pKa	3,5		6
Receptor affinity	+	+ +	+ + +
Pain at injection	+ 40%	± 5%	–

Table 2. Comparison of the pharmacokinetic parameters of diazepam, flunitrazepam and midazolam

	Diazepam	Flunitrazepam	Midazolam
Protein binding [%]	97	80	97
Distribution volume [ml/kg]	700–1700	2500–4600	1100–1700
Clearance [ml/kg/min]	0.2–0.5	1.9–5.6	6.4–11.1
T 1/2 elimination [h]	24–57	14–21	1.7–2.6

Posture and Circadian Rhythm

Klotz and Ziegler studied the temporal changes of midazolam in 6 subjects and found consistent variations of the mean values of the clearance [2]. Midazolam clearance was significantly higher in the morning when they were supine than when they were sitting and walking (616 versus 317 ml/min). As a matter of fact, supine position can increase hepatic blood flow by about 40–60%. Moreover, in the same conditions of sitting and walking, clearance of midazolam in the morning was lower than in the evening (317 versus 463 ml/min). This might be caused by a circadian rhythm in enzyme activities per se or by their modification by steroid rhytmicity.

The same authors performed a chronopharmacokinetic study with prolonged infusion of midazolam [3]. Supine position was maintained throughout the study. In all subjects, small but clinically irrelevant fluctuations of plasma concentrations were observed. The authors concluded that hepatic elimination of midazolam is relatively stable under controlled and constant conditions.

Hepatic Metabolism

A 6% sub-population of poor metabolizers with defective hepatic metabolism may exist for midazolam [4]. These findings are probably of no clinical importance when single doses of midazolam are given as it would still be rapidly redistributed. However, when the drug is infused or given by intermittent injection, as in the ICU, a patient with a prolonged midazolam half life might show a marked cumulative effect with a delayed recovery. This 6% incidence is very similar to the frequency of poor metabolisers in the oxidation of debrisoquine and sparteine but it is very unlikely that metabolis of midazolam is controlled by the sparteine/debrisoquine gene locus [5].

Age

To study the influence of age on midazolam kinetics, Avram et al. [6] have injected 0.2 mg/kg midazolam IV for induction in women of 2 age groups. They found little changes in midazolam kinetics with age. T½ elimination, total clearance and the volume of distribution were not significantly different between the young patients aged from 22 to 33 and the older aged from 50 To 60. No difference was noted concerning awakening times or plasma concentrations.

On the other hand, Greenblatt et al. [7] found a significant difference of the total clearance (7.8 versus 4.4 ml/min.kg) and T½ elimination between young and old males. Harper et al. [8] have found the same difference between young and elderly patients aged more than 50. T½ elimination was 4.1 hours in the elderly group compared with 2.4 hours in the young group. The total clearance was respectuely 402 ml/kg·hour versus 325 ml/kg·hour. The total volume of distribution was not significantly different. They conclude that T½ elimination was sprolonged with age, secondary to a decreasing clearance.

Obesity

The total volume of distributionis greater (2.7 versus 1.7 l/kg) in the obese subjects even after correction for total weight. T½ elimination was then prolonged (8.4 versus 2.7 hours) due to the increased volume of distribution [7].

Chronic Renal Failure

Renal disease does not alter the distribution, elimination or clearance of unbound midazolam but decreases significantly its protein binding (93.5 versus 96.1%). Moreover, chronic renal failure patients are more susceptible to the sedative effects of midazolam [9].

Hypovolemia

Midazolam pharmacodynamics and pharmacokinetics were studied during acute hypovolemia in dogs [10]. 7 dogs received 10 mg/kg IV midazolam twice, 4 days apart. Hypovolemia corresponded to the withdrawal of 1/3 blood volume. Hypovolemia was accompanied by significantly longer t 1/2 beta and lower clearance than during normovolemia. A similar percentage of decrease of blood pressure and cardiac output was measured in hypovolemic and normovolemic states but the absolute values of blood pressure and cardiac output were significantly lower in the hypovolemic state. Moreover, the hypotensive effects of midazolam were potentiated by hypovolemia [10].

Surgery

The nature of operation also influences the pharmacokinetics of midazolam. The total volume of distribution is significantly greater in major surgery (intra-abdominal or intra-thoracic surgery) compared with minor surgery (gynecological or endoscopic) although total clearance is not statistically modified [8]. $T\frac{1}{2}$ elimination is then statistically prolonged (3.8 hours versus 2.4). Clearance rate of midazolam after cardiopulmonary bypass (CPB) is not different from values reported in healthy volunteers [11]. Midazolam keeps its short duration of action after CPB [12].

Anesthesia

Method of administration· After oral administration, the correlation between the effect and the concentration of midazolam and its metabolite is better than with midazolam alone [13]. At identical plasma concentrations of midazolam, the oral dose produces more marked effect than the intravenous administration because of the influence of the α-hydroxymetabolite which is formed by first-pass metabolism [14].

The $T\frac{1}{2}$ elimination of midazolam after IM administration is prolonged as compared with IV administration [14]. This is probably due to a slow IM depot release of midazolam whichis slower than the plasma elimination rate representing the rate-limiting step in the elimination of midazolam after im administration.

With a continuous midazolam infusion at 5 mg/hour during 26 hours for sedation of the intubated but spontaneously breathing patients, the pharmacokinetic parameters of midazolam were comparable with values obtained after IV single bolus injections in surgical patients [15]

Epidural anesthesia: During caesarean section performed under epidural analgesia, Kanto et al. [16] found a greater clearance (13.2 ml/min/kg) and a shorter $T\frac{1}{2}$ elimination (68 minutes) of midazolam compared with the usual pharmacokinetic parameters. The increased hepatic blood flow in the supine position (40–60%) and the increased hepatic blood flow in sympathetic blockade (epidural) may influence the increased hepatic extraction ratio.

Intravenous anesthetic drugs: Persson et al. [17] have studied the pharmacokinetics of midazolam in total IV anaesthesia. Midazolam plasma clearance (483 ml/min), apparent volume of distribution (1.94 l/kg) and terminal half life (3.1 h) were in agreement with other reports studied in volunteers. There is no obvious evidence that the concomitant use of other anesthetic drugs influence the pharmacokinetics of midazolam. Moreover, there is no influence of the benzodiaze-pine antagonist (flumazenil) on the kinetics of midazolam [18].

Concomitant Drug Therapy

On the one hand, induction of benzodiazepine oxidation can be achieved by rifampicin and chronic ethanol use. On the other hand, inhibition of benzodia-zepine oxidation is induced by cimetidine, acute ethanol use, oral contracep-tives, disulfiram, isoniasid and propranolol.

Midazolam Pharmacodynamic Parameters

Table 3 shows the relation between the benzodiazepine receptor occupancy and the theoretical observed pharmacological effect. Table 4 compares the potency of the pharmacological effects of midazolam and diazepam. For midazolam, there is a relationship between the plasma concentration and the clinical effect. This relation has been demonstrated not only for the pharmacodynamic effects studied by psychometric tests, but also for the EEG and for the level of anesthe-sia.

Table 3. Relation between the benzodiazepine receptor occupancy and the pharmacological ef-fect

Receptor occupancy	Pharmacological effect
0	
	Anticonvulsivant effect
20%	Anxiolysis
	Sedation
	Amnesia
50%	Hypnosis

Table 4. Comparison of the pharmacological effects of midazolam (MDZ) and diazepam (DZP)

Amnesia	MDZ > DZP
Anxiolysis	DZP > MDZ
Sedation	MDZ > DZP
Anticonvulsivant effect	DZP > MDZ
Myorelaxant effect	DZP > MDZ

Psychometric Tests

On the basis of performance tests, there is a close relationship between plasma midazolam concentration and tracing test, reaction time test, self-rating by subjects and investigator's assessment [13]. The relation between the logarithm of the plasma midazolam concentration and the clinical effect shows a progressive increasing effect above 50 ng/ml followed by a linear relation between 100 and 400 ng/ml. Above 400 ng/ml, there data are lacking because the tests could not be performed.

EEG

The relationship between the plasma concentration of either diazepam or midazolam to pharmacodynamic EEG activity of diazepam and midazolam is characterised by an increase in fractional EEG activity in the 13–30 Hz range [19].

Anesthesia

Allonen et al. [20] has observed that the threshold level of midazolam effect is 40 ng/ml and that the sedative effects are visible in all the tests when the plasma level is superior to 80 ng/ml. The midazolam plasma concentration for amnesia is around 100 ng/ml [21]. When the plasma level is superior to 100 ng/ml, the subjects often fall asleep but are still arousable. Peak concentrations are associated with reversible effects such as dizziness, muscle relaxation, ataxia [20]. So, if adequate sedation during spontaneous ventilation is needed in the pre-, per- or post-operative period, a plasma midazolam level between 100 and 200 ng/ml seems to be the target. Adequate sedation in the postoperative period with an endotracheal tube needs a mean plasma midazolam concentration superior to 250 ng/ml in pediatric patients [22]. 300 ng/ml of midazolam was associated with adequate sedation during surgery [23]. The minimal plasma level producing a deep hypnotic effect with an EEG-median of less than 5/second is 500 ng/ml [24]. After total IV anesthesia induced and maintained with midazolam and alfentanil in healthy patients, the mean plasma level of midazolam at the time of extubation was 165 ± 38 ng/ml. Patients were able to give their name and date of birth at 104 ± 38 ng/ml of plasma midazolam concentration and were able to solve simple arithmetic problems at 96 ± 42 ng/ml [17].

Conclusion

There is a correlation between the plasma midazolam concentration and the clinical effect. In healthy patients, in the absence of drug tolerance, 100 ng/ml of midazolam seems to be the minimum effective target concentration to obtain amnesia and sedation. A concentration above 500 ng/ml is not justified because of a plateau effect.

Computer Simulation for Midazolam

Allonen showed a good agreement between steady state plasma levels and the theoretical concentrations calculated with a computer program but he found no correlation between the concentration in the peripheral compartment and the measured dynamic effects [20]. On the basis of pharmacokinetic analysis, Lauven et al. [24] by using the BET (Bolus, Elimination, Transfer) infusion technique were able to establish a controlled infusion scheme to attain nearly constant of plasma target level midazolam from the beginning of their infusion without initial overshoot in healthy volunteers. Hence, computer simulation could help to design the midazolam infusion regimen to generate and maintain a target concentration.

A computer simulation program, developed with LOTUS 1-2-3 and running on IBM personal computer is now available [25]. It incorporates a database which contains records of multiple-compartment pharmacokinetic models for several intravenous anesthetic drugs, including midazolam. On request, this program provides the graph for the theoretical drug distribution and for the infusion rate required to maintain the target concentration.

Table 5 gives an example of the loading doses injected over different time periods needed to generate 3 different levels of midazolam target concentrations (0.1, 0.3, 0.5 μg/ml). These loading doses have been calculated with the SPINA program and the turn over rates of the pharmacokinetic model studied by Persson in surgical patients [17]. Figure 1 shows the 3 continuous exponentially declining infusions calculated to maintain the 3 target levels by compensating the distribution and elimination of midazolam during a 3-hour period.

However, some variability remains between the pharmacokinetic parameters of the existing pharmacokinetic models. Figure 2 shows the theoretical decrease of the plasma midazolam concentration after the administration of a bolus of 0.1 mg/kg injected over 2 minutes and calculated with the 2 models of midazolam

Table 5. List of the theoretical loading doses (μg/kg) to provide a target concentration of 0.1, 0.3 or 0.5 μg/ml calculated with the model of Persson et al. [17]

0.1 μg/ml	0.3 μg/ml	0.5 μg/ml	Duration (min)
47.10	141.30	235.50	0
47.18	141.55	235.92	0.1
47.52	142.57	237.62	0.5
47.95	143.85	239.76	1
48.81	146.43	244.05	2
49.68	149.03	248.38	3
50.55	151.65	252.74	4
51.43	154.28	257.14	5
52.31	156.94	261.57	6
54.11	162.32	270.53	8
55.92	167.76	279.61	10
60.56	181.68	302.80	15
65.33	195.98	326.64	20

FLOW RATE (mcg/kg/min)

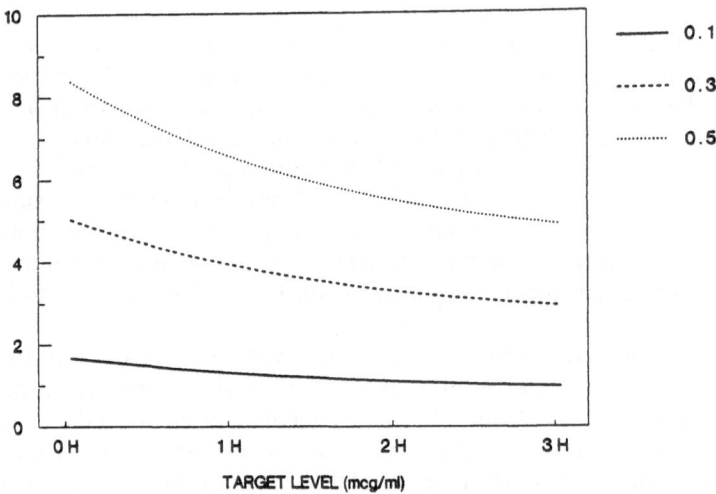

TARGET LEVEL (mcg/ml)

Fig. 1. Infusion regimens to maintain 3 target levels of 0.1, 0.3, 0.5 µg/ml of midazolam. These curves are calculated with the turn-over rates constants of the pharmacokinetic model of Persson et al. studied in surgical patients. (From [17])

PLASMA LEVEL (mcg/ml

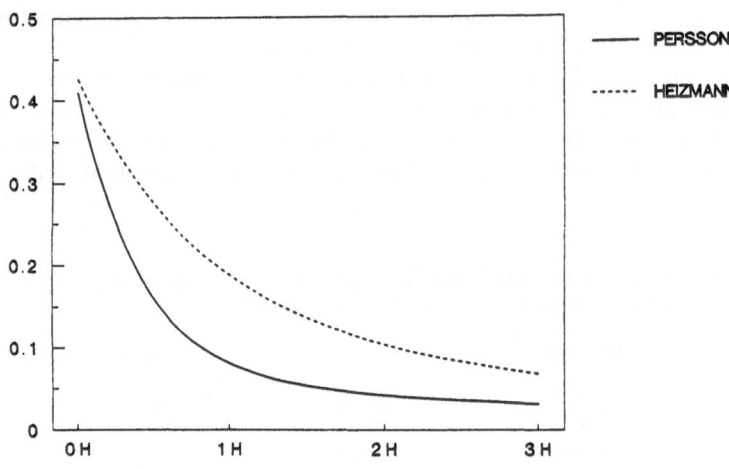

Fig. 2. Decrease of the theoretical midazolam plasma concentration after a bolus of 0.1 mg/kg using the turn-over rates constants of the pharmacokinetic model of Persson et al. studied in surgical patients [17] and the pharmacokinetic model of Heizmann et al. studied in healthy adult volunteers [26].

included in the database of SPINA. After the loading dose, the peak plasma concentration of midazolam is very similar whatever the selected pharmacokinetic model. Thereafter, the decrease of the plasma concentration is not parallel.

It is slower with the pharmacokinetic model of Heizmann et al. [26] studied in volunteers than with the pharmacokinetic model of Persson et al. [17] studied in surgical patients.

Conclusions

The science of pharmacokinetics is often considered as a purely mathematical approach to the quantitation of drug disposition in the body. The mathematical complexity that has developed in pharmacokinetics to project the phases in drug absorption, distribution and elimination has prevented many clinicians from developing a basic understanding of this science. But with the development of computer simulation programs, it becomes possible to predict the theoretical concentration of the anesthetic drugs.

Among all the available parenteral benzodiazepines, no major differences in the profile of their clinical pharmacological effects have been demonstrated. Their diversity is essentially apparent with regard to their pharmacokinetics which in turn determines their pharmacodynamic duration of action.

At present, the benzodiazepine with the most appropriate pharmacokinetic profile is midazolam, because its total body clearance is much higher than that of any other injectable benzodiazepine. So, computer simulation and the pharmacokinetic-pharmacodynamic relationship of midazolam is more reliable than with the other benzodiazepines. Computer drug simulation, associated with or without a computer controlled infusion system, could help the anesthetist to achieve the range of the therapeutic drug concentration generally associated with sedation or hypnosis. This can easily be performed in healthy surgical patients for whom single injection or short infusion of midazolam are generally administered.

On the contrary, in ICU patients, the drug administration is longer and many pharmacokinetic parameters may be affected by several factors such as liver function impairment, alteration of liver blood flow, plasma protein binding, drug interactions, drug distribution, hypovolemia and body position. Moreover, during long term infusion, the development of pharmacodynamic tolerance to the sedative effects of the benzodiazepines may yield to a great pharmacodynamic variability. Consequently, computer simulation with standard pharmacokinetic parameters is not justified in ICU patients; it is better to adapt the rated midazolam infusion to the wanted level of sedation. In case of excessive CNS depression, a control of the plasma concentration or the injection of the antagonist drug flumazenil may help the physician to differentiate excessive sedation from a neurological problem.

References

1. Reves JG, Fragen RJ, Vinik R, Greenblat DJ (1985) Midazolam: pharmacology and uses. Anesthesiology 62:310–324
2. Klotz U, Ziegler G (1982) Physiologic and temporal variation in hepatic elimination of midazolam. Clin Pharmacol Ther 323, 1:107–112

3. Klotz U, Reimann IW (1984) Chronopharmacokinetic study with prolonged infusion of midazolam. Clin Pharmacok 5:469–474
4. Dundee JW, Collier PS, Carlisle RJT, Harper KW (1986) Prolonged midazolam elimination half life. Br J Clin pharmac 21:425–429
5. Klotz U, Mikus G, Zekorn C, Eichelbaum M (1986) Pharmacokinetics of midazolam in relation to polymorphic sparteine oxidation. Br J Clin Pharmac 22:618–620
6. Avram MJ, Fragen RJ, Caldwell NJ (1983) Midazolam kinetics in women of 2 age groups. Clin Pharmacol Ther 34, 4:506–508
7. Greenblatt DJ, Abernethy DR, Locniskar A, et al (1984) Effect of age, gender, and obesity on midazolam kinetics. Anesthesiology 61:27–35
8. Harper KW, Collier PS, Dundee JW, et al (1985) Age and nature of operation influence the pharmacokinetics of midazolam. Br J Anaesth 57:866–871
9. Vinik HR, Reves JG, Greenblatt DJ, Abernethy DR (1983) The pharmacokinetics of midazolam in chronic renal failure patients. Anesthesiology 59:390–394
10. Adams P, Gelman S, Reves JG, Greenblatt DJ, Alvis M, Bradley E (1985) Midazolam pharmacodynamics and pharmacokinetics during acute hypovolemia. Anesthesiology 63:140–146
11. Cheng EY, Westphal LM, White PF, Sladen RN, Rosenthal MH (1986) Use of a midazolam infusion for sedation following aortocoronary bypass surgery. Anesthesiology 65:3a, a67
12. Lowry KG, Dundee JW, Mc Clean E, Lyons SM, Carson IW, Orr IA (1985) Pharmacokinetics of diazepam and midazolam when used for sedation following cardiopulmonary bypass. Br J Anaesth 57:883–885
13. Crevoisier C, Ziegler WH, Eckert M, Heizmann P (1983) Relationship between concentration plasma and effect of midazolam after oral and iv administration. Br J Clin Pharmac 16:51s–61s
14. Raeder JC, Nilsen OG (1988) Prolonged elimination of midazolam after IM administration. Acta Anaesthesiol Scand 464–466
15. Driessen JJ, Dirksen MSC, Rutten JMS, et al (1989) Continuous infusion of midazolam during anaesthesia and postoperative sedation after maxillofacial surgery. Acta Anaesthesiol Scand 33:116–121
16. Kanto J, Aaltonen L, Erkkola R, Aarimaa L (1984) Pharmacokinetics and sedative effects of midazolam in connection with caesarean section performed under epidural analgesia. Acta Anaesthesiol Scand 28:116–118
17. Persson A, Nilsson A, Hartvig P, Tamsen A (1987) Pharmacokinetics of midazolam in total IV anaesthesia. Br J Anaesth 59:548–556
18. Raeder JC, Nilsen OG, Hole A (1988) Pharmacokinetics of midazolam and alfentanil in outpatient general anesthesia. Acta Anaesthesiol Scand 32:467–472
19. Greenblatt DJ, Ehrenberg JG, Gunderman J et al (1989) Pharmacokinetic and EEG study of iv diazepam, midazolam and placebo. Clin Pharmacol Ther 45:356–365
20. Allonen H, ZIegler G, Klotz U (1981) Midazolam kinetics. Clin Pharmacol Ther 30, 5:653–661
21. Dundee JW, Wilson DB (1980) Amnesic action of midazolam. Anaesthesia 35:459–461
22. Lloyd-Thomas AR, Booker PD (1986) Infusion of midazolam in paediatric patients after cardiac surgery. Br J Anaesth 58:1109–1115
23. Nilsson A, Tamsen A, Persson P (1986) Midazolam-fentanyl anesthesia for major surgery. Plasma levels of midazolam during prolonged total intravenous administration. Anaesthesia 30:66069
24. Lauven PM, Stoeckel H, Schwilden H (1982) A microprocessor controlled infusion scheme for midazolam to achieve constant plasma levels. Anaesthesist 31:15–20
25. Barvais L, Coussaert E, Cantraine F, d'Hollander A (1989) The pharmacokinetics of intravenous anesthetic drugs given by infusion: SPINA – a software program. Eur J Anesthesiol 6:435–447
26. Heizmann P, Eckert M, Ziegler WH (1983) Pharmacokinetics and bioavailability of midazolam in man. Br J Clin Pharmac 16:43S–49S

The Use of Neuromuscular Blocking Agents in Intensive Care

B. J. Pollard

Introduction

Patients undergoing treatment on an Intensive Care Unit (ICU) may require as one component of their management a period of artificial ventilation of the lungs. Being intubated and having ventilation controlled is a traumatic experience and the great majority of patients therefore require sedation. Specific sedative agents, e.g. benzodiazepines, are useful in order to reduce anxiety and make the patient sleep. In addition, specific analgesic agents are often required and members of the opioid family are commonly prescribed for this purpose. These latter agents also possess other desirable properties, including respiratory depression and sedation. The use of one or a combination of these agents, therefore, is important and the actual choice is a matter of personal preference, patient requirements and unit policy.

In addition to these sedative agents a muscle relaxant may also be prescribed as part of the therapy. There has been a considerable alteration in the use of this family of drugs. Ten years ago over 90% of ICU's used a muscle relaxant on a frequent basis [1] (usually pancuronium). A study published in 1986, however, suggested that this number had decreased to about 16% [2]. Why has there been this decline? The answer must lie in a changing attitude towards their need. When the muscle relaxants were introduced into intensive care they rapidly acquired a place in the "sedation" of patients. Common regimes were to administer a combination of pancuronium and an opiate (often phenoperidine) by intermittent i.v. bolus doses. Confusion then developed over the exact function of each component and it is not difficult to see how the use of pancuronium became more important than the sedative agent, because a paralysed patient would remain immobile and more easily allow nursing and other procedures to be undertaken. If the sedative were administered without the muscle relaxant movements coughing, etc., might hinder management. The confusion therefore would seem to have been between immobility and sedation. Furthermore, many people held the mistaken view that muscular paralysis was a calm and pleasant state.

The turning point seems to have come following an editorial in the Lancet in 1981, which drew attention to the problems of paralysis in the conscious patient [3]. It began to become clear that pharmacological paralysis was not the pleasant, pain-free state which had been assumed. This was further reinforced by a number of published recollections of medical colleagues who had received a period of intensive care [4, 5]. On pharmacological grounds, it may be thought surprising that neuromuscular blocking agents were regarded in the same category as sedative agents [6]. It may also be thought that once attention had been drawn to this error the situation should improve. There remains, however, a worrying misconception of the properties of the neuromuscular blocking agents. As recently as 1989 a study was reported which sought to canvas the views of the pharmacological knowledge of a group of I.C.U. nursing and medical staff [7]. The findings indicated that approximately 5–10% thought that pancuronium possessed analgesic properties and approximately 50–70% that it possessed anxiolytic properties. The problem has therefore not gone away.

The response of the profession seems to have been to stop the routine use of neuromuscular blocking agents in ICU patients and to rely solely on sedative agents, anaesthetic agents and opiates [2]. It would appear that this is not entirely possible however, and this is exemplified by Cohen and Kelly's findings [8]. They noted that despite attempting to rely principally on a continuous infusion of alfentanyl together with bolus doses of midazolam, 7 out of the 16 patients studied additionally required the administration of a muscle relaxant to facilitate controlled ventilation. To attempt to stop the routine use of neuromuscular blocking agents would therefore seem not to be the most logical solution. Rather better to improve education so that the drugs are used more sensibly.

Indications for the Use of Neuromuscular Blocking Agents in Intensive Care

There are a number of situations where the use of a neuromuscular blocking agent is useful or even essential.

Tracheal Intubation

It is possible to intubate the trachea without the use of a neuromuscular blocking agent if the patient is already weak or under the influence of a generous dose of an anesthetic agent. Local analgesia of the pharynx or larynx may also be employed. The administration of a neuromuscular blocking agent, however, allows easier and less traumatic intubation [8], it is also particularly important when the airway has to be secured without delay or when there is a risk of regurgitation of gastric contents. In the latter situations succinylcholine is the agent of choice (with cricoid pressure) unless there is a specific contraindication to its use.

Facilitation of Procedures

There are a number of procedures where a completely immobile patient is either highly desirable or even essential. In order to obtain the best high quality CT images the use of a neuromuscular blocking agent has been recommended [9]. Other procedures including NMR imaging and rigid bronchoscopy also benefit and a neuromuscular blocking agent should usually be used in these circumstances.

To Assist Ventilation

Even though adequately sedated, there are a number of patients who cannot tolerate mechanical ventilation. This may lead to coughing and bucking and making respiratory attempts out of phase with the ventilator's cycle. The result of this is quite considerable swings in intrathoracic pressure. This is reflected in large swings in the intracranial pressure (ICP), a situation which is particularly undesirable in the neurosurgical or head injured patient. In addition, there may be considerable changes in blood pressure, also undesirable in the critical care patient. Thirdly, excess strain will be put on abdominal wall suture lines which may lead to wound dehiscence. In neurosurgical patients and those patients who cannot otherwise tolerate mechanical ventilation, the use of a neuromuscular blocking agent is therefore highly desirable.

Critical Gas Exchange

In the more critically ill patient who has greatly reduced lung compliance and in whom there are difficulties in achieving adequate gas exchange during mechanical ventilation with the use of sedative agents alone, the addition of a neuromuscular blocking agent is useful. The abolition of tone in the thoracic musculature results in a small increase in compliance which may improve ventilation. The energy consumption of striated muscle will also fall, thus decreasing the patient's oxygen requirements and carbon dioxide production, albeit by a small amount.

Allow the Reduction of Sedative Agent

In the light of what has previously been discussed, this is clearly a controversial issue. There is no doubt that when reliance is placed on sedative agents alone, some patients require very high doses. This may result in delays in weaning. If a neuromuscular blocking agent is employed, then it should be possible to use less sedation and thus accelerate the weaning process (unless this is further delayed by an excess of neuromuscular blocking agent!). The difficulty then arises of ensuring that adequate sedation is achieved. This should nowadays be easier, using infusions, than the previous techniques of intermittent bolus doses. There is still one problem, however, which has not been solved, namely the difficulty of assessing sedation in the paralysed patient. This important topic does not lie within the remit of this article.

Disadvantages of Using Relaxants

Just as there are two sides to every coin, so there are disadvantages to the use of neuromuscular blocking agents. There are no absolute contraindications, save those of known or suspected allergy to the drug. Each patient must therefore be considered on his or her own merits and the advantages weighed against the disadvantages for that patient.

Difficulties with Neurological Assessment

In a patient who has a complete neuromuscular blockade it is clearly not possible to assess a number of neurological parameters. Spontaneous movement or movement to command are not possible. Conscious level will be affected by the sedative agent in use and its infusion rate, but gross changes should be apparent, some of which might be difficult to determine in the presence of a neuromuscular blocking agent. What is particularly important is that focal or localising neurological signs may be missed in the paralyzed patient, leading to delay in treatment. This could be serious in some circumstances, e.g. expansion of subdural hematoma. Bearing in mind the advantages of neuromuscular blockade in patients with raised ICP, the clinician is here faced with a dilemma which can only be resolved by consideration of each individual case on its own merits. If a neuromuscular blocking agent is used, it should be discontinued at suitable intervals to allow the assessment of the patient, or the degree of blockade adjusted such that incomplete paralysis is present. Atracurium or vecuronium would seem, therefore, to be the agents of choice under these circumstances.

Disconnection

It may be argued that in the event of a patient becoming disconnected from the ventilator it is possible in the absence of a neuromuscular blocking agent he may be able to breathe spontaneously for a short while and thus maintain gas exchange. This will clearly not be possible if the patient has received a neuromuscular bleeking agent. The critical nature of ventilatory function in most ICU patients, however, makes it doubtful whether or not much benefit would be obtained from attempts at spontaneous ventilation. This is likely to be depressed by the disease process or by the administration of other agents. Furthermore, the use of ventilators without disconnection alarms is extremely inadvisable. This therefore would seem to remain principally a theoretical disadvantage.

Awareness

This has already been discussed above. The injudicious use of a muscle relaxant may mask inadequate sedation.

Incidence of the Thrombo-Embolism

In ICU patients who receive a neuromuscular blocking agent there is an increased incidence of pulmonary emboli [10].

Choice of Relaxant

Depolarizing Agents

The only member of this family now in regular clinical use is succinylcholine. Succinylcholine, having the shortest onset time of any of the muscle relaxants, finds its main use in situations where it is necessary to rapidly intubate a patient who might have a full stomach. This situation is most likely to occur in the newly admitted patient, and it is wise to assume that all critically ill patients are at risk from regurgitation at all times. Many of the conditions which precipitate admission to the ICU are associated with delayed gastric emtying. Once the trachea is intubated it is unusual to administer repeat doses of succinylcholine to maintain neuromuscular blockade. Succinylcholine possesses a number of unwanted actions which are of importance in ICU. The principal problems are the rise in serum potassium and the rise in ICP following its administration. The former is of great importance if the serum potassium is already elevated and the latter in patients with already raised intracranial pressure. The majority of its other side effects, e.g. muscle pains, are not so important in intensive care.

Nondepolarizing Agents

When considering long term use in intensive care, it is a member of this family which is selected. It is probably true to say that all of the nondepolarizing relaxants have been used at some time in ICU patients, although only a few have found regular use.

Pancuronium: This synthetic neuromuscular blocking agent has been the most popular for use in ICU. The reasons for this probably lie in its minimal cardiovascular action in patients with existing cardiovascular instability. Its intrinsic sympathomimetic and vagolytic actions prevent a fall in blood pressure and may even result in the blood pressure rising. In most critical care patients this is advantageous, although an occasional patient does exhibit a marked tachycardia. It is administered in intermittent bolus doses rather than by infusion. Its route of excretion is by both liver and kidney and it might be expected therefore to be an ideal drug in patients with organ impairment, possessing two routes of excretion. A case of prolonged paralysis in a patient with renal failure has, however, been reported [11].

Tubocurarine: This naturally occurring substance is a popular relaxant for use in anaestesia. It has never found a great following in intensive care principally due to its propensity to lower the blood pressure. It is a moderately potent ganglion blocking agent and will release histamine.

Alcuronium: This agent is a synthetic derivative of a naturally occurring alkaloid and enjoyed a moderate popularity in intensive care for some years. Although possessing fewer cardiovascular side effects than tubocurarine, its cardio-stability was not as great as pancuronium. Its principal disadvantage is that it is primarily excreted through the kidneys and therefore may have a prolonged action in patients with renal impairment, a situation which is not uncommon in ICU patients [12].

Atracurium: The use of this intermediate acting neuromuscular blocking agent in intensive care has risen quite dramatically within the last few years. It has minimal cardiovascular side effects. Its short duration of action means that administration by intermittent bolus injection is not really practical and therefore it is given by a continuous infusion. Its major advantage is its novel mode of breakdown, by the Hoffmann elimination reaction, which is independent of liver or kidneys. Thus, in the critically ill patient, who may have quite marked impairment of kidney or liver function, there will be no prolongation of the action of atracurium. The reversal of neuromuscular blockade is predictable and reliable, and following discontinuation of an infusion of atracurium, neuromuscular blockade can be expected to have fully disappeared in approximately one hour [13]. This of course makes it a particularly valuable agent for intensive care, as neurological assessment can be easily planned with the knowledge that there will be no neuromuscular blockade to complicate the issue. Furthermore, there is no delay in weaning, a problem which might result from the use of one of the longer-acting agents.

There is one potential problem with atracurium, namely the existance of the metabolite laudanosine, which has been shown to possess cerebral excitatory activity in certain laboratory animals [14]. Evidence for the accumulation of laudanosine in patients who have received a continuous infusion of atracurium for some time is growing [15], but the significance of this is unclear and it seems likely that it will prove to be of little clinical relevance.

Vecuronium: Like atracurium, this intermediate acting agent has good cardiostability and requires to be administered by continuous intravenous infusion. This clinical profile is regarded by many as almost identical to atracurium. It differs in two principal ways however. The first is that the molecule does not self-destruct as does atracurium and so accumulation is possible in patients with renal impairment and has certainly been reported [16]. The second is that there are no metabolites with any pharmacological activity and this is therefore not the concern with vecuronium. The choice between vecuronium and atracurium would seem to be principally one of personal preference, although the possibility of accumulation with vecuronium must always be borne in mind.

Pipacurium and Doxacurium: There is little information as to the use of these two new agents in intensive care. They would appear to possess a longer duration of action that pancuronium, yet have greater cardiovascular stability. It is likely that they will acquire some place in intensive care in the future.

Monitoring Neuromuscular Blockade in Intensive Care

In order to use any drug as efficiently as possible its effects should be monitored and recorded so that the dose or method of administration can be adjusted accordingly. The use of neuromuscular blocking agents in intensive care is no exception. Whichever neuromuscular blocking agent is in use, therefore, it is important to use a form of monitoring so that the dose or infusion rate can be tailored to the response. This prevents inadequate blockade with its inherent disadvantages, or excessive blockade with possibly delated recovery. The best method of monitoring neuromuscular blockade in ICU patients has still not really been fully resolved. The patient is already surrounded by a plethora of equipment, and so the use of complex EMG systems may be regarded as an unwanted intrusion. From the author's own personal experience, the most appropriate way is with the use of a simple hand held nerve stimulator. The muscular response can then be assessed at convenient intervals by either visual or tactile means. The Train of Four is used in our ICU, although there is no reason why one of the other techniques, e.g. doubleburst stimulation, could not be used instead. A suitable level of neuromuscular blockade is with the first or first and second twitches of the Train of Four present. If there is not response to Train of Four stimulation the infusion rate is decreased and if there are three or more switches the infusion rate is increased. This regime has been found to produce very satisfactory conditions in a great many patients on our ICU. There are two problems with the use of a nerve stimulator in ICU patients. The first relates to electrode position, which should be kept as constant as possible. Most ECG type electrodes are suitable for use as nerve stimulation electrodes but it is advisable to change them daily. The second and principal problem, however, is that of variation in response. This appears to be due mainly to the accumulation of tissue edema which is present in many ICU patients. This reduces the intensity of what was previously supramaximal stimulus by virtue of the increased tissue thickness between the skin surface and the nerve trunk. It may be overcome in most patients by exerting moderate pressure over the site of the electrodes for one to two minutes before stimulating.

Specific Situations

Myasthenia Gravis

It is often unnecessary to use a neuromuscular blocking agent in these patients, because they are already weak. It is possible, however, to use a neuromuscular blocking agent as part of their ICU management [17] and the agent of choice would seem to be atracurium. It must be remembered that maintenance requirements for a constant neuromuscular blockade are of the order of 20% of those for a normal adult [17].

Tetanus

The use of a neuromuscular blocking agent is positively indicated in these patients in order to reduce their muscle spasms and allow controlled ventilation. Tetanus is accompanied by periods of gross cardiovascular instability and so the choice of a relaxant with minimal cardiovascular action, e.g. atracurium or vecuronium, is beneficial.

Conclusions

It can therefore be seen that neuromuscular blocking agents are a valuable adjunct to the treatment of intensive care patients. The most logical agent is atracurium by continuous infusion. Whichever agent is used though, it is recommended that neuromuscular function is monitored by some means. Of even greater importance is the necessity to ensure that pharmacological paralysis is not confused with sedation and that all patients who receive a neuromuscular blocking agent are adequately sedated. If these points are adhered to, then there is no reason why the use of neuromuscular blocking agents in intensive care patients should not be recommended.

References

1. Merriman HM (1981) The techniques used to sedate ventilated patients: A survey of methods used in 34 ICUs in Great Britain. Intensive Care Med 7:217-224
2. Bion JF, Ledingham I McA (1987) Sedation in intensive care - a postal survey. Intensive Care Med 13:215-216
3. Editorial (1981) Paralysed with fear. Lancet 1:427
4. Shovelton DS (1979) Reflections on an intensive therapy unit. Br Med J 1:737-738
5. Donald I (1976) At the receiving end. A doctor's personal recollections of second-time cardiac valve replacement. Scottish Med J 21:49-57
6. Miller-Jones CMH, Williams JH (1980) Sedation for ventilation. A retrospective study of fifty patients. Anesthiology 35:1104-1107
7. Loper KA, Butler S, Nessly M, Wild L (1989) Paralysed with pain: the need for education. Pain 37:315-316
8. Cohen AT, Kelly DR (1987) Assessment of alfentanyl by intravenous infusion as long-term sedation in intensive care. Anesthesiology 42:545-548
9. Hutchins WW, Vogalzang RL, Fuld IL, Foley MJ (1984) Utilization of temporary muscle paralyses to eliminate CT motion artifact in the critically ill patient. J Comp Assist Tomogr 8:181-183
10. Sykes MK, McNichol MW, Campbell EJM (1976) Respiratory failure, 2nd edn. Blackwell, Oxford
11. Sangala W, Dixon J (1987) Pancuronium and renal failure. Anaesthesiology 42:36
12. Smith CI, Hunter JM, Jones RS (1987) Prolonged paralysis following an infusion of alcuronium in a patient with renal disfunction. Anesthesiology 42:522-525
13. Criffiths RB, Hunter JM, Jones RS (1986) Atracurium infusions in patients with renal failure on an ITU. Anesthesiology 41:375-381
14. Chapple DJ, Miller AJ, Ward JB, Wheatly PL (1987) Cardiovascular and neurological effects of laudanosine. Studies in mice and rats and in conscious and anaesthetised dogs. Br J Anaesth 59:218-225

15. Yate PM, Plynn PJ, Arnold RW, Weatherly EC, Simmonds RJ, Dopson T (1987) Clinical experience and plasma laudanosine concentrations during the infusion of atracurium in the intensive therapy unit. Br J Anaesth 59:211–217
16. Slater RM, Pollard BJ, Doran BRH (1988) Prolonged neuromuscular blockade with vecuronium in renal failure. Anesthesiology 43:250
17. Pollard BJ, Harper NJN, Doran BRH (1989) Use of continuous prolonged administration of atracurium in the ITU to a patient with myasthenia gravis. Br J Anesth 61:95–97

Pain and Sedation in the Pediatric Patient: The 1990 Approach to a Very Old Problem

D. A. Rosen and K. R. Rosen

Introduction

The child presenting to the Pediatric Intensive Care Unit (PICU) is experiencing disease symptoms, pain, and anxiety. The physician tends to focus on the disease process often overlooking the pain and anxiety, buth the child cannot overlook them as easily. The young patient's anxiety is strongly aroused by the strange surroundings and lack of familiar faces. Pain is immediate and intrusive.

If a physician forgot to give an appropriate dose of an antibiotic to a child with an infection, he/she would feel remiss. But if the physician performed a painful procedure on a child without an adequate dose of analgesics, this would be regarded with less concern. It is unfortunate but true that many physicians hold themselves accountable for infection control but not for pain control and sedation.

The lesser concern about pain and anxiety may arise from the belief that these states are abstract and difficult to measure. In fact, there is no need for that to be the case. On the nursing flow sheet, the patient's temperature is recorded on a regular basis. When it rises above 40 degrees, the physician begins a septic work-up and a rational course of antibiotics. Pain can be approached in the same manner by using a pain thermometer or a pain scale. When a rise is noted, the physician should immediately respond with a pain workup and initiate some form of analgesia. Just as the septic workup may lead the physician to modify the antibiotics, so the pain workup may lead to a modification of the analgesia.

The purpose of this paper is to review the state of the art of pediatric pain control and sedation so that the practicing clinician can more easily deal with these issues that impact the child so strongly - included is a review of the literature and a description of the clinical practice of the authors at the University of Michigan Departments of Anesthesia and Pediatrics.

Pain

Because serious research on pain has begun only recently, knowledge in this area is limited. Pediatric research has been particularly limited because of the difficulty of studying pain in children. But progress is beginning to be made. Dr. Bonica in adult research and Dr. McGrath [1] in pediatric research have stimulated considerable clinical interest. The initial studies in pediatric pain management by Beyer, Mather, and Mackie and more recently by Shecter have focused on whether pain medication was ordered or given, not on how well the pain was controlled [2–4]. The Beyer and Schecter studies also contrasted the pediatric data to the adult data. They discovered that, although adult patients may not receive adequate pain medications, children receive even less [3, 4].

Though the interest hurdle has been crossed, there still remain many methodological issues in the study of pain in the pediatric patient. Pain is a subjective experience with many external variables and is very difficult to quantify. Standardized self-reporting pain scales and questionnaires that have been developed for the adult population are rarely effective in the young patient. Scoring systems based on objects that the child can relate to are vital in order to accurately quantify the pain. Systems based on poker chips, a series of line face drawings, or the CHEOPS scoring system seem to work well [5]. At the University of Michigan, the "Oucher" developed by Beyer has been used effectively [6]. The "Oucher" is a line from 0–100 with faces of children in various degrees of pain next to it. The child who is older can relate to pain on a graded score from 0–100 while the child who is not capable of that level of abstraction can point to a picture. Unfortunately, unlike a variable such as temperature, there is no easy way to measure pain using the "Oucher" without the child's cooperation. Pain evaluation systems – for example, the one developed by Hannallah and Broadman called the Objective Pain – Discomfort Scale (OPS) – use a scoring system to rate pain in terms of observed and measured behavior [7]. The major problem with this type of rating system is that variables other than pain may interfere with the values obtained.

Though the experience of pain in the adult cannot be denied, it is not uncommon to deny the experience in the child. Beyer examined the patterns of postoperative analgesic use in adults and children following cardiac surgery [3]. Her study identified 5 rationalizations for why the child is denied pain medications. Four of these rationalizations placed the blame on the child:

1. different cardiac pathology
2. children have less pain
3. children require less medication
4. children do not communicate about pain.
   Only one rationalization placed the blame on the reluctance of caregivers to administer the drugs;
5. caregivers fear potent analgesics in children.

A popular belief still maintains that though the child might feel pain, the neonate does not. The work by Anand has put this common myth ro rest [8]. He documented that the human neonate possesses the pathways for pain at cortical as well as subcortical levels and that the neurochemical pathways for pain are also present. The neonate demonstrates the same physiologic responses to pain as an adult, and when measured, the hormonal, metabolic, and cardiorespiratory changes are frequently greater than those observed in adults. Anand also looked at the catecholamine response, endorphins, glucose, and lactate of neonates undergoing major surgery. He was able to identify three different groups. The group with the lowest levels of catecholamine and endophin response had received the most profound pain relief, which consisted of a high-dose narcotic technique followed by a continuous infusion of narcotic. The group with the highest catecholamine and endorphin response had received a standard inhalational anesthetic followed by PRN postoperative pain control [9]. The significance of his findings is further amplified by the fact that the group with the lower stress response appeared to have a lower incidence of morbidity and mortality.

A study by Parfrey et al., also proposed that uncontrolled pain may affect mortality [10]. Their study notèd that children in pain during a sickle cell crisis had a higher incidence of unexplained death as compared to those who were not in pain.

The Importance of Pain Control

At the University of Michigan the approach we take to the pediatric patient is referred to as the "battery theory". The child is conceptualized as a battery with a limited amount of power. When the medical staff is presented with the child, there is no way of knowing how much power is in the battery or whether it is new or old. What is known is that whenever the child is stressed, the battery will discharge, and when the battery is empty, the next stressful event will produce a poor outcome. It is essential to provide pain control to reduce stress because, unfortunately, we do not know how to recharge the battery.

Because the interpretation of stimuli as pain occurs by transmission of impulses at many levels, many different approaches can be taken to pain control. In the ICU, where monitoring capabilities are not limited, the options available are increased to include epidural, intrathecal, and continuous infusion.

Narcotics

In the ICU, narcotics provide the mainstay of pain control. They act by binding to specific opioid receptors in the nervous system labeled μ, $\varkappa$, σ, δ and ε [11, 12]. The receptors produce the desired anlagesic effect but are also responsible for undesirable side effects such as respiratory depression, dysphoria, and hallucinations. The various analgesics have different potentials for binding to these receptors. Therefore, when unwanted psychotropic effects are being elicited, the physician can change from one narcotic to another until the effects are eliminated.

Epidural Administration

The primary route of administration of narcotic analgesics in the PICU is intravenous, but there are other options available as well. Intrathecal and epidural applications have become popular alternative routes [13, 14]. Narcotics applied in this manner have significant differences when compared to intravenous administration. Their duration of action and onset of effect are related to their lipid solubility. Drugs with less lipid solubility such as morphine tend to have a delayed onset (20–60 minutes) but a prolonged duration (8–18 hours). Those with high-lipid solubility such as fentanyl have onset times of less than 10 minutes and analgesia lasting only 1–6 hours. The advantage of epidural applications is that they produce profound analgesia with no hemodynamic side effects and minimal sedation. The disadvantage is that they can produce an array of side effects. These side effects appear to be closely related to the dose of medication. They include pruritus, urinary retention, nausea and vomiting, and respiratory depression. Respiratory depression occurring hours after the injection is especially troublesome. Although this effect has been reported in children, it occurs at a much lower incidence than in adults [15]. When the side effects occur, an important question must be asked. Is the child with these effects also experiencing pain? If the child is not in pain, naloxone should be administered slowly so as to relieve the symptoms without causing the pain to break through. Our experience has been that this can be accomplished with one or two small doses. We have not had to place a child on a naloxone infusion, as is commonly done in the adult setting.

The simplest approach to placing the narcotics in the epidural space in the child is the caudal approach. We have found that epidural morphine administered by this route is effective for pain occurring in the lower extremities and at more distant sites such as the thoracic region [13]. We postulate that caudally applied morphine is effective at a distant site because the low-lipid solubility of morphine does not cause it to act locally but rather to ascend into the brain where it binds to morphine receptors.

Our initial approach was to do a caudal every time installation of the narcotic was needed. Technology has now produced small (24 gauge) catheters which can be left in place permitting the narcotics to be given on an intermittent or continuous basis. The development of these catheters has also increased the variety of drugs that can be used. The catheters can be inserted from the caudal space to whatever dermatome is needed. Lypophylic agents can then be continuously infused to produce pain relief locally without the side effects associated with narcotic spread to higher brain centers.

Unfortunately, there are situations where epidural or intrathecal narcotics should not or cannot be administered. These include the presence of sepsis, the presence of infection at the insertion site, or anatomical deformities that prevent insertion. Also, in the pediatric population it is not uncommon for the insertion site to become soiled, resulting in the need for alternative methods of pain control.

Intravenous Administration

When a bolus of narcotic is injected, the aim is to produce a plasma concentration that is adequate to provide analgesia but, except in the intubated and ventilated patient, not so high as to produce ventilatory depression. In the nonventilated, conscious child in pain in the PICU, patient controlled analgesia (PCA) is a reliable technique, as it is in adults [16]. A simple question developed by Dr. Lynn Broadman at the Children's Hospital National Medical Center in Washington, D.C., can be used to determine whether the child is capable of using the PCA machine. Broadman found that if a child can accurately place the expected pain from a mosquito bite, a bee sting, and a bicycle crash on a pain scoring system then he/she is capable of using the PCA machine. The PCA approach to pain relief is effective not only because it provides the child with good analgesia, but also because it gives the child some control over his/her own care providing some relief for the feeling of helplessness that patients often feel in the PICU.

For those children who are intubated and ventilated, analgesia can reliably be produced by continuous infusion of narcotics. The goal of this approach is to achieve plasma levels high enough to suppress the response to noxious stimulation.

Addiction

A child who is under-treated for pain is more likely to become addicted than one who is made comfortable. The under-treated child may become obsessed with receiving the next dose of pain medication in order to achieve some relief. When evaluating patients, it is important to distinguish between addiction and dependency. Dependency is easily controlled simply by tapering the narcotic. The incidence of addiction in the University of Michigan PICU is less than 0.01%. All of the children who did become addicted had been maintained on narcotic infusion at a level sufficient to suppress any response to noxious stimulation for prolonged periods of time (> 1 month). The addiction was dealt with easily by converting the child from the intravenous narcotic to an equivalent dose of methadone and then tapering the methadone. We find that often when children are requiring excessively high doses of narcotics in order to be comfortable, the problem is not addiction but rather the binding of the narcotic at opioid receptors other than the μ sites. Binding to Sigma receptors appears to be responsible for much of this phenomenon. Methadone in children seems to have very little Sigma binding activity.

Regional Pain Control

Narcotics are not the only approach that can be used for pain relief in the intensive care setting. Regional blocks using local anesthetics should also be considered. The development of indwelling catheters has opened up many new horizons in this area. Catheters placed in the brachial plexus or femoral plexus can provide continuous analgesia to the extremities, while catheters placed in the epidural or subarachnoid space can provide more widespread pain control. A new approach to pain relief in the thoracic or upper abdomen has been the placement of intrapleural catheters [17]. These have been inserted in an open fashion at the time of surgery or percutaneously when chest surgery has not been performed. Local anesthetics applied in this manner by continuous infusion or intermittent bolus can provide profound analgesia.

Summary

There is never a reason to make a child suffer. Therefore, the physician must make a rational approach toward pain management. Questions need to be asked such as: What is the duration of the pain? Will it be short as might be experienced with an invasive procedure or will it be more long lasting as in surgical recovery? What level of pain relief is desired? There are occasions when pain is a valuable diagnostic tool and can be critical for the accurate assessment of the child's disease. This does not mean that the child should be totally deprived of all relief but that a technique should be used that will allow breakthrough of pain. An example of this might be the use of a sympathectomy to attenuate the pain. Another approach is a block with low concentrations of local anesthetic, which would provide post-operative pain relief yet would not block the pain response to something intense like a compartment syndrome.

Pain and sedation are frequently not isolated needs. There are times when the child wants pain relief but wishes also to be awake, alert, and functioning. At other times it is desirable for the patient to be well-sedated with the pain management. The approach must be titrated so that either of these options is possible.

Because pain is complex and personal, it can be influenced by many factors. One of those factors is the anxiety produced in the child by the unfamiliarity of the clinical surroundings. This anxiety needs to be controlled because it may intensify the pain experience. The careful choice of a sedative agent can enhance the efficacy of the analgesics.

Sedation

Approaches to sedation in the Intensive Care Unit have been changing. Two studies on adults separated by only 6 years demonstrate remarkable differences. In 1981, Merriman noted that 91% of patients received muscle relaxant in the ICU [18]. A 1987 study by Bion and Ledingham noted that this had fallen to 16% [19]. While this area has never been specifically studied in the pediatric population, issues of sedation have become increasing important. As noted earlier, sedation is needed not only for comfort but also to insure cooperation with procedures, invasive lines, and simply lying in bed. Protocols that work in adults frequently must be modified to achieve the same success in children.

Ideal Sedative

The ideal sedative should have many properties. It needs to be a rapid-acting drug that will sedate the child in minutes, but it must be short-acting so that it may be titrated to the clinical setting. To be short acting, it needs to have minimal metabolites. As a short-acting drug, it will need to be given by continuous infusion so that sedation can be maintained. A continuous infusion drug must not be sclerosing to the veins. Because it is used in all clinical situations, it should have minimal hemodynamic effects, and because it will be given to intubated as well as nonintubated children, it needs to have minimal respiratory depression. The drug must not demonstrate tolerance or have addictive potential since the duration of critical illness is variable. Because the child is growing, nutritional needs are usually greater than for the adult; and, therefore, the drug should allow for feeding the patient through the stomach and alimentary tract instead of a central IV. Finally, because sedation will frequently need to be initiated prior to securing venous access, the drug needs to be effective by parenteral as well as nonparenteral routes. The ideal sedative with all the above characteristics does not exist, but midazolam comes closer than other drugs in most clinical situations.

Continuous Midazolam Infusion

Midazolam infusions are initiated by bolusing the patient with 0.25 mg/kg over 3–5 minutes. The bolus is immediately followed by the initiation of a continuous infusion that is started at 0.4 mcg/kg/min. The dose is then titrated up and down as the clinical setting requires. Initially the infusions should be kept in the low range 0.4–2.0 mcg/kg/min [20, 21]. Supplemental medications are often needed because children frequently experience pain in addition to anxiety. After a short while, if the infusion rate needs to be increased, it can be extended up to 4.0 mcg/kg/min. However, in order to maintain its effectiveness, the infusion should be kept at the lowest dose possible. An effective method for titrating sedation is to use a sedation scale, which is filled out on an hourly basis and rates the effectiveness of the sedation (Table 1).

We recommend increasing the infusion when a child gets to a score of 4 but, more importantly, decreasing it when a score of 2 is achieved.

Midazolam infusion has been successfully used to sedate children of all ages. However, because most problems with cooperation in the PICU are noted in children under 4 years of age, most work has been reported for children in that age group. Midazolam infusions have been used to provide sedation from minutes to months at a mean infusion rate of 0.92 mcg/kg/min with a median rate that tends to vary from day to day [20].

Table 1. Sedation scale

1	2	3	4	5
Asleep, does not open eyes with minor stimulation	Drowsy, eyes closed, responds to minor stimulation	Calm, lying with eyes open	Active, moving about controlled fashion, tubes & lines not at risk	Wild & uncontrollable, tubes & lines at risk

In the University of Michigan PICU, midazolam infusion was first used for children recovering from airway-related illness, primarily croup and epiglottitis. As its use has been extended to other processes, the need for supplemental medications during the infusion has steadily increased. The primary reason that supplemental medications are given is to treat an underlying painful process occurring simultaneous with the need for sedation.

Advantages of Midazolam Infusion

Adverse hemodynamic effects are much less common in the pediatric patient receiving midazolam infusion than has been noted in the adult population. Spontaneous respiration with or without an endotracheal tube is also possible. Another positive effect of midazolam infusion is that it permits continued use of the alimentary tract for nutrition throughout the sedation period, if it is delivered through a nasogastric tube. There have been no reports of aspiration resulting from feeding during midazolam sedation.

Metabolic parameters appear to be positively affected in children on continuous midazolam infusions. Oxygen consumption has been reported to fall 39% and CO_2 production 5%, whereas the respiratory quotient rose 5% [20]. Clinical experience at the University of Michigan has confirmed that midazolam positively affects the supply-demand ratio in very sick children. Following recovery from a serious illness, those pediatric patients who have been on midazolam infusions appear to have a better psychological profile than those who have not.

Midazolam infusions also affect nursing efficiency in the PICU. Because the drug is given continuously, the nurse has to spend less time away from the patient getting sedative medications. Parental acceptance is high because the child is able to respond rather than lie paralyzed or tightly restrained. Some of the children we place on midazolam infusions are patients who might be expected to have seizures because of their condition. None of them has ever had a seizure, however, which suggests that the midazolam has anti-seizure potential. Although this effect has never been studied in children, Galvin reports that midazolam is an effective anti-seizure medication in adults [22].

Another significant advantage of midazolam in the pediatric patient is that it can be given by non-intravenous routes. Because of its pharmacology, it is water soluble as it is dispensed and rapidly becomes lipid soluble as the pH normalizes to physiologic pH. Frequently, sedation is required in the pediatric patient prior to securing intravenous access. Midazolam has been shown to be effective by a variety of routes [23–25]. The ability for reversal by a specific antagonist flumazanil also makes midazolam most attractive [26].

Breakthrough in Sedation with Continuous Infusion of Midazolam

During midazolam infusion, it is important to titrate the medication closely against the patient's sedation level, keeping the infusion rate as low as possible.

This will prevent tolerance to the drug and may alleviate some of the psycho-tropic reactions that have been observed in children on high doses over a pro-longed period of time. The drug to use for breakthrough in sedation should be carefully chosen. If the breakthrough is thought to be due to pain, opioids should be selected because intravenous midazolam does not possess analgesic properties. There appears to be considerable differences in the sedative effects of the different opioids in patients under midazolam sedation. A recent article by Vinik et al., documented the synergism between midazolam and alfentanil [27] while another study by Tverskoy et al. showed no synergism with morphine [28].

Shortcomings of Midazolam Infusion

As effective as midazolam infusions appear to be, there are cases when they have failed. Careful examination of these cases show that the primary reason for ini-tial failure has been absence of a loading dose - the infusion had been started without the bolus dose being given. In other cases, the problem occurs when an infusion is interrupted for some reason, such as to correct a medication incom-patibility. When the medication is restarted without a bolus, the sedation control is frequently difficult to obtain. We now recommend doubling the infusion rate and changing the medication over to oral 35-45 minutes before stopping the IV medication. Another common cause of failure is excessively high infusion rates usually resulting from medication errors. Infusion rates starting at greater then 4 mcg/kg/min produce acute tolerance in the child after about 48 hours.

Other problems with midazolam infusion use in the pediatric patient are:

1. In the U.S., the preservative in the drug is benzyl alcohol. Benzyl alcohol has been shown to cause death in neonates from grey baby syndrome. Fortunate-ly, the level of benzyl alcohol necessary to produce this syndrome is high (>98 mg/kg/day). A midazolam infusion 24 times the therapeutic range would have to be given to reach this threshold. However, a recent article in Pediatrics by Jardine and Rogers contends that any benzyl alcohol in preterm infants may place them at risk for kernicterus and intraventricular hemorr-hage [29].
2. Drug levels don't always correlate with sedation. Investigators have reported patients not sedated at concentrations >3000 ng/mL and others not awaken-ing at concentrations <80 ng/mL [30–32].
3. Acute tolerance appears to be more of a problem than chronic tolerance. Those pediatric patients at the University of Michigan who have been main-tained on prolonged midazolam infusions (72 weeks) can be maintained at an appropriate level of sedation without having to steadily increase the infusion rate.
4. Finally, the clinician must be aware that there is no pain relief from midazo-lam, so patients experiencing pain must be administered concomitant analge-sics.

Withdrawal

Withdrawal reactions from the long-acting benzodiazapines have been reported [33, 34]. Withdrawal symptoms from abrupt cessation of midazolam infusion are suspected in one case at the University of Michigan and also in cases reported from Great Britain [35]. Unfortunately, none of the cases are clear cut, and all patients had some confounding variables which may have been presenting withdrawal-like symptoms. The only active metabolite of midazolam is α-hydroxy midazolam which has a shorter duration than the parent compound [36]. Except for one unclear case, we have never seen withdrawal symptoms in our patients even though we do not wean the midazolam following an infusion. However, about 50% of our patients receive a long-acting sedative after stopping the infusion so we might not see withdrawal symptoms even if they did exist.

Sedation During Extracorporeal Membrane Oxygenation

At the University of Michigan, adequate sedation and control of pain has been possible in every situation except one. Sedation of the child during extracorporeal membrane oxygenation (ECMO) remains an uncertain area. Children well sedated on midazolam infusion have become unsedateable on midazolam within 15 minutes of being placed on ECMO. This occurs because of the affinity of the membrane oxygenator in the ECMO circuit to actively remove the drug from the plasma concentration [37]. The capacity of the membrane oxygenator for midazolam has not been fully appreciated. Increasing the midazolam does little good because it appears that the affinity for the oxygenator is greater than the endogenous receptor for the drug.

During ECMO it is not uncommon for painful procedures to be performed. Narcotics must be chosen very carefully because the oxygenator's affinity for them may be even greater than for the sedatives. Patients who were well controlled on fentanyl infusions have become wild after being placed on ECMO with a new unprimed oxygenator. The University of Michigan lab has worked on the fentanyl kinetics in the ECMO circuit and found that the fentanyl is very tightly bound to the SciMed membrane oxygenator [38]. This binding allows prior saturation of the membrane oxygenator before initiating ECMO so that a steady fentanyl level can be easily maintained and the patient kept pain free throughout the ECMO experience.

All too often, advance planning has not been done with regards to pain and sedation during ECMO. In this setting we use morphine to provide pain relief because it is not bound by the membrane oxygenator. Along a similar line, we use lorazepam to provide sedation because significantly less lorazepam is removed by the membrane oxygenator than midazolam [39].

Summary

We have reviewed the problems of pain control and sedation in the pediatric intensive care unit and have provided some new approaches to these problems.

Areas that call out for further research are: new routes of administration that do not require parenteral administration; new drugs with durations that can be closely correlated with the clinical need; and new drugs that can provide analgesia or sedation without the unwanted side effects of present drug protocols. Investigators are already examining a new classification of drugs called alpha agonist, which have the ability to produce analgesia by inhibiting substance P. Clearly we are in the infancy of optimal pain and sedation control, but with the present increased interest in this area, progress should be rapid.

References

1. McGrath PJ, Unruh A (1987) Pain in children and adolescents. Elsevier Science, Amsterdam
2. Mather L, Mackie J (1983) The incidence of postoperative pain in children. Pain 15:271–282
3. Beyer JE, DeGood DE, Ashley LC, et al (1983) Patterns of postoperative analgesia use with adults and children following cardiac surgery. Pain 17:71–81
4. Schecter NL, Allen DA, Hanson K (1986) Status of pediatric pain control: A comparison of hospital analgesic usage in children and adults. Pediatrics 77:11-15
5. McGrath PJ, Johnson G, Goodman JT, Schillinger J, Dunn J, Chapman JA (1985) CHEOPS: A behavioral scale for rating postoperative pain in children. In: Fields, Dubner, Cervero (eds) Advances in pain research and therapy, 9th edn. Raven Press, New York, pp 395-402
6. Beyer JE (1984) The oucher: A user's manual and technical report. University of Virginia Alumni Patent Foundation, Charlottesville
7. Hannallah RS, Broadman LM, Belman AB, Abramowitz MD, Epstein BS (1987) Comparison of caudal and ilioinguinal/iliohypogastric nerve blocks for control of post-orchidopexy pain in pediatric ambulatory surgery. Anesthesiology 66:832-834
8. Anand KJS, Hickey PR (1987) Pain and its effects in the human neonate and fetus. N Engl J Med 317:1321–1329
9. Anand KJS, Sippell WG, Aynsley-Green A (1987) Randomised trial of fentanyl anesthesia in preterm babies undergoing surgery. Effects on the stress response. Lancet 1 62–66
10. Parfrey NA, Moore W, Hutchins DMJ (1984) Is pain crisis a cause of death in sickle cell disease. Clin Pathol 84:209–212
11. Snyder SH (1984) Drug and neurotransmitter receptors in the brain. Science 224:22–31
12. Wood PL (1982) Multiple opiate receptors: support for unique mu, delta and Kappa sites. Neuromarmacoloty 21:487–497
13. Rosen KR, Rosen DA (1989) Caudal epidural morphine for control of pain following open heart surgery in children. Anesthesiology 70:418–421
14. Jones SE, Beasley JM, Macfarlane DW, David JM, Hall-Davies G (1984) Intrathecal morphine for postoperative pain relief in children. Br J Anaesth 56:137–140
15. Krane EJ (1988) Delayed respiratory depression in a child after caudal epidural morphine. Anesth Analg 67:79–82
16. Gaukroger PB, Tomkins DP, Vander Wait JH (1988) Use of patient-controlled analgesia (PCA) in children. J Pediatr Surg 23(12):1227-1228
17. McIlvaine WB, Know RF, Fennessey PV, Goldstein M (1988) Continuous infusion of bupivacaine via intrapleural catheter for analgesia after thoracotomy in children. Anesthesiology 69:261–264
18. Merriman HM (1981) The techniques used to sedate ventilated patients. A survey of methods used in 34 ICUs in Great Britain. Intensive Care Med 7(5):217–224
19. Bion JF, Ledingham IM (1987) Sedation in intensive care – a postal survey. Intensive Care Med 13(3):215–216

20. Rosen DA, Rosen KR (1990) Benzodiapapine usage in the pediatric intensive care unit. Intens Care Med (in press)
21. Silvasi DL, Rosen DA, Rosen KR (1988) Continuous intravenous midazolam infusion for sedation in the pediatric intensive care unit. Anesth Analg 67:286–288
22. Galvin GM, Jelinek GA (1987) Midazolam: an effective intravenous agent for seizure control. Arch Emerg Med 4:169–172
23. Crevoisier C, Ziegler WH, Eckert M, Heizmann P (1983) Relationship between plasma concentration and effect of midazolam after oral and intravenous administration. Br J Clin Pharmacol 16:51–61S
24. Wilton NCT, Leigh J, Rosen DA, Pandit R (1988) Preanesthetic sedation of preschool children using intranasal midazolam. Anesthesiology 69:972–975
25. DeJong PC, Verburg MP (1988) Comparison of rectal to intramuscular administration of midazolam and atropine for premedication of children. Acta Anaesthesiol Scand 32(6):485–489
26. Burnstein S (1988) The uses of midazolam and flumazanil in intensive care resuscitation. 16(suppl) 5100–5106
27. Vinik HR, Bradley EL Jr, Kissin I (1989) Midazolam-alfentanil synergism for anesthetic induction in patients. Anesth Analg 69:231–237
28. Tverskoy M, Fleyshman G, Ezry J, Bradley EL Jr, Kissin I (1989) Midazolam-morphine sedative interaction in patients. Anesth Analg 68:282–285
29. Jardine DS, Rogers K (1989) Relationships of benzyl alcohol to kernicterus, intraventricular hemorrhage, and mortality in preterm infants. Pediatric 83:153–160
30. Persson MP, Nilsson A, Hartvig P (1988) Relation of sedation and amnesia to plasma concentration of midazolam in surgical patients. Clin Pharmacol Ther 43: 324–331
31. Lloyd-Thomas AR, Booker PD (1986) Infusion of midazolam in paediatric patients after cardiac surgery. Br J Anaesth 58:1109–1115
32. Oldenhof H, deJong M, Steehock A, Janknegt R (1988) Clinical pharmacokinetics of midazolam in intensive care patients, a wide interpatient variability. Clin Pharmacol Ther 43:3, 263–269
33. Mackinnon GL, Parker WA (1982) Benzodiazepine withdrawal syndrome: A literature review and evaluation. Am J Drug Alcohol Abuse 9:19
34. Committee on Safety of Medicines (1988) Benzodiazepines, dependence and withdrawal syndrome. Curr Probl:21
35. Sury MRJ, Russel GN, Thornington R, Vivori E (1989) Acute benzodiazepine withdrawal after midazolam infusions in children. Crit Care Med 17:301–302
36. Ziegler WH, Schalch E, Leishman B, Eckert M (1983) Comparison of the effects of intravenously administered midazolam, triazolam and their hydoxymetabolites. Br J Clin Pharmacol 16:63–69S
37. Silvasi DL, Rosen D, Rosen KR (1989) Absorption of midazolam by the SciMed membrane oxygenator (Abstract). Anesth Analg 68:S261
38. Rosen D, Rosen K, Davidson B, Broadman L (1988) Fentanyl uptake by the SciMed membrane oxygenator. J Cardiothor Anesth 619–626
39. Leong P, Rosen D, Rosen K (1990) Uptake of lorazepam by SciMed oxygenator membrane. Anesth Analg 70:Suppl (in press)

Liver Metabolism of Analgesic Agents

G. R. Park and K. Quinn

Introduction

The importance of the liver in the metabolism of analgesic agents has long been recognized. Important changes in the elimination of these drugs may occur in critically ill patients. Changes in liver blood flow are particularly important since hypotension, anesthesia and surgery [1], trauma, sepsis, hypoxia and possibly inotropic therapy lead to significant alterations, resulting in large changes in the clearance of these drugs. To date there has been little systematic study of commonly used drugs in *acute* hepatic insufficiency, a common accompaniment of serious illness. Furthermore the concurrent administration of some of the many drugs used to treat such illness including benzodiazepines, cimetidine etc. may interfere with the liver enzymatic activity, decreasing or increasing the rate of metabolism. Of all of the analgesics in common use in the critically ill, morphine is the commonest in use worldwide. This review will predominately concentrate on the altered metabolism of morphine in critically ill humans although the newer synthetic opiates will also be discussed.

Morphine

Widely different alterations in the pharmacokinetics of morphine have been demonstrated in several disease states which might be encountered in patients requiring intensive care some of which are shown in Table 1. It is commonly administered by continuous intravenous infusion. Stanski et al. [5] have shown both normal and abnormal morphine clearance in cirrhosis. This difference was thought to be related to the differences in the severity of the hepatic dysfunction

Table 1. Changes in the pharmacokinetics of unchanged morphine in different disease states

Disease [Ref.]	Clearance	Volume of distribution	Elimination half-life
Cirrhosis [2]	Decreased	Unchanged	Increased
Uremia [3]	Unchanged	Decreased	Unchanged
Septic shock [4]	Decreased	Unchanged	Increased

in the two groups studied. MacNab et al. [4] have demonstrated that in septic shock the clearance of morphine is reduced, a feature he attributed to a reduction in hepatic blood flow.

Metabolism of Morphine (Fig. 1)

Morphine is principally metabolised to morphine-3-glucuronide and morphine-6-glucuronide, with a small amount metabolised to normorphine and subsequently normorphine-3-glucuronide. Codeine is metabolised to codeine-6-glucu-

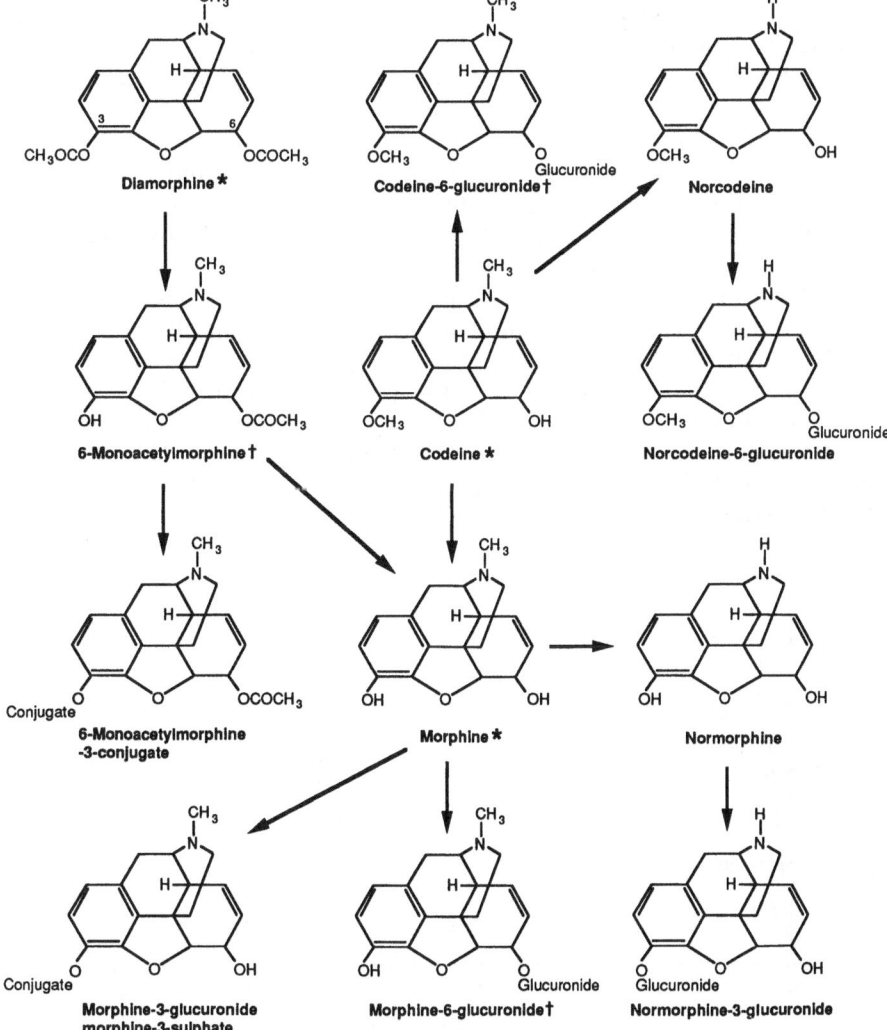

Fig. 1. From [24]

ronide and norcodeine (with subsequent metabolism to norcodeine-6-glucuronide), but a significant quantity is metabolised to morphine.

Importance of the Assay Method

The ability to measure morphine concentrations at pharmacological doses in man has been a recent event since the radioimmunoassay (RIA) was introduced for morphine by Spector and co-workers in 1971 [6]. RIA techniques are very sensitive but suffer from lack of specificity by measuring metabolites and morphine analogues. Dependent upon the site of conjugation with bovine serum albumin to make morphine immunogenic, the major metabolites morphine-3-glucuronide and morphine-6-glucuronide can have a cross-reactivity of between 1 to 150% of the parent compound in displacing radiolabelled ligand from the antibody binding site. More recently the removal of morphine metabolites by solid phase extraction prior to RIA has successfully resolved the problem of analytical specificity [7].

The assay of morphine in plasma by gas chromatography (GLC) was described by Edlund [8]. Separation, precision and sensitivity of the assay were excellent and with a reported limit of detection of 1 ng/ml. However this technique does not directly measure metabolites.

High performance liquid chromatography methods (HPLC) require no derivatization for either the separation or detection of morphine. In addition HPLC methods utilizing electrochemical detection can increase the sensitivity for morphine by 100 times compared to ultra-violet detection techniques. Using this method morphine and its metabolites were quantified amperometrically by the electrochemical oxidation of the phenolic hydroxyl group [9]. This method gave linear, quantitative results covering a wide range of morphine concentrations (1–400 ng/ml) with acceptable coefficients of variation.

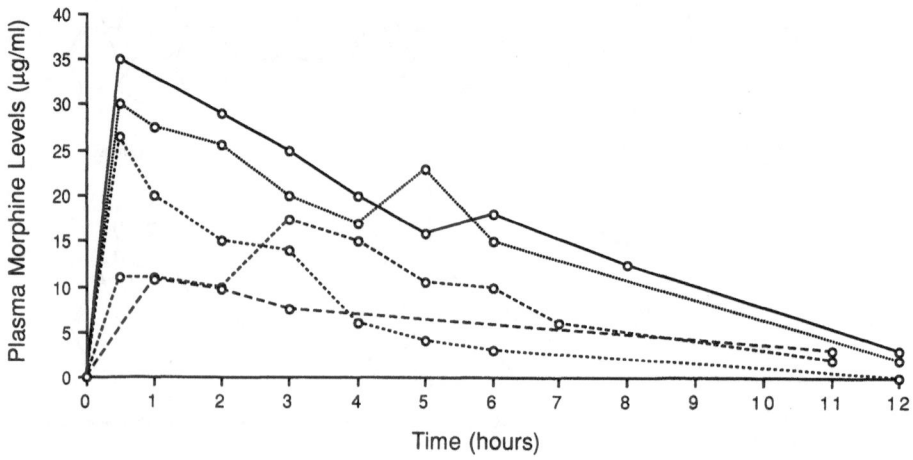

Fig. 2. From [25]

Early Postoperative Studies in Patients Following Liver Transplantation: In an attempt to elucidate the effects of surgery and ischemia on the metabolism of morphine we studied patients immediately following liver transplantation. This particular model was used because the recently transplanted liver has been damaged by two operations (one for removal from the donor and the other the recipient operation) with an intervening period of ischemia whilst the liver is transported. The first study was performed once cardiorespiratory stability has been achieved immediately following liver transplantation whilst the patient was in the Intensive Care Unit. Morphine sulfate, 2.5 mg, was given intravenously and the plasma sampled for 24 hours. Morphine concentrations were analyzed using RIA. The results are shown in Fig. 2 and demonstrate a secondary peak, a feature previously attributed to the entero-hepatic recirculation. However, in these patients this is unlikely since a T-Tube was in place in the common bile duct and due to the early postoperative ileus most of the bile would have drained through this externally.

A further study was performed in 7 patients following liver transplantation and used a larger intravenous bolus of morphine sulfate (10 mg). The plasma and urine were analysed using high performance liquid chromatography. On this occasion a bi-exponential decay was observed with no second peaks. Though the distribution and elimination half lives for morphine were similar to previous studies a greater total apparent volume of distribution was observed, reflecting an increased plasma clearance of morphine than has been previously reported. The concentration of morphine glucuronides remained high 24 hours following the administration of morphine although the clinical significance of this remains to be established. The metabolism of morphine was virtually complete with 4.5% unchanged morphine recovered in the urine 24 hours following drug administration.

Intraoperative Studies in Two Children During Liver Transplantation: A further study was performed to attempt to identify the reason for the second peak [10]. Two children with end-stage biliary atresia, and therefore almost total absence of biliary drainage re-studied immediately following induction of anesthesia but before surgery commenced (60 minutes later). At induction of anesthesia 1 mg/ kg of morphine sulfate was administered intravenously and plasma sampled until surgery started. During the operation and in the immediate postoperative period morphine was not administered, fentanyl being used for escape analgesia, allowing a further sample to be obtained at 24 hours. In both children morphine clearance was higher than had been previously reported and this was associated with the rapid production of both morphine-3-glucuronide and morphine-6-glucuronide. In the first child who had normal renal function plasma concentrations of these metabolites were decreasing by the end of the 60 minute period and were totally undetectable by 24 hours. The second child had unrecognized renal dysfunction at the time of operation and although morphine clearance was rapid, high concentrations of morphine-6-glucuronide and morphine-3-glucuronide were present at 60 minutes and 24 hours later. During the perioperative period this child's renal function deteriorated with long periods of anuria. Postoperatively the first child was rapidly rousable and required multiple increments of fentanyl to facilitate artificial ventilation. The second child however remained unconscious and did not require any additional opioid analgesia until a diuresis was induced. No second peaks were observed and it would appear those seen in the early study are artefacts due to the cross reactivity of the RIA with metabolites. The prolonged narcosis seen in this child was attributed to morphine-6-glucuronide.

Importance of Morphine-6-glucuronide

Shimomura et al. [11] demonstrated that this substance administered parenterally to rats has an analgesic potency 4 times and a duration of action twice that of morphine. Direct intracisternal administration of morphine-6-glucuronide revealed an analgesic potency 44 times that of morphine. Others [12] have also demonstrated the clinical effects of prolonged narcosis due to morphine-6-glucuronide in critically ill patients with renal failure. Ball et al. [13] have also demonstrated that morphine clearance is directly related to creatinine clearance, although the assay method used in this study was an RIA which may cross-react with morphine-6-glucuronide. Although this work supported the clinical observations, that in renal failure the effects of morphine are prolonged, it is likely that this is due to the accumulation of metabolites rather than the parent drug. Recently, morphine-6-glucuronide has been shown to be a highly active analgesic agent in patients with chronic pain [14] and to be present in cerebrospinal fluid after both oral and intramuscular administration of morphine [15].

Site of Morphine Metabolism

Anhepatic Studies in Humans: The presence of extra-hepatic sites for liver metabolism have long been postulated. Animal work, principally in dogs [16], has demonstrated that the liver is likely to be the primary site of morphine metabolism but other metabolic sites may be present. We have studied 7 adult patients during the anhepatic period of orthotopic liver transplantation and measured the concentrations of any metabolites produced. At the beginning of the anhepatic period 10 mg of morphine were injected as a single intravenous bolus and the plasma and urinary concentrations of morphine, morphine-3-glucuronide, morphine-6-glucuronide and normorphine were measured using HPLC. Insignificant concentrations of morphine metabolites were found in the plasma and the urine whilst there was no functional liver tissue but these markedly increased when the new donor liver was reperfused. This suggests that in these patients the liver is the primary site for morphine metabolism although other insignificant sites may exist.

In Vitro Metabolism of Morphine by the Kidney: In an attempt to identify if the kidney is a site for the glucuronidation of morphine the in vitro ability of human liver and kidney microsomes to metabolise morphine was studied. The liver tissue was obtained from the patient's own liver (which was therefore severely diseased) during liver transplantation. Renal tissue was obtained from unaffected parts of the kidney during removal for an upper or lower pole tumours. Microsomes were obtained from this tissue and incubated with morphine. Glucuronidation was found to be preserved in 6 out of 11 microsomal specimens demonstrating the validity of the method. In only 3 of the 6 incubates of microsomes from the kidney were we able to identify small quantities of morphine-3-glucuronide. Whilst in the liver morphine-3-glucuronide and morphine-6-glucuronide were produced. This confirms that the liver is the major source of morphine metabolism even when severely damaged by disease. The kidney plays a more minor role in its metabolism.

Importance of Liver Blood Flow

MacNab et al. [14] have shown in 6 shocked patients that plasma clearance of morphine is reduced. They also measured liver blood flow, using indocyanine green, and demonstrated a decrease in this in the shocked group. There was however no correlation between magnitude of the decrease of liver blood flow and the clearance of morphine. We have further investigated the influence of liver blood flow on morphine elimination in patients with portal hypertension, but normal liver function due to schistosomiasis. Twelve patients were studied, 6 before portacaval anastomosis and 6 afterwards. In the first group the elimination half-life was shorter, and clearance greater than in the second group, confirming the importance of liver blood flow in the metabolism of morphine.

Morphine Mixtures

Papaveretum is a mixture of alkaloids including morphine, codeine, narcotine, thebaine and papaverine. Although we understand the metabolism of the principle agent little is known of the other agents in animals or volunteers let alone the critically ill. These alkaloids can be expected to be active in humans.

Synthetic Opiates

Meperidine

This opiate has been used by continuous infusion to provide analgesia to postoperative patients but it is less frequently used in critically ill patients and little information on its activity exists. It is metabolized principally to normeperidine and thence to normeperidineic acid (Fig. 3). In patients with cirrhosis and viral hepatitis the clearance of meperidine is decreased and the elimination half-life increased. The volume of distribution and degree of protein binding are, however, unchanged. The prolonged half-life of meperidine in such patients has been attributed to metabolic dysfunction of the liver [17]. In renal failure the concen-

CH₃—CH₂—O—C
Meperidine

N-demethylation   hydrolysis

Normeperidine   hydrolysis   Meperidinic acid

Major biotransformation pathways
for pethedine (meperidine) in man

Norameperidinic acid   **Fig. 3.** From [26]

tration of the principle metabolite can increase leading to toxicity, this is principally seen in the central nervous system when fits may develop.

Phenoperidine

Despite widespread use of this agent within the United Kingdom particularly for
those suffering from head injury little is known of its metabolism. It is principally metabolized within the liver to meperidine. In patients with liver disease
phenoperidine has a prolonged elimination half-life and a reduced clearance
[18]. Similar constraints to those of meperidine apply about its use in renal failure.

Table 2. Pharmacokinetics of different opiates in adults

Drug [ref.]	Vdss (L/kg)	CL (L/kg/h)	$t^{1/2}_\beta$ (h)
Alfentanil [19]	0.39	0.20	1.63
Fentanyl	4.8	1.3	3.09
Morphine [5]	3.2	0.90	2.9
Meperidine [20]	3.7	0.84	3.7

$Vdss$ = volume of distribution at steady-state; CL = total body clearance; $t^{1/2}_\beta$ = elimination
half-life.

Fentanyl

Fentanyl has a high extraction ratio and might therefore be expected to have altered pharmacokinetics in the presence of hepatic cirrhosis. This has not been shown to be so and may be a reflection of its large volume of distribution. Table 2 demonstrates the pharmacokinetic differences between the opiates when used during anesthesia. These may dramatically change in the critically ill. When they are in use for a long period it is important to remember redistribution. Flow-limited drugs may change to being dependent upon elimination for termination of effect. So far as is known fentanyl does not have any active metabolites.

Alfentanil

This is a new short acting opiate currently undergoing investigation as an analgesic for use by continuous intravenous infusion in critically ill patients. The small volume of distribution results in a short elimination half life which should result in rapid recovery. It is metabolized by N- and O-dealkylation in the liver with the resulting metabolites being inactive. Decreased clearance has been seen in patients with cirrhosis with an increase in plasma elimination half life from 1.63 to 3.6 hours [21]. Using the post liver transplant model described for morphine we have shown similar large alterations in its pharmacokinetics with the elimination half-life increasing to almost 12 hours. Sear et al. have shown 9 fold variations in plasma clearance when alfentanil is infused into critically patients reflecting changes in hepatic blood flow [22].

Pharmacogenetics: Genetic polymorphism has been reported with alfentanil which may account for some of the wide individual variability in plasma clearance rates. Recent work suggests (3–10%) of the caucasian population are slow metabolisers of alfentanil [23]. More recent studies have failed to demonstrate this abnormality both in vitro using human liver microsomes and in 3 human volunteers. One of these volunteers was known to have an abnormal cytochrome P450 but despite this demonstrated normal alfentanil pharmacokinetics.

Conclusion

The liver is the major site of opiate metabolism. Deterioration in its metabolic abilities will be seen when it is affected by disease or alterations in liver blood flow. In these instances accumulation and toxicity of these agents will be seen. There is an increasing awareness of the activity of metabolites previously thought to be inactive. These will accumulate if renal failure is part of the patients illness. Some metabolites appear to be analgesic whilst others exhibit potentially dangerous toxicity. When clinicians treat seriously ill patients they should consider as yet undescribed unwanted effects commonly used drugs or their metabolites when unusual situations occur.

Acknowledgement: Mr. K. Quinn was in receipt of a grant from Addenbrooke's Hospital Trust Fund during the preparation of this manuscript.

References

1. Gelman SI (1976) Disturbances in hepatic blood flow during anesthesia and surgery. Arch Surg 111:881–883
2. Mazoit JX, Sandouk P, Zelanoui P, Schermann JP (1987) Pharmacokinetics of morphine in normal and cirrhotic subjects. Anesth Analg 66:293–298
3. Chauvin M, Sandouk P, Scherrmann JM, et al (1987) Morphine pharmacokinetics in renal failure. Anesthesiology 66:327–331
4. MacNab MSP, Macrae DJ, Guy E, Grant LS, Feely J (1986) Profound reduction in morphine clearance and liver blood flow in shock. Intensive Care Med 12:366–369
5. Stanski DR, Greenblatt DJ, Lowenstein E (1978) Kinetics of intravenous and intramuscular morphine. Clin Pharmacol Ther 24:52–59
6. Spector S, Vessel ES (1971) Disposition of morphine in man. Science 174:421–422
7. Quinn K, Galloway DB, Leslie ST, Ness C, Robertson S, Shill A (1988) Determination of morphine in human plasma by radioimmunoassay utilising a preliminary liquid solid extraction. J Pharm Biomed Anal 6:15–22
8. Edlund PO (1981) Gas chromatography with mass fragmentography for morphine and its congeners. J Chromatogr 206:109
9. Svensson CK, Woodruff MN, Baxter JG, Lalka D (1986) Free drug concentration monitoring in clinical practice. Clin Pharmacokin 1:450–469
10. Shelly MP, Cory EP, Park GR (1986) Pharmacokinetics of morphine in two children before and after liver transplantation. Br J Anaesth 58:1218–1223
11. Shimomura K, Kamata O, Ueki S, et al (1971) Analgesic effects of morphine glucuronides. Toh J Exp Med 105:45–52
12. Osbourne RJ, Joel SP, Slevin ML (1986) Morphine intoxication in renal failure: The role of morphine-6-glucuronide. Br Med J 292:1548–1549
13. Ball M, McQuay HU, Moore RA, et al (1985) Renal failure and the use of morphine in intensive care. Lancet 1:784
14. Osbourne R, Joel S, Trew D, Slevin M (1988) Analgesic activity of morphine-6-glucuronide. Lancet 1:828
15. Hand CW, Blunnie WP, Clattey LP, McShane AJ, McQuay HJ, Moore RA (1987) Potential analgesic contribution from morphine-6-glucuronide in CSF. Lancet 1:1207–1208
16. Jacqz E, Ward S, Johnson R, Schenker S, Gerkens J, Branch R (1986) Extrahepatic glucuronidation of morphine in the dog. Drug Metab Disp 14:627–630
17. McHorse TS, Wilkinson GR, Johnson RF, Shenker MD (1975) Effect of acute viral hepatitis in man on the disposition and elimination of meperidine. Gastroenterology 68:775–780
18. Isherwood CN, Calvey TN, Williams NE, Chan K, Murray KR (1984) Elimination of phenoperidine in liver disease. Br J Anaesth 56:843–846
19. Bower S, Hull CJ (1982) Comparative pharmacokinetics of fentanyl and alfentanil. Br J Anaesth 54:871–877
20. Mather LE, Tucker GT, Pflug A, Lindop MJ, Wilkinson C (1975) Meperidine kinetics in man. Clin Pharm Ther 17:21–30
21. Ferrier C, Mary J, Bouttard Y, et al (1985) Alfentanil pharmacokinetics in patients with cirrhosis. Anesthesiology 62:480–484
22. Sear JW, Fisher A, Summerfield RJ (1987) Is alfentanil by infusion useful for sedation on the ITU. Eur J Anaesth S1:55–61
23. McDonnell TE, Bartkowski RR, Kahn C (1982) Evidence for polymorphic oxidation of alfentanil in man. Anesthesiology 61:A284
24. Bodenham A, Shelly M, Park G (1988) The altered pharmacokinetics and pharmacodynamics of drugs commonly used in critically ill patients. Clin Pharmac 14:347–373

25. Shelly M, Quinn K, Park G (1986) Pharmacokinetic study of morphine in the postoperative period following liver transplantation: a preliminary communication. In: Band P, Stewart J, Towson T (eds) Advances in the management of chronic pain. The international symposium on pain control. Purdue Frederick, Toronto
26. Intussi CF, Umans JG (1983) Pethidine and its active metabolite norpethidine. Clin Anaesth

Fluids and Electrolytes – Endocrine Function

The Kidney – The Innocent Bystander

M. H. Rosenthal

Introduction

One of Sir William Osler's quotes states that "Patients don't die of their disease, they die of the physiologic abnormalities of their disease." Nowhere is this sentiment more appropriate than in reviewing the implication of acute renal insufficiency as a complication of other disease processes. The majority of renal insufficiency occurring in critically ill patients is not a primary process, but rather a sequelae of associated systemic disease or therapy. Such renal insufficiency, if requiring dialysis, often proves fatal. The purpose of this discussion is to examine those situations that may lead to renal insufficiency, the etiologies of such an insult and approaches that may be used in an attempt to normalize or attenuate kidney failure.

Etiology

The majority of instances of developing renal insufficiency may be attributed to hemodynamically mediated hypoperfusion [1]. Commonly caused by hypovolemia, renal circulatory impairment may also result from cardiac failure, sepsis, increased vascular resistance, (i.e., hypertension, toxemia of pregnancy) localized renal arterial pathology, pharmacologic therapy or humoral factors including excess levels of sympathomimetic amines, renin and vasoconstrictor prostaglandins or deficiencies in angiotensin II. In evaluating oliguria as a warning of renal compromise, the clinician must also recognize the implications of altered anti-diuretic hormone, atrial natriuretic peptide and aldosterone activity and the potential for their role in such processes as positive pressure ventilation, cardiopulmonary bypass and stress. Intravascular hypovolemia is likely the leading cause of decreased cardiac output and, thus renal hypoperfusion, in medical and surgical critically ill patients. Obvious causes including hemorrhage, excess urine, gastrointestinal losses or perspiration may be easy to identify, yet, of equal incidence, if not more likely, is the loss of intravascular volume due to altered capillary permeability with loss of fluid into the interstitium, often referred to as the "third-space". This increase in permeability accompanies sepsis, allergic reactions, activation of bradykinin, complement and leukotrienes and spanchnic circulatory insufficiency. Relative hypovolemia may also occur with a decrease in vascular resistance. The use of diuretics as well as vasodilator drugs may also result in an absolute or relative hypovolemia, respectively.

In addition to hemodynamic mediators, renal insults can also occur due to post-renal obstruction, disseminated intravascular coagulopathy (DIC), and intrinsic and extrinsic nephrotoxins. Specific identification of renal insufficiency in patients with end-stage liver disease and respiratory failure is warranted. Hepatorenal syndrome is postulated to arise as a result of insufficient renal blood flow and altered circulating humoral factors both of which cause decreased glomerular perfusion [2]. It is the therapeutic maneuvers in respiratory failure that are often implicated in developing renal failure including diuresis, fluid restriction and positive pressure ventilation [3]. Once again renal hypoperfusion is implicated.

Pathophysiology

To understand the pathophysiology responsible for renal insufficiency in the context of hypoperfusion requires a review of those mechanisms that interact to produce ultrafiltration of urine. Figure 1 diagrammatically depicts a partial nephron unit demonstrating the blood supply to the glomerular capillary bed. The afferent renal arteriole brings blood into the glomerulus and the efferent arteriole, in turn, removes it. The ultrafiltration of plasma to produce urine is most significantly dependent on the capillary hydrostatic pressure (CHP) present in the glomerular capillary. This CHP is dependent on the pressure-flow relationship of renal perfusion. Optimal conditions would involve sufficient cardiac output, aorto-renal flow, afferent renal arteriolar dilatation and efferent renal arteriolar constriction.

The afferent arteriole will constrict as a consequence of the action of renin, alpha-1 vasoconstrictor agents and vasoconstrictor prostaglandins (thromboxane) and dilate as a result of beta-2 and dopaminergic stimulation and vasodila-

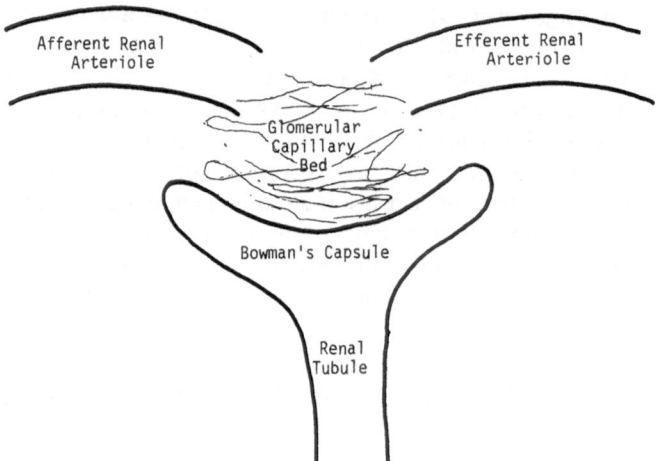

Fig. 1. The circulatory components of the glomerulus

tor prostaglandins (prostacyclin, prostaglandin E1 and E2). Constriction of the efferent arteriole appears to be principally controlled by levels of angiotensin II. Given the importance of the renin-angiotensin system in regulating CHP and ultrafiltration Fig. 2 is displayed to outline the components of this system and to assist in understanding the implications of both renal hypoperfusion and liver failure. Angiotensin I, although of no direct hemodynamic consequence, is a necessary intermediary for angiotensin II production as well as inhibiting further release of renin. Thus, with hepatic insufficiency, the failure to produce renin substrate (angiotensinogen) results in both excess renin production and lack of angiotensin II, both of which adversely affect CHP. It is also appropriate at this point to note a potential detrimental role for angiotensin converting enzyme (ACE) inhibitors, such as captopril, in escalating renal insufficiency. These drugs, commonly used for systemic afterload reduction and control of hyperten-

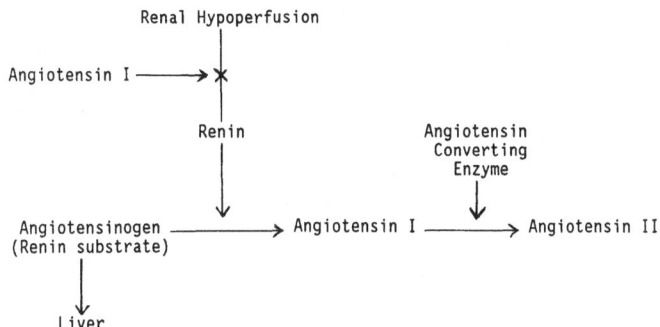

Fig. 2. Renin-angiotensin mechanism

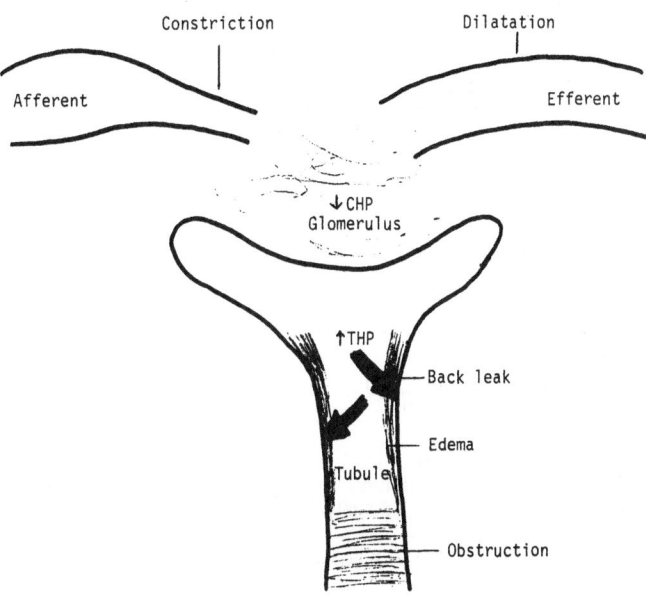

Fig. 3. Factors influencing glomerular ultrafiltration

sion, may also decrease CHP and ultrafiltration by decreasing angiotensin II production.

In addition to the above vascular mechanisms involved in hemodynamically mediated renal insufficiency, tubular obstruction may also result in impaired production of urine. Glomerular and tubular ischemia results in the potential for large quantities of casts and other cellular debris, that will obstruct the tubules and collecting ducts. Additionally tubular ischemia may alter epithelial permeability allowing for the "back-leak" of filtrate into peritubular spaces compressing the tubules. The effect of both the intraluminal obstruction and peritubular edema could be to raise tubular hydrostatic pressure and, thus compromise the filtration hydrostatic pressure (P_F) gradient (CHP – THP) producing loss of glomerular function. Figure 3 summarizes the above described mechanisms that likely co-exist in producing renal compromise.

The evaluation of renal function is critical in identifying the existence, severity and possible pathophysiologic mechanisms involved in renal dysfunction. Table 1 outlines the commonly used laboratory studies and where appropriate normal values as well as those frequently encountered in pre-renal states and acute tubular necrosis (ATN).

Perhaps the most sensitive indicator of tubular function to differentiate the pre-renal versus tubular necrotic status of the kidney is the fractional excretion of sodium (Fe_{Na}). Equations 1, 2 and 3 below outline the calculations for creatinine clearance (CrCl), fractional excretion of any substance (x) (Fe_x) and the Fe_{Na}.

$$CrCl = \frac{Urine\ Cr \cdot Urine\ Volume}{Plasma\ Cr} \tag{1}$$

$$Fe_x = \frac{Clearance\ of\ X}{CrCl} \cdot 100 \tag{2}$$

$$Fe_{Na} = \frac{Urine\ Na \cdot Plasma\ Cr}{Urine\ Cr \cdot Plasma\ Na} \cdot 100 \tag{3}$$

Table 1. Laboratory values

	Normal[a]	Pre-renal	ATN
Urine Na [mEq/L]	20–40	<20	>40
Blood urea nitrogen [mg/dl]	5–25	↑	↑
Serum creatinine [mg/dl]	0.5–1.4	↑	↑
BUN/Cr ratio	5–15	>15	<10
Urine/serum osmolality	1.5–4	>1.8	<1.1
Creatinine clearance [ml/min]	90–120	↓	↓
Fractional excretion of Na$^+$ [%]	1.2	<1	>2

[a] Note variations due to laboratory and procedural differences. Check own lab for normal values.

In addition to these studies examination of urine sediment, urine hemoglobin and myoglobin, creatine phosphokinase, evidence of disseminated intravascular coagulation, X-ray evaluations and scans, cystoscopy and renal biopsies may be indicated given the clinical scenario surrounding the kidney failure. Of considerable import is a critical and sensitive evaluation of hemodynamics both to assist in evaluating etiology as well as guiding therapy.

Therapy

Therapy to prevent, modify or attenuate acute renal insufficiency involves removal of any offending factors including sepsis, hemoglobin, myoglobin, contrast material and nephrotoxic pharmacology. Beyond this, optimizing renal perfusion and maintaining tubular urine flow form the basis for therapy. Table 2 lists the principle nephrotoxins that may be related or contributory to renal compromise and should be avoided or at least cautiously monitored and justified.

Renal perfusion is best assured by adhering to the principle set forth by Starling at the turn of the century utilizing the monitoring techniques that best define existing hemodynamic pathophysiology. Although a complete discussion of such an approach is beyond the scope of this presentation, Fig. 4a, b outlines a concept for forming a clinical impression of the pathophysiology surrounding the cardio-vascular dysfunction (4a) and applying this to a selection of appropriate therapy (4b) [4].

The rapid assessment of this treatment will serve both to confirm or deny the initial diagnosis, as well as to guide further intervention. In addition to maintaining an adequate cardiac output, steps should be taken to avoid afferent arteriolar constriction and efferent dilatation, as well as the maintenance of adequate renal perfusion pressure. The latter may require supernormal values for cardiac output or in rare circumstances vasopressor therapy. Recognition of the need for higher levels of mean arterial pressure may be necessary in patients with long histories of systemic hypertension, particularly if renal arterial disease is prevalent. Avoidance or reversal of afferent arteriolar constriction can often be facilitated by the use of dopamine at dopaminergic stimulating doses (2-3 mcg/kg/min) [5, 6].

Table 2. Current nephrotoxins

Pencillinase-R antibiotics	Mercurials
Aminoglycosides	Acetominophen
Amphotericin	Ibuprofen
Cyclosporin	Indomethacin
Salicylates	Phenylbutazone
Polymixin	Allopurinol
Radiocontrast dyes	
Myoglobin	
Hemoglobin	
Gold	

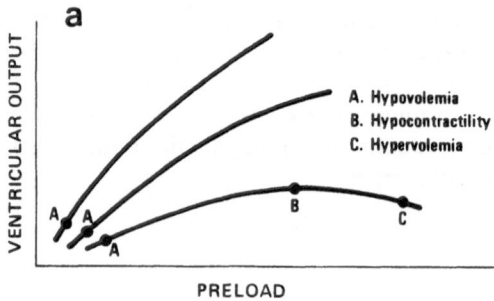

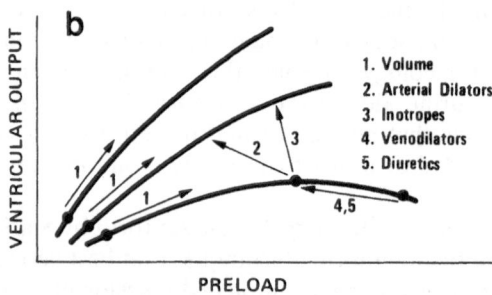

Fig. 4. a The Starling mechanism used to estimate the pathophysiology of hemodynamic insufficiency. b Therapy for hemodynamic insufficiency based on estimations of pathophysiologic mechanisms

Awareness of the increasing α-1 vasoconstricting affects of higher doses of dopamine [7] may warrant consideration of the choice of alternative inotropic support while maintaining the afferent dilator response to lower dopamine dosage. Several agents used in critically ill patients are known to block dopaminergic receptors, thus potentially counteracting the benefits of "low-dose" dopamine. These include the butyrophenones, phenothiazine and metoclopramide. As mentioned earlier avoidance of ACE inhibitors is wise to minimize any potential harm from decreased angiotensin II and accompanying efferent renal arteriolar dilatation.

The provision of adequate tubular urine flow with the production of urine in at least 0.5 ml/kg/hr quantities is often assured by maneuvers to optimize perfusion. Yet, oliguria may persist and the need to improve urine flow in order to maintain proper fluid and electrolyte balance, as well as removal of toxins and to minimize tubular obstruction may require further therapy. Commonly this results in the administration of a potent diuretic such as furosemide. In so doing the clinician has the responsibility to insure adequacy of preload and ventricular output prior to the administration of an agent having both venodilatory and diuretic effects. Such a response to furosemide, if not recognized, commonly results in renal hypoperfusion and deterioration of renal function. Controversy exists as to the direct renal effects of furosemide beyond those of loop diuresis. Evidence points to an increase in vasodilator metabolites of arachidonic acid (PGE2, prostacyclin) with resultant increase in afferent arteriolar blood flow [8]. Although intriguing as to its therapeutic potential hesitancy to increase the use of such an agent should exist based on discussion above. When indicated, some reports have favored a continuous infusion of 2–10 mg/hr of furosemide rather than bolus therapy to produce a more constant diuretic response [9]. Alternative agents such as bumetidine, ethacrynic acid or the synergistic addition of thiazides should be considered, if responses to higher furosemide doses (80–120 mg) are inadequate.

Beyond these therapies there exists a number of furhter options whose efficacy remains unproven and some purely experimental. The controversy regarding the selection of crystalloid or colloid solutions for fluid resuscitation was based on the supposition that lung water accumulation or pulmonary edema might be influenced by selection of one or the other of these groups of solutions [10, 11]. Many, including the author, now believe that lung water (LW) accumulates without regard for such a selection nor the level of capillary oncotic pressure (COP) [12]. This is most apparent in those disease states accompanied by altered capillary permeability. Just as many used the Starling equilibrium shown in Fig. 5 to theorize the importance of maintaining COP to minimize LW, similar consideration arose indicating that a decrease in COP in the glomerular capillaries might favor ultrafiltration.

Examination of this concept both in man [13] and animals [14] has suggested a benefit for crystalloid solutions in improving glomerular filtration and maintaining renal function following hypoperfusion episodes. Figure 6 and equation 4

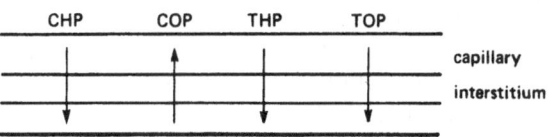

Fig. 5. The Starling equilibrium of pressures controlling the transvascular movement of liquid

CHP = Capillary hydrostatic pressure
COP = Capillary oncotic pressure
THP = Tissue hydrostatic pressure
TOP = Tissue oncotic pressure

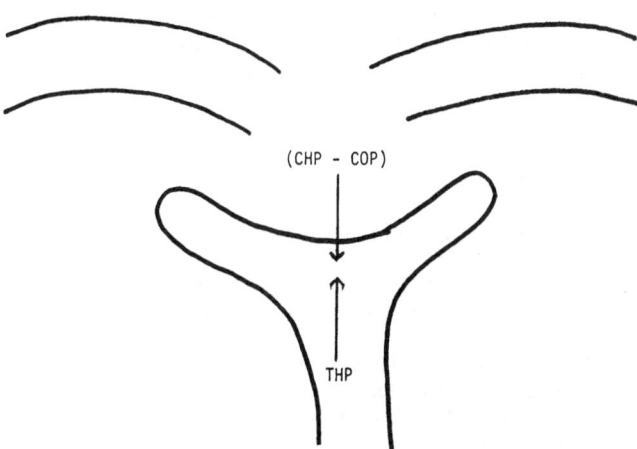

Fig. 6. Determinants of ultrafiltration pressure

summarize the interaction of hydrostatic and oncotic forces potentiating glomerular ultrafiltration.

$$P_F = (CHP - COP) - THP \qquad (4)$$

P_F = Ultrafiltration pressure; CHP = Capillary hydrostatic pressure; COP = Capillary oncotic pressure; THP = Tubular hydrostatic pressure.

A further area of interest and speculation surrounds the existence of a "no-reflow" phenomenon [15] in which ischemia of tissues results in a failure of reperfusion after successful central hemodynamic resuscitation. Originally this concept postulated the development of endothelial swelling due to increased intracellular sodium and water secondary to ischemia. This swelling might then result in microvascular obstruction with persistent ischemia and necrosis. Attempts have been made utilizing this theory to alleviate the swelling and obstruction with hyperosmotherapy using hypertonic mannitol. Studies of the brain [16], myocardium [17] and kidney [18] have demonstrated modest benefit using such an approach. More recently investigators have introduced calcium induced vasospasm as an explanation for this microcirculatory failure [19]. They suggest that calcium channels open as a result of ischemic induced depolarization with increased intracellular ionized calcium facilitating muscular contraction. If such existed in the terminal arterioles, vasospasm could dominate. Studies demonstrating increased tolerance to ischemia in the brain [20] and kidney [21] using calcium channel blockers has led to enthusiasm for this therapy and investigation continues. Other areas of research continue to examine such approaches as prostaglandin E1 [22] as an afferent arteriolar dilator and hypertonic saline as a more efficient plasma expander.

The emphasis in this discussion is based on the frequency of hemodynamic compromise leading to renal insufficiency. As discussed earlier obstructive phenomena, nephrotoxic agents, hormonal imbalance and associated diseases and therapy must also be considered in attempting to prevent or reverse renal dysfunction. The kidney as an "innocent bystander" often becomes insufficient when the clinician's concern for the treatment of a primary process neglects to recognize the implications to renal function of both the disease and chosen therapy. A multi-organ focus must be maintained lest success in treatment of the primary disease be accompanied by fatal secondary complications.

References

1. Myers BD, Moran SM (1986) Hemodynamically mediated acute renal failure. N Engl J Med 314:97–105
2. Papper S (1980) Hepatorenal syndrome. Contr Nephrol 23:55–74
3. Rosenthal MH (1986) Hemodynamic effects of pulmonary insufficiency. Int Anesth Clin 24:145–148
4. Rosenthal MH, Pearls RG (1987) Shock. In: Donegan (ed) Anesthesia in emergency surgery. Churchill-Livingstone
5. Veda S, Yano S, Sakanashi M (1982) In-vitro evidence for dopaminergic receptors in human renal artery. J Cardiovasc Pharm 4:76–81

6. Barnado DE, Baldus WP, Maher FT (1970) Effects of dopamine on renal function in patients with cirrhosis. Gastroenterology 58:524–531
7. Beregovich J, Blanchi C, Rubler S, et al (1974) Dose-related hemodynamic and renal effects of dopamine in congestive heart failure. Am Heart J 87:550–556
8. Gerber JG (1983) Role of prostaglandins in the hemodynamic and tubular effects of furosemide. Fed Proc 42:1707–1710
9. Krasna MJ, Scott GE, Scholz PM, et al (1986) Postoperative enhancement of urinary output in patients with acute renal failure using continuous furosemide therapy. Chest 89:294–295
10. Rackow EC, Fein IA, Leppo J (1977) Colloid osmotic pressure as a prognostic indicator of pulmonary edema and mortality in the critically ill. Chest 72:709–713
11. Holcroft JW, Trunkey DD (1974) Extravascular lung water following hemorrhagic shock in the baboon. Ann Surg 180:408–417
12. Pearl RG, Halperin BD, Mihm FG, Rosenthal MH (1988) Pulmonary effects of crystalloid and colloid resuscitation from hemorrhagic shock in the presence of oleic acid induced pulmonary capillary injury in the dog. Anesthesiology 68:12–20
13. Carey LC, Lowery BD, Cloutier CT (1971) Hemorrhagic shock. Curr Probl Surg Jan
14. Siegal DC, Cochin A, Geocaris T, Moss GS (1973) Effects of saline and colloid resuscitation on renal function. Ann Surg 177:51–57
15. Cournand A, Riley RL, Bradley ES, et al (1943) Studies of the circulation in clinical shock. Surgery 13:964–972
16. Ames A, Wright RL, Kowada M, et al (1968) Cerebral ischemia II, the no-reflow phenomenon. Am J Pathol 52:437–444
17. Powell WJ, DiBona DR, Flores J, et al (1976) Effects of hyperosmotic mannitol in reducing ischemic cell swelling and minimizing myocardial necrosis. Circulation 53:145–149
18. Flores J, DiBona DR, Bleck CH, et al (1972) The role of cell swelling in ischemic renal damage and the protective effect of hypertonic solute. J Clin Invest 51:118–126
19. Bolton TB (1984) Mechanism of action of transmitters and other substances on smooth muscle. Physiol Rev 59:606–628
20. Steen PA, Gisvold SE, Milde JH, et al (1985) Nimodipine improves outcome when given after complete cerebral ischemia in primates. Anesthesiology 62:406–414
21. Wooley JL, Barker GR, Jacobsen WK, et al (1988) Effect of the calcium entry blocker verapamil on renal ischemia. Crit Care Med 16:48–51
22. Johnston HH, Herzog JP, Lauler DP (1967) Effect of prostaglandin E1 on renal hemodynamics, sodium and water excretion. Am J Physiol 213:939–951

Acute Hypophosphatemia

G. Conti, M. Rocco, and A. Gasparetto

Introduction

Hypophosphatemia (i.e. a plasmatic inorganic phosphate level lower than 2.5 mg/dl) is commonly detected in patients hospitalized for various causes: In particular, hypophosphatemia has been frequently reported in patients suffering from pulmonary disease of infectious origin [1–3]. However, the isolated observation of a mild hypophosphatemia has often a limited clinical meaning. On the contrary, severe hypophosphatemia (i.e. Pi below 1.5 mg/dl) can represent a real emergency.

In normal conditions, 85% total body amount is fixed to the bone tissues, and only 15% is found in the soft tissues or in the plasma. Moreover, the large majority of this amount is intracellular (where phosphorus is the main anion) and only 1‰ of the total body amount of phosphorus is present in the plasma. This is the amount that we can investigate, performing a dosage of plasmatic inorganic phosphorus (Pi) (Normal values: 2.5–4.5 mg/dl). Phosphorus is generally absorbed from milk, milk products and meat at jejunum level. This process is normally increased by vitamin D metabolites and decreased by an excessive intake of calcium. The excretion is through the kidneys.

Major Causes of Hypophosphatemia

They are (Table 1):

1. Insufficient phosphorus intake often observed during long term malnutrition or in an experimental setting of weight loss and phosphorus depletion.
2. Insufficient digestive absorption as can be observed in patients suffering from long therm diarrhea or vomiting. A similar mechanism can be supposed in long-term treatment with high dose magnesium and aluminium hydroxide as antiacid therapy [4, 5].
3. Urinary depletion: this is caused by the loss of the mechanism of tubular reabsorption, as observed during hyperparathyroidism, metal intoxication, osmotic diuresis or other conditions of polyuria.
4. Intracellular transfer: this is generally observed during two clinical situations, after administration of I.V. glucose and insulin and during respiratory

Table 1. Major causes of hypophosphatemia

(A) Reduced intake:
- Malnutrition
- Anorexia nervosa

(B) Reduced intestinal absorption:
- Intestinal dysfunction
- Extense intestinal resection
- Cancer (?)
- Mg, Al hydroxide as antiacid therapy

(C) Increased urinary loss:
- Hyperparathyroidism
- Osmotic diuresis
- Toxic tubulopathies

(D) Intracellular transfer:
- Glucose + insulin
- Respiratory alkalosis
- Hypercaloric nutrition

(E) Chronic alcoholism

(F) Extensive burns

---

alkalosis. The insulin administration produces an intracellular transfert of both glucose and Pi; on the other hand respiratory alkalosis increases the activity of the phosphofructokinase enzyme. This mechanism, well known for many years [6], is probably involved in the hypophosphatemia often observed during neurologic hyperventilation, acetylsalicylic acid overdose or acute pneumopathies.

5. Chronic alcoholism represents a clinically relevant cause of hypophosphatemia; however, apart from the malnutritional state that is often observed in this situation, little is known on the exact pathogenetic mechanisms.

6. Extensive burns: there also, the exact mechanism is not clear [7].

7. Hyperalimentation after malnutrition. The administration of large amounts of carbohydrates and amino acids after long-term malnutrition seems to produce a violent increase of the cellular anabolic processes, causing an important of Pi for energetic purposes [8].

Consequences of Hypophosphatemia

Phosphate has a central role in many energetic cellular processes, even as a direct energetic carrier (ATP) or as enzymatic cofactor in fundamental metabolic functions. Moreover, its presence and function are ubiquitous. This explains that virtually all organ functions are involved during severe hypophosphatemia. We shall briefly analyze only the effects frequently observed in the critically ill patients.

Effects on Red Blood Cells

Phosphate plays a central role in the red cell physiology. Moreover, the red blood cell concentration of phosphorus is controlled by a simple mechanism of passive diffusion with the plasma, so that any reduction in plasma Pi level induces a rapid reduction of the erythrocytes Pi concentration. This determines an important perturbation of the glycolytic mechanisms, mainly by the reduction of glucose-6-phosphate, fructose-6-phosphate, ATP and 2-3 diphosphoglicerate (DPG). The latter phenomenon is particularly dangerous because 2-3 DPG reduction decreases P50, and thus oxygen delivery to the tissues [9, 10].

Effects on Muscles

Skeletal muscle dysfunction during hypophosphatemia has been reported already 20 years ago by Lotz et al. [11] who described important general weakness in humans, after experimental phosphate depletion. Apart from the myopathy caused by chronic phosphate depletion [12], acute severe hypophosphatemia can produce a clinical syndrome characterized by hypotony and generalized muscular weakness, sometimes so important that it mimicks Guillain-Barré syndrome [13]. The proposed pathogenetic mechanisms are based upon an important reduction of the ATP containt, with consequent alterations in mitochondria energetic transport chain and complete alterations of the intracellular energetic and ionic homeostatic mechanisms.

Cardiovascular Effects

The cardiovascular effects of severe hypophosphatemia have been documented both in clinical [14] and in experimental conditions [15, 16]: O'Connor et al. [14] analyzed the cardiac performance in 7 critically ill hypophosphoremic patients and by measuring cardiac output and cardiac stroke work were able to detect an important reduction in myocardial contractility. Phosphorus level was then corrected to normal within 8 hours by a continuous infusion and the hemodynamic pattern at the same loading conditions showed an increase in left ventricular stroke work.

An experimental study, by Kreusser et al. [16] offers some explanations about the pathophysiology of these cardiovascular alterations. In phosphate diet-free induced hypophosphatemia these authors observed a severe reduction in ATP, CPK and inorganic phosphate in the myocardium associate with a 25% loss of contractile strength and a reduced response to epinephrine. In other therms, it is highly probable that severe hypophosphatemia impairs the myocardial contractility also by damaging the mitochondrial energetic transport chain. Although hypophosphatemic cardiomiopathy is not an accepted clinical entity, these results underline the importance of maintaining normal plasma phosphorus level in patients with reduced cardiac reserve.

Respiratory Effects

Impressive clinical and experimental data suggest that hypophosphatemia impairs the contractile properties of the respiratory muscles producing or aggravating acute respiratory failure (ARF) or impairing the weaning from mechanical ventilation. In 1977 Newmann et al. [17] reported two clinical observations of ARF during hypophosphatemia, promptly reversed by phosphate administration. Often the weaning from mechanical ventilation has been obtained only after correction of hypophosphatemia [18, 19]. The proposed mechanisms are multiple, but there is strong evidence that the reduction in muscular strength and diaphragmatic contractility may play a central role in ARF and ventilator dependance during hypophosphatemia.

Aubier et al. [20] recently observed an important diaphragmatic impairment in a group of ARF patients with severe hypophosphatemia by measuring the transdiaphragmatic pressure generated during bilateral supramaximal electrical simulation of the phrenic nerves. The correction of the hypophosphatemia with a 4 hours IV administration of 10 mmol of phosphorus resulted in a dramatic improvement in the transdiaphragmatic pressure after phrenic nerve stimulation (from 9.75 ± 3.8 to 17.25 ± 6.5 cmH$_2$O).

The role of hypophosphatemia in respiratory muscle weakness has been confirmed also by Gravelyn et al. [21] who compared the maximal inspiratory and expiratory pressure (MIP, MEP) in a group of hypophosphatemic medical and surgical patients, compared with a similar population of normophosphatemic patients. The majority of the hypophosphatemic patients (16 of 23), but none of the normophosphatemic patients showed signs of muscular weakness, defined by a MIP < 40 cmH$_2$O and a MEP < 70 cmH$_2$O. Moreover, phosphate repletion led to a increases in MIP from 37 ± 26 to 48 ± 24 cmH$_2$O and MEP from 60 ± 20 to 68 ± 19 cmH$_2$O. This study documents the incidence of respiratory muscle weakness not only in mechanically ventilated ICU patients but also in patients from medical or surgical departments, underlining the importance of hypophosphatemia.

Although the incidence of "primary" hypophosphatemia-induced ARF is probably low, hypophosphatemia can be a cofactor ARF. It is therefore important to maintain normal plasma phosphate levels in patients requiring mechanical ventilation.

Treatment of Hypophosphatemia

In patients who are not critically ill, a symptom-free hypophosphatemia can be easily corrected by diet (milk or derivates) or by discontinuation of substances able to reduce the intestinal absorption of phosphate. By contrast, severe hypophosphatemia should always be corrected by intravenous administration of phosphate salts. The most used salts are mono or bi-K-phosphate administered as an IV infusion at a rate ranging from 0.5 mMol/kg during 4 hours [22] to 0.3 mmol/kg during 12 hours [23]. The plasma levels of phosphate, calcium and potassium must be routinely controlled during the infusion to avoid the risk of cardiac arrhythmia. Particular attention must be paid to diabetic patients suffering from ketoacidosis, as the large majority of the accidents observed during phosphate administration has been observed in this situation [24, 25]. Nearly all patients with diabetic ketoacidosis develop hypophosphatemia during treatment with insulin and large amounts of fluid, but only a small percentage have a real phosphate depletion, preexisting to the treatment, and only this situation requires phosphate salts administration [26]. Indeed the systematic administration of phosphate salts has no beneficial effect on the duration of acidosis, glucose utilization or erythrocyte metabolic alterations. Finally, it is important to remind that phosphate salts should not be administered in patients suffering from hypercalcemia (risk of metastatic precipitations of calcium) and renal failure.

Acknowledgements: We are indebted to Miss Nadine Bedfert for her kind collaboration in the manuscript preparation.

References

1. Betro MG, Pain RW (1972) Hypophosphatemia in a hospital population. Br Med J 1:273-276
2. Larson I, Rebel K, Sorbo B (1983) Severe hypophosphatemia: a hospital survey. Acta Med Scand 24:221-223
3. Fisher J, Magid N, Kallmann C, et al (1983) Respiratory illness and hypophosphatemia. Chest 83:504-508
4. Lotz M, Zisman E, Bartter F (1968) Evidence for a phosphorus depletion syndrome in man. N Engl J Med 278:408-414
5. Dent CE, Winter CS (1974) Ostheomalacia due to phosphate depletion form excessive aluminium hydroxide ingestion. Br Med J 1:551-554
6. Mostellar ME, Tuttle EP (1964) Effects of alkalosis on plasma concentration and urinary excretion of inorganic phosphate in man. J Clin Invest 43:138-149
7. Nordstrom H, Lennquist S (1977) Hypophosphatemia in severe burns. Acta Chir Scand 143:395-399
8. Hill GL, Guinn EJ, Dudrick SJ (1976) Phosphorus distribution in hyperalimentation induced hypophosphatemia. J Surg Res 20:727-731
9. Lichtman M, Miller DR, Cohen J, Waterhouse C (1971) Reduced red cell glycolysis, 2-3 DPG and ATP concentration and increased hemoglobin-oxygen affinity caused by hypophosphatemia. Ann Intern Med 74:562-568
10. Travis SF, Sugerman HJ, Ruberg RL, et al (1974) Alterations of red cells glycolitic intermediates and oxygen transport as a consequence of hypophosphatemia in patients receiving intravenous hyperalimentation. N Engl J Med 285:723-728
11. Lotz M (1964) Osteomalacia and debility resulting from phosphorus depletion. Trans Assoc Am Phys 77
12. Knochel JP (1982) Neuromuscular manifestations of electrolyte disorders. Am J Med 72:521-535
13. Weintraub MI (1976) Hypophosphatemia mimicking acute Guillain-Barré-Strohl syndrome. A complication of parenteral hyperalimentation. JAMA 235:1040-1041
14. O'Connor LR, Wheller WS, Bethune JE (1977) Effects of hypophosphatemia on myocardial performance in man. N Engl J Med 287:901-903
15. Fuller TJ, Nichols WW, Brenner BJ, Peterson JC (1978) Reversible depression in myocardial performance in dogs with experimental phosphorus deficiency. J Clin Invest 62:1194-2000
16. Kreusser W, Vetter HO, Mittman U, et al (1982) Hemodynamics and myocardial metabolism of phosphorus depleted dogs: effects of catecholamines and angiotensin II. Eur J Clin Invest 12:219-228

17. Newmann JH, Neff TA, Ziporin P (1977) Acute respiratory failure associated with hypophosphatemia. N Engl J Med 296:1101–1103
18. Brown EL, Jenkins B (1980) A case of respiratory failure complicated by acute hypophosphatemia. Anaesthesia 35:42–45
19. Augusti A, Torres A, Estopa R, Agusti-Vidal A (1984) Hypophosphatemia as a cause of failed weaning: the importance of metabolic factors. Crit Care Med 12:142–143
20. Aubier M, Murciano D, Lecocguic Y, et al (1985) Effects of hypophosphatemia on diaphragmatic contractility in patients with acute respiratory failure. N Engl J Med 313:420–424
21. Gravelyn TR, Brophy N, Siegert C, Peters-Goldon M (1988) Hypophosphatemia associated respiratory muscle weakness in a central inpatients population. Am J Med 84:870–876
22. Kingston M, Al'Sibai MB (1985) Treatment of severe hypophosphatemia. Crit Care Med 13:16–18
23. Vannatta JB, Wang R, Papper S (1981) Efficacy of intravenous phosphorus in the severely hypophosphatemia patient. Arch Inter Med 9:772–774
24. Chernow B, Rainey TG, Georges LP, O'Brian JP (1981) Iatrogenic hyperphosphatemia: a metabolic consideration in critical care medicine. Crit Care Med 9:772–774
25. Winter RJ, Harris CJ, Philips LS, Creen OC (1979) Diabetic ketoacidosis induction of hypocalcemia and hypomagnesemia by phosphate therapy. Am J Med 67:897–900
26. Knochel JP (1985) Deranged phosphorus metabolism. In: Sedin DW, Giebish G (eds) The kidney: physiology and pathophysiology. Raven Press, New York, pp 1397–1416

Atrial Natriuretic Factor: Clinical Implications*

A. Mebazaa and D. Payen

Introduction

The discovery of Atrial Natriuretic Factor (ANF) was one of the important events in physiology during the past 10 years. Its diuretic and vasorelaxant actions help explain the blood volume balances of the organism. The discovery of ANF and its functions has led to a totally new concept: the cardiac muscle has an endocrine function.

History

In 1981, a young American investigator, de Bold, discovered ANF by an elegant investigation [1]. The results of his experiments facilitated the understanding and the linking of the results of two series of studies done in parallel; the histological analyses which indentified granules in the cardiac atrial walls, and the physiological analyses which focused on an unidentified "third factor".

Histological Studies

In 1956, Hish noted the presence of granules in the atrial cardiocyte of mammals [2]. At that time, Cantin et al. showed that these cells secrete peptides but not catecholamines or renin. Using electron microscopy in 1976, the French group directed by Hatt established the first connection between the number of cardiocyte granules and the sodium intake: water and sodium restrictions for five days was related to an increase in the number of granules in atrial myocytes [3].

Physiological Studies

Two famous physiologists, Gauer and Henry, demonstrated the relation between cardio-pulmonary blood volume during a controlled-temperature immersion and a rapid and intense natriuresis. Their result could not be fully explained by

---

* This work was supported in part by Institutional Grant Program of University Paris VII and UER Lariboisière-Saint-Louis.

glomerular filtration rates and aldosterone modifications. They hypothetized the existence of a "third factor", probably hormonal, to explain their results [4].

Experiment of de Bold

Extracts of rat atrium intravenously injected into anesthetized rats caused an intense and short-term diuresis and natriuresis, whereas the same injection with ventricular extracts did not [1]. The linkage between atrial granules and natriuresis was demonstrated, thus identifying a "third factor". A new hormone was born which was named Atrial Natriuretic Factor, and the heart became an "endocrine gland".

Following this discovery, several authors have suggested that the heart synthesizes and releases other hormones, in particular, components of the renin-angiotensin system (RAS), since angiotensinogen, renin, and converting enzymes are present in myocardial cells [5].

The Atrial Natriuretic Factor

Current international nomenclature recommends the use of one of the following names: Atrial Natriuretic Factor (Ser99-Tyr126) or ANF (99-126). This active peptide has aprecursor: the pre-proANF. In humans, the pre-proANF contains 151 amino-acids (aa), and is the product of the expression of only one gene, localized on the short arm of chromosome 1. The pre-proANF becomes the propeptide ANF (1-126) containing 126 aa which constitutes the form stored in atrial granules. In the presence of a release stimulus, such as atrial distension, the propeptide is hydrolysed before secretion, giving an active, circulating peptide of 28 aa: the ANF (Ser99-Tyr126).

The biological activity of ANF (99-126) varies according to the structure. Thus, the rupture of the disulfure bridge Cys105-Cys121 linking the two NH_2 and COOH branches induces a loss of ANF activity (99-126). This bridge is therefore necessary for biological activity.

The half-life of ANF is very short; about 3 to 4 minutes in humans [6]. Recent studies have proven the existence of two types of ANF receptors:

1. the heavy molecular weight receptors, specific of ANF (99-126) and directly coupled to the guanylate cyclase, which explains a large part of ANF's activity mediated by the cyclic GMP (cGMP);
2. the light molecular weight receptors, non-selectives, called clearance sites, to which the ANF but also fragments of the ANF, are attached (99-126).

The clearance sites appear to be coupled to endopeptidases. The whole system could explain the very short half-life of ANF.

Using electron microscopy, ANF was first detected in granules containing about 600 per atrial cell. Granules were localized at both poles of the nucleus in the Golgi apparatus (Fig. 1). The absence of granules in the ventricle of normal hearts indicated that ANF was only synthesized by atria. In reality, it was re-

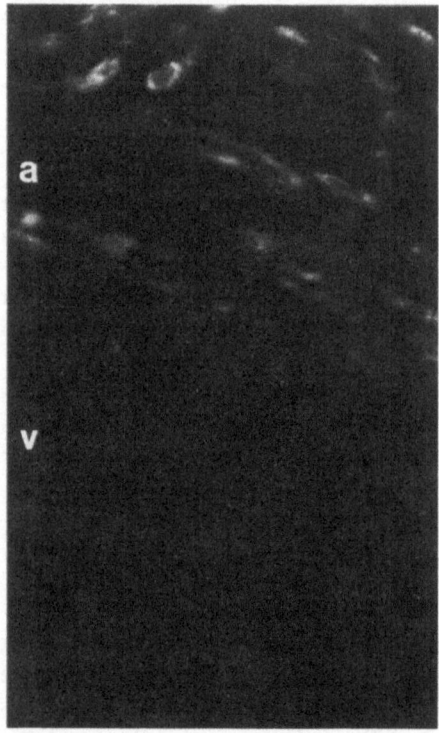

Fig. 1. Indirect immunofluorescence labeling of immunoreactive atrial natriuretic factor (ANF) in normal adult rat heart. Note the differences in the staining of the left atrium (a) as compared with the left ventricle (v). (In collaboration with JL Samuel, U127 Inserm, Paris, France)

cently shown that normal left ventricles of adult rats contains 1.5% of the ANF synthesized by atria. It was demonstrated in rats, that both fetal and hypertrophied ventricles largely contain more ANF after volume or pressure overload than normal adult rats. Our data suggest both the presence of ANF and RAS in coronary walls of hypertrophied ventricles. Their release might regulate ventricular afterload during hypertrophy.

In the adult human, ANF is for the most part missing from normal ventricles. However, is fetus was well as during certain cardiac pathologies of adults, ventricular synthesis of ANF could be high. Thus, in patients with severe cardiomyopathies, during the precardiac transplantation phase, the concentration of ventricular ANF rises. Mercadier et al. suggested, as with isomyosin transcription, a reexpression of the ANF fetal gene during ventricular hypertrophy [7]. Several authors have suggested that the synthesis and the secretion of ANF by the hypertrophied ventricle could participate in the circulating "pool" of ANF. Apart from the heart, ANF has also been found in the lungs, the hypophysis and the hypothalamus. The hormone found in the hypothalamus is called Brain ANF or B-ANF.

ANF Effects on Kidney and Peripheral Vessels

In normal subjects, ANF is released essentially during volume loading and thus tends to maintain a volemic balance. This effect resulted from two different effects:

1. a reduction of plasma volume, through its diuretic and natriuretic properties and
2. a vasodilatation.

Effects on the Kidney

Just as its name indicates, ANF is a natriuretic and a diuretic hormone which increases glomerular filtration, renal vascular resistances and filtration fractions. Thus, it has been suggested that ANF reacts through a double mechanism: a pre-glomerular vasorelaxation and a post-glomerular vasoconstriction, which explains the increase in glomerular filtration, despite a slightly-modified or lowered renal blood flow.

In 10 normal subjects, Weidman et al. have shown that the perfusion of ANF increased glomerular filtration (+15%) without any change in renal bood flow, allowing for a large increase in the glomerular filtration fraction (+37%). Natriuresis, chloride excretion and free water clearance were also increased [6].

Using autoradiographic methods, renal receptors for ANF and active sites were localized in glomerular capillaries, and in the vasa recta of the medulla and the papilla. Actions of ANF on the kidney are mediated by guanylate cyclase coupled to the ANF receptor. An injection of ANF increases by 2-fold the cGMP found in the collecting tubules and by 50-fold in the glomeruli, without any change in the proximal tubules. Moreover, under the same circumstances, ANF inhibits adenylate cyclase in the same sites.

Vascular Effects

A direct vasodilatator effect of ANF has been observed on coronary, renal, internal mammary arteries and on the aorta, and is associated with a rise in cGMP. Large vessels seem to be more sensitive to ANF than small ones. When arteries are preconstricted *in vitro* by norepinephrine or angiotensin II, ANF provokes a dose-dependent relaxation of the smooth muscles, similar to that observed with nitred vasodilatators. Nevertheless, vasoconstriction produced by hyperpolarization with KCl remains unchanged by ANF. Venous effects seem to be much less i.e., most veins appear insensitive. A venoconstriction of an isolated human saphenous vein induced by norepinephrine is not relaxed by ANF. The induced arterial hypotension observed after ANF injection was attributed to a cardiac output decrease essentially mediated by a direct negative inotropic effect of ANF. Nevertheless, this result was not observed in healthy human subjects i.e., the injection of ANF had no negative inotropic effects. At this time, cardiac output and blood pressure decreases seem to be due to a decrease in preload secondary to an increase in venous return [8].

In the pulmonary circulation, ANF seems to play a distinct role. First, ANF receptors are present in pulmonary vessels. Very recently Springall et al. proved that the lung was capable of secreting ANF [9]. On vascular preparations of pigs *in vitro*, ANF has a relaxant effect 10 times greater on the pulmonary artery than on the renal artery. Lastly, during its transpulmonary passage, ANF is captured by the vascular endothelium. Moreover, ANF could have a physiological role during hypoxia: it has been shown that ANF rises during hypoxia, and inhibits the hypoxic pulmonary vasoconstriction. The authors therefore suggest that the right heart and especially the right atrium (RA) influence the pulmonary circulation to reduce the right ventricular afterload and consequently its stroke work.

Pharmacological Interactions

Anesthesic Drugs

Morphine was the first substance recognized to have a secreting effect on ANF in rats [10]. The mechanism appeared mediated by cardiac morphine receptors since naloxone (receptor antagonist) prevents or reduces morphine induced ANF release. This effect was not confirmed in humans using fentanyl. The injection of an IV bolus of 250 micrograms of fentanyl in patients, 12 hours after cardiac surgery, paradoxically showed a 30% decrease of pANF [11].

In rats Horky et al. [12], tested other anesthetic agents: ketamine, diethyl-ether and chloralhydrate raise pANF, while sodium pentobarbital and urethane leave it unchanged. The authors suggest that these anesthetic drugs react indirectly by the reflex increase of catecholamine concentrations.

Taking into consideration these results, the utmost of care must be used when studying pANF during anesthesia. An interval of time, at least one hour, must be allowed between the last injection of an anesthesic drug and the first blood sampling for pANF.

Alpha- and Beta-Agonists

Data about a direct effect of α- and β-adrenoreceptors agonists are controversial. In humans, vasopressors do not raise pANF, except when atrial pressures are increased suggesting that vasopressor agents have no direct effects on ANF release.

Nevertheless, α- and β-receptors could mediate ANF secretion while injection of α_1 agonist (methoxamine) increases ANF secretion. β-adrenergic receptors can also mediate the secretion of ANF. In humans, injection of dobutamine increased ANF release; however in this study heart rate increased significantly, so that it is difficult to attribute ANF release only to β-receptor stimulation [13]. Conversely, it is interesting to note that perfusion of dopamine at 2 mcg/kg/min in premature infants does not change pANF.

Calcium Agonists

Stimulation of calcium channels by a known agonist: BAY K 8644, induces an important ANF release through the increase of intracellular calcium concentrations which appears to be an important factor in ANF secretion.

Factors Controlling ANF Secretion

The Old Concept: Volume Loading

Several animal and human studies have shown that volume expansion raises pANF. Thus, Dietz was the first to prove *in vitro* in an isolated heart-lung preparation that distension of the atria increases ANF secretion [14]. The first experiments *in vivo* were performed by Lang et al. who separately administered 2 and 8 ml of a normal saline solution to two groups of anesthetized rats. The increase in right atrial pressure (RAP) induced in one minute a slight increase in pANF in the first group, and a large increase in the second group. They therefore concluded that ANF secretion is linked to a RAP increase [15]. Conversely, the sodium hypertonic surcharge *per se,* without volume loading, does not modify ANF secretions.

The circulating ANF is very probably released from both atria. In humans, most of the studies were done on the RA, easier to explore demonstrating the role of RA distension. But histologic examinations reveal the presence of ANF granules in the RA was well as in the left atria (LA). Recently left atrial secretion of ANF has been confirmed in humans. pANF increases between inferior vena cava and pulmonary artery (PA), due to the coronary sinus blood containing high concentrations of ANF (10-fold the peripheral concentrations). After PA, pANF decreases significantly in the pulmonary veins (PV), due to an ANF uptake by the lungs. Between the PV and the aorta, pANF increases in relation to a direct passage in the cavity of ANF from different parts of the left atrial wall [16].

Several studies on humans confirm the role of LA distension on ANF secretion [17]. In patients suffering from a mitral stenosis with a chronic dilatation of the LA and an elevated pANF, transcutaneous mitral valvuloplasty decreases intraluminale LA pressure (LAP II) with a rapid fall in pANF. These studies also give new information: even if atrial distension is chronic the ANF secretion can be rapidly inhibited when distension is released.

Two liters of an isotonic saline solution perfused in healthy volunteers in a supine position raised RAP and elevated ANF concentrations about 30%. This observation explains the elevated pANF observed in several pathological or physiological conditions such as: congestive heart failure, arterio-venous fistula, non-decompensated hepatic cirrhosis, chronic renal failure, the syndrome of inappropriate secretion of ADH, primary aldosteronism, and pregnancy. Treatment of these pathologies returns the pANF level to normal.

An elevation of pANF can also be observed after RAP increases at constant intravascular volumes. The redistribution of blood from the peripheral compartment towards the intra-thoracic compartment results from water immersion up to the neck, a change in position from upright to supine and an increase in Lower Body Positive Pressures (LBPP) with a G-suit [18].

The role of atrial pressure increases in ANF secretion was superbly confirmed by Schwab et al. in two patients with Jarwik 7 artificial hearts. The device was implanted between native PA and aorta, and the native atria, preserving 95% of the latter. The decrease in the artificial heart's output induced a large increase in both the RAP and the pANF [19].

Conversely, total or partial hypovolemia will decrease pANF. In rats, water restriction for more than 3 days decreases pANF as well as the messenger RNA in atrial tissue. In humans, rapid deflation of the G-suit, and moving from supine to upright positions induces a movement of blood from the central compartment towards the periphery which decreases both atrial pressure and pANF. These results are important because they confirm the presence of a complete endocrine loop control system of ANF secretion.

New Concepts: Transmural Pressure and Tachycardia

Very recently, two studies have clarified the understanding of the secreting mechanism of ANF as follows:

1. atrial distension and not intraluminal pressure *per se* is the principal stimulus for ANF secretion suggesting that "atrial volume" is not necessarily related to "intraluminal atrial pressure",
2. atrial tachycardia alone may induce ANF secretion.

Atrial Distension: Few studies among those cited earlier have shown a strong correlation between intraluminal RAP (Il RAP) and pANF. The atrial intraluminal pressure/distention relationship suggests a minor role of atrial compliance and of external pressure. Several authors have suggested that intraluminal pressure itself does not reflect atrial distension, because of parietal atrial elastic properties and the pericardium. If this is the case, then the transmural RAP (Tm RAP) would be more related to RA volume than intraluminal pressure.

In 6 open chest dogs, Mancini et al. [20] have performed the two following procedures:

1. a tamponade by instillation into the pericardium of 150 to 250 ml of gelatin fluid over a 30 minute period,
2. a rapid vascular expansion by 1 liter of Ringer's solution during 5 minutes without tamponade and with tamponade.

In the first situation, despite a significant increase in the Il RAP, pANF did not vary. In the second situation, pANF rose during the volemic expansion phase but stabilized or even decreased during tamponade in spite of a greater increase in Il RAP. Although the authors, having only measured Il RAP, suggested that tamponade raised both pericardial pressures and Il RAP, which led to a decrease in transmural atrial pressure. They then showed a dissociation between Il RAP and ANF secretion. Using the same animal model, Edwards et al. [21] confirmed this result. They monitored pericardial pressure, Il RAP and pulmonary capillary pressures and calculated Tm pressures. During the tamponade procedure, Il RAP increased, but Tm RAP and the pANF did not vary. During simultaneous stenosis of the aorta and the PA, the Tm RAP and Il RAP increased in parallel inducing an increase in pANF.

The existence of a threshold for ANF release was suggested by two studies: Zioris et al. [22] created a tamponade in 8 dogs for two hours which was followed by a rapid decompression leading to a sudden Tm pressure increase. With a Tm pressure of less than 5 mmHg, no increase in pANF was noted. The increase in ANF release was observed only when the Tm pressure was higher than 5 mmHg. Stone et al. [23] studied 15 open chest dogs: The Il RAP was 8 mmHg with a Tm RAP of 2 mmHg. A RA pericardotomy was performed simultaneously with a vascular expansion adapted to return RAP Il at 8 mmHg. Tm pressure was then increased under these conditions from 2 to 8 mmHg with a significant increase in pANF. The authors using this protocol proved that ANF secretion was absent until the Tm pressure reached 4 mmHg, suggesting the existence of a secreting threshold of ANF. The Tm RAP/pANF relationship was clearly demonstrated in humans using PEEP and/or a G-suit to modify Tm RAP. A strong exponential correlation between Tm RAP and pANF was obtained [24].

PEEP and pANF: The antidiuretic effect of mechanical ventilation with positive pressure and notably with PEEP is constant. The mechanism of this phenomenon remains open to debate. An inhibition of ANF secretion was proposed to explain the antidiuretic and antinatriuretic effects of PEEP. Several studies have shown a decrease in pANF under PEEP [25] without any relation with renal function alterations. Clinical studies where performed on patients under controlled ventilation for acute respiratory failure. A PEEP of 10 cm H_2O, which increases Il RAP and could decrease Tm RAP induced a decrease in pANF. The authors suggest therefore that the antinatriuretic effect of PEEP can be partially explained by pANF decreases.

We studied patients with normal lungs during mechanical ventilation. The application of a PEEP of 15 cm H_2O resulted in an antidiuresis and antinatriuresis, an Il RAP increase and a slight increase in pANF. G-suit inflation increased Il RAP, Tm RAP and ANF release. Nevertheless, the pANF increase during G-suit inflation did not correct the PEEP-induced antidiuresis. We therefore concluded that antidiuresis and antinatriuresis during PEEP cannot be explained by ANF release inhibition [18].

Tachycardia: In 1985, Schiffrin et al. [26] have showed an increase in pANF during atrial tachycardia and suggested that this result could explain the frequent polyuria observed after supraventricular tachycardia. Several other studies using supraventricular tachycardias (SVT) have shown a constant and significant increase in pANF. Moreover in human heart transplants, the same results were seen, suggesting a minor role of cardiac innervation. However, two questions remain to be asked:

1. is the rate heart itself independent of RAP increases the mechanism of ANF release?, and
2. is this ANF release related to the polyuria observed in supraventricular tachycardia?

During SVT, both atrial pressure and pANF increase significantly, returning to normal parameters as soon as SVT is stopped. It is difficult to separate the effect of tachycardia alone from the effects of RAP increases of ANF release. Some arguments suggest that ANF is released by increasing the contraction rate of atrial cells. Recently, two groups of patients with dilatation of mitral stenosis were separated: Group I with sinus rhythm, and Group II with atrial fibrillation [17]. After dilatation of mitral stenosis, despite a similar fall in LAP in the two groups, pANF significantly decreased except only in the Group 1. The authors suggested that atrial fibrillation raises the contraction rate of atrial cells inducing ANF secretion. This has been recently confirmed after reduction of atrial fibrillation and flutter which induced a decrease in pANF despite the absence of atrial pressure changes.

Although dissociation between the "distension" and the "tachycardia" is difficult to obtain, the exact role of atrial tachycardia was proven in humans. In 8 patients, RAP was raised after inflating a G-suit. Then, at the time the G-suit was quickly deflated, the heart rate was raised from 80 to 150 beats/minute for 5 minutes using atrial pacing. Despite a decrease in both Tm RAP and LAP, the tachycardia multiplied by 2-fold pANF in these patients [27].

The inconsistent polyuria observed during tachycardia does not seem to be linked to a pANF increase, and no correlation has been found between variations in pANF and appearance of pulyuria.

Cardiac Innervation: It is now well documented that cardiac nerves are not essential for ANF secretion. Secretion of ANF after LAP increases in conscious dogs, with a denervated heart, is similar to that obtained in intact dogs. In humans, this result was confirmed in heart transplant patients. Three days after a heart transplantion, the increase in Il RAP from 10 to 27 mmHg increases pANF by 5-fold. Compared with healthy volunteers, heart transplant patients subjected to water immersion, have a similar pANF increase.

Despite adequate hemodynamic conditions, all heart transplant patients have a higher pANF than normal, peaking at 4 days, and which remains 2 to 5 times higher than normal for several years [28]. Several hypothesis have been formulated besides the one regarding cardiac denervation:

1. the role of immunosuppressor treatment;
2. the decrease in ANF clearance by the corticosteroids;
3. the rise in atrial parietal tension (Laplace's law); and finally,
4. the heart rejection.

We can conclude from these experimental and human studies that cardiac innervation is not required for ANF secretion.

Conclusion

Although the ANF recent discovery represents a fundamental step in sodium and water homeostasis understanding. Its clinical implication remains unclear. Nevertheless, in both atria, it is demonstrated that volume distension more than elevated intraluminal pressure is the most important stimulus for ANF release. Moreover, recent studies have demonstrated the role of atrial contraction rate in ANF release. Tachycardia over 130 beats/min induces an ANF release even if Tm atrial pressures decrease. Finally, the integrity of cardiac nerves is not necessary for physiological ANF release. The exact role in human physiology and pathophysiology especially for renal excretion of sodium and water remains to be elucidated before pharmacologic development. The last concept flowing from ANF research is that the heart should be now considered as an endocrine organ.

References

1. De Bold AJ, Borenstein HR, Veress AT, Sonnenberg HA (1981) A rapid and potent natriuretic response to intravenous injection of atrial myocardial extracts in rats. Life Sci 28:89–94
2. Kish B (1956) Electron microscopy of the atrium of the heart: Guinea pig. Exp Med Surg 14:99–112
3. Marie JP, Guillemot H, Hatt PY (1976) Le degré de granulation des cardiocytes auriculaires. Etude planimétrique au cours de différents apports d'eau et de sodium chez le rat. Pathol Biol 24:549–554
4. Gauer OH, Henry JP (1963) Circulatory basis of fluid control. Physiol Rev 43:423–481
5. Mebazaa A, Chevalier B, Mercadier JJ, Echter E, Rappaport L, Swynghedauw B (1989) A review of the renin-angiotensin system in the normal heart. J Cardiovasc Pharmacol 14(suppl 4):S16–S20
6. Weidmann P, Hasler L, Gnadinger MP et al (1986) Blood levels and renal effects of atrial natriuretic peptide in normal man. J Clin Invest 77:734–742
7. Mercadier JJ, Zongazo MA, Wisnewsky C, Butler-Brown G, Gros D, Carayon A, Schwartz K (1989) Atrial natriuretic factor messenger ribonucleic acide and peptide in the human heart during ontogenic development. Biochem Biophys Res Commun 159:777–782
8. Indolfi C, Piscione F, Volpe M, et al (1989) Cardiac effects of atrial natriuretic peptide in subjects with normal left ventricular function. Am J Cardiol 63:353–357
9. Springall DR, Bhatnagar M, Wharton J, et al (1988) Expression of the atrial natriuretic peptide gene in the cardiac muscle of rat extrapulmonary and intrapulmonary veins. Thorax 43:44–52
10. Gutkowska J, Racz K, Garcia R, Thibault G, Kuchel O, Genest J, Cantin M (1986) The morphine effect on plasma ANF. Eur J Pharmacol 131:91–94
11. Payen DM, Leclerc D, Caraco JJ, Viossat J, Chabrier P, Braquet P (1986) Evidence for fentanyl alteration of plasma atrial natriuretic factor-right atrial pressure relationship after cardiac surgery. Anesthesiology 65(suppl):A510
12. Horky K, Gutkowska J, Garcia R, Thibault G, Genest J, Cantin M (1985) Effect of different anesthetics on immunoreactive atrial natriuretic factor concentrations in rat plasma. Bioch Biophys Res Commun 129:651–657
13. Payen D, Greck E, Eurin J, Maistre F, Laborde F, Echter E (1987) Evidence for dobutamine-induced atrial natriuretic factor release. Circulation 76(suppl IV):IV 71
14. Dietz JR (1984) Release of natriuretic factor from rat heart-lung preparation by atrial distension. Am J Physiol 247:R1093–R1096
15. Lang RE, Tholken H, Ganten D, Luft FC, Ruskoaho H, Unger T (1985) Atrial natriuretic factor a circulating hormone stimulated by volume loading. Nature 314:264–266

16. Singer DRJ, Buckley MG, Mac Gregor GA, Khaghani A, Banner NR, Yacoub MH (1986) Raised concentrations of plasma atrial natriuretic peptides in cardiac transplant recipients. Br Med J 293:1391

17. Dussaule JC, Vahanian A, Michel PL, Soulier I, Czekalski S, Acar J, Ardaillou R (1988) Plasma atrial natriuretic factor and cyclic GMP in mitral stenosis treated by balloon valvulotomy, effect of atrial fibrillation. Circulation 78:276-285

18. Fratacci MD, Greck E, Froidevaux R, Bellec C, Dupuy P, Eurin J, Payen D (1988) Antidiuresis during PEEP is not mediated by an inhibiting of atrial natriuretic factor release. Anesthesiology 69(suppl):A184

19. Schwab TR, Edwards BS, De Vries WC, Burnett JC (1986) Atrial endocrine function in humans with artificial hearts. N Engl J Med 315:1398-1401

20. Mancini GBJ, Mac Gillem MJ, Bates ER, Weder AB, Deboe SF, Grekin RJ (1987) Hormonal responses to cardiac tamponade: inhibition of release of atrial natriuretic factor despite elevation of atrial pressures. Circulation 76:844-890

21. Edwards BS, Zimmerman RS, Schwab TR, Heublein DM, Burnett JC (1988) Atrial stretch, not pressure, is the principal determinant controlling the acute release of atrial natriuretic factor. Circ Res 62:687-692

22. Zioris H, Karayannacos P, Zerva C, Alevizou-Terzaki V, Pavlatos F, Skalkeas G (1989) Atrial natriuretic peptide levels during and after acute cardiac tamponade in dogs. J Am Coll Cardiol 13:936-940

23. Stone JA, Wilkes PRH, Keane PM, Smith ER, Tyberg JV (1989) Pericardial pressure attenuates release of atriopeptin in volume-expanded dogs. Am J Physiol 256:H648-H654

24. Payen D, Greck E, Fratacci MD, Eurin J (1988) Transmural right atrial pressure is a major stimulus for atrial natriuretic factor (pANF) release in man. Circulation 78(suppl II):II 588

25. Kharash ED, Yeo KT, Kenny MA, Buffington CW (1988) Atrial natriuretic factor may mediate the renal effects of PEEP ventilation. Anesthesiology 69:862-869

26. Schiffrin EL, Gutkowska J, Kuchel O, Cantin M, Genest J (1985) Plasma concentration of atrial natriuretic factor in a patient with paroxysmal atrial tachycardia. N Engl J Med 312:1196

27. Mebazaa A, Maistre G, Payen D (1990) Direct effect of atrial tachycardia on release of atrial natriuretic factor in man. J Am Coll Cardiol (in press)

28. Farge D, Guillemain R, Payen D, et al (1989) Plasma atrial natriuretic factor and other water and sodium regulating hormones after human heart transplantation. Transplant Proc 21:2573-2575

Endocrine Disturbances in the Critically Ill: The Role of Growth Hormone and Cortisol

H. J. Voerman, R. J. M. Strack van Schijndel, and L. G. Thijs

Introduction

In critically ill patients a wide variety in metabolic changes is observed. Metabolic rate increases and proteolysis for energy production are thought to result from both alterations in production of mediators and from hormonal changes.

The metabolic and hormonal response to severe illness has been divided in an early and a late response. The early response lasts up to 48 hours and shows an increase in concentrations of vasopressin, epinephrine, norepinephrine, dopamine, ACTH, growth hormone (GH) and prolactin. Secondary effects include an increase in cortisol, aldosterone and glucagon levels and a decrease in insulin secretion. The late response is characterised by an increase in insulin concentration, not appropriate to the level of hyperglycemia thus indicating insulin resistance. The hormonal response to illness is dependent on the severity of the underlying disorder. Different patterns of the various hormones are observed in trauma patients, patients with the sepsis syndrome and patients with septic shock [1]. The increased levels of catecholamines, glucagon and cortisol lead to a change in the use of the body energy stores resulting in an increase in glucose and free fatty acid levels. Administration of these catabolic hormones to healthy subjects results in hormonal and metabolic changes identical to those seen in the critically ill [2].

GH, which promotes fat oxidation, is increased during stress. Insulin, which promotes the storage of lipids and carbohydrates is reduced in the early phase but increased in the late phase of a critical illness. As there is a failure to increase glucose uptake despite hypergycemia and hyperinsulinemia, insulin resistance exists.

Thyroid function tests can be influenced by critical illness. Low, normal as well as high thyroxin levels have been found. Triiodothyronine levels are reduced and reverse T3 increased. When levels of non-proteinbound T4 and T3 are measured, normal to low levels are observed. Extensive discussions on this subject have recently been published and will therefore not be discussed in this review [3].

With the ability to synthesize human GH new interest in the metabolic action of GH has emerged. GH increases lipolysis but promotes muscle anabolism and may therefore ameliorate the protein loss seen in critically ill patients.

The use of corticosteroids in critically ill patients, especially those with the sepsis syndrome has been controversial for many years. In large trials no beneficial effect of administration of high-dose corticosteroids could be documented. However, a subgroup of patients with low cortisol concentrations correlating with a severe mortality has been described. Substitution therapy in this group might be indicated, but no conclusive studies have been published.

In this review we will attempt to summarize the changes in GH and cortisol secretion in the critically ill and their implications for therapy.

Growth Hormone

Physiology

GH is a single-chain polypeptide (mol. weight of 21500), secreted by somato-throphic cells in the anterior pituitary gland. In plasma it is bound to a specific binding globulin. GH secretion is regulated by both stimulatory (GH releasing hormone: GHRH) and inhibitory (somatostatin) factors of hypothalamic origin [4, 5]. GH is secreted in a pulsatile manner over a 24 hour period in humans [6]. This may be important for the biological action of these hormones. The rate of protein formation remains elevated for many hours after a single dose of GH, so that constant plasma levels are not required [7]. The pulsatile nature of the GH secretion results from both GHRH- and somatostatin activity at the pituitary level. The secretory pattern differs with age and sex [8]. During the day GH secretion is low and only a few peaks occur [9] while at night most of the GH release occurs [10]. In the aged the nightly increase in secretion is often absent.

Many neuropeptides, such as opoids and vasoactive intestinal polypeptide (VIP) influence GH secretion. Administration of morphine may alter GH concentration and/or pulse frequency in the critically ill. Many other agents may alter the release of GHRH and/or somatostatin from the hypothalamus. Dopamine and α-adrenergic agonists stimulate GH release, while β-receptor agonists inhibit GH release and cholinergic blockade inhibits GH secretion [11].

GH has an important role in production of linear growth. It stimulates the synthesis of proteins and nucleic acids. Exogenous GH administration produces hypoglycemia. A refractory period of 24–48 hour exists for this insulin-like effect [7]. This response is only seen in GH deficient animals and requires protein synthesis. When administered for a longer period of time GH stimulates glucose production by the liver and induces insulin resistance in the peripheral tissues resulting in an elevated glucose concentration. This is known as the diabetogenic effect of GH. On the other hand, infusion of a glucose load in healthy volunteers results in a reduction of GH levels. GH raises the level of free fatty acids and glycerol in the blood and thus indirectly affects fat oxidation [12]. When GH is administered during starvation the lipolytic effects are more pronounced [13]. The fasting state itself is related to increased GH levels [4].

Many effects of GH are thought to be mediated by Insulin-like Growth factor I (IGF-I), which is synthesised in the liver. However, GH has been shown to have direct effects on protein synthesis independent of IGF-I. IGF-I is not only regulated by GH but by nutrition as well.

Role in Disease

Generally it is assumed that GH levels are increased in the critically ill patient. This increase is observed despite concentrations of plasma glucose which would inhibit its secretion in the healthy person. Table 1 summarizes some studies concerning changes in GH concentration in patients with injury and sepsis.

Table 1. Growth hormone levels in humans during/after injury and sepsis

Reference	Number of patients	Age	Diagnosis	Sampling method	Growth hormone ng/ml
[52]	5	20–34	Sandfly fever	24 hrs, every 60 min.	normal 1–3 night 9–10 infection: 10–19
[15]	13	46–80	critically ill	basal and after glucose	5.2±2.2[a] 3.2±1.2
[53]	7	30–59	postoperative	between 08.00–09.00 on admission (day 0) and 1, 2, 4, and 8 days after surgery	day 0: 2.3±0.7 day 1: 5.2±1.8 day 2: 5.9±2.1 day 4: 2.6±0.6 day 8: 2.4±1.0
[54]	8	33–74	postoperative	fasting levels	max. 25
[55]	13	–	critically ill	basal levels	5.2±2.2 3.2±1.2
[56]	14	–	trauma	on admission	58.8 range: 6.6–180
[57]	9	18–49	burns	basal	acute: 1.7±0.2 recoverd: 1.8±0.3
[58]	22	–	burns	09.00	mild: 4.3 (1–11.1)[b] moderate: 4.8 (0.6–14.8) severe: 5.4 (1.0–12.7)
[35]	5	–	sepsis	basal	2.5±2.9
[59]	13	28–54	postoperative	before and after surgery	day 0: 1.9 (1.0–2.8) day 1: 15.2 (1.2–100) day 2: 3.7 (1.0–10.1)
[60]	25	9–65	trauma	daily	range: max 150[a]
[61]	19	10–54	head injury	on admission	0.8±1.4
[62]	26	14–85	postoperative	before direct p.o. 24 hr p.o.	1.4±0.5 10.1±9.6 0.9±0.4
[41]	13	21–34	after endotoxin administration	2, 4, and 8 hrs after endotoxin	2 hrs: 16.8±2.1 4 hrs: 7.3±1.2 8 hrs: 8.4±1.6
[63]	7	23–65	during surgery		before: 1.1±0.4 peak (60 min.): 23.9±6.5

Values given as mean and SD or range in ng/ml.
[a] mU/ml; [b] mg/L.

From these data it is clear that a variable response exists. Only a few studies showed an increase in GH, mainly during or shortly after the insulting event. None of the studies showed a sustained increase in GH levels. In some studies GH levels were measured in patients during or directly after surgery. As the type of anesthesia can influence the GH secretion interpretation of these data is difficult. Another study design consists of the measurement of GH after administration of glucose or arginine. In healthy volunteers glucose infusion inhibits GH secretion, while arginine is a powerful stimulus of GH secretion. In critically ill patients glucose infusion often leads to a paradoxal increase in GH concentration. However suppression of GH or lack of response have also been observed [14]. These variable results could be due to different levels of stress or severity of illness in the patients studied. An absence of response is correlated with an increased mortality [15].

The value of this 'stress' test can be questioned. What is the significance of a rise in GH concentration after glucose infusion? It may indicate that reserve function is normal and that basal secretion is inhibited. This view is supported by the low baseline values in most studies. On the other hand a paradoxical increase could be due to a timing coincident of the glucose load and a spontaneous secretory peak [16]. Especially in situations with an increase in GH pulses this phenomenon can play a role.

Pulse Characteristics

In most studies no increase in GH concentration was found and levels varied greatly (Table 1). These large variations in GH concentration could be the result of the pulsatile nature of GH secretion. No data have been published on the pulsatile pattern of GH secretion in the critically ill. Animal studies indicate a reduction in pulsatile secretion after endotoxin administration [17]. Tumour necrosis factor (TNF) inhibits GH secretion in vitro [18]. To elucidate the pattern of pulsatile hormone secretion in the critically ill, we measured GH levels during 24 hour periods in patients with septic shock. After informed consent was obtained, blood samples were drawn every 20 minutes. Diabetic patients were excluded because diabetes is known to alter GH secretion. The patients were in the age group of 50–70 years. In healthy volunteers of this age GH secretion is low.

Table 2. Growth hormone and cortisol patterns in 8 patients with septic shock

Blood levels	Range	Number of peaks/24 h	Height	Interval between peaks (min)	Peak width (min)
Growth hormone (ng/ml)					
3.3±2.5	0.1–34.52	9±2.8	5.2±3.4	136±23	89±19
Cortisol (nmol/L)					
640±461	272–3505	5.5±2.3	909±1056	198±63	164±71

Integrated GH secretion is 3.44 ± 0.30 ng/ml, pulse duration 108 ± 8 min, pulse aplitude 4.99 ± 1.10 ng/ml and no more than 2 GH peaks occur during 24 hours [8]. In the patients with septic shock average levels of GH were not or just slightly increased, pulse amplitude was unchanged, but pulse frequency increased markedly to 9 pulses a day and pulse duration decreases to 89 ± 19 min (Table 2). The shortened pulse duration could be due to an increase in metabolic clearance. Due to the pulsatile secretion a wide range of GH concentrations is observed during the study period and could explain the variations observed in other studies. Single measurements cannot be used to evaluate GH levels and a less frequent sampling method only allows to study large variations in GH secretion.

All but one patient showed an increase in pulse frequency. Several mechanisms other than the severe illness itself could be responsible for the observed increase in pulse frequency. Dopamine could be involved as it increases pulse frequency in diabetic subjects [19]. In normal man plasma GH concentration varies during dopamine infusion. Both increases and absence of change have been observed. In vitro dopamine was not able to stimulate GH release by pituitary cells, so the effect of dopamine remains uncertain. All our patients received dopamine to maintain blood pressure. Other drugs may be of importance as well. Benzodiazepines, frequently used in mechanically ventilated patients for sedation can increase GH concentrations [20]. Theophylline and other phosphodiesterase inhibitors decrease the GH response to GHRH and block in vitro the effect of GH on protein synthesis [7]. While studying pulsatile secretion attention should also be given to the type of feeding as well. Total parenteral nutrition may blunt the GH peak response, not in number but in hight [21].

Growth Hormone Administration in the Critically Ill

Despite the small increase in (pulsatile) GH secretion, and increases in insulin levels, catabolism is not abolished in critically ill patients. It is well known that

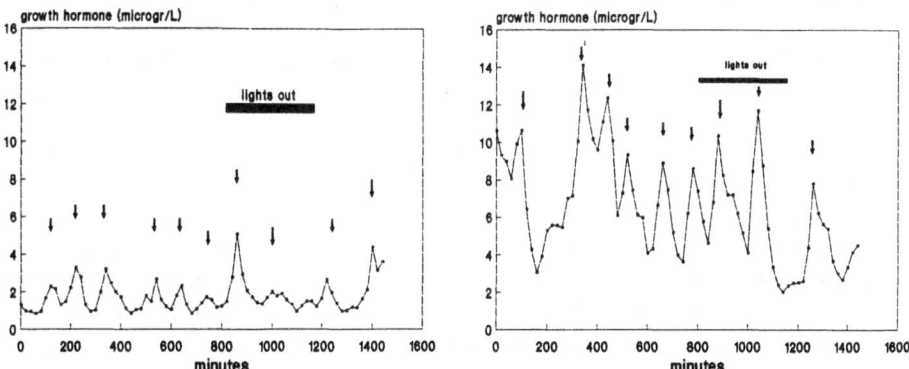

Fig. 1. 24-hour profile of growth hormone in 2 patients with septic shock. Secretory peaks are indicated by arrows

even aggressive metabolic support is unable to induce a positive nitrogen balance in critically ill septic patients. Furthermore low levels of GH may contribute to the loss of immunocompetence which can be observed in the critically ill [22].

For this reason several investigators studied the influence of human GH on nitrogen balance in catabolic states or during feeding with a hypocaloric, hyponitrogenous feeding [23–33]. In most studies a positive nitrogen balance was induced or a decrease in urea production noticed. This response was dose related [29]. Only early studies reported an increase in nitrogen loss, no change or variable response during GH treatment, especially when given intravenously [30, 31]. Factors probably contributing to this variable response could be differences in nutrition (parenteral or enteral nutrition and amount of calories administered) and the use of human as well as bovine GH [29]. Bovine GH, used in some studies, is now known to have an unpredictable anabolic activity in humans [26]. GH administration reduces nitrogen excretion and decreases muscle catabolism by promoting protein synthesis in patients after surgery, during starvation or on a hypocaloric nutrition. When administering GH during prolonged starvation a decrease in urea nitrogen excretion is observed, but the lipolytic effect is more pronounced [13]. IGF-I levels increased in most studies after administration of human GH.

The induction of a positive nitrogen balance is thought to parallel a decrease in muscle catabolism and thus preservation of muscle mass. Some studies were not able to show a positive nitrogen balance accompanied by a reduction of muscle breakdown [24, 34]. The septic state has not been studied extensively, and doubt exists on the effectiveness of GH in the septic patient. A decrease in urea production, but no increase in the concentration of IGF-I have been observed [23, 35]. It is not known to which extent IGF-I is a permissive factor for the anabolic action concerning nitrogen balance and muscle breakdown. Studies in acromegalic subjects clearly show little correlation between GH concentration and IGF-I level. Factors contributing to the diminished response of exogenous GH in sepsis could be hepatic dysfunction and the absence or inadequate nutrition during some studies. We were able to observe an episode of septic shock in a patient treated with human GH. In this patient no muscle breakdown was observed during the septic episode and nitrogen balance remained positive despite an unchanged IGF-I level. It is clear that the influence of GH on nitrogen balance and muscle catabolism in sepsis and septic shock deserves further study.

GH administration in the critically ill patient not only affects protein metabolism. In surgical patients GH may accelerate the formation of granulation tissue and thus wound healing [36]. Thyroid hormone levels increase after GH administration, due to extrathyroidal conversion of T4 to T3. Other effects of GH are a decline in the secretion of calcium, phosphorus and potassium [7]. Hypophosphatemia and hypocalcemia are common in the critically ill. GH administration leads to a positive calcium and phosphate balance. The effects of GH on potassium level varies, as increases as well as decreases in potassium concentration have been noted during treatment [25]. GH causes retention of potassium by the kidney, but an increase in glucose and insulin levels could reduce potassium concentration. Early studies suggest that the net result of GH on potassium balance depends on the level of potassium intake. Above a critical point potassium retention is observed [26]. The retention of sodium and water due to GH administration results in a positive fluid balance [25].

GH administration influences myocardial and renal function. An increase in myocardial contractility was observed after GH administration in normal volunteers and in a patient with hypopituitarism [37, 38]. Long term administration in an animal model resulted in myocardial hypertrophy. GH effects kidney function by enhancing both GFR en RPF, mediated by IGF-I [39]. GH appears to enhance erythropoiesis and increases plasma concentrations of all the components of the factor VIII complex, within three hours after an intravenous dose [22]. Psychological side effects are euphoria, mood elevation and an increase in appetite [29].

Conclusion

GH levels in critically ill patients are only slightly increased; this is probably due to an increase in pulse frequency. GH administration to catabolic patients or during hypocaloric feeding results in a decrease in nitrogen loss and a positive nitrogen balance. Its influence on muscle metabolism remains to be elucidated. The effects of GH in patients with sepsis or septic shock remains to be elucidated.

Cortisol

Cortisol Secretion in the Critically Ill

Cortisol, one of the major glucocorticoids, is essential for the survival of the stressed patient. In critically ill patients the adrenal gland is capable of autoregulating as a shift from mineralocorticoids and adrenal androgens to glucocorticoid secretion is observed [40]. Hypoxia contributes to this autoregulation by inhibition of aldosterone secretion.

Cortisol, like GH, has a prominent circadian secretory pattern. Cortisol release decreases through the afternoon and evening. Frequent sampling detects a series of secretory bursts with intervals of 40 minutes to hours [6].

After administration of endotoxin to healthy volunteers cortisol levels raise for 4 to 8 hours [41]. The extent and duration of the increased cortisol secretion in the critically ill are related to the severity of the insult [1, 40, 42, 43]. In patients undergoing minor surgery the circadian rhythm can alter: the amplitude increases and a phase shift may occur. After major surgery the circadian rhythm disappears and the cortisol level remains elevated for several days [43].

Although cortisol concentrations are thought to increase during stress, normal and low cortisol concentrations have been found in critically ill patients. Normal cortisol levels may represent a relative adrenal insufficiency, and reduced cortisol levels have been associated with an increase in mortality [3, 44]. An inverse relation between cortisol level and injury severity score has also been reported [42]. Other studies failed to correlate a normal or decreased cortisol level with an increased mortality and observed high cortisol levels to be associated with a poor outcome [45].

In earlier animal studies similar results were obtained, as both low and high levels of cortisol were found related to an increased lethality [46].

Several factors contribute to the variation in cortisol level during a critical illness. Hemorrhagic shock can result in a progressive decrease in adrenal blood flow and hence corticosteroid secretion. Furthermore, in the terminal stage of hemorrhagic shock degeneration and necrosis of the adrenal cortex can be observed, and contribute to the decrease in cortisol level. When single plasma cortisol levels are obtained, sampling errors may contribute to the 'normal' cortisol levels observed. In some patients secretory episodes may increase but 'baseline' levels of cortisol remain unchanged.

In order to study the variability in cortisol levels we measured blood cortisol levels every 20 min for 24 hours in 8 patients with septic shock (Table 2). Cortisol levels varied more than 300% during the day (Fig. 2). No circadian rhythm was observed and clear secretory peaks occurred. As cortisol levels vary enormously it is clear that 'on admission' or random levels do not represent average cortisol levels and are of limited value.

Administration of Corticosteroids in Critically Ill Patients

Glucocrticoids have been advocated in the treatment of septic shock, but their use remains controversial. Corticosteroids inhibit phospholipase A_2 and the secretion of endorphins, both of which may contribute to the hypotension in endotoxin shock [3]. Endotoxin is known to have an 'anti-glucocorticoid effect', which may induce 'relative' adrenal insufficiency in septic patients [3]. As corticosteroids may induce an acute rise in β-adrenergic receptors and support the cardiovascular system, their administration may be beneficial in septic shock

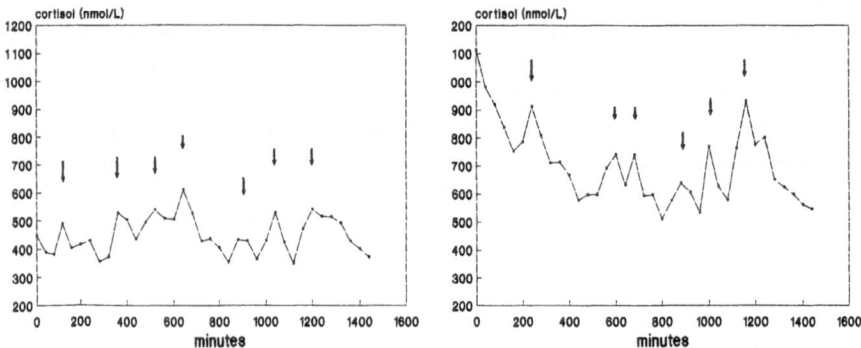

Fig. 2. 24-hour profile of cortisol secretion in two patients with septic shock. Secretory peaks are indicated by arrows

[47]. Early initiation of corticosteroid therapy was thought to be an essential component of a beneficial response. However, in a study in baboons it became clear that even delayed treatment can be beneficial [48].

Several studies, based upon the experience in animals, have been undertaken to study the effects of high dose glucocorticoids in patients with sepsis and septic shock [49–51]. These trials showed no benefits of high doses of corticosteroids in sepsis and septic shock. In the treated group resolution of secondary infections was lower than in the control group and more deaths related to secondary infections were observed [49, 51]. Large doses of steroids are known to have a detrimental effect on host defence mechanism and thus could be responsible for this increase [46]. Treatment with corticosteroids impeded the reversal of ARDS and increased the mortality rate in patients with ARDS [50]. These clinical trials have shown that high doses of glucocorticosteroids are not indicated in the treatment of sepsis and septic shock. In patients with gram-negative sepsis a beneficial effect may exist, but this should be clarified by further clinical investigation.

In all trials large doses of glucocorticoids were administrated. Some of the adverse effects could be dose-related as well. The effects of smaller doses have not been studied. As corticosteroids have a cardiovascular effect we studied 6 patients who remained dependent on vasoactive drugs to preserve mean arterial pressure (MAP). All patients had received vasoactive drugs for at least 6 days when 100 mg hydrocortisone was administered intravenously. Within 1 hour MAP rose from 64 to 90 mmHg and vasoactive drugs could be tapered down. These changes were thought to be due to an increase in systemic vascular resistance. Another study showed, although again a high dose was applied, a beneficial effect of corticosteroids in critically ill patients with a low cardiac output as well [47]. The effects of corticosteroids in low doses than applied in earlier studies remain to be elucidated, especially in septic patients who remain dependent on vaso-active drugs and have 'normal' cortisol concentrations.

Conclusion

Cortisol concentrations vary in critically ill patients. Low as well as high levels have been found to correlate with an increase in mortality. The large variations in cortisol levels observed could in part be due to the pulsatile nature of cortisol secretion irrespective of the persistence of the circadian rhythm. High doses of corticosteroids are not indicated in the treatment of septic shock, but its role in gram-negative septic shock and in septic patients who remain dependent on vasoactive drugs remains to be clarified.

References

1. Siegel JH, Cerra FB, Coleman B, Giovannini I, Shetye M, Border JR, McMenamy RH (1979) Physiological and metabolic correlations in human sepsis. Surgery 86:163–193
2. Gelfand RA, Matthews DE, Bier DM, Sherwin RS (1984) Role of counterregulatory hormones in the catabolic responce to stress. J Clin Invest 74:2238–2248

3. Teich S, Sharpe S, Chernow B (1985) Endocrine function in the critically ill. Clin Anaesthesiol 3:999–1026
4. Thorner MO, Vance ML, Evans WS, et al (1986) Physiological and clinical studies of GFR and GH. Rec Progress in Horm Res 42:589–640
5. Frohman LA, Jansson J-O (1986) Growth hormone-releasing hormone. Endocrin Rev 7:223–253
6. Weigle DS (1987) Pulsatile secretion of fuel-regulatory hormones. Diabetes 36:764–775
7. Kostyo KL, Reagan CR (1976) The biology of growth hormone. Pharmac Ther 2:591–604
8. Ho KY, Evans S, Blizzard RM, et al (1987) Effects of sex and age on the 24-hour profile of growth hormone secretion in man: importance of endogenous estradiol concentrations. J Clin Endocrinol Metab 64:51–58
9. Quabbe H-J, Schilling E, Helge H (1966) Pattern of growth hormone secretion during a 24-hour fast in normal adults. J Clin Endocrinol 26:1173–1177
10. Hunter WM, Rigal WM (1966) The diurnal pattern of plasma growth hormone concentration in children and adolescents. J Endocrinol 34:147–153
11. Dieguez C, Page D, Scanlon MF (1988) Growth hormone neuroregulation and its alterations in disease states. Clin Endocrin 28:109–143
12. Goodman HM, Grichting G (1983) Growth hormone and lipolysis: a reevaluation. Endocrinology 113:1697–1702
13. Felig P, Marliss EB, Cahill GF (1971) Metabolic response to human growth hormone during prolonged starvation. J Clin Invest 50:411–421
14. Rayfield EJ, George DT, Beisel WR (1974) Altered growth hormone homeostasis during acute bacterial sepsis in the rhesus monkey. J Clin Endocrinol Metab 38:746–754
15. Dahn MS, Jacobs LA, Lange MP, Smith S, Mitchell RA (1986) Endocrine mediators of metabolism associated with injury and sepsis. JPEN 10:253–257
16. Edge JA, Human DH, Matthews DR, Dunger DB (1989) Spontaneous growth hormone (GH) pulsatility in the major determinant of GH release after thyrotropin-releasing hormone in adolescent diabetics. Clin Endocrinol 30:397–404
17. Kasting NW, Martin JB (1982) Altered release of growth hormone and thyrotropin induced by endotoxin in the rat. Am J Physiol 243:E332–E337
18. Walton PE, Cronin MJ (1989) Tumor necrosis factor-alpha inhibits growth hormone secretion from cultured anterior pituitary cells. Endocrinology 125:925–929
19. Lorenzi M, Karam JH, McIlroy MB, Forsham PH (1980) Increased growth hormone response to dopamine infusion in insulin-dependent diabetic subjects. J Clin Invest 65:146–153
20. Grandison L (1983) Actions of benzodiazepines on the neuroendocrine system. Neuropharmacology 22:1505–1510
21. Barber AE, Marano MA, Fong Y, et al (1989) Circadian rhythms of growth hormone and cortisol in parenterally fed man. Clin Nutr 8 (suppl):50
22. Williams TC, Frohman LA (1986) Potential therapeutic indications for growth hormone and growth hormone releasing hormone in conditions other than growth retardation. Pharmacotherapy 6:311–318
23. Gottardis M, Hackl JM (1988) Die Beeinflussung des katabolen Stoffwechsels bei septischen Patienten und Schädel-Hirn-Traumatisierten durch Gabe von humanem Wachstumhormon. Infusionstherapie 15:112–117
24. Manson JMck, Smith RJ, Wilmore DW (1988) Growth hormone stimulates protein synthesis during hypocaloric parenteral nutrition. Ann Surg 208:136–142
25. Ziegler TR, Young LS, Manson JM (1988) Metabolic effects of recombinant human growth hormone in patients receiving parenteral nutrition. Ann Surg 208:6–16
26. Soroff HS, Pearson E, Green NL, Artz CP (1960) The effect of growth hormone on nitrogen balance at various levels of intake in burned patients. Surgery 111:259–273
27. Ponting GA, Halliday D, Teale JD, Sim AJW (1988) Postoperative positive nitrogen balance with intravenous hyponutrition and growth hormone. Lancet 1:438–439
28. Manson JMcK, Wilmore DW (1986) Positive nitrogen balance with human growth hormone and hypocaloric intravenous feeding. Surgery 100:188–197
29. Wilmore DW, Myolan JA, Bristow BF, Mason AD, Pruitt BA (1974) Anabolic effects of human growth hormone and high caloric feedings following thermal injury. Surg Gynecol Obstet 138:875–884

30. Soroff HS, Rozin RR, Mooty J, Lister J, Raben MS, MacAuley AJ, Paddock J (1967) Role of human growth hormone in the response to trauma I. Metabolic effects following burns. Ann Surg 166:739-752

31. Johnston IDA, Hadden DR (1963) Effect of human growth hormone on the metabolic response to surgical trauma. Lancet 1:584-586

32. Ward HC, Halliday D, Sim AJW (1987) Protein and energy metabolism with biosynthetic human growth hormone after gastrointestinal surgery. Ann Surg 206:56-61

33. Manson JM, Smith RJ, Wilmore DW (1988) Growth hormone stimulates protein synthesis during hypocaloric parenteral nutrition: role of hormonal-substrate environment. Ann Surg 208:136

34. Okamura K, Okuma T, Horochi Y, Myauchi Y (1989) The effect of human growth hormone on protein metabolism in rats with hypocaloric intravenous feeding. Clin Nutr 8 (suppl):106

35. Dahn MS, Lange MP, Jacobs LA (1988) Insulin-like growth factor 1 production is inhibited in human sepsis. Arch Surg 123:1409-1414

36. Jorgensen PH, Andreassen TT (1988) The influence of biosynthetic human growth hormone on biomechanical properties and collagen formation in granulation tissue. Horm Metabol Res 20:490-493

37. Thuessen L, Christiansen JS, Sorensen KE, Jorgensen JOL, Orskov H, Henningsen P (1988) Increased myocardial contractility following growth hormone administration in normal man. Dan Med Bull 35:193-196

38. Cuneo RC, Wilmshurst P, Lowy C, McGauley G, Sonksen PH (1989) Cardiac failure responding to growth hormone. Lancet 1:838-839

39. Hischberg R, Kopple JD (1987) Effects of growth hormone on GFR and renal plasma flow in man. Kidney Int 32 (suppl) 22:S21-S24

40. Wade CE, Lindberg JS, Cockrell JL, Lamiell JM, Hunt MM, Ducey J, Jurney TH (1988) Upon-admission adrenal steroidogenesis is adapted to the degree of illness in intensive care patients. J Clin Endocrinol Metab 67:223-227

41. Kimball HR, Lipsett MB, Odell WD, Wolff SM (1968) Comparison of the effect of the pyrogens, etiocholanolone and bacterial endotoxin on plasma cortisol and growth hormone in man. J Clin Endocrin 28:337-342

42. Stoner HB, Frayn KN, Barton RN, Threfall CJ, Little RA (1979) The relationship between plasma substrates and hormones and the severity of injury in 277 recently injured patients. Clin Science 56:563-573

43. Q McIntosh TK (1987) Prolonged alterations in plasma cortisol circadian rythms following trauma in baboons. Am J Physiol 252:R548-R553

44. McKee JI, Finlay WEI (1983) Cortisol replacement in severely stressed patients. Lancet 1:484

45. Jurney TH, Cockrell JL, Lindberg JS, Lamiel JM, Wade CE (1987) Spectrum of serum cortisol response to ACTH in ICU patients. Chest 92:292-295

46. Beisel WR, Rapoport MI (1969) Inter-relations between adrenocortical functions and infectious illness. N Engl J Med 280:541-546 en 596-604

47. Ogawa R (1989) Corticosteroids enhance cardiac response to catecholamines in critically ill patients. Proceedings 5th world congress on intensive and critical care medicine. Kyoto, p 89

48. Hinshaw LB, Archer LT, Bellar-Todd BK, Benjamin B, Flournoy DJ, Passey R (1981) Survival of primates in lethal septic shock following delayed treatment with steroid. Circ Shock 8:291-300

49. Bone RC, Fisher CJ, Clemmer TP, Slotman GJ, Metz CA (1987) A controlled clinical trial of high dose methylprednisolone in the treatment of severe sepsis and septic shock. N Engl J Med 317:653-658

50. Bone RC, Fisher CJ, Clemmer TP, Slotman GJ, Metz CA (1987) Early methylprednisolone treatment for septic syndrome and the adult respiratory distress syndrome. Chest 92:1032-1036

51. The Veterans Administration Systemic Sepsis Cooperative Study Group (1987) Effect of high-dose glucocorticoid therapy on mortality in patients with clinical signs of systemic sepsis. N Engl J Med 317:659-665

52. Bunner DL, Morris E, Smallridge RC (1984) Circadian growth hormone and prolactin blood concentration during a self limited viral infection and arteficial hyperthermia in man. Metabolism 33:337–341
53. Goschke H, Bar E, Girard J, Leutenegger A, Niederer W, Oberholzer M, Wolff G (1978) Glucagon, insulin, cortisol, and growth hormone levels following major surgery: their relationship to glucose and free fatty acid elevations. Horm Metab Res 10:465–470
54. Wright PD, Johnston IDA (1975) The effect of surgical operation on growth hormone levels in plasma. Surgery 77:479–486
55. Dahn MS, Mitchell RA, Smith S, Lange MP, Whitcomb MP, Kirkpatrick JR (1984) Altered immunologic function and nitrogen metabolism associated with depression of plasma growth hormone. JPEN 8:690–694
56. Carey LC, Cloutier CT, Lowery BD (1971) Growth hormone and adrenal cortical response to shock and trauma in the human. Ann Surg 174:451–458
57. Wilmore DW, Orcutt TW, Mason AD, Pruitt BA (1975) Alterations in hypothalamic function following thermal injury. J Trauma 15:697–703
58. Alberti KGMM, Batstone GF, Foster K, Johnston DG (1980) Relative role of various hormones in mediating the metabolic response to injury. JPEN 4:141–146
59. Charters AC, Odell WD, Thompson JC (1969) Anterior pituitary function during surgical stress and convalescence. Radioimmunoassay measurement of blood TSH, LH, FSH, and growth hormone. J Clin Endocrinol 2963:63–71
60. Josten KU, Stoekel H, Lauwen P, Mosebach KO, Schulte am Esch J, Rommelsheim K (1980) Das Verhalten der hGH-Sekretion bei Schwerverletzten. Anaesth Intensivther Notfallmed 15:213–223
61. Hackl JM (1980) Verhalten des Wachstumshormons bei schwerem Schädel-Hirn-Trauma mit sekundären Hirnstammschäden. Infusionstherapie 5:237–247
62. Noel GL, Suh HK, Stone JG, Frantz AG (1972) Human prolactin and growth hormone release during surgery and other conditions of stress. J Clin Endocrinol Metab 35:840–851
63. Ichikawa Y, Kawagoe M, Nishikai M, Yoshida K, Homma M (1971) Plasma corticotropin (ACTH), growth hormone (GH), and 11- OCHS (hydroxycorticosteroid) response during surgery. J Clin Lab Metab 78:882–890

Evaluation of Intensive Care

Intensive Care for Patients with the Acquired Immunodeficiency Syndrome and Respiratory Failure Caused by *Pneumocystis carinii* Pneumonia: The View from San Francisco General Hospital

J. M. Luce and R. M. Wachter

Introduction

Pneumonia caused by *Pneumocystis carinii* is the most common opportunistic infection in patients with the acquired immunodeficiency syndrome (AIDS), occuring in 80 percent of such patients during the course of their illness [1]. *Pneumocystis carinii* pneumonia (PCP) also is the most common cause of death in AIDS patients, carrying a one-month mortality rate of 20% despite frequently successful therapy with trimethoprim-sulfamethoxazole or parenteral pentamidine [2, 3]. Since most patients who die from PCP do so because of respiratory failure, the question of whether these patients should receive intensive care unit (ICU) admission for endotracheal intubation and mechanical ventilation comes up commonly. The question also carries immense ethical and economic importance, given that intensive care costs upwards of $ 2,000 per day in the United States and accounts for 10% of the country's health care budget. We will review the intensive care of AIDS patients with PCP and respiratory failure.

Early Approaches to Intensive Care

Early in the AIDS epidemic, a period spanning the years 1981 through 1983 in the United States, data to guide physicians and patients in making decisions about intubation and mechanical ventilation for severe PCP were unavailable. As a result, patients and their physicians seemed inclined to pursue aggressive therapy, and those of us working in the ICUs at San Francisco General Hospital (SFGH) assumed that we would have to open and staff more beds for AIDS patients. This was in keeping both with the unknown short and long term prognoses of PCP in such patients and with the practice of offering ICU admission to other patients, including those with hematologic malignancies and bone marrow transplants, whose prognoses in the setting of respiratory failure was understood to be poor [4, 5].

Between 1984 and 1987, six groups of investigators [6–11] reported inhospital mortality rates of from 86 to 100% in AIDS patients with PCP who received mechanical ventilation (Fig. 1). At SFGH, we noted that 36 of 42 of intubated AIDS patients died before hospital discharge; this yielded a mortality rate of 86% in the years 1981 through 1985 [10]. The long term prognosis of these patients also appeared to be poor, with only one patient alive at one year. Patient

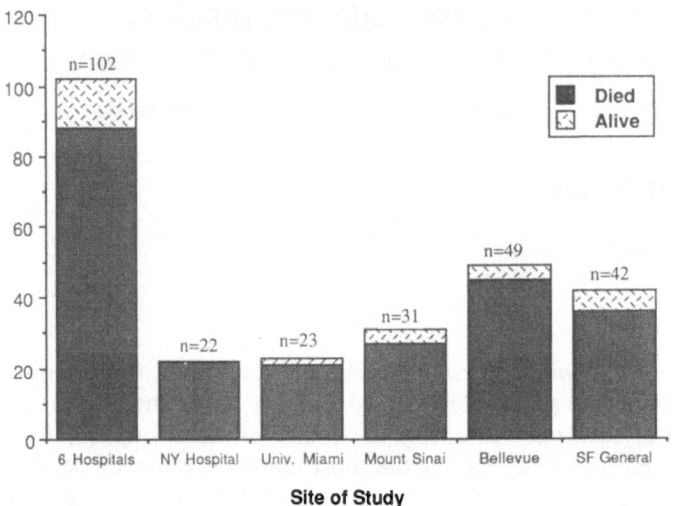

Fig. 1. Outcome studies demonstrating results of intensive care admission for patients with the acquired immunodeficiency syndrome and *Pneumocystis carinii* pneumonia, 1981–1986

age, therapy, or episode of PCP did not appear to influence mortality, although it did increase for patients admitted to the ICU after five or more days of hospitalization. The negative effect of prolonged earlier hospitalization presumably reflected the patient's failure to respond to treatment for PCP.

Based on these data, a consensus emerged among patients and physicians that life-sustaining therapy was not indicated for AIDS patients with severe PCP. This consensus was reflected in a study that documented the desire of AIDS patients in San Francisco to discuss the pros and cons or intensive care with their physicians [12] and in a poll of physicians at SFGH and the University of California, San Francisco (UCSF) that revealed both that physicians held such discussions as early as possible with AIDS patients and that the physicians would decline ICU admission if they themselves had PCP [13].

In a separate study, we verified that SFGH and UCSF physicians discussed life-sustaining treatment with 88% of their AIDS patients, compared with 82% of patients with stage III lung cancer, 54% of patients with hepatic cirrhosis and varices, and 43% of patients with severe congestive heart failure [14]. Furthermore, we found that do-not-resuscitate (DNR) orders were written for 52% of a sample of AIDS patients at our hospitals, compared with 47% of patients with advanced lung cancer, 16% of patients with cirrhosis, and 5% of patients with heart failure. The finding that discussions were initiated and DNR orders were written more often for patients with AIDS and cancer than for patients with cirrhosis and heart failure suggested that physicians viewed the first two conditions as more hopeless than the last two. This occurred despite the fact that when the physicians were asked, they acknowledged that all four diseases actually had similar prognoses.

In terms of the utilization of intensive care services, the major result of this consensus on the part of patients and physicians was that ICU admissions for

AIDS patients with severe PCP fell precipitously at SFGH between 1984 and 1986 [10] (Fig. 2). Overall admissions of AIDS patients to SFGH and inhospital diagnostic procedures for PCP increased just as dramatically during the same period. The decline in ICU admissions was providential from an economic standpoint because budgetary limitations and deficiencies in nurse recruitment forced SFGH to reduce its numbers of ICU beds in the mid-1980s. The in-

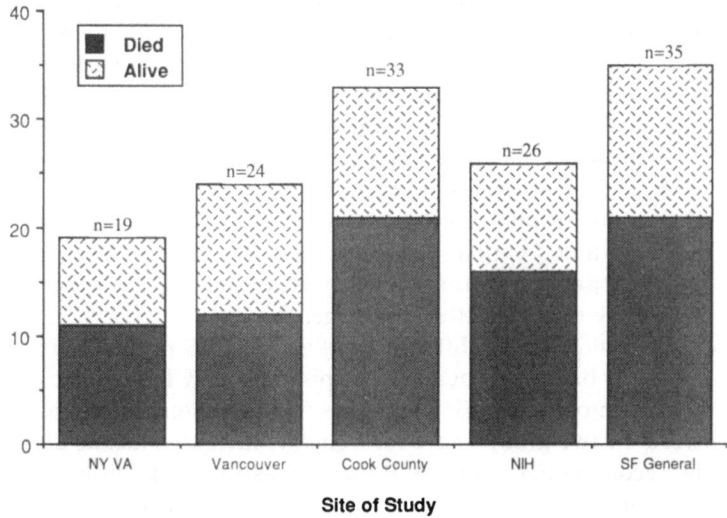

Fig. 2. Outcome studies demonstrating results of intensive care admission for patients with the acquired immunodeficiency syndrome and *Pneumocystis carinii* pneumonia, 1987–1989

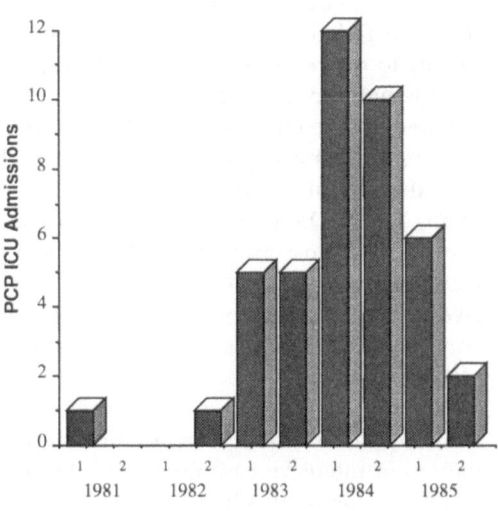

Fig. 3. Intensive care unit (ICU) admission for *Pneumocystis carinii* pneumonia (PCP) and respiratory failure (RF) at San Francisco General Hospital, 1981–1985

creased need for ICU beds for AIDS patients that had been anticipated earlier in the epidemic seemed to have been unfounded.

In 1988 and 1989, however, four groups of investigators reported an improved mortality ranging from 50 to 65% for AIDS patients with PCP who received mechanical ventilation [15-18] (Fig. 3). Because of all these reports were retrospective and none contained extensive clinical data, the possibility that selection of healthier patients for ICU admission had led to the apparent improvement could not be ignored. Nor could the possibility of publication bias, that is, the tendency of journal editors to publish more optimistic papers following more the pessimistic earlier reports. More important, no study involved a sample size adequate to answer detailed questions about outcome variables.

To meet these shortcomings, we examined the course of 35 AIDS patients with PCP and respiratory failure who were cared for in the SFGH ICUs from 1986 through 1988 and compared them with the 42 patients in the 1981 through 1985 cohort [19]. We found that only 21 of the 35 patients in the new cohort had died in the hospital, for an inhospital mortality of 60% compared with the 86% mortality noted earlier. The long term prognosis of patients in the new cohort remained poor, however, with only 9% of patients from the new group predicted to be alive one year after discharge.

We could find no differences in ages, AIDS risks factors (predominantly homosexual behavior), number of episodes of PCP, or other demographic factors to explain our findings. Vital signs and laboratory values also did not differ between the two groups, save for a slightly increased lactate dehydrogenase level in the second cohort. Anti-PCP therapy also was similar between the two groups, save for the fact that only two of 42 (5%) patients in the first cohort received corticosteroids compared with 26 of the 35 (74%) in the second. Despite this difference between groups and anecdotal evidence of the beneficial effects of corticosteroids in severe PCP [16, 20], survivorship among the second cohort patients who did or did not receive corticosteroids was not statistically different. These data, coupled with a prospective, randomized trial [21] at our institution that also failed to show a beneficial effect of corticosteroids in PCP, leave us unable to prove the value of this therapy.

Although no apparent demographic, clinical, or therapeutic variables accounted for the changing outcome, the possibility of a change in the *Pneumocystis carinii* organisms or in host factors such as immunologic status still must be considered. But whether or not such a secular trend exists, the short term programs for AIDS patients who require mechanical ventilation clearly has improved. The most dramatic sign of this improvement is that patients and physicians at SFGH and UCSF appear more optimistic about the outcome of intensive care for patients with severe PCP. Presumably as a reflection of this new consensus, ICU admissions of such patients at SFGH have increased fourfold in recent years (Fig. 4).

Awareness of the improved short term prognosis of AIDS patients with PCP who require mechanical ventilation may be primarily responsible for this new pattern of intensive care utilization, but it comes at a time when attitudes about AIDS in general also have changed. Once a mystery that defied medical investigation, AIDS now is extensively studied and reasonably well-understood. And

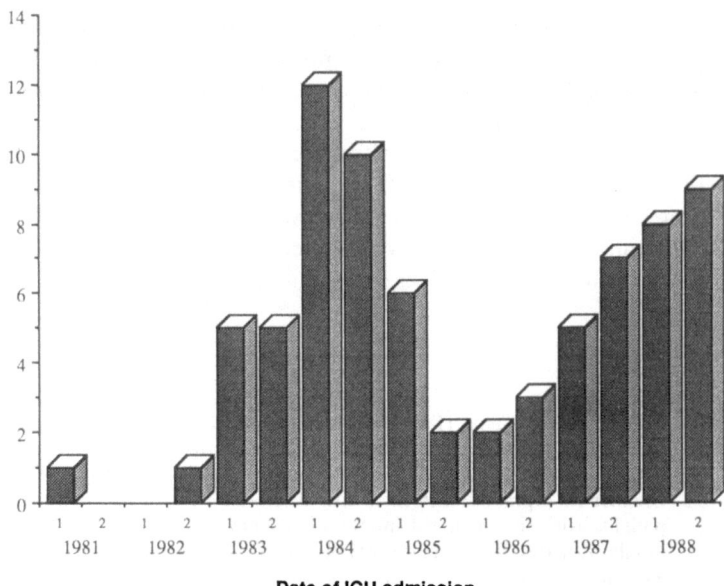

Date of ICU admission

Fig. 4. Intensive care unit (ICU) admissions for *Pneumocystis carinii* pneumonia and respiratory failure at San Francisco General Hospital, 1981–1988

although it still kills some patients quickly, AIDS is seen by many as a chronic condition that can be treated, if not yet cured. Indeed, AIDS increasingly is regarded as the most extreme manifestation of infection with the human immunodeficiency virus (HIV), and asymptomatic HIV carriers are receiving prophylaxis with zidovudine, aerosolized pentamidine, and other therapies once reserved for AIDS patients. In the words of a *San Francisco Chronicle* article recently written, for all HIV-infected patients "the struggle now is to stay alive."

How this struggle impacts upon the ICUs at SFGH and other hospitals in the United States has yet to be determined. One possibility is that anti-HIV and anti-PCP prophylaxis will lead to a decrease in ICU admissions. Equally possible is that those AIDS patients who do develop PCP will be more immunologically deplete and therefore require more intensive care. But whatever scenario unfolds, it seems likely that a large number of the 20,000 or more San Franciscans who already are infected with HIV will be candidates for intubation and mechanical ventilation in the future. And given current attitudes about the treatability of AIDS, we expect that many of these patients and their physicians will seek admission to the ICUs at SFGH.

From the start of the AIDS epidemic, we have argued that patients with severe PCP should be informed of their options regarding the use of life-sustaining treatments and allowed to make their own choices [10, 22, 23]. Although it is ethically permissible for physicians not to offer these treatments if doing so would be futile, the new data from our and other institutions suggest that intensive care for AIDS patients with severe respiratory failure due to PCP cannot be described as such. Nor can physicians overlook the fact that ICU admission still is routinely afforded to patients with other conditions, including those mentioned earlier, whose short term prognosis may be poorer than that of patients with AIDS. Unless further research indicates that the improved outcome of AIDS patients with severe PCP is not sustained, or unless rationing of intensive care services to all patients with poor long term prognoses is enacted, we believe that ICU utilization for AIDS patients will markedly increase in the United States. Given that 1,500,000 Americans are already infected with HIV, the clinical, ethical, and economic consequences of this increase will be a major challenge in the years ahead.

References

1. Kovacs JA, Hiemenz HW, Macher AM, et al (1984) Pneumocystis carinii pneumonia: a comparison between patients with the acquired immunodeficiency syndrome and patients with other immunodeficiencies. Ann Intern Med 100:663-671
2. Brenner M, Ognibene FP, Lack EE, et al (1987) Prognostic factors and life expectancy of patients with the acquired immunodeficiency syndrome and Pneumocystis carinii pneumonia. Am Rev Respir Dis 136:1199-1220
3. Zaman MK, White DA (1988) Serum lactate dehydrogenase levels and Pneumocystis carinii pneumonia. Diagnostic and prognostic significance. Am Rev Respir Dis 137:796-800
4. Schuster DP, Marion JM (1983) Precedents for meaningful recovery during treatment in a medical intensive care unit: outcome in patients with hematologic malignancy. Am J Med 75:402-408
5. Crawford SW, Schwartz DA, Petersen FB, Clark JG (1988) Mechanical ventilation after marrow transplantation: risk factors and clinical outcome. Am Rev Respir Dis 137:682-687
6. Murray JF, Garay SM, Hopewell PC, Mills J, Snider GL, Stover DG (1987) NHLBI Workshop summary: pulmonary complications of the acquired immunodeficiency syndrome: an update. Am Rev Respir Dis 135:504-509
7. Stover DE, White DA, Romano PA, Gellene RA, Robeson WA (1985) Spectrum of pulmonary diseases associated with the acquired immunodeficiency syndrome. Am J Med 78:429-437
8. Schein RM, Fischl MA, Pitchenik AE, Sprung CL (1986) ICU survival of patients with the acquired immunodeficiency syndrome. Crit Care Med 14:1026-1027
9. Rosen MJ, Cucco RA, Teirstein AS (1986) Outcome of intensive care in patients with the acquired immunodeficiency syndrome. J Int Care 1:55-60
10. Wachter RM, Luce JM, Turner J, Volberding P, Hopewell PC (1986) Intensive care of patients with the acquired immunodeficiency syndrome: outcome and changing patterns of utilization. Am Rev Respir Dis 134:891-896
11. Baggott LA, Baggott BB (1987) Pneumocystis carinii pneumonia in AIDS patients in intensive care (abstract). Chest 92:132S
12. Steinbrook R, Lo B, Moulton J, Saika G, Hollander H, Volberding PA (1986) Preferences of homosexual men with AIDS for life-sustaining treatment. N Engl J Med 314:457-460
13. Wachter RM, Cooke M, Hopewell PC, Luce JM (1988) Attitudes of medical residents regarding intensive care for patients with the acquired immunodeficiency syndrome. Arch Intern Med 148:149-152
14. Wachter RM, Luce JM, Hearst N, Lo B (1989) Decisions about resuscitation: inequities among patients with different diseases but similar prognoses. Ann Intern Med 111:525-532
15. El-Sadr W, Simberkoff MS (1988) Survival and prognostic factors in severe Pneumocystis carinii pneumonia requiring mechanical ventilation. Am Rev Respir Dis 137:1264-1267
16. Montaner JSG, Russell JA, Ruedy J, Lawson L (1989) Acute respiratory failure secondary to Pneumocystis carinii pneumonia in the acquired immunodeficiency syndrome: a potential role for systemic corticosteroids. Chest 95:881-884

17. Friedman Y, Franklin C, Rackow EC, Weil MH (1989) Improved survival in patients with acquired immunodeficiency syndrome, Pneumocystis carinii pneumonia, and severe respiratory failure. Chest (in press)
18. Rogers PL, Lane HC, Henderson DK, Parrillo J, Masur H (1989) Admission of AIDS patients to a medical intensive care unit: causes and outcome. Crit Care Med 17:113-117
19. Wachter RM, Russi MB, Hopewell PC, Luce JM (1989) The improving survival rate after intensive care for P. carinii pneumonia and respiratory failure (abstract). Fifth International Conference on AIDS, Montreal, Canada
20. Mac Fadden DK, Hyland RH, Inouye T, Edelson JD, Rodriguez CH, Rebuck AS (1987) Corticosteroids as adjunctive therapy in treatment of Pneumocystis carinii pneumonia in patients with acquired immunodeficiency syndrome. Lancet 2:1477-1479
21. Clement M, Edison R, Turner J, et al (1989) Corticosteroids as adjunctive therapy in severe Pneumocystis carinii pneumonia. A prospective placebo-controlled trial. Am Rev Respir Dis 139:A250
22. Wachter RM, Luce JM, Turner J, Volberding P, Hopewell PC (1986) Intensive care of patients with the acquired immunodeficiency syndrome: outcome and changing patterns of utilization. Am Rev Resp Dis 134:891-896
23. Wachter RM, Luce JM, Lo B, Raffin TA (1989) Life-sustaining treatment for patients with AIDS. Chest 95:647-652

Intensive Care for HIV Infected Patients: The View from Brussels St Pierre Hospital

P. Hermans, M. C. Payen, and P. Dechamps

Introduction

The role of ICU management in HIV infected patients is not easy to define. In the earlier stage of the epidemic, the very high mortality of the patients in spite of aggressive resuscitation technique, has led the AIDS physicians to consider ICU admission with reluctance. By now, a change in attitude has occured, and is mostly due to the improved prognosis and the lower morbidity of HIV infection when Zidovudine (AZT) therapy is possible.

We report our experience with HIV infected patients admitted into ICU at St Pierre University Hospital in Brussels. Moreover, major advances have been achieved in treating severe opportunistic infections except for atypical mycobacterial infections or cryptosporidiosis. Primary and secondary prophylaxis associated with better methods of diagnosis could also increase the survival of patients with AIDS. Nevertheless, the medical staff of institutions caring for a great number of patients with AIDS must define their attitudes regarding ICU utilization.

Patients

St Pierre University Hospital, Brussels, is one of the leading centers in Belgium treating 40 to 45% of all AIDS cases. Initially our HIV population consisted of the epidemic on African cases [1] and now mostly of homosexuals (39%), heterosexuals (41%), intravenous drug users (13%). Since 1987, treatment with AZT has been proposed to all our AIDS cases after acute treatment of their opportunistic infection. In addition, AZT therapy is also proposed to patients with severe AIDS-related conditions and low lymphocytes T4 cells level (less than 200 cells/mm^3). Therefore, two periods can be defined in the management of HIV infected patients: before AZT (1982–1986) and after AZT (1987–1989) [2].

To assess the importance of intensive care in the management of HIV infected patients, we reviewed the records of all HIV seropositive patients who were admitted to our ICU between January 1, 1982 and November 15, 1989. We defined demographic data, clinical manifestations, HIV staging following the CDC classification, ICU admission criteria, therapeutic requirements and clinical outcome.

A total of 46 patients were admitted to the ICU, 29 men (28 caucasians and 1 black) and 17 women (2 caucasians and 15 blacks). Among the men, there were 22 homosexuals, 2 transfused, 4 heterosexuals and 1 IV drug user. Among the women, 15 were contaminated through heterosexual contact, 1 was transfused and 1 was IV drug user. The mean age was 39 years (median 36.5 – range: 20 to 71). There were 38 AIDS patients (CDC IV, B, C1, D, E), 3 ARC patients (CDC IV, A, C2), 5 CDC II and III and 1 patient who presented an HIV seroconversion. One patient was admitted three times and 3 patients were admitted twice. We have thus records of 51 ICU admissions. Reasons for admission were respiratory failure (17, 33%), neurological problems (15, 29%), postoperative surveillance (6, 12%), hypovolemic or septic shock (7, 13%), metabolic problems (1, 2%), suicide attempts (4, 8%) and CIVD (1, 2%). One patient was admitted 3 times for respiratory failure and died during the third hospitalisation. The 3 patients who were admitted twice had various admission criteria and did not die during their hospitalisation.

Results

The diagnoses made during the hospitalisation are summarized in the Table 1. It is striking to note that Pneumocystis carinii pneumopathy was not the first diagnosis. This is due to the type of population, characterized by an elevated rate of cerebral toxoplasmosis and esophageal candidiasis.

Among the 46 patients, 13 (27%) died in the ICU and 33 patients were discharged. Among those 33 patients, 7 (14%) died in the hospital and 26 (55%) left

Table 1. Diagnosis of HIV related conditions

Diagnosis	No. of Patients
Opportunistic Infections and Cancers	
– Pneumocystis carinii pneumopathy	10 (19%)
– Esophageal candidiasis	12 (23%)
– Cerebral toxoplasmosis	11 (21%)
– Severe mucocutaneous herpes	10 (19%)
– Cryptococcal meningitis	4 (8%)
– Tuberculosis (generalized and pulmonary)	10 (19%)
– Kaposi's sarcoma	2 (4%)
– Lymphoma	2 (4%)
– Miscellaneous	3 (6%)
Other Conditions	
– Pyogenic pneumopathies	9 (18%)
– Septicemia	5 (10%)
– Pyogenic meningitis	2 (4%)
– Neuro-syphilis	1 (2%)
– Suicide attempts	2 (4%)
– Arterial embolism	3 (6%)
– Cerebral angioma	1 (2%)
– Extradural hematoma	1 (2%)

the hospital. Thus the overall mortality rate is 41%. Among the survivors, 8 (17%) were lost of follow up, 8 (17%) are still alive and 11 (24%) died within a median period of 16 months.

The immediate cause of death can be summarized as follows: respiratory failure under mechanical ventilation (4, 20%), neurological problems (4, 20%), postoperative complications (1, 5%), shock (1, 5%) and "multiple organ failure" (10, 50%).

We also reviewed the management in the ICU: among the 51 admissions, there were 18 intubations (35%), 30 central venous catheter (60%) and 4 Swan-Ganz catheters (8%), 3 radial catheters (6%), 38 urinary bladder catheterism (73%), 18 enteral nutrition (35%), 13 surgical procedures (26%) and 1 parenteral nutrition (2%). Interestingly the physician decided to discontinue the ICU management in 9 patients with uncontrolled multiple organ failure.

The two periods of time, before and after availability of AZT therapy (1982–1986 vs 1987–1989), were compared. During the first period, 19 patients were admitted into the ICU (4 respiratory failures, 6 neurological problems and 9 others), 6 were intubated and 5 died. During the second period, there were 32 admissions (13 respiratory failures, 9 neurological problems and 10 others), 12 were intubated and 15 patients died. There was no statistically significant difference for any parameter (Table 2). Since the total number of hospitalisations was not recorded before 1987, we were unable to calculate the rate of ICU admission before and after the introduction of AZT.

Discussion

Our results show a lower mortality rate of HIV infected patients in the ICU than reported by other centers [3–5]. This could be related to an improvement of the therapeutic armamentarium or to a bias in the recruitment of our patients.

Recent data suggest that the prognosis can be linked to the type of hospital. Indeed, among American hospitals, patients are better managed by physicians who have a greater experience of the disease [6]. In this setting, St Pierre University Hospital has the most important Belgian AIDS unit characterized by a multidisciplinary approach [7], which could have provided optimal patient care.

Table 2. ICU admissions according to the period before and after zidovudine availability

	1982–1986	1987–1989	Total
Causes of admission			
– Respiratory failure	4	13	17
– Neurologic disorders	6	9	15
– Other causes	9	10	19
Patients under mechanical ventilation	6	12	18
In-hospital mortality	5	15	20
Mean duration in ICU (days)	11	8	9

In addition, major progress in early diagnosis of infections (such as Pneumocystis carinii by immunofluorscence) and alternative therapies for opportunistic infections have been recently introduced. Indeed corticoids are increasingly used in PCP with severe respiratory failure [8]. Even if the benefit has not been proved by extended controlled trials, the great majority of our severely ill patients received corticoids in uncontrolled manner.

Admittedly, some of our ICU patients were only moderately disabled by conditions such as suicide attempts, postoperative states and transient metabolic disturbances. It we exclude these patients (13 out 51 admissions), the mortality rate is 50%. If only mechanically ventilated patients are considered, we find that 13 of these 20 patients died (65%). This mortality rate is similar to those of other centers [3–5].

Since 1987, due to the availability of antiretroviral drugs and particularly Zidovudine, the decision regarding ICU admission for HIV patients has been reconsidered. Indeed, under AZT therapy, the median survival has been prolonged from 8 to 22 months. This longer survival among AZT treated patients is observed after PCP but also after cerebral toxoplasmosis [9] (the two most life-threatening opportunistic infections among AIDS patients).

Although a better management of patients with AIDS has been achieved, it remains a fatal disease. Physicians and health care workers must take in account the ethical problems and the emotional charge of the management of these patients. Several studies have attempted to define a rational use of ICU based upon objective variables. Nonetheless, these attitudes may change during time according to new therapeutic approaches. The first major study published on ICU utilization for patients with AIDS has been performed at the San Francisco General Hospital (SFGH). Between March 1981 and December 1985, 82 patients were admitted to the ICU. The overall in-hospital mortality of the patients with AIDS admitted to the ICUs (4 units with a total bed capacity of 38) was 69%. Death rate of AIDS patients in the ICU was 52% compared with 12% of the other patients admitted during the same period. Indications for intensive care were: 45 (52%) patients with respiratory failure required mechanical ventilation, 4 (5%) patients presented with other opportunistic lung infections and were intubated, 9 (10%) patients with a Pneumocystis carinii who did not require assisted ventilation, 9 (10%) patients after surgical procedures and 19 (24%) patients admitted for different reasons (sepsis, hypotension, seizure, drug overdose, asthma, ...) for a total of 86 admissions for 82 patients. It clearly appeared that mortality rate was higher in the subgroup of patients requiring mechanical ventilation (87%) than among patients without mechanical ventilation (43%). During the study period, the rates of ICU to hospital admissions for AIDS patients firstly increased to 15% but subsequently decreased to 3%.

The experience at the SFGH is summarized in the results of a questionnaire on physician attitudes toward ICU care completed by 76% of their medical house staff. Seventy-three percent of the physicians estimated that intubation for AIDS patients with Pneumocystis carinii pneumonia and respiratory failure is never or rarely indicated. Moreover, 89% of the clinicians would discuss ICU care with the patients whenever possible on admission or as soon as possible.

A French study published in 1987 showed similar results. Between January 1982 and August 1986, 150 patients with HIV infection were admitted to the ICU (166 admissions). The overall in-hospital mortality rate was also 69% and 52% of the patients died on the ICU. Indications for intensive care were not defined for the whole group. The average duration in the ICU was 23.5 days. Mechanical ventilation was required for 94 patients (57%). Only mechanical ventilation and a prolonged duration in hospital before ICU admission (more than 8 days) were associated with a higher in-hospital mortality rate: 88% and 70% respectively.

Two studies [8, 10] led to reassess the physician's pessimistic attitude on intensive care for AIDS patients with Pneumocystis carinii pneumonia (PCP) and respiratory failure. Moreover, the authors of the editorial underlined the better knowledge of the disease, the earlier recognition of PCP, the improvement of the armamentarium, the potential benefit of corticosteroids, the benefit of Zidovudine administration and the therapeutic advantages of prophylaxis on the survival. They concluded that the AIDS physicians may have better reasons than ever for recommending ICU utilization for AIDS patients with opportunistic lung infections.

All these changes could partially explain the lack of significant differences in ICU admissions when we compared the periods before and after availability of AZT therapy.

However, ICU management should consider life expectancy and patient's confort. We think that patients who are at the very end-stage of their disease (generalised Kaposi's sarcoma, profuse uncontrolled Cryptosporidium diarrhea, bilateral blindness, ...) should be allowed to die with dignity, with the support of family and friends.

Acknowledgements: The authors thank B. Sommereijns for her help in data management and comments on statistical analysis, Prof. N. Clumeck (Division of Infections Diseases) and Prof. A. Cornil (Division of Intensive Care) from St Pierre University Hospital, Brussels, Belgium.

References

1. Clumeck N, Sonnet J, Taelman H (1984) Acquired immunodeficiency syndrome in African patients. N Engl J Med 310:492–497
2. Weerts D, Cauchie E, De Wit S, Clumeck N (June 1988) One year experience on azidothymidine administered 6 hourly in 40 patients with AIDS or AIDS-related complex. IV International Conference on AIDS, Stockholm. Abstract No 3604
3. Wachter RM, Luce JM, Turner J, Volberding P, Hopewell C (1986) Intensive care of patients with the AIDS. Am Rev Respir Dis 134:891–896
4. Luce JM, Wachter M, Hopewell C (1988) Intensive care of patients with the AIDS. Time of reassessment. Am Rev Respir Dis 137:1261–1263
5. Regnier B, Wolff M, Katlama C (1987) Résultats et limites de la réanimation chez les patients atteints de SIDA. In: Goulon M (ed) Réanimation et médecine d'urgence. Expansion Scientifique Française, Paris, France, pp 274–283
6. Bennet CL, Garfinkle JB, Greenfield S, et al (1989) The relation between hospital experience and in-hospital mortality for patients with AIDS-related PCP. JAMA 261:2975–2979

7. Clumeck N, Hermans P, De Wit S (1988) Current problems in the management of AIDS patients. Eur J Clin Microbial Infect Dis 7:2–10
8. Gallacher P, Gallacher W, Mc Fadden D (1989) Treatment of acute Pneumocysits carinii pneumonia with corticosteroids in a patient with acquired immunodeficiency syndrome. Crit Care Med 17:104–105
9. Clumeck N, De Wit S, Hermans P, Magrez P (1988) The benefit of Zidovudine on the long-term survival of AIDS patients with CNS toxoplasmosis. 28th ICAAC, Los Angeles, USA, Abs No 1474, pp 372
10. El-Sadr W, Simberkoff MS (1988) Survival and prognostic factors in severe Pneumocystis carinii pneumonia requiring mechanical ventilation. Am Rev Respir Dis 137:1264–1267

Intensive Care for Complications of Malignant Disease: Presentation and Outcome

C. J. Hinds and E. H. S. Yau

Introduction

In recent years there have been many important advances in the management of malignant disease and as a result cancer is no longer inevitably fatal. Although there have been some significant developments in the management of solid tumors, the most dramatic improvements in long term outcome have been seen in patients with hematological and lymphoreticular malignancies, a significant proportion of whom can now be cured with aggressive chemotherapy [1, 2]. There have also been important improvements in supportive care; in particular the administration of platelet concentrates has reduced the incidence of fatal thrombocytopenic hemorrhage and the development of specialist nursing techniques, combined with the more effective use of anti-microbial agents has greatly reduced the mortality from intercurrent infection.

Patients with malignant disease are prone to a wide variety of acute life-threatening disturbances related either to the effects of the tumor or to complications of its treatment. Dangerous complications directly caused by the tumor include pleural or pericardial effusions, renal failure induced by ureteric compression, pancytopenia due to marrow invasion, airway obstruction, metabolic disturbances (eg, uremia or hypercalcemia), various neurological syndromes and massive hemorrhage from an ulcerated lesion. Infection is the commonest life-threatening complication of treatment and is usually a result of immunosuppression caused by chemotherapy, radiotherapy or steroids. Sometimes bleeding, most often due to thrombocytopenia caused by bone marrow suppression, is of sufficient severity to warrant admission to an intensive care unit. Other dangerous complications of anti-cancer treatment which are encountered less frequently on the intensive care unit include cardiomyopathy induced by irradiation or cytotoxic agents, pulmonary fibrosis related to chemotherapy or radiotherapy, graft versus host (GVH) reactions and tumor lysis syndrome. Recently a case of multiple organ failure has been described following the administration of interleukin-2 and lymphokine-activated killer cells for the treatment of metastatic hypernephroma [3].

The majority of these disorders are potentially reversible and in view of the improved long term prognosis it is appropriate to admit selected cases to the intensive care unit, provided that the prospects for cure or worthwhile palliation of the underlying malignancy are considered to be reasonable.

Patients with malignant disease may also benefit from elective admission to the intensive care unit (ICU) following extensive surgical procedures such as pelvic exenteration, total cystectomy, pulmonary resection, esophago-gastrectomy and partial hepatectomy, particularly if they are high risk cases by virtue of co-existent medical disorders. Intensive care may also be required for complications developing postoperatively.

Clinical Presentation of Critically Ill Patients with Malignant Disease

Although a significant proportion of patients admitted to general ICU will have malignant disease (23% in one series) the majority of such cases are surgical and only a small percentage (less than 6%) will have life threatening complications of hematological malignancy [4, 5].

Infection

Overwhelming infection is a frequent complication and an important cause of death in patients with cancer [6], particularly those with hematological malignancy [7], in whom it is the commonest factor precipitating admission to the ICU [5, 8, 9].

The increased susceptibility of patients with malignancy to infection may be related to reduced or abnormal granulocytes, decreased antibody production, impaired cellular immunity or a combination of these factors. Moreover mucocutaneous barriers in the alimentary canal and tracheobronchial tree can be disrupted by treatment with cytotoxic agents, drainage tracts may become obstructed by tumor, the patient is often subjected to a variety of invasive procedures and colonisation with gram negative organisms, as well as fungi, is encouraged by antibiotic treatment. In general immune competence is relatively intact prior to treatment and the majority of those with impaired cellular and humoral immunity have received chemotherapy, radiotherapy or corticosteroids.

Neutropenia is by far the most important cause of impaired immunity in patients with hematological malignancy and there is an inverse correlation between the granulocyte count and both the incidence and the severity of infection [10]. Although the incidence of infectious complications increases as the granulocyte count falls below $1 \cdot 10^9/L$ it is not until the count is less than $0.5 \cdot 10^9/L$ that the risk rises dramatically. The mortality rate from infection is related both to the duration of the neutropenia and to whether the neutrophil count rises or falls [7], a factor which also seems to have an important influence on outcome in those receiving intensive care [8]. The most pronounced immune suppression is seen in patients in relapse, probably largely as a result of previous courses of chemotherapy. Bone marrow transplantation is now established as a useful form of treatment for some patients with acute leukemia but is a technique associated with an extremely high risk of infectious complications.

The commonest sites of infection in immunocompromised patients are the lung, and mucosal surfaces; frequently infection is disseminated with bacterial or fungal septicemia [6]. Infections of the central nervous system are unusual,

except in those with impaired cell mediated immunity who may develop crypto-
coccal meningitis, but they may occur secondary to a generalised bacteremia
(especially due to Staph. aureus) or fungemia. Genitourinary infections are also
infrequent except in patients with pelvic tumors, the elderly and those with urinary catheters.

Septic Shock

Hypotension is second only to respiratory failure (see below) as a cause of admission of cancer patients to the ICU. Although in a few cases the fall in blood
pressure is precipitated by complications such as gastrointestinal hemorrhage or
cardiac failure, by far the most frequent diagnosis is septic shock [5, 9, 11, 12]. In
our series of 60 patients with hematological malignancy 39 had septic shock,
most often in association with respiratory failure [8], and in a group of adult
patients dying with acute leukemia the overall incidence of fatal bacterial septicemia was 47% [6]. The commonest source of infection is the lung [6], although
occasionally septic shock occurs without pulmonary involvement in which case
it may originate from the gastrointestinal tract, the genito-urinary tract, the skin
or the soft tissues. In some cases the site of infection cannot be identified.

Respiratory Failure

In one series of patients dying with neoplastic disease respiratory failure was the
primary cause of death in 19% and respiratory insufficiency (including aspiration) was a contributory factor in a further 3% [13]; as might be anticipated,
respiratory failure is the commonest indication for the admission of patients
with malignant disease to an ICU [5, 8, 9, 14, 15]. Although respiratory failure
does occur in patients with solid tumors, particularly carcinomas of the lung
and, less frequently, the breast, it is seen most often in those with hematological
malignancies [16–18] and is the commonest acute complication of bone marrow
transplantation requiring intensive therapy [19].

The lung appears to be particularly susceptible to infection during periods of
immunosuppressive chemotherapy [20] and by far the commonest cause of respiratory failure in cancer patients is pneumonia [5, 8, 16, 21]. Similarly pneumonia
is a common complication of bone marrow transplantation and the more widespread use of aggressive chemotherapy for the treatment of solid tumors has led
to an increased incidence of pulmonary complications in these patients. Mortality rates are high when patients with hematological malignancy develop lung
infiltrates and pneumonia complicating bone marrow transplantation is also associated with a high mortality [20, 22].

Non-infectious causes of respiratory failure in patients with malignant disease
include chemotherapy induced lung damage, radiation pneumonitis, infiltration
of the lungs with tumor cells, pulmonary leukostasis, intrapulmonary hemorrhage, pulmonary edema and pulmonary embolus. Tracheo-bronchial compression by tumor can produce life-threatening airway obstruction requiring me-

chanical ventilation and this is often precipitated by diagnostic surgical procedures, such as mediastinotomy, performed under general anesthesia. Very occasionally transtracheal aspiration in a patient with a coagulopathy can precipitate uncontrollable hemorrhage with hematoma formation and tracheal compression of sufficient severity to require emergency endotracheal intubation or tracheostomy. In some patients pleural effusions, fluid overload or cardiac failure [5] may contribute to the onset of respiratory failure, while others require mechanical ventilation for postoperative respiratory insufficiency.

Standard techniques, including transtracheal aspiration, often fail to establish the etiology of lung disease in immunosuppressed patients, particularly in those with diffuse bilateral involvement. If the patient fails to respond to empirical antimicrobial therapy more invasive measures are therefore often undertaken in an attempt to establish the diagnosis. This may involve percutaneous needle aspiration, needle biopsy, trephine drill biopsy, transbronchial lung biopsy or open lung biopsy. The hazards of such procedures are increased in many patients with malignant disease because of associated problems such as thrombocytopenia, coagulopathy, poor lung function and impaired tissue healing [23]. There is also a risk of pneumothorax which may precipitate respiratory failure requiring admission to the ICU [8].

In mechanically ventilated patients with respiratory failure open lung biopsy is probably the most reliable means of establishing the diagnosis (a specific diagnosis can be established in about 70% of immunosuppressed patients with pulmonary infiltrates) [23] and is probably the safest technique. Although there is a significant risk of pneumothorax, hemostasis can be secured under direct vision and with the use of automatic stapling devices the likelihood of postoperative intrapleural hemorrhage is negligible [24]. Morbidity and mortality directly attributable to open lung biopsy is low [24]. In one series [24] pneumothorax was seen in only 7%, and there were no cases of persistent air leak, while wound dehiscence and hemoptysis each ocurred in only 1 patient (2%). Prolonged mechanical ventilation was required for respiratory failure which was present preoperatively in 14 of 42 patients. Although the deaths of 2 patients might have been hastened, none could be directly attributed to the surgical procedure.

In many cases patients are admitted to the ICU with a diagnosis of adult respiratory distress syndrome (ARDS) [12, 14, 16]. The development of this clinical syndrome in cancer patients is most often related to pulmonary infection, systemic sepsis and/or disseminated intravascular coagulation; occasionally pulmonary aspiration is implicated. ARDS may also follow aggressive chemotherapy and is probably related to the release of a variety of mediators from necrotic tumor cells, sometimes combined with the development of disseminated intravascular coagulation [25]. Often this situation is accompanied by other manifestations of the 'tumor lysis syndrome' (see below). Some would include radiation pneumonitis, chemotherapy induced lung damage, diffuse pulmonary infiltration with tumor and extensive intraparenchymal hemorrhage as causes of ARDS. Acute respiratory distress has also been described as a complication of hyperleucocytic granulocytic leukemias [26] and treatment of leukemia with cytosine arabinoside has been implicated in the development of a frequently fatal non-cardiogenic pulmonary edema [27].

Patients with malignant disease who develop acute respiratory failure are more susceptible to sepsis than those without cancer [17] and pneumonia is commonly associated with septicemia. In our series [8] 50 of the 60 patients with hematological malignancy admitted to the ICU were in respiratory failure; 9 had pneumonia alone, 3 pneumonia complicated by pneumothoraces which had occurred after endoscopic transbronchial biopsy and 34 – that is more than half the total number of patients – had both pneumonia and septicemic shock. Although the patient may be admitted with respiratory failure, death is usually associated with progressive and intractable hypotension [5], often accompanied by coagulation disorders, acidosis and multiple organ failure [21].

Hemorrhage

Hemorrhage is a common cause of acute deterioration in patients with malignancy. This is particularly true for those with acute leukemia in whom hemorrhage contributes to 23% of deaths [6] and precipitates 16% of ICU admissions [28]. In one series of patients with all types of cancer, bleeding was the cause of death in 11% and a contributory factor in a further 25% [13]. There are a number of causes of the increased susceptibility of patients with malignancy to bleeding including thrombocytopenia, platelet dysfunction, disseminated intravascular coagulation, coagulation factor abnormalities, vitamin K deficiency and liver impairment.

Metabolic Disturbances

Tumor Lysis Syndrome: Treatment of sensitive tumors with cytotoxic agents can produce rapid lysis of malignant cells, resulting in severe hyperuricemia, hyperphosphatemia, hyperkalemia, hypocalcemia, metabolic acidosis, acute renal failure, and, in some cases, ARDS. The syndrome is most frequently seen in those with lymphoid malignancies and acute lymphoblastic leukemia, especially of the Burkitt type.

Hypercalcemia: This may occur in up to 10% of patients with malignant disease [29], although the incidence varies depending on the type of malignancy. It is particularly common in those with squamous cell carcinoma of the bronchus, breast cancer and hematological malignancies (especially multiple myeloma and lymphomas). Although the disorder is potentially life-threatening, it is easily diagnosed and normally readily reversible; admission to ICU is usually unnecessary.

Primary Cardiovascular Disturbances

These are responsible for the death of about 7% of cancer patients [13]. A variety of complications of malignancy, or its treatment, can precipitate acute disorders of cardiovascular function, many of which can be life-threatening and may therefore warrant admission to the ICU.

Superior Vena Cava Obstruction (SVCO): This dangerous medical emergency is caused by mediastinal tumor extension, most often bronchogenic carcinoma or, less frequently malignant lymphoma. With aggressive management (initially with steroids, followed by radiotherapy or, less often, chemotherapy) 25% of patients who present with SVCO survive at least 1 year [30].

Cardiac Tamponade: This is a rare but potentially lethal complication of malignancy, usually due to direct involvement of the pericardium by metastatic tumor. The commonest causes are bronchogenic carcinoma and breast cancer, although, rarely, a primary tumor of the pericardium may be responsible. Irradiation of the chest may also occasionally be complicated by the formation of a pericardial effusion.

Constrictive Pericarditis: This may be caused by local tumor extension around the heart or may follow radiotherapy.

Arrhythmias: Some cytotoxic agents can precipitate acute arrhythmias, especially in patients with pre-existing cardiac disorders. Adriamycin and Amsacrine (m-AMSA) are most often implicated.

Cardiomyopathy: A more serious complication of treatment with adriamycin is the development of a cardiomyopathy; the mortality is high. Cyclophosphamide is a commonly used alkylator, which is not cardiotoxic in standard doses. With the larger doses now being used in patients undergoing bone marrow transplantation, however, delayed cardiotoxicity has been reported.

Gastrointestinal Disorders

Acute gastroenterological problems may be due to the direct effects of the tumor, complications of treatment or infection.

Intra abdominal tumors may cause bowel obstruction, perforation or hemorrhage, and the management of these is usually surgical. Treatment with chemotherapy or radiotherapy may also precipitate perforation or hemorrhage, especially if the bowel wall was previously infiltrated with tumor. Chemotherapy induced toxicity may also manifest as severe diarrhea or a paralytic ileus, the latter being well described following vincristine.

Neutropenic enterocolitis is a recently recognized complication in patients undergoing aggressive chemotherapy for neoplastic diseases, especially hematological malignancies. Inflammation and damage to the bowel wall seem to be caused by a variety of factors, including cytotoxic agents, leukemic infiltration and bacterial invasion [31]. In one autopsy series 10-12% of leukemic patients were found to have histological evidence of neutopenic enterocolitis [31].

Renal Disorders

There are many causes of acute renal failure in patients with neoplastic disease and these are listed in Table 1. Patients with isolated renal impairment will not usually require admission to an ICU.

Neurological Disorders

A variety of acute neurological disturbances may arise in patients with malignant disease (Table 2) but these are a relatively unusual cause of admission to intensive care.

Hyperviscosity Syndrome

Increased blood viscosity may occur in patients with Waldenstrom macroglobulinemia and myeloma, and can cause mucosal bleeding, neurological disturbances, retinopathy and cardiac failure. Plasma exchange can be life-saving but patients will not necessarily require admission to an ICU.

Table 1. Causes of renal impairment in patients with malignancy

Pre-renal	– Hypovolemia:
	Hemorrhage
	Dehydration
	– Circulatory collapse
	– Renal vascular obstruction
Renal	– Tumor infiltration
	– Complications of tumors:
	Paraproteinemia: myeloma
	Hypercalcemia
	Immune complex disease
	Disseminated intravascular coagulation
	Hyperuricemia
	– Treatment related:
	Cisplatin
	Methotrexate
	Antibiotics (especially aminoglycosides)
	Tumor lysis syndrome
	Radiation nephritis
	– Septicemia
Post-renal	– Obstructive:
	Bladder outlet
	Urethral
	Ureteric
	Retroperitoneal fibrosis

Table 2. Causes of neurological disturbances in patients with malignancy

Direct effect:	Intracranial tumors
	Spinal tumors
	Leptomeningeal syndromes
Remote:	Paraneoplastic syndromes
Infective:	Abscess
	Meningoencephalitis
Vascular:	Hemorrhage
	Thrombosis
Treatment-related:	Radiotherapy
	Chemotherapy
	– Systemic: peripheral
	neuropathy
	– Intrathecal: convulsions
	arachnoiditis
	encephalopathy

Graft Versus Host Disease

More intensive treatment with higher doses of cytotoxic agents and radiotherapy, often in association with bone marrow transplantation has been increasingly used in the past decade in an attempt to increase tumor cell kill. This has been accompanied by an increased incidence of complications, including the development of graft vs host disease (GVHD) in those who have received allogeneic transplants. GVHD may present acutely or in a more chronic form. Clinically the patient suffers from severe skin rashes, florid diarrhea and hepatic adnormalities. In some cases there is progressive airway obstruction with acute bronchitis or bronchospasm and an increased risk of lower respiratory tract infection. Recently it has been recognized that a progressive, necrotizing bronchiolitis obliterans may occur in association with chronic GVHD [22]. The incidence of GVHD varies, but may be as high as 45–75%, and the mortality is significant.

Postoperative Intensive Care

The extensive surgical procedures now sometimes undertaken as part of the radical treatment of cancer are inevitably associated with considerable postoperative morbidity and mortality. Pelvic exenteration, for example, is a prolonged and traumatic procedure, frequently accompanied by considerable blood loss; many therefore recommend routine postoperative intensive care for such cases [32–34] and it has been suggested that such a policy can contribute to significant reductions in mortality [32, 33]. The potential benefits of admitting cancer patients to an ICU following major surgery are the same as those for any high risk postoperative patient; they include continuous hemodynamic monitoring to assist optimal volume replacement and preserve renal function, the early identification of cardiovascular and respiratory disturbances and the availability of facilities for respiratory support, including mechanical ventilation. Moreover, the patient will receive constant skilled nursing care and effective analgesia can be assured [34].

Elective postoperative intensive care following major surgery is in most ICU the commonest indication for admitting patients with malignant disease. In one ICU in a major cancer hospital, just over 70% of admissions were from the surgical services and gastrointestinal, thoracic and urological surgery patients accounted for 56% of all admissions [11].

Outcome

As might be anticipated, mortality rates are high when patients with malignant disease develop an acute illness severe enough to warrant admission to an ICU [5, 8, 9, 11, 12, 14–19, 21, 35–37]. An overall hospital mortality rate of about 70–80% can be expected in patients admitted to ICU with acute complications of hematological malignancies [5, 8, 9, 12, 15] or bone marrow transplantation [9, 19]. In our series of 60 patients with life-threatening medical complications of hematological malignancy 22% (13 patients) survived to leave hospital but the median duration of survival of those who have since died was only 11 months (range 5 months–46 months). Nevertheless, five patients are still alive 8, 7, 6, 5 and 3 years after leaving hospital (giving an overall median survival time of 44 months).

Lower mortality rates (23–55%) have been reported in series which have included patients with all types of malignancy, including solid tumors [11, 14, 37], as well as surgical cases [4, 11]. Mortality will also be lower when significant numbers of patients with metabolic abnormalities are admitted, since most of these survive [14]. In a recent publication Sculier et al. [37] reported that 77% of cancer patients admitted to an ICU with medical emergencies survived. Their patient population was, however, unusual since the commonest causes of admission in descending order of frequency, were hypercalcemia, thromboembolic disease, cardiac arrhythmias, encephalopathies and 'diffuse pneumopathies'.

In-hospital mortality rates are particularly high (80–96%) when patients with malignant disease develop respiratory failure [5, 8, 9, 12, 14, 15, 17–19, 21, 36] and the long term prognosis for those who do survive to leave hospital is often poor [16, 35, 36]. In one series of cancer patients with respiratory failure 26% survived to be extubated but only 7% lived for six months or more [16] and in a group of patients with hematological malignancy the median duration of survival of the 18% who were discharged from hospital was 12 months [36]. In our series the hospital mortality of those with respiratory failure was identical to that of these latter authors (82%) but the median duration of survival was longer (44 months) including 2 patients who are still alive, 8 years and 6 years later. When patients with lung cancer require mechanical ventilation for respiratory failure the chances of long term survival are remote; Ewer et al. [35] reported that of 46 such patients 7 were weaned from ventilatory support and survived for at least 24 hours, but only 4 were discharged from hospital and of these 3 died within 4 months.

Not only are mortality rates high in critically ill cancer patients, but it must be recognized that in most cases transfer of a patient to the ICU involves a quantum increase in the commitment of resources, rather than simply a continuation of supportive care [11]. Moreover, the decision to institute intensive care crystallises fears of impending death and the prospect of removal to a strange environment with unfamiliar staff is frightening. Subsequently, the delivery of intensive care inevitably involves mental and physical distress for the patients and their relatives, especially when treatment is unsuccessful. Both for a humane approach to the management of malignant disease, and to ensure that limited resources are used appropriately, it is therefore important to select those patients most likely to benefit from ICU and to limit further extraordinary measures when the outlook is clearly hopeless. Such decisions can be extremely difficult, but should be based on the best possible understanding of the factors which determine both the immediate and long term outcome in critically ill patients with malignant disease. It is also important to consider the quality of life of survivors when evaluating the results of intensive care. Of the 5 patients in our series who are still alive 3 describe their health as good or very good, one as fair and only one as poor; 3 are working full-time, 1 is retired through age and all state that they would wish to receive intensive care again under similar circumstances. We also assessed the patients' perception of their quality of life using a previously described 11-item Perceived Quality of Life scale [38]. The median score in our 5 patients was 88 (range 49–94) which compares favourably with a mean score of 75 ± 18 in survivors from a general medical ICU and a mean score of 79 ± 14 obtained from a group of well elderly patients living in the community. These findings emphasise the importance of being able to identify those patients who might benefit from intensive care because those who do survive long-term may enjoy an excellent quality of life.

A number of authors have therefore attempted to identify features associated with a poor prognosis. For example, Poe et al. [39] found that in immunocompromised patients with pulmonary infiltrates the need for mechanical ventilation within 72 hours, an initial room air $PaO_2 < 50$ mmHg and corticosteroid therapy were the dominant independent variables, in that order, to significantly predict mortality. Indeed no patient survived who had a room air $PaO_2 < 50$ mmHg, was receiving corticosteroids and was mechanically ventilated. In patients with hematological disorders admitted to an ICU pneumonia, the necessity for mechanical ventilation, residual malignancy, sepsis and shock all had a significantly adverse effect on outcome [9] and following bone marrow transplantation septic shock was invariably rapidly fatal [19]. We also found that septic shock occurring in patients with hematological malignancy was associated with a poor prognosis; the mortality of the 39 patients requiring inotropes (including "low dose" dopamine) was high (35 deaths) and only 3 of the 30 who received inotropic doses of dopamine, dobutamine or adrenaline were discharged from hospital alive [8]. The combination of pneumonia and septic shock had a particularly poor prognosis (32 of 34 patients died) and no such patient who received inotropes survived [8].

It is well recognized that patients who survive a critical illness usually show an early improvement in response to treatment and this also appears to be the case for those with malignant disease. It has been suggested, for example, that recovery is unlikely when patients with respiratory failure complicating hematological malignancy require mechanical ventilation for more than a few days [5] and in one series of patients with lung cancer no patient ventilated for more than 6 days could be weaned from respiratory support [35]. Moreover, the duration of artificial ventilation correlated strongly with a poor prognosis [35]. Others have remarked that if there are no signs of improvement within 72 hours the chances of recovery are low [17] and following bone marrow transplantations mortality was 100% in patients requiring mechanical ventilation for more than 7 days [19]. Some authors, however, have found no significant difference between the duration of mechanical ventilation in survivors and non-survivors [16, 36].

The importance of the number of organ systems involved in determining outcome has been demonstrated by a number of investigators. Snow et al. [16], for example, reported a mortality rate of 91% in cancer patients when respiratory failure was complicated by renal failure and commented that "the most striking predictor of mortality was dysfunction of increasing numbers of critical organ systems". In another series mortality was 100% when patients with malignant disease developed respiratory failure complicated by just one other organ system failure [17] and in patients admitted with acute complications of bone marrow transplantation those with less than 3 system failure always survived, while multiple organ failure was significantly associated with death in the ICU [19]. In our series we found that in the 14 patients who had respiratory failure requiring mechanical ventilation, but in whom three or fewer systems were affected, the mortality was 57%. Conversely when 4 or more systems were involved none of the patients who required IPPV survived. When patients without respiratory failure were included we found that those who died in hospital had significantly more systems affected (median 5, range 2–7) than those who were discharged (median 3, range 1–4) [8].

The outcome of a critical illness is related not only to the number of organ systems which fail, but also to the severity of the acute physiological disturbance and the patients previous health status. These factors can be quantified by calculating an 'acute physiology score' from the most abnormal values of selected physiological variables and combining this with points awarded for age and chronic health status to derive the Apache II score. This scoring system has now been extensively validated and correlates closely with outcome for large groups of critically ill patients [40]. This close relationship between Apache II score and outcome was clearly apparent in our patients with hematological malignancy but within each of six score bands hospital mortality was consistently higher than previously reported in a mixed population of critically ill patients [40], rising to a mortality of 100% in score bands above 30. Moreover no patient with an Apache II score greater than 26 survived to leave hospital, similar to Johnson's observation that all those granulocytopenic patients with scores greater than 23 on admission to the ward or the intensive care unit died [15]. It is recognized, however, that the relationship between the Apache score and outcome depends on the nature of the patients acute illness and most of our patients were suffering from respiratory failure, septic shock or both, conditions known to be associated with a higher than average mortality, even in those without cancer [40]. Knaus et al.

therefore recommend calculating a predicted risk of death for each individual patient by weighting the Apache II score according to their diagnostic category. The predicted risk of death for the group can then be estimated by summing the individual risks and dividing by the total number of patients. In our patients with hematological malignancy the mean predicted risk of death in survivors was 34.8% (range 6.6–56.7%) and in non-survivors 66.6% (range 16.6–97.1%) ($P < 0.05$ – comparison of two proportions); no patient with a predicted risk of death greater than 60% survived. For the whole group of 60 patients the mean predicted risk of death was 59.7% (range 6.6 to 97.1%) compared with an actual mortality of 78% ($P = 0.004$ – comparison of two proportions), suggesting that hospital mortality rates for patients with hematological malignancy are significantly higher than those in a general population of critically ill patients. This conclusion is supported by observing that our mortality rates are remarkably similar to those reported by other authors in patients with hematological malignancy (see above). Moreover, a number of other studies [14, 15, 17] have also indicated that mortality rates for those with malignant disease are higher than for other medical ICU patients with an acute illness of equivalent severity.

The nature and progress of the underlying malignancy would be expected to be of considerable importance in determining the final outcome. It is recognized that a significant number of critically ill cancer patients (10–21%) die on the general ward shortly after discharge from the ICU [5, 8, 11, 19] in most instances when it has become clear that the underlying malignancy has not been controlled and the decision has been made to limit further aggressive treatment. In our series of patients with hematological malignancy the admission Apache II scores and number of systems affected in patients who died on the ward were no different from those of the patients who left hospital alive, confirming the importance of the progress of the underlying malignancy, rather than the severity of the acute illness, as a determinant of hospital discharge [8]. Similarly Dragsted et al. [4] analyzed outcome in a large series of patients admitted to their ICU and found that, although the in-unit mortality was not influenced by the presence of malignancy, the mortality during the ensuing hospital stay was significantly greater in those with cancer.

More specifically in patients with hematological malignancy and respiratory failure the chances of survival may be greater in those with chronic lymphatic leukemia than in those with acute myelogenous leukemia and those with Hodgkin's disease may be more likely to surivive than those with non-Hodgkin's lymphoma [36]. We also noted a tendency for a worse prognosis in patients with acute myeloid leukemia (AML) and non-Hodgkin's lymphoma (NHL) than in those with acute lymphoblastic leukemia (ALL), although this was not statistically significant [8]. Snow et al. [16] had no 6 month-survivors amongst those with ALL, AML or adenocarcinoma of the lung, and all their patients with respiratory failure following bone marrow transplantation died while receiving mechanical ventilation. In contrast our 5 patients who are still alive include 1 AML and 1 ALL, as well as 1 CML, 1 NHL and 1 HL. In those who have relapsed or who have failed to achieve complete remission after an induction course of chemotherapy cure is unlikely [41]. In our experience the mortality of patients who had relapsed (21 of 22) was significantly higher than those on first presentation

(26 of 35), and all 3 patients in remission survived. Others, however, have not found any differences in survival between those undergoing primary treatment and those with relapsed malignancy [36].

In most patients a successful outcome depends on recovery of bone marrow function following effective chemotherapy, while persistent neutropenia appears to adversely affect survival. In our series all long term survivors either had adequate neutophil counts throughout or showed an appreciable recovery of bone marrow function whilst in the ICU. Conversely 36 of the 47 patients who died in hospital were leucopenic at the time of death. Similarly, Torrecilla et al. [19] reported that only 1 of 8 neutropenic patients admitted to intensive care following bone marrow transplantation survived, and his white count returned to normal whilst on the intensive care unit. Others [9] have also suggested that reversal of granulocytopenia during intensive care increases the likelihood of survival. On the other hand, Peters et al. [36] could not demonstrate any difference in total leucocyte or neutrophil counts between survivors and non-survivors in patients with hematological malignancy complicated by respiratory failure. Moreover Johnson et al. [15] could find no correlation between the duration of leukopenia and mortality in a group of granulocytopenic patients with hematological malignancy receiving ICU or ward based care.

In conclusion the in hospital mortality of critically ill patients with life-threatening medical complications of malignant disease appears to be higher than that of an equivalent population of patients without cancer, and long term survival rates are disappointingly low. Nevertheless, for some patients intensive care is life-saving, and in a few the prospects for long term survival are good. Moreover the quality of life of those who do survive long term can be excellent. We suggest that in those with medical complications of hematological malignancy an Apache II score of greater than 30, the dysfunction of an increasing number of organ systems, failure to recover from neutropenia after chemotherapy, and unresponsive malignant disease, particularly in patients who have relapsed, are all indicative of a poor prognosis. In such cases clinicians, in consultation with other members of staff and the patients' relatives should consider discontinuing aggressive supportive treatment.

References

1. Scott RB (1957) Leukaemia. Lancet 1:1053–1058
2. Bassan R, Rohatiner AZS, Gregory W, Amess J, Binils R, Barnett MJ, Lister TA (1987) The treatment of acute myelogenous leukaemia. Haematol Blood Transf 31:35–36
3. Sculier JP, Bron D, Verboven M, Klastersky J (1988) Multiple organ failure during interleukin-2 administration and LAK cells infusion. Intensive Care Med 14:666–667
4. Dragsted L, Qvist J, Madsen M (1989) Outcome from intensive care II. A 5-year study of 1308 patients: short term outcome. Eur J Anaesthesiol 6:131–144
5. Schuster DP, Marion JM (1983) Precedents for meaningful recovery during treatment in a medical intensive care unit. Outcome in patients with hematological malignancy. Am J Med 75:402–408
6. Chang HY, Rodriguez V, Narboni G, et al (1976) Causes of death in adults with acute leukaemia. Medicine 55:259–268

7. Bodey GP, Bolivar R, Fainstein AV (1982) Infectious complications in leukemic patients. Sem Hematol 19:193-226

8. Lloyd-Thomas AR, Wright I, Lister TA, Hinds CJ (1988) Prognosis of patients receiving intensive care for life threatening medical complications of haematological malignancy. Br Med J 296:1025-1029

9. Anger B, Schmeiser T, Sigel H, Heimpel H (1987) Intensive care therapy for patients with hematological diseases. Haematol Bluttransfus 30:519-523

10. Bodey GP, Buckley M, Sathe YS, et al (1966) Quantitative relationships between curculating leukocytes and infection in patients with acute leukemia. Ann Intern Med 64:328-340

11. Turnbull AD, Carlon G, Baron R, Sichel W, Young C, Howland W (1979) The inverse relationship between cost and survival in the critically ill cancer patient. Crit Care Med 7:20-23

12. Lloyd-Thomas AR, Dhaliwal HS, Lister TA, Hinds CJ (1986) Intensive therapy for life-threatening medical complications of haematological malignancy. Intensive Care Med 12:317-324

13. Ambrus JL, Ambrus CM, Mink IB, Pickern JW (1975) Causes of death in cancer patients. J Med 6:61-64

14. Hauser MJ, Tabak J, Baier H (1982) Survival of patients with cancer in a medical critical care unit. Arch Intern Med 142:527-529

15. Johnson MH, Gordon PW, Fitzgerald FT (1986) Stratifaction of prognosis in granulocytopenic patients with haematologic malignancies using the APACHE-II severity of illness score. Crit Care Med 14:693-697

16. Snow RM, Miller WC, Rice DL, Ali MK (1979) Respiratory failure in cancer patients. JAMA 241:2039-2042

17. Cox SC, Norwood SM, Duncan CA (1985) Acute respiratory failure: Mortality associated with underlying disease. Crit Care Med 13:1005-1008

18. Goldiner PL, Pinilla J, Turnbull A (1976) Acute respiratory failure in patients with advanced lymphoma. In: Lacker MJ (ed) Hodgkins disease. Wiley & Sons, New York, pp 371-376

19. Torrecilla C, Cortes JL, Chamorro C, Rubio JJ, Galdos P, De Villota ED (1988) Prognostic assessment of the acute complications of bone marrow transplantation requiring intensive therapy. Intensive Care Med 14:393-398

20. Fanta CH, Pennington JE (1981) Fever and new lung infiltrates in the immunocompromised host. Clin Chest Med 2:19-39

21. Estopa R, Marti AT, Kastanos N, et al (1984) Acute respiratory failure in severe hematological disorders. Crit Care Med 12:26-29

22. Krowka MJ, Rosenow EC, Hoagland HC (1985) Pulmonary complications of bone marrow transplantation. Chest 87:237-246

23. Greenman RL, Goodall PT, King D (1975) Lung biopsy in immunocompromised hosts. Am J Med 59:488-496

24. Leight GS, Michaelis LL (1978) Open lung biopsy for the diagnosis of acute, diffuse pulmonary infiltrates in the immunosuppressed patient. Chest 73:477-482

25. Hewlett RI, Archie F, Wilson (1977) Adult respiratory distress syndrome (ARDS) following aggressive management of extensive acute lymphoblastic leukaemia. Cancer 39:2422-2425

26. Vernant JP, Brun B, Mannoni P, Dreyfus B (1979) Respiratory distress of hyperleukocytic granulocytic leukemias. Cancer 44:264-268

27. Haupt MH, Hutchins GM, Moore GW (1981) Ara-C lung: Noncardiogenic pulmonary oedema complicating cytosine arabinoside therapy of leukaemia. Am J Med 70:256-261

28. Ersek MT (1984) Clinical reviews in critical care. The adult leukemia patient in the intensive care unit. Heart Lung 13:183-193

29. Sherwood LM (1980) The multiple causes of hypercalcemia in malignant disease. N Engl J Med 303:1412-1413

30. Armstong BA, Perez CA, Simpson JR, Hederman MA (1987) Role of irradiation in the management of superior vena cava syndrome. Int J Radiat Oncol Biol Phy 13:531-539

31. Baniel J, Lombrozo R, Ziv Y, Wolloch Y (1988) Neutopenic enterocolitis. Acta Chir Scand 154:71-73

32. Girtanner RE, DeCampo T, Alleyn JN, Averette HE (1981) Routine intensive care for pelvic exenterative operations. Surg Gynecol Obstet 153:657–659
33. Averette HE, Lichtinger M, Sevin BU, Girtanner RE (1984) Pelvic exenteration: A 15 year experience in a general metropolitan hospital. Am J Obstet Gynecol 150:179–184
34. Hinds CJ, Watson JD (1985) Intensive care. In: Shepherd JH, Monaghan JH (eds) Clinical gynaecological oncology. Blackwell Scientific Publications, Oxford, pp 351–368
35. Ewer MS, Ali MK, Atta MS, et al (1986) Outcome of lung cancer patients requiring mechanical ventilation for pulmonary failure. JAMA 256:3364–3366
36. Peters SG, Meadows JA, Gracey DR (1988) Outcome of respiratory failure in haematologic malignancy. Chest 94:99–102
37. Sculier JP, Ries F, Verboven N, Coune E, Klatersky J (1988) Role of intensive care unit in a medical oncology department. Eur J Cancer Clin Oncol 24:513–517
38. Patrick DL, Danis M, Southerland LI, Hong G (1988) Quality of life following intensive care. J Gen Intern Med 3:218–223
39. Poe RH, Wahl GW, Qazi R, et al (1986) Predictors of mortality in the immunocompromised patient with pulmonary infiltrates. Arch Intern Med 146:1304–1308
40. Knaus WA, Draper EA, Wagner DP, Zimmerman JE (1985) APACHE II: A severity of disease classification system. Crit Care Med 13:818–829
41. Lister TA, Rohatiner AZS (1982) The treatment of acute myelogenous leukaemia in adults. Sem Hemat 19:172–191

Audit in Intensive Care

J. Bion

Introduction

The term "audit" is of Latin origin, and implied public examination of fact. In an industrial context it refers to verification of accounts and assessment of performance – cost effectiveness. Medical audit is more difficult to define because of the diversity of activities which represent health care, and audit therefore means different things to different people. There are however certain common elements of medical audit, which may be defined as "the systematic and public examination of factors which affect the delivery of good medical care". This activity has always been a normal part of medical practice in the form of morbidity and mortality meetings, consensus conferences, and in the conduct of medical research. However, the definition raises questions which should themselves be the subject of research: what systems or standards are needed, and how can they be derived? Who should monitor results and have access to data? What factors should we measure and how? What do we mean by good medical care? Does the process of audit itself improve medical care? Simplistic phrases such as 'value for money' ignore the fact that health care systems are complex structures, even when the relationship between purchaser and provider is apparently clearly defined as in private practice.

Audit is conventionally divided into Input, Process and Outcome. Input refers to the structure, staffing and funding of a system. Process audit is best for considering the elements of good care and can be used to examine compliance with protocols, but definitions and standards are often not clear an may not be universally accepted. Outcome has the advantage of clear end-points but does not examine how results were obtained; it may allow the development of predictive indices if the outcome event is sufficiently common. The majority of clinicians use outcome audit to examine the process of care, and then extrapolate from this to identify deficiencies in service input such as inadequate funding. The problem with this approach is that the further one moves from the original facts, the greater the risk of misinterpretation.

A good example of the type of problems affecting poorly constructed audit programmes is the use of Diagnosis-Related Groups (DRGs) to compare costs and average length of hospital stay for patients cared for by different clinicians. "Efficient" consultants with low costs and short hospital stays might merely be shifting responsibilities to the community services. Similarly, "inefficient" consultants might be caring for patients with more severe disease. The costs of identifying patients with unneccessarily prolonged hospital stays was reported to be $ 53000 in one study from the USA [1]. One method of resolving this difficulty is to simplify data collection and to introduce a measure of severity of disease which is applicable across diagnostic groups. This is of particular importance in intensive care, where there is a considerable diversity of disease but relatively few patients in each diagnostic category.

Audit in Intensive Care

Intensive care audit is complicated by the absence of a satisfactory definition of intensive care, by the inhomogeneity of the patient population, and by the apparent failure of many therapeutic techniques to influence survival. The high cost of intensive care and completing demands for limited resources make audit even more important, since it may help to identify areas of practice which could be improved, with a reduction in the marginal costs of care.

Intensive care is however at an advantage over many other clinical specialities in the development of systems of audit, in that it is a data-rich environment with a relatively common and clearly defined outcome measure: death. Mortality rates vary from 8% to 35% [2], sufficiently frequent for useful statistical analysis. Other outcome measures should include the quality of survival, records of morbodity, and of patients' and relatives' satisfaction with the care they received. The fate of patients denied access to intensive care when resources are not available should also be recorded. Process audit should examine, compliance with established standards when these can be defined, a record of costs, and some estimate of factors such as the compassion with which care was delivered, since death may in itself not always be an inappropriate outcome.

Outcome Audit

The next step is to determine the factors which influence outcome from intensive care. They may be categorised as relating to the patient, the disease, and the treatment. They include the patient's physiological reserve, the diagnosis, the severity of disease, the specificity of treatment and the rapidity with which it was applied. The first three factors form part of the scoring system which is known as the APACHE II score – Acute Physiology and Chronic Health Evaluation. This was devised by Dr Knaus and his colleagues from Washington [3], and is currently undergoing further refinement to produce a modified third version. When compared with hospital mortality, the APACHE score is a potent predictor of outcome for groups of patients. The intensity of treatment, though not its specificity, can be measured using the Therapeutic Intervention Scoring System (TISS) [4], which was originally designed to measure costs.

The use of these two systems allows comparisons to be made between groups of patients in terms of their predicted and actual outcomes and to observe the effect of severity of disease on other variables. Comparisons can then be made of different ICUs [2], different methods of care [5, 6], different treatment regimes [7], and quality of survival in relation to cost [8].

The prediction of individual outcome is much more difficult, and raises practical and ethical difficulties which are related in part to misconceptions about scoring systems in general. First, it must be remembered that scoring systems represent a form of medical technology and must therefore be examined for their effect on clinical practice before random introduction. Second, they may also be considered as medical tests, and therefore have false positive and false negative rates which must be understood by the user. Third, no system should be regarded as having an immutable monopoly of the truth; such an approach would result in self-justifying prophecies, and would deny the possibility of therapeutic advances. The aim should be to reduce prognostic uncertainty, not to abolish the need for human intervention.

The importance of prognostic uncertainly and its effect on clinical management were examined in a study from the Massachusetts General Hospital [9]. The authors asked attending medical staff to estimate the chance of survival of 1,831 consecutive admissions to intensive and coronary care, and then recorded lenght of stay, costs, and actual outcome. The patients attracting the highest charges were those with the least expected outcomes: the survivors expected to die, and the non-survivors expected to live. By refining prognostic accuracy and providing a guide to response to therapy, scoring systems may help to reduce inappropriately prolonged treatment.

Accuracy of Scoring Systems

Scoring systems are themselves assessed for accuracy in the same manner as any laboratory test. Individual values of the "separator variable" (the score) are categorised according to outcome once this is known. This produces two bell-shaped distribution curves which will overlap unless the test distinguishes perfectly between survivors and non-survivors. The next step is to determine the values of the score at which the test may be said to be "positive" – that is, to predict death. It is usual to choose a cut-off value which divides the non-survivors into two equal groups, the 50% rule. A two-by-two table is then constructed using this cut-off value, of "predicted" and actual outcomes, and from this the sensitivity (true positive rate, non-survivors) and specificity (true negative rate, survivors) can be calculated. By changing the cut-off value, different sensitivities and specificities can be calculated, and plotted as a ration to produce what is known as a receiver-operator characteristic curve, the shape of which provides a visual guide to the accuracy of the scoring system.

The problem of predictive accuracy becomes clearer when the relationship between severity score and outcome is analysed for different diseases. Knaus has shown that there is a close correlation between APACHE score and survival for sepsis, but that the curve is shifted to the right for heart failure, and is flat for diabetic ketoacidotic coma [10]. This "right shift" is an index of our understanding of pathophysiology and thus of therapeutic specificity. In order to compensate for this effect on predictive power of the APACHE system, Knaus and his colleagues incorporate weights for different diagnoses. The problem with this approach is that it is often difficult to identify a single diagnosis in patients with multiple organ failure. It also requires recalibration of the weights with advances in medical techniques.

Dynamic Systems and Catastrophe theory

An alternative approach is to develop a dynamic system which incorporates a measure of reversibility of physiological disturbance. This has the advantage of following established clinical practice by observing the response to treatment rather than using a "treatment-free" value for prediction. The similar methods have been used: the proportional change in APACHE score from admission to day four of intensive care [11], or a sequential system incorporating organ-system failures [12]. In the first of these studies, it was shown that patients with moderately severe levels of physiological disturbance on admission required a mean fall of 22% in severity score for survival to occur, while for the most severely ill the reduction required was 45%, suggesting a degree of hysteresis in the relationship between severity of illness and survival. The most appropriate model of this relationship may be the cusp model of catastrophe theory (Fig. 1), in which either of two states may exist for the same values of the control factors. As increasing severity of illness is superimposed on limited physiological reserve, the degree of therapeutic support must be increased in order to preserve organ-sys-

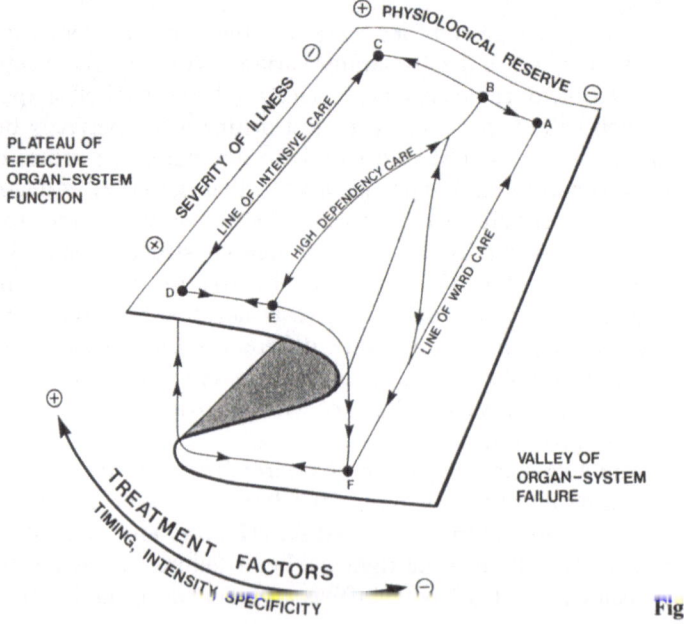

Fig. 1

tem function. Failure to do this results in the patient following the "line of ward care" towards progressive organ-system failure. Abrupt changes of state occur when movements over the fold take place, representing for example the cardiac arrest-resuscitation cycle. This type of model will become more useful if we can measure more precisely physiological reserve, severity of illness, and treatment; and attach values to these variables at which certain levels of care are required. This might also help to reduce the admission rate of low-dependency patients who do not need intensive care services.

Long-term Outcome and Costs

In general, patients who survive to home have a good quality of life and a near-normal life expectancy [13]. Certain subgroups can be identified however: patients with impaired health before admission, and those with admission APACHE and TISS scores greater than 26 and 151 respectively, had a reduced quality of life following discharge [8]. Although the cost per survivor may be high (\$ 40000), when expressed as cost per year of extended life the investment seems reasonable (\$ 1420) [14].

Conclusions

Clinicians and nurses must minimize the high financial and human costs of intensive care by developing systems of measurement which will improve clinical practice. Systems which allow prediction of outcome show that organ-system support can improve survival provided that specific treatments produce a sufficient reduction in physiological disturbance. The failure of nonspecific support to alter outcome is due to the fact that we do not understand the basic pathophysiology of conditions such as sepsis, or the factors which govern tissue repair and healing.

References

1. McSherry CK (1976) Quality assurance: the cost of utilisation review and the educational value of medical audit in a university hospital. Surgery 80:122–129
2. Knaus WA, Draper EA, Wagner DP, Zimmerman JE (1986) An evaluation of outcome from intensive care units in major medical centers. Ann Intern Med 104:410-8
3. Knaus WA, Draper EA, Wagner DP, Zimmerman JE (1985) APACHE II: a severity of disease classification system. Crit Care Med; 10:818–829
4. Cullen DJ, Civetta JM, Briggs BA, Ferrara LC (1974) Therapeutic intervention scoring system: a method for quantitative comparison of patient care. Crit Care Med 2:57–60
5. Bion JF, Edlin SA, Ramsay G, McCabe S, Ledingham IMcA (1985) Validation of a prognostic score in critically ill patients undergoing transport. Br Med J 291:432-4
6. Bion JF, Wilson IH, Taylor PA (1988) Transporting critically ill patients by ambulance: audit by sichness scoring. Br Med J 296:170
7. Watt I, Ledingham IMcA (1984) Mortality amongst multiple trauma patients admitted to an intensive therapy unit. Anaesthesia 39:973–981

8. Sage WM, Rosenthal MH, Silverman JF (1986) Is intensive care worth it? – an assessment of input and outcome for the critically ill. Crit Care Med 14:777–782
9. Detsky AS, Stricker SC, Mulley AG, Thibault GE (1981) Prognosis, survival and the expenditure of hospital resources for patients in an intensive care unit. N Engl J Med 305:667–672
10. Wagner DP, Knaus WA, Draper EA (1986) Physiologic abnormalities and outcome from acute disease. Evidence for a predictable relationship. Arch Intern Med 146:1389–1396
11. Bion JF, Aitchison TC, Edlin SA, Ledingham IMcA (1988) Sichness scoring and response to treatment as predictors of outcome from critical illness. Intensive Care Med 14:167–172
12. Chang RWS, Jacobs S, Lee B, Pace N (1988) Predicting deaths among intensive care unit patients. Crit Care Med 16:34–42
13. Zaren B, Bergstrom R (1989) Survival compared to the general population and changes in health status among intensive care patients. Acta Anaesthesiol Scand 33:6–12
14. Thoner J (1987) Outcome and costs of intensive care. A follow-up study on patients requiring prolonged mechanical ventilation. Acta Anaesthesiol Scand 31:693–698

Long-term Outcome of Premature Babies

A. Calame and C. L. Fawer

Introduction

Better knowledge of fetal and neonatal physiology, improvement in both Obstetrics and Neonatal Intensive Care, together with progress in technology and a better health organization have accounted for a reduction in perinatal mortality over the last 25 years.

If perinatal mortality is easily recorded and provides useful parameters for evaluation and comparison, perinatal morbidity and long-term outcome are much more difficult to define and assess. With the introduction of Neonatal Intensive Care and the concomitant decline in mortality, the quality of survival became a major concern of all neonatologists. The main reasons to set up follow-up programs were the control of the quality of intensive care, the establishment of the true long-term prognosis of high risk newborn infants and the evaluation of changing patterns in outcome of Neonatal Intensive Care, in relation to periods of time and changes in neonatology.

Perinatal and Early Neonatal Care

Improvement in neonatal care depends not only on technical advances but also on better coordination and continuity of perinatal care. During pregnancy, the precise monitoring of the fetus should allow, even for the smallest infants, an optimal birth, with the best timing and the correct type of delivery.

Numerous studies have been performed in order to identify perinatal factors that might predict outcome in extremely low birth weight infants [1-8]. Despite the fact that data comes from various centers that have developed their own perinatal policy, their main conclusions are fairly similar. The most powerful predictors could be related to maturation, stabilization and neonatel complications. They included a lower gestational age, the five munites Apgar score, the need for ventilation, hypoxemia, acidosis, hypercapnia, and pneumothorax, sepsis and seizures. All these factors are known to have potential adverse effects on the developing brain.

Morphologic and Hemodynamic Characteristics of the Developing Brain

1. In very premature infants, there is a persisting immature vascular rete in the subependymal matrix. The small vessels of the germinal layer have a very thin

wall, which will be more exposed to insults and may rupture, leading to a germinal layer hemorrhage.

2. The intracerebral arterioles have very little elastine. This might compromise their ability to vasoconstrict or vasodilate, impairing autoregulation.
3. The deep vein drainage system in the developing brain is far more extensive than has usually been considered. Virtually, the whole white matter area of the hemispheres drains into the terminal vein. The venous part of the brain circulation should not been neglected since, in the post-ischemic changes, the non-reflow phenomenon depends on venous blood stagnation.
4. The arterial blood supply is characterized by a basal ganglia-orientated circulation and the watersheds in the periventricular white matter. The lesions of periventricular leukomalacia (PVL) will develop in these relatively avascular areas [9].

The ability of the brain to keep its perfusion constant in view of a varying perfusion pressure is termed the cerebral autoregulation. This phenomenon is also present in the newborn but the range of autoregulation is narrower. In very immature infants, normotension may be dangerously close to the lower limit of autoregulation. It has been therefore suggested that abolition of autoregulation may be a crucial pathogenic element of hemorrhage as well as ischemia [10, 11].

Brain Injury and Cerebral Ultrasound

Since 1979, real-time ultrasonography has been used in many units. It has now become an invaluable routine procedure. If the validity for the diagnosis of intracerebral hemorrhage has been rapidly recognized by most centers, its use for the detection of PVL has been much more controversial. However, with careful correlation studies between ultrasound appearances, consistent with leukomalacia and post-mortem observations [12, 13], the accurate diagnosis of leukomalacia has been recently achieved.

Classification of Cerebral Ultrasound Findings

The classification of ultrasound changes has varied over time with the equipment and with the investigators experience. To achieve a precise diagnosis, the timing of cranial ultrasound is essential. Furthermore, each lesion (hemorrhage or PVL) should be described with regards to the size, localisation, extent and evolution of ultrasound changes. Our ultrasound findings were classified as shown in Fig. 1:

1. constantly normal scans;
2. grade I-II-III hemorrhage [14];
3. transient echogenicity resolving usually in less than 15 days;

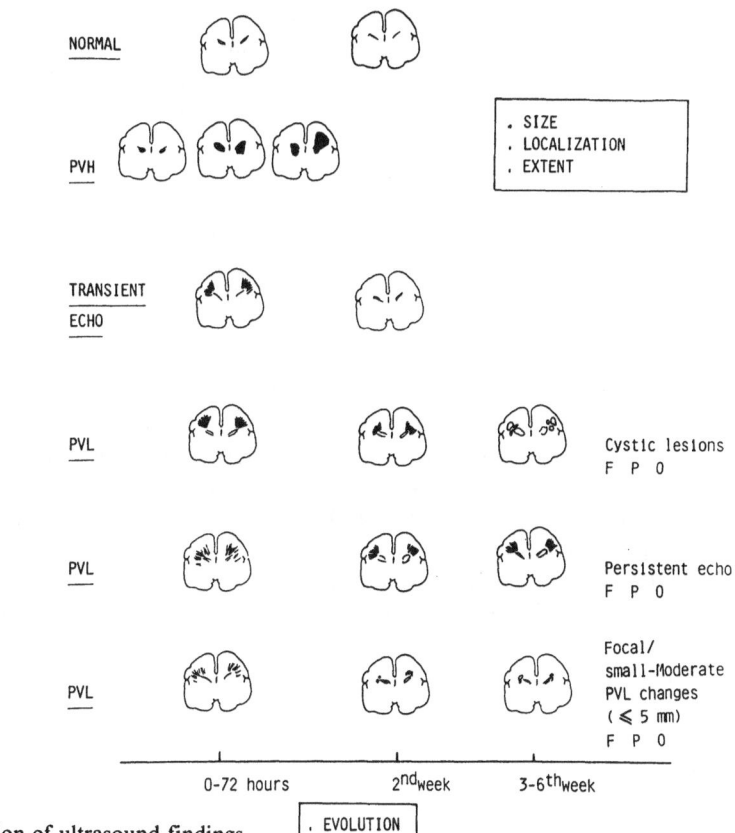

Fig. 1. Classification of ultrasound findings

4. periventricular leukomalacia leading to cystic formations, localized in frontal parietal and occipital areas;
5. persistant echogenicity lasting more than two weeks and usually associated with a slight ventricular enlargement;
6. focal, small or moderate changes of PVL appearing as tiny cysts or localized echogenicity.

All these types of lesions except transient echogenicities have been considered for the establishment of the prognosis.

Validity of Ultrasound in the Prediction of Later Neurodevelopmental Outcome

Very recently, several authors investigated the predictive value of ultrasound. These studies referred to different ultrasonographic definitions and the assessment of outcome is based on various parameters. Despite these differences, comparison between specificity and sensitivity are quite similar and in agreement with our own findings (specificity 100%, sensitivity 80%). The most powerful ultrasound predictors for handicaps were found to be PVL lesions and severe hemorrhagic damage. On the other hand a favourable scan and a normal neurological examination near term were found to be good predictors for normal neurodevelopmental progress [15–19].

In a recent study, we examined at 3½ years of age 154 children born with 34 weeks' gestation or less (22 were not fully examined but none of them did present a major handicap). They were allocated in the following groups according to the ultrasound findings. Group 1: normal scan (n = 70), Group 2: isolated hemorrhage (n = 18), Group 3: post-hemorrhagic hydrocephalus (n = 5), Group 4: perivascular leukomalacia (n = 39). A control group of term infants (n = 28) born after a normal pregnancy and delivery were also examined at 3½ years of age. The neurodevelopmental outcome is illustrated in Fig. 2. The vertical axis represents the Intellectual General Index obtained by the McCarthy children's abilities scales. The normal mean index is 100. Children with normal scan, with isolated hemorrhage and hydrocephalus had similar outcome. Two children presented mild diplegia. Children with PVL had a variable prognosis. In this group, 18 major handicaps were diagnosed.

Figure 3 shows the relation which could be established between the size and extent of the PVL lesions and the type and severity of the handicaps. All children with isolated changes in the frontal areas developed normally. Among children with frontal and parietal lesions, 7 had a major handicap. Children with

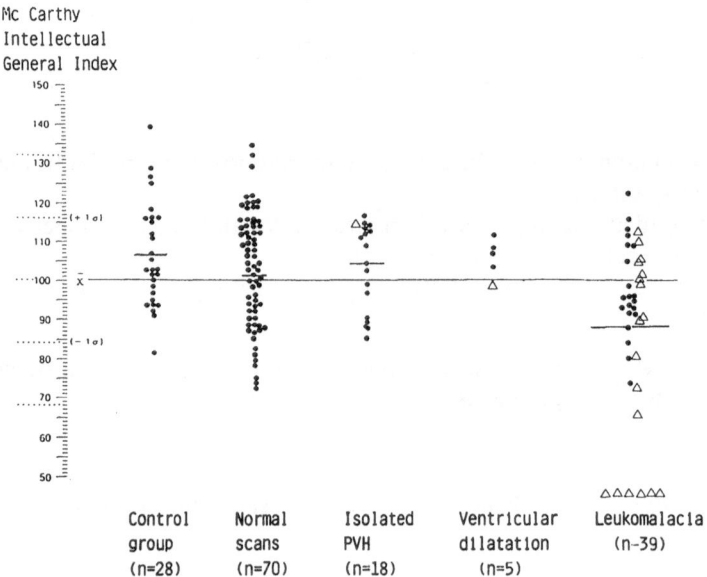

Fig. 2. Neurodevelopmental outcome according to neonatal ultrasound findings (see text for details). ΔMajor handicaps

PVH = perivascular hemorrhage

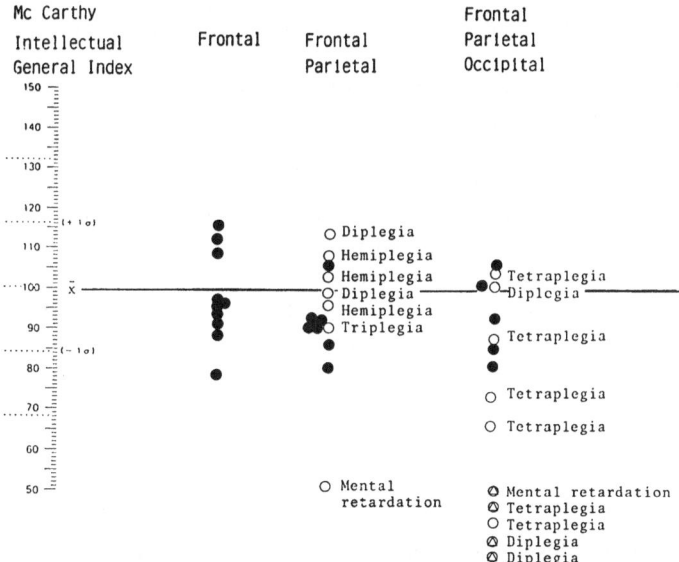

Fig. 3. Relation between the size and extent of PVL lesions and the type and severity of the handicaps. Δ = Visual impairment

extensive lesions in frontal, parietal, and occipital regions had a poor prognosis as most of them developed a multiple handicap (cerebral palsy, visual impairment or mental retardation).

Assessment of Cerebral Circulation

The evaluation of cerebral circulation in the neonatal period is essential to improve our understanding of etiopathogenic mechanisms underlying brain injury. Recently, Doppler ultrasound method for recording blood flow velocities has been used to investigate cerebral hemodynamics [20, 21]. In several reports, particular importance could be derived for fluctuations in cerebral blood flow, abrupt increases in flow or decreases in flow [22].

In a prospective study performed among preterm infants, we compared Doppler parameters obtained before the detection of ultrasound changes with the measurements in a control group (normal scans). Systolic velocities and areas under the velocity curve, parameters directly proportional to cerebral blood flow were found to be higher in the infants who were going to develop hemorrhage and PVL changes.

When interpretating these results, two hypothesis can be formulated:

1. the increase in velocities might be due to CO_2 reactivity (infants with cerebral lesions had a higher mean PCO_2 at the time of Doppler recordings);
2. this higher flow might also represent the post-insult hyperperfusion phenomenon which has been reported in experimental models [23, 24].

Comprehensive Assessment of Preterm Infants for Long-term Prognosis

In addition to ultrasound findings, the evaluation of recovery by standardized neurological examinations [25] is an essential part of the comprehensive assessment around term. Furthermore abnormal EEG recording appears to provide a sensitive early guide to the severity and prognosis of lesions [26–28]. Finally, auditory brainstem evoked potentials represent, now, the procedure of first choice to detect neurosensory hearing loss before hospital discharge [29, 30]. In conclusion, a comprehensive assessment at term allows the detection of neurological dysfunctions which might indicate a therapeutic program and will help the neonatologist when discussing with parents at discharge.

Changing Patterns in Outcome of Neonatal Intensive Care

The routine use of brain ultrasound in our units has clearly showed since 1982 a decrease in the incidence of cerebral lesions (Fig. 4). Simultaneously, the incidence of major handicaps has also decreased (Fig. 5).

These encouraging observations can be attributed to numerous factors:

1. a better coordination in perinatal care with an active collaboration between obstetricians and neonatologists (–, i.e. in utero transfer);

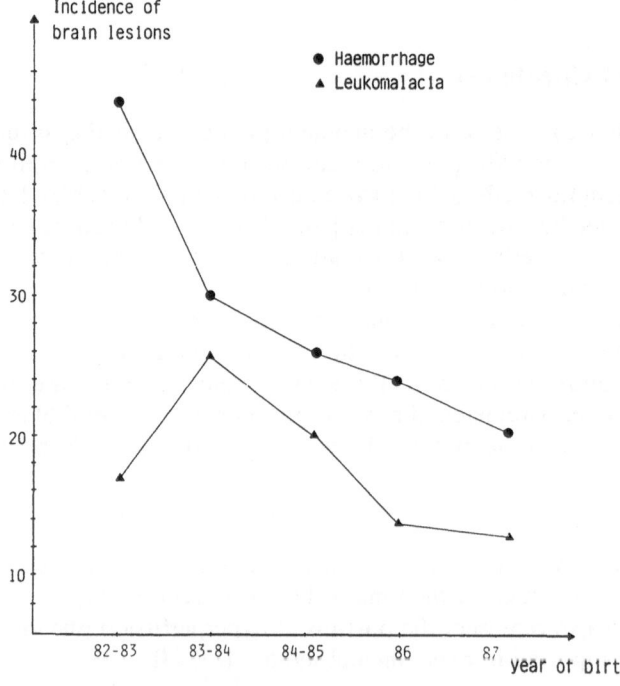

Fig. 4. Incidence of cerebral lesions among premature infants ≤ 34 weeks gestation (1982–1987)

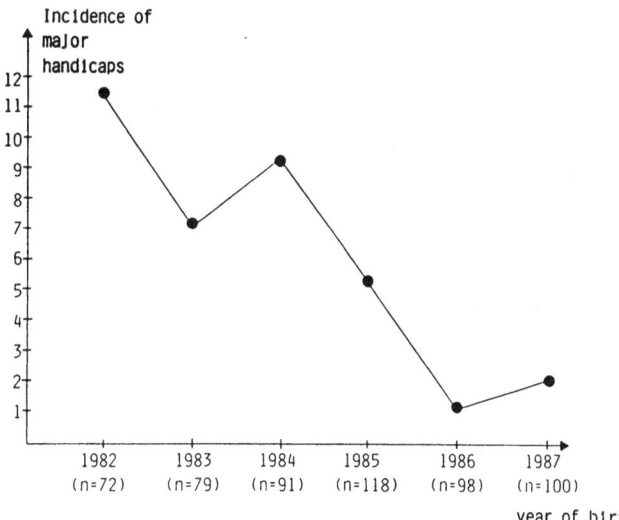

Fig. 5. Incidence of major handicaps among preterm infants ≤ 34 weeks gestation (1982–1987)

2. immediate resuscitation of the neonate by a well-trained neonatal team resulting in a rapid and optimal stabilization of the premature infants and
3. improvement in Neonatal Care.

One of the major, but the most difficult task of medicine is to find out the right marker for evaluating not only gains that are hoped to be achieved, but also subsequent disadvantages or even harmful effect. Assessment of Neonatal Intensive Care is important. It should include the establishment of the true long term prognosis of high risk newborn infants. As there is constant improvement in perinatal medicine, relevant and updated questions should be asked. Regular reappraisal of the quality of care will define guidelines for better neonatal management and prevention of neurodevelopmental sequelae as well as for a rational health policy.

References

1. Driscoll JM, Driscoll Y, Steir ME, et al (1982) Mortality and morbidity in infants less than 1001 grams birth weight. Pediatrics 69:21–26
2. Haas G, Asprions B, Leidig E, Buchwald-Saal M, Mentzel H (1986) Obstetrical and neonatal risk factors in very low birth weight infants related to their neurological development. Eur J Pediatr 145:341–346
3. Hack M, Fanaroff AA (1986) Changes in the delivery room care of the extremely small infant (<750 g). Effect on morbidity and outcome. N Engl J Med 314:660–664
4. Skouteli HN, Dubowitz LMS, Levene MI, Miller G (1985) Predictors for survival and normal neurodevelopmental outcome of infants weighing less than 1001 grams at birth. Dev Med Child Neurol 27:588–595
5. Watkins A, Szamonowicz W, Yu VVY (1988) Significance of seizures in very low-birth-weight infants. Dev Med Child Neurol 30:162–169
6. Yu VYH, Downe L, Astbury J, Bajuk B (1986) Perinatal factors and adverse outcome in extremely low birthweight infants. Arch Dis Child 61:554–558

7. Yu VYH, Loke HL, Bajuk B, Szymonowicz W, Orgill AA, Astbury J (1986) Prognosis for infants born at 23 to 28 weeks gestation. Br Med J 293:1200–1203
8. Zarfin J, Van Aerde J, Perlman M, Pape K, Chipman M (1986) Predicting survival of infants of birth weight less than 801 grams. Crit Care Med 14:768–772
9. Pape KE, Wigglesworth JS (1979) Haemo·hage, ischaemia and the perinatal brain. Clinics in Developmental Medicine 68/70. William Heinemann Medical Books
10. Jorch G, Jorch N (1987) Failure of autoregulation of cerebral blood flow in neonates studied by pulsed Doppler ultrasound of the internal carotid artery. Eur J Pediatr 146:468–472
11. Lou HC, Lassen NA, Griis-Hansen B (1979) Impaired autoregulation of cerebral blood flow in the distressed newborn infants. J Pediatr 94:118–121
12. De Vries LS, Wigglesworth JS, Regev R, Dubowitz LMS (1988) Evolution of periventricular leukomalacia during the neonatal period and infancy: correlation of imaging and postmorten findings. Early Hum Dev 17:205–219
13. Fawer CL, Calame A, Perentes E, Anderegg A (1985) Periventricular leukomalacia: a correlation study between real-time ultrasound and autopsy findings. Neuroradiol 27:292–300
14. Levene MI, Fawer CL, Lamont RF (1982) Risk factors in the development of intraventricular haemorrhage in the preterm neonates. Arch Dis Child 57:410–417
15. Bozynski MEA, Nelson MN, Genaze D, et al (1988) Cranial ultrasonography and the prediction of cerebral palsy in infants weighing < 1200 grams at birth. Dev Med Child Neurol 30:342–348
16. Cooke RWI (1987) Early and late cranial ultrasonographic appearances and outcome in very low birthweight infants. Arch Dis Child 62:931–937
17. Graham M, Levene MI, Trounce JQ, Rutter N (1987) Prediction of cerebral palsy in very low birthweith infants: prospective ultrasound study. Lancet 2:593–596
18. Nwaesei CG, Allen AC, Vincer MJ, et al (1988) Effect of timing of cerebral ultrasonography on the prediction of later neurodevelopmental outcome in high-risk preterm infants. J Pediatr 112:970–975
19. Stewart A, Hope PL, Hamilton P, et al (1988) Prediction in very preterm infants of satisfactory neurodevelopmental progress at 12 months. Dev Med Child Neurol 30:53–63
20. Archer LNJ, Evans DH (1988) Doppler assessment of the neonatal cerebral circulation. In: Levene MI, Bennett MJ, Punt J (eds) Fetal and neonatal neurology and neurosurgery. Churchill Livingstone, Edinburgh London Melbourne New York, pp 162–168
21. Levene MI (1987) Cerebral blood flow. In: Neonatal neurology. Current Reviews in Paediatrics 3. Churchill Livingstone, Edinburgh London Melbourne New York, pp 23–41
22. Volpe JJ (1987) Neurology of the newborn, 2nd edn. Saunders, Philadelphia
23. Ames A, Wright RL, Kowada M (1968) Cerebral insult: II. the no-reflow phenomenon. Am J Pathol 52:437–453
24. Hossman KA, Sakaki S, Kimoto K (1976) Cerebral uptake of glucose and oxygen in the cat brain after prolonged ischaemia. Stroke 7:301–305
25. Amiel-Tison C (1976) A method for neurologic evaluation within the first year of life. Current problems in pediatrics. Chicago: Year Book Medical Publishers, vol VII, pp1–50
26. Connell J, Oozeer R, Regev R, De Vries LS, Dubowitz LMS, Dubowitz V (1987) Continuous four-channel EEG monitoring in the evaluation of echodense ultrasound lesions and cystic leucomalacia. Arch Dis Child 62:1019–1024
27. Connell J, De Vries L, Oozeer R, Regev R, Dubowitz LMS, Dubowitz V (1988) Predictive value of early continuous electroencephalogram monitoring in ventilated preterm infants with intraventricular hemorrhage. Pediatrics 82:337–343
28. Watanabe K, Hakamada S, Kuroyanagi T, Takeuchi T (1983) Electroencephalographic study of intraventricular hemorrhage in the preterm newborn. Neuropediatrics 14:225–230
29. Lary S (1988) Brainstem evoked potentials. In: Levene MI, Bennett MJ, Punt J (eds) Fetal and neonatal neurology and neurosurgery. Churchill Livingstone, Edinburgh London Melbourne New York, pp 197–205
30. Majnemer A, Rosenblatt B, Riley P (1988) Prognostic significance of the auditory brainstem evoked response in high-risk neonates. Dev Med Child Neurol 30:43–52

Long-term Outcome from Intensive Care

L. Dragsted

Introduction

As an evaluation of intensive care treatment, outcome seems to be the best: for the patient, as for the doctor, outcome counts. Unfortunately, the outcome, either defined as the initial and final level of health or defined in a comparison between the observed and the optimal result is extremely difficult to measure. It is difficult to obtain reproducible results, and several factors might influence outcome measures.

The criteria of mortality and morbidity are notoriously insufficient and the indices of patient satisfaction are often deceptive. The major problem is the very notion of the outcome of a stay in the ICU (or a hospitalization). The outcome is not a final, but an intermediate result of the state of health of an individual at a specific moment of his life. This intermediate result allows one to forecast the future of the patient, but with considerable uncertainty. Middle and long term consequences of many surgical and medical treatments are unpredictable. Evaluation of medical activities, like intensive care medicine, implies evaluation of diagnostic and therapeutic procedures. There are many methods for the evaluation of medical activities; the best known being the comparative controlled trials. This has never been applied to critically ill patients, as it has been considered unethical.

The evaluation of medical activities like intensive care is of considerable interest for it allows an evaluation of the efficacy of medical strategies by analyzing the effects of successive decisions taken during ICU stay and the whole hospitalization. Alterations in the level of health induced by the treatment do not all go in the same direction. The rational of medical activities is not linear. The reasons of the patient, of the patients family, and of the doctor often differ, their rational are multiple, which might lead to a therapeutical/diagnostical decision.

Evaluation of intensive care medicine must deal, not with the analysis of the rational of the doctor, but with the utility value that the patients give to the intensive care medicine. For example, the utility of a therapeutic procedure, established after a comparative trial, is often evaluated by the five year survival rate. If the trial compares e.g. a medical and a surgical treatment, the survival rates will often be different. If the survival rate of operated patients is lower than the medically treated patients, say for half of the 5 year period, and afterwards is greater, surgery will be preferred by the doctors. However, the patient might prefer a greater likelihood of survival in the beginning of the 5 year period.

An evaluation of intensive care medicine may be expected to have the following consequences.

1. An improvement of procedures which might lead to an improvement in the quality of ICU-care.
2. Modifications in teaching.
3. Reduction of the economic costs for the society.
4. An increased efficiency as an effect of a better control of the organization.

The short-term outcome, either stated as the in-unit or the in-hospital mortality, is still the most commonly used measure for the efficacy of intensive care medicine. For many patients and their families the expected life time (or life expectancy) and the quality of life are more important measures for the benefit of intensive care treatment than the survival rate. However, the unavailability of disease adjusted actuarial data for various diagnostic sub groups makes prediction of expected life time for patients with chronic diseases inaccurate. Survival rates have been the easiest accessable and therefore the most of used measure. Survival rates are objective data, and in most European countries reliable informations on living status can be obtained. It is also possible to follow a group of patients over a greater time period (e.g. establish five year survival rates for diagnostic sub groups like the outcome measure in patients with cancer). If wanted, the observed survival rate can be compared with the estimated survival rate in the background population, using a Kaplan-Meier estimation or the life table method [1], or compared with the observed survival rate in the normal population. This comparison can demonstrate the net gain or loss of expected lifetime for the study group. The interpretation of a detected difference, however, might prove difficult, e.g. if the age and sex composition of the groups compared is not nearly identical [2].

Survival in itself is an unsatisfactory measure. Among survivors from intensive care medicine, functional status, including employment, and quality of life are more than, or just as important as survival rate to the survivor.

It would be optimal to determine patients quality of life rather than their functional level, but quality of life is a poorly defined concept. It is a mixture of social circumstances, behavior (ambulation, self care, social interactions), and the satisfaction of basic needs [3], but so far there have not been any generally accepted methods to measure these factors. Existing studies of quality of life in long-term ICU survivors have used working status, mental status, or health status.

Functional status or health status has been assessed for various diagnostic sub groups with a variety of systems. A health status measure must be appropriate to the users' need, reliable, with a high internal consistency, and validity. If the measure is intended for large scale studies, the time factor in completing the measure will be as important as the methods for collecting data. The most used systems (or best validated) are the Health Index Score, the Activities of Daily Living, The Sickness Impact Profile [4] and the Perceived Quality of Life [5]. These systems, however, have only been used in small study groups of ICU patients and the results are thus difficult to compare.

Some Existing Studies

Long-term Outcome

During the last 15 years several studies have dealt with the long-term outcome for ICU patients. The results are impossible to compare as the starting point and the duration of the follow up differ in the studies.

The patient populations in the ICUs studied are not comparable as they are not stratified using the same system. A high proportions of patients aged 70 years and above, however, seem to be a common finding.

Campion et al. followed 1832 MICU/CCU patients for 12 months after hospital discharge [6]. The patients were aged 55 years and above. During the follow up time the mortality was 32% and major risk factors were age and chronic health. In a Swedish study by Zaren 980 general ICU patients were followed for 24 months after ICU admission and their mortality rate compared with that of the general population [7]. The study showed an initial increase in the mortality, but after one year the mortality rate had stabilized and was nearly identical to that of the general population. Unfortunately, comparisons between the observed and expected survival rates were obliged to show difference because the follow up started at ICU admission thereby including patients, dying during hospital stay. It remains unclear whether the study demonstrated a true difference in observed and expected mortality rates. The cumulative mortality was 32% (includes the mortality during ICU and hospital stay) during the follow-up period.

Parno et al. [8] found no differences between the 2-year post-hospital survival rate of 558 ICU patients and 124 non-ICU patients. These two groups do not appear to be comparable in age and sex distribution, and the selection of the non-ICU patients has not been detailed. Accordingly, differences in age and sex distribution cast doubt on their observation of a similar two year-survival rate of 81% in the two groups. A Danish study [2] has described the 5 year survival rate of 926 general ICU patients, discharged alive from the hospital. The observed 5 year survival rate was found to be significantly lower than the expected survival rate in an age and sex adjusted normal population. Mortality during the follow up period was 42% and the excess mortality five times higher than expected. In a study of patients with respiratory failure, Nunn [9] found that 17 of 47 survivors died during a 4 year period after discharge from the hospital, while only four deaths were expected according to the life tables. He also found a reduced life expectancy among the survivor compared to healthy persons of same age.

Though the studies vary in type of unit, patient age and casemix, they seem to agree on which are the major risk factors for death after hospital discharge. Nearly all studies state that increasing age and chronic diseases especially cancer, were the most important risk factors for post hospital mortality.

Functional Level (Quality of Life)

Most often, studies of ICU outcome state the results in survival rates, simply because duration of survival is easily measured; only few studies have used functional status a measure to evaluate outcome. Using functional status as an end-result require the patients' pre-hospital functional status for comparison. The results obtained in existing studies are not comparable, as the methods, the patients and the follow-up time vary from one study to another.

Cullen et al. [10] followed the most critically ill surgical patients (Cullen class. IV) for one year after ICU admission. They found that the majority of surviving patients were functioning at their pre-hospital level of daily activities after one year. Survival rate and quality of life was found to be independent of age, but this might be due to the small sample size. Parno et al. [11] followed ICU patients for two years after hospital discharge and they showed that among the ICU survivors responding to the follow-up, 85% were able to perform daily activities and 66% were working. In a one year study of 228 ICU patients LeGall et al. [12] demonstrated with the use of the Chronic Health Evaluation part of the APACHE I system that increasing age and previous health status were important indicators for functional outcome. In a Danish study Dragsted and Qvist [13] followed 1308 ICU patients for twelve months after ICU admission. Among the survivors, 44% reported that they had returned to their normal pre-hospital activity level, and 26% reported limited activity level at one year. Increasing age and chronic diseases were found to influence the functional outcome significantly. However, among the eldest patients (70 years and above) 30% of the survivors had returned to normal activity level while almost 40% recorded limited activity level at one year. Goldstein et al. [14] followed 2213 MICU/CCU patients for one year and demonstrated that most survivors regained their pre-admission functional status with 60% of the previously employed returning to work. However, post-hospital mortality was high and was related to prior functional status.

In conclusion, long-term outcome from intensive care, in terms of survival and in terms of quality of life, is still insufficiently studied. However, a review of existing studies indicates that patients who survive their critical illness, do have a realistic hope of regaining normal activity level and an acceptable life expectancy. Major determinants for long-term outcome appear to be age and the influence of existing chronic diseases.

References

1. Berkson J, Gage RP (1950) Calculations of survival rates for cancer. Proc Staff Meet Mayo Clin 25:270–286
2. Dragsted L, Qvist J, Madsen (1990) Outcome from intensive care IV: A 5-year study of 1308 patients: Long-term outcome. Eur J Anaesthesiol (in press)
3. Sage WM, Rosenthal MH, Silverman JF (1986) Is intensive care worth it? An assessment of input and outcome for the critically ill. Crit Care Med 14:777–782
4. McDowell I, Newell C (1987) Measuring health. A guide to rating scales and questionnaires. Oxford University Press
5. Patrick DL, Danis M, Southerland LI, Hong G (1988) Quality of life following intensive care. J Gen Intern Med 3:218–223
6. Campion EW, Mulley AG, Goldstein RL, et al (1981) Medical intensive care for the elderly: A study of current use costs, and outcomes. JAMA 246:2052–2056

7. Zarén B (1987) Prognosis of outcome of intensive care patients. Ph. D. thesis. University of Uppsala
8. Parno JR, Teres P, Lemeshow S, et al (1982) Hospital changes and long-term survival of ICU patients versus non-ICU patients. Crit Care Med 10-569-574
9. Nunn JF, Milledge JS, Singaraya J (1979) Survival of patients ventilated in an intensive therapy unit. Br Med J 1:1525-1527
10. Cullen DJ, Keene R, Waternaux C, Kensman JM, Caldera DL, Peterson H (1984) Severity of illness, outcome analysis, and cost of intensive care for critically ill patients in major issues in critical care medicine. In: Parillo UE, Ayres SM (eds) Williams & Williams
11. Parno JR, Teres D, Lemeshow S, Brown RB, Avrunin JS (1984) Two-year outcome of adult intensive care patients. Med Care 22:167-176
12. LeGall JR, Brun-Buisson C, Trunet P, Latournerie J, Chantereau S, Rapin M (1982) Influence of age, previous health status, and severity of illness on outcome from intensive care. Crit Care Med 10:575-577
13. Dragsted L, Qvist J (1989) Outcome from intensive care III. A 5-year study of 1308 patients activity level. Eur J Anaesthesiol 6:385-396
14. Goldstein RL, Campion EW, Thibault GE, Mulley AG, Skinner E (1986) Functional outcome following medical intensive care. Crit Care Med 14:783-788

Subject Index